Contemporary Orthodontics

Seventh Edition

Henry W. Fields, Jr., DDS, MS, MSD

Professor Emeritus
Division of Orthodontics
College of Dentistry
The Ohio State University
Chief, Orthodontics
Nationwide Children's Hospital
Columbus, Ohio

Brent E. Larson, DDS, MS

Professor and Director
Division of Orthodontics
University of Minnesota
Minneapolis, Minnesota

David M. Sarver, DMD, MS

Adjunct Professor, Orthodontics
University of Alabama at Birmingham
Birmingham, Alabama
University of North Carolina
Chapel Hill, North Carolina
Sarver Orthodontics
Vestavia Hills, Alabama

William R. Proffit, DDS, PhD

Deceased, September 30, 2018
Professor Emeritus (formerly Kenan Distinguished Professor)
Department of Orthodontics
School of Dentistry
University of North Carolina
Chapel Hill, North Carolina

ELSEVIER

ELSEVIER
3251 Riverport Lane
St. Louis, Missouri 63043

CONTEMPORARY ORTHODONTICS,
SEVENTH EDITION ISBN: 978-0-323-93071-0

Senior Content Strategist: Kelly Skelton
Senior Content Development Specialist: Kevin Travers
Senior Content Development Manager: Meghan Andress
Publishing Services Manager: Deepthi Unni
Senior Project Manager: Kamatchi Madhavan
Book Designer: Ryan Cook

Printed in India by Manipal Technologies Limited
Udayavani Building, Press Corner, Manipal,
Karnataka, India-576104

Last digit is the print number: 9 8 7 6 5 4 3 2

In Memoriam, William R. Proffit, 1936–2018

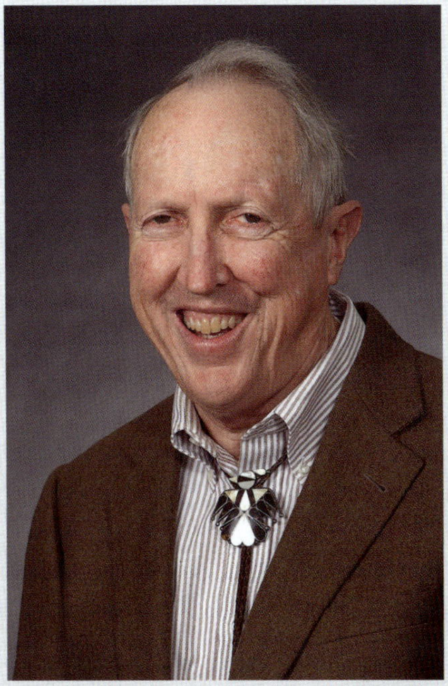

(Courtesy UNC Adams School of Dentistry)

Bill, Prof, or Bob, to a select few, died in 2018 at 82 years old. As mentioned in the Preface, he conceived of this book, and the first edition was published in 1986. He was involved in the first six editions as the senior author and the unifying voice. In this edition, his influence and words remain clearly evident but not as powerful as a single voice. For these reasons, depending on the chapter, he is included as an author to recognize his continuing contributions to this seventh edition. In many ways, we are still the same team trying to achieve the same things.

List of Contributors

Regina L. Blevins, DDS, MS
Adjunct Facuty
Division of Orthodontics
University of Minnesota
Minneapolis, Minnesota, United States
Orthodontist
Minnesota Orthodontics
Inver Grove Height
Minnesota, United States

Toru Deguchi, DDS, MSD, PhD
Professor
Division of Orthodontics and Prosthodontics
Chair
Department of Rehabilitative and Reconstructive Dentistry
University of Louisville School of Dentistry
Louisville, Kentucky, United States

Benjamin W. Fields, PhD
Clinical Child and Adolescent Psychologist
Big Lots Behavioral Health Services
Nationwide Children's Hospital
Columbus, Ohio, United States
Clinical Assistant Professor
Department of Psychiatry and Behavioral Health
The Ohio State University
Columbus, Ohio, United States

Henry W. Fields, Jr., BA, DDS, MS, MSD
Emeritus Professor
Division of Orthodontics
The Ohio State University College of Dentistry
Columbus, Ohio, United States
Chief, Section of Orthodontics
Nationwide Children's Hospital
Columbus, Ohio, United States

Ching-Chang Ko, DDS, MS, PhD
Professor
Vig-Williams Chair of Orthodontics
Division of Orthodontics
The Ohio State University College of Dentistry
Columbus, Ohio, United States

Kaitrin Kramer, DDS, PhD, MS
Craniofacial Orthodontist
Department of Plastic and Reconstructive Surgery
Nationwide Children's Hospital
Columbus, Ohio, United States
Assistant Professor
Division of Orthodontics
The Ohio State University College of Dentistry
Columbus, Ohio, United States

Brent E. Larson, DDS, MS
Professor and Director
Division of Orthodontics
University of Minnesota
Minneapolis, Minnesota, United States

Matthew E. Larson, DDS, MS
Adjunct Clinical Professor
Division of Orthodontics
University of Minnesota
Minneapolis, Minnesota, United States
Orthodontist
Larson Orthodontic Specialists
Eau Claire, Wisconsin, United States

Benjamin T. Pliska, DDS, MSc, FRCD(C)
Associate Professor
Oral Health Sciences
University of British Columbia
Vancouver, British Columbia, Canada

William Proffit, DDS, PhD†
Professor Emeritus (formerly Kenan Distinguished Professor)
Department of Orthodontics
School of Dentistry
University of North Carolina
Chapel Hill, North Carolina, United States

David M. Sarver, DMD, MS
Adjunct Professor
Orthodontics
University of Alabama at Birmingham
Birmingham Alabama, Alabama, United States
University of North Carolina
Chapel Hill, North Carolina, United States
Sarver Orthodontics
Vestavia Hills, Alabama

†Deceased, September 30, 2018.

Preface

This is the seventh edition of *Contemporary Orthodontics*. The first edition was published in 1986—nearly 40 years ago. We have tried to keep the focus the same. Dental students can learn basic growth and development, the etiology of orthodontic problems, and some treatment methods. New residents can be introduced to orthodontic dilemmas, perspectives, and treatment alternatives based on evidence. Practitioners can be updated and reflect on their orthodontic care, the evolving orthodontic discipline, and the treatment provided by colleagues.

What is new? Lots! We have a smaller author team because of the death of Bill Proffit. Bill created the foundation of this book when he was building the self-instruction orthodontic curriculum at the University of Florida and then enhanced it at the University of North Carolina starting in 1975. Over the next decade, we joined him as faculty and residents and later colleagues. We worked together on more projects than just this book. His strength was to organize and simplify a problem, its essence, and solutions. He was trained as a physiologist as well and liked gadgets and quantifiable results but was not averse to speculating on data. He was a relentless worker, motivator, and thinker. Our part in this partnership, which continues in his stead, was and is to explore, reflect, challenge, distill, and make orthodontics available to all with an interest and desire to learn. Marked by Bill as we were, we strive to make sense of this exciting discipline that still has more questions than answers.

In addition to new topics and images, we have added more contributors: Matthew Larson, Regina Blevins, Kaitrin Kramer, Benjamin T. Pliska, Ching-Chang Ko, Toru Deguchi, and Benjamin W. Fields, whose contributions are listed in the Table of Contents and the chapter headings. They have helped us add:

- An artificial intelligence perspective and potential.
- Data evaluation and priority.
- A voice for standard metrics in orthodontic research.
- Social and behavioral problems related to orthodontics.
- An overview of common craniofacial problems.
- Obstructive sleep apnea as a diagnostic and treatment-related issue.
- Revised diagnosis and treatment planning with more specific guidance.
- Systematic diagnostic checklists.
- Updated informed consent as understanding.
- Clear tray aligners and hybrid treatment for adolescents and adults.
- Expanded biomechanics related to clear tray aligners.
- More discussion of skeletal anchorage options and applications.
- 3D options for orthognathic surgery planning.

This is a book that attempts to rely on evidence and is moderately referenced, but more than previous editions. We intend that the conclusions are evidence informed. With the remembrance of Bill and his guidance and in the traditions set in previous editions, we carry on.

Henry W. Fields, Jr.
Brent E. Larson
David M. Sarver

Acknowledgments

We thank those who provided resources and aid not recognized in print. The residents of the Orthodontic classes of 2024 at the Ohio State University College of Dentistry Division of Orthodontics and the University of Minnesota Division of Orthodontics, and the Division of Pediatric Dentistry Class of 2024 at Ohio State University College of Dentistry and Nationwide Children's Hospital supplied critiques, ideas, and images to support this publication.

Our new authors, who are acknowledged in the Table of Contents and chapter headings included, Drs. Ching-Chang Ko, Kaitrin Kramer, Benjamin W. Fields, Benjamin T. Pliska, Matthew Larson, Toru Deguchi, and Regina Blevins. They expanded our breadth and depth of knowledge. As always, Dr. Tim Shaughnessy provided sources of images and cases, and Dr. Joen Iannucci provided radiologic support information and advice.

Dr. Tessa Streeter proofread sections of the text in an extremely thorough and timely manner to enhance our responses to the publisher.

We appreciate the support of Elsevier, who has worked with us for seven editions.

Thank you.

Henry W. Fields, Jr.
Brent E. Larson
David M. Sarver

Contents

Section 3: Biomechanics, Mechanics, and Contemporary Orthodontic Appliances

Section 4: Treatment in Preadolescent Children: What Is Different?

Section 5: Growth Modification

Section 6: Comprehensive Orthodontic Treatment in the Early Permanent Dentition

SECTION 1

The Orthodontic Problem

This section of the book addresses important questions that are the intellectual and scientific background for the practice of orthodontics:

Why do we provide orthodontic treatment?
Who needs treatment?
How do people benefit from it?
How prevalent are orthodontic problems?
How do children, adolescents and adults grow and develop
How are these problems related to growth of the head and face?
How are these problems related to eruption of the teeth?
Can we identify the etiology of these orthodontic problems?
How do we make decisions about treatment based on the evidence?

You need to consider the answers to these questions before you can appropriately diagnose orthodontic problems, plan the treatment that will provide maximum benefit to the patient, and carry out that treatment. The answers, to the best of our ability to provide them now, are in chapters1–5.

1

Malocclusion and Dentofacial Abnormalities in Contemporary Society

HENRY W. FIELDS JR., WILLIAM R. PROFFIT AND CHING-CHANG KO

CHAPTER OUTLINE

The Changing Goals of Orthodontic Treatment

The Development of Orthodontics

Crowded, irregular, and protruding teeth have been a problem for some individuals since antiquity and attempts to correct this disorder go back at least to 1000 BC. Primitive (and surprisingly well-designed) orthodontic appliances have been found in both Greek and Etruscan materials.[1] As dentistry developed in the 18th and 19th centuries, a number of devices for the "regulation" of the teeth were described by various authors and apparently used sporadically by the dentists of that era.

After 1850 the first texts that systematically described orthodontics appeared, the most notable being Norman Kingsley's *Oral Deformities*.[2] Kingsley, who had a tremendous influence on American dentistry in the latter half of the 19th century, was among the first to use extraoral force to correct protruding teeth. He was also a pioneer in the treatment of cleft palate and related problems. Kingsley also wrote about the importance of the artistic form of the face and recognized the importance of facial esthetics.

Despite the contributions of Kingsley and his contemporaries, the emphasis in orthodontics remained the alignment of the teeth and the correction of facial proportions. Little attention was paid to bite relationships, and because it was common practice to remove teeth for many dental problems, extractions for crowding or malalignment were frequent. In an era when an intact dentition was a rarity, the details of occlusal relationships were considered unimportant.

To make good prosthetic replacement teeth, it was necessary to develop a concept of occlusion, and this occurred in the late 1800s. As the concepts of prosthetic occlusion developed and were refined, it was natural to extend this to the natural dentition. Edward H. Angle (Fig. 1.1), whose influence began to be felt about 1890, can be credited with much of the development of a concept of occlusion in the natural dentition. Angle's original interest was in prosthodontics, and he taught in that department in dental schools in Pennsylvania and Minnesota in the 1880s. His increasing interest in dental occlusion and in the treatment necessary to obtain normal occlusion led directly to his development of orthodontics as a specialty, with himself as the "father of modern orthodontics."

Angle's classification of malocclusion in the 1890s was an important step in the development of orthodontics because it not only subdivided major types of malocclusion but also included the first clear and simple definition of normal occlusion in the natural dentition. Angle's postulate was that the upper first molars were the key to occlusion and that the upper and lower molars should be related so that the mesiobuccal cusp of the upper molar occludes in the buccal groove of the lower molar. If the teeth were arranged on a smoothly curving line of occlusion (Fig. 1.2) and this molar relationship existed (Fig. 1.3), then normal occlusion

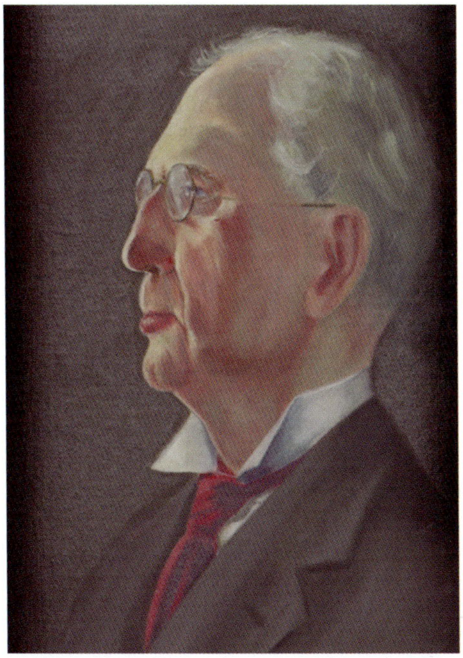

• **Fig. 1.1** Edward H. Angle in his 50s, as the proprietor of the Angle School of Orthodontia. After establishing himself as the first dental specialist, Angle operated proprietary orthodontic schools from 1905 to 1928 in St. Louis, Missouri; New London, Connecticut; and Pasadena, California, in which many of the pioneer American orthodontists were trained.

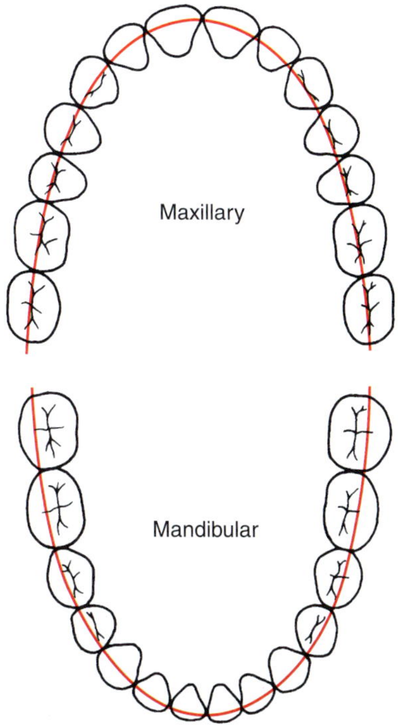

• **Fig. 1.2** The line of occlusion is a smooth (catenary) curve passing through the central fossa of each upper molar and across the cingulum of the upper canine and incisor teeth. The same line runs along the buccal cusps and incisal edges of the lower teeth, thus specifying the occlusal as well as interarch relationships once the molar position is established.

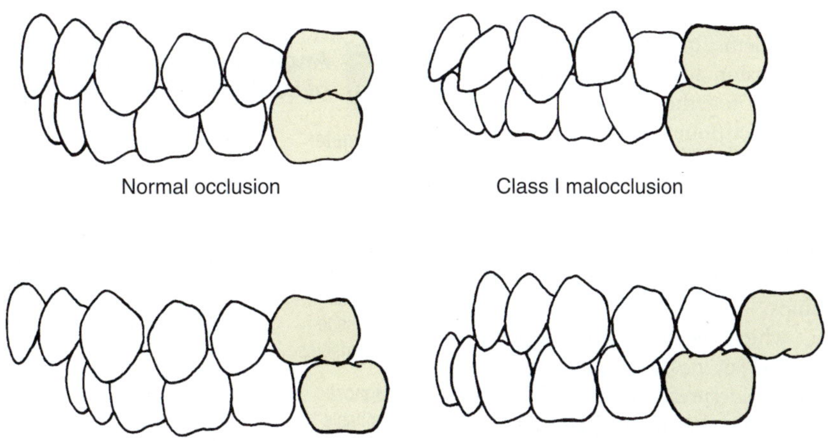

• **Fig. 1.3** Normal occlusion and malocclusion classes as specified by Angle. This classification was quickly and widely adopted early in the 20th century. It is incorporated within all contemporary descriptive and classification schemes.

would result.[3] This statement, which 100 years of experience has proved to be correct except when there are aberrations in the size of teeth, brilliantly simplified normal occlusion.

Angle then described three classes of *malocclusion*, based on the occlusal relationships of the first molars:

- Class I: Normal relationship of the molars, but line of occlusion incorrect because of malposed teeth, rotations, or other causes
- Class II: Lower molar distally positioned relative to upper molar, line of occlusion not specified
- Class III: Lower molar mesially positioned relative to upper molar, line of occlusion not specified

Note that the Angle classification has four classes: normal occlusion, Class I malocclusion, Class II malocclusion, and Class III malocclusion (see Fig. 1.3). Normal occlusion and Class I malocclusion share the same molar relationship but differ in the arrangement of the teeth relative to the line of occlusion. The line of occlusion may or may not be correct in Class II and Class III malocclusion.

With the establishment of a concept of normal occlusion and a classification scheme that incorporated the line of occlusion, by the early 1900s orthodontics was no longer just the alignment of irregular teeth. Instead, it had evolved into the treatment of malocclusion, defined as any deviation from the ideal occlusal scheme described by Angle. Because precisely defined relationships required a full complement of teeth in both arches, maintaining an intact dentition became an important goal of orthodontic treatment. Angle and his followers strongly opposed extraction for orthodontic purposes. With the emphasis on dental occlusion that followed, however, less attention came to be paid to facial proportions and esthetics. Angle abandoned extraoral force because he decided this was not necessary to achieve proper occlusal relationships. He solved the problem of dental and facial appearance by simply postulating that the best esthetics always were achieved when the patient had ideal occlusion.

As time passed, it became clear that even an excellent occlusion was unsatisfactory if it was achieved at the expense of proper facial proportions. Calvin Case was an advocate of carefully considering protrusion and extraction treatment in order to achieve the best dentofacial harmony for the individual. With that he also realized that tipping and root movement could also bring different esthetic results.[4]

Not only had some realized that the teeth needed to be related to the face, Dr. Paul Simon believed that the dentition was invariably related to the skull. His theory that the canine was related to the orbital plane was examined by Broadbent using skulls and a craniostat. It was found to be too variable to be of use as an orthodontic landmark for the dentition.[5] But, as orthodontics was developing as a profession some were examining more than just the alignment of the teeth, with the addition of lip protrusion and facial esthetics.

Not only were there esthetic problems, it often proved impossible to maintain an occlusal relationship achieved by prolonged use of heavy elastics to pull the teeth together as Angle and his followers had suggested. So, early practitioners discovered retention issues as well.

Under the leadership of Charles Tweed in the United States and Raymond Begg in Australia (both of whom had studied with Angle), extraction of teeth was reintroduced into orthodontics in the 1940s and 1950s to enhance facial esthetics and achieve better stability of the occlusal relationships.

Cephalometric radiography, which enabled orthodontists to measure the changes in tooth and jaw positions produced by growth and treatment, came into widespread use after World War II. These radiographs made it clear that many Class II and Class III malocclusions resulted from faulty jaw relationships, not just malposed teeth. By use of cephalometrics, it was also possible to see that jaw growth could be altered by orthodontic treatment. In Europe, the method of "functional jaw orthopedics" was developed to enhance growth changes, while in the United States, extraoral force came to be used for this purpose. At present, both functional and extraoral appliances are used internationally to control and modify growth and form. Obtaining correct or at least improved jaw relationships became a goal of treatment by the mid-20th century.

The changes in the goals of orthodontic treatment, which now focus on facial proportions and the impact of the dentition on facial appearance, have been codified in the form of the soft tissue paradigm.[6]

Modern Treatment Goals: The Soft Tissue Paradigm

A paradigm can be defined as "a set of shared beliefs and assumptions that represent the conceptual foundation of an area of science or clinical practice." The soft tissue paradigm states that both the goals and limitations of modern orthodontic and orthognathic treatment are determined by the soft tissues of the face, not by the teeth and bones. This reorientation of orthodontics away from the Angle paradigm that dominated the 20th century is most easily understood by comparing treatment goals, diagnostic emphasis, and treatment approach in the two paradigms (Table 1.1). With the soft tissue paradigm, the increased focus on clinical examination rather than examination of dental casts and radiographs leads to a different approach to obtaining important diagnostic information, and that information is used to develop treatment plans that would not have been considered without it.

More specifically, what difference does the soft tissue paradigm make in planning treatment? There are several major effects:

1. The primary goal of treatment becomes esthetic and proportional soft tissue relationships and adaptations, not Angle's ideal occlusion. This broader goal is not incompatible with Angle's ideal occlusion, but it acknowledges that to provide maximum benefit for the patient, ideal occlusion (in terms of a nonextraction ideally aligned dentition) cannot always be the major focus of a treatment plan. Soft tissue relationships, both the 3D proportions of the facial soft tissue and the protrusive/retrusive relationships of the dentition to the lips and face, are the major determinants of facial appearance. Soft tissue adaptations to the position of the teeth (or lack of it) determine whether the orthodontic result will be stable and esthetic. Dentofacial appearance affects social interactions, but also

TABLE 1.1 Angle Versus Soft Tissue Paradigms: A New Way of Looking at Treatment Goals

Parameter	Angle Paradigm	Soft Tissue Paradigm
Primary treatment goal	Ideal dental occlusion	Normal soft tissue proportions and adaptations
Secondary goal	Ideal jaw relationships	Functional occlusion
Hard and soft tissue relationships	Ideal hard tissue proportions produce ideal soft tissues	Ideal soft tissue proportions define ideal hard tissues
Diagnostic emphasis	Dental casts, cephalometric radiographs	Clinical examination of intraoral and facial soft tissues
Treatment approach	Obtain ideal dental and skeletal relationships, assume the soft tissues will be all right	Plan ideal soft tissue relationships and then place teeth and jaws as needed to achieve this
Function emphasis	TMJ in relation to dental occlusion	Soft tissue movement in relation to display of teeth
Stability of result	Related primarily to dental occlusion	Related primarily to soft tissue pressure and equilibrium effects

TMJ, Temporomandibular joint.

perceptions of individuals' ability to learn and be employed. Keeping this in mind while planning treatment is critically important for complete success.

2. The secondary goal of treatment becomes *functional occlusion.* What does that have to do with soft tissues? Temporomandibular (TM) dysfunction, to the extent that it relates to dental occlusion, is best thought of as the result of injury to the soft tissues around the temporomandibular joint (TMJ) caused by clenching and grinding the teeth, whatever the source of the injury and associated pain and dysfunction. Given that, an important goal of treatment is to arrange the occlusion to minimize the chance of injury. In this also, Angle's ideal occlusion is not incompatible with the broader goal, but deviations from the Angle ideal may provide greater benefit for some patients and should be considered when treatment is planned.
3. The thought process that goes into "solving the patient's problems" is reversed. In the past, the clinician's focus was on dental and skeletal relationships, with the tacit assumption that if these were correct, soft tissue relationships would take care of themselves. With the broader focus on facial and oral soft tissues, the thought process is to establish what these soft tissue relationships should be and then determine how the teeth and jaws would have to be arranged to meet the soft tissue goals. Why is this important in establishing the goals of treatment? It relates very much to why patients and parents seek orthodontic treatment and what they expect to gain from it. Most want an appearance so they can function as productive and self-assured members of society.

The following sections of this chapter provide some background on the prevalence of malocclusion, what we know about the need for treatment of malocclusion and dentofacial abnormalities, and how soft tissue considerations, as well as teeth and bone, affect both need and demand for orthodontic treatment. It must be kept in mind that orthodontics is shaped by biological, psychosocial, and cultural determinants. For that reason, when defining the goals of orthodontic treatment, one has to consider not only morphologic and functional factors, but a wide range of psychosocial and bioethical issues as well. All these topics are discussed in much greater detail in the following chapters on diagnosis, treatment planning, and treatment.

The Usual Orthodontic Problems: Epidemiology of Malocclusion

Angle's "normal occlusion" more properly should be considered the ideal without a facial context. In fact, perfectly interdigitating teeth arranged along a perfectly regular line of occlusion are quite rare. For many years, epidemiologic studies of malocclusion suffered from considerable disagreement among investigators about how much deviation from the ideal should be accepted within the bounds of normal. By the 1970s, a series of studies by public health or university groups in most developed countries provided a reasonably clear worldwide picture of the prevalence of the various types of malocclusion by degree of severity.

In the United States, two large-scale surveys carried out by the US Public Health Service (USPHS) covered children ages 6 to 11 years from 1963 to 1965 and youths ages 12 to 17 years in 1969 and 1970.[7,8] As part of a large-scale national survey of health care problems and needs in the United States in 1989 through 1994 (Third National Health and Nutrition Examination Survey [NHANES III]), estimates of malocclusion again were obtained. This study of 14,000 individuals was statistically designed to provide weighted estimates for approximately 150 million persons in the sampled racial or ethnic and age groups. The data provide reasonably current information for US children and youths and include the first good data set for malocclusion in adults, with separate estimates for the major racial (White and Black) and one ethnic group (Mexican American).[9]

The characteristics of malocclusion evaluated in NHANES III included the irregularity index, which is a measure of incisor alignment (Fig. 1.4); the prevalence of midline diastema larger than 2 mm (Fig. 1.5); and the prevalence of posterior crossbite (Fig. 1.6). In addition, overjet (Fig. 1.7) and overbite or open bite (Fig. 1.8) were measured. Overjet reflects Angle's Class II and Class III molar relationships. Because overjet can be evaluated much more precisely than molar relationship in a clinical examination, molar relationship was not evaluated directly.

Data for these characteristics of malocclusion for the children (age 8–11), youth (12–17) and adults (18–50) are provided for the US population, taken from the NHANES III study, and are displayed graphically in Figs. 1.9–1.13.

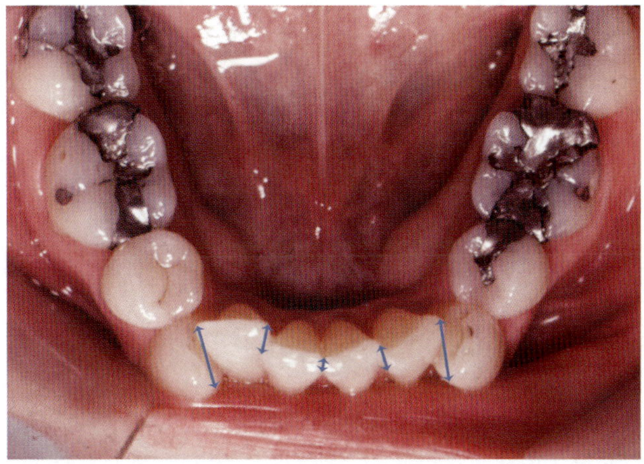

• **Fig. 1.4** Incisor irregularity usually is expressed as the irregularity index: the total of the millimeter distances from the anatomic contact point on each incisor tooth to the anatomic contact point that it should touch, as shown by the blue lines. For this patient, the irregularity index is 10 (mm).

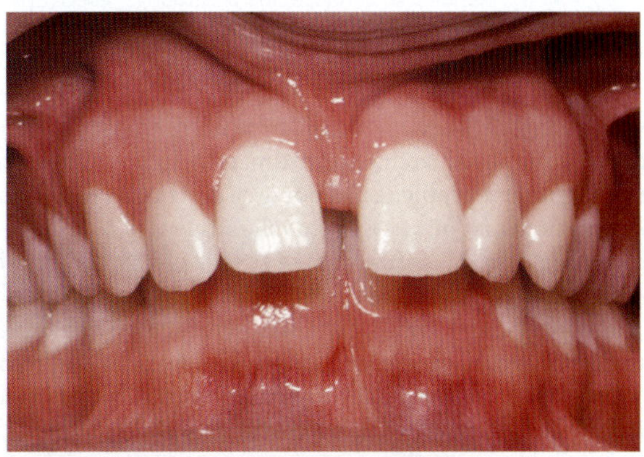

• **Fig. 1.5** A space between adjacent teeth is called a *diastema*. A maxillary midline diastema is relatively common, especially during the mixed dentition in childhood, and disappears or decreases in width as the permanent canines erupt. Spontaneous correction of a childhood diastema is most likely when its width is less than 2 mm, so this patient is on the borderline and may need future treatment.

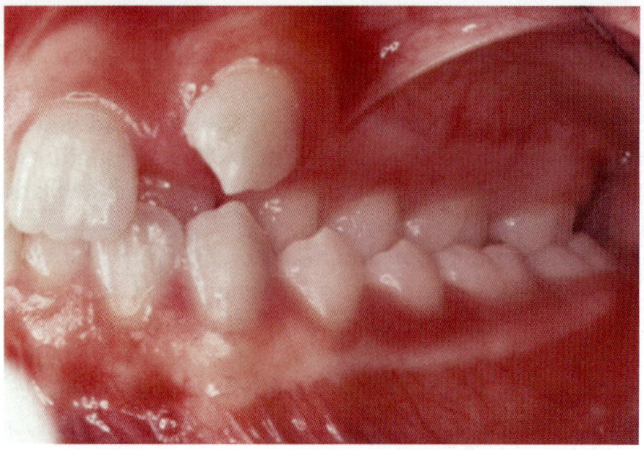

• **Fig. 1.6** Posterior crossbite exists when the maxillary posterior teeth are lingually positioned relative to the mandibular teeth, as in this patient. Posterior crossbite most often reflects a narrow maxillary dental arch but can arise from other causes. This patient also has a one-tooth anterior crossbite, with the lateral incisor trapped lingually.

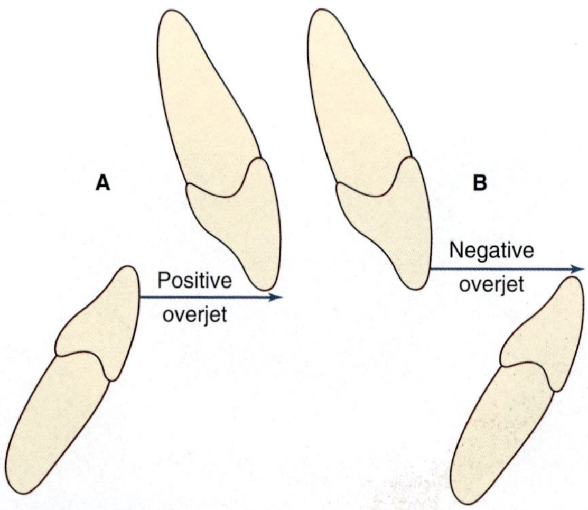

• **Fig. 1.7** Overjet is defined as horizontal overlap of the incisors, measured from the facial surface of the most prominent mandibular incisor to the facial surface of the most prominent maxillary incisor. Normally the incisors are in or near contact, with the upper incisors ahead of the lower by only the thickness of their incisal edges (i.e., positive overjet of +2 to 3 mm). If the lower incisors are in front of the upper incisors, with overjet measured from the same facial surfaces, the condition is called *reverse or negative overjet* or *anterior crossbite*.

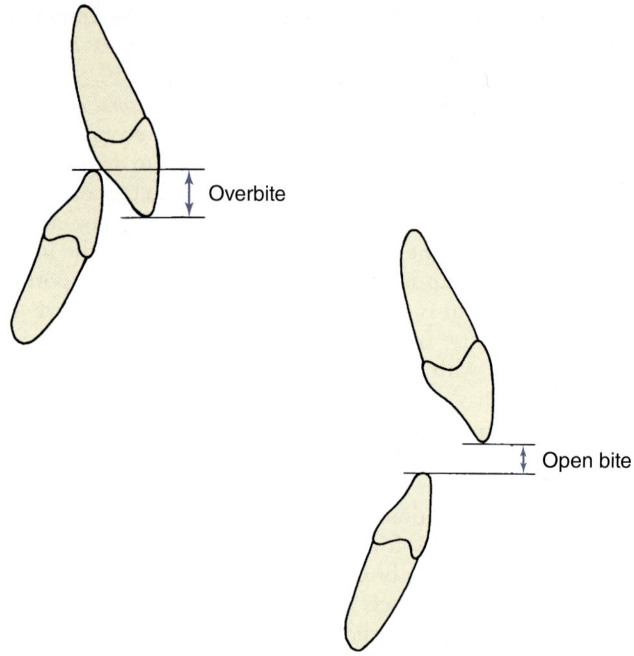

• **Fig. 1.8** Overbite is defined as the vertical overlap of the incisors. Normally, the lower incisal edges contact the lingual surface of the upper incisors at or above the cingulum (i.e., normally there is a 1- to 2-mm overbite). In open bite, there is no vertical overlap, and the vertical separation of the incisors is measured to quantify its severity and given a negative value of, say -3 mm.

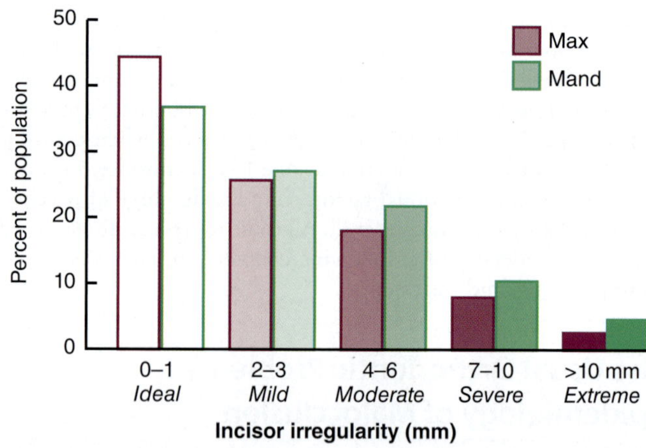

• **Fig. 1.9** Incisor irregularity in the US population, 1989–94. Of the population, 20%–25% have moderately irregular (usually crowded) incisors, and nearly 15% have severe or extreme irregularity. Note that irregularity in the lower arch is more prevalent at any degree of severity.

Note in Fig. 1.9 incisor irregularity is common and usually more so in the lower arch. Approximately 15% have severe or extreme alignment problems. Major arch expansion or extraction of some teeth would be necessary to align them.

In the age 8 to 11 group, just over half of US children have well-aligned incisors. The rest have varying degrees of malalignment and crowding (Fig. 1.10). The percentage with excellent alignment decreases in the age 12 to 17 group as the remaining permanent teeth erupt, then remains essentially stable in the upper arch but worsens in the lower arch for adults.

Racial and ethnic differences are apparent from the data. Mexican Americans are more likely to have severe maxillary crowding, but they and Whites have the most severe mandibular crowding (Fig. 1.11). A midline diastema larger than 2 mm is present in 26% of US children. This amount of space can be an esthetic problem and can cause space problems with eruption of the lateral incisors. Although this space tends to close, over 6% of youths and adults still have a noticeable diastema that compromises the appearance of the smile (see Fig. 1.5). Blacks are more than twice as likely to have a midline diastema as Whites or Mexican American.

Occlusal relationships must be considered in all planes of space. Lingual posterior crossbite (i.e., upper teeth lingual to lower teeth) is the major deviation from the normal transverse or coronal dental relationship. According to the NHANES III data,[9] it occurs in 7% to 8% of the US population. Posterior crossbites are near 7% in childhood, 8% in youth and 9% in adults (see Fig. 1.10).

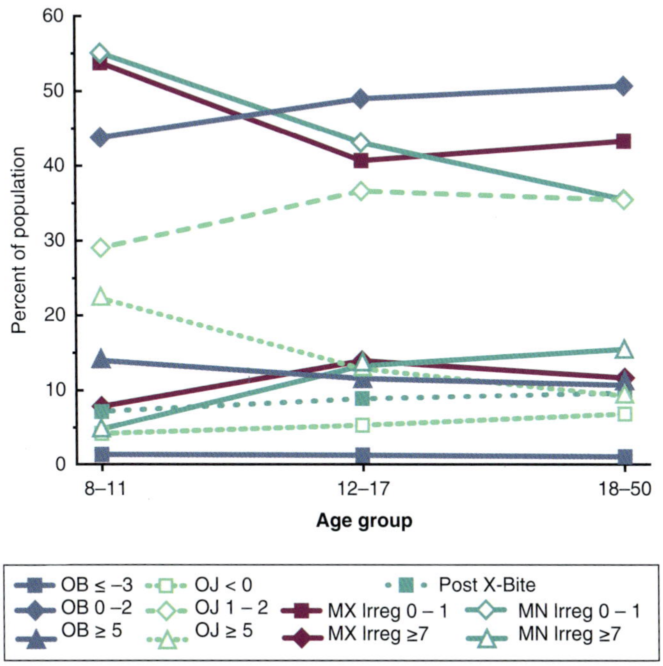

• **Fig. 1.10** Changes in the prevalence of types of malocclusion from childhood to adult life, United States, 1989–94. Note the increase in incisor irregularity, decrease in severe overjet and increase in negative overjet as children mature, both of which are related to more mandibular than maxillary growth. Posterior crossbites gradually increase with maturity. Open bites appear to be stable in number, while normal overbites increase and deep overbites decrease.

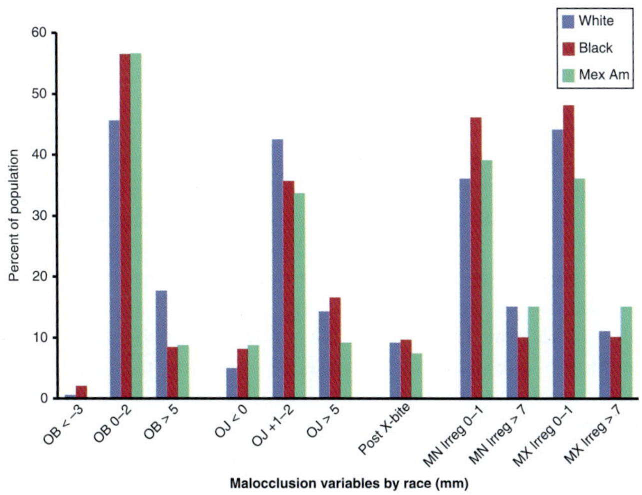

• **Fig. 1.11** Incisor irregularity by racial or ethnic groups. The percentage of the Mexican American population with severe crowding is equal or greater than the other two groups for both the maxilla and mandible followed by Whites. ideal alignment is lowest for Whites in the mandible and Mexican Americans in the maxilla. This may reflect the low number of Mexican Americans with orthodontic treatment at the time of the NHANES III survey. Posterior crossbites are similar in all groups. Increased overjet is more frequent in Blacks and negative overjet is more frequent in Blacks and Mexican Americans. Vertically, deep bites are a common White trait and open bites more common in Blacks.

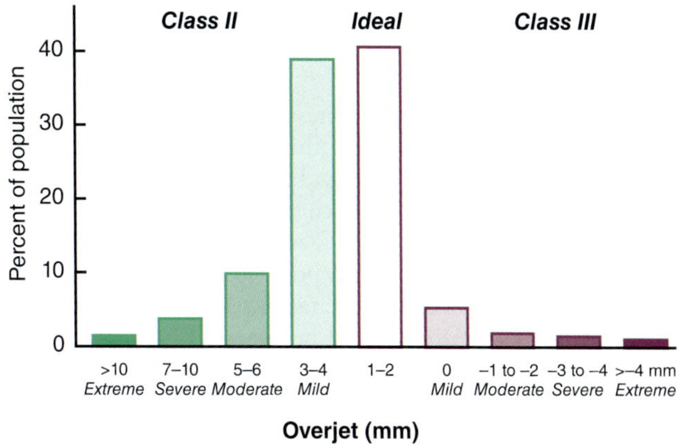

• **Fig. 1.12** Overjet (Class II) and reverse overjet (Class III) in the US population, 1989–94. Only one-third of the population have ideal anteroposterior incisor relationships, but overjet is only moderately increased in another one-third. Increased overjet accompanying Class II malocclusion is much more prevalent than reverse overjet accompanying Class III.

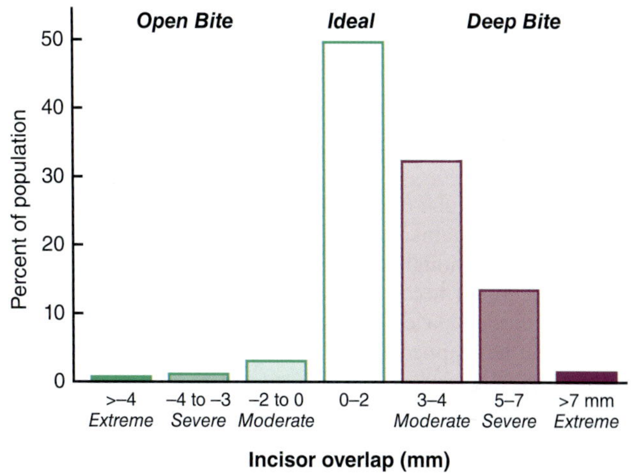

• **Fig. 1.13** Open bite and deep bite relationships in the US population, 1989–94. Half the population have an ideal vertical relationship of the incisors. Deep bite is much more prevalent than open bite, but vertical relationships vary greatly among racial groups (Fig. 1.11).

Posterior crossbite differs little among the racial and ethnic groups (see Fig. 1.11).

Normal overjet is 2 mm. Increased positive overjet or reverse overjet (negative) indicates anteroposterior deviations in the Class II or Class III direction, respectively, with Class III being much less prevalent (Fig. 1.12). Overjet of 5 mm or more, suggesting Angle's Class II malocclusion, occurs in 22% of children, 13% of youths, and 9% of adult, while 0 mm or <0 mm overjet increases over time (Fig. 1.10). This reflects the greater postnatal growth of the mandible than the maxilla, which is discussed in Chapter 2. Class II problems are more prevalent in Black and White groups and Class III problems are more prevalent in Mexican American and Black groups (Fig. 1.11).

Vertical deviations from the ideal overbite of 2 mm are frequent (Fig. 1.13). More people in the US have deep bites than open bites. Open bites appear to remain stable, while deep bites become less severe (see Fig. 1.10). There are striking differences between the racial or ethnic groups in vertical dental relationships. Severe deep bite is nearly twice as prevalent in Whites as Blacks or Mexican Americans, whereas open bite of greate than 3 mm is more prevalent in Blacks (see Fig. 1.11). This almost surely reflects the slightly different craniofacial proportions of the Black population groups (see Chapter 5 for a more complete discussion). In contrast to the higher prevalence of anteroposterior problems, vertical problems are less prevalent in Latinx than either Blacks or Whites.

From the survey data, it is interesting to calculate the percentage of American children and youths who would clearly fall into Angle's Class I, II and III groups. From this perspective, 30+% at most have Angle's normal occlusion. Class II malocclusions (approximately 15-20+%); and Class III (less than ~5%). The remainder are variations of antero-posterior discrepancies.

Differences in malocclusion characteristics between the United States and other countries would be expected because of differences in racial and ethnic composition. Although the available data are not as extensive as for American populations, it seems clear that Class II problems are most prevalent in Whites of northern European descent (for instance, 25% of children in Denmark are reported to have Class II malocclusion), whereas Class III problems are most prevalent in Asian populations (3%–5% in Japan, nearly 2% in China), with another 2% to 3% pseudo–Class III (i.e., shifting into anterior crossbite because of incisor interferences). African populations are by no means homogenous, but from the differences found in the United States between Blacks and Whites, it seems likely that Class III and open bite are more frequent in African than European populations and deep bite less frequent.

Why Is Malocclusion So Prevalent?

Crowded and irregular teeth now occur in a majority of the population; skeletal remains indicate that this was unusual until relatively recently, although not unknown (Fig. 1.14). Because the mandible tends to become separated from the rest of the skull when long-buried skeletal remains are unearthed, it is easier to be sure what has happened to alignment of teeth than to occlusal relationships. The skeletal remains suggest that all members of a group might tend toward a Class III or, less commonly, a Class II jaw relationship. Similar findings are noted in present population groups (crowding and malalignment of teeth) that are uncommon in ancient skeletal remains. The majority of the group may have mild anteroposterior or transverse discrepancies, as in the Class III tendency of South Pacific islanders[10] and buccal crossbite (X-occlusion) in aboriginal people of Australia.[11]"

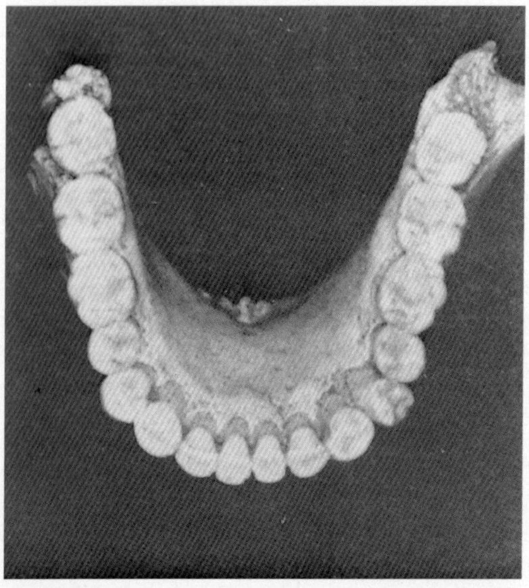

• **Fig. 1.14** Mandibular dental arches from specimens from the Krapina cave in Yugoslavia, estimated to be approximately 100,000 years old. Note the excellent alignment in this specimen. Near-perfect alignment or minimal crowding was the usual finding in this group. (From Wolpoff WH. *Paleoanthropology*. Alfred A Knopf; 1998.)

Although 1000 years is a long time relative to a single human life, it is a very short time from an evolutionary perspective. The fossil record documents evolutionary trends over many thousands of years that affect the present dentition, including a decrease in the size of individual teeth, in the number of the teeth, and in the size of the jaws. For example, there has been a steady reduction in the size of both anterior and posterior teeth over at least the last 100,000 years (Fig. 1.15). The number of teeth in the dentition of higher primates has been reduced from the usual mammalian pattern (Fig. 1.16). The third incisor and third premolar have disappeared, as has the fourth molar. At present, the human third molar, second premolar, and second incisor often fail to develop, which indicates that these teeth may be on their way out. Compared with other primates, modern humans have quite underdeveloped jaws.

It is easy to see that the progressive reduction in jaw size, if not well matched to a decrease in tooth size and number, could lead to crowding and malalignment. It is less easy to see why dental crowding should have increased quite recently, but this seems to have paralleled the transition from primitive agricultural to modern urbanized societies. Cardiovascular disease and related health problems appear rapidly when a previously unaffected population group leaves agrarian life for the city and civilization. High blood pressure, heart disease, diabetes, and several other medical problems are so much more prevalent in developed than underdeveloped countries that they have been labeled "diseases of civilization."

There is some evidence that malocclusion increases within well-defined populations after a transition from rural villages to the city. Corruccini, for instance, reported a higher prevalence of crowding, posterior crossbite, and buccal segment discrepancy in urbanized youths compared with rural Punjabi youths of northern India.[12] One can argue that malocclusion is another condition made worse by the changing conditions of modern life, perhaps resulting in part from less use of the masticatory apparatus with softer foods now. Under primitive conditions, of course, excellent function of the jaws and teeth was an important predictor of the ability to survive and reproduce. A capable masticatory apparatus was essential to deal with uncooked or partially cooked meat and plant foods. Watching an Australian aboriginal man using every muscle of his upper body to tear off a piece of kangaroo flesh from the barely cooked animal, for instance, makes one appreciate the decrease in demand on the masticatory apparatus that has accompanied civilization (Fig. 1.17). An interesting proposal by anthropologists is that the introduction of cooking, so that it did not take as much effort and energy to masticate food, was the key to the development of the larger human brain. Without cooked food, it would not have been possible to meet the energy demand of the enlarging brain. With it, excess energy is available for brain development and robust jaws are unnecessary.[13]

Determining whether changes in jaw function have increased the prevalence of malocclusion is complicated by the fact that both dental caries and periodontal disease, which are rare on the primitive diet, appear rapidly when the diet changes. The resulting dental pathology can make it difficult to establish what the occlusion might have been in the absence of early loss of teeth,

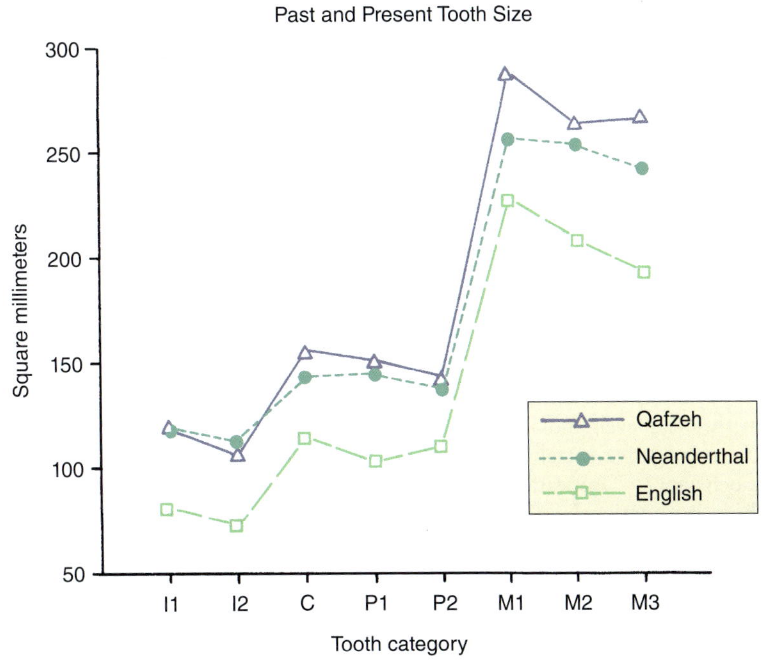

• **Fig. 1.15** The generalized decline in the size of human teeth can be seen by comparing tooth sizes from the anthropologic site at Qafzeh, dated 100,000 years ago; Neanderthal teeth, 10,000 years ago; and modern human populations. (Redrawn from Kelly MA, Larsen CS, eds. *Advances in Dental Anthropology*. Wiley-Liss; 1991.)

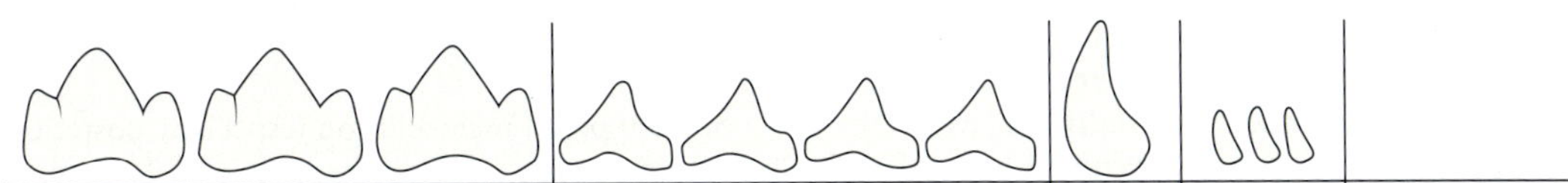

Molars (M)	Premolars (PM)	Canines (C)	Incisors (I)	
M-3	PM-4	C-1	I- 3	Basic mammalian
M-3	PM-3	C-1	I- 2	Prosimian
M-3	PM-2	C-1	I- 2	Higher ape
M-3 (2)	PM-(1-2)	C-1	I- (1-2)	Man

• **Fig. 1.16** Reduction in the number of teeth has been a feature of primate evolution. In the present human population, third molars are so frequently missing that it appears a further reduction is in progress, and the relatively high prevalence of missing maxillary lateral incisors and mandibular second premolars suggests evolutionary pressure on these teeth.

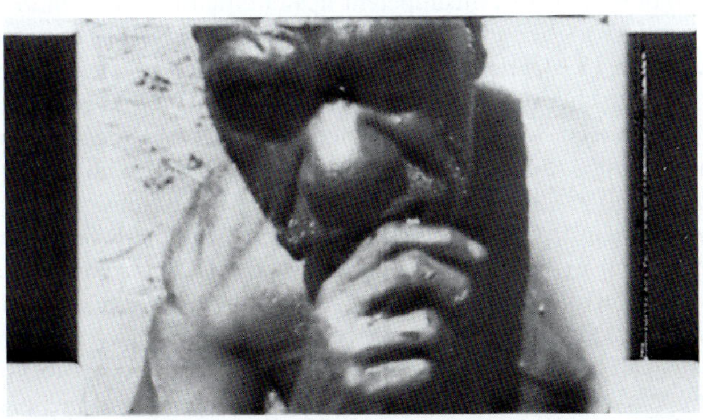

• **Fig. 1.17** A frame from a 1960s movie of an Australian aboriginal man eating a kangaroo prepared in the traditional (barely cooked) fashion. Note the activity of muscles, not only in the facial region, but throughout the neck and shoulder girdle. (Courtesy M. J. Barrett.)

gingivitis, and periodontal breakdown. The increase in malocclusion in modern times certainly parallels the development of modern civilization, but a reduction in jaw size related to disuse atrophy is hard to document. Although it is difficult to know the precise cause of any specific malocclusion, we do know in general what the etiologic possibilities are, and these are discussed in some detail in Chapter 5.

What difference does it make if you have a malocclusion? Let's now consider the reasons for orthodontic treatment.

Who Needs Treatment?

Protruding, irregular, or maloccluded teeth have been reported to cause three types of problems for the patient: (1) social discrimination because of facial appearance; (2) problems with oral function, including difficulties in jaw movement (muscle incoordination or pain), temporomandibular dysfunction (TMD), and problems with mastication, swallowing, or speech; and (3) greater susceptibility to trauma and periodontal disease, or tooth decay. Below we examine the evidence.

Psychosocial Problems

A number of studies in recent years have confirmed what is intuitively obvious: that severe malocclusion is likely to be a social handicap. The usual caricature of an individual who is not too bright often includes protruding upper incisors. A witch not only rides a broom, she has a prominent lower jaw that would produce a Class III malocclusion. Simply revealing malaligned teeth can reduce facial attractiveness. Well-aligned teeth and a pleasing smile carry positive status at all social levels and ages, whereas irregular or protruding teeth carry negative social cues, imply reduced intelligence and ethical behavior.[14–16] Appearance can and does make a difference in teachers' expectations and therefore in student progress in school, in employability, and in competition for a mate. This places the concept of "handicapping malocclusion" in a broader and more important context. If the way you interact with other individuals is affected constantly by your teeth, your dental handicap is far from trivial. There is no doubt that social responses conditioned by the major deviations from the usual appearance of the face and teeth can severely affect quality of life and self-esteem in a way that compromises an individual's whole adaptation to life.[17]

It is interesting that psychic distress caused by dental or facial abnormalities is not directly proportional to the anatomic severity of the problem. An individual with anomalies (e.g., with a distorted nose and scarred lip after cleft lip or palate repair) can anticipate a consistently negative response.[18] An individual with an apparently less severe problem (e.g., a deficient chin or protruding maxillary incisors) is sometimes treated differently because of this, but sometimes not. It seems to be easier to cope with a defect if other people's responses to it are consistent than if they are not. Unpredictable responses produce anxiety and can have strong deleterious effects.[19] The impact of a physical abnormality on an individual also will be strongly influenced by that person's self-esteem. The result is that the same degree of anatomic abnormality can be merely a condition of no great consequence to one individual but a genuinely severe problem to another.

In short, it seems clear that the major reason people seek orthodontic treatment is to minimize psychosocial problems related to their dental and facial appearance.[20] These problems are not "just cosmetic." They can have a major effect on the quality of life,[21] and the evidence presented in the final section of this chapter documents that orthodontic treatment can improve it.

Oral Function

Although severe malocclusion surely affects oral function, oral function adapts to form surprisingly well. It appears that malocclusion usually affects function not by making it impossible but by making it difficult, so that extra effort is required to compensate for the anatomic deformity. For instance, everyone uses as many chewing strokes as it takes to reduce a food bolus to a consistency that is satisfactory for swallowing, so if chewing is less efficient in the presence of malocclusion, either the affected individual uses more effort to chew or settles for less well-masticated food before swallowing it. Tongue and lip posture adapt to the position of the teeth so that swallowing rarely is affected (see Chapter 5). Similarly, almost everyone can move the jaw so that proper lip relationships exist for speech, so distorted speech is rarely noted even though an individual may have to make an extraordinary effort to produce normal speech. New data appears to indicate that Cl III malocclusions and anterior open bites severe enough to require orthognathic surgery can distort speech sounds and respond positively to surgical correction.[22,23] As methods to quantify functional adaptations of this type are developed, it is likely that more effects of malocclusion on speech function will be appreciated.

The relationship of malocclusion and adaptive function to TMD, manifesting with pain in and around the TMJ, is understood much better now than only a few years ago. The pain may result from pathologic changes within the joint but more often is caused by muscle fatigue and spasm. Muscle pain almost always correlates with a history of clenching or grinding the teeth as a response to stressful situations or of constantly posturing the mandible to an anterior or lateral position.

Some dentists have suggested that even minor imperfections in the occlusion serve to trigger clenching and grinding the teeth. If this were true, it would indicate a real need for perfecting the occlusion in everyone, to avoid the possibility of developing facial muscle pain. Because the number of people with at least moderate degrees of malocclusion (50% to 75% of the population) far exceeds the number with TMD (5% to 30%, depending on which symptoms are examined), it seems unlikely that dental occlusion alone is enough to cause hyperactivity of the oral musculature. A reaction to stress usually is involved. Some individuals react by clenching and grinding their teeth; others develop symptoms in other organ systems. An individual almost never has both ulcerative colitis (also a common stress-induced disease) and TMD.

Some types of malocclusion (especially posterior crossbite with a shift on closure, anterior open bite and Cl II and Cl III relationships) correlate positively with TMJ problems and other types do not, but even the strongest correlation coefficients are only 0.3 to 0.4. This means that for the great majority of patients, there is no association between malocclusion and TMD[24] or previous orthodontic treatment and TMD.[25] Therefore, orthodontics as the primary treatment for TMD almost never is indicated, but in special circumstances (see Chapter 18) it can be a useful adjunct to other treatment for the muscle pain.

Relationship to Injury and Dental Disease

Malocclusion, particularly protruding maxillary incisors, beyond 5 mm of overjet with incompetent lips can increase the likelihood of an injury to the teeth (Fig. 1.18).[26] About 15% to 18% of youth aged 12 to 18 experience permanent incisor trauma.[27] The majority of these children will incur only minor chips in the enamel.[28] For that reason, reducing the chance of injury when incisors protrude is not a strong argument for early treatment of all Class II problems (see Chapter 13), but with previous trauma and age younger than 9 years, the risk of additional trauma is 8.4 times higher than in children with no history of trauma.[29] For such a child, retracting the incisors (but not growth modification) is indicated. Extreme overbite, so that the lower incisors contact the palate, can cause significant tissue damage leading to early loss of the upper incisors and also can result in extreme wear of incisors. Both of these effects can be avoided by orthodontic treatment (see Chapters 11 and 12).

It is certainly possible that malocclusion could contribute to both dental decay and periodontal disease by making it

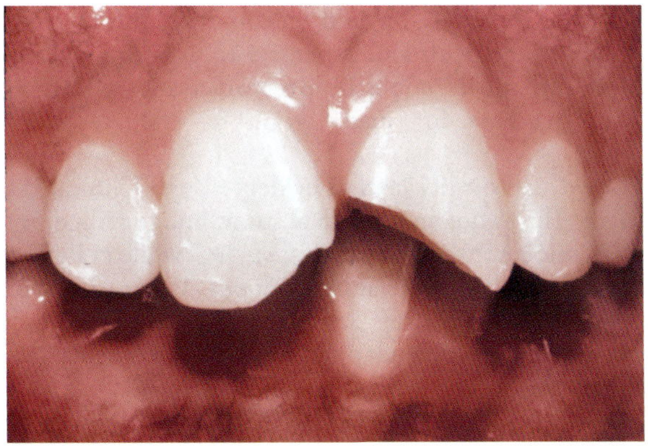

• **Fig. 1.18** Fractured maxillary central incisors in a 10-year-old girl. There is almost one chance in three of an injury to a protruding incisor, though fortunately the damage is rarely this severe. Most of the accidents occur during normal activity, not in sports.

harder to care for the teeth properly or by causing occlusal trauma. There is some weak evidence that malocclusion may be tied to periodontal health, but this may be dependant on overall oral health status and the association does not mean causation.[30] An individual's willingness and motivation determine oral hygiene much more than how well the teeth are aligned, and presence or absence of dental plaque is the major determinant of the health of both the hard and soft tissues of the mouth. If individuals with malocclusion are more prone to tooth decay, the effect is small compared with hygiene status. Occlusal trauma, once thought to be important in the development of periodontal disease, now is recognized to be a secondary, not a primary, etiologic factor. There is only a tenuous link between untreated malocclusion and major periodontal disease later in life.

Could orthodontic treatment itself be an etiologic agent for oral disease? Long-term studies have shown no indication that orthodontic treatment increased the chance of later periodontal problems.[31] The association between early orthodontic and later periodontal treatment appears to be only another manifestation of the phenomenon that one segment of the population seeks dental treatment while another avoids it. Those who have had one type of successful dental treatment, such as orthodontics in childhood, are more likely to seek another such as periodontal therapy in adult life.

In summary, it appears that both psychosocial and functional handicaps can produce significant need for orthodontic treatment. The evidence is less clear that orthodontic treatment reduces the development of later dental disease.

Generating and Assessing Data

Evidence-Based Selection

If treatment is needed, how do you decide what sort of treatment to use? The present trend in health care is strongly toward evidence-based treatment—that is, treatment procedures should be chosen on the basis of clear evidence that the selected method is the most successful approach to that particular patient's problem(s). The better the evidence, the easier the decision.

Meta-analysis, Systematic Reviews and Clinical Practice Guidelines: The Best Evidence

Orthodontics traditionally has been a specialty in which the opinions of leaders were important, to the point that professional groups coalesced around a strong leader. Angle, Begg, and Tweed societies still exist, and new ones whose primary purpose is to promulgate their leaders' opinions are still being formed in the 21st century. As any professional group comes of age, however, there must be a focus on evidence-based rather than opinion-based decisions. That very much includes orthodontics.

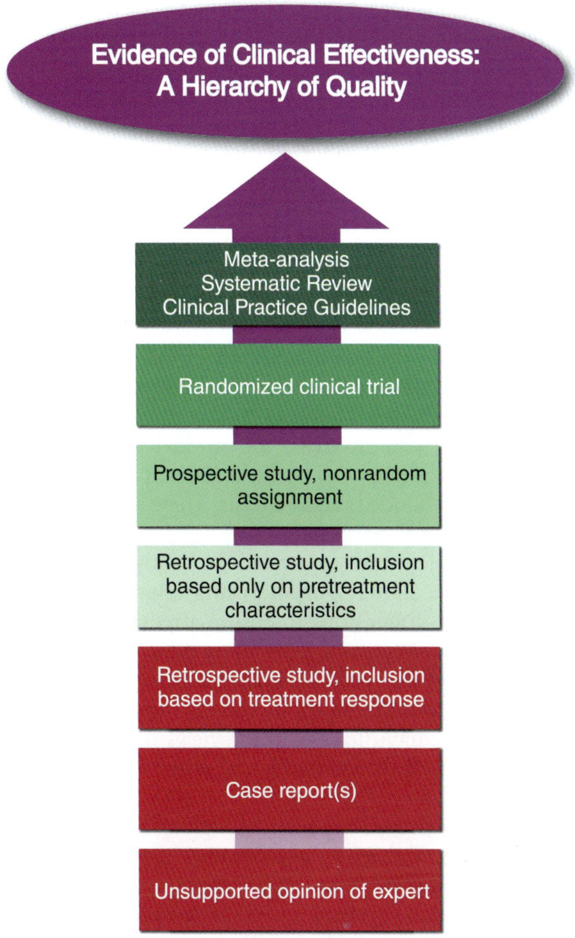

• **Fig. 1.19** Evidence of clinical effectiveness: a hierarchy of quality. Note that systematic reviews, by themselves, can have a wide range of quality.

As Fig. 1.19 illustrates, a hierarchy of quality exists in the evidence available to guide clinical decisions. It reflects, more than anything else, the probability that an accurate conclusion can be drawn from the group of patients who have been studied. The unsupported opinion of an expert is the weakest form of clinical evidence. Often, the expert opinion is supported by a series of cases that were selected retrospectively from clinical practice records.

The problem with that, of course, is that the cases are likely to have been selected because they show the expected outcome. A clinician who becomes an advocate of a treatment method is naturally tempted to select illustrative cases that show the desired outcome, and if even they try to be objective, it is difficult to avoid introducing bias. When outcomes vary, as they often do, picking the cases that came out the way they were supposed to and discarding the ones that didn't is a great way to make your point (and usually invalid). Information based on selected cases, therefore, must be viewed with considerable reservation. One important way to control bias in reporting the outcomes of treatment is to be sure that *all* of the treated cases are included in the report.

For this reason, the gold standard for evaluating clinical procedures is the randomized clinical trial, in which patients are randomly assigned in advance to alternative treatment procedures. The great advantage of this method is that random assignment, if the sample is large enough (i.e., has enough power), should result in a similar distribution of all variables between (or among) the groups. Even variables that were not recognized in advance should be controlled by this type of patient assignment—and in clinical work, important variables often are identified only after the treatment has been started or even completed. Clinical trials in orthodontics are referred to throughout this book.

In randomized clinical trials, the studied individuals come from unbiased samples guided by inclusion and exclusion criteria and allocated on a blinded random basis. These studies are expensive and demanding to perform.

Systematic reviews are generated by studying a group of studies aimed at a similar purpose using criteria that evaluate the studies for all dimensions to ensure a reduced or low level of bias. These reviews can be even more effective when proper tools are used to evaluate the sample, methods and data (which have their own recommended methods), otherwise they can be harmful. The conclusions of the reviews draw conclusions, qualify the quality of the evidence, and point to future research directions.

If the group of studies is similar enough and uses comparable samples, methods, and reported outcomes, they can be statistically evaluated and weighted. Again, methods must be appropriate and tools must be available to evaluate these meta-analyses. This is an even higher level of analysis.

Orthodontic research is an excellent example of an area in which numerous small studies have been carried out toward similar ends, but differences in protocols and outcome variables were different enough to make comparisons difficult. That is why orthodontics should move to a core outcomes set that includes patient satisfaction so better comparisons can be made and we can approach bigger data sets. Meta-analyses are no substitute for new data collected with precise protocols, and including poorly done studies in a meta-analysis carries the risk of confusing rather than clarifying the issue.[32] Nevertheless, applying meta-analysis to clinical questions has considerable potential to reduce uncertainty about the best treatment methods.

An important caveat for meta-analyses is that the emphasis on statistical significance should not lead to overlooking the difference between statistical and clinical significance. Statistical significance evaluates the chance that a difference in the data set would be due just to the random variation that affects any group of treatment responses; clinical significance evaluates whether a difference of this magnitude would have any practical effect on the provision of treatment. Not all statistical differences are clinically significant, and sometimes differences that do not reach statistical significance nevertheless may indicate a clinical advance. That is why effect size or the quantification of differences between treatments introduced by Cohen is important.[33]

Unfortunately, randomized trials and meta-analysis cannot be used in many situations for ethical or practical reasons. For instance, a randomized trial of extraction versus nonextraction orthodontic treatment would encounter ethical concerns, would be very difficult and expensive to organize and manage if ethical difficulties could be overcome, and would require following patients for many years to evaluate long-term outcomes.

Another high quality level of evidence is the Clinical Practice Guideline. This is not an individual study, but a method to move from systemic reviews to the clinical setting, while evaluating the benefits and harms of the treatment options. This method includes expert panels and consensus development in an interdisciplinary manner. Again, recommendations are formulated using accepted tools.

Retrospective Studies: Control Group Required

Another acceptable way to replace opinion with evidence is by careful retrospective study of treatment outcomes under well-defined conditions. The best way to know—often the only way to know—whether a treatment method really works is to compare treated patients with an untreated control group. For such a comparison to be valid, the two groups must be equivalent before treatment starts. If the groups were not equivalent, they can be statistically adjusted, so you can say with confidence that posttreatment differences were due to the treatment.

There are difficulties in setting up control groups for orthodontic treatment. The principal ones are that the controls must be followed over a long period of time, equivalent to the treatment time, and that sequential radiographs usually are required. Radiation exposure for untreated children is problematic. At present, it is very difficult to get permission to expose children to x-rays that will be of no benefit to them personally. This means the longitudinal growth studies in the mid-20th century that used a series of cephalometric radiographs of untreated children cannot be repeated now. In the absence of newer data, they still are being used to provide control data in studies involving growth modification—although it is well established that in the United States and almost all other countries, children now grow larger and mature more quickly than at the time of those studies (see Fig. 3.7). When historic controls are the best that are available, it is better to have them than nothing, but the limitations must be kept in mind. Growth magnitudes and timing, along with so much else, have changed in the last 70 years.

A final important consideration is that what clinicians consider the important aspects of outcomes of treatment may or may not coincide with how patients perceive the outcome. In orthodontics, it is apparent that the appearance of the teeth on smile is a key outcome for patients. Fortunately, what the patients think now receives more attention than it did all the way through the 20th century, and data for the acceptable range of tooth display have become available recently.[15] Patient and practitioners often hold different viewpoints regarding the same dental feature and these perspectives must be weighed carefully. This has been demonstrated in many studies. Patient-centered treatment does not mean the patient is always right, but it does mean that the patient's point of view must be kept in mind both when treatment is planned and when its success is evaluated. But, practitioners cannot accept patient-generated treatment plans that do not meet the standard of care.

The era of orthodontics as an opinion-driven specialty is clearly at an end. In the future, it will be evidence informed, which is all for the best. This means evidence that is applied to maximize the results for *this* patient given their esthetic, functional, physical, behavioral, and financial preferences and limitations AND given the ability and experience of the practitioner. Limited care for an adolescent may be just as appropriate as comprehensive care for an adult and vice versa given these constraints.

In the meantime, clinical decisions must still be made using the best information currently available. When the latest new method appears with someone's strong recommendation and a series of case reports in which it worked very well, it is wise to remember the aphorism "Enthusiastic reports tend to lack controls; well-controlled reports tend to lack enthusiasm."

In this and the subsequent chapters, recommendations for treatment are based insofar as possible on solid clinical evidence. When this is not available, the authors' current opinions are provided and labeled as such.

Artificial Intelligence in Orthodontics

At present, the application of artificial intelligence (AI) in orthodontics is still in its infancy. However, AI applications to digital orthodontics is obvious, and there are increasing AI tools available for practitioners. It is important to understand AI terminologies (machine learning versus deep learning), principles (algorithms such as convolutional neuron network), and clinical applications. Digital dentistry is important because it allows AI to impact a traditional practice.

Traditional orthodontic workflow. Orthodontists need to perform many tasks while focusing on important information that will lead to the correct decisions and actions. These skills are critical for treatment success. Many are repetitive and include taking patient records, analyzing the records, summarizing diagnoses and treatment plans, placing appliances, adjusting orthodontic mechanics and forces, finishing and retention. In a conventional practice, clinicians execute these tasks themselves by chairside observation, writing a treatment plan and then performing treatment like bending wires, and so on.

Digital orthodontics. Recent digital technology has revolutionized these tasks. Hardware such as digital cephalometric and panoramic radiography, cone beam computer tomography (CBCT), intra-oral 3D scanners and printers have helped in gathering digital data. Software has been useful in representing these data like digital electronic records, graphic tracings, and 3D imaging renditions for analysis.

Digital workflow. Transition from traditional workflow to digital dentistry requires a change in clinical setup and workflow, which involves the use of advanced technologies and software to plan, design and execute orthodontic treatment. Digital radiographs allow for faster image acquisition, reduced radiation exposure, and the ability to store and transmit images electronically with the immediate reconstruction of digital images, on a computer screen. The use of 3D CBCT can render 3D images, which adds information that helps locate, plan, and treat anomalies within tissues like impacted teeth, supernumerary teeth, craniofacial anomalies and facial asymmetries.

Optical scanning technology has become increasingly prevalent in acquiring three-dimensional information for contemporary orthodontics. The 3dMDface System (3dMD LLC, Atlanta, US) allows acquisition of 3D surface topology and the color texture of a patient's face. The 3D scan provides higher resolutions for quantitative assessment of facial expression and animation. Researchers have applied the method to study surgical outcomes of reconstruction of patients with congenital orofacial anomalies.

The intra-oral scanner is the most popular technology, which replaces conventional impressions. Many orthodontic offices have already adopted intra-oral scan as a routine procedure so the images can be transmitted and printed quickly and accurately.

Orthodontic diagnosis and treatment planning. Operations of traditional practice and contemporary digital orthodontics share the same purpose, which is to provide optimal diagnosis and treatment planning for patient care. Since the 1920s orthodontists have accumulated data to describe malocclusion, faces, and growth patterns. From the data, problem lists and treatment plans were generated. As large data bases were accumulated, bioinformatics applications began assisting clinicians in making medical diagnoses and predicting outcomes. In orthodontics, diagnosis and treatment planning of every patient includes data classification, imaging analysis, treatment, and monitoring progress. Because there are 5 million people undergoing orthodontic treatment in the United States per year, these processes are repeated 5 million times annually. This is a repetitive process and artificial Intelligence (AI) is particularly useful for dealing with repetitive and tedious jobs.

Artificial intelligence (AI). Today, AI can suggest options for decisions, prioritization, and planning. There are two types of AI, commonly defined as weak and strong AI. Weak AI, also known as narrow AI, refers to artificial intelligence designed to perform a specific task or set of tasks.[34,35] These tasks include identifying objects in images. However, it does not possess the broad, adaptable intelligence associated with human cognition. Most current orthodontic AI applications (classification, regression, image segmentation, and landmark identification), are weak AI.

On the other hand, strong AI, also known as artificial general intelligence (AGI), refers to AI that exhibits human-like cognitive abilities and can learn and reason in a manner that is indistinguishable from human intelligence.[36,37] A sophisticated multimodel AI for diagnosis and treatment planning could be classified in this category.

AI applications. Specific neural network algorithms should be selected according to the types of input data and outcome predictions (Fig. 1.20). Neural networks can be applied to a wide range of data types and tasks, making them a powerful tool for artificial intelligence and machine learning. Those data types include tabular data, images, and text. Although neural networks are flexible for many data types, it is important to use a suitable neural network in order to effectively and efficiently learn underlying patterns from the corresponding data. In this section, we will discuss various AI algorithms and their related data types for different clinical applications.

Supervised machine learning. A major subset of AI algorithms is "Machine Learning" (ML), which focuses on the development of algorithms and statistical models that allow computer systems to learn and make predictions or decisions without being explicitly programmed. ML algorithms can be broadly categorized into supervised learning, unsupervised learning, and reinforcement learning. Tabulated data with predetermined features (e.g., orthodontic crowding, overjet, overbite, and cephalometric measures) are most suitable for training machine learning. For example, an important part of orthodontic treatment is to determine whether to extract or not to extract permanent teeth. Researchers have used supervised machine learning algorithms to study extraction decisions. The predictability ranges from 80% to 95%, depending

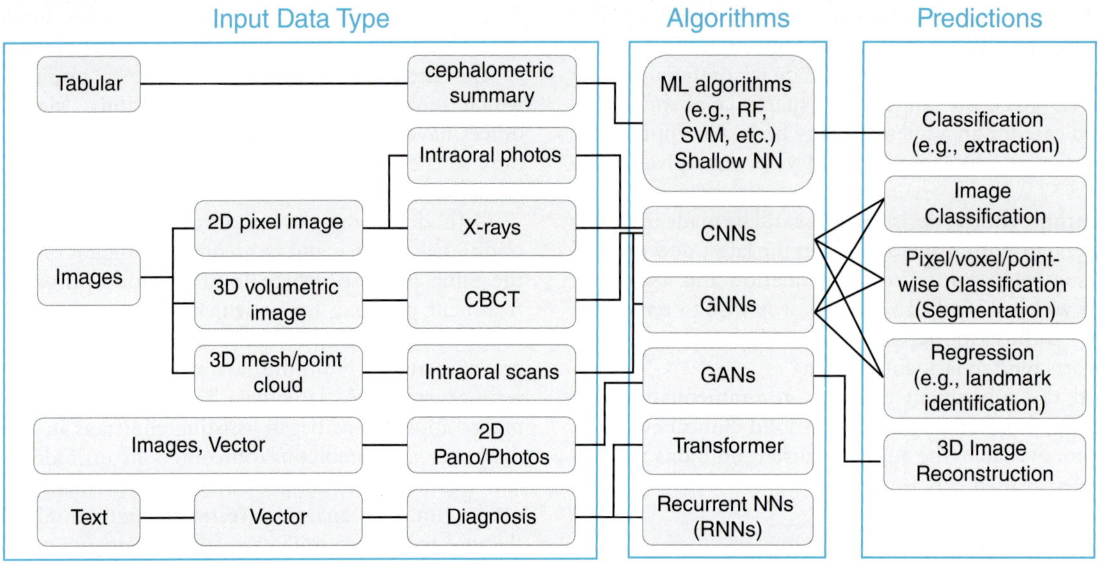

• **Fig. 1.20** Neural networks can be applied to a wide range of data types and tasks, but they must be used with the appropriate data types to be productive and obtain the required outcomes. *CBCT*, Cone Beam Computer Tomography; *ML*, Machine Learning; *RF*, Radio Frequency; *SVM*, Support Vector Machine; *NN*, Neural Network; *CNN*, Convolutional Neural Network; *GNN*, Graph Neural Network; *GAN*, Generative Adversarial Network; *RNN*, Recurrent Neural Network.

upon the method of sample collections and the type and amount of information provided. A critical factor is what is really the right answer or "ground truth." Is the ground truth one practitioner's opinion or the opinion of multiple expert practitioners or a true gold standard? A method with diverse providers would require bigger data for the machine to learn. It is possible that an AI model, trained from a diverse population, could predict extractions across different practice settings.

Unsupervised machine learning. The examples of unsupervised machine learning (no predetermined ground truth) are clusterings of shapes such as the shape of the mandibular condyle or a pattern classification of craniofacial form. Shape analysis is the automatic analysis of geometric shapes. When analyzing ten unilateral cleft palatal defects, the first three geometric descriptors (principal components) are: volume, curvature, and transverse dimension of the cleft (Fig. 1.21.) A complete shape descriptor is a representation that can be used to completely reconstruct the defective object.

Deep learning. Deep learning is a subset of machine learning that focuses on training artificial neural networks with multiple layers to learn and extract complex patterns and representations from data. It is inspired by the structure and function of the human brain, particularly the interconnected network of neurons. Traditional machine learning algorithms often require manual adjustments, where humans handcraft relevant features from the data. In deep learning, however, neural networks are designed to automatically learn hierarchical representations of data through multiple layers of interconnected nodes, called neurons or units. Each layer of neurons performs transformations on the input data, gradually extracting higher-level features and representations.

Deep learning has the potential, if managed carefully, to make an impact on orthodontics. This is possible due to the ability of deep neural networks to automatically learn and discover intricate patterns and representations directly from raw data, eliminating the need for manual adjustments. Artificial neural networks (ANNs) are a core element of deep learning algorithms. Recurrent neural network (RNN) and convolutional neural network (CNN) are the most common network architectures in deep learning. The most obvious practical examples are auto-landmarking of cephalometric images and analysis, automatic analysis of panoramic X-rays, auto-segmentations of CBCT images and intra-oral scan surfaces.

Convolutional neural network (CNN). A deep network AI model was reported to automatically detect cephalometric landmarks based on X-ray cephalograms from various manufacturers and CBCT-generated cephalograms.[38] The mean radial error of the average value of all landmarks was 1.42 mm. This type of software could streamline orthodontic data gathering and analysis (Phimentum [Newton, MA] and CephPro3D Largev [Beijing, China]).

There is an industrial software that can automatically label tooth numbers and perform pathological and non-pathological detection, including impacted teeth, caries, third molars, periapical anomalies, missing teeth, supernumerary teeth, retained deciduous teeth, residual root, residual crown, alveolar bone resorption, low/high-density jaw anomalies, dental implant, crown, filling, and root canal treatment (Fig. 1.22). This could allow orthodontists to formulate diagnostic conclusions supplemented by an AI assistant's second opinion, significantly reducing the risk of missed diagnoses.

CBCTs consist of voxels in a sequential order. CNN can be used to automatically segment a CBCT into the foreground teeth and background craniofacial bones. Sheng and coworkers derived a sophisticated CNN algorithm from 4125 annotated CBCTs. They showed that the AI model can precisely auto-segment orofacial bone and teeth. Some commercial software can automatically segment and reconstruct the teeth, maxilla, mandible, maxillary sinus, inferior alveolar canal, airway, and soft tissue profiles (Fig. 1.23).

Applying similar algorithms to a canine impaction case, Fig. 1.24 shows where the canine is trapped between the roots of the central and lateral incisors. The original (unsegmented) CBCT shows a blurred image of the impacted canine. The auto-segmentation offers clinicians the information to guide canine eruption with minimum damage to the roots of incisors.

Another example of CNN applications is to automatically determine dental crowding using clinical intraoral photos. Using

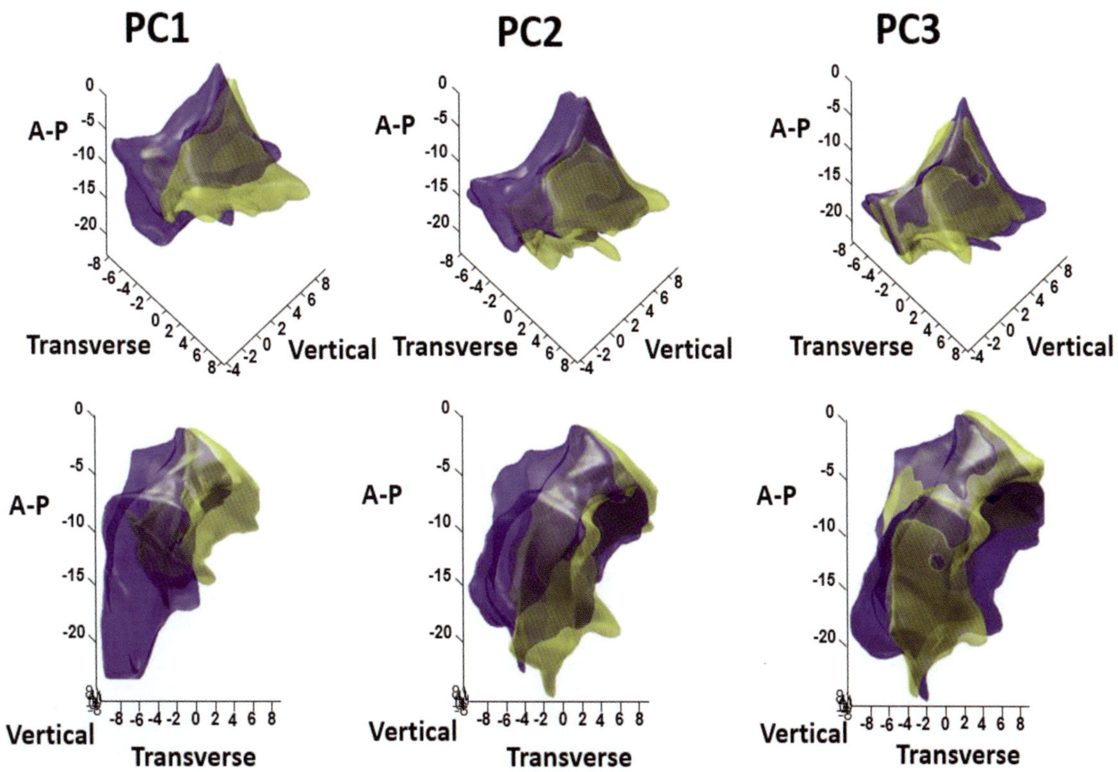

• **Fig. 1.21** Principal components (PC) of shape analysis of the defect in the unilateral palatal cleft. PC1: Volume of the cleft; PC2: Curving of the cleft; PC3: Transverse of the cleft.

835 patients and maxillary occlusal photos, residual neural network (Resnet) returned 84% predicted crowding with an error ≤3 mm. Although the Resnet model applying CNN to measure crowding of images is promising, future research will use standardized photos and the exclusion of confounding areas of the image to reduce prediction errors. The previous work suggests CNN's capability of learning orthodontic features, which may improve workflow efficiency in orthodontic treatment and education.

Graphic neural network (GNN). 3D surface data from the intra-oral scanner consists of a discrete set of points in space. These data, do not possess a sequential order nor do the neighboring points have a uniform relationship. This format is more suitable for GNN, which deals with geographic features. Many companies (e.g., Align Tech, ULab System, 3M-UNITEK, Henry Schein) have their own AI program for tooth segmentation. They can use this technology to manufacture products such as aligners. In addition, automated landmark identification of individual teeth from the intra-oral scan has allowed defining tooth orientation and anatomic features.[38,39] Researchers have utilized these technologies to quantify tooth movement from clinical data sets and compare outcomes between different orthodontic modalities. Murphy et al.[40] found that clear aligner achieved smaller movements than that of the conventional bracket-wire system. These evidence-based studies using big data are becoming available with the use of these AI tools.

It appears the future of AI in orthodontics, when supervised, can be a productive clinical tool in terms of options for diagnosis and treatment planning. It can also provide new information regarding treatment methods not previously available as long as the ground truth is available for development and testing.

Demand for Treatment

Epidemiologic Estimates of Orthodontic Treatment Need

Psychosocial and facial considerations, not just the way the teeth fit, play a role in defining orthodontic treatment need. For this reason, it is difficult to determine who needs treatment and who does not just from an examination of dental casts or radiographs. Nevertheless, it seems reasonable that the severity of a malocclusion correlates with need for treatment, and as we will discuss in more detail here, there is good evidence to support that correlation. This assumption is necessary when treatment need is estimated for population groups.

Several indices for scoring how much the teeth deviate from the normal, as indicators of orthodontic treatment need, were proposed in the 1970s but not widely accepted for the screening of potential patients. There are now two major methods for scoring the severity of malocclusion: the peer assessment rating (PAR) system, developed in the United Kingdom, and the American Board of Orthodontics (ABO) discrepancy index, developed in the United States. It is important to keep in mind that these systems consider just the dentition, not skeletal or facial characteristics.

PAR scores are calculated from measurements of maxillary and mandibular anterior alignment (crowding and spacing), buccal segment occlusion (anteroposterior, transverse, and vertical), overjet or reverse overjet, overbite, and midline discrepancies, with use of a weighting scale for each characteristic.[41] ABO index scores are calculated similarly, with the difference primarily that it adds three cephalometric measurements.[42] The PAR analysis is valuable as a

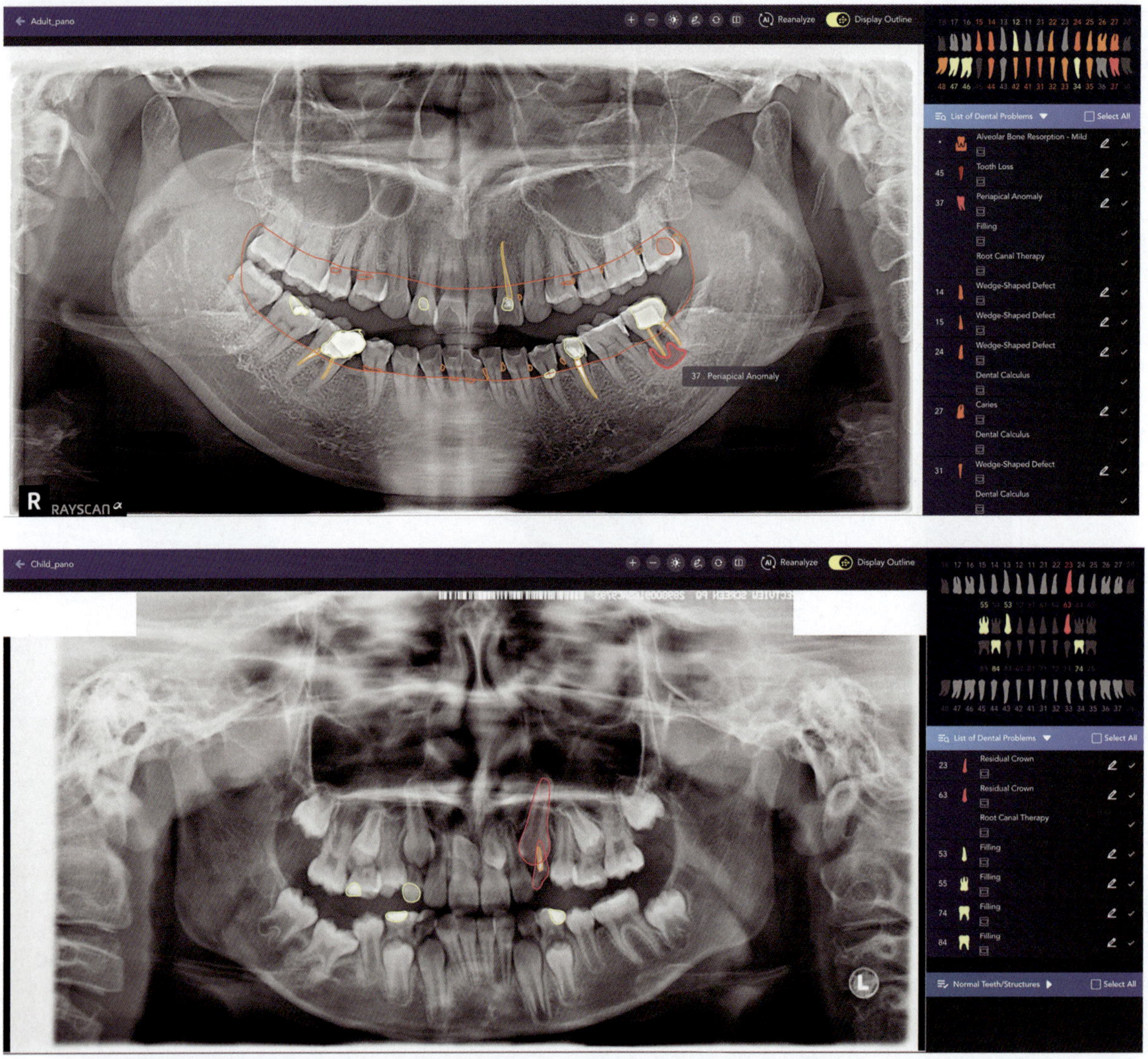

• **Fig. 1.22** AI programs can identify pathologic and nonpathologic elements of images to serve as a second opinion for examination data. (Courtesy of DeepCare Inc.)

pre- and posttreatment tool to measure both conditions and the improvement. The ABO index evaluates the final result of treatment against a standard. Both systems have been shown to correlate reasonably well with expert opinions of orthodontic treatment need.

The Index of Treatment Need (IOTN), developed by Brook and Shaw in the United Kingdom,[43] was designed to evaluate need for treatment. It places patients in five grades from "no need for treatment" to "treatment required" that correlate reasonably well with clinician's judgments of need for treatment. The index has a dental health component derived from occlusion and alignment (Box 1.1 outlines the criteria and an esthetic component derived from comparison of the patient's dental appearance versus standard photographs (Fig. 1.25). An AI method trained and tested on novel images demonstrated sensitivity = 0.77, specificity = 0.88, PPV = 0.89 and NPV = 0.75 assigning the esthetic component as 1–5 or 6–10, essentially no treatment need vs treatment need.[44] There is a surprisingly good correlation between treatment need assessed by the dental health and esthetic components of IOTN.[45]

With some allowances for the effect of missing teeth, it is possible to calculate the percentages of US children and youths who would fall into the various IOTN grades from the NHANES III data set.[46] Fig. 1.26 shows the percentage of youths age 12 to 17 in the three major racial or ethnic groups in the US population estimated with IOTN to have mild, moderate, or severe treatment need and the percentage who had treatment at that time. As the graph shows, the number of White youths who received treatment was considerably higher than the number of Black or Mexican American children ($P < 0.001$). Treatment almost always produces an improvement but may not totally eliminate all the characteristics of malocclusion, so the effect is to move some individuals from the severe to the mild treatment need categories. The higher proportion of severe malocclusion among Blacks probably reflects more treatment in the White group, which moved them down the severity scale, rather than the presence of more severe malocclusion in the Black population.

How do the IOTN scores compare with what parents and dentists think relative to orthodontic treatment need? The existing (rather weak) data suggest that in typical American neighborhoods, about 35% of adolescents are perceived by parents and peers as needing orthodontic treatment. Note that this is larger than the number of children who would be placed in IOTN grades 4 and 5 as having severe problems and definitely needing

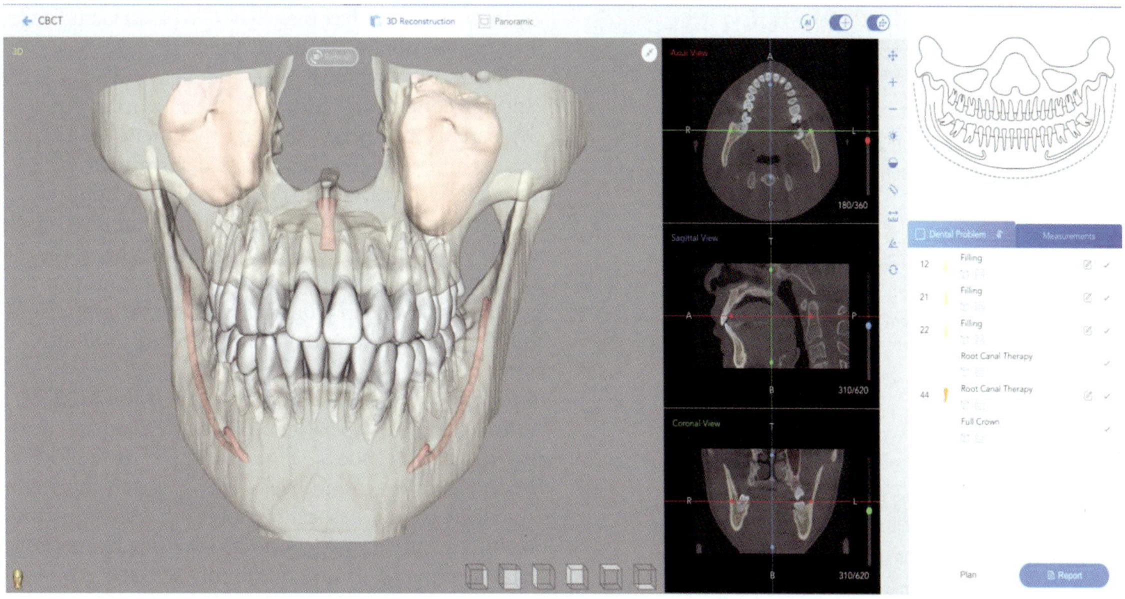

• **Fig. 1.23** By segmenting the teeth and other structures, like the maxilla, mandible, sinus and some nerves from the background, structures can be more apparent for evaluation. (Courtesy of DeepCare Inc.)

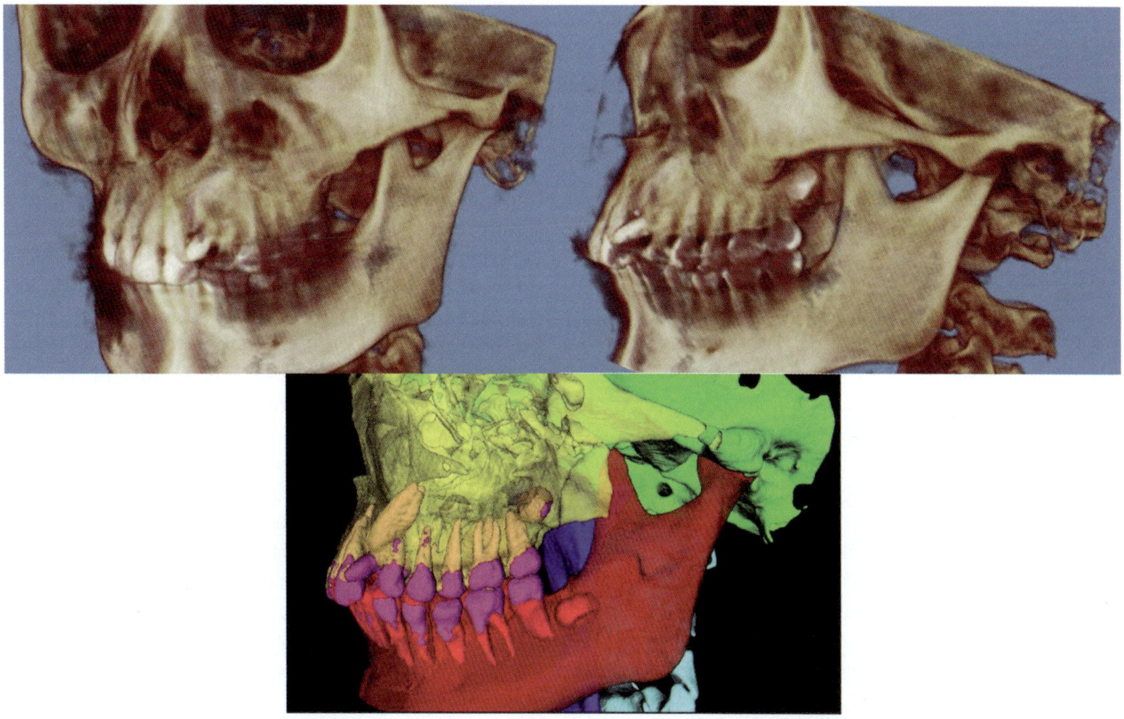

• **Fig.1.24** Here is a contrast of two images. The upper image is from a standard CBCT and the lower segmented image that provides an enhanced view of the impacted maxillary left canine. This makes determining the status of the tooth and surrounding teeth as well as potential methods and direction of traction more discernable.

treatment, but smaller than the total of grades 3, 4, and 5 for moderate and severe problems.

Dentists usually judge that only about one-third of their patients have normal occlusion, and they suggest treatment for about 55% (thereby putting about 10% in a category of malocclusion with little need for treatment). It appears that they include all the children in IOTN grade 3 and some of those in grade 2 in the group who would benefit from orthodontics. Presumably, facial appearance and psychosocial considerations are used in addition to dental characteristics when parents judge treatment need or dentists decide to recommend treatment.

Who Seeks Treatment?

Demand for treatment is indicated by the number of patients who actually make appointments and seek care. Not all patients with malocclusion, even those with extreme deviations from the norm, seek orthodontic treatment. Some do not recognize that they have

• BOX 1.1 Index of Treatment Needs (IOTN) Treatment Grades

Grade 5 (Extreme/Need Treatment)

5.i	Impeded eruption of teeth (except third molars) due to crowding, displacement, the presence of supernumerary teeth, retained deciduous teeth, and any pathologic cause.
5.h	Extensive hypodontia with restorative implications (more than one tooth per quadrant) requiring preprosthetic orthodontics.
5.a	Increased overjet greater than 9 mm.
5.m	Reverse overjet greater than 3.5 mm with reported masticatory and speech difficulties.
5.p	Defects of cleft lip and palate and other craniofacial anomalies.
5.s	Submerged deciduous teeth.

Grade 4 (Severe/Need Treatment)

4.h	Less extensive hypodontia requiring prerestorative orthodontics or orthodontic space closure (one tooth per quadrant).
4.a	Increased overjet greater than 6 mm but less than or equal to 9 mm.
4.b	Reverse overjet greater than 3.5 mm with no masticatory or speech difficulties.
4.m	Reverse overjet greater than 1 mm but less than 3.5 mm with recorded masticatory or speech difficulties.
4.c	Anterior or posterior crossbites with greater than 2 mm discrepancy between retruded contact position and intercuspal position.
4.l	Posterior lingual crossbite with no functional occlusal contact in one or both buccal segments.
4.d	Severe contact point displacements greater than 4 mm.
4.e	Extreme lateral or anterior open bites greater than 4 mm.
4.f	Increased and complete overbite with gingival or palatal trauma.
4.t	Partially erupted teeth, tipped, and impacted against adjacent teeth.
4.x	Presence of supernumerary teeth.

Grade 3 (Moderate/Borderline Need)

3.a	Increased overjet greater than 3.5 mm but less than or equal to 6 mm with incompetent lips.
3.b	Reverse overjet greater than 1 mm but less than or equal to 3.5 mm.
3.c	Anterior or posterior crossbites with greater than 1 mm but less than or equal to 2 mm discrepancy between retruded contact position and intercuspal position.
3.d	Contact point displacements greater than 2 mm but less than or equal to 4 mm.
3.e	Lateral or anterior open bite greater than 2 mm but less than or equal to 4 mm.
3.f	Deep overbite complete on gingival or palatal tissues but no trauma.

Grade 2 (Mild/Little Need)

2.a	Increased overjet greater than 3.5 mm but less than or equal to 6 mm with competent lips.
2.b	Reverse overjet greater than 0 mm but less than or equal to 1 mm.
2.c	Anterior or posterior crossbite with less than or equal to 1 mm discrepancy between retruded contact position and intercuspal position.
2.d	Contact point displacements greater than 1 mm but less than or equal to 2 mm.
2.e	Anterior or posterior open bite greater than 1 mm but less than or equal to 2 mm.
2.f	Increased overbite greater than or equal to 3.5 mm without gingival contact.
2.g	Prenormal or postnormal occlusions with no other anomalies.

Grade 1 (No Need)

1.	Extremely minor malocclusions, including contact point displacements less than 1 mm.

a problem; others feel that they need treatment but cannot afford it or cannot obtain it.

Both the perceived need and demand vary with social and cultural conditions. More children in urban areas are thought (by parents and peers) to need treatment than children in rural areas. Family income is a major determinant of how many children receive treatment (Fig. 1.27). This appears to reflect two things: not only that higher income families can more easily afford orthodontic treatment, but also that good facial appearance and straight teeth are associated with more prestigious social positions and occupations. The higher the aspirations for a child, the more likely the parents are to seek orthodontic treatment for him or her.

Why do they seek treatment for their children? We have already noted that psychosocial handicaps are the major reason. Another way to put this issue is "Does having a less than ideal smile affect the way people act and live?" This question was examined by the American Dental Association's Health Policy Institute in 2015.[47] An online survey was conducted by the Harris Poll, and nearly 15,000 responses from a randomly selected group of individuals age 18 and older were analyzed. The study group was evaluated as a whole, by economic status (low, middle, and high household income), and by age (18–34, 35–49, 50–64, and 65 or older). This national data set tells an interesting story related to dental esthetics. Twenty-nine percent of low-income adults and 28% of young adults (18–34) believed the appearance of their mouth and teeth affected their ability to interview for a job. That is over one-fourth of these groups. Twenty-five percent of all adults said they avoid smiling, 23% feel embarrassed, and 20% experience anxiety because of the condition of their mouth and teeth. But low-income and young adults felt the greatest impact, with a minimum of 30% in each of these two groups indicating that they experienced a problem related to the appearance of their teeth very often or occasionally. Finally, 82% of all responders agreed with the statement "It is easier to get ahead in life if I have straight, bright teeth."

So, although the need for treatment and its assessments and benefits are usually determined with carefully quantified dental morphologic and degrees of craniofacial deformity, poor dental esthetics is enough to clearly impair people. Often, we lose track of that simple truth by trying to justify orthodontic treatment at a higher and seemingly more significant level. In fact, people value straight teeth because it makes their lives easier and better.

Because it is widely recognized now that severe malocclusion can affect an individual's entire life, every US state now provides at least some orthodontic treatment for low-income families through its Medicaid program. Nevertheless, Medicaid and related programs support only a tiny fraction of the population's orthodontic care. From that perspective, it is interesting that even in the lowest income group, almost 5% of youths and over 5% of adults report having received treatment; 10% to 15% at intermediate income levels have received treatment. This indicates the importance placed on orthodontic treatment by families who judge that it is a factor in social and career progress for their children.

The effect of financial constraints on demand can be seen most clearly by the response to third-party payment plans. When third-party copayment is available, the number of individuals seeking orthodontic treatment rises considerably, but even when all costs are covered, some individuals for whom treatment is recommended do not accept it. It seems likely that under optimal economic conditions, demand for orthodontic treatment will at least reach the 35% level thought by the public to need treatment.

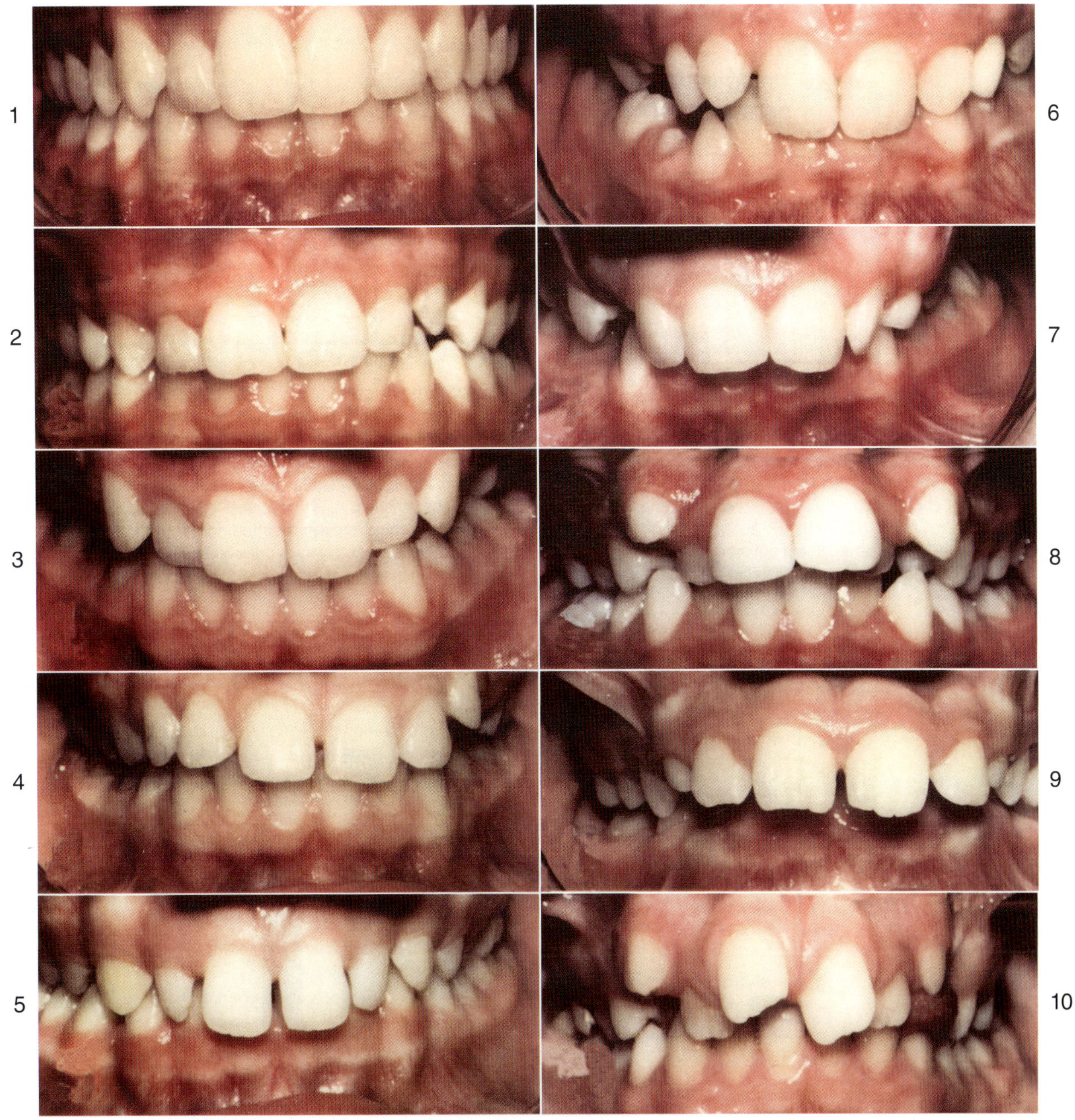

• **Fig. 1.25** The representative standard photographs of the Index of Treatment Need (IOTN) esthetic index. The score is derived from matching the esthetics of the malocclusion being observed to the appropriate standard photograph. Number 1 is the most attractive and number 10 the least attractive arrangement. Grades 8–10 indicate definite need for orthodontic treatment; 5–7, moderate or borderline need; 1–4, no or slight need.

In higher socioeconomic areas in the United States, 35% to more than 50% of children and youths now are receiving orthodontic care. In Switzerland, where high average incomes and supplemental social programs mean that essentially all citizens who want treatment can get it, 56% of the 2012 population aged 15 to 24 years were receiving or had received orthodontic treatment.[48] Acceptance of treatment is at similar levels in the Scandinavian countries for the same reasons.

Orthodontic treatment for adults was rare until the latter half of the 20th century. In the 1960s, only 5% of all orthodontic patients in the United States were adults (age 19 or older). By 1990, about 25% of all orthodontic patients were adults (18 or older) (Fig. 1.28). It is interesting to note that the absolute number of adults seeking orthodontic treatment remained constant for the next decade while the number of younger patients grew, so by 2000 the proportion of adults in the orthodontic patient population had dropped to about 20%. By 2010 it had increased again to over 25% of the total, and the most recent survey by the American Association of Orthodontists (2017) indicated a little over 25% were being treated.

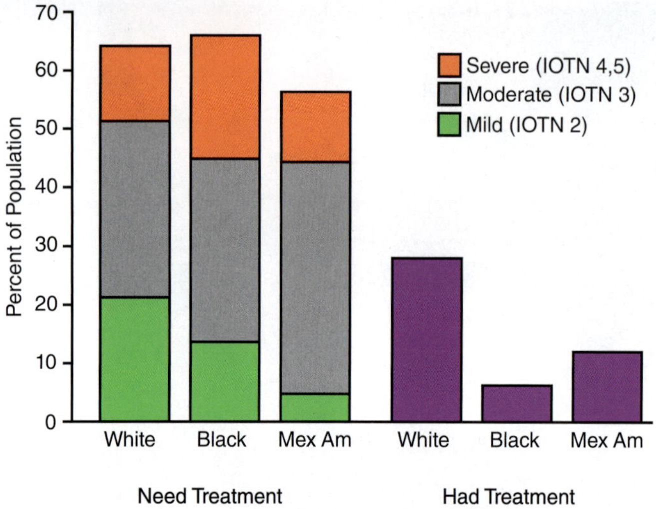

• **Fig. 1.26** Orthodontic need by severity of the problem for White, Black and Mexican American youths age 12–17 in the United States, 1989–94, and the percentage of each group who reported receiving previous orthodontic treatment. Approximately 12–20% have severe malocclusions. The greater number of Whites who received treatment probably accounts for the greater proportion of mild and moderate problems in the White population.

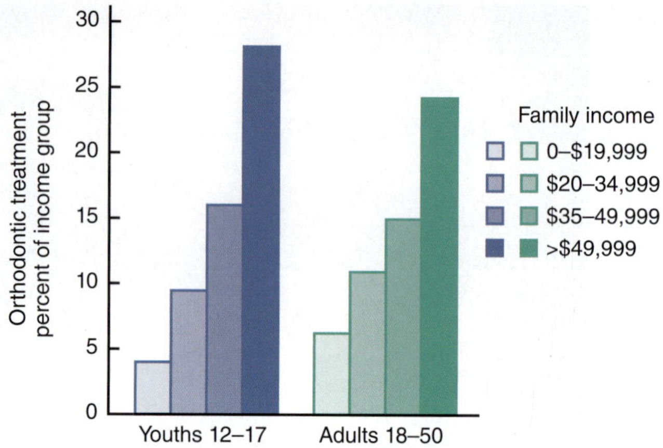

• **Fig. 1.27** The percentage of the US population, 1989–94, who received orthodontic treatment, as a function of family income. Although severe malocclusion is recognized as an important problem and all states offer at least some coverage to low-income children through their Medicaid programs, this funds treatment for a very small percentage of the population. Nevertheless, nearly 5% of the lowest income group and 10%–15% of intermediate income groups reported some orthodontic treatment. This reflects the importance given to orthodontic treatment—it is sought even when it stretches financial resources in less-affluent families.

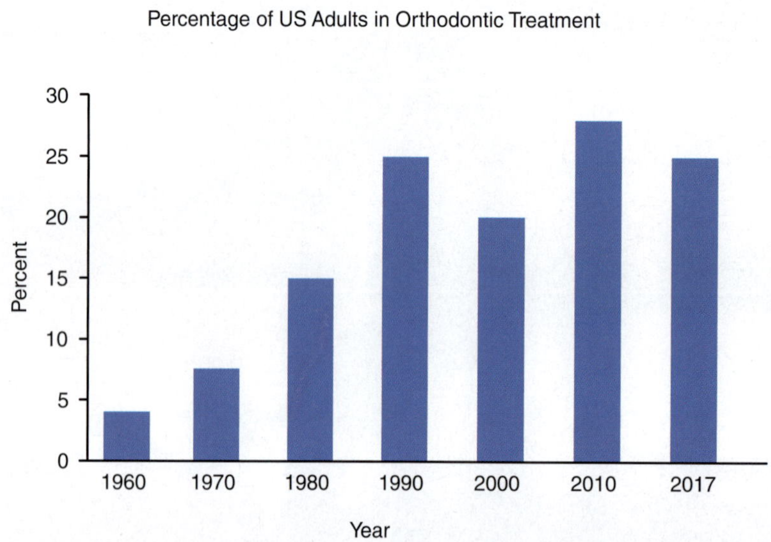

• **Fig. 1.28** From the mid-20th century, when almost no adults received orthodontic treatment, to the 1990s, there was an almost steady rise in the number of adult patients. In the 1980s, a "baby bust" period, the increasing number of adult patients was the major source of the overall increase in orthodontics, whereas in the 1990s, a "baby boom" period, the number of adult patients increased a little but most of the growth involved treatment of children, so the adult percentage declined. There was a further increase in the number of adults in treatment and their percentage of the total patient population in the first decade of the 21st century, bringing the percentage back to 25%–30%.

Many adult patients indicate that they wanted treatment earlier but did not receive it, often because their families could not afford it; now they can. Wearing braces as an adult is more socially acceptable than it was previously. Clear aligners have made orthodontic treatment even more acceptable to many patients. Recently, an increased number of older adults (40 and over) have sought orthodontics, usually in conjunction with other treatment, to save their teeth, and the majority of that oldest subgroup were male (every other age group from childhood on has more females). As the population ages, these older adults are likely to be the fastest growing group who seek orthodontic treatment.

Many of the children and adults who seek orthodontic treatment today have dentofacial conditions that are within the normal range of variation, at least by definitions that focus tightly on obvious degrees of handicap. Does that mean treatment is not indicated for those with lesser problems? Today, medical and dental interventions that are intended to make the individual either "better than well" or "beyond normal" are called *enhancements*.

Typical medical and surgical enhancements are drugs to treat erectile dysfunction, face lifts, and hair transplants. In dentistry, a good example of enhancement is tooth bleaching.

In this context, orthodontics often can be considered an enhancement technology. It is increasingly accepted that appropriate care for individuals should often include enhancement to maximize their quality of life. If you really want it because you are convinced you need it, perhaps you really do need it—whether it is orthodontics or many other types of treatment. Medicaid and Medicare and many insurance companies now have accepted the reality that at least some enhancement procedures have to be accepted as reimbursable medical expenses. Similarly, when orthodontic benefits are included in insurance coverage, the need for treatment is no longer judged just by the severity of the malocclusion. The bottom line: Enhancement is appropriate dental and orthodontic treatment, just as it is in other contexts.

A key question, of course, is "Does orthodontic treatment really increase quality of life and self-esteem?" A number of studies have documented improvement in quality-of-life scores and self-esteem in children and adolescents,[49] and reports have shown quality-of-life effects after orthodontic treatment in children of African, European, and Asian descent.[50–52] Multiple studies have shown that this is true for adults as well, and the range of improvements in quality of life extend further than one might have thought. For instance, a Brazilian study showed that adults with ideal smiles are considered to be more intelligent and have a greater chance of finding a job,[53] and a systematic review documented patient satisfaction after orthodontic treatment combined with orthognathic surgery.[54] The data can be summarized succinctly: If your dental and facial appearance differs significantly from that of your group, you benefit socially from correcting it.

Orthodontics has become a more prominent part of dentistry in recent years, and this trend is likely to continue. The vast majority of individuals who had orthodontic treatment feel that they benefited from the treatment and are pleased with the result. Not all patients have dramatic changes in dental and facial appearance, but nearly all recognize an improvement in both dental condition and psychologic well-being.

References

1. Corruccini RS, Paciani E. "Orthodontistry" and dental occlusion in Etruscans. *Angle Orthod.* 1989;59:61–64.
2. Kingsley NW. *Treatise on Oral Deformities as a Branch of Mechanical Surgery.* Appleton; 1880.
3. Angle EH. *Treatment of malocclusion of the teeth and fractures of the maxillae. Angle's System.* 6th ed. SS White Dental Mfg Co; 1900.
4. Baker CR. Orthodontic profile: calvin suvenil case. *Am J Orthod Dentofacial Orthop.* 1990;98:26–30A.
5. Broadbent BH. Investigatioin of the orbital plane. The Dental Cosmos. *LXIX.* 1927:797–805.
6. Sarver DM. Interactions of hard tissues, soft tissues, and growth over time, and their impact on orthodontic diagnosis and treatment planning. *Am J Orthod Dentofacial Orthop.* 2015;148:380–386.
7. Kelly JE, Sanchez M, Van Kirk LE. *An Assessment of the Occlusion of Teeth of Children.* National Center for Health Statistics; 1973. DHEW Publication No. (HRA) 74-1612.
8. Kelly J, Harvey C. *An Assessment of the Teeth of Youths 12-17 Years.* National Center for Health Statistics; 1977. DHEW Pub No. (HRA) 77-1644.
9. Brunelle JA, Bhat M, Lipton JA. Prevalence and distribution of selected occlusal characteristics in the US population, 1988-91. *J Dent Res.* 1996;75:706–713.
10. Baume LJ. Uniform methods for the epidemiologic assessment of malocclusion: results obtained with the World Health Organization standard methods (1962 and 1971) in South Pacific populations. *Am J Orthod.* 1974;66:251–272.
11. Brown T, Abbott AA, Burgess VB. Longitudinal study of dental arch relationships in Australian aboriginals with reference to alternate intercuspation. *Am J Phys Anthropol.* 1987;72:49–57.
12. Corruccini RS. Anthropological aspects of orofacial and occlusal variations and anomalies. In: Kelly MA, Larsen CS, eds. *Advances in Dental Anthropology.* Wiley-Liss; 1991.
13. Wrangham R. *Catching Fire: How Cooking Made Us Human.* Basic Books; 2009.
14. Shaw WC, Rees G, Dawe M, et al. The influence of dentofacial appearance on the social attractiveness of young adults. *Am J Orthod.* 1985;87:21–26.
15. Perrini S, Rossini G, Castroflorio T, et al. Laypeople's perceptions of frontal smile esthetics: a systematic review. *Am J Orthod Dentofacial Orthop.* 2016;150:740–750.
16. Papio MA, Fields HW, Beck FM, Firestone AR, Rosenstiel SF. The role of dental and background facial attractiveness on facial attractiveness and perceived integrity, social and intellectual attractiveness. *Am J Orthod Dentofacial Orthop.* 2019;1256:464–474.
17. Dimberg L, Arnrup K, Bondemark L. The impact of malocclusion on the quality of life among children and adolescents: a systematic review of quantitative studies. *Eur J Orthod.* 2015;37:238–247.
18. Meyer-Marcotty P, Gerdes AB, Reuther T, et al. Persons with cleft lip and palate are looked at differently. *J Dent Res.* 2010;89:400–404.
19. Macgregor FC. Social and psychological implications of dentofacial disfigurement. *Angle Orthod.* 1979;40:231–233.
20. Lin F, Ren M, Yao L, et al. Psychosocial impact of dental esthetics regulates motivation to seek orthodontic treatment. *Am J Orthod Dentofacial Orthop.* 2016;150:476–482.
21. Gavric A, Mirceta D, Jakobovic M, et al. Craniodentofacial characteristics, dental esthetics-related quality of life, and self-esteem. *Am J Orthod Dentofacial Orthop.* 2015;147:711–718.
22. Lathrop-Marshall H, Keyser MMB, Jhingree S, et al. Orthognathic speech pathology: impacts of Class III malocclusion on speech. European. *J Orthop.* 2022;44:340–351.
23. Keyser MMB, Lathrop H, Jhingree S, et al. Impacts of skeletal anterior open bite malocclusion on speech. *FACE.* 2022;3(2):339–349.
24. Macfarlane TV, Kenealy P, Kingdon HA, et al. Twenty-year cohort study of health gain from orthodontic treatment: temporomandibular disorders. *Am J Orthod Dentofacial Orthop.* 2009;192:e1–e8.
25. McNamara Jr JA, Seligman DA, Okeson JP. Occlusion, orthodontic treatment, and temporomandibular disorders: a review. *J Orofac Pain.* 1995;9(1):73–90. Winter.
26. Thiruvenkatachari B, Harrison J, Worthington H, O'Brien K. Early orthodontic treatment for Class II malocclusion reduces the chance of incisal trauma: results of a Cochrane systematic review. *Am J Orthod Dentofacial Orthop.* 2015;148:47–59.
27. Petti S, Glendor U, Andersson L. World traumatic dental injury prevalence and incidence, a meta-analysis - One billion living people have had traumatic dental injuries. *Dent Traumatol.* 2018;34:71–86.
28. Koroluk LD, Tulloch JFC, Phillips C. Incisor trauma and early treatment for Class II division 1 malocclusion. *Am J Orthod Dentofacial Orthop.* 2003;123:117–125.
29. Glendor U, Koucheki B, Halling A. Risk evaluation and type of treatment of multiple dental trauma episodes to permanent teeth. *Endod Dent Traumatol.* 2000;16:205–210.
30. Bollen AM, Cunha-Cruz J, Bakko DW, et al. The effects of orthodontic therapy on periodontal health: a systematic review of controlled evidence. *Am J Orthod Dentofacial Orthop.* 2008;135:413–422.
31. Jonsson T, Karlsson KO, Ragnarsson B, et al. Long-term development of malocclusion traits in orthodontically treated and untreated subjects. *Am J Orthod Dentofacial Orthop.* 2010;137:277–284.
32. Papageorgiou SN. Meta-analysis for orthodontists: part II—Is all that glitters gold? *J Orthod.* 2014;41:327–336.
33. Cohen J. *Statistical Power Analysis for the Behavioral Sciences.* Routledge Academic; 1988.

34. Goodfellow I, Bengio Y, Courville A. *Deep learning*, MIT Press; 2016.
35. Silver D, Huang A, Maddison CJ, et al. Mastering the game of Go with deep neural networks and tree search. *Nature*. 2016;529(7587): 484–489.
36. Christiano PF, Leike J, Brown T, Martic M, Legg S, Amodei D. Deep reinforcement learning from human preferences. In: Advances in Neural Information Processing Systems. *Curran Associates*; 2018:4299–4308.
37. Marcus G. *Deep Learning: A Critical Appraisal*. 2018. arXiv preprint arXiv:1801.00631.
38. Lian C, Wang L, Wu T-H, Wang F, Yap P-T, Ko CC, Shen D. Deep multi-scale mesh feature learning for automated labeling of raw dental surfaces from 3D intraoral scanners. *IEEE Trans Med Imaging, IEEE Xplore*. 2020;39(7):2440–2450. https://doi.org/10.1109/TMI.2020.2971730. PMID: 32031933.
39. Wu T-H, Lian C, Lee S, et al. Two-stage mesh deep learning for automated tooth segmentation and landmark localization on 3D intraoral scans. *IEEE Trans Med Imaging*. 2022;41(11):3158–3166. https://doi.org/10.1109/TMI.2022.3180343.
40. Murphy SJ, Lee S, Scham JC, et al. Comparison of maxillary anterior tooth movement between Invisalign and fixed appliances. *AJODO*. 2023 Jul;164(1):24–33.
41. Firestone AR, Beck FM, Beglin FM, Vig KWL. Evaluation of the peer assessment rating (PAR) index as an index of orthodontic treatment need. *Am J Orthod Dentofacial Orthop*. 2002;122: 463–469.
42. Cangialosi TJ, Riolo ML, Owens Jr SA, et al. The ABO discrepancy index: a measure of case complexity. *Am J Orthod Dentofacial Orthop*. 2004;125:270–278.
43. Brook PH, Shaw WC. The development of an index for orthodontic treatment priority. *Eur J Orthod*. 1989;11:309–332.
44. Stetzel L, Foucher F, Jang SJ, et al. Artificial intelligence for predicting the aesthetic component of the index of orthodontic treatment need. *Bioengineering*, 2024;11(9):861. https://doi.org/10.3390/bioengineering11090861.
45. Richmond S, Shaw WC, O'Brien KD, et al. The relationship between the Index of Treatment Need and the consensus opinion of a panel of 74 dentists. *Brit Dent J*. 1995;178:370–374.
46. Proffit WR, Fields HW, Moray LJ. Prevalence of malocclusion and orthodontic treatment need in the United States: estimates from the NHANES III survey. *Int J Adult Orthodon Orthognath Surg*. 1998;13:97–106.
47. American Dental Association, Health Policy Institute. Oral health and well-being in the United States. Available at https://www.ada.org/en/science-research/health-policy-institute/oral-health-and-well-being
48. Stadelmann P, Zemp E, Weiss C, et al. Dental visits, oral hygiene behaviour, and orthodontic treatment in Switzerland. *Schweiz Monatsschr Zahnmed*. 2012;122:104–126.
49. Liu Z, McGrath C, Haag U. The impact of malocclusion/orthodontic treatment need on the quality of life: a systematic review. *Angle Orthod*. 2009;79:585–591.
50. Isiekwe GI, Sofola OO, Olanrewaju O, et al. Dental esthetics and oral health-related quality of life in young adults. *Am J Orthod Dentofacial Orthop*. 2016;150:627–636.
51. Gavrik A, Mirceta D, Jakobovic M, et al. Craniofacial characteristics, dental esthetics-related quality of life, and self-esteem. *Am J Orthod Dentofacial Orthop*. 2015;147:711–718.
52. Choi SH, Kim JS, Cha JY, Hwang CJ. Effect of malocclusion severity on oral health-related quality of life and food intake ability in a Korean population. *Am J Orthod Dentofacial Orthop*. 2016;149:384–390.
53. Pithon MM, Nascimento CC, Barbosa GC, Coqueiro RD. Do dental esthetics have any influence on finding a job? *Am J Orthod Dentofacial Orthop*. 2014;146:423–429.
54. Pacheco-Pereira C, Abreu LG, Dick BD, et al. Patient satisfaction after orthodontic treatment combined with orthognathic surgery: a systematic review. *Angle Orthod*. 2016;86:495–508.

2

Concepts of Growth and Development

WILLIAM R. PROFFIT, HENRY W. FIELDS JR., KAITRIN KRAMER, BENJAMIN FIELDS, AND F. THOMAS MCIVER

CHAPTER OUTLINE

A thorough background in craniofacial growth and development is necessary for every dentist. Even for those who never work with children, it is difficult to comprehend conditions observed in adults without understanding the developmental processes that produced these problems. For those who interact professionally with children—and almost every dentist does so at least occasionally—it is important to distinguish normal variation from the effects of abnormal or pathologic processes. Because dentists and orthodontists are heavily involved in the development of not just the dentition but the entire dentofacial complex, a conscientious practitioner may be able to manipulate facial growth for the benefit of the patient. It is not possible to do so without a thorough understanding of both the pattern of normal growth and the mechanisms that underlie it.

The very terms *growth* and *development* can cause difficulties in understanding. Growth and development, although closely related, are not synonymous. In conversational English, *growth* usually refers to an increase in size but tends to be linked more to change than anything else. Only if growth meant change, after all, could someone seriously speak of a period of economic recession as one of "negative economic growth." Some tissues grow rapidly and then shrink or disappear, so a plot of physical growth versus time may include a negative phase. On the other hand, if growth is defined solely as a process of change, the term becomes almost meaningless. In this chapter, the term growth usually refers to an increase in size or number.

As a general term, *development* connotes an increasing degree of organization, often with unfortunate consequences for the natural environment. With reference to growth, the term *development* is used almost always to refer to an increase in complexity, and it is used in that way in this chapter. Development carries an overtone of increasing specialization, so that one price of increased development is a loss of potential. Growth is largely an anatomic phenomenon, whereas development is physiologic and behavioral.

Although dentists work with the physical features of the teeth and face, a major reason for orthodontic treatment is its psychosocial effects. Furthermore, patient cooperation is necessary, and eliciting it in children of different ages requires a knowledge of social and behavioral development. Both physiologic and psychosocial development are important subjects for this chapter. For convenience, not because they are innately more important, physical growth concepts are presented first, and then behavioral developmental factors are reviewed.

Growth: Pattern, Variability, and Timing

In studies of growth and development, the concept of pattern is important. In a general sense, pattern (as in the pattern from which articles of clothing of different sizes are cut) reflects

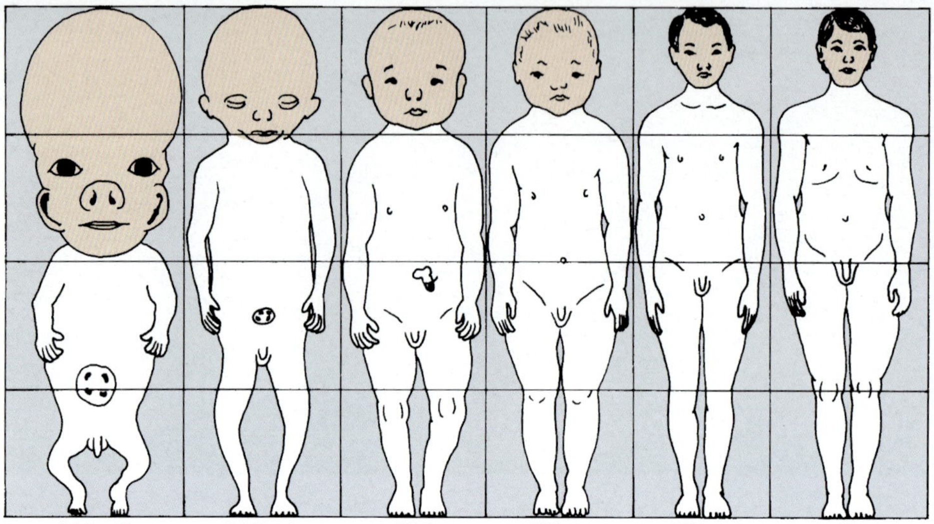

• **Fig. 2.1** Schematic representation of the changes in overall body proportions during normal growth and development. After the third month of fetal life, the proportion of total body size contributed by the head and face steadily declines. (Redrawn from Robbins WJ, et al. *Growth*. Yale University Press; 1928.)

proportionality, usually of a complex set of proportions rather than just a single proportional relationship. Pattern in growth also represents proportionality, but in a still more complex way, because it refers not just to a set of proportional relationships at a point in time but to the change in these proportional relationships over time. In other words, the physical arrangement of the body at any one time is a pattern of spatially proportioned parts. However, there is a higher level pattern, the pattern of growth, which refers to the changes in these spatial proportions over time.

Fig. 2.1 illustrates the change in overall body proportions that occurs during normal growth and development. In fetal life, at about the third month of intrauterine development, the head takes up almost 50% of the total body length. At this stage, the cranium is large relative to the face and represents more than half the total head. In contrast, the limbs are still rudimentary, and the trunk is underdeveloped. By the time of birth, the trunk and limbs have grown faster than the head and face, so that the proportion of the entire body devoted to the head has decreased to about 30%. The overall pattern of growth thereafter follows this course, with a progressive reduction of the relative size of the head to about 12% in the adult. At birth the legs represent about one-third of the total body length, whereas in the adult they represent about half. As Fig. 2.1 illustrates, there is more growth of the lower limbs than the upper limbs during postnatal life. All of these changes, which are a part of the normal growth pattern, reflect the "cephalocaudal gradient of growth." This simply means that there is an axis of increased growth extending from the head toward the feet.

Another aspect of the normal growth pattern is that not all the tissue systems of the body grow at the same rate (Fig. 2.2). Obviously, as the relative decrease in head size after birth shows, the muscular and skeletal elements grow faster than the brain and central nervous system. The overall pattern of growth reflects the growth of the various tissues making up the whole organism. To put it differently, one reason for gradients of growth is that different tissue systems that grow at different rates are concentrated in various parts of the body.

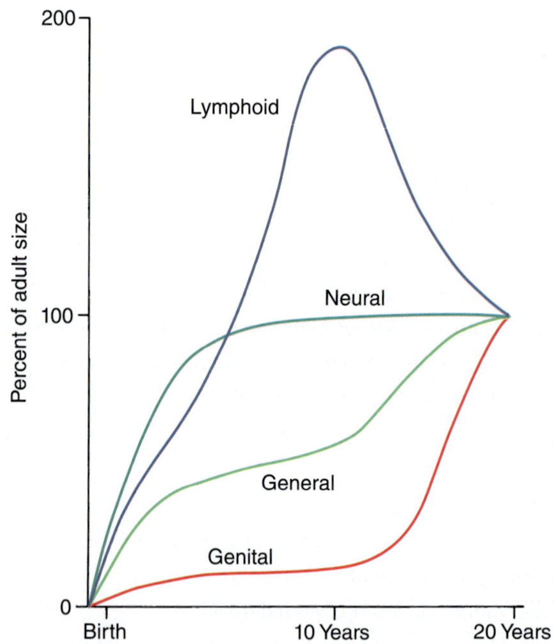

• **Fig. 2.2** Scammon's curves for the growth of the four major tissue systems of the body. As the graph indicates, growth of the neural tissues is nearly complete by 6 or 7 years of age. General body tissues, including muscle, bone, and viscera, show an S-shaped curve, with a definite slowing of the rate of growth during childhood and an acceleration at puberty. Lymphoid tissues proliferate far beyond the adult amount in late childhood and then undergo involution at the same time that the growth of the genital tissues accelerates rapidly. From Scammon RD. The measurement of the body in childhood. In: Harris JA, ed. *The Measurement of Man*. University of Minnesota Press; 1930.

Even within the head and face, the cephalocaudal growth gradient strongly affects proportions and leads to changes in proportion with growth (Fig. 2.3). When the skull of a newborn infant is compared proportionally with that of an adult, it is easy to see that the

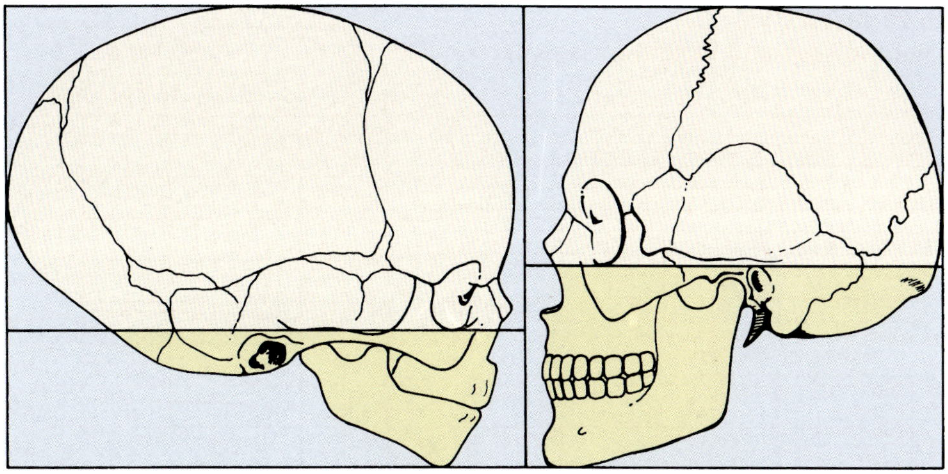

• **Fig. 2.3** Changes in proportions of the head and face during growth. At birth, the face and jaws are relatively underdeveloped compared with their extent in the adult. As a result, there is much more growth of facial than cranial structures postnatally. (Redrawn from Lowery GH. *Growth and Development of Children*. 6th ed. Year Book Medical Publishers; 1973.)

infant has a relatively much larger cranium and a much smaller face. This change is an important aspect of the pattern of facial growth. Not only is there a cephalocaudal gradient of growth within the body, but there is also one within the face. From that perspective, it is not surprising that the mandible, being farther away from the brain, tends to grow more and later than the maxilla, which is closer.

An important aspect of a pattern is its predictability. Patterns repeat, whether in the organization of different-colored tiles in the design of a floor or in skeletal proportions changing over time. The proportional relationships within a pattern can be specified mathematically, and the only difference between a growth pattern and a geometric one is the addition of a time dimension. Thinking about patterns in this way allows one to be more precise in defining what constitutes a change in pattern. Change, clearly, would denote an alteration in the predictable pattern of mathematical relationships. A change in growth pattern would indicate some alteration in the expected changes in body proportions.

A second important concept in the study of growth and development is variability. Obviously, all people are not alike in the way that they grow, as in everything else. It can be difficult but clinically very important to decide whether an individual is merely at the extreme of the normal variation or falls outside the normal range.

Rather than categorizing growth as normal or abnormal, it is more useful to think in terms of deviations from the usual pattern and to express variability quantitatively. One way to do this is to evaluate a given child relative to peers on a standard growth chart (Fig. 2.4). Although charts of this type are commonly used for height and weight, the growth of any part of the body can be plotted in this way. The "normal variability," as derived from large-scale studies of groups of children, is shown by the solid lines on the graphs. An individual who stood exactly at the midpoint of the normal distribution would fall along the 50% line of the graph. One who was larger than 90% of the population would plot above the 90% line; one who was smaller than 90% of the population would plot below the 10% line.

These charts can be used in two ways to determine whether the growth is normal or abnormal. First, the location of an individual relative to the group can be established. A general guideline is that a child who falls outside the range of 97% of the population should receive special study before being accepted as just an extreme of the normal population. Second and perhaps more important, growth charts can be used to follow a child over time to evaluate whether there is an unexpected change in the growth pattern. Pattern implies predictability. For the growth charts, this means that a child's growth should be generally plotted along the same percentile line at all ages. If the percentile position of an individual relative to their peer group changes, especially if there is a marked change (see Fig. 2.4B), the clinician should suspect some growth abnormality and should investigate further. Inevitably, there is a gray area at the extremes of normal variations, at which it is difficult to determine if the growth is normal.

A final major concept in physical growth and development is timing. Variability in growth arises in several ways: from normal variation, from influences outside the normal experience (e.g., serious illness), and from timing effects. Variation in timing arises because the same event happens for different individuals at different times—or, viewed differently, the biological clocks of different individuals are set differently.

Variations in growth and development because of timing are particularly evident in human adolescence. Some children grow rapidly and mature early, completing their growth quickly and thereby appearing on the high side of developmental charts until their growth ceases and their contemporaries begin to catch up. Others grow and develop slowly and so appear to be behind, even though, given time, they will catch up with and even surpass children who once were larger. All children undergo a spurt of growth at adolescence, which can be seen more clearly by plotting changes in height or weight (Fig. 2.5), but the growth spurt occurs at different times in different individuals.

Growth effects because of timing variation can be seen particularly clearly in girls, in whom the onset of menstruation (menarche) gives an excellent indicator of the arrival of sexual maturity. The process of sexual maturation is accompanied by a spurt in growth. When the growth velocity curves for early-, average-, and late-maturing girls are compared in Fig. 2.6, the marked differences in size among these girls during growth are apparent. At age 11, the early-maturing girl is already past the peak of the adolescent growth spurt, whereas the late-maturing girl has not even begun to grow rapidly. This sort of timing variation occurs in many aspects of both growth and development and can be an important contributor to variability.

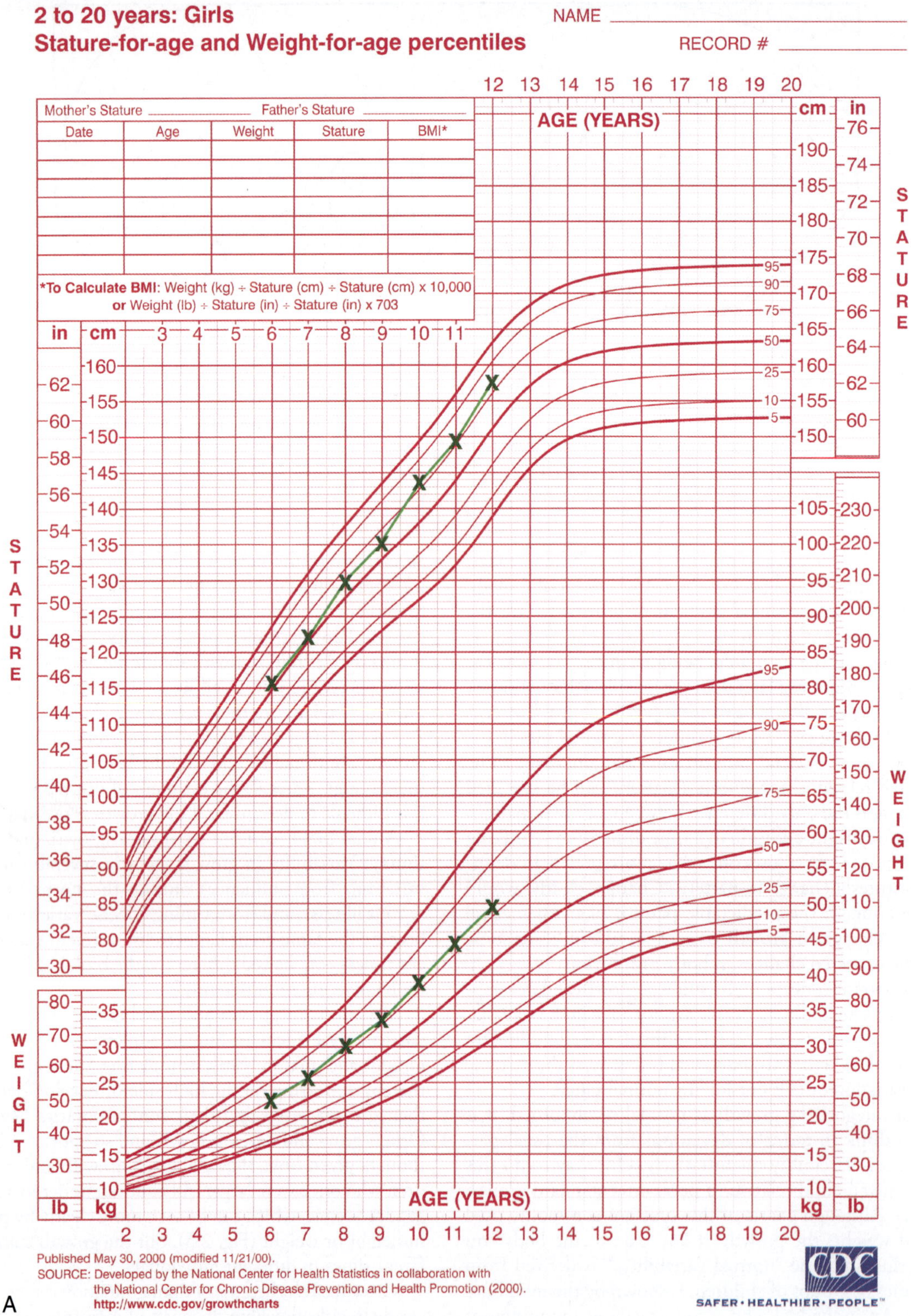

A

• **Fig. 2.4** (A) Growth of a normal girl plotted on the chart for females. Note that this girl remained at about the 75th percentile for height and weight over this entire period of observation. *Continued*

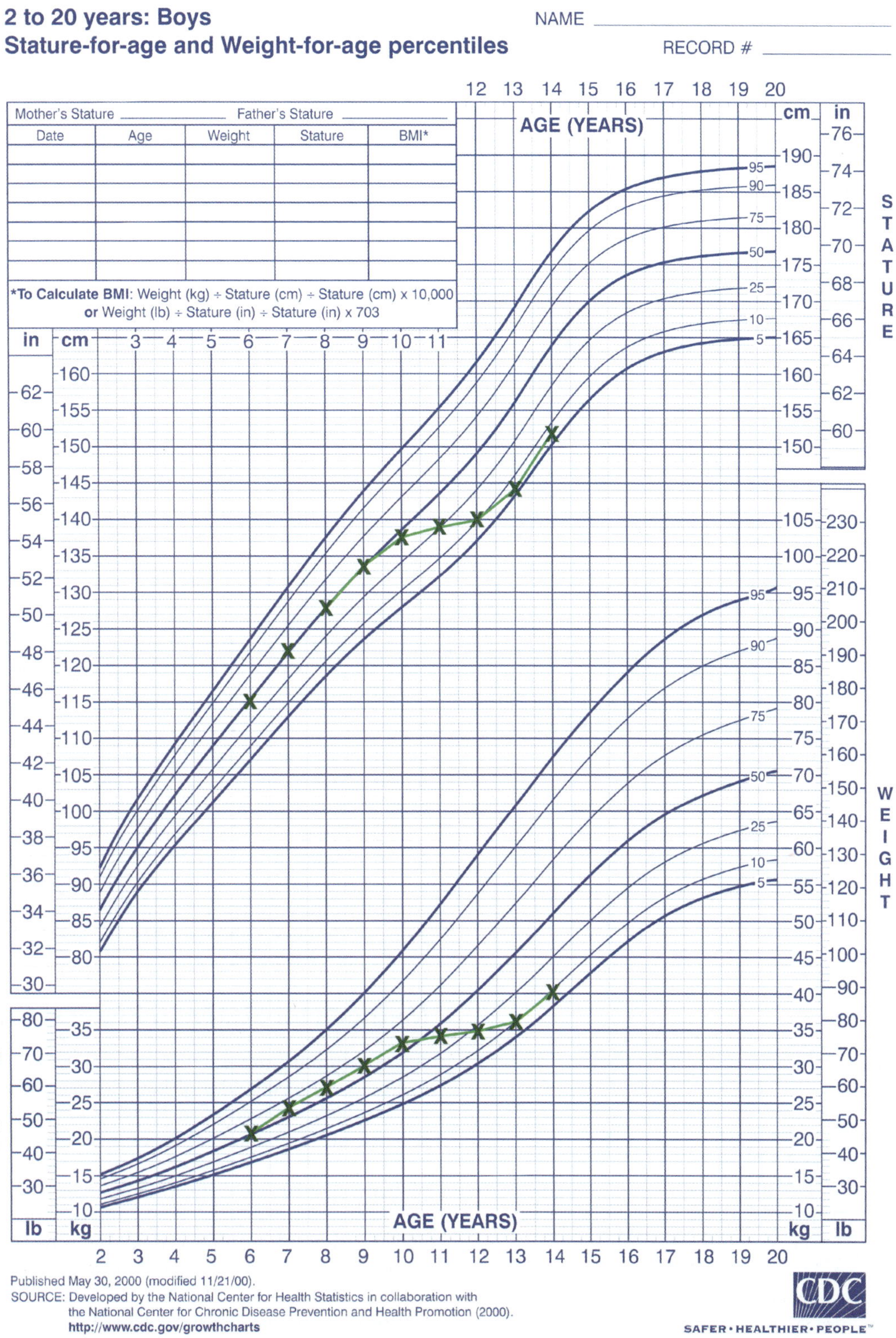

B

• **Fig. 2.4, cont'd** (B) Growth of a boy who developed a medical problem that affected growth, plotted on the male chart. Note the change in pattern (crossover of lines on the chart) between ages 10 and 11. This reflects the impact of serious illness beginning at that time, with partial recovery after age 13 but a continuing effect on growth. (Data from Hamill PV, et al. National Center for Health Statistics, 1979; charts developed by the National Center for Health Statistics in collaboration with the National Center for Chronic Disease Prevention and Health Promotion, published May 30, 2000, revised November 21, 2000—the latest available) (Charts available from http://www.cdc.gov/growthcharts/.)

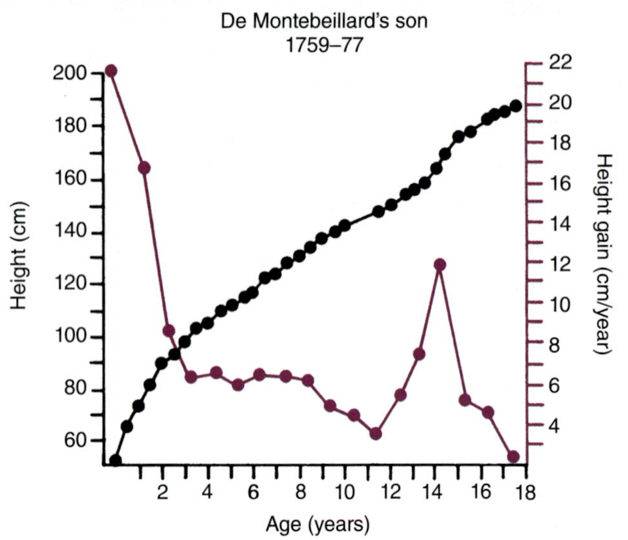

• **Fig. 2.5** Growth can be plotted in either height or weight at any age *(black line)* or the amount of change in any given interval (*maroon line*, showing the same data as the *black line*). A curve like the black line is called a *distance curve*, whereas the maroon line is a *velocity curve*. Plotting velocity rather than distance makes it easier to see when accelerations and decelerations in the rate of growth occurred. These data are for the growth of one individual, the son of a French aristocrat in the late 18th century, whose growth followed the typical pattern. Note the acceleration of growth at adolescence, which occurred for this individual at about age 14. (Data from Scammon RE. The first seriatim study of human growth. *Am J Phys Anthropol*. 1927;10(3):329-336.)

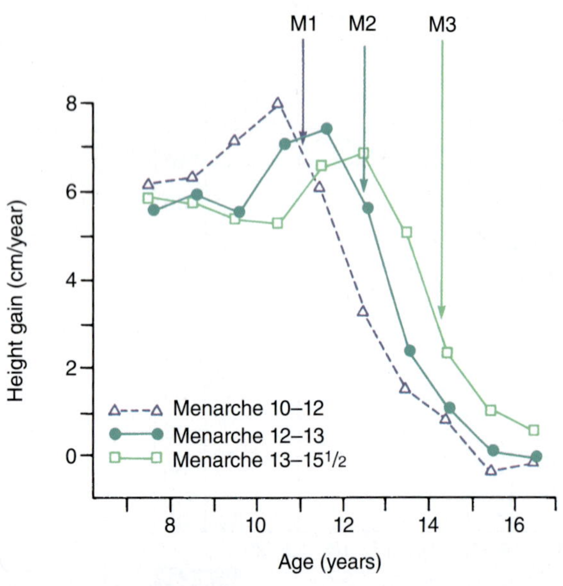

• **Fig. 2.6** Growth velocity curves for early-, average-, and late-maturing girls. It is interesting to note that the earlier the adolescent growth spurt occurs, the more intense it appears to be. Obviously, at age 11 or 12, an early-maturing girl would be considerably larger than one who matured late. In each case, the onset of menstruation (menarche) (*M1, M2*, and *M3*) came after the peak of growth velocity.

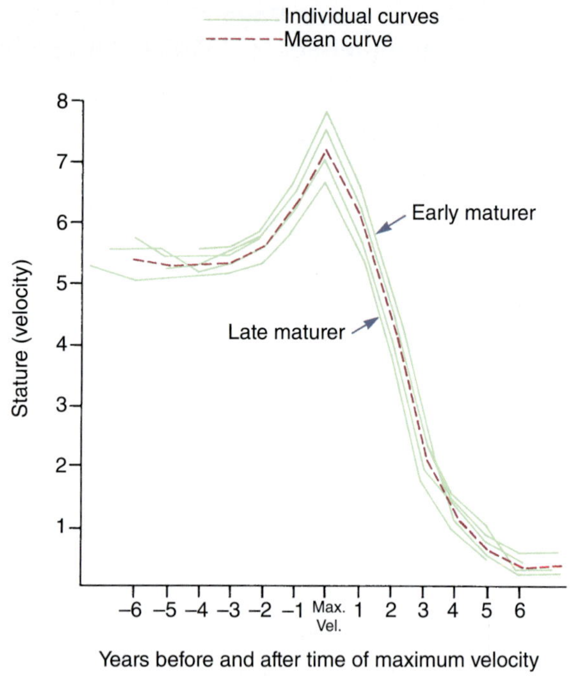

• **Fig. 2.7** Velocity curves for four girls with quite different times of menarche, replotted using menarche as a zero time point. It is apparent that the growth pattern in each case is quite similar, with almost all of the variations resulting from timing.

Although age is usually measured chronologically as the amount of time since birth or conception, it is also possible to measure age biologically, in terms of progress toward various developmental markers or stages. Timing variability can be reduced by using developmental age rather than chronologic age as an expression of an individual's growth status. For instance, if data for gain in height for girls are replotted, using maximum height velocity as a reference time point (Fig. 2.7), it is apparent that girls who mature early, at an average time, or late really follow a very similar growth pattern. This graph substitutes the stage of growth for chronologic age to produce a biological time scale and shows that the pattern is expressed at different times chronologically but not physiologically. The effectiveness of biological or developmental age in reducing timing variability makes this approach useful in evaluating a child's growth status.

Methods for Studying Physical Growth

Before beginning the examination of growth data, it is important to have a reasonable idea of how the data were obtained. There are two basic approaches to studying physical growth. The first is based on techniques for measuring living animals (including humans), with the implication that the measurement itself does no harm and that the animal will be available for additional measurements at another time. The second approach uses experiments in which growth is manipulated in some way. This implies that the subject of the experiment will be available for study in some detail, and the detailed study may be destructive. For this reason, such experimental studies are largely restricted to nonhuman species.

Measurement Approaches

Acquiring Measurement Data

Craniometry

The first of the measurement approaches for studying growth, with which the science of physical anthropology began, is craniometry, based on measurements of skulls found among human skeletal remains. Craniometry was originally used to study the Neanderthal and Cro-Magnon peoples whose skulls were found in European caves in the 18th and 19th centuries. From such skeletal material, it has been possible to piece together a great deal of knowledge about extinct populations and to get some idea of their pattern of growth by comparing one skull with another. Craniometry has the advantage that rather precise measurements can be made on dry skulls; it has the important disadvantage for growth studies that, by necessity, all these growth data must be cross-sectional. *Cross-sectional* means that although different ages are represented in the population, the same individual can be measured at only one point in time.

Anthropometry

It is also possible to measure skeletal dimensions in living individuals. In this technique, called *anthropometry*, various landmarks established in studies of dry skulls are measured in living individuals simply by using soft tissue points overlying these bony landmarks. For example, it is possible to measure the length of the cranium from a point at the bridge of the nose to a point at the greatest convexity of the rear of the skull. This measurement can be made on either a dried skull or a living individual, but results would be different because of the soft tissue thickness overlying both landmarks. Although the soft tissue introduces variation, anthropometry does make it possible to follow the growth of an individual directly, making the same measurements repeatedly at different times. This produces longitudinal data: repeated measures of the same individual. The best data of that type come from Farkas's anthropometric studies in the late 20th century, which provided valuable new data for human facial proportions and their changes from childhood to adolescence and adult life.[1]

Cephalometric Radiology

The third measurement technique, cephalometric radiology, is of considerable importance not only in the study of growth but also in the clinical evaluation of orthodontic patients. The technique depends on precisely orienting the head before making a radiograph, with equally precise control of magnification. This approach can combine the advantages of craniometry and anthropometry. It allows a direct measurement of bony skeletal dimensions because the bone can be seen through the soft tissue covering in a radiograph, but it also allows the same individual to be followed over time. Growth studies are done by superimposing a tracing or digital model of a later cephalogram on an earlier one, so that the changes can be measured. Both the locations and amounts of growth can be observed in this way (Fig. 2.8). Cephalometric superimposition techniques are described in detail in Chapter 6.

The disadvantage of a standard cephalometric radiograph is that it produces a two-dimensional (2D) representation of a three-dimensional (3D) structure, and so, even with precise head positioning, not all measurements are possible. To some extent, this can be overcome by making more than one radiograph at different orientations and using triangulation to calculate oblique distances. The general pattern of craniofacial growth was known from craniometric and anthropometric studies before cephalometric radiography was invented, but much of the current picture of craniofacial growth is based on cephalometric studies.

Three-Dimensional Imaging

New information is now being obtained with the application of 3D imaging techniques. Computed axial tomography (CAT or, more commonly, computed tomography [CT]) allows 3D reconstructions of the cranium and face, and this method has been applied in the last 35 years to plan surgical treatment for patients with facial deformities (Fig. 2.9). Recently, cone beam computed tomography (CBCT) rather than axial CT has been applied to scans of the head and face. This significantly reduces both the radiation dose and the cost. CBCT allows scans of patients with radiation exposure that are much closer to the dose from cephalograms. CBCT also reduces flaws within 2D imaging such as head position, superimposition of anatomical structures, and magnification errors. The superimposition of 3D images is much more difficult than the superimpositions used with 2D cephalometric radiographs, but methods have been developed to address the time and difficulty involved (Fig. 2.10).[2]

Magnetic resonance imaging (MRI) also provides 3D images that can be useful in studies of growth, with the advantage that there is no radiation exposure with this technique. This method has already been applied to the analysis of the growth changes produced by functional appliances,[3] but it shows soft tissues more clearly than hard tissues, just the reverse of radiographic images.

Three-dimensional photography now makes possible much more accurate measurements of facial soft tissue dimensions and changes (Fig. 2.11). A more detailed examination of 3D changes

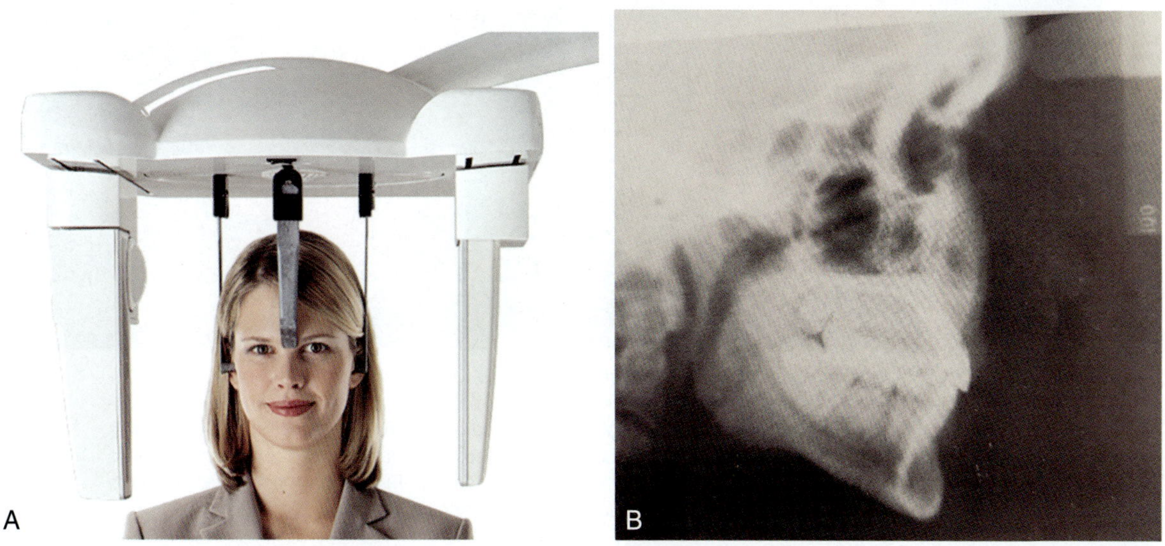

• **Fig. 2.8** (A) A cephalometric radiograph merits this name because of the use of a head-positioning device to provide precise orientation of the head. This means that valid comparisons can be made between external and internal dimensions in members of the same population group or that the same individual can be measured at two points in time because the head orientation is reproducible. (B) This radiograph (a cephalogram) was taken in natural head position (NHP) (see Chapter 6 for a description of this head-positioning technique).

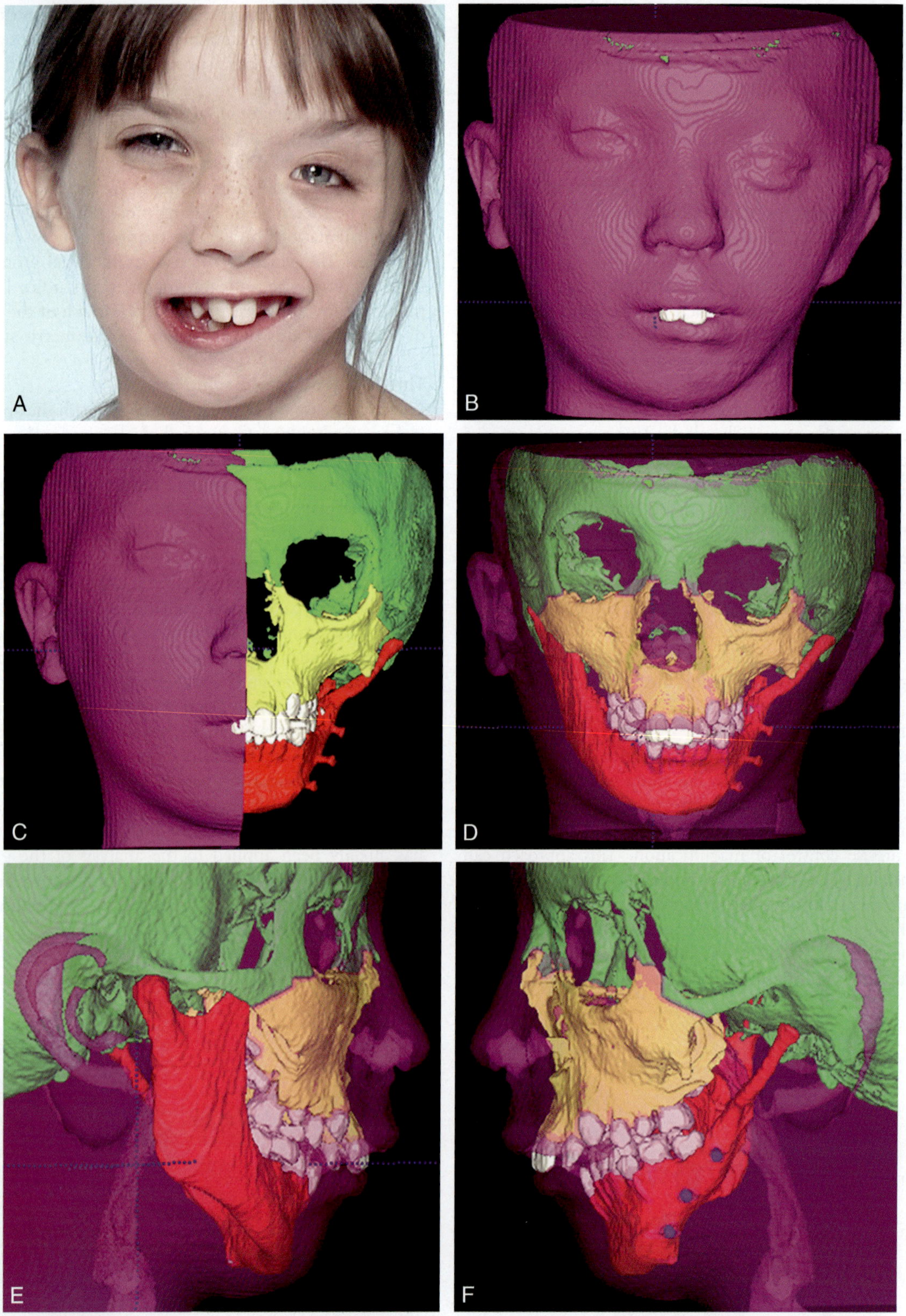

• **Fig. 2.9** Computed tomography (CT) scans are the best way to determine the details of skeletal deformities. These views of a 9-year-old girl (A) with severe hemifacial microsomia (and previous surgical treatment to build up the affected side of the mandible) illustrate that CT scans can show both skin contours and bony relationships from any aspect. Color can be added to different structures to make it easier to visualize them (B), and surface layers can be made transparent (as in C–F) to reveal the skeletal structures beneath. Views of this type greatly facilitate surgical treatment planning. (Courtesy Dr. L. Cevidanes.)

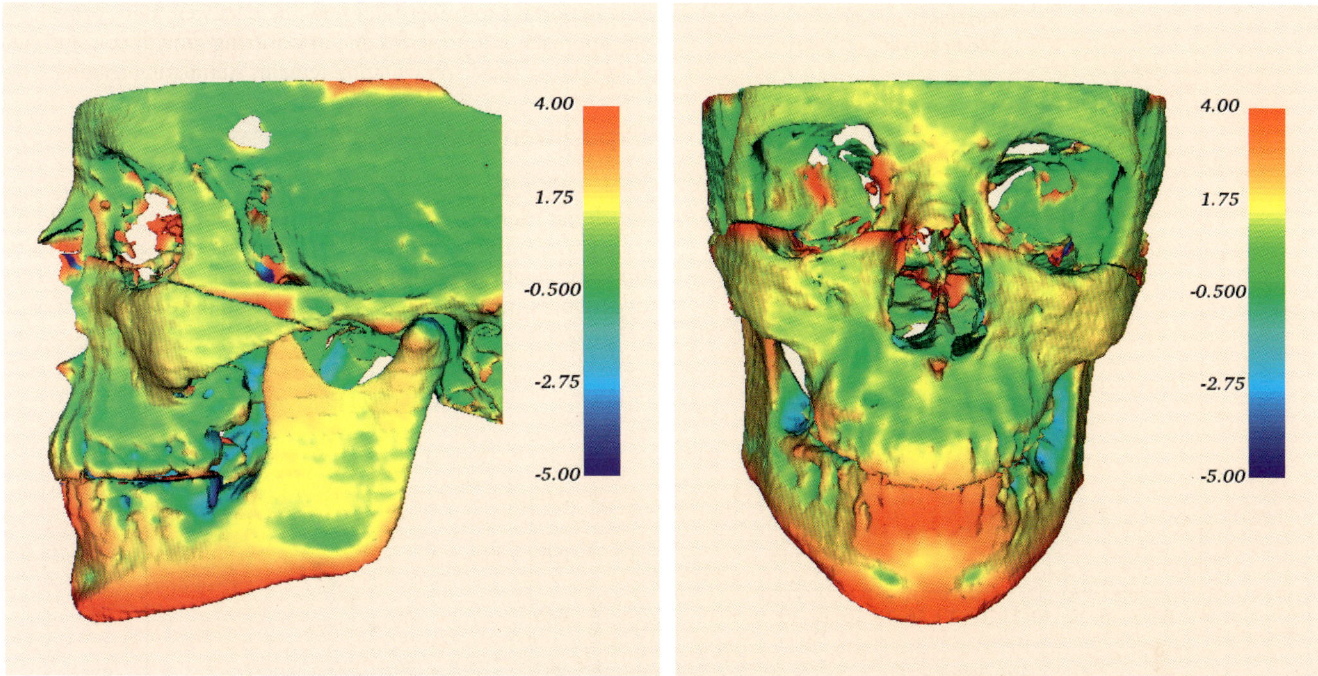

• **Fig. 2.10** Superimposition of computed tomography (CT) images is much more difficult than superimposition of cephalometric tracings but more accurately detects the amount of change and can be used to see changes in exquisite detail. These images are superimposed on the cranial base; a color map is used to show the change from the initial image of an adolescent with a normal growth pattern at age 12 to the same individual at age 14. In the color map, green shows areas of little or no change; deepening shades of red indicate 3–4 mm of movement away from the cranial base; and shades of blue (seen here only on the front of the mandibular ramus) indicate areas that moved closer to the cranial base. The map shows the downward and forward movement of the mandible at a time, as you would expect, of more mandibular than maxillary growth and resorption of the front of the ramus that lengthens the body of the mandible to provide space for eruption of the second molars. Note that the zygomatic arches and the maxillary teeth moved forward a small amount while the bony area just above the maxilla stayed largely in the same place. Understanding growth changes from carefully examining superimposition images such as these is much easier than deciphering the meaning of a series of measurements and gives a broader view of the skeletal changes due to growth.

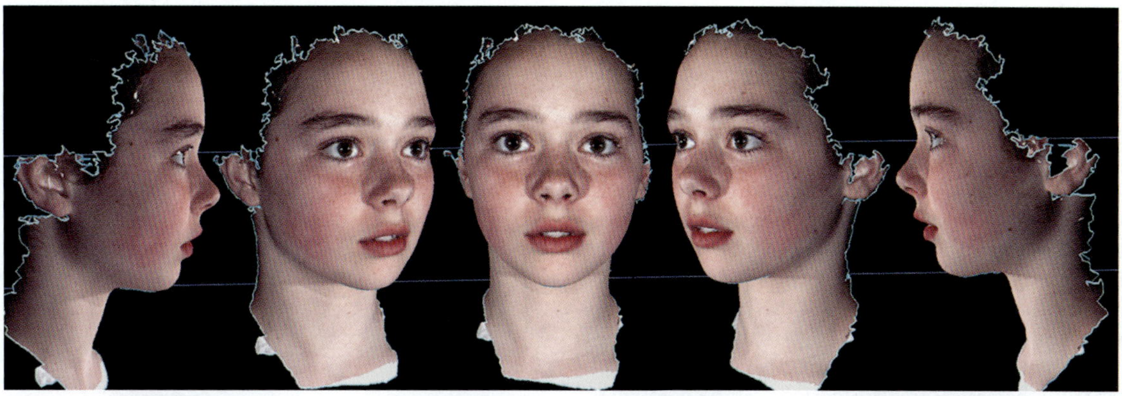

• **Fig. 2.11** Images from a single photograph with a 3dMD camera. Both profile and oblique and frontal views can be captured at the same head position, and measurements of soft tissue dimensions and proportions can be made with great accuracy at any orientation of the face, which makes a camera that provides such three-dimensional views a valuable research tool.

in growing patients almost surely will add to current knowledge of growth patterns in the near future.

Analysis of Measurement Data

Both anthropometric and cephalometric data can be expressed cross-sectionally rather than longitudinally. Obviously, it would be much easier and quicker to do a cross-sectional study, gathering data once for any individual and including subjects of different ages, rather than spending many years on a study in which the same individuals are measured repeatedly. For this reason, most studies are cross-sectional. When this approach is used, however, variability within the sample can conceal details of the growth

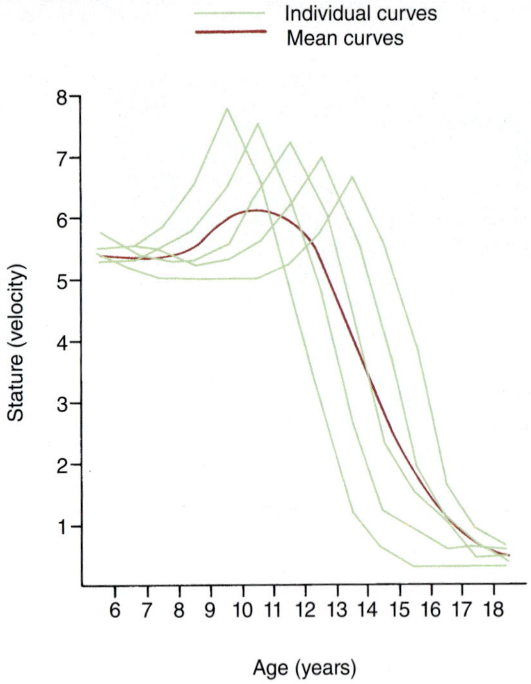

• **Fig. 2.12** If growth velocity data for a group of individuals with different timings for their adolescent growth spurt are plotted on a chronologic scale, it is apparent that the average curve is not an accurate representation of the pattern of growth for many individuals. This smoothing of individual variation is a characteristic of cross-sectional data and a major limitation in the use of the cross-sectional method for studies of growth. Only by following individuals through time in a longitudinal study is it possible to see the details of growth patterns.

pattern, particularly when there is no correction for timing variation (Fig. 2.12). Fluctuations in the growth curve that may occur for nearly every individual would be seen in a cross-sectional study only if they occurred at the same time for each person, which is unlikely. Longitudinal studies are efficient in the sense that a great deal of information can be gained from a relatively small number of subjects, fewer than would be needed in a cross-sectional study. In addition, the longitudinal data highlight individual variations, particularly variations caused by timing effects.

Measurement data can be presented graphically in a number of different ways, and frequently it is possible to clarify growth changes by varying the method of display. For example, we have already seen that growth data can be shown either by plotting the size attained as a function of age, which is called a "distance" curve, or as a "velocity" curve, showing not the total length but the increment added each year (see Fig. 2.5). Changes in the rate of growth are much more easily seen in a velocity curve.

Various other mathematical transformations can be used with growth data to make them easier to understand. For instance, the growth in weight of any embryo at an early stage follows a logarithmic or exponential curve because the growth is based on the division of cells; the more cells there are, the more cell divisions can occur. If the same data are plotted using the logarithm of the weight, a straight-line plot is attained (Fig. 2.13). This demonstrates that the rate of multiplication for cells in the embryo remains more or less constant.

More complex mathematical transformations were used many years ago by D'Arcy Thompson[4] to reveal similarities in proportions and growth changes that had not previously been suspected (Fig. 2.14). To correctly interpret data after mathematical transformation, it is important to understand how the data were transformed, but the approach is a powerful one in clarifying growth concepts, and Thompson's classic presentation remains stimulating reading.

Experimental Approaches

Vital Staining

Much has been learned about skeletal growth using the technique called *vital staining*, in which dyes that stain mineralizing tissues (or occasionally, soft tissues) are injected into an animal. These dyes remain in the bones and teeth and can be detected later after

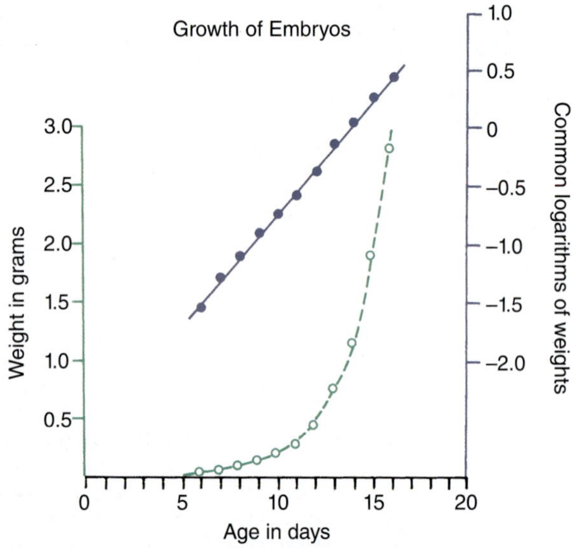

• **Fig. 2.13** Data for the increase in weight of early embryos, with the raw data plotted in green and the same data plotted after logarithmic transformation in blue. At this stage the weight of the embryo increases dramatically, but, as shown by the straight line after transformation, the rate of multiplication of individual cells remains fairly constant. When more cells are present, more divisions can occur, and the weight increases faster. (From Lowery GH. *Growth and Development of Children*. 8th ed. Year Book Medical Publishers; 1986.)

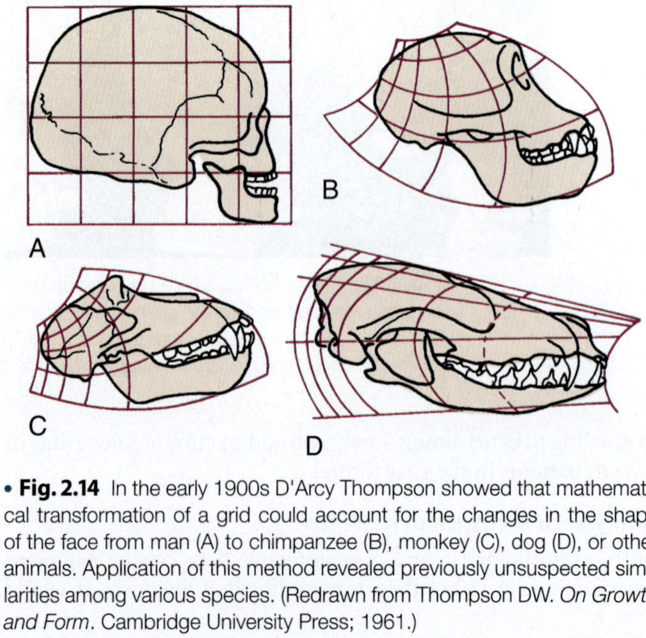

• **Fig. 2.14** In the early 1900s D'Arcy Thompson showed that mathematical transformation of a grid could account for the changes in the shape of the face from man (A) to chimpanzee (B), monkey (C), dog (D), or other animals. Application of this method revealed previously unsuspected similarities among various species. (Redrawn from Thompson DW. *On Growth and Form*. Cambridge University Press; 1961.)

death. This method was originated by the great English anatomist John Hunter in the 18th century. Hunter observed that the bones of pigs that occasionally were fed textile waste were often stained in an interesting way. He discovered that the active agent was a dye called *alizarin*, which is still used for vital staining studies. Alizarin reacts strongly with calcium at sites where bone calcification occurs. Because these are the sites of active skeletal growth, the dye marks the locations at which active growth was occurring when it was injected. Bone models rapidly, and areas from which bone is being removed can also be identified by the fact that vital stained material has been removed from these locations (Fig. 2.15). Highly detailed vital staining studies of bony changes in craniofacial development in experimental animals, from work done at the US National Institute of Dental and Craniofacial Research, are available.[5]

Although studies using vital stains are not possible in humans, vital staining can occur inadvertently. Many children born in the late 1950s and early 1960s were treated for recurrent infections with the antibiotic tetracycline. It was discovered too late that tetracycline is an excellent vital stain that binds to calcium at growth sites in the same way as alizarin. The discoloration of incisor teeth that results from tetracycline given when the teeth are mineralizing has been a serious esthetic problem for some individuals (Fig. 2.16). Although this does not commonly occur now, it is still seen occasionally.

With the development of radioactive tracers, it has become possible to use almost any radioactively labeled metabolite that becomes incorporated into the tissues as a sort of vital stain. The location is detected by the weak radioactivity given off at the site where the material was incorporated. The gamma-emitting isotope technetium 99m (^{99m}Tc) can be used to detect areas of rapid bone growth in humans, but these images are more useful in the diagnosis of localized growth problems such as condylar hyperplasia (see Chapter 6) than for studies of growth patterns. For most studies of growth, radioactively labeled materials in the tissues of experimental animals are detected by the technique of

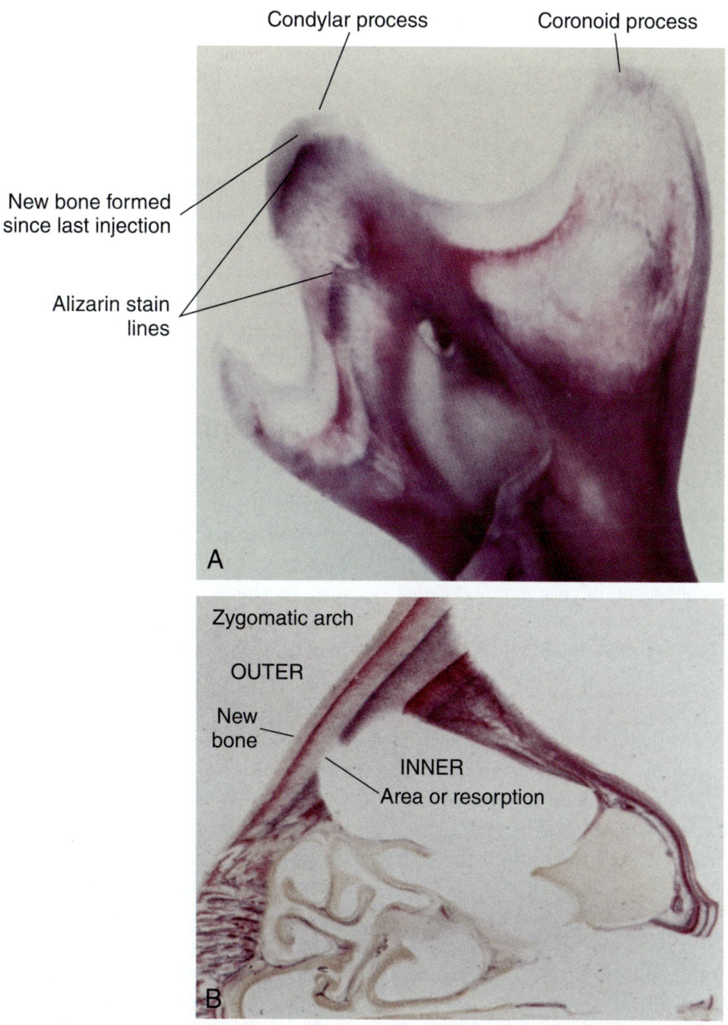

• **Fig. 2.15** (A) The mandible of a growing rat that received four injections of alizarin (red-blue-red-blue) at 2-week intervals and was killed 2 weeks after the last injection (so that the bone formed since then is white). Modeling of the bone as it grows blurs some of the lines of intensely colored bone created by each injection, but the red-blue sequential lines in the condylar process can be seen clearly. (B) Section through the zygomatic arch from the same animal. The zygomatic arch grows outward by apposition of bone on the outer surface and removal from the inner surface. The interruptions in the staining lines on the inner surface clearly show the areas where the bone is being removed. What was once the outer surface of the zygomatic arch becomes the inner surface a relatively short time later and then is removed.

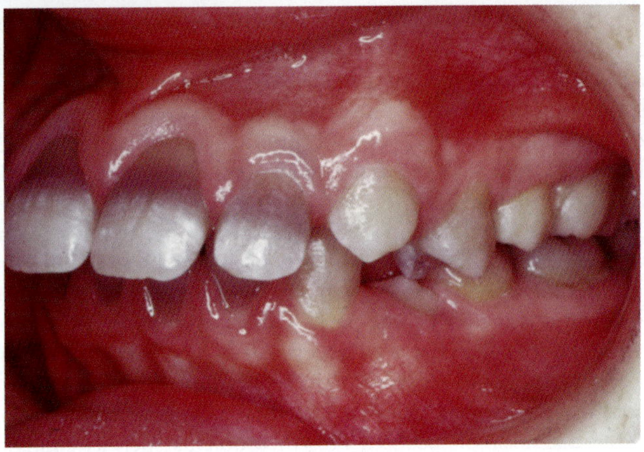

• **Fig. 2.16** Tetracycline staining in the teeth of a boy who received large doses of tetracycline because of repeated upper respiratory infections in early childhood. From the location of the staining, it is apparent that tetracycline was not administered in infancy but was given in large doses beginning when the crowns of the central incisors were about half formed or at approximately 30 months.

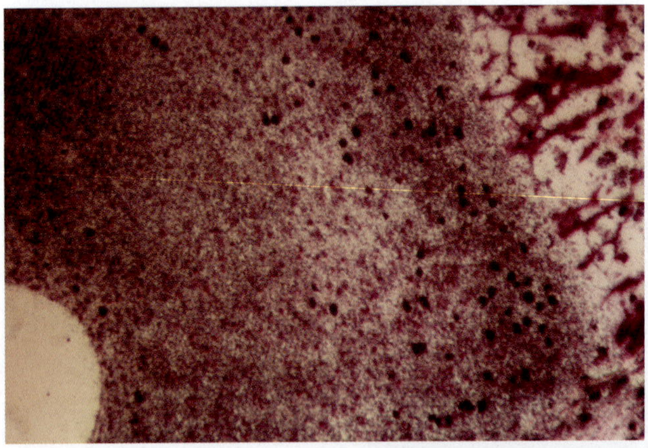

• **Fig. 2.17** An autoradiograph of fetal rat bones growing in organ culture, with carbon 14 (^{14}C)–proline and tritium (^{3}H)–thymidine incorporated in the culture medium. Thymidine is incorporated into DNA, which is replicated when a cell divides, so labeled nuclei are those of cells that underwent mitosis in culture. Because proline is a major constituent of collagen, cytoplasmic labeling indicates areas where proline was incorporated, primarily into extracellularly secreted collagen.

autoradiography, in which a film emulsion is placed over a thin section of tissue containing the isotope and is then exposed in the dark by the radiation. After the film has been developed, the location of the radiation that indicates where growth is occurring can be observed by looking at the tissue section through the film (Fig. 2.17).

Implant Radiography

Another experimental method applicable to studies of humans is implant radiography. In this technique, inert metal pins are placed in bones anywhere in the skeleton, including the face and jaws. These metal pins are well tolerated by the skeleton, become permanently incorporated into the bone without causing any problems, and are easily visualized on a cephalogram (Fig. 2.18). If they are placed in the jaws, a considerable increase in the accuracy of a longitudinal cephalometric analysis of growth patterns can be achieved. This method of study was developed by

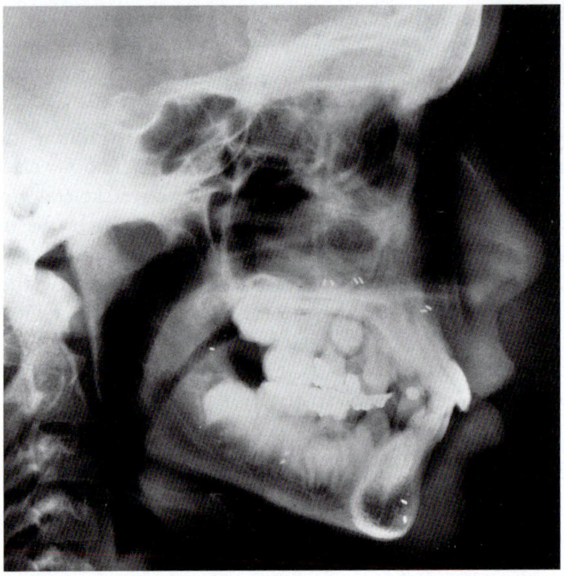

• **Fig. 2.18** Lateral cephalometric radiograph from the archives of Björk's implant studies showing a subject with six maxillary and five mandibular tantalum implants. (Courtesy Department of Orthodontics, University of Copenhagen, Denmark.)

Professor Arne Björk and coworkers at the Royal Dental College in Copenhagen, Denmark, and was used extensively by workers there (see Chapter 4). It provided important new information about the growth pattern of the jaws.

With 21st-century technology, precise evaluation of dentofacial growth in humans using implant cephalograms has largely been superseded by 3D imaging via CBCT or MRI, but it still can be helpful to use implants to provide landmarks for superimposition.

Genetic Influences on Growth

Rapid advances in molecular genetics are providing new information about growth, its control, and links to the development of orthodontic problems. It has now been shown that homeobox *Msx* and *Dlx* genes, which are known to be critically important in the establishment of the body plan, pattern formation, and morphogenesis, are expressed differentially not only in the development of the teeth but also in the growth of the mandible. Msx-1 predominates in tooth formation and is expressed in mesenchyme during tooth development, whereas Msx-2 is expressed in both epithelial and mesenchymal components of the developing tooth germ.[6–8] Dlx-1 and Dlx-2 are expressed in the dental mesenchyme and in the epithelium of the maxillary and mandibular arch mesenchyme, and other homeobox gene groups have been shown to play a role in dental and facial development.[9] An association between a specific genotype for muscle myofibril anchor proteins and class II and deep bite malocclusions has been demonstrated.[10]

The proper function of families of growth factors and their cognate receptors is essential in regulating embryonic processes of cell growth and organ development, as well as a myriad postnatal processes that include growth, wound healing, bone remodeling, and homeostasis. The US National Institute of Dental and Craniofacial Research has recently announced the establishment of a consortium to accelerate the understanding of craniofacial developmental biology through interactive projects including global and specific gene expression patterns, genome-wide association patterns, and transcriptional profiling over the course of embryonic and postnatal development in animal models and humans.[11] Essentially, this is a project toward the use of "big data" to better understand complex genetic interactions. It seems likely that interactive research of this type by groups of investigators will lead to the development of gene therapy for developmental problems.

Interaction between different tissues within the craniofacial complex creates yet another level of regulation of growth and development. One example of this is the convergence of the development of the muscles that attach to the mandible and the bony areas to which they attach. Although many genes are involved in determining mandibular size, genetic alterations in muscle development and function translate into changes in the forces on areas of bone where muscles attach, and this leads to the modification of skeletal areas such as the coronoid process and gonial angle area of the mandible. Genetic alterations that affect muscle also would affect these skeletal areas. To understand this, it is necessary to identify the specific genes involved and to deduce how their activity is modified, but it is already apparent that gene expression can be upregulated or downregulated by mechanical stresses.

Another good example of complex, tightly regulated tissue interactions is found in the development of a tooth and the beginning of eruption. Tooth formation begins with the differentiation of ameloblasts (which form the outer enamel layer of the crown of a tooth) and odontoblasts (which form the dentin layer) within the rapidly calcifying alveolar bone, while multipotential cells continue to be present within the forming crown. As crown formation continues, the dental follicle, a fibrous sac containing the developing tooth, signals the differentiation of osteoblasts from precursors and the differentiation of odontoclasts (resorb dentin) and osteoclasts (resorb bone) from monocytes. This process is mediated by a number of signaling factors including CSF-1, MCSP-1, and OPG/RANK/RANKL. Mature osteoclasts resorb bone over the crown allowing the eruptive movement initiated by the dental follicle. The expression of these factors is time sensitive and correlates with the formation of the tooth root, which initiates the occlusal movement characteristic of eruption into the oral cavity.[12]

There has been significant progress in understanding the genetics of human eruption problems, and the identification of a genetic mutation leading to primary failure of eruption (PFE) in 2009 made it possible for the first time to diagnose an orthodontic problem from examination of DNA from a sample of blood or saliva.[13] PFE is discussed further in Chapters 3 and 12.

An exciting prospect for the future is a better understanding of how patients with orthodontic problems that are known to have a genetic component (class III malocclusion being the best example) will respond to treatment. Chromosomal loci associated with class III malocclusion have been identified. There are multiple subtypes of class III, and a necessary first step is better characterization of these phenotypes. Establishing phenotypic markers (distinct clinical characteristics) makes it possible to establish definitive correlations with modes of inheritance and is necessary for linkage studies that will clarify the genetic basis for the problem.

It is unlikely that genetic analysis will ever be applicable to planning treatment for the majority of orthodontic problems, but it could yield valuable information about the best approach to some of the most difficult skeletal malocclusions, predicting how a patient will respond to treatment and perhaps the application of gene therapy to growth problems.

The Nature of Skeletal Growth

At the cellular level, there are only three possibilities for growth. The first is an increase in the size of individual cells, which is referred to as *hypertrophy*. The second possibility is an increase in the number of cells, which is called *hyperplasia*. The third is the *secretion of extracellular material*, thus contributing to an increase in size independent of the number or size of the cells themselves.

In fact, all three of these processes occur in skeletal growth. Hyperplasia is a prominent feature of all forms of growth. Hypertrophy occurs in a few special circumstances but is a less important mechanism than hyperplasia in most instances. Although tissues throughout the body secrete extracellular material, this phenomenon is particularly important in the growth of the skeletal system, where extracellular material later mineralizes.

The fact that the extracellular material of the skeleton becomes mineralized leads to an important distinction between the growth of the soft or nonmineralized tissues of the body and the hard or calcified tissues. Hard tissues are bones, teeth, and sometimes cartilages. Soft tissues are everything else. In most instances, cartilage, particularly the cartilage significantly involved in growth, behaves like soft tissue and should be thought of in that group rather than as hard tissue.

Growth of soft tissues occurs by a combination of hyperplasia and hypertrophy. These processes go on everywhere within the tissues, and the result is what is called *interstitial growth*, which simply means that it occurs at all points within the tissue. Although the secretion of extracellular material can also accompany interstitial growth, hyperplasia primarily and hypertrophy secondarily are its characteristics. Interstitial growth is characteristic of nearly all soft tissues and of uncalcified cartilage within the skeletal system.

In contrast, when mineralization takes place so that hard tissue is formed, interstitial growth becomes impossible. Hyperplasia, hypertrophy, and secretion of extracellular material are all still possible, but in mineralized tissues, these processes can occur only on the surface, not within the mineralized mass. Direct addition of new bone to the surface of existing bone can and does occur through the activity of cells in the periosteum—the soft tissue membrane that covers the bone. Formation of new cells occurs in the periosteum, and extracellular material secreted there is mineralized and becomes a new bone. This process is called the *direct* or *surface apposition* of bone. Interstitial growth is a prominent aspect of overall skeletal growth because a major portion of the skeletal system is originally modeled in cartilage. This includes the basal part of the skull, as well as the trunk and limbs.

Fig. 2.19 shows the cartilaginous and neural development of the face and cranium at 8 and 12 weeks of intrauterine development. Cartilaginous skeletal development occurs most rapidly during the third month of intrauterine life. A continuous plate of cartilage extends from the nasal capsule posteriorly all the way to the foramen magnum at the base of the skull. It must be kept in mind that cartilage is a nearly avascular tissue whose internal cells are supplied by diffusion through the outer layers. This means that the cartilage must be thin. At early stages in the development of the fetus (the fetal stage begins at the start of the third month), its extremely small size makes a chondroskeleton feasible, but with further growth such an arrangement is no longer possible without an internal blood supply.

During the fourth month in utero, there is an ingrowth of blood vascular elements into various points of the chondrocranium (and the other parts of the early cartilaginous skeleton). These areas become centers of ossification, at which cartilage is transformed

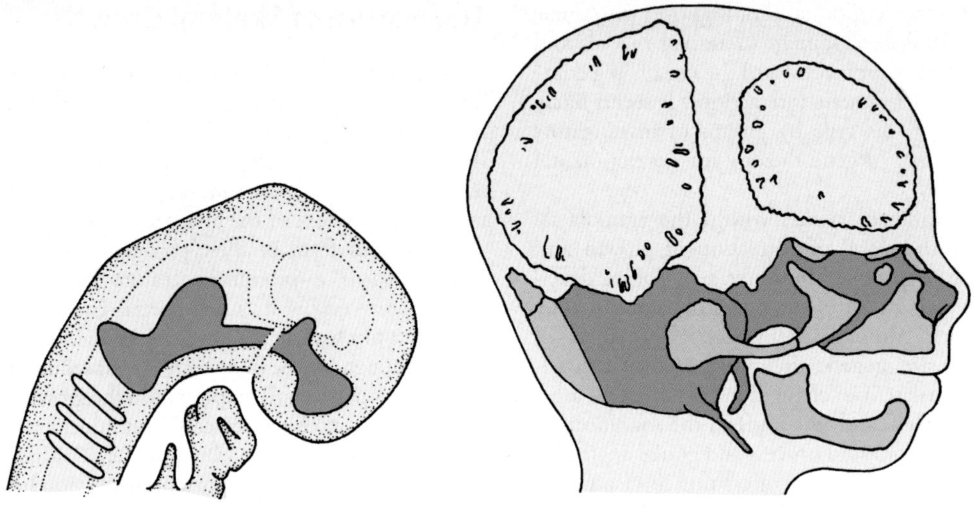

A B

• **Fig. 2.19** Development and maturation of the chondrocranium (cartilage, *light blue; bone, dark blue*). (A) Diagrammatic representation at about 8 weeks. Note that an essentially solid bar of cartilage extends from the nasal capsule anteriorly to the occipital area posteriorly. (B) Skeletal development at 12 weeks. Ossification centers have appeared in the midline cartilage structures, and in addition, intramembranous bone formation of the jaws and braincase has begun. From this point on, bone replaces the cartilage of the original chondrocranium rapidly so that only the small cartilaginous synchondroses connecting the bones of the cranial base remain.

into bone in the process called *endochondral ossification*, and islands of bone appear in the sea of surrounding cartilage (see Fig. 2.19B). The cartilage continues to grow rapidly but is replaced by bone with equal rapidity. The result is that the amount of bone increases rapidly and the relative (but not the absolute) amount of cartilage decreases. Eventually, the old chondrocranium is represented only by small areas of cartilage interposed between large sections of bone, which assume the characteristic form of the ethmoid, sphenoid, and basioccipital bones. Growth at these cartilaginous connections between the skeletal bones is like growth in the limbs.

In the long bones of the extremities, areas of ossification appear in the center of the bones and at the ends, ultimately producing a central shaft called the *diaphysis* and a bony cap on each end called the *epiphysis*. Between the epiphysis and diaphysis is a remaining area of uncalcified cartilage called the *epiphyseal plate* (Fig. 2.20A). The epiphyseal plate cartilage of the long bones is a major center for their growth, and in fact, this cartilage is responsible for almost all growth in the length of these bones. The periosteum on the surfaces of the bones also plays an important role in adding to thickness and reshaping the external contours.

Near the outer end of each epiphyseal plate is a zone of actively dividing cartilage cells. Some of these, pushed toward the diaphysis by proliferative activity beneath, undergo hypertrophy, secrete an extracellular matrix, and eventually degenerate as the matrix begins to mineralize and then is rapidly replaced by bone. If the rate at which cartilage cells proliferate is equal to or greater than the rate at which they mature, growth will continue. Eventually, however, toward the end of the normal growth period, the rate of maturation exceeds the rate of proliferation, the last of the cartilage is replaced by bone, and the epiphyseal plate disappears. At that point, the growth of the bone is complete, except for surface changes in thickness, which can be produced by the periosteum.

Endochondral ossification also occurs at the mandibular condyle, which superficially looks like half an epiphyseal plate (Fig. 2.20B and C). As we will see, however, the cartilage of the condyle does not behave like an epiphyseal plate—and the difference is important in understanding mandibular growth.

Not all bones of the adult skeleton were represented in the embryonic cartilaginous model, and it is possible for bone to form by secretion of bone matrix directly within connective tissues without any intermediate formation of cartilage. Bone formation of this type is called *intramembranous ossification*. This type of bone formation occurs in the cranial vault and both jaws (Fig. 2.21).

Early in embryonic life (which is discussed in some detail later at the beginning of Chapter 5), the mandible of higher animals develops in the same area as the cartilage of the first pharyngeal arch—Meckel cartilage. Unlike other bones of the cranium, the development of the mandible begins as a condensation of mesenchyme just lateral to Meckel cartilage and proceeds entirely by intramembranous bone formation (Fig. 2.22). Meckel cartilage disintegrates and largely disappears as the bony mandible develops. Remnants of this cartilage are transformed into a portion of two of the small bones that form the conductive ossicles of the middle ear but not into a significant part of the mandible. Its perichondrium persists as the sphenomandibular ligament. The condylar cartilage develops initially as an independent secondary cartilage, which is separated by a considerable gap from the body of the mandible (Fig. 2.23). Early in fetal life, it fuses with the developing mandibular ramus.

The maxilla forms initially from a center of mesenchymal condensation in the maxillary process. This area is located on the lateral surface of the nasal capsule, the most anterior part of the chondrocranium, but endochondral ossification does not contribute directly to the formation of the maxillary bone. An accessory cartilage, the zygomatic or malar cartilage, which forms in the developing malar process, disappears and is totally replaced by bone well before birth, unlike the mandibular condylar cartilage, which persists.

Whatever the location for intramembranous bone formation, interstitial growth within the mineralized mass is impossible, and

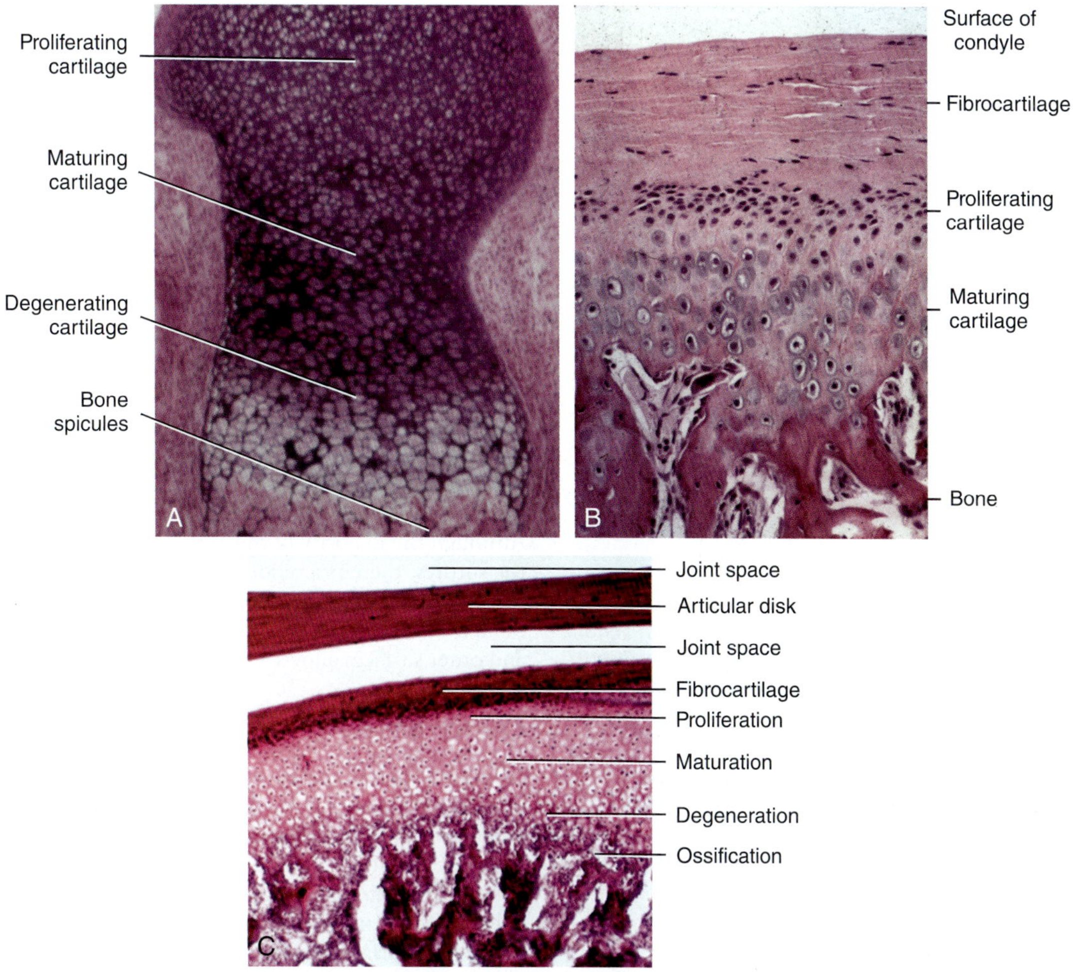

• **Fig. 2.20** (A) Endochondral ossification at an epiphyseal plate. Growth occurs by proliferation of cartilage, occurring here at the top. Maturing cartilage cells are displaced away from the area of proliferation, undergo hypertrophy, degenerate, and are replaced by spicules of bone, as seen in the bottom. (B and C) Endochondral ossification in the head of the condyle. A layer of fibrocartilage lies on the surface, with proliferating cells just beneath. Maturing and degenerating cartilage cells can be seen toward the area of ossification.

the bone must be formed entirely by apposition of new bone to free surfaces. Its shape can be changed through the removal (resorption) of bone in one area and the addition (apposition) of bone in another (see Fig. 2.15). This balance of apposition and resorption, with new bone being formed in some areas while old bone is removed in others, is an essential component of the growth process. It has two components: *modeling* and *remodeling*.

Bone modeling adapts structure to function by changing bone size and shape to maintain bone strength as the loading of the bone changes. This is mediated by the independent activities of osteoblasts and osteoblasts. This process also includes bone drift, such as the relocation of the mandibular ramus during growth (described in detail later). Bone remodeling occurs via osteocyte apposition and osteoclast resorption in the same area without changing the shape of bone. An excellent example of remodeling is the process that takes place with tooth movement, but internal remodeling of bony structures occurs in a continuous cycle.[14] Keeping this distinction between modeling and remodeling in mind can make it easier to understand the bony changes that occur during growth that are discussed in the following sections of this chapter, where these terms are *not* used interchangeably.

Sites and Types of Growth in the Craniofacial Complex

To understand growth in any area of the body, it is necessary to understand (1) the sites or location of growth, (2) the type of growth occurring at that location, (3) the mechanism of growth (i.e., how growth changes occur), and (4) the determinant or controlling factors in that growth.

In the following discussion of sites and types of growth in the head and face, it is convenient to divide the craniofacial complex into four areas that grow rather differently: the cranial vault, the bones that cover the upper and outer surface of the brain; the cranial base, the bony floor under the brain, which also is the dividing line between the cranium and the face; the nasomaxillary complex, made up of the nose, maxilla, and associated small bones; and the mandible. The sites and types of growth are discussed in the following section of this chapter. The mechanism and determinants for growth in each area, as they are viewed from the perspective of current theories of growth control, are discussed later.

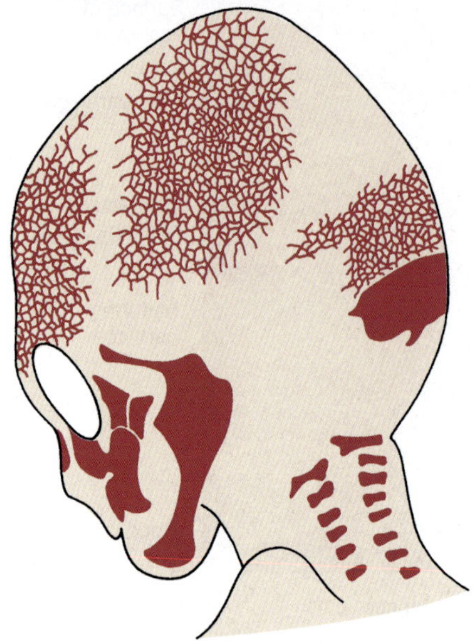

• **Fig. 2.21** The bones of the skull of a 12-week-old fetus, drawn from a cleared alizarin-stained specimen. (Redrawn from Sadler TW, Langman J. *Langman's Medical Embryology*. 9th ed. Lippincott Williams & Wilkins; 2003.)

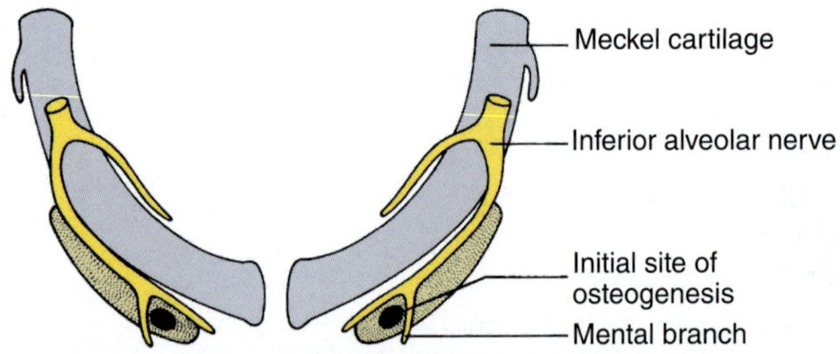

• **Fig. 2.22** Diagrammatic representation of the relation of initial bone formation in the mandible to Meckel cartilage and the inferior alveolar nerve. Bone formation begins just lateral to Meckel cartilage and spreads posteriorly along it without any direct replacement of the cartilage by the newly forming bone of the mandible. (Redrawn from Ten Cate AR. *Oral Histology: Development, Structure, and Function*. 5th ed. Mosby; 1998.)

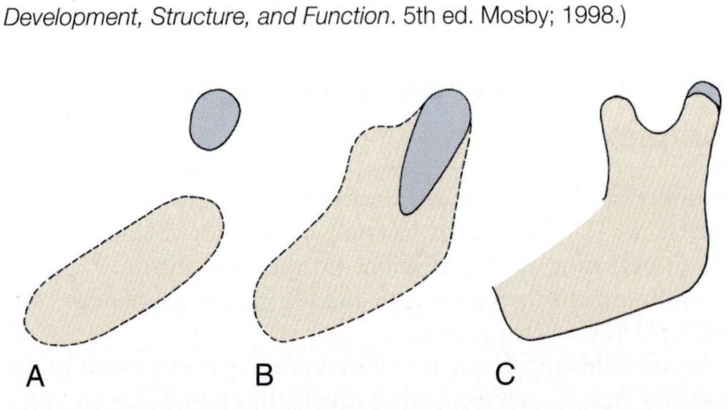

• **Fig. 2.23** The condylar cartilage *(blue)* develops initially as a separate area of condensation from that of the body of the mandible and is only later incorporated within. (A) Separate areas of mesenchymal condensation at 8 weeks. (B) Fusion of the cartilage with the mandibular body at 4 months. (C) Situation at birth (reduced to scale).

Cranial Vault

The cranial vault is made up of a number of flat bones that are formed directly by intramembranous bone formation without cartilaginous precursors. From the time that ossification begins at several locations that foreshadow the eventual anatomic bony units, the growth process is entirely the result of periosteal activity at the surfaces of the bones. Modeling (addition of new bone) and growth occur primarily at the periosteum-lined contact areas between adjacent skull bones, the *cranial sutures*, but periosteal activity also produces modeling changes on the inner and outer surfaces of these platelike bones.

At birth, the flat bones of the skull are rather widely separated by loose connective tissues (Fig. 2.24). These open spaces, the fontanelles, allow a considerable amount of deformation of the skull at birth. This is important in allowing the relatively large head to pass through the birth canal (see Chapter 3 for more detail). After birth, the apposition of bone along the edges of the fontanelles eliminates these open spaces quickly, but the bones remain separated by a thin, periosteum-lined suture for many years, eventually fusing in adult life.

Despite their small size, the apposition of new bone at these sutures is the major mechanism for growth of the cranial vault. Although the majority of the growth in the cranial vault occurs at the sutures, there is a tendency for the bone to be removed from the inner surface of the cranial vault, while at the same time new bone is added on the exterior surface. This modeling of the inner and outer surfaces allows for changes in contour during growth.

Cranial Base

In contrast to the cranial vault, the bones of the base of the skull (the cranial base) are formed initially in cartilage, and these cartilage models are later transformed into bone by endochondral ossification. The situation is more complicated, however, than in a long bone with its epiphyseal plates. The cartilage modeling is particularly true of the midline structures. As one moves laterally, growth at sutures and surface remodeling becomes more important.

As indicated previously, ossifications appear early in embryonic life in the chondrocranium, indicating the eventual location of the basioccipital, sphenoid, and ethmoid bones that form the cranial base. As ossification proceeds, bands of cartilage called *synchondroses* remain between the centers of ossification (Fig. 2.25). These important growth sites (and centers) are the synchondrosis between the sphenoid and occipital bones, or *spheno-occipital synchondrosis;* the *intersphenoid synchondrosis* between two parts of the sphenoid bone; and the *spheno-ethmoidal synchondrosis* between the sphenoid and ethmoid bones. Histologically, a synchondrosis looks like a two-sided epiphyseal plate (Fig. 2.26). Synchondrosis has an area of cellular hyperplasia in the center with bands of maturing cartilage cells extending in both directions, which will eventually be replaced by bone.

A significant difference from the bones of the extremities is that immovable joints develop between the bones of the cranial base, in considerable contrast to the highly movable joints of the extremities. The cranial base is thus rather like a single long bone, except that there are multiple epiphyseal plate–like synchondroses. Immovable joints also occur between most of the other cranial and facial bones, the mandible being the only exception. The periosteum-lined sutures of the cranium and face, containing no cartilage, are quite different from the cartilaginous synchondroses of the cranial base.

Maxilla (Nasomaxillary Complex)

The maxilla develops postnatally entirely by intramembranous ossification. Because there is no cartilage replacement, growth

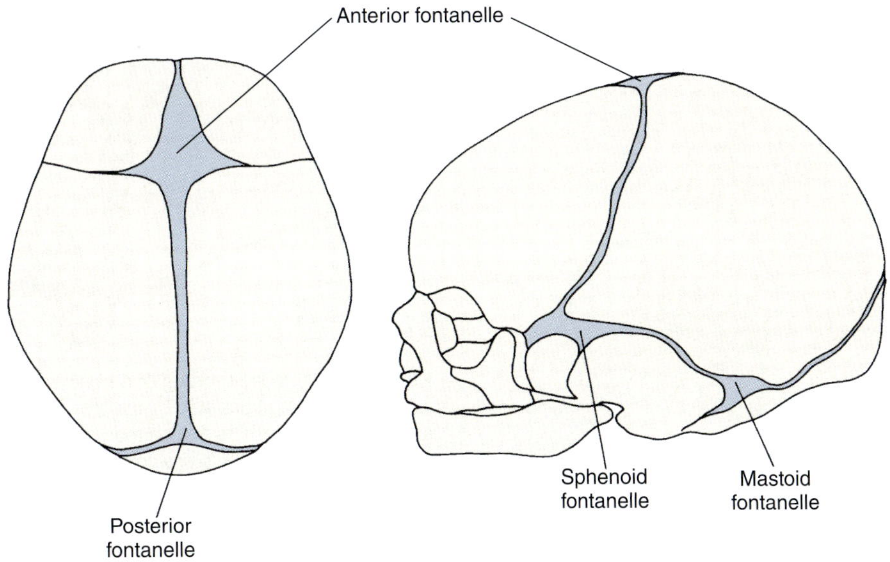

• **Fig. 2.24** The fontanelles of the newborn skull *(blue)*.

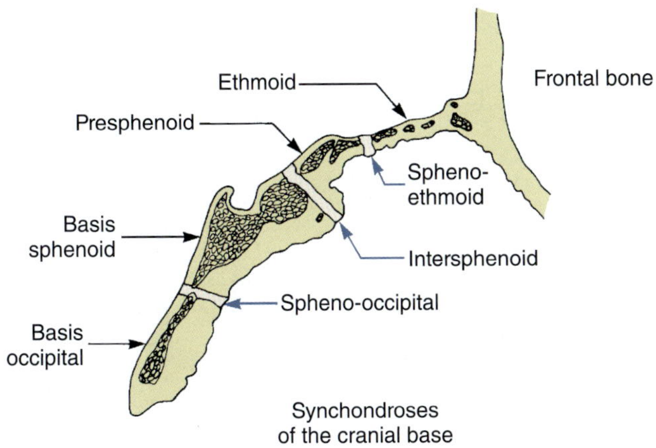

• **Fig. 2.25** Diagrammatic representation of the synchondroses of the cranial base, showing the locations of these important growth sites.

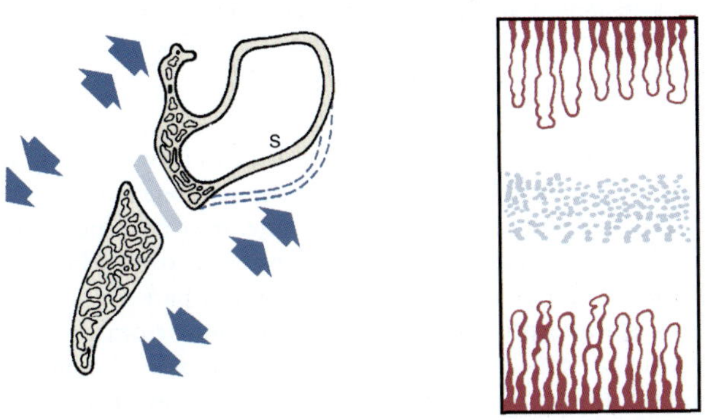

• **Fig. 2.26** Diagrammatic representation of growth at the spheno-occipital synchondrosis. A band of immature proliferating cartilage cells is located at the center of the synchondrosis, a band of maturing cartilage cells extends in both directions away from the center, and endochondral ossification occurs at both margins. Growth at the synchondrosis lengthens this area of the cranial base. Even within the cranial base, bone remodeling on surfaces is also important—it is also the mechanism by which the sphenoid sinus(es) enlarges, for instance.

occurs in two ways: (1) by apposition of bone at the sutures that connect the maxilla to the cranium and cranial base and (2) by surface modeling. In contrast to the cranial vault, however, surface changes in the maxilla are quite dramatic and as important as changes in the sutures. In addition, the maxilla is moved forward by the growth of the cranial base behind it.

The growth pattern of the face requires that it grow "out from under the cranium," which means that as it grows, the maxilla must move a considerable distance downward and forward relative to the cranium and cranial base. This is accomplished in two ways: (1) by a push from behind created by cranial base growth and (2) by growth at the sutures. Because the maxilla is attached to the anterior end of the cranial base, lengthening of the cranial base pushes it forward. Up until about age 6, displacement from cranial base growth is an important part of the maxilla's forward growth. Failure of the cranial base to lengthen normally, as in achondroplasia (see Fig. 5.27) and several congenital syndromes, creates a characteristic midface deficiency. At about age 7, cranial base growth stops, and then sutural growth is the only mechanism for bringing the maxilla forward.

As Fig. 2.27 illustrates, the sutures attaching the maxilla posteriorly and superiorly are ideally situated to allow its downward and forward repositioning. As the downward and forward movement occurs, the space that would otherwise open at the sutures is filled in by the proliferation of bone at these locations. The sutures remain the same width, and the various processes of the maxilla become longer. Bone apposition occurs on both sides of a suture, so the bones to which the maxilla is attached also become larger. Part of the posterior border of the maxilla is a free surface in the tuberosity region. Bone is added at this surface, creating additional space into which the primary and then the permanent molar teeth successively erupt.

It is interesting to note that as the maxilla grows downward and forward, its front surfaces are modeled, and bone is removed from most of the anterior surface. Note in Fig. 2.28 that almost the entire anterior surface of the maxilla is an area of resorption, not apposition.

To understand this seeming paradox, it is necessary to comprehend that two quite different processes are going on simultaneously.

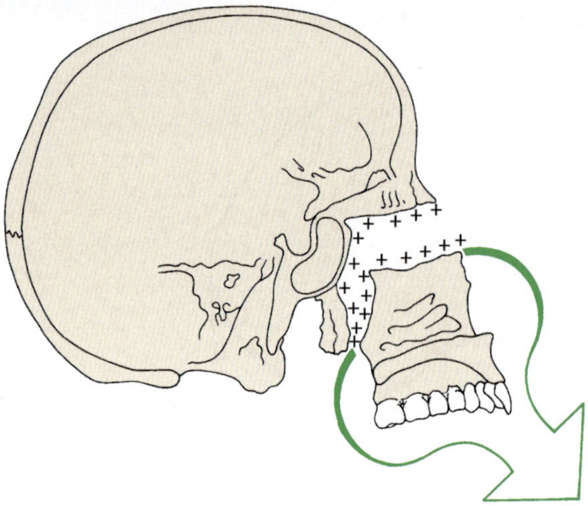

• **Fig. 2.27** As the growth of surrounding soft tissues translates the maxilla downward and forward, opening up space at its superior and posterior sutural attachments, new bone is added on both sides of the sutures. (Redrawn from Enlow DH, Hans MG. *Essentials of Facial Growth*. WB Saunders; 1996.)

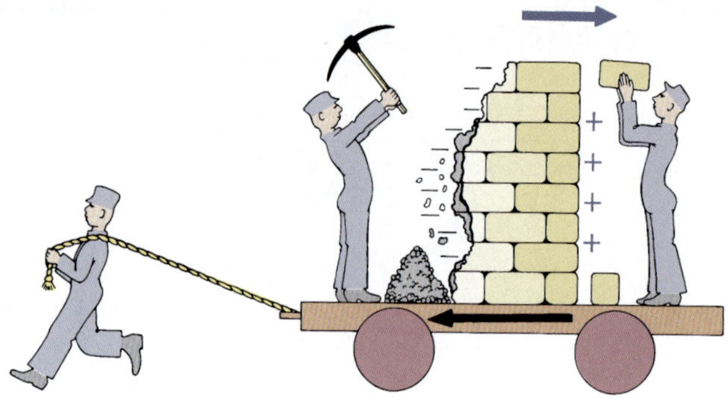

• **Fig. 2.29** Surface modeling of a bone in the opposite direction to that in which it is being translated by the growth of adjacent structures creates a situation analogous to this cartoon, in which the wall is being rebuilt to move it backward at the same time the platform on which it is mounted is being moved forward. (Redrawn from Enlow DH, Hans MG. *Essentials of Facial Growth*. WB Saunders; 1996.)

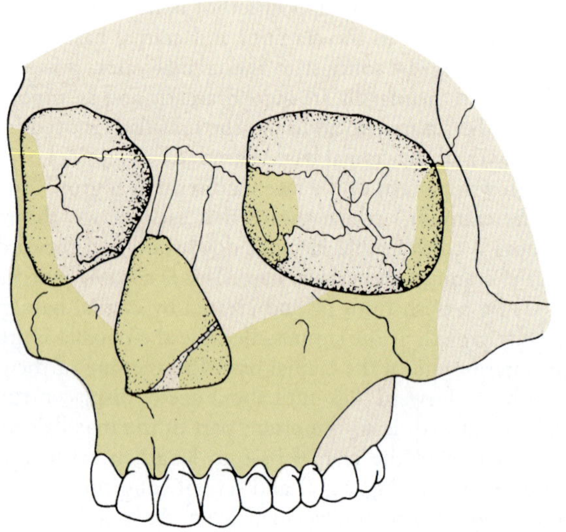

• **Fig. 2.28** As the maxilla is carried downward and forward, its anterior surface tends to resorb. Resorption surfaces are shown here in dark yellow. Only a small area around the anterior nasal spine is an exception. (Redrawn from Enlow DH, Hans MG. *Essentials of Facial Growth*. WB Saunders; 1996.)

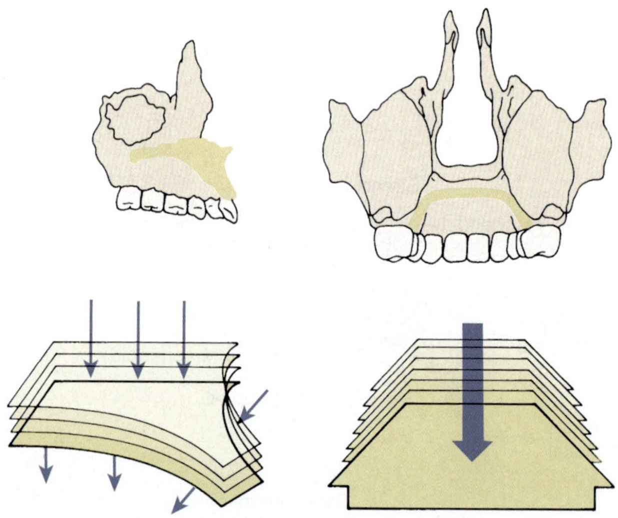

• **Fig. 2.30** Modeling of the palatal vault (which is also the floor of the nose) moves it in the same direction as it is being translated; bone is removed from the floor of the nose and added to the roof of the mouth. On the anterior surface, however, bone is removed, partially canceling the forward translation. As the vault moves downward, the same process of bone remodeling also widens it. (Redrawn from Enlow DH, Hans MB. *Essentials of Facial Growth*. WB Saunders; 1996.)

The overall growth changes are the result of both a downward and forward translation of the maxilla and simultaneous surface modeling. The whole bony nasomaxillary complex is moving downward and forward relative to the cranium, being translated in space. Enlow, whose careful anatomic studies of the facial skeleton underlie much of our present understanding, illustrated this in cartoon form (Fig. 2.29). The maxilla is like the platform on wheels, being rolled forward, while at the same time, its surface, represented by the wall in the cartoon, is being reduced on its anterior side and built up posteriorly, moving in space opposite to the direction of overall growth.

It is not necessarily true that modeling changes oppose the direction of translation. Depending on the specific location, translation and modeling may either oppose each other or produce an additive effect. The effect is additive, for instance, on the roof of the mouth. This area is carried downward and forward along with the rest of the maxilla, but at the same time, bone is removed on the nasal side and added on the oral side, thus creating an additional downward and forward movement of the palate (Fig. 2.30). Immediately adjacently, however, the anterior part of the alveolar process is a resorptive area, so removal of bone from the surface here tends to cancel some of the forward growth that otherwise would occur because of translation of the entire maxilla.

Mandible

In contrast to the maxilla, both endochondral and periosteal activity are important in the growth of the mandible, and displacement created by cranial base growth that moves the temporomandibular joint plays a negligible role (with rare exceptions; see Fig. 4.10). Cartilage covers the surface of the mandibular condyle at the

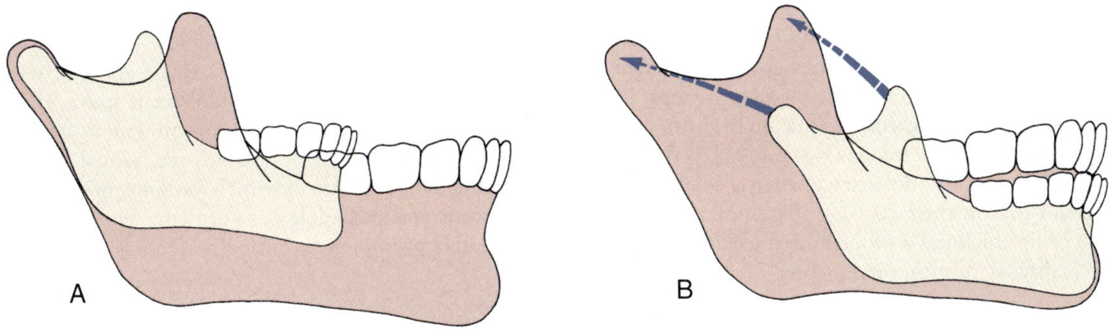

• **Fig. 2.31** (A) Growth of the mandible, as viewed from the perspective of a stable cranial base. The chin moves downward and forward. (B) Mandibular growth, as viewed from the perspective of vital staining studies, which reveal minimal changes in the body and chin area, while there is exceptional growth and modeling of the ramus, moving it posteriorly. The correct concept is that the mandible is translated downward and forward and grows upward and backward in response to this translation, maintaining its contact with the skull.

temporomandibular joint. Although this cartilage is not like the cartilage at an epiphyseal plate or a synchondrosis, hyperplasia, hypertrophy, and endochondral replacement do occur there. All other areas of the mandible are formed and grow by direct surface apposition (modeling).

The overall pattern of growth of the mandible can be represented in two ways, as shown in Fig. 2.31. Depending on the frame of reference, both are correct. If the cranium is the reference area, the chin moves downward and forward. On the other hand, if data from vital staining experiments are examined, it becomes apparent that the principal sites of growth of the mandible are the posterior surface of the ramus and the condylar and coronoid processes. There is little change along the anterior part of the mandible. From this frame of reference, Fig. 2.31B is the correct representation.

As a growth site, the chin is almost inactive. It is translated downward and forward, as the actual growth occurs at the mandibular condyle and along the posterior surface of the ramus. The body of the mandible grows longer by periosteal apposition of bone only on its posterior surface, while the ramus grows higher by endochondral replacement at the condyle accompanied by surface modeling. Conceptually, it is correct to view the mandible as being translated downward and forward while increasing in size by growing upward and backward. The translation occurs largely as the bone moves downward and forward along with the soft tissues in which it is embedded.

Nowhere is there a better example of modeling resorption than the backward movement of the ramus of the mandible. The mandible grows longer by apposition of new bone on the posterior surface of the ramus. At the same time, large quantities of bone are removed from the anterior surface of the ramus (Fig. 2.32). In essence, the body of the mandible grows longer as the ramus moves away from the chin, and this occurs by the removal of bone from the anterior surface of the ramus and the deposition of bone on the posterior surface. Based on this, what was the posterior surface at one time becomes the center at a later date and eventually may become the anterior surface as modeling proceeds.

In infancy the ramus is located at about the spot where the primary first molar will erupt. Progressive posterior modeling creates space for the second primary molar and then for the sequential eruption of the permanent molar teeth. More often than not, however, this growth ceases before enough space has been created for the eruption of the third permanent molar, which becomes impacted in the ramus.

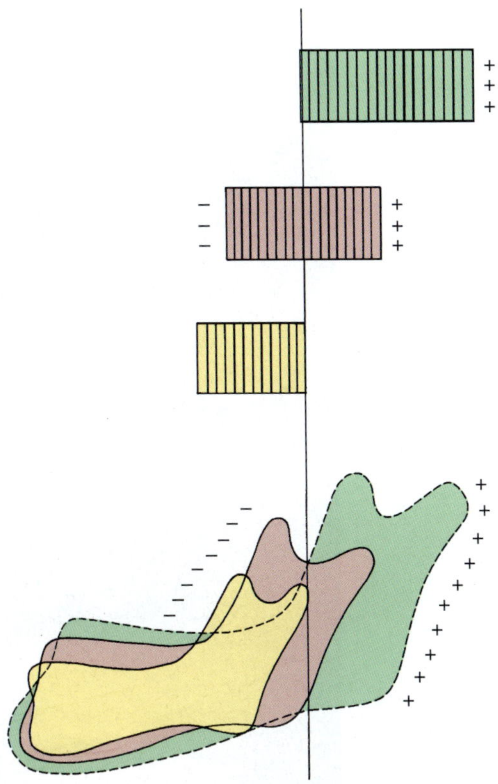

• **Fig. 2.32** As the mandible grows in length, the ramus is extensively modeled, so much so that bone at the tip of the condylar process at an early age can be found at the anterior surface of the ramus some years later. Given the extent of surface remodeling changes, it is an obvious error to emphasize endochondral bone formation at the condyle as the major mechanism for growth of the mandible. (Redrawn from Enlow DH, Hans MB. *Essentials of Facial Growth*. WB Saunders; 1996.)

Further aspects of the growth of the jaws, especially in relation to the timing of orthodontic treatment, are discussed in Chapter 4.

Facial Soft Tissues

An important concept is that the growth of the facial soft tissues does not perfectly parallel the growth of the underlying hard tissues. Let us consider the growth of the lips and nose in more detail.

Growth of the Lips

The lips trail behind the growth of the jaws before adolescence, then undergo a growth spurt to catch up. Because lip height is relatively short during the mixed dentition years, lip separation at rest (often termed *lip incompetence*) is maximal during childhood and decreases during adolescence (Fig. 2.33). Lip thickness reaches its maximum during adolescence, then decreases (Fig. 2.34)—to the point that in their 20s and 30s, some people may consider the loss of lip thickness a problem and seek treatment to increase it. This is discussed further in Chapter 7.

Growth of the Nose

Growth of the nasal bone is complete at about age 10. Growth thereafter is only of the nasal cartilage and soft tissues, both of which undergo a considerable adolescent spurt. The result is that the nose becomes much more prominent in adolescence, especially in boys (Fig. 2.35). The lips are framed by the nose above and chin below, both of which become more prominent with adolescent and postadolescent growth, while the lips do not, so the relative prominence of the lips decreases. This can become an

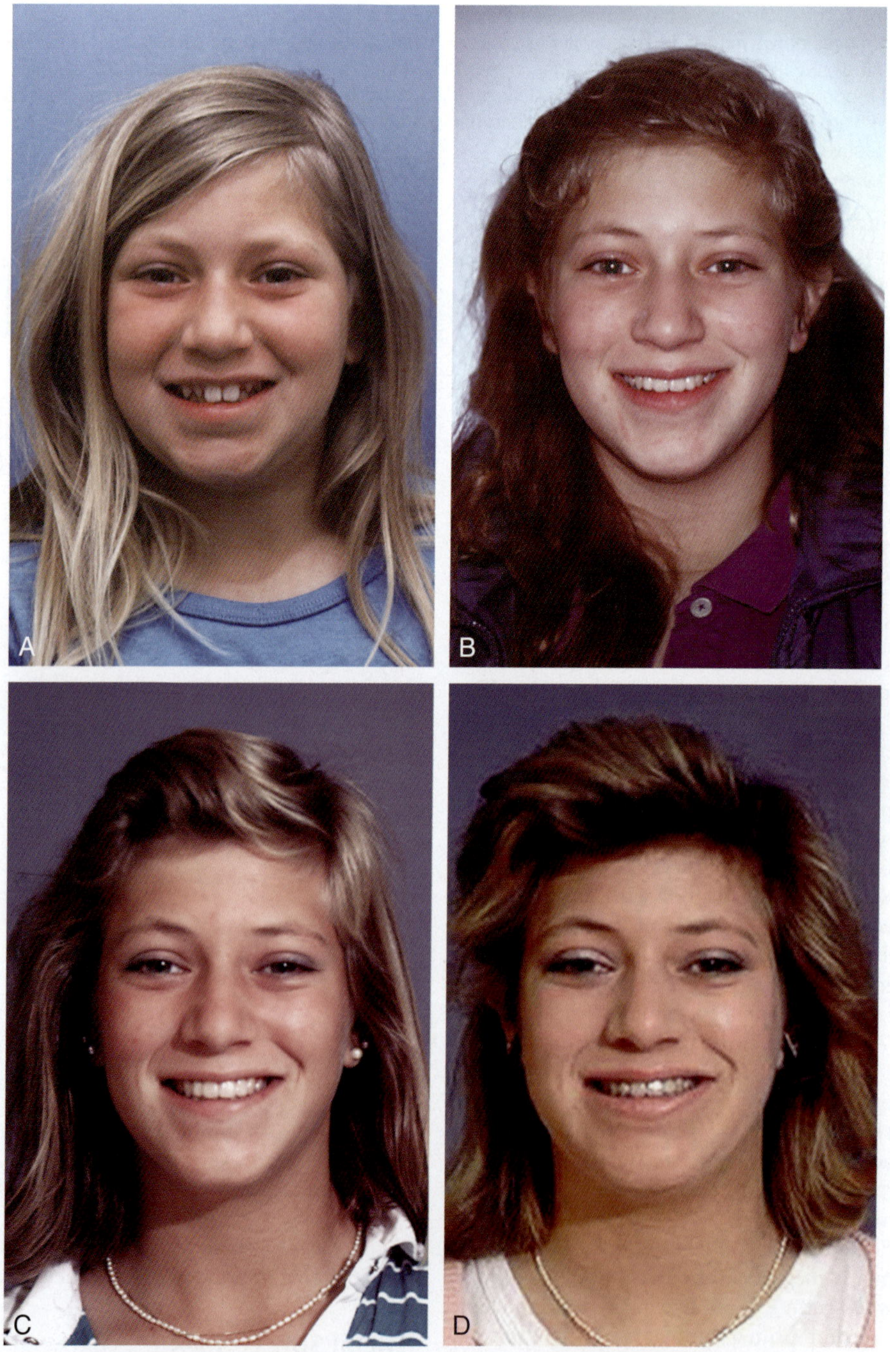

• **Fig. 2.33** Growth of the lips trails behind growth of the facial skeleton until puberty, then catches up and tends to exceed skeletal growth thereafter. As a result, lip separation and exposure of the maxillary incisors is maximal before adolescence and decreases during adolescence and early adult life. (A) Age 11 years, 9 months, prior to puberty. (B) Age 14 years, 8 months, after the adolescent growth spurt. (C) Age 16 years, 11 months. (D) Age 18 years, 6 months.

important point in determining how much lip support should be provided by the teeth at the time orthodontic treatment typically ends in late adolescence.

Changes in the facial soft tissues with aging, which also must be taken into consideration in planning orthodontic treatment, are covered in Chapter 4.

Theories of Growth Control

It is true that growth is strongly influenced by genetic factors, but it also can be significantly affected by the environment in the form of nutritional status, degree of physical activity, health or illness, and a number of similar factors. Because a major part of the need for orthodontic treatment is created by disproportionate growth of the jaws, to understand the etiologic processes of malocclusion and dentofacial deformity, it is necessary to learn how facial growth is influenced and controlled. Great strides have been made in recent years in improving the understanding of growth control. Exactly what determines the growth of the jaws, however, remains unclear and continues to be the subject of intensive research.

Three major theories in recent years have attempted to explain the determinants of craniofacial growth: (1) bone, like other

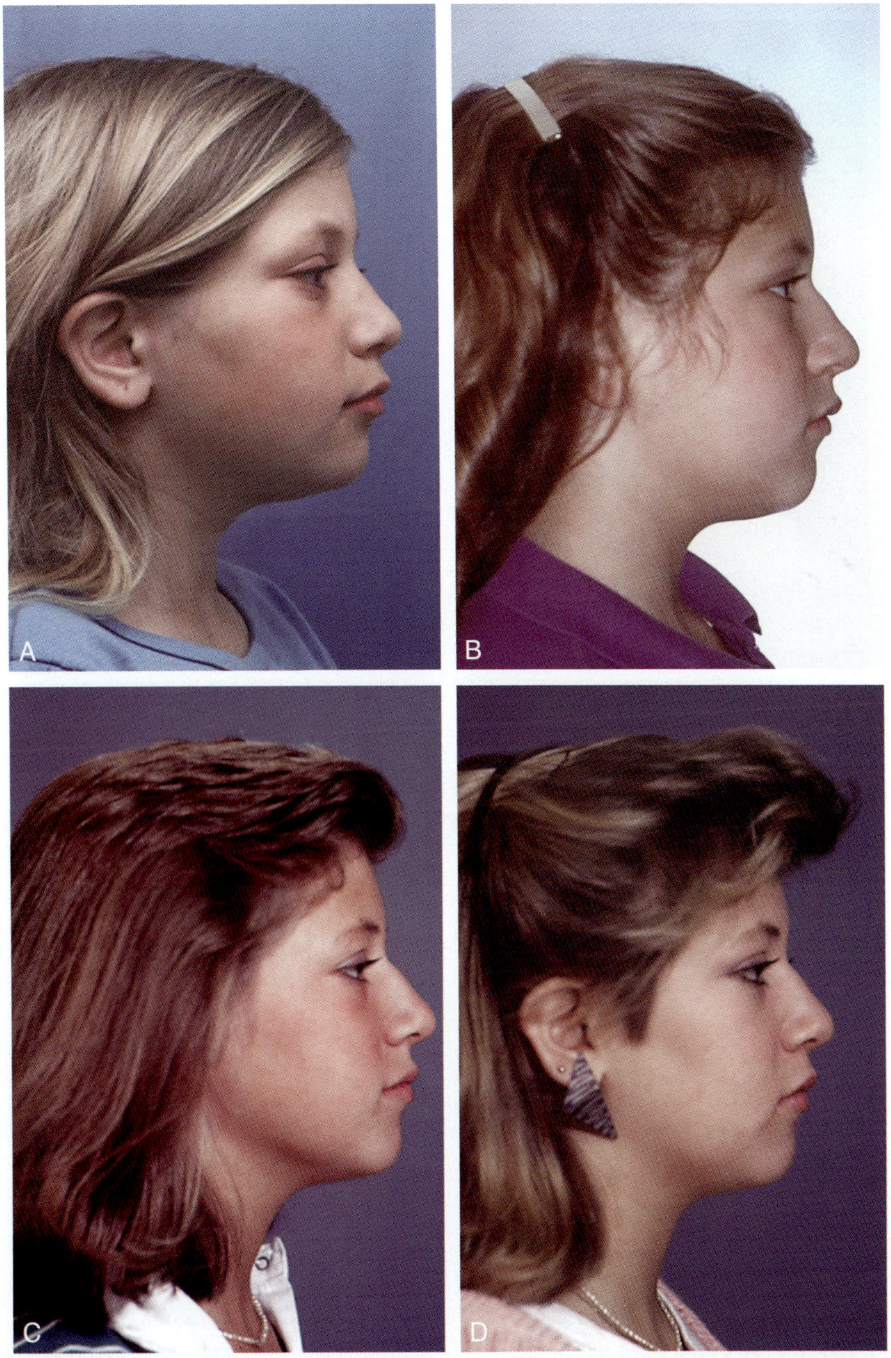

• **Fig. 2.34** Lip thickness increases during the adolescent growth spurt and then decreases (and therefore is maximal at surprisingly early ages). For some girls, loss of lip thickness is perceived as a problem in their early 20s. (A) Age 11 years, 9 months, prior to puberty. (B) Age 14 years, 8 months, after the adolescent growth spurt. (C) Age 16 years, 11 months. (D) Age 18 years, 6 months.

tissues, is the primary determinant of its own growth; (2) cartilage is the primary determinant of skeletal growth, while bone responds secondarily and passively; and (3) the soft tissue matrix in which the skeletal elements are embedded is the primary determinant of growth, and both bone and cartilage are secondary followers.

The major difference in the theories is the location at which genetic control is expressed. The first theory implies that genetic control is expressed directly at the level of the bone; therefore its locus should be the periosteum. The second, or cartilage, theory suggests that genetic control is expressed in the cartilage, while bone responds passively to being displaced as cartilage grows. Indirect genetic control, whatever its source, is called *epigenetics*. The third theory assumes that genetic control is mediated to a large extent outside the skeletal system and that the growth of both bone and cartilage is controlled epigenetically, occurring only in response to a signal from other tissues. In contemporary thought, the truth is to be found in some synthesis of the second and third theories; the first, although it was the dominant view until the 1960s, has largely been discarded.

Level of Growth Control: Sites Versus Centers of Growth

Distinguishing between a *site* of growth and a *center* of growth clarifies the differences between the theories of growth control.

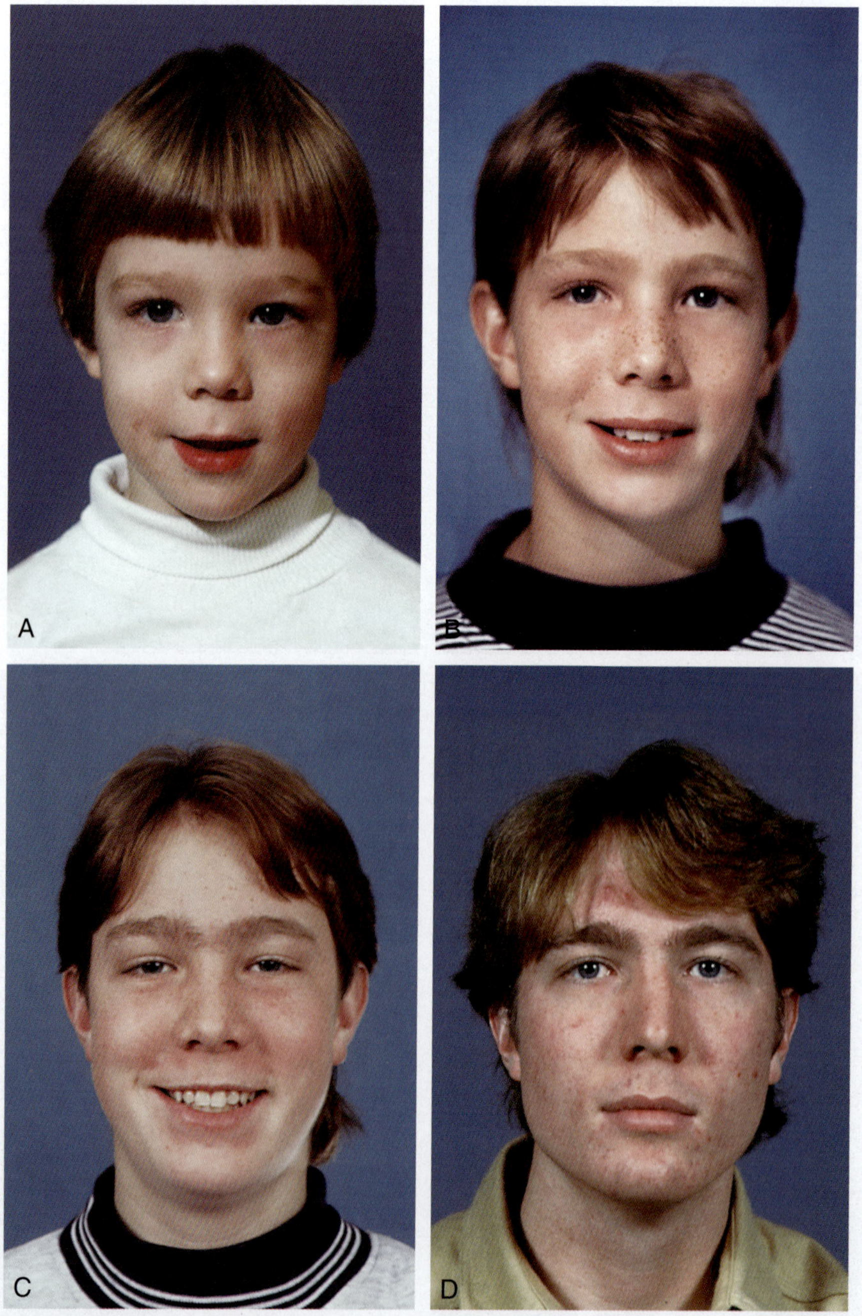

• **Fig. 2.35** The nasal bone grows up until about age 10, but after age 10, growth of the nose is largely in the cartilaginous and soft tissue portions. Especially in boys, the nose becomes much more prominent as growth continues after the adolescent growth spurt (and this process continues into the adult years). (A) Age 4 years, 9 months. (B) Age 12 years, 4 months. (C) Age 14 years, 8 months. (D) Age 17 years, 8 months.

A site of growth is merely a location at which growth occurs, whereas a center is a location at which independent (genetically controlled) growth occurs. All centers of growth also are sites, but the reverse is not true. A major impetus to the theory that the tissues that form bone carry with them their own stimulus to do so came from the observation that the overall pattern of craniofacial growth is remarkably constant. This constancy of the growth pattern was interpreted to mean that the major sites of growth were also centers. In particular, the sutures between the membranous bones of the cranium and jaws were considered growth centers, along with the sites of endochondral ossification in the cranial base and at the mandibular condyle. Growth, in this view, was the result of the expression at all these sites of a genetic program. The mechanism for translation of the maxilla, therefore, was considered to be the result of pressure created by the growth of the sutures so that the maxilla was literally pushed downward and forward.

If this theory were correct, growth at the sutures should occur largely independently of the environment and it would not be possible to change the expression of growth at the sutures very much. While this was the dominant theory of growth, few attempts were made to modify facial growth because orthodontists "knew" that it could not be done.

It is clear now that sutures, and the periosteal tissues more generally, are not primary determinants of craniofacial growth. Two lines of evidence lead to this conclusion. The first is that when an area of the suture between two facial bones is transplanted to another location (to a pouch in the abdomen, for instance), the sutural tissue does not continue to grow. This indicates a lack of innate growth potential in the sutures. Second, growth at sutures will respond to outside influences under a number of circumstances. If cranial or facial bones are mechanically pulled apart at the sutures, new bone will fill in, and the bones will become larger than they would have been otherwise (see Fig. 2.27). If a suture is compressed, growth at that site will be impeded. Thus sutures must be considered areas that respond to stimuli and are not primary determinants. The sutures of the cranial vault, lateral cranial base, and maxilla are sites of growth but are not growth centers.

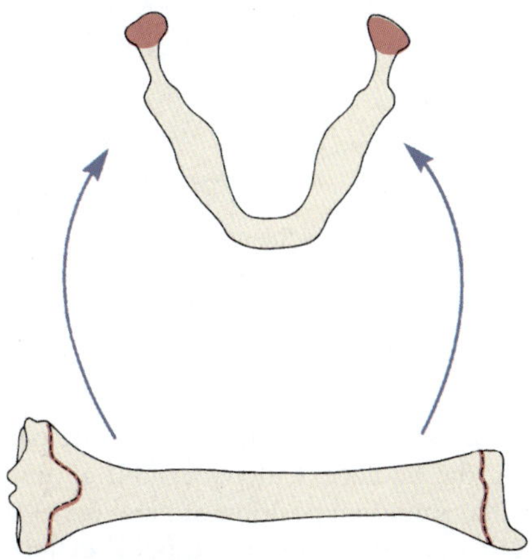

• **Fig. 2.36** The mandible was once viewed conceptually as being analogous to a long bone that had been modified by (1) removal of the epiphysis, leaving the epiphyseal plates exposed, and (2) bending of the shaft into a horseshoe shape. If this analogy were correct, of course, the cartilage at the mandibular condyles should behave like true growth cartilage. Modern experiments indicate that although the analogy is attractive, it is incorrect.

Cartilage as a Determinant of Craniofacial Growth

The second major theory is that the determinant of craniofacial growth is the growth of cartilage. The fact that, for many bones, cartilage does the growing while bone merely replaces it makes this theory attractive for the bones of the jaws. If cartilaginous growth were the primary influence, the cartilage at the condyle of the mandible could be considered a pacemaker for the growth of that bone and the modeling of the ramus and other surface changes could be viewed as secondary to the primary cartilaginous growth.

One way to visualize the mandible is by imagining that it is like the diaphysis of a long bone, bent into a horseshoe with the epiphyses removed, so that there is cartilage representing "half an epiphyseal plate" at the ends, which represents the mandibular condyles (Fig. 2.36). If this were the true situation, then indeed the cartilage at the mandibular condyle should act as a growth center, behaving basically like an epiphyseal growth cartilage. From this perspective, the mechanism of downward and forward growth of the mandible would be a "cartilage push" from growth at the condyle.

Growth of the maxilla is more difficult but not impossible to explain on a cartilage theory basis. Although there is no cartilage in the maxilla itself, there is cartilage in the nasal septum, and the nasomaxillary complex grows as a unit. Proponents of the cartilage theory hypothesize that the cartilaginous nasal septum serves as a pacemaker for other aspects of maxillary growth. Note in Fig. 2.37 that the cartilage is located so that its growth could easily be the model for downward and forward translation of the maxilla. If the sutures of the maxilla served as reactive areas, they would respond to the nasal cartilage growth by forming new bone when the sutures were pulled apart by forces from the growing cartilage. A small area of cartilage would have to influence a large area of sutures, but such a pacemaker role is certainly possible. The mechanism for maxillary growth would be at first a forward push from lengthening of the cranial base, then a forward pull from the nasal cartilage.

Two kinds of experiments have been carried out to test the idea that cartilage can serve as a true growth center. These involve an analysis of the results of transplanting cartilage and an evaluation of the effect on growth of removing cartilage at an early age.

Transplantation experiments demonstrate that not all skeletal cartilage acts the same when transplanted. If a piece of the

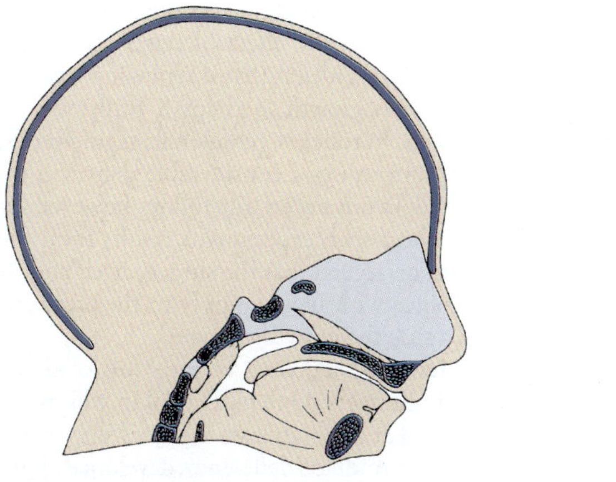

• **Fig. 2.37** Diagrammatic representation of the chondrocranium at an early stage of development, showing the large amount of cartilage in the anterior region that eventually becomes the much smaller cartilaginous nasal septum—not because it shrank, but because adjacent tissues grew more.

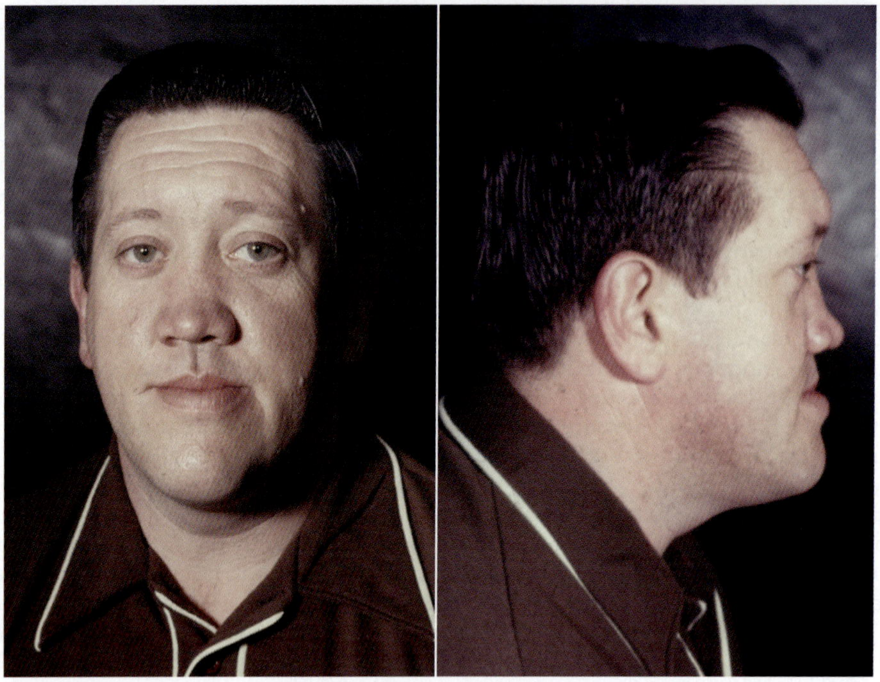

• **Fig. 2.38** Profile view of a man whose cartilaginous nasal septum was removed at age 8, after an injury. The obvious midface deficiency developed after the septum was removed.

epiphyseal plate of a long bone is transplanted, it will continue to grow in a new location or in culture, indicating that these cartilages do have innate growth potential. Cartilage from the spheno-occipital synchondrosis of the cranial base also grows when transplanted, but not as well. It is difficult to obtain cartilage from the cranial base to transplant, particularly at an early age when the cartilage is actively growing under normal conditions. Perhaps this explains why it does not grow in vitro as much as epiphyseal plate cartilage. In early experiments, transplanting cartilage from the nasal septum gave equivocal results—sometimes it grew, sometimes it did not. In more precise later experiments, however, nasal septal cartilage was found to grow nearly as well in culture as epiphyseal plate cartilage.[15] Little or no growth was observed when the mandibular condyle was transplanted, and cartilage from the mandibular condyle showed significantly less growth in culture than the other cartilages.[16] From these experiments, the other cartilages appear capable of acting as growth centers, but the mandibular condylar cartilage does not.

Experiments to test the effect of removing cartilages are also informative. The basic idea is that if removing a cartilaginous area stops or diminishes growth, perhaps it really was an important center for growth. In rodents, removing a segment of the cartilaginous nasal septum causes a considerable deficit in the growth of the midface. It does not necessarily follow, however, that the entire effect on growth in such experiments results from the loss of the cartilage. It can be argued that the surgery itself and the accompanying interference with blood supply to the area, not the loss of the cartilage, cause the growth changes.

There are few reported cases of early loss of the cartilaginous nasal septum in humans. One individual in whom the entire septum was removed at age 8 after an injury is shown in Fig. 2.38. It is apparent that a midface deficiency developed, but one cannot confidently attribute this to the loss of the cartilage. Nevertheless, the loss of growth in experimental animals when this cartilage is removed is great enough to lead most observers to conclude that the septal cartilage does have some innate growth potential and that its loss makes a difference in maxillary growth. Binder syndrome, also known as nasomaxillary hypoplasia, is a rare congenital condition affecting the midface. Patients exhibit an underdeveloped nose and maxilla, abnormal position of nasal bones with a flatted nose, absent anterior nasal spine, and class III malocclusion.[17]

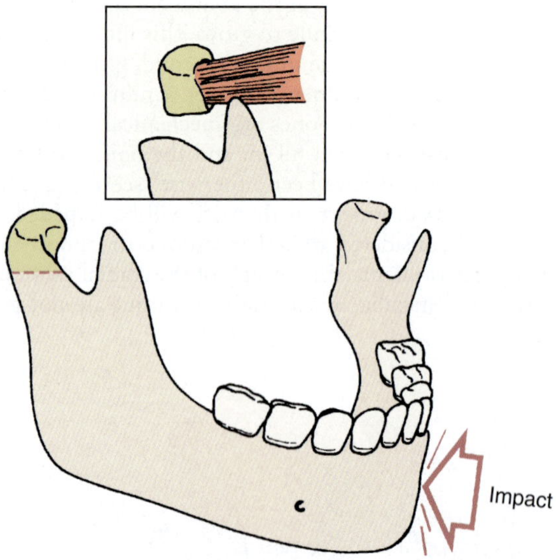

• **Fig. 2.39** A blow to one side of the mandible may fracture the condylar process on the opposite side. When this happens, the pull of the lateral pterygoid muscle distracts the condylar fragment, including all the cartilage, and it subsequently resorbs.

The neck of the mandibular condyle is a relatively fragile area. When the side of the jaw is struck sharply, the mandible often fractures just below the opposite condyle. When this happens, the condyle fragment is usually retracted well away from its previous location by the pull of the lateral pterygoid muscle (Fig. 2.39). The condyle has literally been removed when this occurs, and it resorbs over a period of time. Condylar fractures occur relatively frequently in children. If the condyle were an important growth center, one would expect to see severe growth impairment after such an injury at an early age. If so, surgical intervention to locate the condylar segment and put it back into position would be the logical treatment.

Two excellent studies carried out in Scandinavia disproved this concept. Both Gilhuus-Moe[18] and Lund[19] demonstrated that after fracture of the mandibular condyle in a child, there was an excellent chance that the condylar process would regenerate to approximately its original size and a small chance that it would overgrow after the injury. In experimental animals and in children, after a fracture, all of the original bone and cartilage resorb, and a new condyle regenerates directly from the periosteum at the fracture site (Fig. 2.40). Eventually, at least in experimental animals, a new layer of cartilage forms at the condylar surface. Although there is no direct evidence that the cartilage layer itself regenerates in children after condylar fractures, it is likely that this also occurs in humans.

However, in 15% to 20% of the Scandinavian children studied who sustained a condylar fracture, there was a reduction in growth after the injury. This growth reduction seems to relate to the amount of trauma to the soft tissues and the resultant scarring in the area. The mechanism by which this occurs is discussed in the following section.

In summary, it appears that epiphyseal cartilages and (probably) the cranial base synchondroses can and do act as independently growing centers, as can the nasal septum (perhaps to a lesser extent). Transplantation experiments and experiments in which the condyle is removed lend no support to the idea that the cartilage of the mandibular condyle is an important growth center and neither do studies of the cartilage itself in comparison to primary growth cartilage. It appears that growth at the mandibular condyles is much more analogous to growth at the sutures of the maxilla—which is entirely reactive—than to growth at an epiphyseal plate.

Functional Matrix Theory of Growth

If neither bone nor cartilage is the determinant for the growth of the craniofacial skeleton, it would appear that the control would have to lie in the adjacent soft tissues. This point of view was introduced formally in the 1960s by Melvin Moss in his "functional matrix theory" of growth and was reviewed and updated by him in the 1990s.[20] While granting the innate growth potential of cartilages of the long bones, his theory holds that neither the cartilage of the mandibular condyle nor the cartilaginous nasal septum is a determinant of jaw growth. Instead, he theorized that growth of the face occurs as a response to functional needs and neurotrophic influences and is mediated by the soft tissue in which the jaws are embedded. In this conceptual view, the soft tissues grow, and both bone and cartilage react to this form of epigenetic control.

The growth of the cranium illustrates this view of skeletal growth very well. There can be little question that the growth of the cranial vault is a direct response to the growth of the brain. The pressure exerted by the growing brain separates the cranial bones at the sutures, and new bone passively fills in at these sites so that the braincase fits the brain.

This phenomenon can be seen readily in humans in two experiments of nature (Fig. 2.41). First, when the brain is very small, the cranium is also very small, and the result is microcephaly (which is now seen much more frequently because of Zika virus infections in pregnant females that interfere with neural growth in the fetus). In this case, the size of the head is an accurate representation of the size of the brain. A second natural experiment is hydrocephaly. In this case, reabsorption of cerebrospinal fluid is impeded, the fluid accumulates, and intracranial pressure builds up. The increased intracranial pressure impedes the development of the brain, and as a result, there is a small brain and intellectual impairment, but this condition also leads to an enormous growth of the cranial vault. Uncontrolled hydrocephaly may lead to a cranium two or three times its normal size, with enormously enlarged frontal, parietal, and occipital bones. This is perhaps the clearest example of a "functional matrix" in operation. Another excellent example is the relationship between the size of the eye and the size of the orbit. An enlarged eye or a small eye will cause a corresponding change in the size of the orbital cavity. In this instance, the eye is the functional matrix.

Moss theorized that the major determinant of the growth of the maxilla and mandible is the enlargement of the nasal and oral cavities, which grow in response to functional needs. The theory does not make it clear how functional needs are transmitted to the tissues around the mouth and nose, but it does predict that the cartilages of the nasal septum and mandibular condyles are not important determinants of growth and that their loss would have little effect on growth if the proper function could be obtained. From the view of this theory, however, the absence of normal function would have wide-ranging effects.

We have already noted that in 75% to 80% of human children who sustain a condylar fracture, the resulting loss of the condyle does not impede mandibular growth. The condyle regenerates very nicely. What about the 20% to 25% of children in whom a growth deficit occurs after a condylar fracture? Could some interference with function be the reason for the growth deficiency?

The answer clearly seems to be "yes." It has been known for many years that mandibular growth is greatly impaired by ankylosis at the temporomandibular joint (see Fig. 2.39 and 2.40), defined as fusion across the joint so that motion is prevented (which totally stops growth) or limited (which impedes growth). Mandibular ankylosis can develop in a number of ways. For instance, one possible cause is a severe infection in the area of the joint, leading to the destruction of tissues and ultimate scarring (Fig. 2.42). Another cause, of course, is trauma, which can result in a growth deficiency if there is enough soft tissue injury to lead to scarring that impedes motion as the injury heals. This mechanical restriction impedes translation of the mandible as the adjacent soft tissues grow and leads to decreased growth.

It is interesting and potentially quite significant clinically that under some circumstances, bone can be induced to grow at surgically created sites by the method called *distraction osteogenesis* (Fig. 2.43). The Russian surgeon Ilizarov discovered in the 1950s that if cuts were made through the cortex of a long bone of the limbs, the arm or leg could then be lengthened by tension to separate the bony segments. Current research shows that the best results are obtained if tension across the bone injury site starts after a few days of initial healing and callus formation, not immediately, and if the segments are separated at a rate of 0.5 to 1.5 mm/day. Surprisingly, large amounts of new bone can form at the surgical site, lengthening the arm or leg by several centimeters in some cases. Distraction osteogenesis is now widely used to correct limb deformities, especially after injury, but also in patients with congenital conditions and craniofacial anomalies such as maxillary hypoplasia or micrognathia.

The bone of the mandible is quite similar in its internal structure to the bone of the limbs, even though its developmental course is rather different. Lengthening the mandible via distraction osteogenesis is clearly possible (Fig. 2.44), and major changes in mandibular length (a centimeter or more) are managed best in

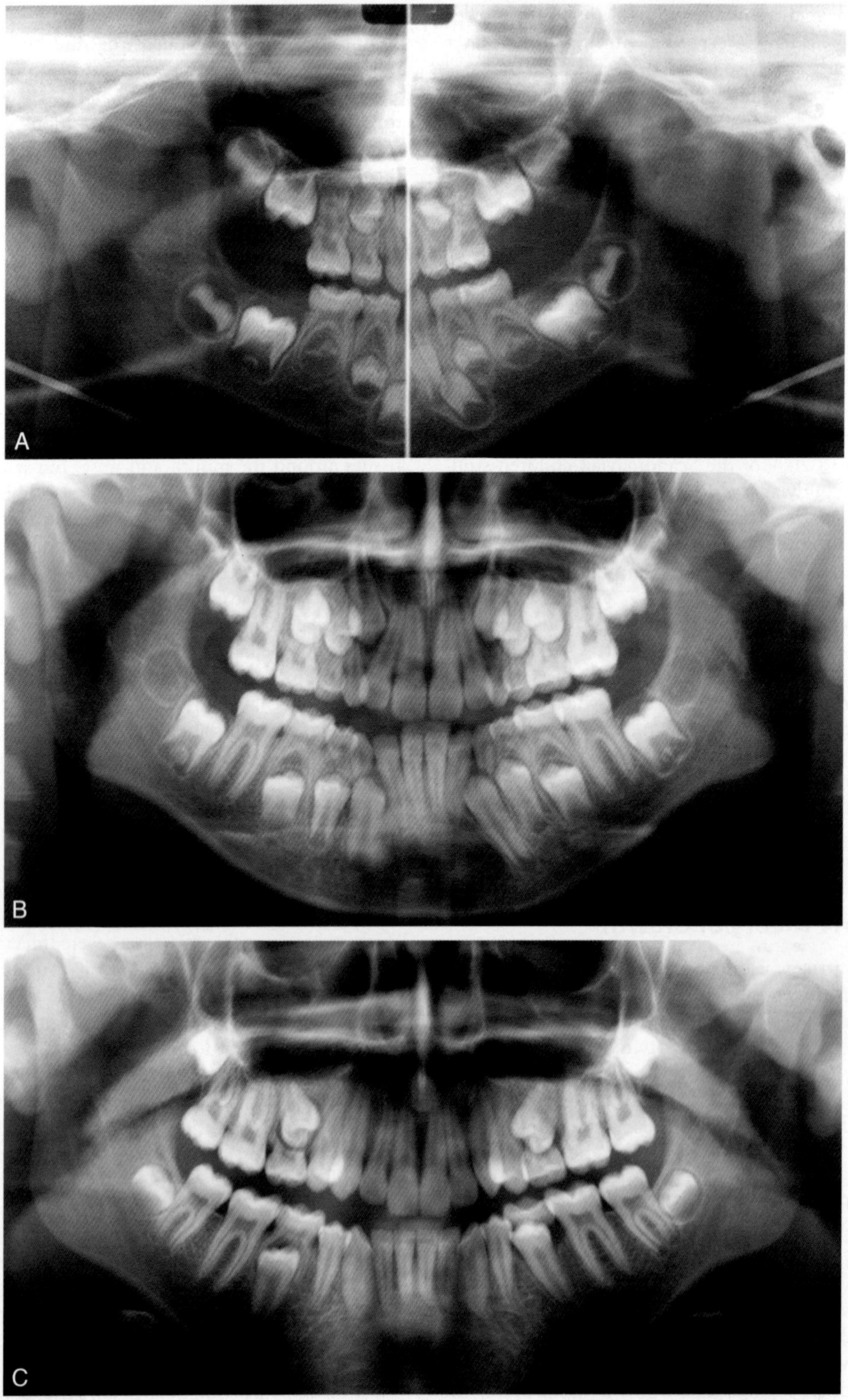

• **Fig. 2.40** After a condylar fracture and resorption of the condyle, regeneration of a new condyle is quite possible in humans. Whether it occurs is a function of the severity of the soft tissue injury that accompanied the fracture. (A) Age 5, at the time mandibular asymmetry was noticed on a routine dental visit. Note that the left condylar process is missing. The history included a fall at age 2 with a blow to the chin that created a condylar fracture, with no regeneration up to that time. (B) Age 8, after treatment with an asymmetric functional appliance that led to growth on the affected side and a reduction in the asymmetry. (C) Age 14, at the end of the adolescent growth spurt. Regeneration of a condyle on the affected side is apparent in (B) and (C).

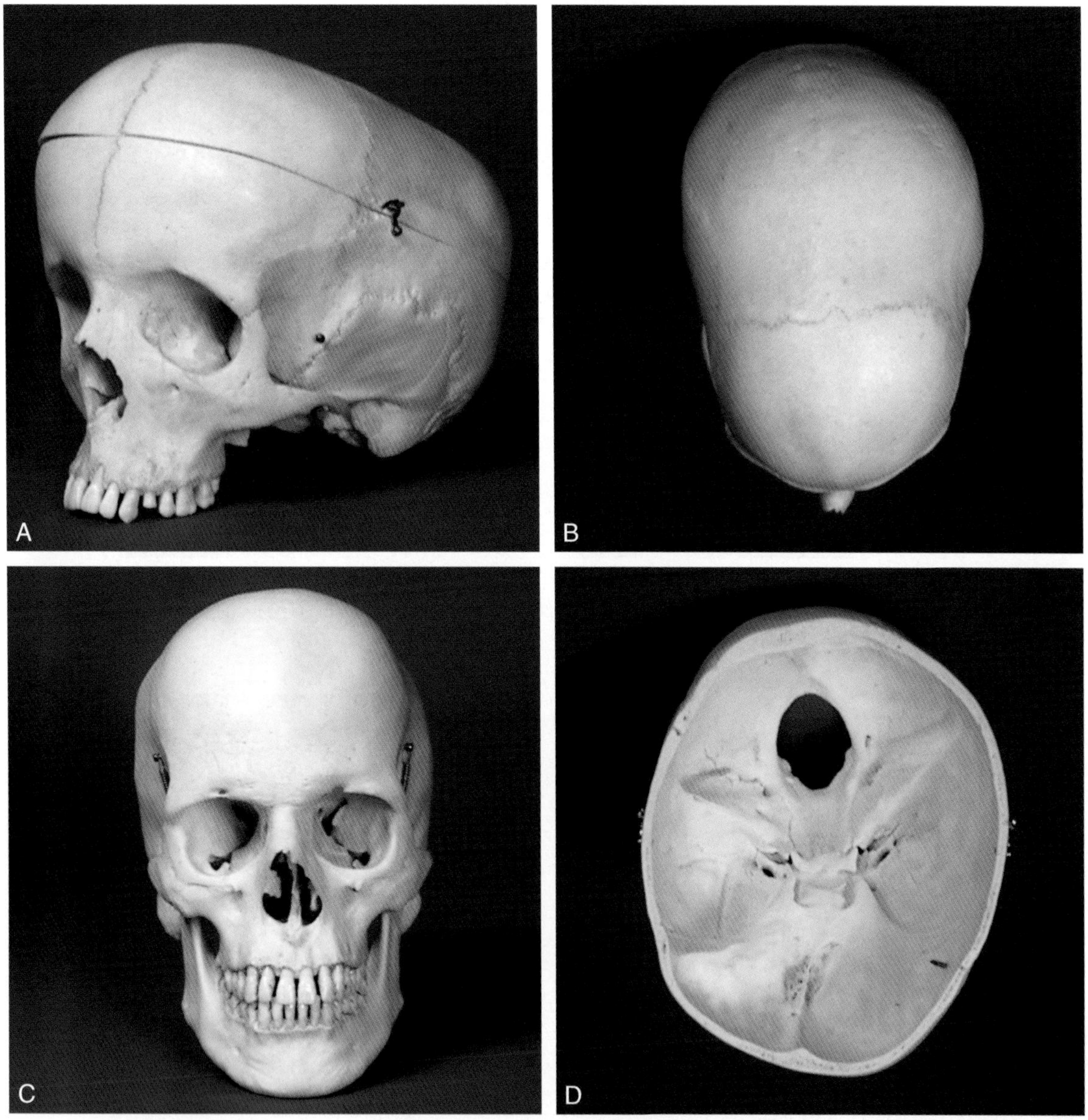

• **Fig. 2.41** (A) The skull of a young child who had hydrocephaly. Note the tremendous enlargement of the braincase in response to the increased intracranial pressure. (B and C) Superior and front views of the skull of an individual with scaphocephaly, in which the midsagittal suture fuses prematurely. Note the absence of the midsagittal suture and the extremely narrow width of the cranium. In compensation for its inability to grow laterally, the brain and braincase have become abnormally long posteriorly. (D) The cranial base of an individual with premature fusion of sutures on the right side, leading to a marked asymmetry that affected both the cranium and cranial base.

this way. Precise positioning of the jaw is not possible, so conventional orthognathic surgery remains the preferred way to treat mandibular deficiency. In a sense, inducing maxillary growth by separating cranial and facial bones at their sutures is a distraction method. Manipulating maxillary growth by influencing growth at the sutures has been a major part of orthodontic treatment for many years, and this can be done at later ages with surgical assistance as a distraction osteogenesis procedure. The current status of distraction osteogenesis as a method to correct deficient growth in the face and jaws is reviewed in some detail in Chapter 22.

In summary, it appears that the growth of the cranium occurs almost entirely in response to growth of the brain (Table 2.1). Growth of the cranial base is primarily the result of endochondral growth and bony replacement at the synchondroses, which have independent growth potential but are perhaps influenced by the growth of the brain. Growth of the maxilla and its associated structures occurs from a combination of growth at sutures and modeling of the surfaces of the bone. The maxilla is translated downward and forward as the face grows, and new bone fills in at the sutures. The extent to which the growth of cartilage of the nasal septum leads to translation of the maxilla remains unknown, but both the surrounding soft tissues and this cartilage probably contribute to the forward repositioning of the maxilla. Growth of the mandible occurs by both endochondral proliferation at the condyle and apposition and resorption of bone at surfaces. It seems clear that the mandible is translated in space by the growth of muscles and other adjacent soft tissues and that the addition of new bone at the condyle is in response to the soft tissue changes.

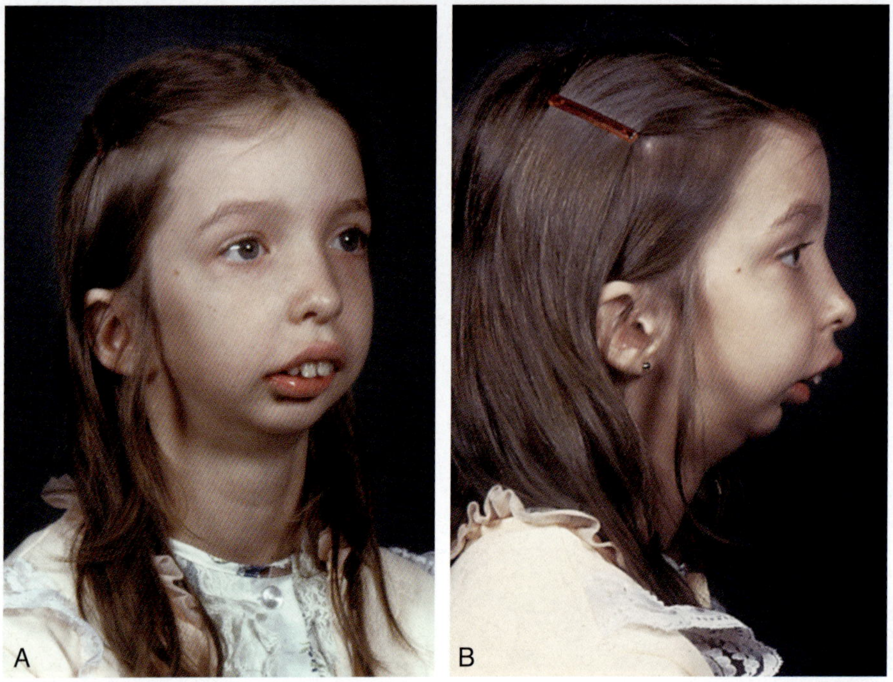

• **Fig. 2.42** Oblique (A) and profile (B) views of a girl in whom a severe infection of the mastoid air cells involved the temporomandibular joint and led to ankylosis of the mandible. The resulting restriction of mandibular growth is apparent.

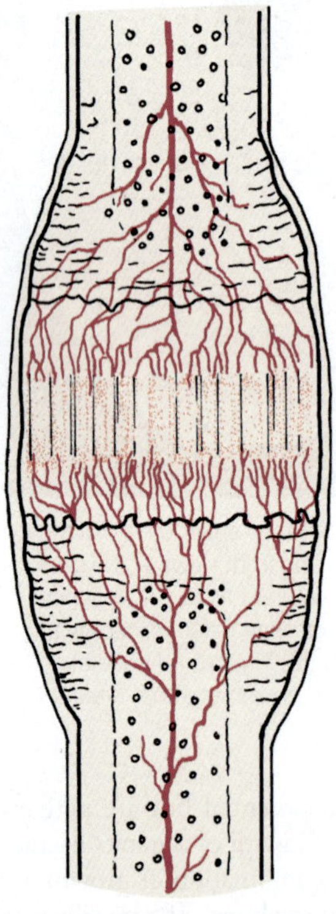

• **Fig. 2.43** Diagrammatic representation of distraction osteogenesis in a long bone. The drawing represents the situation after bone cuts through the cortex, undisturbed initial healing for 3–5 days (latency period), and then a few days of distraction. In the center, there is a fibrous radiolucent interzone with longitudinally oriented collagen bundles in the area where the lengthening of the bone occurs. Proliferating fibroblasts and undifferentiated mesenchymal cells are found throughout this area. Osteoblasts appear at the edge of the interzone. On both sides of the interzone, a rich blood supply is present in a zone of mineralization. Beneath that, a zone of remodeling exists. This sequence of formation of a stretched collagen matrix, mineralization, and remodeling is typical of distraction osteogenesis. (Redrawn from Samchukov M, et al. In: McNamara J, Trotman C, eds. *Distraction Osteogenesis and Tissue Engineering*. The University of Michigan Center for Human Growth and Development; 1998.)

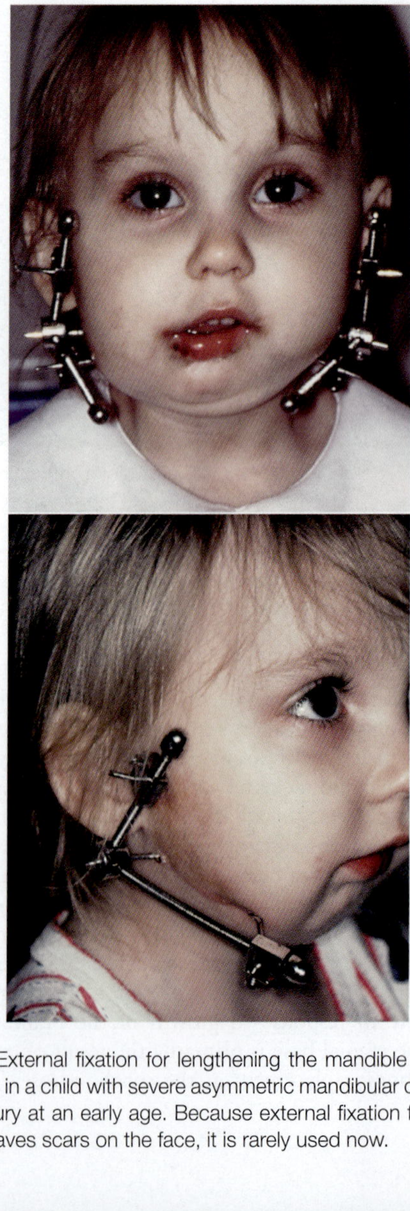

• **Fig. 2.44** External fixation for lengthening the mandible by distraction osteogenesis in a child with severe asymmetric mandibular deficiency secondary to injury at an early age. Because external fixation for mandibular distraction leaves scars on the face, it is rarely used now.

TABLE 2.1 Growth of Craniofacial Units

Growth	Cranial Vault	Cranial Base	Maxilla	Mandible
Sites	Sutures (major) Surfaces (minor)	Synchondroses Sutures (laterally)	Sutures Surfaces: apposition remodeling	Condyle Ramus Other surfaces
Centers	None	Synchondroses	None	None
Type (mode)	Mesenchymal	Endochondral Mesenchymal (lateral only)	Mesenchymal	Endochondral (condyle only) Mesenchymal
Mechanism	Pressure to separate sutures	Interstitial growth at synchondroses	Cartilage push (cranial base) Soft tissue pull Cartilage pull? (nasal septum)	Soft tissue pull (neurotrophic?)
Determinant	Intracranial pressure (brain growth)	Genetic (at synchondroses) Cartilage pull (at lateral sutures)	Soft tissue pull (neurotrophic?)	Soft tissue pull (neurotrophic?)

Cognitive, Social, Emotional, and Behavioral Development in Dentistry

Physical growth can be considered the outcome of an interaction between genetically controlled cell proliferation and environmental influences that modify the genetic program. Similarly, behavior can be viewed as the result of an interaction between innate or instinctual behavioral patterns and behaviors learned after birth. In animals, it appears that the majority of behaviors are instinctive, although even lower animals are capable of a degree of learned behavior. In humans, on the other hand, it is generally conceded that the great majority of behaviors are learned.

For this reason, it is less easy to construct stages of behavioral development in humans than stages of physical development. The higher proportion of learned behavior means that what might be considered environmental effects can greatly modify behavior. On the other hand, there are human instinctual behaviors (e.g., the avoidance of pain), and—in a sense—the outcome of behavior hinges on how the instinctual behavioral urges have been modified by learning. As a general rule, the older the individual, the more complex the behavioral pattern and the more important the learned overlay of behavior will be.

In this section, a brief overview of behavior development and types of learning are simplified and presented. Comments are made that are relevant to the dental, but often more specifically, orthodontic situations. Then commonly encountered social, cognitive, and behavioral-based situations are discussed.

Orthodontic treatment often begins between the ages of 7 and 11, corresponding to what Swiss psychologist Jean Piaget termed the "concrete operational stage" of cognitive development. At these ages, children are developing an improved ability to reason and use logical processes, especially regarding objects that can be handled and manipulated. However, their ability to reason on a more abstract level, beyond what can be seen and touched at the present time, remains limited.

As a result of this cognitive development, children at this age are becoming more like adults in some of the ways they understand the world but are still cognitively different from adults. For the dentist, presenting ideas as abstract concepts, rather than illustrating them with tangible, visible objects, can present a major barrier to communication. Instructions for care—if a child this age is expected to actively participate in their care—must be illustrated with concrete examples (Fig. 2.45). For example, it would likely be too abstract for an orthodontist to merely say, "This is your retainer. You need to wear it every night to keep your teeth straight." More appropriate, concrete instructions, after adjusting it for fit, might be, "This is your retainer. You put it in your mouth like this, and take it out like that, now you try it. Put it in every evening right after dinner, and wear it until the next morning. Brush it like this with your toothbrush and your parents' dishwashing soap to keep it clean. Do not use hot water—it will melt it!" Actually demonstrating the physical process and/or providing visual instructions for the patient to take home may also help to promote compliance with the prescribed process.

For most children the ability to deal with abstract concepts and abstract reasoning develops by about age 11, at which time early adolescence has begun. At this stage, which Piaget termed the "formal operational stage" of development, the child's thought process begins to resemble that of an adult, in that the child is capable of understanding abstract concepts outside of what is immediately present, including concepts such as health, disease, and preventive treatment. When working with children at this stage of development, the dentist can begin to provide information in a manner that more closely resembles how one would provide information to an adult, and—in fact—can negatively impact the treatment relationship by "talking down" to a child by using the concrete approach needed with a younger child. Successful communication, in other words, requires a feel for the child's stage of intellectual development (Fig. 2.46).

In addition to the ability to deal with abstractions, adolescents have developed cognitively to the point that they can think about

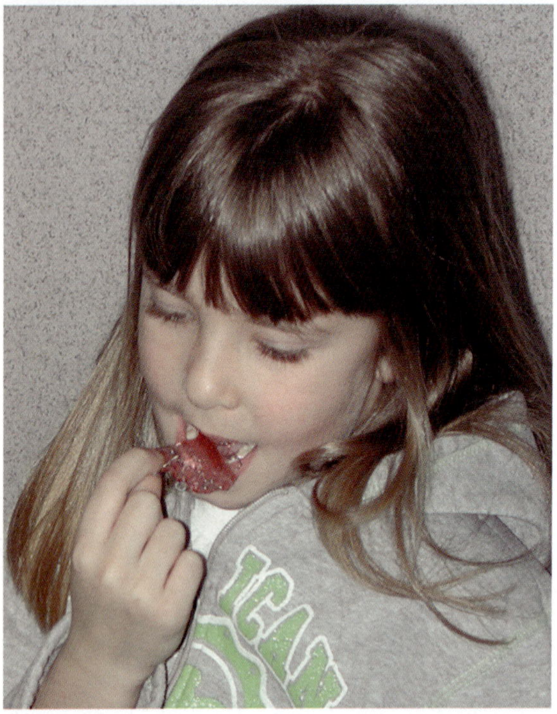

• **Fig. 2.45** Instructions for a young child who will be wearing a removable orthodontic appliance must be explicit and concrete. Children at this stage cannot be motivated by abstract concepts but are influenced by improved acceptance or status from the peer group.

thinking. They are now aware that others think, often presuming that they and others are thinking about the same thing, and are increasingly impacted by their peer group—a dynamic that should be appreciated by the dentist working with a child and adolescent population.

It is particularly important for the dentist to assess sources of adolescent motivation. These patients' desire for treatment can ultimately impact both adherence and outcome, and, in fact, orthodontic treatment in most adolescents should be instituted only if the patient wants it—not just to please the parent. Adolescents demonstrate both a stronger desire for independence in decision-making, as well as an increased ability to dictate their independence. In addition, it appears that parents' ability to assess adolescents' desire for orthodontic treatment is limited, meaning that the dentist's ability to effectively communicate with the young patients is crucial.[21] Although functional impairment related to malocclusion is a driver of and justification for treatment, adolescents' own desire for orthodontic treatment is most commonly driven by esthetic concerns and associated emotional distress, with masticatory impairment being a much less frequent concern.[21,22]

As orthodontic treatment has become more common, adolescents have less concern about being singled out simply because they have braces on their teeth but are—perhaps not surprisingly—very susceptible to suggestions from their peers about how the braces should look. In some settings, this has led to pleas by older adolescents for tooth-colored brackets (to make them less visible and more esthetic). For younger patients, brightly colored ties, elastics, and retainers have been popular (because everybody is wearing them). At present, both children and adolescents place metal appliances with colored elastic ties in the most acceptable category, equal to the "esthetic" appliances often favored by adults. This is convenient for practitioners because they can use the most durable and cost-effective appliances for children and most adolescents and be on safe ground.[23]

The challenge for the dentist is not to try to impose change on reality as perceived by adolescents but rather to understand that perceived reality and introduce other information that may help the adolescent test the veracity or relative importance of those perceptions. A teenage patient may protest to their orthodontist that they do not want to wear a particular appliance because others will think it makes them "look weird." In this situation, telling the patient that they should not be concerned, because many of their peers also are wearing this appliance, would likely do little to encourage them to wear it. A more useful approach, in which the dentist does not deny the point of view of the patient, is to acknowledge the possibility of negative peer reactions and then ask the patient to give it a try for a specified time. If their peers do respond as the teenager predicts, then a different but potentially less effective treatment technique can be discussed. In most cases, however, the teenager's experience will demonstrate either

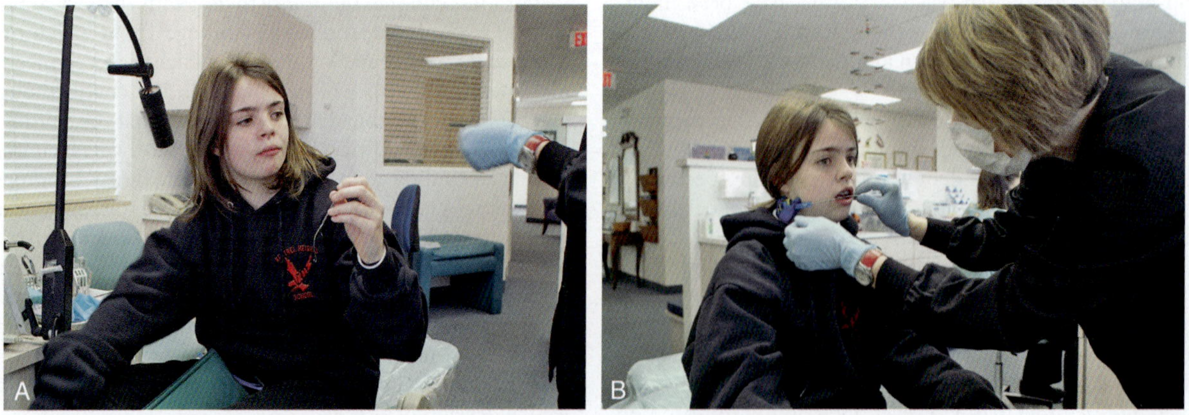

• **Fig. 2.46** (A and B) Instructions for this girl as to how to put her headgear on and take it off are important, but at her stage of development, she can and must understand why she needs to wear it while her jaws are growing. It would be a mistake to talk to her as one would to a younger child.

that peers do not respond negatively to the appliance or that the patient can successfully cope with the peer response. Wearing interarch elastics while in public often plays out in such a manner.

Sometimes, teenage patients may require guidance to help them accurately assess the view of their peer audience. Experience with 13-year-old Beth illustrates this point. Following the loss of a maxillary central incisor in an accident, treatment for Beth included a removable partial denture to replace the tooth. She and her parents had been told on several occasions that it would be necessary to wear the removable appliance until enough healing and growth had occurred to permit treatment with a temporary fixed bridge and finally an implant. At a routine recall appointment, Beth asked if the bridge could be placed now. Realizing that this must be a significant concern for Beth, the dentist commented "Beth, wearing this partial must be a problem. Tell me more about it." Beth replied, "It's embarrassing." Inquiring further, the dentist asked, "When is it embarrassing?" Beth said, "When I spend the night at other girls' homes and have to take it out to brush my teeth." However, when asked about the particular response of her peers when they see her removing the partial denture, Beth replied, "They think it's cool." Perhaps having realized that her concern was not validated by her own reported experience, Beth said nothing more about making the fixed bridge, and the conversation moved to the vacation that Beth's family was planning.

This illustration indicates how it is possible to provide guidance toward a more accurate evaluation of the attitude of the peer audience and thus allow teenagers to solve their own problems. This approach on the part of the dentist neither argues with the teenager's reality nor uncritically accepts it. One role of an effective dental professional is to help teenagers test the reality that actually surrounds them. To be received, the dentist's message must be presented in terms that correspond to the stage of cognitive and psychosocial development that a particular child has reached. It is the job of the orthodontist as well as the family dentist to carefully evaluate the development of the child and to adapt their language so that concepts are presented in a way that the patient can understand. The adage "different strokes for different folks" applies strongly to children, whose variations in intellectual and psychosocial development affect the way they receive orthodontic treatment, just as their differing stages of physical development do.

Learning and the Development of Behavior

The basic mechanisms of learning appear to be essentially the same at all ages. As learning proceeds, more complex skills and behaviors appear, but it is difficult to define the process in distinct stages—a continuous flow model appears more appropriate. It is important to remember that this discussion is about the development and maintenance of behavioral patterns, not the acquisition of knowledge or intellectual skills in the academic sense. Essentially, "learning," as discussed herein, is the process by which people come to do the things they do and is a function of the interaction between the person and their environment.

There are three general mechanisms by which learning occurs and behavioral responses develop: (1) classical conditioning, (2) operant conditioning, and (3) observational learning.

Classical Conditioning (Learning by Association)

Classical conditioning was first described by the Russian physiologist Ivan Pavlov, who discovered in the 19th century during his studies of reflexes that previously unrelated or unassociated stimuli (events) could come to produce reflexive or automatic behavior. Pavlov's classic experiments involved the presentation of food to a hungry animal, along with a neutral or unrelated stimulus—for example, the ringing of a bell. The presentation of food normally elicits salivation in hungry animals by a reflex mechanism, which does not have to be learned or "conditioned" over time but rather occurs automatically; thus food functions as an "unconditioned stimulus" in this example. However, if a bell is rung just before the presentation of food, the auditory stimulus of the ringing bell will become associated with the stimulus of food, and in a relatively short time, the ringing of a bell by itself will elicit salivation. The bell has changed from a neutral stimulus to a "conditioned stimulus," in that it produces the reaction of salivation only due to its learned association with the unconditioned stimulus. Classical conditioning, then, operates by the simple process of association of one stimulus with another (Fig. 2.47). For that reason, this mode of learning is sometimes referred to as *learning by association.*

Classical conditioning occurs readily with young children and can impact a young child's behavior in the dental office, particularly in children prone to anxiety, who tend to demonstrate a higher level of reactivity to lower levels of fear-provoking stimuli,[24] such as some of the sights and sounds common in a dental office. By the time a child is brought for the first visit to a general dentist—and certainly by the time a child is likely to present for orthodontic treatment—it is highly likely that they will have had many experiences with pediatricians or other medical personnel, at least some of which are likely to have caused pain or physical discomfort (e.g., vaccinations; oral/nasal examinations). When a child experiences pain, the reflex reaction is crying and withdrawal. In classical conditioning terms, the sensation of pain is an unconditioned stimulus, but a number of aspects of the setting in which the pain occurs can come to be associated with this unconditioned stimulus.

For instance, it is unusual for a child to encounter people who are dressed in long white coats outside of a medical setting. If the unconditioned stimulus of painful treatment comes to be associated with the stimulus of white coats, a child may cry and withdraw immediately at the first sight of a white-coated dentist or dental assistant. In this case, the child has learned to associate the unconditioned stimulus of pain with the conditioned stimulus of a white-coated adult, and the mere sight of the white coat is enough to produce the reflex behavior initially associated with pain.

Associations of this type can become generalized. Painful and unpleasant experiences associated with medical treatment can become associated with elements of the general environment of a physician's office, so that the atmosphere of a waiting room, receptionist, and other waiting children may produce crying and withdrawal after several experiences in the physician's office, even if there is no sign of a white coat.

Due to this impact of learning via association, it has been theorized that behavior management in the dentist's office may be easier if the dental office looks different than the typical pediatrician's office or hospital clinic. Indeed, research suggests that younger children generally prefer a dental setting in which the clinic is decorated rather than plain,[25] though this preference likely becomes less salient as patients progress into adolescence. Despite the previously discussed example of "white coat anxiety," which is useful for illustrating the process of classical conditioning, it appears that *most* children and adolescents are tolerant of—and may even prefer—white coat dental attire or scrubs, though younger, anxious children, in particular, may prefer colored coats to white ones.

It may also help if the child's first visit to a dental provider is different from previous visits to the physician. Treatment that

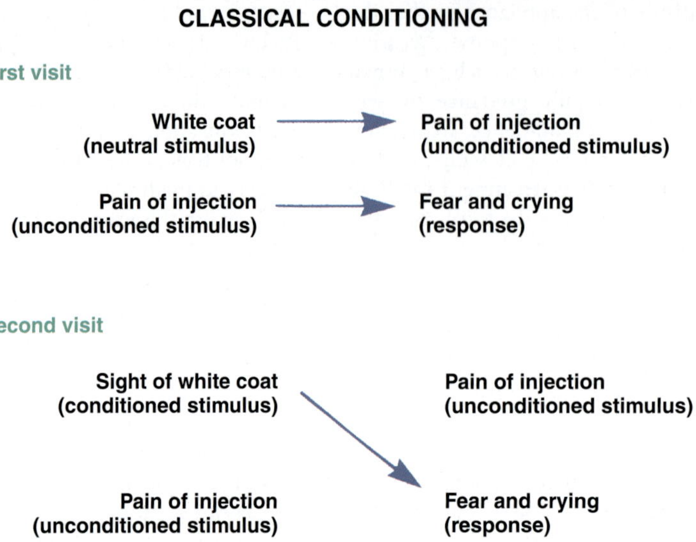

• **Fig. 2.47** Classical conditioning causes an originally neutral stimulus to become associated with one that leads to a specific reaction. If individuals in white coats are the ones who give painful injections that cause crying, the sight of an individual in a white coat soon may provoke an outburst of crying.

might produce pain should be avoided if at all possible on the first visit to the dental office. The association between a conditioned and an unconditioned stimulus is strengthened or reinforced every time they occur together. Every time a child is taken to a hospital clinic where something painful is done, the association between pain and the general atmosphere of that clinic becomes stronger, as the child becomes more certain of their conclusion that bad things happen in such a place. Conversely, if the association between a conditioned and an unconditioned stimulus is not reinforced, the association between them will become less strong, and eventually, the conditioned response will no longer occur. This phenomenon is referred to as the *extinction of the conditioned behavior*. This is the basis for a "happy visit" to the dentist following a stressful visit. Once a conditioned response has been established, it is necessary to reinforce it only occasionally to maintain it. If the conditioned association of pain with the doctor's office is strong, it can take many visits without unpleasant experiences and pain to extinguish the associated crying and avoidance.

The opposite of generalization of a conditioned stimulus is discrimination. The conditioned association of a medical office with pain can easily be generalized to a dental office setting. However, if a child is taken into other office settings that are somewhat different from the one where painful things happen—a dental office, for instance, where painful injections are not necessary—discrimination between the two types of offices will soon develop, and the generalized response to any office as a place where painful things occur will be extinguished.

Conditioning (Learning by Consequences)

Principles of operant conditioning, which can be viewed conceptually as a significant extension of classical conditioning, were introduced by psychologist B.F. Skinner, who contended that these principles could explain more complex and conscious behaviors than could be explained via classical conditioning. Although it is not possible to explore operant conditioning in great detail here, a brief overview is presented as an aid in understanding the acquisition of behavior that children and adolescents are likely to demonstrate, both in the dentist's or orthodontist's office and elsewhere.

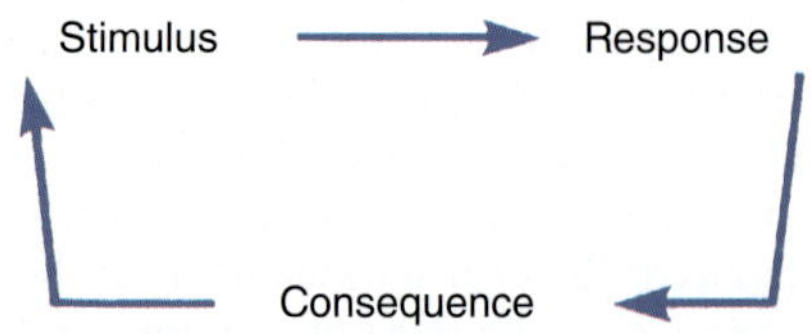

• **Fig. 2.48** Operant conditioning differs from classical conditioning in that the consequence of a behavior is considered a stimulus for future behavior. This means that the consequence of any particular response will affect the probability of that response occurring again in a similar situation.

The basic principle of operant conditioning is that the consequence that follows a behavior will alter the probability of that behavior occurring again in a similar situation (Fig. 2.48). Principles of operant conditioning are always at play, whether or not we are aware of the impact they are exerting on behavioral patterns. That said, these principles can also be utilized intentionally to increase or decrease salient behaviors. The general rule, summarized by psychologist Edward Thorndike's "law of effect," is that if the consequence of a certain response is perceived as pleasant or desirable, the individual is more likely to demonstrate that response again in the future. On the other hand, if a particular response produces an undesirable consequence, the probability of the individual engaging in that response in the future is diminished.

Four basic concepts are essential to understanding operant conditioning, each distinguished by the nature of the consequence (i.e., whether a stimulus is presented or removed in response to a behavior) and the consequence's impact on subsequent behavior (i.e., whether it increases or decreases the likelihood of that behavior occurring again) (Fig. 2.49).

	Probability of Response Increases	Probability of Response Decreases
Pleasant stimulus (S_1)	I S_1 Presented Positive reinforcement or reward	III S_1 Withdrawn Omission or time-out
Unpleasant stimulus (S_2)	II S_2 Withdrawn Negative reinforcement or escape	IV S_2 Presented Punishment

• **Fig. 2.49** The four basic types of operant conditioning.

The first concept is *positive reinforcement*. In positive reinforcement, a stimulus or consequence occurs following a behavior, with the result being that the behavior is more likely to occur again in the future. For example, consider the adolescent patient who recently had their braces removed and receives several compliments from peers about how nice their teeth look when they notice them smiling; the patient may then begin to smile more frequently. In this case, the patient's smile and the ability to show their teeth have been positively reinforced by the stimulus of their peers providing positive attention. Note that stimuli need not be *intuitively* desirable to positively reinforce behavior. Consider the example of the restless pediatric patient, admonished by a frustrated dentist to stay still, who responds to the clinician's exasperated instructions by deliberately moving even more in their chair. In this example, though few patients would find the dentist's stern feedback to be truly desirable, it still functions to positively reinforce and increase this particular child's restless behavior.

A second concept of operant conditioning, *negative reinforcement*, involves the removal or "subtraction" (thus the term "negative") of a stimulus following behavior and is characteristic of situations in which a particular behavior results in avoidance or escape from an undesirable stimulus. As with positive reinforcement, negative reinforcement increases the likelihood of the behavior occurring in the future. Note that negative reinforcement is not a synonym for punishment, another type of operant conditioning discussed below.

A child who views a visit to the hospital clinic as an unpleasant experience may throw a temper tantrum at the prospect of having to go there. If this behavior (response) succeeds in allowing the child to escape the visit to the clinic, the behavior has been negatively reinforced and is more likely to occur the next time a visit to the clinic is proposed. The same can be true, of course, in the dentist's office. If behavior considered unacceptable by the dentist and their staff nevertheless succeeds in allowing the child to escape from dental treatment, this behavior has been negatively reinforced and is more likely to occur the next time the child is in the dental office.

Negative reinforcement can also impact adherence to treatment between visits. Consider the example of the patient who is reminded by their orthodontist, following suboptimal treatment progress, to wear their intraoral elastics on a regular basis. The child leaves the dental visit intending to do so, but after wearing elastics for a day, the child experiences increased pain. As a result, the child again discontinues the use of their elastics, resulting in a decrease in pain. In this case, the child ceasing to comply with the dentist's instructions has been negatively reinforced by the removal of the pain stimulus.

In dental practice, it is important to reinforce desired behavior, and it is equally important to avoid reinforcing behavior that is not desired. Thus it is important to establish achievable goals for a given treatment visit—based both on clinical need and the particular patient's presentation and history of behavior at dental appointments—to avoid, if possible, premature discontinuation of a visit. However, even the most reasonable and well-intentioned plans for a treatment visit may ultimately prove unachievable—particularly when working with pediatric patients. In this case, revising visit goals—to obtain at least some small measure of compliance with the dentist prior to discontinuation of the visit—is advisable, so as to reduce the impact of negative reinforcement on behavior at future visits.

Reinforcement—both positive and negative—increases the likelihood of a response occurring again; two types of *punishment* involve *decreasing* the likelihood of a response. The first of these, *omission* (synonymous with *negative punishment*), involves the removal of a pleasant stimulus after a particular behavior, thereby reducing the chances that the behavior occurs in the future. For example, if a child who throws a temper tantrum has their favorite toy taken away for a short time as a consequence of this behavior, the probability of similar misbehavior is decreased. Because children are likely to regard attention from others as a very pleasant stimulus, withholding attention or engagement ("ignoring") following undesirable behavior is a use of omission or negative punishment that can be useful in reducing unwanted behavior.

Positive punishment—most commonly referred to simply as "punishment"—occurs when an unpleasant stimulus is presented after a particular behavior, decreasing the probability that the behavior that prompted the punishment will occur in the future. Punishment, like other concepts of operant conditioning, applies to people at all ages of development—not just with children. For example, if the dentist with their new sports car receives a ticket for driving 50 miles/h down a street marked for 35 miles/h, they more likely to drive at an appropriate speed on that particular street in the future, particularly if they think that the same radar speed trap is still operating.

While knowledge of punishment is useful in understanding the behavioral patterns in which dental patients engage, positive and negative reinforcement are undoubtedly the most suitable types of operant conditioning to be employed in dental practice. Both types of reinforcement function as more direct methods of achieving desirable behavior, rather than attempting to merely suppress undesirable behavior, as both forms of punishment do. In addition, reinforcement techniques are likely to be more readily available to dentists and more acceptable to child and adolescent patients and their parents.

Observational Learning (Modeling)

Another common way that behavior arises is through imitation of behavior observed in a social context. Certainly, much of the behavior a child displays in a dental setting may have been learned from observing siblings, their parents, or other children.

There are two distinct stages in observational learning: *acquisition* of the behavior by observing it and the actual *performance* of that behavior. Children are capable of acquiring almost any behavior that they observe closely and that is not too complex for them to perform at their level of physical and cognitive development. That said, children are exposed to a tremendous range of possible behaviors, many of which they acquire even though a particular behavior may not be performed immediately or ever.

Whether a child will actually perform an acquired behavior depends on several factors. Important among these are the characteristics of the role model. If the model is liked or respected, the child is more likely to imitate them. For this reason, a parent or older sibling is often the object of imitation by the child. For children in the elementary and junior high school age groups, peers within their own age group or individuals slightly older are increasingly important role models, while the influence of parents and older siblings decreases over time. For adolescents, the peer group is the major source of role models.

Another important influence on whether a behavior learned via observation is performed is the expected consequence of the behavior. If a child sees an older sibling refuse to obey their father's command and then sees punishment follow this refusal, they are less likely to defy the father on a future occasion. Regardless, the child probably still has acquired the behavior, and if they should become defiant, are likely to stage it in a similar way.

Observational learning can be an important tool in the management of dental treatment. If a young child observes an older sibling undergoing dental treatment without complaint or uncooperative behavior, they are likely to imitate this behavior. If the older sibling is observed being rewarded for their behavior, the younger child will also expect a reward for behaving well. Because parents are an important role model for young children, parental attitudes toward dental treatment—including parental dental anxiety—can influence children's behavior in the context of dental visits.

Research has demonstrated that one of the best predictors of how anxious a child will be during dental treatment is how anxious the mother is. A mother who is calm and relaxed about the prospect of dental treatment teaches the child by observation that this is the appropriate approach to being treated, whereas an anxious and alarmed mother tends to elicit the same set of responses in their child.[26]

Observational learning can be used to advantage in the design of dental treatment areas. At one time, it was routine for dentists to provide small private cubicles in which all patients, children and adults, were treated. The modern trend in orthodontics, particularly in the treatment of children and adolescents but to some extent with adults also, is an open area with several treatment stations (Fig. 2.50). Sitting in one dental chair and watching the dentist work with someone else in an adjacent chair can provide a great deal of observational learning about what the experience will be like and how to behave during the appointment. Direct communication among patients, answering questions about exactly what happened, can add even further learning. Both children and adolescents do better, it appears, if they are treated in open clinics rather than in private cubicles, and observational learning plays an important part in this.[27] The dentist hopes, of course, that the patient waiting for treatment observes appropriate behavior and responses on the part of the patient who is being treated, which will be the case in a well-managed clinical setting. The potential behavioral benefits of an open dental operatory, of course, must be balanced against multiple other considerations, including patient privacy and infection control, which came to the forefront prominently during the COVID-19 pandemic.

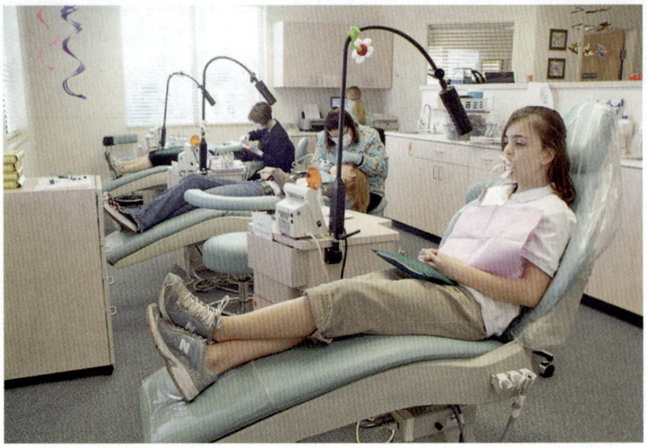

• **Fig. 2.50** The orthodontic treatment room in the pediatric dentistry-orthodontic office with three chairs in an open treatment area. This has the advantage of allowing observational learning for the patients.

In a classic article that still is an excellent summary, Chambers reviewed what we have covered in this section in the context of a child going to the dentist.[28]

Behavior Management in Orthodontic Treatment

A solid understanding of the learning principles discussed previously in this chapter should allow the dentist to flexibly employ these ideas to ameliorate common barriers to treatment progress. Treatment-interfering behaviors may occur at the time of actual dental visits, or between visits.

As mentioned previously, positive and negative reinforcement are likely to offer the most utility in the dental treatment setting, with omission and punishment likely to be more limited in effectiveness and acceptability.

Perhaps the most straightforward means of providing positive reinforcement is via the use of praise or other forms of positive attention (e.g., a "thumbs up" gesture). Take the example of a child beginning a dental exam who is asked to open their mouth wide. When they do as instructed, the dentist praises them by saying, "Nice job opening your mouth! You're making it so easy for me to see all of your teeth." The child then continues to make an effort to keep their mouth wide open for the remainder of the procedure. In this case, the child complying with instructions by opening their mouth wide has been positively reinforced by the stimulus of the dentist providing positive attention.

While social means of providing positive reinforcement are both highly valuable and convenient to utilize, particularly when used in a precise manner (e.g., "I can tell you've worked very hard at wearing your elastics" versus the still reinforcing yet distinctly more vague, "Your teeth look good"), additional reinforcement value can be achieved by presenting some tangible reward (e.g., access to a small prize at the end of a successful appointment).

Timing has a significant impact on the value of a given reinforcer, with a reward that is provided sooner (e.g., at the end of an appointment) having higher reinforcement value than the same reward provided after a delay (e.g., after desirable behavior demonstrated over the course of several treatment visits).

Additionally, it is important to remember that not every reinforcer is equally salient to each patient or retains its value to the same degree over time. Characteristics of the individual, including developmental level and interests, will dictate the precise value of a tangible reward. This can result in wide variability in the value of reinforcers to different members of a patient population, though some generalizations tend to hold true. For example, young children will often be motivated and excited by provision of a reward of trivial value that may serve primarily as a tangible representation of a job well done (e.g., a sticker of a favorite animated character that states "Star Patient!"). On the other hand, older children and adolescents tend to find such rewards minimally reinforcing, as they easily identify that such a reward has no enduring or broader value—there is nothing to *do* with a sticker, after all, except to *stick it* to something.

As rewards for intra-visit behavior are—by definition—provided fairly immediately, there are often few ways to increase the reinforcement value of a tangible reward for older patients other than by capitalizing on personal salience (thus the value of a "prize basket," in which multiple different potential rewards are available, thereby increasing the chances that something in the basket will strike the fancy of an individual patient), or by increasing the magnitude of the reward (i.e., providing a larger reward—a T-shirt, e.g., rather than a small toy). The challenge, of course, in providing rewards of more monetary value is that they can quickly become cost prohibitive to a dental practice, rendering them impractical for regular use. Fortunately, noncompliance during dental visits, be it rooted in anxiety or otherwise, tends to decrease as children age.

Although rewards for compliance during dental visits are commonly provided, the more significant challenge for the orthodontist may lie in the utilization of positive reinforcement for compliance with treatment *between* treatment visits, particularly as orthodontic treatment often demands active patient and parent involvement beyond simply keeping the teeth clean. The effects of reward on orthodontic treatment compliance have appeared underwhelming, as documented in the scientific literature,[29] though this ineffectiveness may reflect the limitations of rewards that are able to be feasibly provided at relatively infrequent dental appointments. Additional value may lie in the dentist working with the patient's caregiver to implement a system of reinforcement in the home environment, thereby expanding the options for reinforcement and decreasing the time delay between the desired behavior and reward. Instead of an orthodontist providing a prize for consecutive appointments with good hygiene, for example, parents could be encouraged to reward the child's daily attention to oral hygiene with a more proximal reward, such as time on a preferred electronic device. Such intervention is more likely to achieve the desired immediate effect and, when implemented consistently over time, also contribute to positive long-term outcomes, including some that are likely to be highly reinforcing to parents (e.g., lower incidence of caries and shortened duration of treatment, both of which may have financial ramifications).

Negative reinforcement, which also accentuates the probability of any given behavior, is more difficult to use as a behavioral management tool in the dental office, but it can be used effectively if circumstances permit. If a child is concerned about a treatment procedure but behaves well and understands that the procedure has been shortened because of their good behavior, their compliance has been negatively reinforced. In orthodontic treatment, long bonding and banding appointments may go more efficiently and smoothly if the child understands that their helpful behavior has shortened the procedure and reduced the possibility that the procedure will need to be redone.

In addition, consider the example of a child undergoing a dental procedure who is told by the dentist to raise their hand if they are experiencing discomfort that is too intense—a technique referred to as "enhancing control" that has been shown to reduce intraoperative pain.[30,31] When they begin to feel significant pain, the child does as instructed, after which the dentist briefly pauses the procedure, providing relatively immediate relief of the child's discomfort. The child then continues to utilize this behavior during the remainder of the procedure. In this case, the child utilizing the appropriate means of alerting the dentist to their pain has been negatively reinforced by the removal of the pain stimulus.

The other two types of operant conditioning, omission and punishment, should be used sparingly and with caution in the dental office. Because a positive stimulus is removed in omission, the child may react with anger or frustration. When punishment is used, both fear and anger sometimes result. In fact, punishment can lead to a classically conditioned fear response. Obviously, it is a good idea for the dentist and staff to avoid creating fear and anger in a child (or adult) patient.

One mild form of punishment that can be used with children is called voice control. Voice control involves speaking to the child in a firm voice to gain their attention, telling them that their present behavior is unacceptable, and directing them as to how they should behave. This technique should be used with care, and the child should be immediately rewarded for an improvement in their behavior, if only by reinforcing them via specific praise (e.g., in a warm tone stating, "That's exactly how I need you to help me. Great job lying still"). This is likely to be most effective when a warm, caring relationship has been established between the dental team and the patient and parent(s), who might otherwise find the use of voice control to be excessive or off-putting.

In addition to the use of the behavioral shaping tools previously mentioned, various other strategies have been employed in the management of behavior in the dental environment, ranging from other behavioral techniques to more involved and intensive strategies that may involve either physical restraint or medication. Each may have its time and purpose, and careful consideration of risks versus benefits is incumbent upon the practitioner, typically in coordination with parents.

Importantly, a 2022 meta-analysis of behavior management techniques in pediatric dentistry found limited evidence for the superiority of specific behavior management techniques over others, though the nature of the studies included precluded the authors from drawing conclusions regarding the relative effectiveness of techniques at specific ages or levels of development.[32] Rather, all of the reviewed basic behavior management techniques—including audio and audiovisual distraction, tell-show-do (TSD), and live modeling, as well as more novel techniques such as cognitive behavioral interventions that combined systematic desensitization, relaxation, and cognitive restructuring—appeared to be acceptable and effective in addressing anxiety and behavior during dental treatments. Despite the appeal of audiovisual techniques incorporating ubiquitous forms of technology such as mobile phone games, tablets, and other screen-based interventions, there was inadequate evidence to suggest these were superior in effectiveness to more "tried and true" techniques such as TSD.

In sum, empirical evidence appears to underscore the need for clinicians to be competent in utilizing a wide range of behavior management techniques to take into account patients' personalities and parent preferences.[32]

Managing Neurodevelopmental and Psychiatric Conditions in Orthodontic Treatment

Although there is a sizable body of research concerning general dental care for patients with disabilities, research specific to orthodontic care of these patients is relatively scarce. There is evidence, however, that both parents of adolescents with disabilities, as well as orthodontists, express apprehension regarding the prospect of successful orthodontic intervention, often due to concerns regarding behavioral barriers to treatment.[33] Despite these concerns, parents of youth with disabilities often express high levels of motivation for pursuing orthodontic treatment, both to address oral dysfunctionality and for esthetic reasons.[34]

Orthodontic care is one of the few dental treatments that includes active patient (and parent) involvement beyond keeping the teeth clean. Cognitive development is essential to have successful orthodontic care. At the least, patients need to be able to tolerate intraoral record taking and placement and adjustment and removal of appliances, in addition to living with the appliances. That means keeping the appliances intact, cleaning the teeth and appliances, and wearing adjuncts such as elastics. Some children with disabilities develop to a level at which they can tolerate these events; others do not. Depending on the situation, some patients with disabilities can have routine orthodontic treatment and do well. Some should not be treated because the treatment can cause more risk to the patient and their oral tissues than is merited for a largely elective treatment that may have more benefit for the parents than the child. This can be difficult for some parents to appreciate because it is "just braces" that appear so benign. This is especially true when having a pretty smile seems to be one thing that their child can achieve in spite of other disabilities.

Sometimes compromises can be made to meet realistic parental desires and accommodate the patient's abilities while staying within the realm of clinically viable, safe, and ethical orthodontics.

To assess whether a patient's developmental capabilities and behaviors are consistent with the potential provision of orthodontic care, efforts should be made to obtain salient historical information prior to treatment (information regarding patient/parent motivation for treatment is also essential and is discussed in Chapter 6). Relevant details include the presence of developmental delays (e.g., cognitive, speech-language, motor), neurodevelopmental disorders (e.g., autism spectrum disorder, intellectual disability, attention-deficit/hyperactivity disorder [ADHD]), and psychiatric issues (e.g., anxiety, depression, disruptive behavior disorders). Attempting to collect such data—at least in part—via written questionnaire is advisable, particularly as parents may feel uncomfortable discussing these issues in front of their children, and children and adolescents may also feel uncomfortable and/or be unable to provide context due to limited insight or developmental delays. In addition to asking about the presence of developmental, psychiatric, and behavioral concerns, inquiring as to current levels of independent functioning, particularly in regard to completion of daily routines (hygiene tasks, dressing), may provide some additional insight regarding how well the child or adolescent is able to remember and perform responsibilities. It is this information regarding a particular child's daily functioning—rather than a set of developmental norms—that is likely to be most helpful for the orthodontist in delivering information and advising caregivers of their role in treatment.

Specific Considerations for Common Developmental and Psychiatric Issues

Intellectual Disabilities

Intellectual disability (ID) occurs in 1% to 2% of the population and is characterized by deficits in cognitive functioning (i.e., an IQ score of approximately two standard deviations or more below the general population), as well as accompanying deficits in adaptive functioning, which can include adherence to daily health routines.[35] Individuals with ID have been found to exhibit both a more frequent need for orthodontic treatment, as well as a more frequent need for urgent care of this type.[36] In addition, the phenotype of certain populations of individuals with ID, such as those with Down syndrome, may contribute to particularly severe levels of malocclusion.[37]

It is important to note that individuals with ID represent a heterogeneous group in regard to their cognitive deficits and the degree to which they struggle in meeting daily functional challenges, including those that may present in the course of orthodontic treatment. Children and adolescents with severe to profound ID—who make up a very small percentage of individuals with the disorder—are likely to be more immediately identifiable to dental providers, given that they typically demonstrate limited communication skills, require a high degree of caregiver supervision to complete daily tasks, and may suffer from congenital syndromes that may further signal to the provider that these are individuals for whom adjustments in expectations and support will be necessary in the course of treatment. On the other hand, the vast majority of individuals with ID demonstrate relatively lower levels of deficit that—while significant and impairing by definition—may not be as evident to providers in the office setting. Once again, surveying caregivers to determine the patient's historical need for support in successfully meeting daily demands (e.g., hygiene tasks, adhering to a schedule) is likely to provide the most salient information for the orthodontist in determining the level of support the patient will require to complete successful treatment.

Autism Spectrum Disorder

ASD is characterized by social communication deficits and the presence of restricted and repetitive interests and behaviors. Despite these common characteristics, individuals with ASD are highly variable in their presentations and suitability for orthodontic treatment. Some of these children and adolescents make exemplary patients because of their attention to detail and order. Others can be bothered by the presence of the appliances themselves and/or demonstrate extreme sensitivities to sensory stimuli that can make adherence to treatment, both within and between appointments, quite difficult. This challenging treatment interaction often can be successfully met by thoughtful adjustment of the goals and expectations on the part of both the practitioner and parents.

Advanced behavior management techniques such as sedation and general anesthesia are often used to address behavioral barriers to dental treatment with children and adolescents with ASD, though this is typically indicated in situations where the treatment is medically necessary (e.g., to address decay or injury). Such techniques, however, carry a degree of medical risk that may not be justified in the case of orthodontic treatment, much of which is elective.

The social communication deficits present in ASD can range from a child who is completely nonverbal to one who has strong expressive and receptive language skills but who might struggle in the pragmatic aspects of language, including nonverbal communication skills and using language for particular purposes. The degree and quality of the social impairment will dictate what accommodations may need to be considered on the part of the orthodontic team. For example, with a child or adolescent with limited language, communication via nonverbal means such as a picture exchange system may be required, while a patient with more developed language skills may benefit from the dental team simply paying closer attention to using concrete language that avoids the use of figures of speech or sarcasm.[38]

Efforts to increase predictability for patients, and to successfully clarify expectations for behavior prior to treatment visits, can also be made via a variety of methods, including the use of "social stories," which help to prepare individuals with ASD for what to expect and how to interact successfully in a given situation.

Intervention to account for the sensory sensitivities of patients with ASD can largely be boiled down to two general concepts: (1) accommodating the individual's sensitivities by modulating stimuli that may be distressing and (2) increasing the individual's ability to tolerate particular sensory inputs.

In regard to accommodation of sensory sensitivities, modulation of operatory light sources (either by changing the light itself or the amount of light that reaches the patient, as in the case of dark glasses) and use of noise-canceling headphones to mitigate auditory stimuli are some examples of strategies that may be relatively easy to implement. Increasing a patient's sensory threshold typically relies on the implementation of systematic desensitization, wherein the patient is gradually exposed to a distressing stimulus, ultimately leading to habituation or a decreased response to the stimulus over time. Particularly in the case of a patient with ASD, it is important to note that this desensitization process requires repeated and carefully tailored exposures that may be relatively time consuming and whose benefits may be narrow (i.e., habituation to one stimulus in a particular environment may not generalize to other stimuli or environments, even if similar).[38] This process is likely to be more feasible for patients for whom desensitization has already been incorporated into management of their behaviors in other environments (e.g., school). Thus, although both accommodation and desensitization may have their place in orthodontic practice for patients with ASD, it is likely that strategies focusing on accommodation will be more practical and time efficient.

Attention-Deficit/Hyperactivity Disorder

Children and adolescents with ADHD, a relatively common neurodevelopmental disorder, demonstrate functionally impairing symptoms of inattention and/or hyperactive-impulsive behavior that reflect broad deficits in self-regulation and executive functioning. This behavior can be confused with children who have obstructive sleep apnea. From a dental perspective, youth with ADHD demonstrate an increased risk for caries and dental trauma and may demonstrate poorer attention to oral hygiene and more behavior management problems in dental settings than those without the disorder.[39–42]

The most significant challenges in orthodontic treatment of individuals with ADHD are likely to be in addressing difficulties with adherence to treatment, either due to inattention/disorganization (e.g., forgetting to engage in regularly prescribed practices) or deficits in motivation, particularly given that orthodontic treatment typically requires sustained effort to achieve a distant goal. Organizing behavior, across time, to meet such goals is one of the key functional deficits demonstrated in ADHD.

A certain degree of internal motivation to participate in orthodontic treatment is often assumed, particularly in adolescents who may identify aesthetic goals to the orthodontist. However, it is important for both the dentist and parent to understand that normative expectations regarding independent follow-through on daily tasks (such as regularly wearing elastics) may be unrealistic in the context of ADHD. Normalizing for parents that they may need to provide increased and ongoing oversight of treatment for a child or adolescent with ADHD can help to facilitate treatment outcomes and potentially head off frustration on the part of the parent. That said, given the high heritability of ADHD, it is also fairly likely to encounter a child with ADHD whose parent also suffers from the disorder. If this shared risk factor contributes to nonadherence to orthodontic treatment, it is also likely contributing to impairment in other areas of life (e.g., schoolwork completion and adherence to other medical regimens).

It is also important for the orthodontist to understand that performance deficits in youth with ADHD (e.g., not regularly following treatment instructions) are less likely to reflect informational deficits. That is, most orthodontic providers take care to communicate expectations and instructions for care to their patients, and most of these patients—including those with ADHD—can understand this information. The key deficit in ADHD is not what the patient knows but what they *do* with what they know. When understood in this light, it should be clear that simply repeating expectations to a nonadherent patient with ADHD is likely to miss the mark. Instead, reiterating to the parent the appropriateness of providing additional support to the patient, including additional reminders and even additional reinforcement for compliance (e.g., tying daily access to a preferred electronic to adherence to treatment), is more likely to improve outcomes.

Specific Considerations for Gender-Diverse Individuals

Gender identity refers to one's internal sense of being a male, a female, a combination of male and female, or even neither gender; gender-diverse individuals, then, include persons whose gender identity differs from the sex they were assigned at birth, as well as those who identify their gender outside of the male/female binary.[43]

As orthodontists are increasingly likely to treat patients who openly identify as gender diverse, it is important for providers to understand that gender diversity is not, in and of itself, considered pathological or harmful. Gender dysphoria (which is based on distress and impairment related to gender identification) is included as a diagnosis in the fifth edition of the *Diagnostic and Statistical Manual of Mental Disorders*, though the creation of this diagnosis was intended to protect access to care rather than to pathologize the individual.[44]

Many gender-diverse patients demonstrate a willingness to discuss their gender identity with medical providers; however, a substantial number may not, even when they feel it may be relevant in that setting.[45] Previous experiences with discrimination and maltreatment may contribute to this reticence; however, in the case of gender-diverse youth, the desire to shield this information from parents entirely—or disagreement with parents over gender identity—may further impact the information they share with the orthodontist.[46]

Although it is ultimately up to the patient to disclose information regarding gender identity, it does appear that youth often prefer that providers ask directly about gender identity, and that this approach may increase disclosure.[47]

From an orthodontic standpoint, working with gender-diverse patients may require sensitive collaboration, particularly when the patient's desire to achieve certain aesthetic outcomes (consistent with their gender identity) conflicts with traditional treatment approaches. For example, a transgender female (i.e., one who was male sex assigned at birth, but who identifies and presents as a female) may wish to maintain facial convexity, though traditional treatment would suggest more mandibular contribution and a straighter face, which may make the individual appear less feminine. In this case, the orthodontist may need to make treatment compromises that maintain facial convexity.

References

1. Farkas LG. *Anthropometry of the Head and Face.* Raven Press; 1994.
2. Weissheimer A, Menezes LM, Koerich L, et al. Fast three-dimensional superimposition of cone beam computed tomography for orthopaedics and orthognathic surgery evaluation. *Int J Oral Maxillofac Surg.* 2015;44:1188–1196.
3. Cevidanes LH, Franco AA, Gehrig G, et al. Assessment of mandibular growth and response to orthopedic treatment with 3-dimensional magnetic resonance images. *Am J Orthod Dentofacial Orthop.* 2005;128:16–26.
4. Thompson DT. *On Growth and Form.* Cambridge University Press; 1971.
5. Baer MJ, Bosma JF, Ackerman JL. *The Postnatal Development of the Rat Skull.* The University of Michigan Press; 1983.
6. Alappat S, Zhang Z, Chen Y. *Msx* homeobox gene family and craniofacial development. *Cell Res.* 2003;13:429–442. https://doi.org/10.1038/sj.cr.7290185.
7. MacKenzie A, Ferguson MW, Sharpe PT. Expression patterns of the homeobox gene, Hox-8, in the mouse embryo suggest a role in specifying tooth initiation and shape. *Development.* 1992;115(2):403–420.
8. Duverger O, Morasso MI. Role of homeobox genes in the patterning, specification, and differentiation of ectodermal appendages in mammals. *J Cell Physiol.* 2008;216(2):337–346. https://doi.org/10.1002/jcp.21491. PMID: 18459147; PMCID: PMC2561923.
9. Berdal A, Molla M, Hotton D, et al. Differential impact of MSX1 and MSX2 homeogenes on mouse maxillofacial skeleton. *Cells Tissues Organs.* 2009;189:126–132.
10. Zebrick B, Teeramongkolgul T, Nicot R, et al. ACTN3 R577X genotypes associate with Class II and deepbite malocclusions. *Am J Orthod Dentofacial Orthop.* 2014;146:603–611.
11. Brinkley JF, Fisher S, Harris MP, et al. The FaceBase Consortium: a comprehensive resource for craniofacial researchers. *Development.* 2016;143:2677–2688.
12. Bastos VC, Gomez RS, Gomes CC. Revisiting the human dental follicle: from tooth development to its association with unerupted or impacted teeth and pathological changes. *Dev Dyn.* 2022;251(3):408–423.
13. Frazier-Bowers SA, Simmons D, Wright JT, et al. Primary failure of eruption and PTH1R: the importance of a genetic diagnosis for orthodontic treatment planning. *Am J Orthod Dentofacial Orthop.* 2010;137:160e1–160e7. discussion 160–161.
14. Maggoli C, Stagi S. Bone modeling, remodeling and skeletal health in children and adolescents: mineral accrual, assessment and treatment. *Ann Pediatr Endocrinol Metab.* 2017;22:1–5.
15. Copray JC. Growth of the nasal septal cartilage of the rat in vitro. *J Anat.* 1986;144:99–111.
16. Delatte M, Von den Hoff JW, van Rheden RE, et al. Primary and secondary cartilages of the neonatal rat: the femoral head and the mandibular condyle. *Eur J Oral Sci.* 2004;112:156–162.
17. NORD Rare Disease Database. *Binder Type Nasomaxillary Dysplasia.* https://rarediseases.org/rare-diseases/binder-type-maxillonasal-dysplasia/
18. Gilhuus-Moe O. *Fractures of the Mandibular Condyle in the Growth Period.* Scandinavian University Books, Universitatsforlaget; 1969.
19. Lund K. Mandibular growth and remodelling process after mandibular fractures: a longitudinal roentgencephalometric study. *Acta Odontol Scand.* 1974;32(64):3–117.
20. Moss ML. The functional matrix hypothesis revisited. *Am J Orthod Dentofacial Orthop.* 1997;112:8–11. 221–226, 338–342, 410–417.
21. Uhac M, et al. Orthodontic treatment demand in young adolescents – are parents familiar with their children's desires and reasons? *Int J Paediatr Dent.* 2022:383–391.
22. Amaral BA, et al. Relationship between normative and self-perceived criteria for orthodontic treatment need and satisfaction with esthetics and mastication in adolescents. *Am J Orthod Dentofacial Orthop.* 2020;157(1):42–48.
23. Walton W, Fields HW, Johnston WM, et al. Orthodontic appliance preferences of children and adolescents. *Am J Orthod Dentofacial Orthop.* 2010;138:698e1–698e12.
24. Hyde J, Ryan KM, Waters AM. Psychophysiological markers of fear and anxiety. *Curr Psychiatry Rep.* 2019;21(56).
25. Oliveira LB, et al. Children's perceptions of dentist's attire and environment: a systematic review and meta-analysis. *Int J Clin Pediatr Dent.* 2020;13(6):700–716.
26. Gustafsson A. Dental behaviour management problems among children and adolescents—a matter of understanding? Studies on dental fear, personal characteristics and psychosocial concomitants. *Swed Dent J.* 2010(suppl 202):1–46.
27. Farhat-McHayleh N, Harfouche A, Souaid P. Techniques for managing behavior in pediatric dentistry: comparative study of live modeling and tell-show-do based on children's heart rates during treatment. *J Can Dent Assoc.* 2009;75:283.
28. Chambers DW. Managing anxieties of young dental patients. *ASDC J Dent Child.* 1970;37:363–373.
29. Aljabaa AJ, et al. A systematic review of randomized controlled trials of interventions to improve adherence among orthodontic patients aged 12 to 18. *Angle Orthod.* 2015;85(2):305–313.
30. American Academy of Pediatric Dentistry. *Behavior guidance for the pediatric dental patient. The Reference Manual of Pediatric Dentistry.* American Academy of Pediatric Dentistry; 2022:321–339.
31. Thrash WJ, Marr JN, Boone SE. Continuous self-monitoring of discomfort in the dental chair and feedback to the dentist. *J Behav Assess.* 1982;4(3):273–284.
32. Gizani S, et al. Basic behavioral management techniques in pediatric dentistry: a systematic review and meta-analysis. *J Dent.* 2022;126:104303.
33. Mendez SV, et al. Barriers and facilitators in the orthodontic treatment of teenagers with neurodevelopmental disabilities. *Am J Orthod Dentofacial Orthop.* 2022;161(1):115–124.
34. Abeleira MT, et al. Orthodontic treatment for disabled children: a survey of parents' attitudes and overall satisfaction. *BMC Oral Health.* 2014;14:98–106.
35. Patrick ME, Shaw KA, Dietz PM, et al. Prevalence of intellectual disability among eight-year-old children from selected communities in the United States, 2014. *Disabil Health J.* 2021;14(2):101023.

36. Cabrita JP, et al. Prevalence of malocclusion in individuals with and without intellectual disability: a comparative study. *Special Care Dent.* 2017;37(4):181–186.
37. Marques LS, et al. Down syndrome: a risk factor for malocclusion severity? *Braz Oral Res.* 2015(29):1.
38. Nelson TM, Sheller B, Friedman CS, et al. Educational and therapeutic behavioral approaches to providing dental care for patients with autism spectrum disorder. *Special Care Dent.* 2015;35:105–113.
39. Blomqvist M, et al. Oral health, dental anxiety, and behavior management problems in children with attention deficit hyperactivity disorder. *Eur J Oral Sci.* 2006;114:385–390.
40. Chau YCY, et al. Oral health of children with attention-deficit hyperactivity disorder: systematic review and meta-analysis. *J Atten Disord.* 2020;24(7):947–962.
41. Nyquist JM, et al. Executive function as a risk factor for incisor trauma. *Dent Traumatol.* 2018;34:229–236.
42. Reddy ER, et al. Oral health status and caries experience in children diagnosed with attention-deficit hyperactive disorder. *Int. J. Clin. Pediatr. Dent.* 2022;15(4):438–441.
43. Rubin JD, et al. Studying gender diversity. *Trends Cogn Sci.* 2020;24(3):163–165.
44. American Psychiatric Association. *Diagnostic and Statistical Manual of Mental Disorders.* American Psychiatric Association; 2013. https://www.psychiatry.org/psychiatrists/practice/dsm.
45. Sequeira GM, et al. Transgender youth's disclosure of gender identity to providers outside of specialized gender centers. *J Adolesc Health Care.* 2020;66:691–698.
46. Heima M, et al. Dental fear among transgender individuals – a cross-sectional survey. *Spec Care Dentist.* 2017;37(5):212–222.
47. Meckler GD, et al. Nondisclosure of sexual orientation to a physician among a sample of gay, lesbian, and bisexual youth. *Arch Pediatr Adolesc Med.* 2006;160:1248–1254.

3

Early Stages of Development

WILLIAM R. PROFFIT, HENRY W. FIELDS, AND KAITRIN KRAMER

CHAPTER OUTLINE

Late Fetal Development and Birth

By the beginning of the third trimester of intrauterine life, the human fetus weighs approximately 1000 g and, although far from ready for life outside the protective intrauterine environment, can often survive premature birth. During the last 3 months of intrauterine life, continued rapid growth results in a tripling of body mass to about 3000 g. Dental development, which begins in the third month, proceeds rapidly thereafter (Table 3.1). Development of all primary teeth and the permanent first molars starts well before birth.

Although the proportion of the total body mass represented by the head decreases from the fourth month of intrauterine life onward because of the cephalocaudal gradient of growth discussed earlier, at birth the head is still nearly half the total body mass and represents the largest impediment to passage of the infant through the birth canal. Making the head longer and narrower obviously would facilitate birth, and this is accomplished by a literal distortion of its shape (Fig. 3.1). The change of shape is possible because, at birth, relatively large noncalcified fontanelles persist between the flat bones of the calvarium. As the head is compressed within the birth canal, the calvarium can increase in length and decrease in width, assuming the desired tubular form and easing passage through the birth canal.

The relative lack of growth of the lower jaw prenatally also makes birth easier because a prominent bony chin at the time of birth would be a considerable problem in passage through the birth canal. Many a young dentist, acutely aware of the orthodontic problems that can arise later because of skeletal mandibular deficiency, has been shocked to discover how incredibly mandibular deficient their own newborn is and has required reassurance that this is a perfectly normal and indeed desirable phenomenon. Postnatally, the normal mandible grows more than the other facial structures throughout puberty and gradually catches up, producing the eventual balanced adult proportions.

Despite the physical adaptations that facilitate it, birth is a traumatic process. In the best circumstances, arriving into the world requires a dramatic set of physiologic adaptations. For a short period, growth ceases, and often there is a small decrease in weight during the first 7 to 10 days of life. Such an interruption in growth produces a physical effect on skeletal tissues that are forming at the time because the orderly sequence of calcification is disturbed. The result is a noticeable line across both bones and teeth that are forming at the time. However, bones are not visible and are remodeled to such an extent that any lines caused by the growth arrest at birth would soon be covered at any rate.

Teeth, on the other hand, are quite visible, and the extent of any growth disturbance related to birth can be seen in the enamel, which is not remodeled. Almost every child has a "neonatal line" across the surface of the primary teeth, its location varying from tooth to tooth depending on the stage of development at birth (Fig. 3.2). The neonatal line is the first enamel formed postnatally. It is a visual change in the enamel presentation caused by changes in the mineralization of the enamel prisms.[1] Under normal circumstances, the line is so slight that it can be seen only if the tooth surface is magnified, but if the neonatal period is challenging, a prominent area of stained, distorted, or poorly calcified enamel can be the result.

TABLE 3.1 Chronology of Tooth Development, Primary Dentition

	CALCIFICATION BEGINS		CROWN COMPLETED		ERUPTION		ROOT COMPLETED	
Tooth	Maxillary	Mandibular	Maxillary (months)	Mandibular (months)	Maxillary (months)	Mandibular (months)	Maxillary (years)	Mandibular (years)
Central	14 weeks in utero	14 weeks in utero	1½	2½	10	8	1½	1½
Lateral	16 weeks in utero	16 weeks in utero	2½	3	11	13	2	1½
Canine	17 weeks in utero	17 weeks in utero	9	9	19	20	3¼	3¼
First molar	15 weeks in utero	15 weeks in utero	6	5½	16	16	2½	2¼
Second molar	19 weeks in utero	18 weeks in utero	11	10	29	27	3	3

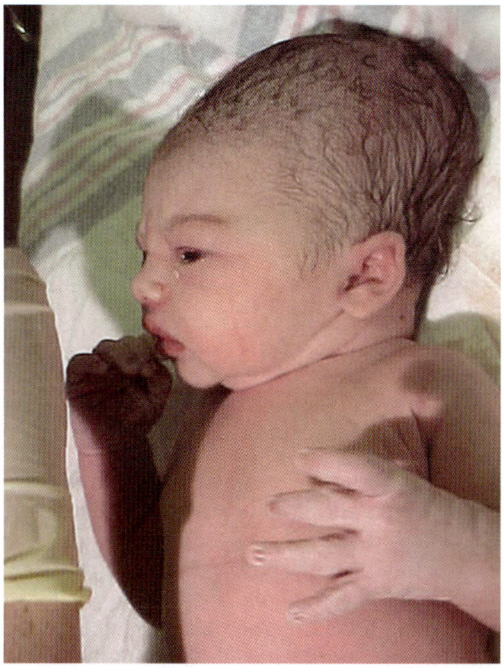

• **Fig. 3.1** This photograph of a newborn infant clearly shows the head distortion that accompanies (and facilitates) passage through the birth canal. Note that the head has been squeezed into a more elliptical or tubular "cone-head" shape, a distortion made possible by the presence of the relatively large fontanelles.

Birth is not the only circumstance that can have this effect on developing teeth. As a general rule, growth disturbances lasting 1 to 2 weeks or more, such as the one that accompanies birth or one caused by a febrile illness later, will leave a visible record in the enamel of teeth forming at the time. Permanent as well as primary teeth can be affected by illnesses during infancy and early childhood.

Infancy and Early Childhood: The Primary Dentition Years

Physical Development in the Preschool Years

The general pattern of physical development after birth is a continuation of the pattern of the late fetal period. Rapid growth continues, with a relatively steady increase in height and weight, although the rate of growth declines dramatically as a percentage of the previous body size (Fig. 3.3).

Influences on Physical Development

Four circumstances merit special attention.

Premature Birth (Low Birth Weight)

Infants weighing less than 2500 g (5 lb 8 oz) at birth are at greater risk of problems in the immediate postnatal period. Extremely low birth weight (ELBW) infants (<1000 g) and extremely premature infants (<28 weeks' gestation) are at high risk for death, disability, and long-term comorbidities even with access to the best specialized neonatal care.[2] Until recent years, children with birth weights below 1500 g (2 lb 5 oz) often did not survive. In fact, birth weight, illness, and day of life (DOL) combine to be better predictors of survival. Eighty percent of deaths in extremely low birth weight infants occur in the first 3 days of life; consequently, once an infant has survived to DOL 4, the likelihood of survival is dramatically increased and depends more on the extent of illness at that point.[3]

If a premature infant survives the neonatal period, however, there is every reason to expect that growth will follow the normal pattern and that the child will gradually overcome the initial hurdle (Fig. 3.4). Premature infants can be expected to be small throughout the first and second years of life. In many instances, by the third year of life, premature and normal-term infants are indistinguishable in attainment of developmental milestones. Although there was concern about a relationship between ELBW and later coronary disease, this has not been supported by recent clinical trials.[4] For the orthodontist, a history of premature birth is not an indicator of problems with childhood or adolescent orthodontic treatment.

Chronic Illness

Skeletal growth is a process that can occur only when the other requirements of the individual have been met. A certain amount of energy is necessary to maintain life. An additional amount is needed for activity, and a further increment is necessary for growth. For a normal child, perhaps 90% of the available energy must be "taken off the top" to meet the requirements for survival and activity, leaving 10% for growth.

Chronic illness alters this balance, leaving relatively less energy available to support growth. Chronically ill children typically fall behind their healthier peers in height and weight, and if the illness persists, the growth deficit is cumulative. An episode of acute illness

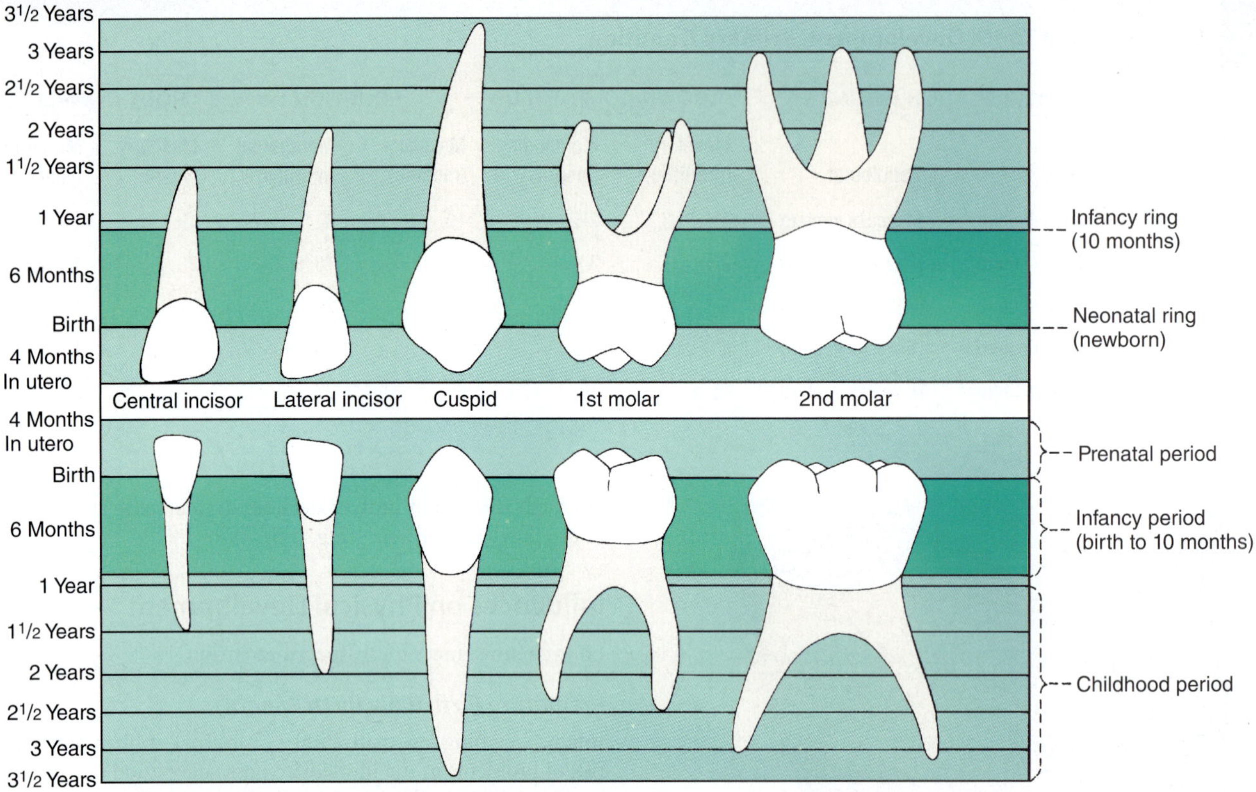

• **Fig. 3.2** Primary teeth shown on a developmental scale that indicates the expected location of the neonatal line. From a chart of this type, the timing of illness or traumatic events that led to disturbances of enamel formation can be deduced from the location of enamel lines on various teeth.

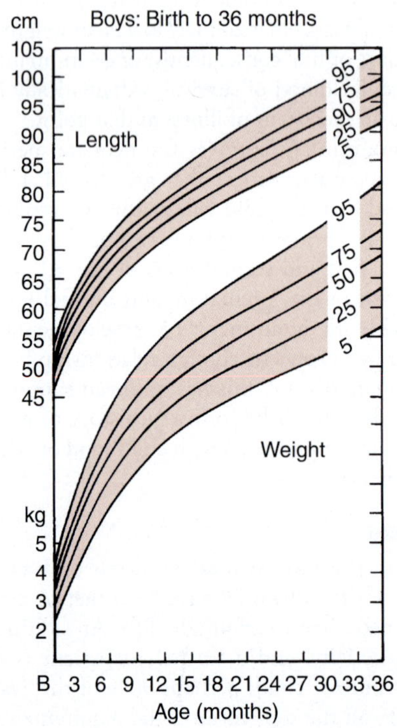

• **Fig. 3.3** Graphs of growth in length and weight in infancy for boys (the curves for girls are almost identical at these ages). Note the extremely rapid growth in early infancy, with a progressive slowing after the first 6 months. (Courtesy The National Center for Health Statistics, Washington, DC.)

leads to a temporary cessation of growth, but if the growth interruption is relatively brief, there will be no long-term effect. The more chronic the illness, the greater the cumulative impact. Obviously, the more severe the illness, the greater the impact at any given time. Children with congenital hormone deficiencies provide an excellent example. If the hormone is replaced, a dramatic improvement in growth and recovery toward normal height and weight often occurs (Fig. 3.5). A congenital heart defect can have a similar effect on growth, and similarly dramatic effects on growth can accompany the repair of the defect.[5] In extreme cases, psychological and emotional stress affects physical growth in somewhat the same way as a chronic illness (Fig. 3.6). Failure to thrive (FTT) describes a child who fails to gain weight or height according to growth charts. A height or weight below the third percentile is considered FTT. FTT can be categorized into organic and nonorganic. Organic FTT occurs when an underlying medical condition contributes to the inability to digest or absorb foods properly, leading to decreased food intake. In nonorganic FTT no medical condition or underlying disease contributes to FTT. Examples include lack of access to food and social or emotional issues.

Nutritional Status

For growth to occur, there must be a nutritional supply in excess of the amount necessary for mere survival. Chronically inadequate nutrition therefore has an effect similar to chronic illness. On the other hand, once a level of nutritional adequacy has been achieved, additional nutritional intake is not a stimulus to more rapid growth. Adequate nutrition, like reasonable overall health, is a necessary condition for normal growth but is not a stimulus to it.

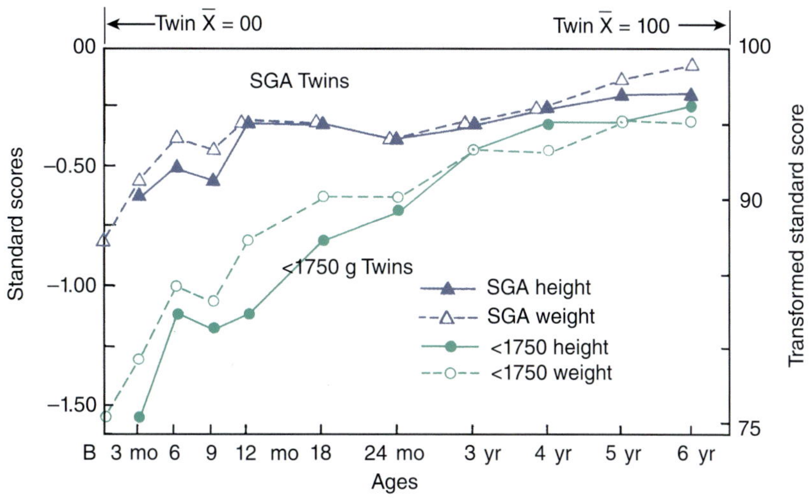

• **Fig. 3.4** Growth curves for two at-risk groups of infants: small-for-gestational-age *(SGA)* twins and twins of less than 1750g birth weight (premature birth). In this graph, 100 is the expected height and weight for normal, full-term infants. Note the recovery of the low birth weight infants over time. (Redrawn from Lowery GH. *Growth and Development of Children*. 8th ed. Year Book Medical Publishers; 1986.)

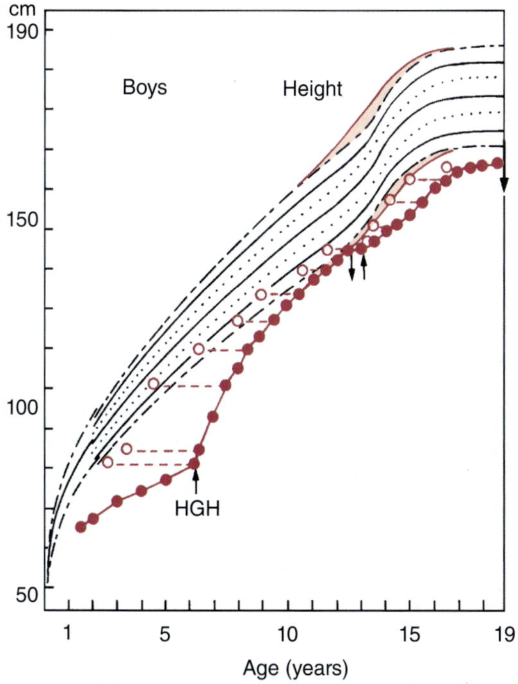

• **Fig. 3.5** The curve for growth in height for a boy with isolated growth hormone deficiency. No treatment was possible until he was 6.2 years of age. At that point, human growth hormone *(HGH)* became available, and it was administered regularly from then until age 19, except for 6 months from 12.5 to 13 years. The beginning and end of the HGH administration are indicated by the *arrows*. The *open circles* represent height plotted against bone age; thus delay in bone age is represented by the length of each horizontal dashed line. The delay was 3.5 years at the beginning of treatment and 0.8 years at 11 to 12 years when catch-up was essentially complete. Note the very high growth rate immediately after treatment started, equal to the average rate of a 1-year-old infant. (Redrawn from Tanner JM, Whitehouse RH. *Atlas of Children's Growth*. Academic Press; 1982.)

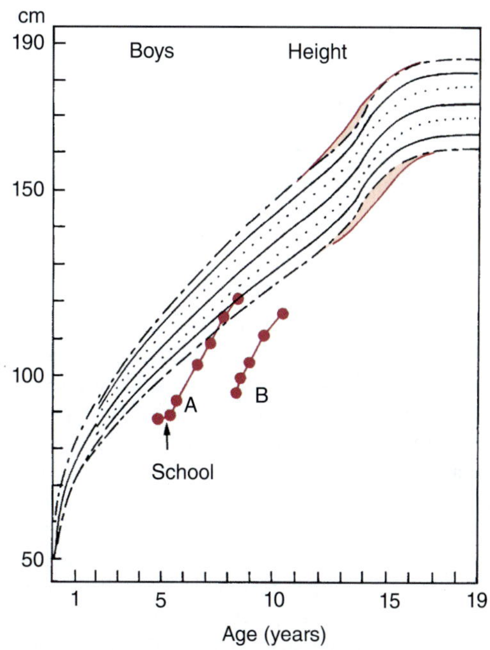

• **Fig. 3.6** The effect of a change in social environment on the growth of two children (A and B) who had an obviously disturbed home environment but no identifiable organic cause for the growth problem. When both children were placed in a special boarding school where presumably their psychosocial stress was lessened, both responded with above-average growth, though the more severely affected child was still outside the normal range 4 years later. The mechanism by which psychosocial stress can affect growth so markedly is thought to be the induction of a reversible growth hormone deficiency, accompanied by disturbance of the nearby appetite center. (Redrawn from Tanner JM, Whitehouse RH. *Atlas of Children's Growth*. Academic Press; 1982.)

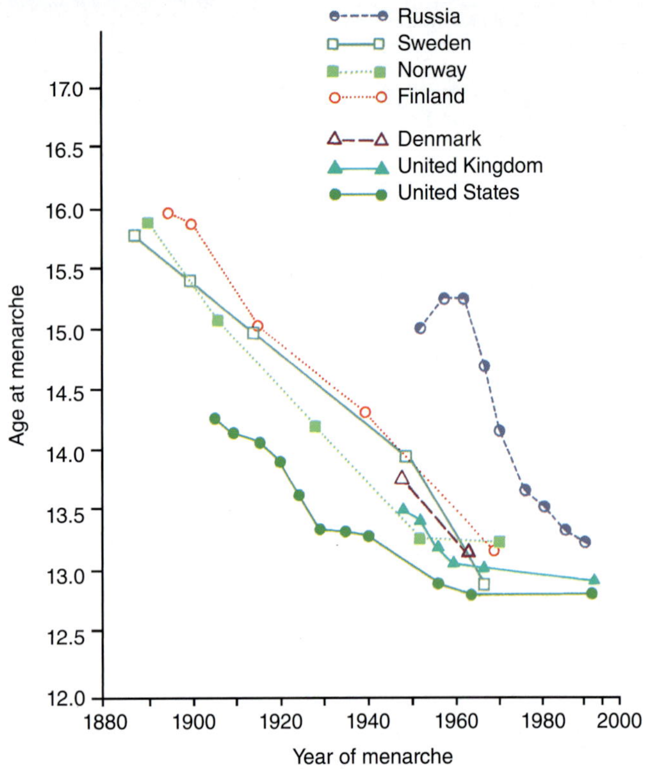

• **Fig. 3.7** Age at menarche declined in both the United States and northern European countries in the first half of the 20th century. On average, children are now larger at any given age than in the early 1900s, and they also mature more quickly. This secular trend seems to have leveled off in the early part of the 21st century. (Data from Tanner JM. *Foetus Into Man*. Harvard University Press; 1978; 1995 U.S. data from Herman-Giddens ME, et al. *Pediatrics*. 1997;99:505–512; 1995 British data from Cooper C, et al. *Br J Obstet Gynaecol*. 1996;103:814–817; Russian data from Dubrova YE, et al. *Hum Biol*. 1995;67:755–767.)

Secular Change in Growth and Development

An interesting phenomenon of the last 300 or 400 years, particularly the 20th century, has been a generalized increase in the size of most individuals. There has also been a lowering in the age of sexual maturation so that children recently have grown faster and matured earlier than they did previously. Since 1900, in the United States, the average height has increased by 2 to 3 inches, and the average age of girls at first menstruation, the most reliable sign of sexual maturity, has decreased by more than 1 year (Fig. 3.7). This "secular trend" toward more rapid growth and earlier maturation continued in most countries throughout the 20th century[6] (e.g., the mean age in Poland from 1982 to 1984 was 13.2 years, and 12.8 years in 1992–94) but seems to be leveling off in the developed countries at present.[7] That still means that signs of sexual maturation now appear in many girls much earlier than the previously accepted standard dates, which have not been updated to match the secular change.

This trend is undoubtedly related to better nutrition, which allows faster weight gain that by itself can trigger earlier maturation. Physical growth requires protein, and it is likely that the amount of protein and appropriate amino acids may be a limiting factor for many populations.[8] Because a secular trend toward earlier maturity has also been observed in populations whose nutritional status does not seem to have improved significantly, nutrition may not be the entire explanation. It has been suggested but not clearly demonstrated that exposure to chemicals in the environment that have estrogenic effects (such as some pesticides or animal feed supplements) may also have played a role.

Secular changes in body proportions, which presumably reflect environmental influences, have also been observed. It is interesting that skull proportions changed during the last century, with the head and face becoming taller and narrower.[9] Some anthropologists feel that such changes are related to the trend toward a softer diet and less functional loading of the facial skeleton (see Chapter 5), but firm evidence does not exist.

These secular changes make comparisons to historical data that have been used as control groups as untreated individuals suspect. Many of these datasets were collected 50 to 70 years ago, and while showing more contemporary leveling off, still show continued changes.

Maturation of Oral Function

The principal physiologic functions of the oral cavity are respiration, swallowing, mastication, and speech. Although it may seem odd to list respiration as an oral function, given that the major portal for respiration is the nose, respiratory needs are a primary determinant of the posture of the mandible and tongue.

At birth, if the newborn infant is to survive, an airway must be established within a few minutes and must be maintained thereafter. As Bosma[10] demonstrated with a classic radiographic study of newborn infants, to open the airway, the mandible must be positioned downward and the tongue moved downward and forward away from the posterior pharyngeal wall. This allows air to be moved through the nose and across the pharynx into the lungs. Newborn infants are obligatory nasal breathers and do not survive without immediate medical support if the nasal passage is blocked at birth. Later, breathing through the mouth becomes physiologically possible. At all times during life, respiratory needs can alter the postural basis from which oral activities begin.

Respiratory movements are "practiced" in utero, although the lungs do not inflate at that time. Swallowing also occurs during the last months of fetal life, and it appears that swallowed amniotic fluid may be an important stimulus to the activation of the infant's immune system. Digit sucking also has been observed in utero.

Once an airway has been established, the newborn infant's next physiologic priority is to obtain milk and transfer it into the gastrointestinal system. This is accomplished by two maneuvers: suckling and swallowing.

The milk ducts of lactating mammals are surrounded by smooth muscle, which contracts to force out the milk stimulated by oxytocin. To obtain milk, the infant's role is to stimulate the smooth muscle to contract and eject milk into their mouth. This is done by suckling when the tongue moves as a wave from front to back and presses the breast against the hard palate. This forces milk out of the milk ducts and into their mouth. The pressing action is largely against the breast since the nipple is only about one-third of the amount of tissue in the infant's mouth. The suction created by the infant is mainly to latch to the breast, stretch out the breast tissue, and hold it in the mouth. The tongue, however, must be placed anteriorly in contact with the lower lip so that milk is in fact deposited on the tongue. This is followed by closure of the nasal passages by the soft palate and the lips. When the milk is squirted into the mouth, it is only necessary for the

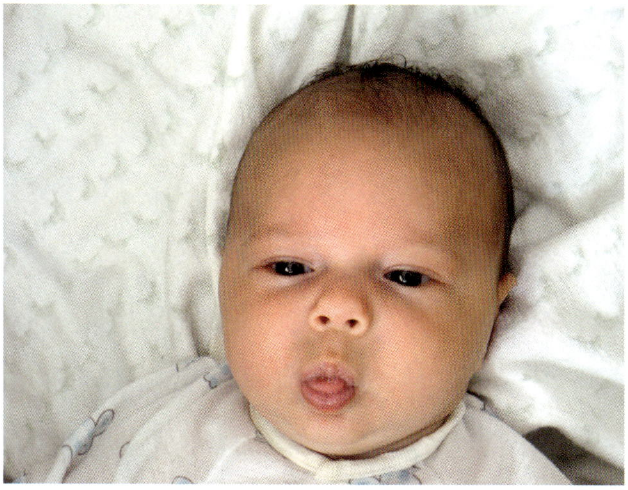

• **Fig. 3.8** Characteristic placement of the tongue against the lower lip in an infant at a few months of age. At this stage of development, tongue contact with the lip is maintained most of the time.

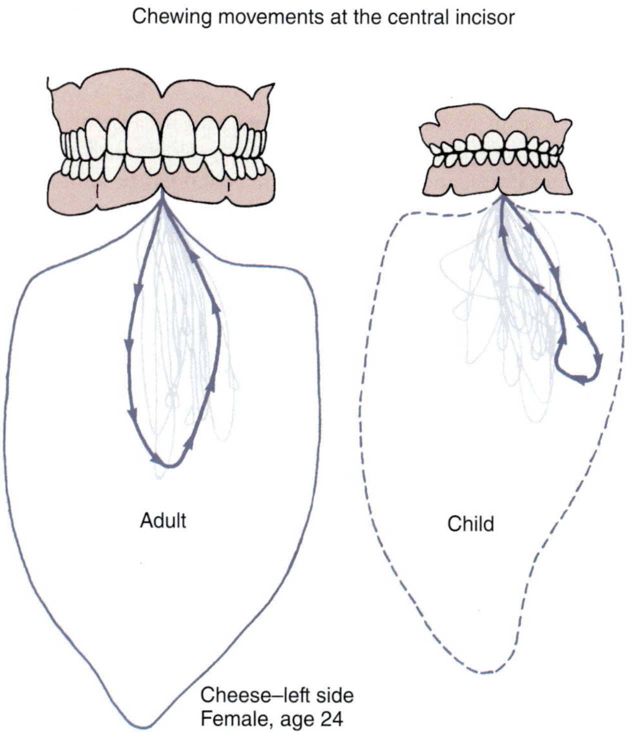

• **Fig. 3.9** Chewing movements of a child contrasted with those of an adult. Children move the jaw laterally on opening, whereas adults open straight down, then move the jaw laterally. (Redrawn from Lundeen HC, Gibbs CH. *Advances in Occlusion*. John Wright's PSG; 1982.)

infant to groove the tongue and allow the milk to flow posteriorly into the pharynx and esophagus. Nutritive sucking depends on this synchronization of sucking, swallowing, respiration, and esophageal function.[11]

This sequence of events defines an infantile swallow, which is characterized by active contractions of the musculature of the lips, a tongue tip brought forward into contact with the lower lip, and little activity of the posterior tongue or pharyngeal musculature. Tongue-to-lower-lip apposition is so common in infants that this posture is usually adopted at rest, and it is frequently possible to gently move the infant's lip and note that the tongue tip moves with it, almost as if the two were glued together (Fig. 3.8). The suckling reflex and the infantile swallow normally disappear during the first year of life.

As the infant matures, there is increasing activation of the elevator muscles of the mandible as the child swallows. As semisolid and eventually solid foods are added to the diet, it is necessary for the child to use the tongue in a more complex way to gather up a bolus, position it along the middle of the tongue, and transport it posteriorly. The chewing movements of a young child typically involve moving the mandible laterally as it opens, then bringing it back toward the midline and closing to bring the teeth into contact with the food (Fig. 3.9). By the time the primary molars begin to erupt, this sort of juvenile chewing pattern is well established. Also, by this time, the more complex movements of the posterior part of the tongue have produced a definite transition beyond the infantile swallow.

Maturation of oral function can be characterized in general as following a gradient from anterior to posterior. At birth, the lips are relatively mature and capable of vigorous suckling activity, whereas more posterior structures are quite immature. As time passes, greater activity by the posterior parts of the tongue and more complex motions of the pharyngeal structures are acquired.

This principle of front-to-back maturation is particularly well illustrated by the acquisition of speech. The first speech sounds are the bilabial sounds /m/, /p/, and /b/, which is why an infant's first word is likely to be "mama" or "papa." Somewhat later, the tongue tip consonants such as /t/ and /d/ appear. The sibilant /s/ and /z/ sounds, which require placing the tongue tip close to but not against the palate, come later still. The last speech sound, /r/, which requires precise positioning of the posterior tongue, often is not acquired until age 4 or 5.

Nearly all modern infants engage in some sort of habitual nonnutritive sucking—sucking a thumb, finger, or a similarly shaped object. Some fetuses have been reported to suck their thumbs in utero, and almost all infants do so during the period from 6 months to 2 years or later. This is culturally determined to some extent; children in parts of the developing world who are allowed ready access to the mother's breast indefinitely rarely suck any other object.[12]

After the primary molars erupt during the second year of life, drinking from a cup replaces drinking from a bottle or continued nursing at the mother's breast, and the number of children who engage in nonnutritive sucking diminishes. When sucking activity stops, a continued transition in the pattern of swallow leads to the acquisition of an adult pattern. This type of swallow is characterized by a cessation of lip activity (i.e., lips relaxed, with the tongue tip placed against the alveolar process behind the upper incisors and the posterior teeth brought into occlusion during swallowing). If sucking habits persist, however, there will not be a total transition to the adult swallow.

Surveys of American children indicate that at age 8 about 60% have achieved an adult swallow, and the remaining 40% are still somewhere in the transition.[13] After sucking habits are extinguished, a complete transition to the adult swallow may require some months. This is complicated, however, by the fact that an anterior open bite, which may well be present if a sucking habit has persisted for a long time, can delay the transition even further because of the physiologic need to seal the anterior space. The relationship of tongue position and the pattern of swallowing to malocclusion is discussed further in Chapter 5.

The chewing pattern of the adult is quite different from that of a typical child. An adult typically opens straight down, then moves the jaw laterally and brings the teeth into contact, whereas a child moves the jaw laterally on opening (see Fig. 3.9). The transition from the juvenile to the adult chewing pattern develops in conjunction with the eruption of the permanent canines, at about age 12. It is interesting to note that adults who do not achieve the normal function of the canine teeth because of a severe anterior open bite retain the juvenile chewing pattern.

Eruption of the Primary Teeth

At birth, neither the maxillary nor the mandibular alveolar process is well developed. Occasionally a "natal tooth" is present, although the first primary teeth normally do not erupt until approximately 6 months of age. The natal tooth may be a supernumerary one, formed by an aberration in the development of the dental lamina but is usually a very early but otherwise normal central incisor. Because of the possibility that it is perfectly normal, such a natal tooth should not be extracted casually. However, if the tooth displays considerable mobility, extraction may be warranted. It is important to counsel the family that there may be a missing incisor in the future as a result of the extraction.

The timing and the sequence of eruption of the primary teeth are shown in Table 3.1. The dates of eruption are relatively variable; up to 6 months of acceleration or delay is within the normal range. Preterm infants typically have some delay,[14] and there is some variance among ethnic groups.[15] The eruption sequence, however, is usually preserved. One can expect that the mandibular central incisors will erupt first, closely followed by the other incisors. After a 3- to 4-month interval, the mandibular and maxillary first molars erupt, followed in another 3 or 4 months by the maxillary and mandibular canines, which nearly fill the space between the lateral incisor and first molar. The primary dentition is usually completed at 24 to 30 months as the mandibular then the maxillary second molars erupt.

Spaces between the teeth are normal throughout the anterior part of the primary dentition but are most noticeable in two locations, called the *primate spaces.* (Most subhuman primates have these spaces throughout life; thus the name.) In the maxillary arch the primate space is located between the lateral incisors and canines, whereas in the mandibular arch the space is between the canines and first molars (Fig. 3.10). The primate spaces are normally present from the time the teeth erupt. Developmental spaces between the incisors are often present from the beginning but become somewhat larger as the child grows and the alveolar processes expand. Generalized spacing of the primary teeth is advantageous for proper alignment of the permanent incisors.

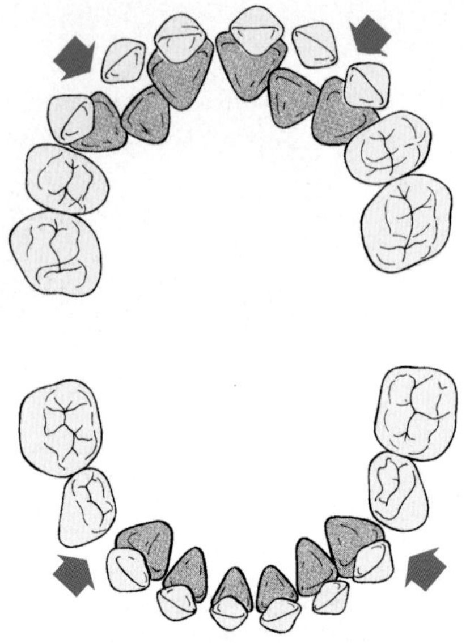

• **Fig. 3.10** The crowns of the permanent incisors (*gray*) lie lingual to the crowns of the primary incisors (*tan*), particularly in the case of the maxillary laterals. *Arrows* point to the primate spaces.

Late Childhood: The Mixed Dentition Years

Physical Development in Late Childhood

Late childhood, from age 5 or 6 to the onset of puberty, is characterized by important social and behavioral changes (see Chapter 2), but the physical development pattern of the previous period continues. The normally different rates of growth for different tissue systems, however, must be kept in mind. The maximum disparity in the development of different tissue systems occurs in late childhood (see Fig. 2.2).

By age 7, a child has essentially completed their neural growth. The brain and the skull (cranial base and calvarium) are essentially as large as they will ever be, and it is unlikely that it would be necessary again to buy the child a larger cap because of growth. Lymphoid tissue throughout the body has proliferated beyond the usual adult levels, and large tonsils and adenoids are common. In contrast, the growth of the sex organs has barely begun and general body growth is only modestly advanced. During early childhood, the rate of general body growth declines from the rapid pace of infancy, then stabilizes at a moderate lower level during late childhood. Both nutrition and general health can affect the level at which stabilization occurs.

Assessment of Skeletal and Other Developmental Ages

In planning orthodontic treatment, it can be important to know how much skeletal growth remains, so an evaluation of skeletal age is frequently needed. This is particularly important when the timing of treatment with use of functional appliances for class II patients is considered, because it is most effective when done during the adolescent growth spurt. A reliable assessment of skeletal age must be based on the maturational status of markers within the skeletal system.

The ossification of the bones of the hand and the wrist was, for many years, the standard for skeletal development (Fig. 3.11). A radiograph of the hand and wrist provides a view of some 30 small bones, all of which have a predictable sequence of ossification. Although a view of no single bone is diagnostic, an assessment of the level of development of the bones in the wrist, hand, and fingers can give an accurate picture of a child's skeletal development status. To do this, a hand-wrist radiograph of the patient is simply compared with standard radiographic images in an atlas of the development of the hand and wrist.[16] It has been shown that stages of hand-wrist development correlate reasonably well with the adolescent spurt in the growth of the mandible. Unfortunately, general practitioners do not have the capability to obtain a hand-wrist radiograph and general dentists and most orthodontists do not engage in this type of radiographic assessment often enough to be reliable. There is also

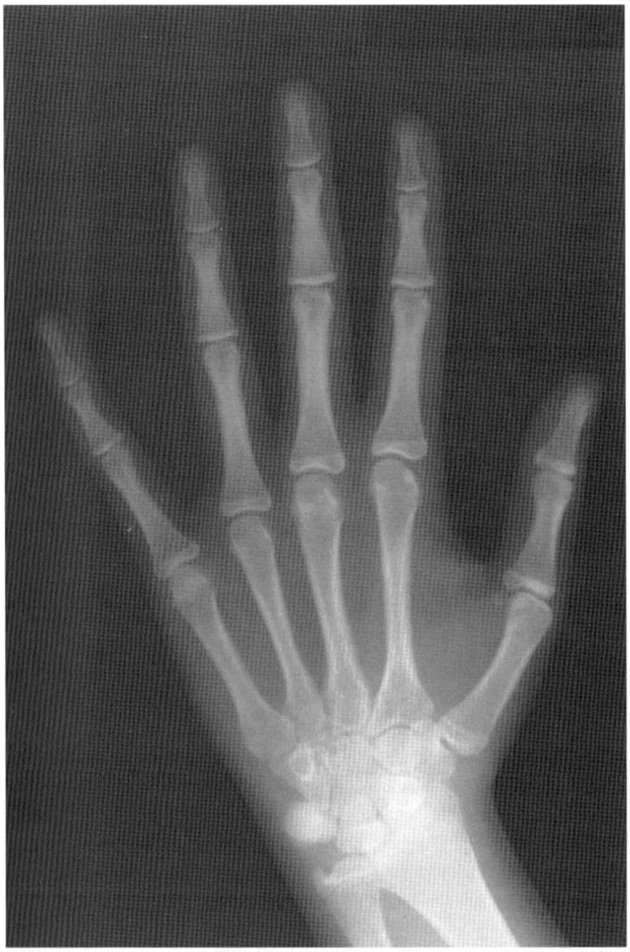

• **Fig. 3.11** A radiograph of the hand and wrist can be used to assess skeletal age by comparing the degree of ossification of the wrist, hand, and finger bones to plates in a standard atlas of hand and wrist development. Knowledge and experience with the technique are required for reliability.

an additional radiation burden for an image that does not precisely address mandibular growth.

A similar assessment of skeletal age based on the cervical vertebrae, as seen in a cephalometric radiograph (the cervical vertebral maturation [CVM] method), has been developed.[17] The characteristics on which vertebral aging is based are described and illustrated in Fig. 3.12. Because cephalometric radiographs are obtained routinely for orthodontic patients, this method has the advantage over hand-wrist radiographs that additional radiation exposure is not needed to judge the probable timing of the adolescent growth spurt of the *mandible*. Although some reports have questioned the reliability of skeletal age derived from the cervical vertebrae,[18] several other studies of CVM have concluded that intraobserver and interobserver reliability are adequate.[19,20]

The question of the validity of the method has been raised by using similar longitudinal datasets of radiographs to evaluate the diagnostic capability of the method. These studies have not been supportive of the method as a strong diagnostic tool.[21,22] with more than one study concluding that chronologic age is as good a predictor as the CVM method.[21,23] A reasonable summary of the current data is that (1) the improvement in assessing growth status relative to peak growth at adolescence from using hand-wrist radiographs, if any, is not worth the extra radiation except in special circumstances, and (2) CVM may not be much better than chronologic age that should be supported by growth data and observations of secondary sexual characteristic development.[21,23,24]

Developmental ages based on any criteria can be established, if there is some scale against which a child's progress can be measured. For instance, one could measure a child's position on a scale of behavior, equating behavior of certain types as appropriate for 5- or 7-year-olds. In fact, behavioral age can be important in the dental treatment of children because it is difficult to render satisfactory treatment if the child cannot be induced to behave appropriately and cooperate. The assessment of behavioral age is covered more completely in the section on social and behavioral development in Chapter 2.

The correlation between developmental ages of all types and chronologic age is quite good, as biological correlations go (Fig. 3.13). For most developmental indicators, the correlation coefficient between developmental status and chronologic age is about 0.8. The ability to predict one characteristic from another varies as the square of the correlation coefficient, so the probability that one could predict the developmental stage from knowing the chronologic age or vice versa is $(0.8)^2 = 0.64$. You would have two chances out of three of predicting one from the other. The correlation of dental age with chronologic age (discussed in detail later) is not quite as good, at about 0.7, which means that there is only about a 50% chance of predicting the stage of dental development from the chronologic age.

It is interesting that the developmental ages correlate better among themselves than the developmental ages correlate with chronologic age. The chances are that a child who is advanced in one characteristic—skeletal age, for instance—is advanced in others as well. The mature-looking and maturely behaving 8-year-old child is quite likely, in other words, also to have an advanced skeletal age and is reasonably likely to have precocious development of the dentition. What will actually occur in any one individual is subject to the almost infinite variety of human variation, and the magnitude of the correlation coefficients must be kept in mind.

Eruption of the Permanent Teeth

Humans are diphyodont meaning they possess two dentitions, the primary and permanent. Since teeth do not increase in size, more teeth and bigger teeth help accommodate the growing jaws. The eruption of any tooth can be divided into several stages. This includes the primary teeth. The physiologic principles underlying eruption that are discussed in this section are not different for the primary teeth, despite the root resorption that eventually causes their loss. The nature of eruption and its control before the emergence of the tooth into the mouth are somewhat different after emergence, and we will consider these major stages separately.

Preemergent Eruption

During the period when the crown of a tooth is being formed, there is a very slow labial or buccal drift of the tooth follicle within the bone, but this follicular drift is not attributed to the eruption mechanism itself. In fact, the amount of change in the position of the tooth follicle is extremely small, observable only with vital staining experiments, and so small that a follicle can be used as a natural marker in radiographic studies of growth. Preemergent eruption begins with the appearance of the dental lamina and continues just prior to the start of root dentin formation. There are multiple

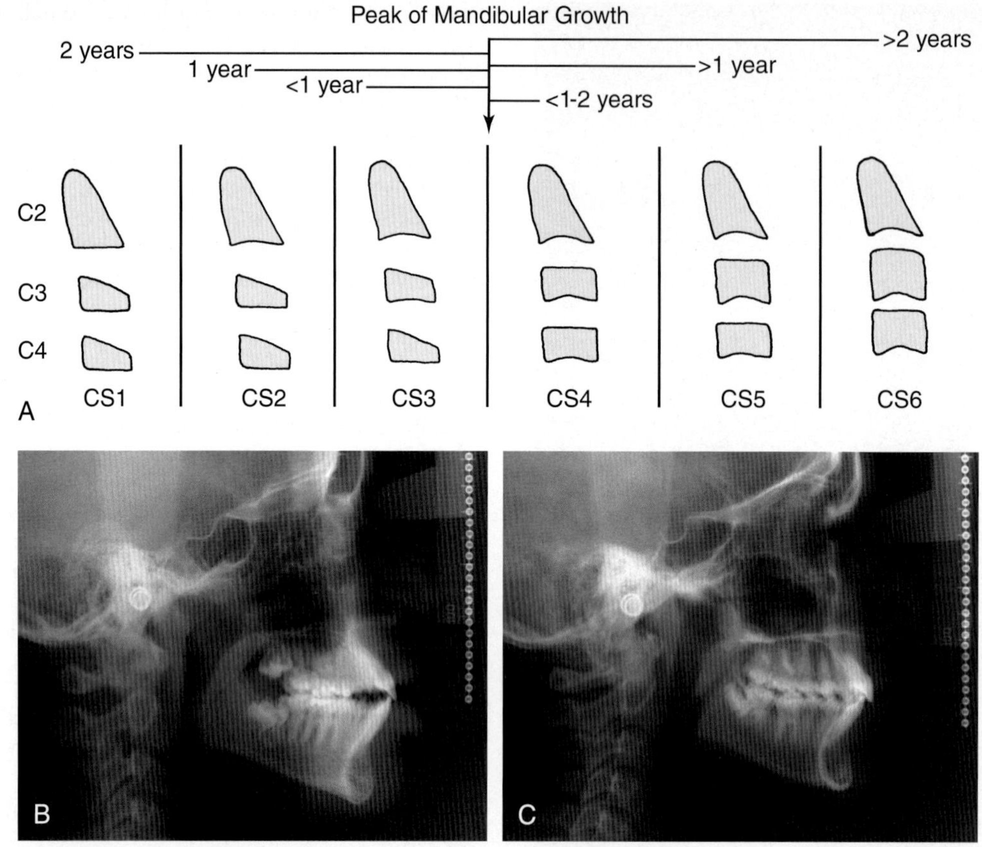

• **Fig. 3.12** Vertebral ages calculated from the image of the cervical vertebrae seen in a lateral cephalometric radiograph. (A) Diagrammatic drawings and relationships of the stages to the peak of mandibular growth. (B) Stage 3, which on average occurs less than 1 year prior to peak growth. (C) Stage 4, typically a year or so beyond peak growth. For a patient with a severe skeletal problem, especially excessive mandibular growth, the best way to determine the cessation of growth is serial cephalometric radiographs. (A, From Baccetti T, Franchi L, McNamara JA Jr. The cervical vertebral maturation (CVM) method for the assessment of optimal treatment timing in dentofacial orthopedics. *Semin Orthod*. 2005;11:119–129.)

signaling factors that control this tightly regulated process.[25] The number of roots and root canals are determined at this stage. Soon after the formation of the root is initiated, the tooth will begin to move occlusally and erupt into the oral cavity. During this occlusal movement, root dentin, cementum, and the periodontal ligament (PDL) are formed. Histological evidence demonstrates a fusion of the oral epithelium and reduced enamel epithelium overlying the erupting crown, contributing to epithelial continuity as the crown erupts. This is why tooth eruption through the gingiva is not coincident with extreme hemorrhaging. This supports the idea that metabolic activity within the PDL is necessary for eruption.

Two processes are necessary for preemergent eruption. First, there must be resorption of bone and primary tooth roots overlying the crown of the erupting tooth; second, a propulsive mechanism then must move the tooth in the direction where the path has been cleared (Fig. 3.14). Although the two mechanisms normally operate in concert, in some circumstances they do not. Investigations of the results of a failure of bone resorption, or alternately a failure of the propulsive mechanism when bone resorption is normal, have yielded considerable insight into the control of preemergent eruption. Loss of the primary tooth is called shedding or exfoliation, mediated by resorption of the bone around the teeth, resorption of the primary roots, and disintegration of the PDL around primary teeth.

Defective bone resorption occurs in a mutant species of mice, appropriately labeled *ia*, for *incisors absent*. In these animals a lack of bone resorption means that the incisor teeth cannot erupt, and they never appear in the mouth. Failure of teeth to erupt because of a failure of bone resorption also occurs in humans, as, for instance, in the syndrome of cleidocranial dysplasia (Fig. 3.15). In children with this condition, not only is resorption of primary teeth and bone deficient but heavy fibrous gingiva and multiple supernumerary teeth also impede normal eruption. The effect is to mechanically block the succedaneous teeth (those replacing primary teeth) from erupting. If the interferences are removed, the teeth often erupt and can be brought into occlusion.

It has been demonstrated experimentally in animals that the rate of bone resorption and the rate of tooth eruption are not controlled physiologically by the same mechanism. For instance, if the tooth bud of a dog premolar is wired to the lower border of the mandible, the tooth can no longer erupt because of this mechanical obstruction, but resorption of overlying bone proceeds at the usual rate, resulting in a large cystic cavity overlying the ligated tooth bud.

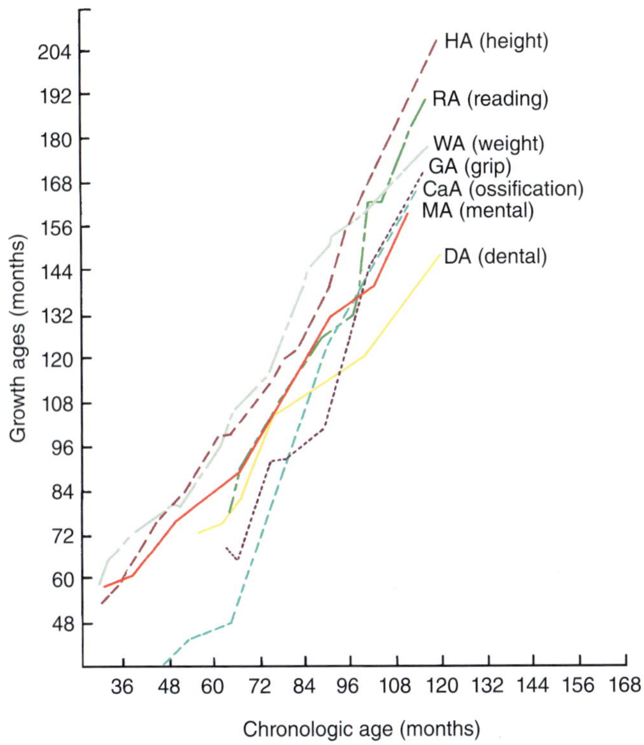

• **Fig. 3.13** Changes in various developmental parameters for one normal child. Note that this child was advanced for their chronologic age in essentially all the parameters and that all are reasonably well correlated. For this individual, as for many children, dental age correlated less well with the group of developmental indicators than any of the others. (Redrawn from Lowery GH. *Growth and Development of Children*. 6th ed. Year Book Medical Publishers; 1973.)

On several occasions, the same experiment has inadvertently been done to a child. If an unerupted permanent tooth is wired to the adjacent bone when a jaw fracture is repaired, as in the child shown in Fig. 3.16, the result is the same as in the animal experiments: the eruption of the tooth stops, but bone resorption to clear an eruption path continues.

It seems clear, therefore, that resorption is the rate-limiting factor in preemergent eruption. Normally, the overlying bone and primary teeth resorb, and the propulsive mechanism then moves the tooth into the space created by the resorption. The signal for resorption of bone over the crown of the tooth is activated by the completion of the crown, which also removes inhibition of the genes that are necessary for root formation as well as inhibition of the layer of osteoclasts that forms just above the top of the crown and creates the eruption path. Because resorption is the controlling factor, active formation of the root is not necessary for continued clearance of an eruption path or for movement of a tooth along it. A tooth will continue to erupt after its apical area has been removed, so the proliferation of cells associated with the lengthening of the root is not an essential part of the mechanism. Normally, the rate of eruption is such that the apical area remains at the same place while the crown moves occlusally, but if the eruption is mechanically blocked, the proliferating apical area will move in the opposite direction, inducing resorption where it usually does not occur (Fig. 3.17). This often causes a distortion of root form, which is called *dilaceration.*

The same pattern of unerupted teeth that do not follow the eruption path that has been cleared for them is also seen in the rare but now well-documented human syndrome called primary failure of eruption (PFE)[26] (see Fig. 12.4). In these patients, however, the reason for the eruption failure is different. The teeth are not mechanically prevented from eruption because when they are surgically exposed, there is no evidence of ankylosis. Instead, it appears that the propulsive mechanism that moves the tooth along the eruption path is defective. A mutation in the parathyroid hormone receptor gene *(PTHR1)* that leads to this condition has been identified, and a genetic test to confirm the diagnosis is possible, but family studies indicate that other genes are involved and the specific mutation that has been identified is not found in all patients.[27] The involved teeth do not respond to orthodontic force and cannot be moved

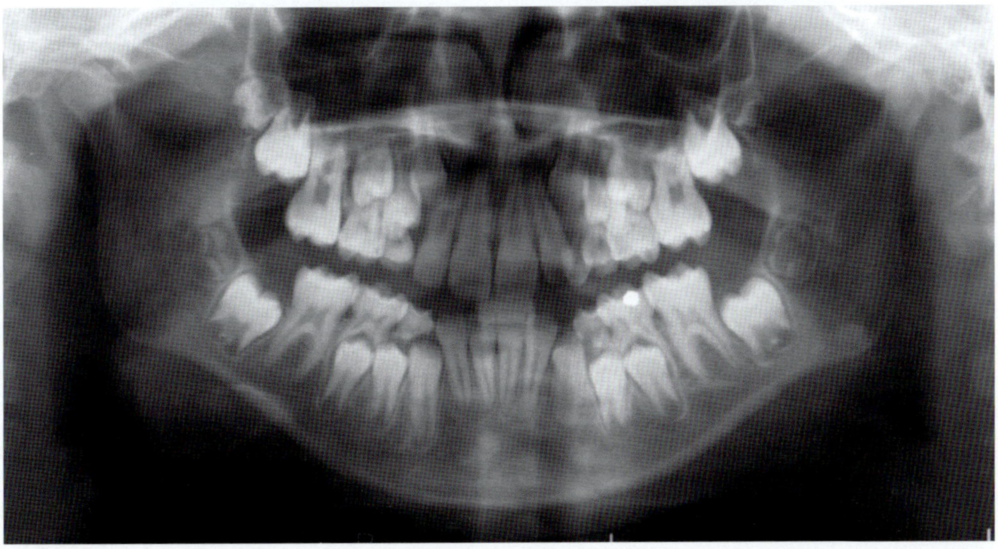

• **Fig. 3.14** Panoramic radiograph of normal eruption in a 10-year-old boy. Note that the permanent teeth erupt as resorption of overlying primary teeth and bone occurs. Resorption must occur to make eruption possible.

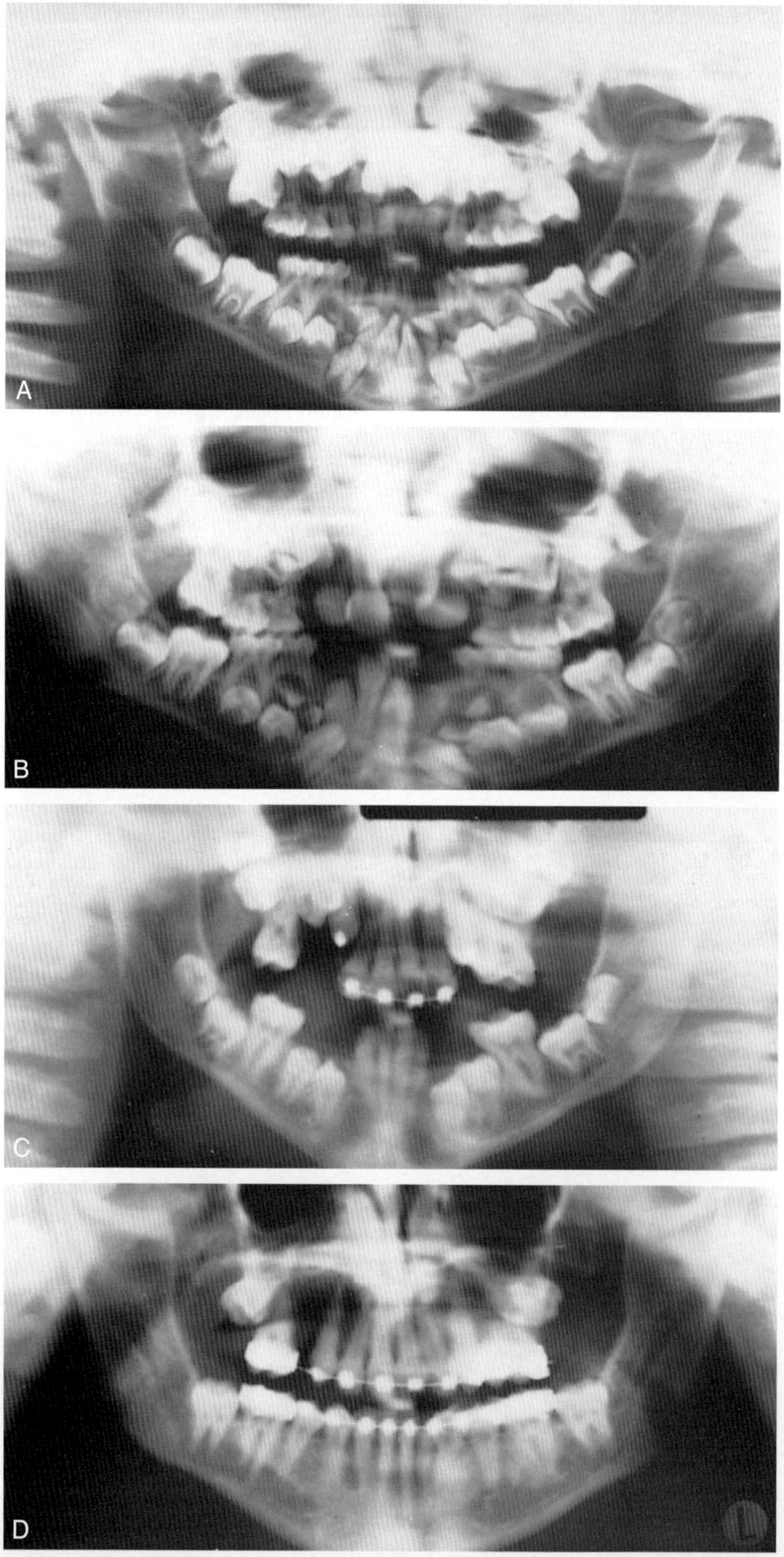

• **Fig. 3.15** (A) Panoramic radiograph of an 8-year-old patient with cleidocranial dysplasia, showing the characteristic features of this condition. In cleidocranial dysplasia, the succedaneous teeth do not erupt because of abnormal resorption of both bone and primary teeth, and the eruption of nonsuccedaneous teeth is delayed by fibrotic gingiva. Supernumerary teeth often are also present, as in this patient, creating additional mechanical obstruction. If the obstruction to eruption is removed, the teeth may erupt spontaneously and can be brought into the arch with orthodontic force if they do not. (B) Age 10, after surgical removal of primary and supernumerary incisors and uncovering of the permanent incisors. (C) Age 14, after orthodontic treatment to bring the incisors into the mouth and surgical removal of primary canines and molars, as well as supernumerary teeth in that area. (D) Age 16, toward the completion of orthodontic treatment to bring the remaining teeth into occlusion. The maxillary right second premolar became ankylosed, but the other teeth responded satisfactorily to treatment.

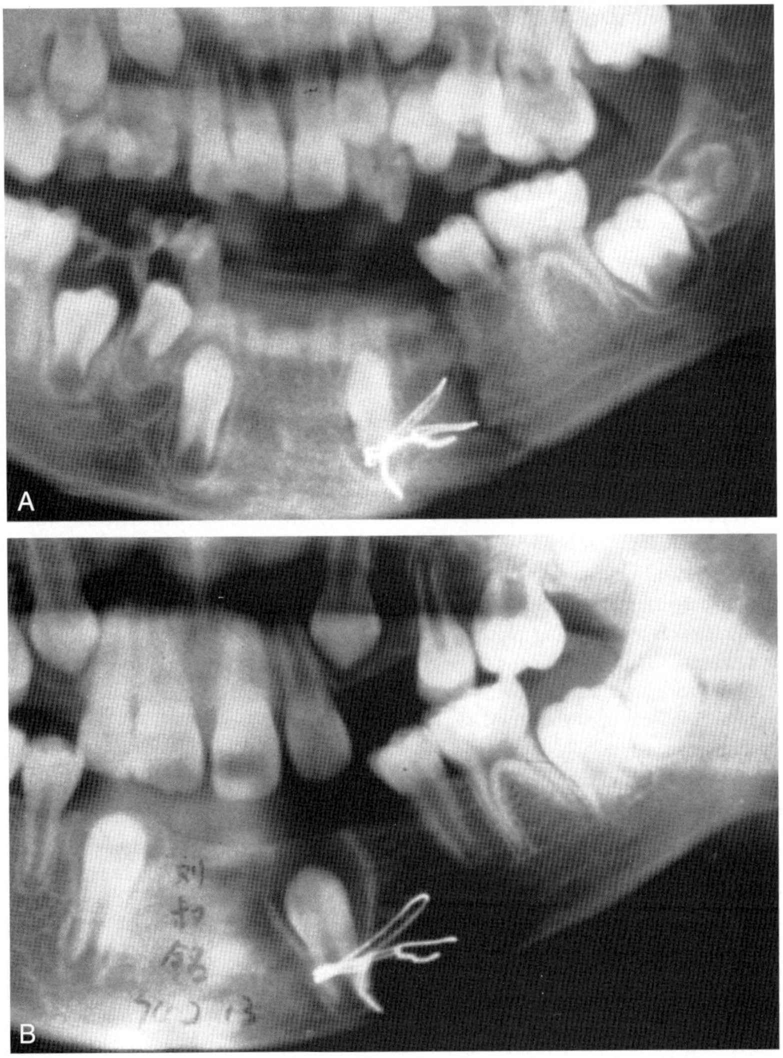

• **Fig. 3.16** Radiographs of a boy whose mandible was fractured at age 10. (A) Immediately after the fracture, when osseous wires were placed to stabilize the bony segments. One of the wires inadvertently pinned the mandibular left canine to the bone, simulating Cahill's experiments with animals. (B) One year later. Note that resorption over the canine has proceeded normally, clearing its eruption path even though it has not moved. (Courtesy Dr. John Lin.)

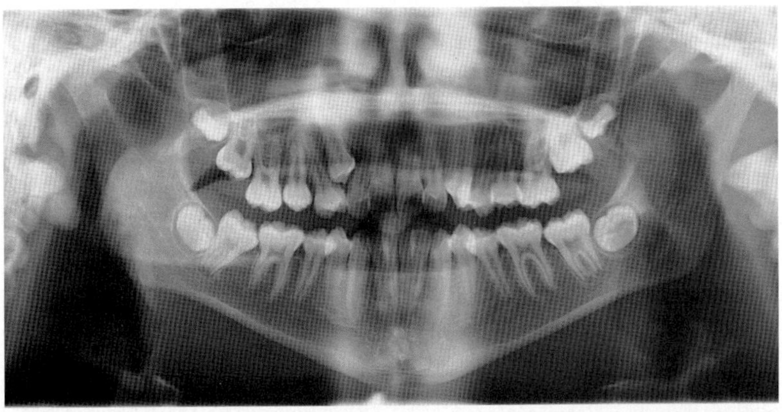

• **Fig. 3.17** In this 11-year-old boy, note the curvature of the root apex of the maxillary right lateral incisor. Deformation of the shape of a tooth root is called *dilaceration* and can occur at various levels of root development and be mid, moderate as shown here, or significantly more severe. It usually occurs as the eruption of a tooth is impeded, but a tooth can continue to erupt normally after dilaceration occurs.

into position, which is evidence of an abnormality in the PDL. The diagnosis and the management of patients with PFE are discussed in Chapter 12.

Despite many years of study, the precise mechanism through which the propulsive force is generated remains unknown. Several studies have shown that the mechanisms of tooth eruptive movement are multifactorial processes. Theories include root formation, bone remodeling, dental follicle, PDL, and molecular determinants. Current research indicates the dental follicle plays a key role in eruptive tooth movement, as the follicle facilitates connective tissue degradation and bony resorption. If the follicle is removed, the eruption is prevented. A classic study by Marks and Cahill in 1984 demonstrated in canine models that if the tooth was removed and replaced by an inert object within an intact follicle, the object would erupt into the oral cavity.[28] The dental follicle mediates bone remodeling through differentiation into osteoblasts and recruitment and activation of osteoclasts, creating an eruptive pathway for the tooth.[29–31] It appears that the mechanism of eruption before the emergence of a tooth into the mouth and the mechanism after a tooth has emerged are different. From animal studies, it is known that substances that interfere with the development of cross-links in maturing collagen also interfere with eruption, which makes it tempting to theorize that cross-linking of maturing collagen in the PDL provides the propulsive force. This seems to be the case after a tooth comes into function, but the collagen fibers are not well organized before the emergence of a tooth into the oral environment—which means that collagen maturation cannot be the primary mechanism to move a tooth along its preemergent eruption path.

Other possibilities for the preemergent propulsive mechanism besides collagen maturation are localized variations in blood pressure or flow, forces derived from contraction of fibroblasts, and alterations in the extracellular ground substances of the PDL similar to those that occur in thixotropic gels.[32]

Postemergent Eruption

Once a tooth has emerged into the mouth, it erupts rapidly until it approaches the occlusal level and is subjected to the forces of mastication. At that point, its eruption slows and then as it reaches the occlusal level of other teeth and is in complete function, eruption all but halts. The stage of the relatively rapid eruption from the time a tooth first penetrates the gingiva until it reaches the occlusal level is called the *postemergent spurt*, in contrast to the following phase of the very slow eruption, termed the *juvenile occlusal equilibrium*.

In the 1990s, new instrumentation made it possible to track the short-term movements of a tooth during the postemergent spurt, and this showed that eruption occurs only during a critical period between 8:00 and midnight or 1:00 a.m. (Fig. 3.18).[33] During the early morning hours and the day, the tooth stops erupting and often intrudes slightly. The day-night differences in eruption seem to reflect an underlying circadian rhythm, probably related to the very similar cycle of growth hormone release. Experiments with the application of pressure against an erupting premolar suggest that eruption is stopped by force for only 1 to 3 minutes, so food contacts with the erupting tooth, even though it is out of contact with its antagonist, almost surely do not explain the daily rhythm.[34] In humans, the eruption of premolars that are moving from gingival emergence toward occlusion has been shown to be affected by changing blood flow in the apical area. This suggests that blood flow is at least a contributing factor in the eruption mechanism up to that point.[35]

The eruption mechanism may be different after emergence—collagen cross-linking in the PDL is more prominent after a tooth

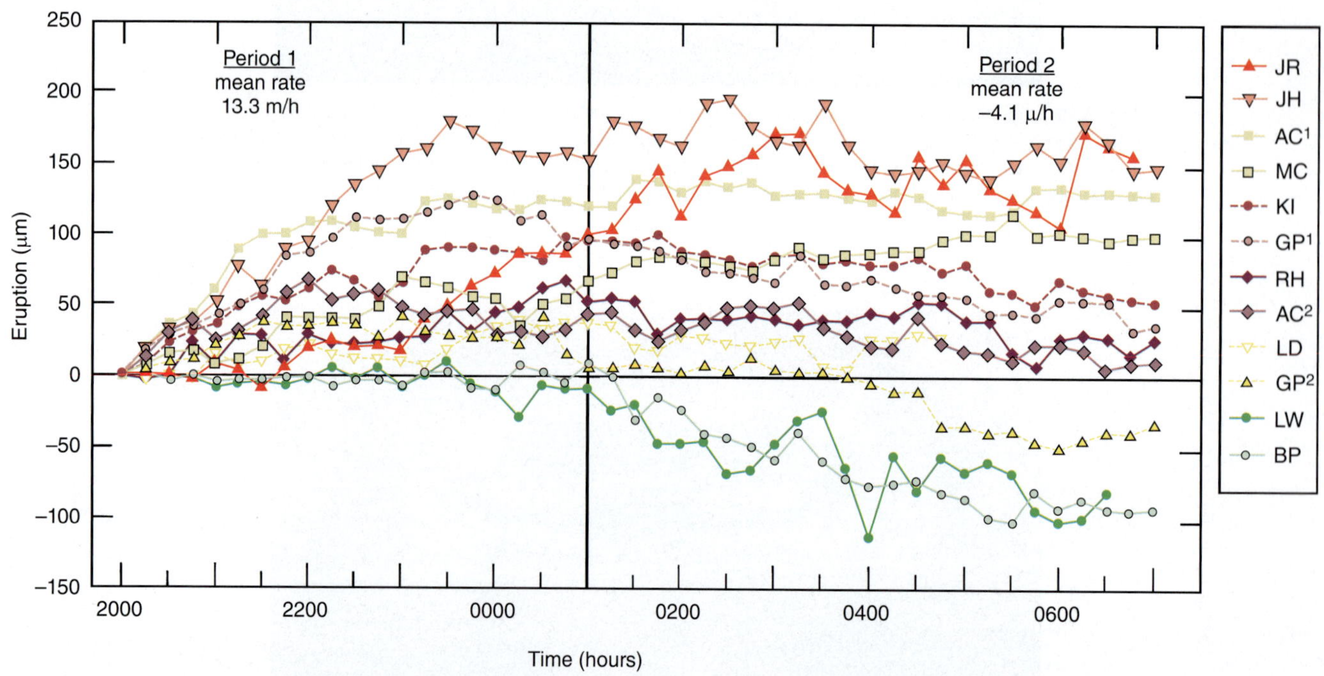

• **Fig. 3.18** Eruption plots for human second premolars observed via a fiber optic cable to a video microscope, which provides 1- to 2-µm resolution, from 8:00 p.m. (2000) to 6 a.m. (0600). Note the consistent pattern of eruption in the early evening, trailing off to no eruption or intrusion toward midnight, with no further eruption after that. It now is clear that eruption occurs only during a few critical hours in the early evening. (Redrawn from Risinger RK, Proffit WR. Continuous overnight observation of human premolar eruption. *Arch Oral Biol*. 1996;41:779–786.)

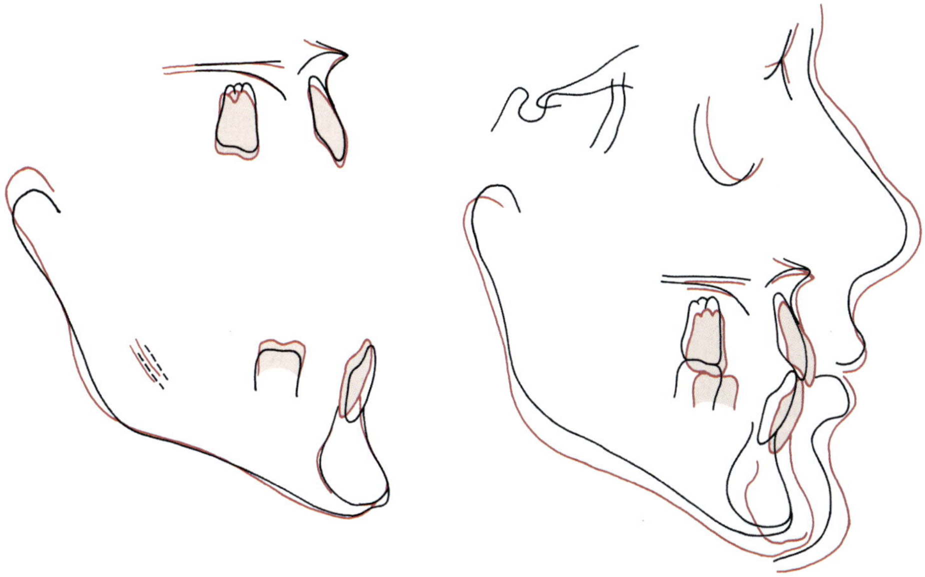

• **Fig. 3.19** The amount of tooth eruption after the teeth have come into occlusion equals the vertical growth of the ramus in a patient who is growing normally. Vertical growth increases the space between the jaws, and the maxillary and mandibular teeth normally divide this space equally. Note the equivalent eruption of the upper and lower molars in this patient between age 10 *(black)* and 14 *(red)*. This is a normal growth pattern.

has come into occlusal function, so shortening of collagen fibers as the mechanism seems more likely—and the control mechanism is certainly different. It seems obvious that as a tooth is subjected to biting forces that oppose eruption, the overall rate of eruption would be slowed, and in fact exactly this occurs. In humans, after the teeth have reached the occlusal level, eruption becomes almost imperceptibly slow, although it continues. During the juvenile equilibrium, teeth that are in function erupt at a rate that parallels the rate of vertical growth of the mandibular ramus (Fig. 3.19). As the mandible continues to grow, it moves away from the maxilla, creating a space into which the teeth erupt. Exactly how eruption is controlled so that it matches mandibular growth, however, is not known, and because some of the more difficult orthodontic problems arise when eruption does not coincide with growth; this is an important area for further study.

Functional loading through mastication stimulates the maturation and arrangement of the PDL fibers. Continued dentin formation and cementum formation occur with a change in movement in the mesial direction. Environmental factors can determine the final position of the teeth within the dental arch. Muscle forces from the cheeks, tongue, and lips can play a role. As previously discussed, prolonged digit sucking can also contribute to final tooth position. Teeth that do not have a tooth to oppose eruption will continue to erupt. This is known as supereruption. If this occurs to a significant amount, the teeth will need to be intruded orthodontically with the use of fixed appliances, auxiliaries, or temporary anchorage devices (TADs) to restore normal vertical occlusion.

The amount of eruption necessary to compensate for jaw growth can best be appreciated by observing what happens when a tooth becomes ankylosed (i.e., fused to the alveolar bone). An ankylosed tooth appears to submerge over a period as the other teeth continue to erupt while it remains at the same vertical level (Fig. 3.20). The total eruption path of a first permanent molar is about 2.5 cm. Of that distance, nearly half is traversed after the tooth has reached the occlusal level and is in function. If a first molar becomes ankylosed at an early age, which fortunately is rare, it can "submerge" to such an extent that the tooth is covered over again by the gingiva as other teeth erupt and bring alveolar bone along with them (Fig. 3.21).

Because the rate of eruption parallels the rate of jaw growth, it is not surprising that a pubertal spurt in the eruption of the teeth accompanies the pubertal spurt in jaw growth. This reinforces the concept that after a tooth is in occlusion, the rate of eruption is controlled by the forces opposing eruption, not those promoting it. After a tooth is in the mouth, the forces opposing eruption are those from chewing, and, perhaps in addition, soft tissue pressures from lips, cheeks, or tongue contacting the teeth. If eruption occurs only during quiet periods, the soft tissue pressures (from tongue position during sleep, for instance) probably are more important in controlling eruption than the heavy pressures during chewing. Light pressures of long duration are more important in producing orthodontic tooth movement (see Chapter 8), so it also seems logical that light but prolonged pressures might affect eruption. What would be the source of this type of pressure? Perhaps the way the tongue is positioned between the teeth during sleep?

When the pubertal growth spurt ends, a final phase in tooth eruption called the *adult occlusal equilibrium* is achieved. During adult life, teeth continue to erupt at an extremely slow rate. If its antagonist is lost at any age, a tooth can again erupt more rapidly, demonstrating that the eruption mechanism remains active and capable of producing significant tooth movement even later in life.

Wear of the teeth may become significant as the years pass. If extremely severe wear occurs, eruption may not compensate for the loss of tooth structure, so that the vertical dimension of the face decreases. In most individuals, however, any wear of the teeth is compensated for by additional eruption, and face height remains constant or even increases slightly in the fourth, fifth, and sixth decades of life (see the section on maturation and aging in Chapter 4).

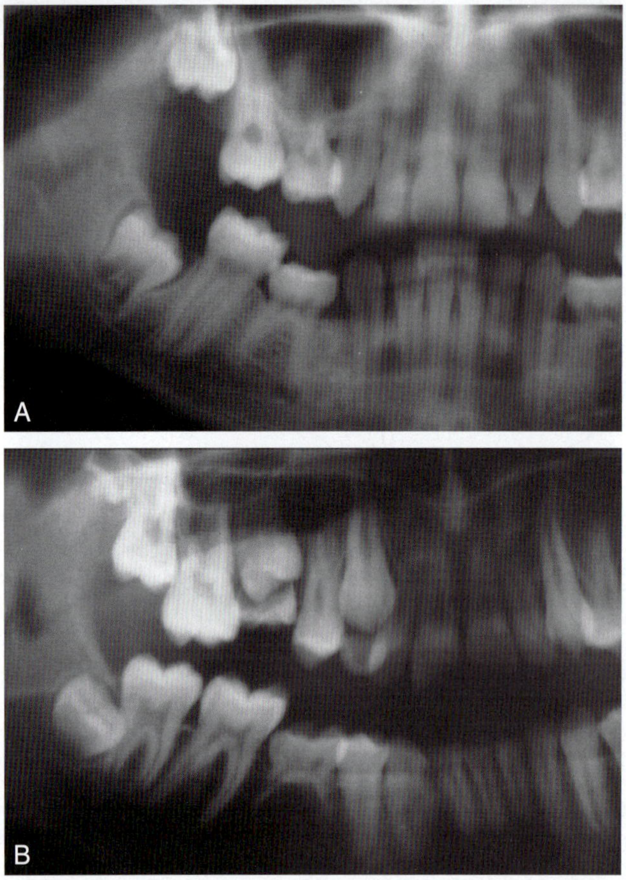

• **Fig. 3.20** (A) In this patient whose premolars were congenitally absent, the primary mandibular right second molar became ankylosed well before eruption of the other teeth was completed. Its apparent submergence is really because the other teeth have erupted past it. Note that the permanent lower first molar has tipped mesially over the submerged primary molar. The primary maxillary second molar has erupted along with the permanent canine and first molar. (B) In this patient an ankylosed primary maxillary second molar has delayed eruption of the second premolar but is resorbing, and the primary mandibular second molar that has no permanent successor also is ankylosed and submerging.

Eruption Sequence and Timing: Dental Age

The transition from the primary to the permanent dentition, which is summarized in Table 3.2, begins at about age 6 with the eruption of the permanent first molars, followed soon thereafter by the permanent incisors. The permanent teeth tend to erupt in groups, and it is less important to know the most common eruption sequence than to know the expected time at which various groups of teeth appear. This information is used in the calculation of dental age, which is particularly important during the mixed dentition years. Dental age is determined from three characteristics. The first is which teeth have erupted. The second and third, which are closely related, are the amount of resorption of the roots of primary teeth and the amount of development of the permanent teeth.

The amount of eruption of permanent teeth at dental age 6 is illustrated in Fig. 3.22. The most common sequence of eruption is the mandibular central incisor, closely followed by the permanent

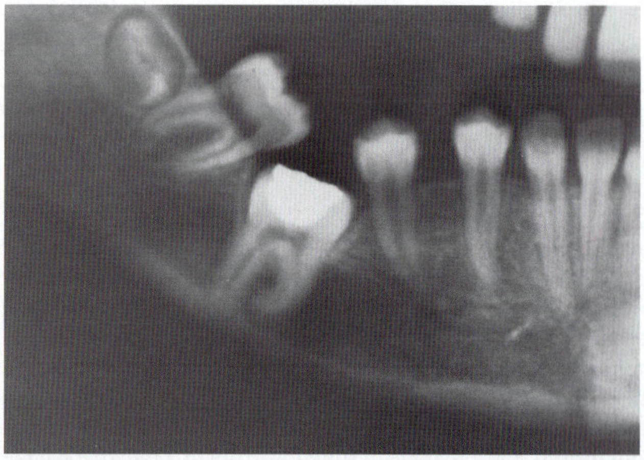

• **Fig. 3.21** The first molar in this 15-year-old girl ceased erupting soon after its emergence into the mouth at age 6 or 7. When the dentist placed an occlusal restoration, the tooth was apparently in or near occlusion, well into the oral cavity. This dramatically illustrates the amount of eruption that must occur after the initial occlusal contact of first molars.

TABLE 3.2 Chronology of Tooth Development, Permanent Dentition

	CALCIFICATION BEGINS		CROWN COMPLETED		ERUPTION		ROOT COMPLETED	
Tooth	Maxillary	Mandibular	Maxillary (years)	Mandibular (years)	Maxillary (years)	Mandibular (years)	Maxillary (years)	Mandibular (years)
Central	3 months	3 months	4½	3½	7¼	6¼	10½	9½
Lateral	11 months	3 months	5½	4	8¼	7½	11	10
Canine	4 months	4 months	6	5¾	11	9	13½	12¾
First premolar	20 months	22 months	7	6¾	10¼	10½	13½	13½
Second premolar	27 months	28 months	7¾	7½	11	11¼	14½	15
First molar	32 weeks in utero	32 weeks in utero	4¼	3¾	6¼	6	10½	10½
Second molar	27 months	27 months	7¾	7½	12½	12	15¾	16
Third molar	8 years	9 years	14	14	20	20	22	22

mandibular first molar and the permanent maxillary first molar. These teeth normally erupt at so nearly the same time, however, that it is within normal variation for the first molars to slightly precede the mandibular central incisors or vice versa. Usually, the mandibular molar will precede the maxillary molar. The beginning eruption of this group of teeth characterizes dental age 6.

At dental age 7, the maxillary central incisors and the mandibular lateral incisors erupt. The maxillary central incisor is usually a year behind the mandibular central incisor but erupts simultaneously with the mandibular lateral incisor. At this age, root formation of the maxillary lateral incisor is well advanced, but it is still about 1 year from the eruption, while the canines and premolars are still in the stage of crown completion or just at the beginning of root formation.

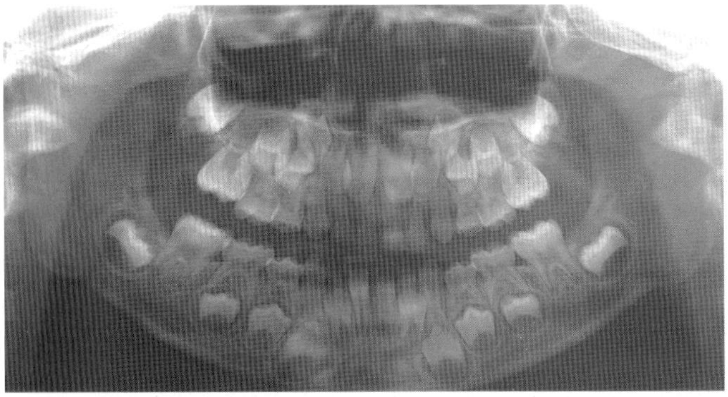

• **Fig. 3.22** This panoramic radiograph of the first stage of eruption of the permanent teeth, at age 6, is characterized by the near-simultaneous eruption of the mandibular central incisors, the mandibular first molars, and the maxillary first molars.

Dental age 8 (Fig. 3.23) is characterized by the eruption of the maxillary lateral incisors. After these teeth come into the arch, there is a delay of 1 to 2 years before any additional permanent teeth appear.

At dental age 9, the mandibular primary canines exfoliate and permanent canines erupt, while the primary first and second molars are present in the mouth (Fig. 3.24). Root development has started on the mandibular second premolar. In the maxillary arch, root development is more advanced on the first premolar than for the canine and the second premolar.

Dental age 10 is characterized by the eruption of the maxillary first premolar and a greater amount of both root resorption of the primary maxillary canines and root development of their permanent successors. The buccal bulge of the maxillary permanent canine should be visible or palpable. At dental age 10, approximately one-half of the root of the mandibular first premolar has been completed, and there is significant root development of the maxillary canine and maxillary and mandibular second premolars.

A tooth usually emerges when about three-fourths of its root has been completed. Thus a signal that a tooth should be appearing in the mouth is root development approaching this level. It takes 2 to 3 years for root formation to be completed after a tooth has erupted into occlusion.

Another indicator of dental age 10, therefore, would be the completion of the roots of the mandibular incisor teeth and near-completion of the roots of the maxillary laterals. By dental age 11,

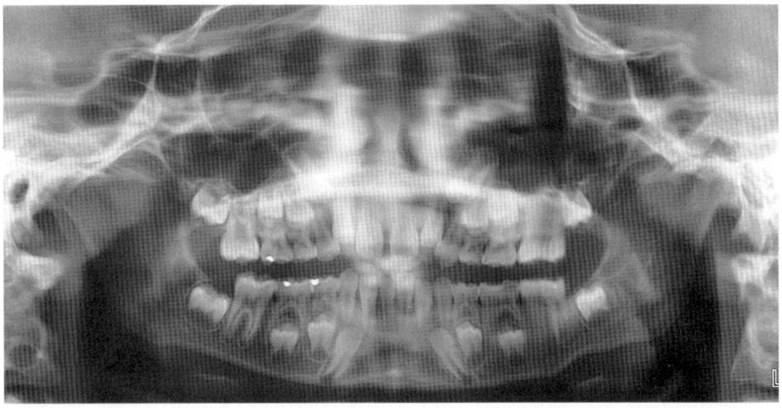

• **Fig. 3.23** Dental age 8 is characterized by eruption of the maxillary lateral incisors.

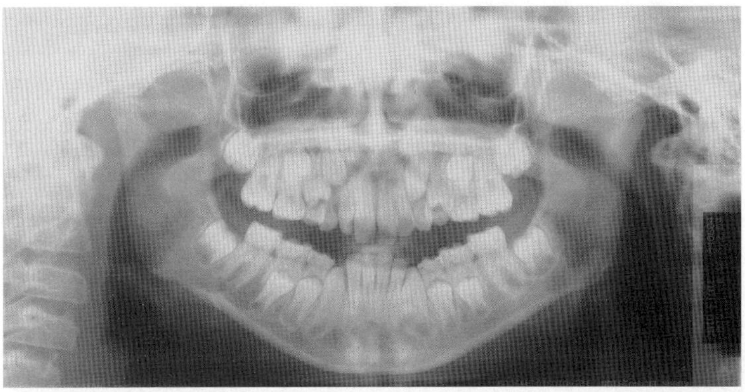

• **Fig. 3.24** At dental age 9, the maxillary lateral incisors have been in place for 1 year, and root formation on other incisors and first molars is nearly complete. Root development of the maxillary canines and all second premolars is advancing; the mandibular canines are erupting.

the roots of all incisors and permanent first molars should be well completed.

Dental age 11 (Fig. 3.25) is characterized by the eruption of another group of teeth: the maxillary canines and mandibular first premolars, which erupt more or less simultaneously. In the mandibular arch, the canine appears ahead of the first premolar. In the maxillary arch, on the other hand, the first premolar usually erupts well ahead of the canine. At dental age 11, the only remaining primary teeth are the maxillary and the mandibular second molars.

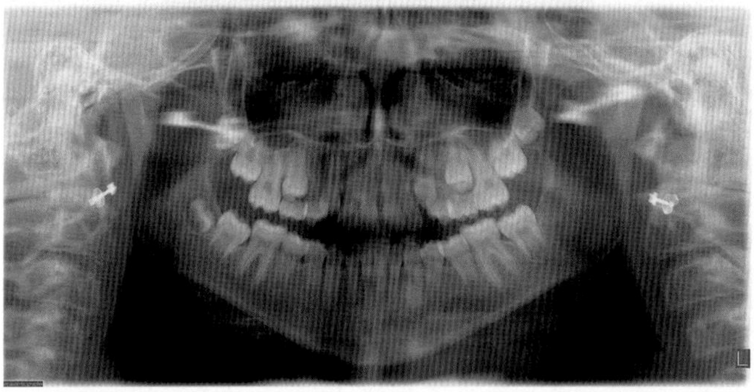

• **Fig. 3.25** Dental age 11 is characterized by the eruption of the maxillary canine following the maxillary first premolars in most cases. The mandibular canines and first premolars are erupted.

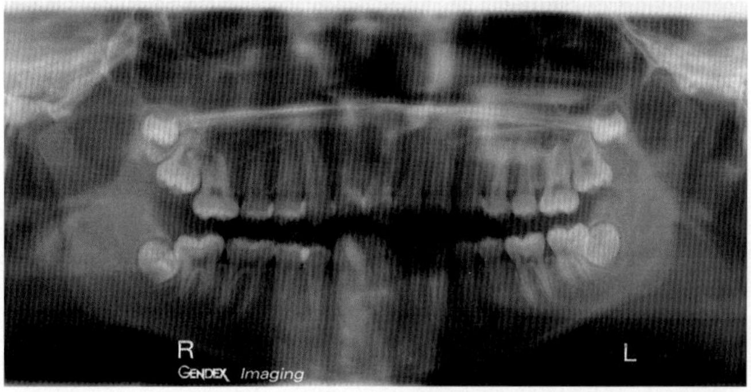

• **Fig. 3.26** Dental age 12 is characterized by eruption of the remaining succedaneous teeth (the maxillary and mandibular second premolars) and typically a few months later, the maxillary and mandibular second molars.

At dental age 12 (Fig. 3.26), the remaining succedaneous permanent teeth erupt. *Succedaneous* refers to permanent teeth that replace primary predecessors; thus a canine is a succedaneous tooth, whereas a first molar is not. In addition, at age 12 the permanent second molars in both arches are nearing eruption. The succedaneous teeth complete their eruption before the emergence of the second molars in most but by no means all normal children. It is usually possible to note the early beginnings of the third molars by age 12, and mineralization of the crown of these teeth begins earlier than that in many children.

Dental ages 13, 14, and 15 are characterized by the extent of completion of the roots of permanent teeth. By dental age 15 (Fig. 3.27), if a third molar is going to form, it should be apparent on the radiographs, and the roots of all other permanent teeth should be complete.

As with all other developmental ages, dental age correlates with chronologic age, but the correlation between dental and chronologic age is one of the weakest. In other words, teeth erupt with a considerable degree of variability from chronologic age standards. It remains true, however, that the teeth erupt in the stages described previously. A child who has precocious dental development might have the mandibular central incisors and first molars erupt at age 5 and could reach dental age 12 by chronologic age 10. A child with slow dental development might not reach dental age 12 until chronologic age 14.

A change in the sequence of eruption is a much more reliable sign of a disturbance in normal development than a generalized delay or acceleration. The more a tooth deviates from its expected position in the sequence, the greater the likelihood of some sort of problem. For example, a delay in the eruption of maxillary canines to age 14 is within normal variation if the second premolars are also delayed, but if the second premolars have erupted at age 12 and the canines have not, something probably is wrong.

Several reasonably normal variations in eruption sequence have clinical significance and should be recognized. These are (1) eruption of second molars ahead of premolars in the mandibular arch, (2) eruption of canines ahead of premolars in the maxillary arch, and (3) unusually large asymmetries in eruption between the right and left sides.

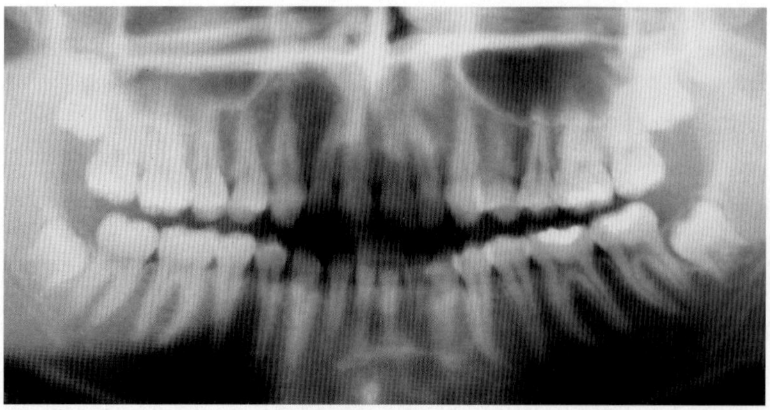

• **Fig. 3.27** By dental age 15, the roots of all permanent teeth except the third molars are complete, and crown formation of third molars often has been completed.

Early eruption of the mandibular second molars can be unfortunate when room to accommodate the teeth is marginal. The eruption of the second molar before the second premolar tends to decrease the space for the second premolar and may lead to its being partially blocked out of the arch. For that reason, when the mandibular second molar erupts early, it may be necessary to open space for the second premolar so that it can complete its eruption.

If a maxillary canine erupts at about the same time as the maxillary first premolar (remember that this is the normal eruption sequence of the lower arch but is abnormal in the upper), the canine probably will be forced labially even if there would have been enough space if it had erupted in the normal sequence. Labial positioning of maxillary canines often occurs when there is an overall lack of space in the arch because this tooth is often the last to erupt normally among the maxillary canine and premolars.

A moderate asymmetry in the rate of eruption on the two sides of the dental arch occurs in almost everyone. A striking illustration of genetic influences on eruption timing is seen in identical twins, who frequently have mirror-image asymmetries in the dentition at the various stages of eruption. For example, if the premolars erupt a little earlier on the left in one of the twins, they will erupt a little earlier on the right in the other. The normal variation is only a few months, however. As a general rule, if a permanent tooth on one side erupts but its counterpart on the other does not within 6 months, a radiograph should be taken to investigate the cause of the discrepancy. Although small variations from one side to the other are normal, large ones often indicate a problem.

It is interesting that an asymmetry in dental age between the two sides of the maxillary arch may be a factor in the development of unilaterally impacted canines. Palatal (but not buccal) canine impaction is more prevalent on the side with delayed development,[36] perhaps because the earlier eruption of the contralateral canine tends to displace the incisors toward the delayed side and decreases space for the eruption of maxillary eruption of that canine. If the delayed canine were positioned buccally, it still could erupt, but if positioned lingually, palatal impaction would be the most likely outcome.

Space Relationships in Replacement of the Incisors

If a dissected skull is examined, in both the maxillary and mandibular arches, the permanent incisor tooth buds lie lingual, as well as apical, to the primary incisors (Fig. 3.28; also see Fig. 3.10). The result is a tendency for the permanent mandibular incisors to erupt somewhat lingually and in a slightly irregular position, even in children who have normal dental arches and normal incisor spacing within the arches. In the maxillary arch, the lateral incisor is likely to be lingually positioned at the time of its emergence and may remain in that position if there is any crowding in the arch. The permanent canines are positioned more nearly in line with the primary canines or slightly facially. If there are problems in eruption, these teeth can be displaced either lingually or labially, but usually they are displaced labially if there is not enough room for them.

The permanent incisor teeth are considerably larger than the primary incisors that they replace. For instance, the permanent mandibular central incisor is about 5.5 mm in width, whereas the primary central it replaces is about 3 mm in width. This is called *incisor liability*. Because the other permanent incisors and canines are each 2 to 3 mm wider than their primary predecessors, spacing between the primary incisors is not only normal, it is critically important (Fig. 3.29). Otherwise, there will not be enough room for the permanent incisors when they erupt. An adult-appearing smile in a child in the primary dentition is an abnormal, not a normal, finding—the spaces are necessary for the alignment of the permanent teeth.

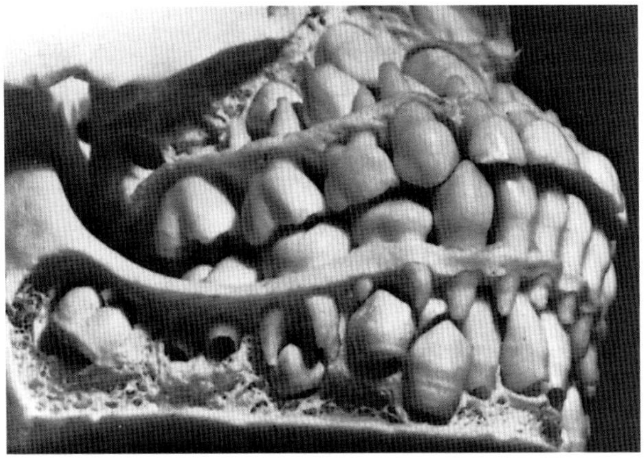

• **Fig. 3.28** This photograph of the dissected skull of a child of approximately 6 years of age shows the relationship of the developing permanent tooth buds to the primary teeth. Note that the permanent incisors are positioned lingual to the roots of the primary incisors, whereas the canines are more labially placed. (From van der Linden FPGM, Deuterloo HS. *Development of the Human Dentition: An Atlas*. Harper & Row; 1976.)

Changes in the amount of space mesial to the canine teeth are shown graphically in Fig. 3.30. Note that a normal child will go through a transitory stage of incisor crowding (up to 2 mm) at age 8 to 9, even if there will eventually be enough room to accommodate all the permanent teeth in good alignment. This is called transitional crowding. Where did the extra space come from? There is no jaw growth in the area where additional space is needed. Moorrees and Chadha showed in a classic study in the 1960s[37] that it comes from three sources:

1. A slight increase in the width of the dental arch across the canines. As growth continues, the teeth erupt not only upward but also slightly outward. This increase is most evident when the lateral incisors erupt. It is small, about 2 mm on average, but it does contribute to the resolution of early crowding of the incisors. More width is gained in the mandibular than the maxillary arch, and more is gained in boys than girls. For this reason, girls have a greater likelihood of incisor crowding, particularly mandibular incisor crowding.
2. Labial positioning of the permanent incisors relative to the primary incisors. Although the permanent incisors may emerge lingually, then drift facially, probably due to tongue pressure. The primary incisors also tend to be quite upright. As the permanent incisors replace them, these teeth lean slightly forward, which arranges them along the arc of a larger circle. Although this change is also small, it contributes 1 to 2 mm of additional space in the average child.
3. Repositioning of mandibular canines. As the permanent incisors erupt, the canines not only widen out but move slightly back into the primate space distal to the canine unless it has been closed by an early mesial shift. The early mesial shift can occur when the permanent first molars erupt and can close the mandibular primate space from the distal.

This primate space, if available, contributes to the slight width increase already noted because the arch is wider posteriorly and provides an extra millimeter of space. Because the primate space in the

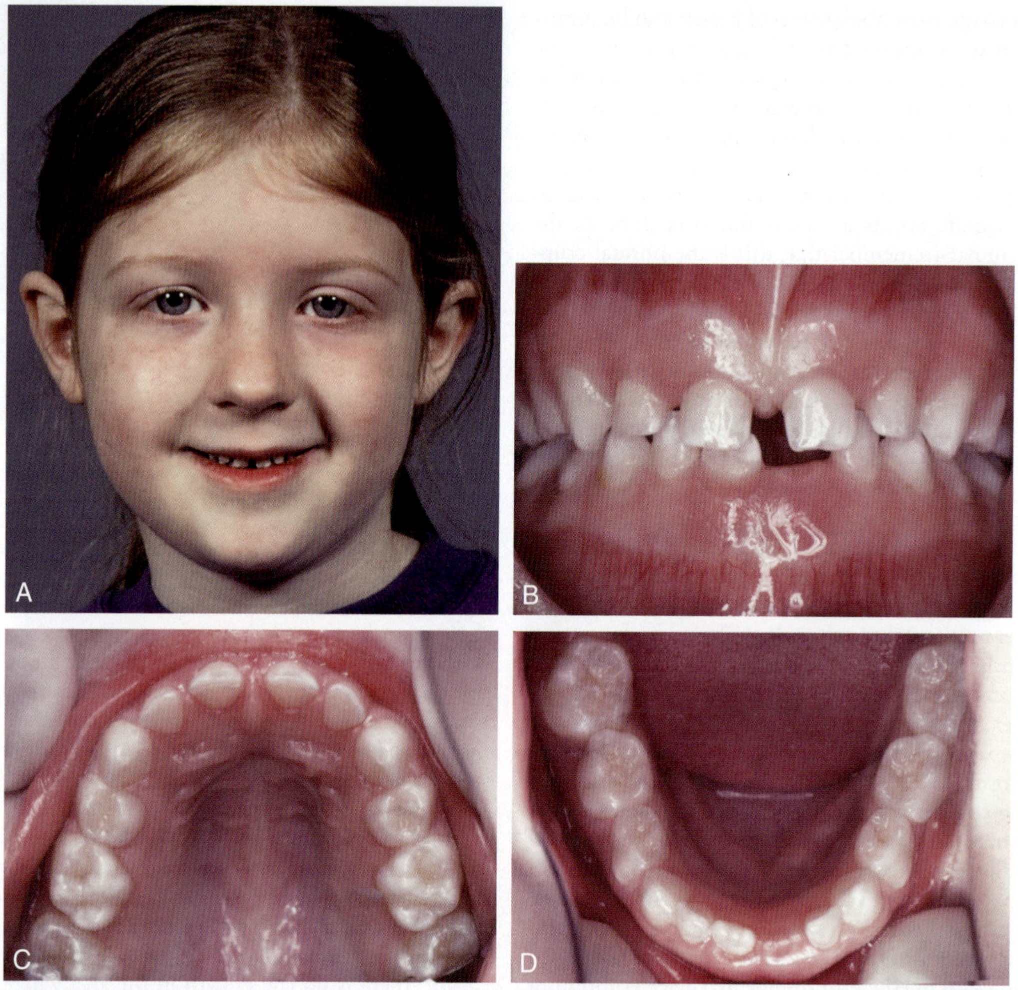

• **Fig. 3.29** (A), Facial and (B–D) intraoral views of a 6-year-old girl, just as the incisor transition is beginning. Spacing of this magnitude between the primary incisors is normal in the late primary dentition and is necessary to provide enough room for alignment of the permanent incisors when they erupt. At age 6, a gap-toothed smile, not a "Hollywood smile" with the teeth in contact, is what you would like to see.

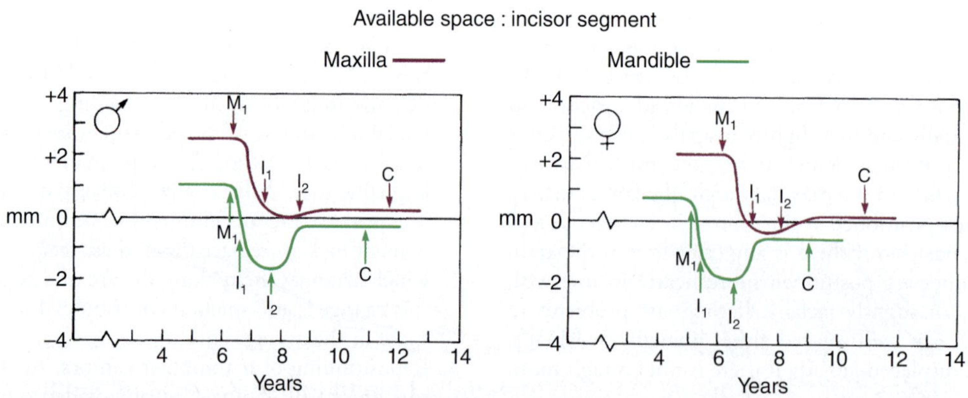

• **Fig. 3.30** Graphical representation of the average amount of space available within the arches in boys *(left)* and girls *(right)*. The time of eruption of the first molar (M_1), central and lateral incisors (I_1 and I_2), and canines *(C)* is shown by *arrows*. Note that in the mandibular arch in both sexes, the space improves as the lateral incisors erupt and the intercanine width improves, but the amount of space for the mandibular incisors in boys and girls is negative for about 2 years prior to that time. This is often referred to as the period of incisor liability. It means that a small amount of crowding in the mandibular arch at this time is normal. (From Moorrees CFA, Chadha JM. Available space for the incisors during dental development—a growth study based on physiologic age. *Angle Orthod*. 1965;35:12–22.)

maxillary arch is mesial to the canine and usually occupied by lateral incisor eruption, there is little opportunity for a similar change in the anteroposterior position of the maxillary canines.

It is important to note that all three of these changes occur without significant skeletal growth in the front of the jaws. The slight increases in arch dimension during normal development are not sufficient to overcome discrepancies of a large magnitude, but in many cases the transitional crowding can be substantial (3–4 mm or more) even when there is sufficient space in the arch perimeter between the mesial surfaces of the permanent first molars. Transitional crowding that is greater than the available arch perimeter between the mesial surfaces of the permanent first molars will either lead to continued crowding or the need to expand the arch dimensions or extract permanent teeth. In fact, crowding of the incisors—the most common form of Angle's class I malocclusion—is by far the most prevalent type of malocclusion.

The mandibular permanent central incisors are almost always in proximal contact from the time that they erupt. In the maxillary arch, however, there may continue to be a space, called a *diastema*, between the permanent maxillary central incisors. A central diastema tends to close as the lateral incisors erupt but may persist even after the lateral incisors have erupted, particularly if the primary canines have been lost or if the upper incisors are flared to the labial. This is another variation in the normal developmental pattern that occurs frequently enough to be almost normal. Because the flared and spaced upper incisors are not very esthetic, this is referred to as the "ugly duckling" stage of development (Fig. 3.31).

The spaces tend to close as the permanent canines erupt. The greater the amount of spacing, the less the likelihood that a maxillary central diastema will totally close on its own. As a general guideline, a maxillary central diastema of 2 mm or less will probably close spontaneously, whereas total closure of a diastema initially greater than 2 mm is unlikely.

Space Relationships in Replacement of Canines and Primary Molars

In contrast to the anterior teeth, the permanent canines are larger than the primary canines and the premolars are smaller than the primary teeth they replace. The primary mandibular second molar is on average 2 mm larger than the second premolar; in the maxillary arch, the primary second molar is 1.5 mm larger (Fig. 3.32).[38] This additional space that came from the transition from the primary second molar to the permanent second premolar is known as the *E space* because the primary second molars were designated as *E* in the United States before the military numbering scheme was widely adopted, and still are in the international tooth numbering scheme. The primary first molar is only slightly larger than the

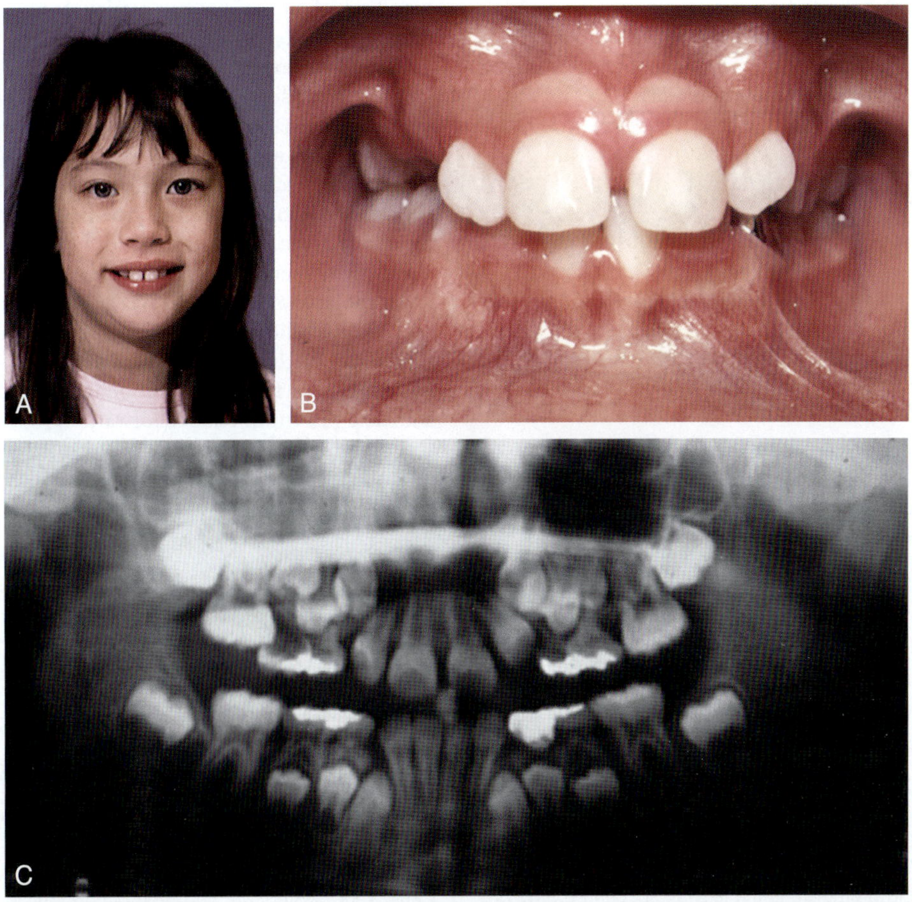

• **Fig. 3.31** In some children, the maxillary incisors flare laterally and are widely spaced when they first erupt, a condition often called the "ugly duckling" stage. (A) Smile appearance, age 9. (B), Dental appearance. (C) Panoramic radiograph. The position of the incisors tends to improve when the permanent canines erupt, but this condition increases the possibility that the canines will become impacted.

first premolar but does contribute an extra 0.5 mm to the mandible. The result is that each side in the mandibular arch on average contains about 2.5 mm of what is called *leeway space;* in the maxillary arch, about 1.5 mm is available on average. But remember that this is just the average, not what would be seen in all patients, so the relative size of the primary and permanent molars should be examined in the panoramic radiograph as decisions about space availability are being made.

When the primary second molars are lost, the permanent first molars move forward (mesially) relatively rapidly into the leeway space, much of which at this point is E space. This decreases both arch length and arch circumference, which are related but not the same thing (Fig. 3.33). Even if incisor crowding is present, the leeway space is normally taken up by the mesial movement of the permanent molars. An opportunity for orthodontic treatment is created at this time because crowding (that substantial 3–4 mm of transitional crowding mentioned earlier) could be relieved by using the leeway space if it were maintained and managed so the molars did not move mesially (see Chapter 11).

Occlusal relationships in the mixed dentition parallel those in the permanent dentition, but the descriptive terms are somewhat different. A normal relationship of the primary molar teeth is the *flush terminal plane* relationship illustrated in Fig. 3.34. In this scenario, the permanent molars are end to end. The primary dentition equivalent of Angle's class II is the *distal step.* A *mesial step* relationship corresponds to Angle's class I. An equivalent of class III is not often seen in the primary dentition because of the normal pattern of craniofacial growth in which mandibular growth lags behind the maxilla. If it is, almost always a large discrepancy in the size of the mandible and maxilla (i.e., a skeletal class III jaw relationship) is present.

At the time the primary second molars are lost, both the maxillary and mandibular molars tend to shift mesially into the leeway space (unless prevented by using the space for transitional crowding), but the mandibular molar normally moves more than its maxillary counterpart. This contributes to the normal transition from a flush terminal plane relationship in the mixed dentition to a class I relationship in the permanent dentition.

Differential growth of the mandible relative to the maxilla is also an important contributor to the molar transition. As discussed earlier, a characteristic of the growth pattern at this age is more growth of the mandible than the maxilla so that a relatively deficient mandible gradually catches up. Conceptually, one can imagine that the upper and lower teeth are mounted on moving platforms and that the platform on which the lower teeth are mounted moves a bit further than the upper platform. This differential growth of the jaws carries the mandible slightly forward relative to the maxilla during the mixed dentition.

If a child has a flush terminal plane molar relationship early in the mixed dentition, about 3.5 mm of movement of the lower molar forward relative to the upper molar is required for a smooth transition to a class I molar relationship in the permanent dentition. About half of this distance can be obtained from the leeway space, which allows greater mesial movement of the mandibular than the maxillary molar. The other half is supplied by differential growth of the lower jaw, carrying the lower molar with it.

Only a modest change in molar relationship can be produced by this combination of differential growth of the jaws and differential forward movement of the lower molar. It must be kept in mind that the changes described here are those that happen to a child experiencing a normal growth pattern. There is no guarantee in any given individual that differential forward growth of the mandible will occur or that the leeway space will close so that the lower molar moves forward relative to the upper molar.

The possibilities for the transition in a molar relationship from the mixed to the early permanent dentition are summarized in Fig. 3.34. Note that the transition is usually accompanied by a one-half-cusp (3–4 mm) relative forward movement of the lower molar, accomplished by a combination of differential growth and tooth movement. A child's initial distal step relationship may change

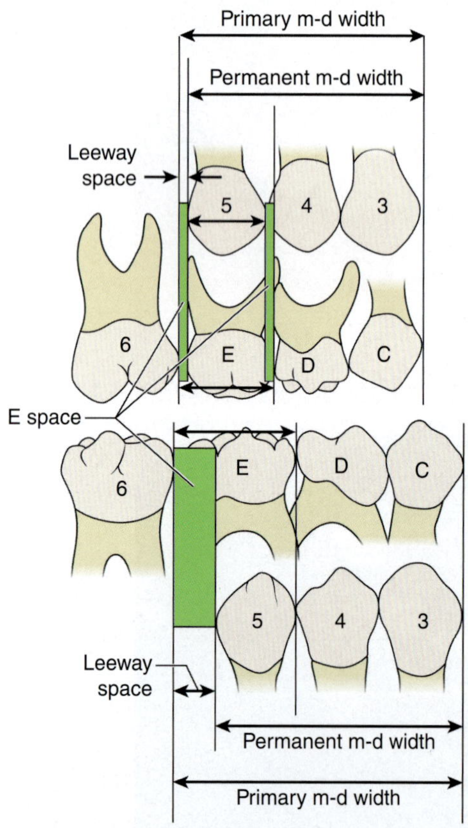

• **Fig. 3.32** The size difference between the primary canine and molars and permanent canine and premolars is the leeway space (*red arrows*). The space noted in green is the E space, the difference in width of the primary second molar and permanent second premolar. The size of the canine and first premolar can impinge on some of the leeway space, especially in the maxillary arch.

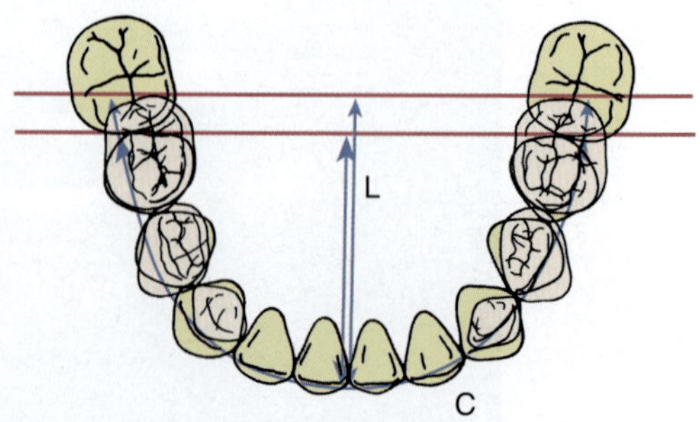

• **Fig. 3.33** Tooth sizes and arch dimensions in the transition to permanent dentition. Both arch length *(L)*, the distance from a line perpendicular to the mesial surface of the permanent first molars to the central incisors, and arch circumference *(C)* decrease as the molars move mesially into the leeway space.

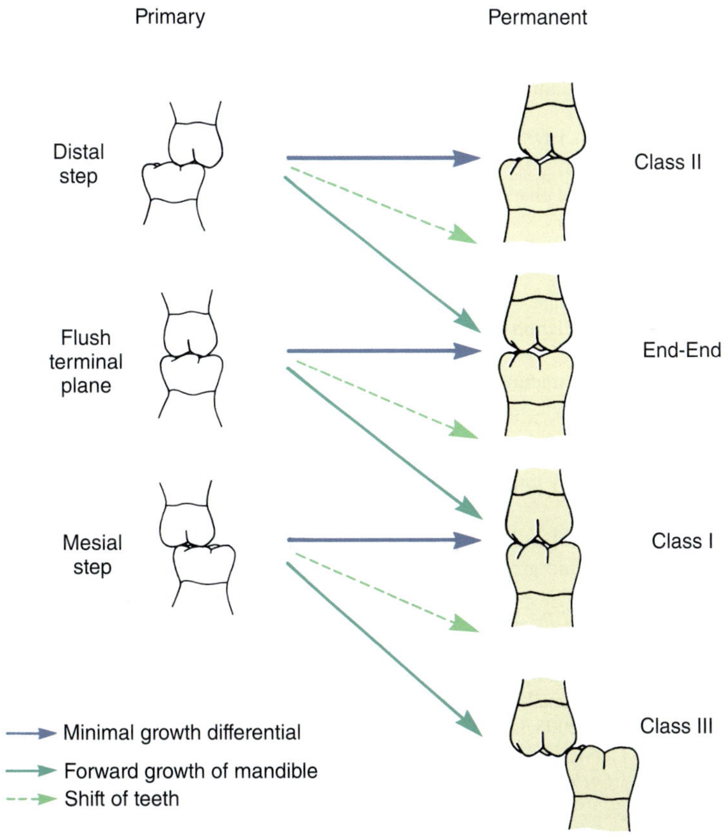

• **Fig. 3.34** Occlusal relationships of the primary and permanent molars. The flush terminal plane relationship, shown in the *middle left*, is the normal relationship in the primary dentition. When the first permanent molars erupt, their relationship is determined by the distal surface of the primary molars and whether there is lower primate space for an early mesial shift. The molar relationship tends to shift at the time the second primary molars are lost and the adolescent growth spurt occurs, as shown by the *arrows*. The amount of differential mandibular growth and molar shift into the leeway space determines the molar relationship, as shown by the *arrows* as the permanent dentition is completed. With good growth and a shift of the molars, the change shown by the *solid black line* can be expected. (Modified from Moyers RE. *Handbook of Orthodontics*. 3rd ed. Year Book Medical Publishers; 1973.)

during the transition to an end-to-end (one-half-cusp class II) relationship in the permanent dentition but is not likely to be corrected all the way to class I. It also is possible that there will be little if any differential forward growth of the mandible, in which case the molar relationship in the permanent dentition probably will remain a full cusp class II.

Similarly, a flush terminal plane relationship, which produces an end-to-end relationship of the permanent molars when they first erupt, can change to class I in the permanent dentition but can remain end-to-end in the permanent dentition if the growth pattern is not favorable.

Finally, a child who has experienced early mandibular growth may have a mesial step relationship in the primary molars, producing a class I molar relationship at an early age. It is quite possible for this mesial step relationship to progress to a half-cusp class III during the molar transition and proceed further to a full class III relationship with continued mandibular growth. On the other hand, if differential mandibular growth no longer occurs, the mesial step relationship at an early age may simply become a class I relationship later.

The bottom line is that the amount and the direction of mandibular growth, not the movement of the permanent molars when the primary second molars are lost, are the key variables in determining the permanent dentition molar relationship.

References

1. Janardhanan M, Umadethan B, BiNiraj K, et al. Neonatal line as a linear evidence of live birth: estimation of postnatal survival of a new born from primary tooth germs. *J Forensic Dent Sci*. 2011;3(1):8–13.
2. Glass HC, Costarino AT, Stayer SA, et al. Outcomes for extremely premature infants. *Anesth Analg*. 2015;120(6):1337–1351.
3. Brandt I. Growth dynamics of low-birth-weight infants. 2nd ed.. In: Falkner F, Tanner JM, eds. *Human Growth*. Vol. 1 Plenum Publishing; 1986.
4. Gomes FM, Subramanian SV, Escobar AM, et al. No association between low birth weight and cardiovascular risk factors in early adulthood: evidence from Sao Paulo, Brazil. *PLoS ONE*. 2013;8(6):e66554.
5. Peterson RE, Wetzel GT. Growth failure in congenital heart disease: where are we now? *Curr Opin Cardiol*. 2004;19:81–83.
6. McDowell MA, Brody DJ, Hughes JP. Has age at menarche changed? Results from the National Health and Nutrition Examination Survey (NHANES) 1999-2004. *J Adolesc Health*. 2007;40:227–231.

7. Rigon F, Bianchin L, Bernasconi S, et al. Update on age at menarche in Italy: toward the leveling off of the secular trend. *J Adolesc Health*. 2010;46:238–244.
8. Semba RD. The rise and fall of protein malnutrition in global health. *Ann Nutr Metab*. 2016;69(2):79–88.
9. Jantz RL. Cranial change in Americans: 1850-1975. *J Forensic Sci*. 2001;46:784–787.
10. Bosma JF. Maturation of function of the oral and pharyngeal region. *Am J Orthod*. 1963;49:94–104.
11. Lau C. Development of infant oral feeding skills: what do we know? *Am J Clin Nutr*. 2016;103(2):616S–621SS.
12. Larsson EF, Dahlin KG. The prevalence of finger- and dummy-sucking habits in European and primitive population groups. *Am J Orthod*. 1985;87:432–435.
13. Gross AM, Kellum GD, Hale ST, et al. Myofunctional and dentofacial relationships in second grade children. *Angle Orthod*. 1990;60:247–253.
14. Pavicin IS, Dumanic J, Badel TE, Vodanovic M. Timing of emergence of the first primary tooth in preterm and full-term infants. *Ann Anat*. 2016;203:19–23.
15. Warren JJ, Fontana M, Blanchette DR, et al. Timing of primary tooth emergence among U.S. racial and ethnic groups. *J Public Health Dent*. 2016;76:259–262.
16. Tanner JM. *Assessment of Skeletal Maturity and Prediction of Adult Height*. WB Saunders; 2001.
17. Baccetti T, Franchi L, McNamara JA, Jr. The cervical vertebral maturation (CVM) method for the assessment of optimal treatment timing in dentofacial orthopedics. *Semin Orthod*. 2005;11:119–129.
18. Gabriel DB, Southard KA, Qian F, et al. Cervical vertebrae maturation method: poor reproducibility. *Am J Orthod Dentofac Orthop*. 2009;136:478.e1–478.e7.
19. Ballrick J, Fields HW, Beck M, Sun Z, Germak J. The cervical vertebrae staging method's reliability in detecting pre and post mandibular growth. *Orthodontic Waves*. 2013;72:105–111.
20. Rainey BJ, Burnside G, Harrison JE. Reliability of cervical vertebral maturation. *Am J Orthod Dentofac Orthop*. 2016;150:98–104.
21. Morris KM, Fields HW, Beck FM, Kim DG. Diagnostic testing of cervical vertebral maturation staging: an independent assessment. *Am J Orthod Dentofacial Orthop*. 2019;156:626–632.
22. Perinetti G, Primozic J, Sharma B, Cioffi I, Contardo L. Cervical vertebral maturation method and mandibular growth peak: a longitudinal study of diagnostic reliability. *Eur J Orthod*. 2018;40(6): 666–672.
23. Gray S, Bennani H, Kieser JA, Farella M. Morphometric analysis of cervical vertebrae in relation to mandibular growth. *Am J Orthod Dentofac Orthop*. 2016;149:92–98.
24. Mellion ZJ, Behrents RG, Johnston LE. The pattern of facial skeletal growth and its relationship to various common indexes of maturation. *Am J Orthod Dentofac Orthop*. 2013;143:845–854.
25. Bei M. Molecular genetics of tooth development. *Curr Opin Genet Dev*. 2009;19(5):504–510.
26. Frazier-Bowers S, Koehler K, Ackerman JL, Proffit WR. Primary failure of eruption: further characterization of a rare eruption disorder. *Am J Orthod Dentofac Orthop*. 2007;131:578e1–578e9.
27. Rhoads SG, Hendricks HM, Frazier-Bowers SA. Establishing the diagnostic criteria for eruption disorders based on genetic and clinical data. *Am J Orthod Dentofac Orthop*. 2013;144:194–202.
28. Marks SC, Jr., Cahill DR. Experimental study in the dog of the non-active role of the tooth in the eruptive process. *Arch Oral Biol*. 1984;29(4):311–322.
29. Wise GE, Frazier-Bowers S, D'Souza RN. Cellular, molecular, and genetic determinants of tooth eruption. *Crit Rev Oral Biol Med*. 2002;13(4):323–335.
30. Bastos VC, Gomez RS, Gomes CC. Revisiting the human dental follicle: from tooth development to its association with unerupted or impacted teeth and pathological changes. *Dev Dyn*. 2022;251(3):408–423.
31. Wise GE, King GJ. Mechanisms of tooth eruption and orthodontic tooth movement. *J Dent Res*. 2008;87(5):414–434.
32. Craddock HL, Youngson CC. Eruptive tooth movement – the current state of knowledge. *Br Dent J*. 2004;197(7):385–391.
33. Risinger RK, Proffit WR. Continuous overnight observation of human premolar eruption. *Arch Oral Biol*. 1996;41:779–789.
34. Trentini CJ, Proffit WR. High resolution observations of human premolar eruption. *Arch Oral Biol*. 1996;41:63–68.
35. Cheek CC, Paterson RL, Proffit WR. Response of erupting human second premolars to blood flow changes. *Arch Oral Biol*. 2002;47:851–858.
36. Naser DH, Abu Alhaija ES, Al-Khateeb SN. Dental age assessment in patients with maxillary canine displacement. *Am J Orthod Dentofacial Orthop*. 2011;140:848–855.
37. Moorrees CF, Chadha JM. Available sfpace for the incisors during dental development—a growth study based on physiologic age. *Angle Orthod*. 1965;35:12–22.
38. Moyers RE, University of Michigan, Center for Human Growth Development. *Standards of Human Occlusal Development*. Center for Human Growth and Development, University of Michigan; 1976.

4

Later Stages of Development

WILLIAM R. PROFFIT, HENRY W. FIELDS, AND KAITRIN KRAMER

CHAPTER OUTLINE

Adolescence: The Early Permanent Dentition Years

Adolescence is the phase of life between childhood and adulthood. More specifically, it is the transitional period during which secondary sexual characteristics appear, the adolescent growth spurt takes place, and profound physiologic changes occur. All these developments are associated with the maturation of the sex organs and the accompanying surge in the secretion of sex hormones.

This period is particularly important in dental and orthodontic treatment because the physical changes at adolescence significantly affect the face and dentition. Major events in dentofacial development that occur during adolescence include the end of the exchange from the mixed to the permanent dentition, an acceleration in the overall rate of facial growth, and differential growth of the jaws.

Initiation of Adolescence

The first events of puberty occur in the brain, and significant recent research findings have clarified the complex interaction between neural, genetic and epigenetic factors (chemical modifications of DNA functions, not sequesnce, that can be inherited or environmentally influenced) that lead to its initiation. The hypothalamic-pituitary-gonadal axis plays a key role in initiating puberty through the pulsatile release of gonadotropin-releasing hormone (GnRH) from neurosecretory cells in the hypothalamus. This stimulates the pituitary gland to produce a variety of these hormones, which in turn activates the release of both estrogens and androgens from the adrenal gland and ovaries or testes (Fig. 4.1). The neurosecretory cells can produce GnRH before puberty and after puberty with epigenetic regulation. There is a general belief that during the prepubertal phase the release of GnRH is under inhibitory control and with the onset of puberty a decrease in inhibitory signals concomitant with excitatory signals initiates puberty.[1] These changes appear to be controlled by transsynaptic activity of neurons in the arcuate nucleus. Most studies looking at the various genes associated with puberty have been done in animals and extrapolated to humans, indicative that a great deal of research is still needed in understanding how and when alterations in epigenetic regulation affect the timing of puberty.

Both the secretory cells in the hypothalamus and their method of action are somewhat unusual. These cells look like typical neurons, but they secrete materials in the cell body, which are carried by cytoplasmic transport down the axon toward a richly vascular area at the base of the hypothalamus near the pituitary gland. The substances secreted by the nerve cells pass into capillaries in this vascular region and are carried a short distance to the pituitary by blood flow. It is unusual in the body for the venous return system to transport substances from one closely adjacent region to another, but here the special arrangement of the vessels seems made to order for this purpose. Accordingly, this special network of vessels, analogous to the venous supply to the liver but on a much smaller scale, is called the *pituitary portal system.*

In the anterior pituitary, the hypothalamic releasing factors stimulate pituitary cells to produce several related but different hormones called *pituitary gonadotropins*. Their function is to stimulate endocrine cells in both the adrenal glands and the developing sex organs to produce sex hormones.

In the male, different cell types in the testes produce both the male sex hormone testosterone and the female sex hormones, and possibly some female hormones are produced in the adrenal cortex. A different pituitary gonadotropin stimulates each of these cell types. In the female, the pituitary gonadotropins stimulate secretion of estrogen by the ovaries, and later progesterone by the same organ; male sex hormones are produced in the adrenal cortex, stimulated by still another pituitary hormone.

Under the stimulation of the pituitary gonadotropins, sex hormones from the testes, ovaries, and adrenal cortex are released into the bloodstream in quantities sufficient to cause the development of secondary sexual characteristics and accelerated growth of the genitalia. The increasing level of the sex hormones also causes other physiologic changes, including the acceleration

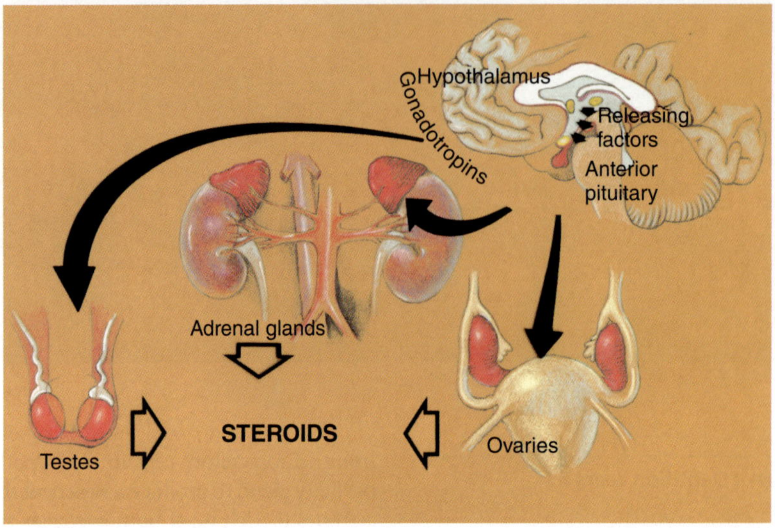

• **Fig. 4.1** Diagrammatic representation of the cascade of endocrine signals controlling sexual development. Releasing factors from the hypothalamus are carried via the pituitary portal circulation to the anterior pituitary gland, where they initiate the release of pituitary gonadotropic hormones. These in turn stimulate cells in the testes, ovaries, and adrenals, which secrete the steroid sex hormones.

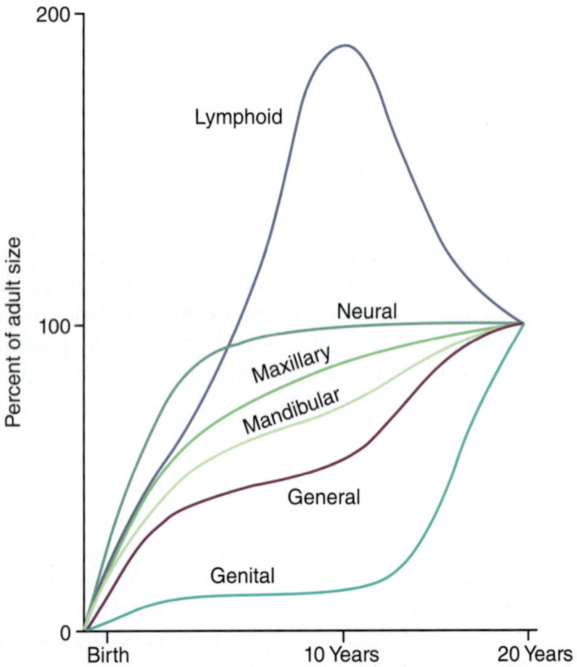

• **Fig. 4.2** Growth curves for the maxilla and mandible shown against the background of Scammon's curves. Note that growth of the jaws is intermediate between the neural and general body curves, with the mandible following the general body curve more closely than the maxilla. The acceleration in general body growth at puberty, which affects the jaws, parallels the dramatic increase in the development of the sexual organs. Lymphoid involution also occurs at this time. (From Scammon RD. The measurement of the body in childhood. In: Harris JA, ed. *The Measurement of Man*. University of Minnesota Press; 1930.)

in general body growth and shrinkage of lymphoid tissues seen in the classic growth curves described in Chapter 2. Neural growth is unaffected by the events of adolescence because it is essentially complete by age 6 to 7. The changes in the growth curves for the jaws, general body, lymphoid, and genital tissues, however, can be considered the result of the hormonal changes that accompany sexual maturation (Fig. 4.2). Eventually, feedback from the levels of circulating sex hormones affects the amount of GnRH hormones and thereby the amount of gonadotropins that are released, so control of this endocrine system is still managed from the hypothalamic level.

The system by which a few neurons in the hypothalamus ultimately control the level of circulating sex hormones may seem curiously complex. The principle, however, is one used in control systems throughout the body and in modern technology. Each of the steps in the control process results in an amplification of the control signal in a way analogous to the amplification of a small musical signal between the signal source and speakers of a stereo system. The amount of pituitary gonadotropin produced is much greater than the amount of gonadotropin-releasing factors produced in the hypothalamus, and the amount of sex hormones produced is many times greater than the amount of the pituitary hormones themselves. The system, then, is a three-stage amplifier. Rather than being a complex biological curiosity, it is better viewed as a rational engineering design. A similar amplification of controlling signals from the brain is used, of course, in all body systems.

Timing of Puberty

There is a great deal of individual variation, but puberty and the adolescent growth spurt occur on average nearly 2 years earlier in girls than in boys (Fig. 4.3). Why this occurs is not known, but the timing of puberty is a highly heritable trait. Although, there is emerging evidence to suggest epigenetic roles in precocious puberty.[1,2] When puberty occurs has an important impact on the timing of orthodontic treatment, which must be done earlier in girls than in boys if the goal is to take advantage of the adolescent growth spurt using growth modification. Because of the considerable individual variation, however, early-maturing boys will reach puberty ahead of slow-maturing girls, and it must be remembered that chronologic age is only one indicator of where an individual stands developmentally. The stage of development of secondary sexual characteristics provides a physiologic calendar of adolescence that correlates with the individual's physical growth status. Not all secondary sexual characteristics are readily visible, of course, but most can be evaluated in a normal fully clothed examination, such as would occur in a dental office.

Puberty for girls can be divided into five stages, based on the extent of sexual development, as described by Tanner.[3] Stage 1 is prepuberty, and there are no visible changes. This usually begins at age 8 for girls. Stage 2 occurs at the beginning of the physical growth spurt in height (between ages 9 and 11), accompanied by the appearance of breast buds and early stages of the development of pubic hair. During stage 3, the peak velocity for height occurs with continued breast development, underarm hair appears, and pubic hair spreads (see Fig. 4.3).

Stage 4 in girls is marked by the onset of menstruation (menarche = M, See Fig. 4.3. Growth in height is slowing, breast fullness continues, and thicker pubic hair is still restricted to a triangle. Stage 5 is the last stage where girls reach adult height at approximately 16, and pubic hair extends to the thighs.

The stages of sexual development in boys are more difficult to define specifically. Puberty begins later and extends over a longer period—about 5 years compared with 3.5 years for girls (see Fig. 4.3). In boys, five stages in development can be correlated with the curve of general body growth at adolescence.

As with girls, stage 1 is normal growth with no physical changes. Stage 2 includes the "fat spurt." The maturing boy gains weight and becomes almost chubby. This probably occurs because estrogen production by the Leydig cells in the testes is stimulated before the more abundant Sertoli cells begin to produce significant amounts of testosterone. During this stage, boys may appear somewhat awkward physically. At this time, the testes and scrotum begin to increase in size and there is pubic hair at the base of the penis.

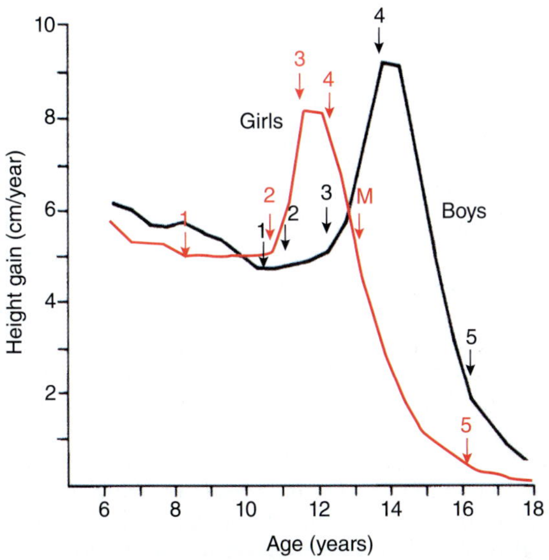

• **Fig. 4.3** Velocity curves for growth at adolescence, showing the difference in timing for girls and boys. Also indicated on the growth velocity curves are the corresponding stages in sexual development (see text). (From Marshall WA, Tanner JM. Puberty. In: Falkner F, Tanner JM, eds. *Human Growth.* Vol 2. 2nd ed. Plenum Publishing; 1986.)

At stage 3, the spurt in height is just beginning. At this stage, there is a redistribution and relative decrease in subcutaneous fat, muscle development begins, and pubic hair spreads as the testes and penis grow. Wet dreams begin as do intermittent voice changes.

Stage 4 coincides with the peak velocity in height. At this time, armpit hair appears, and facial hair appears on the upper lip. A spurt in muscle growth also continues, and pubic hair distribution appears more adult but has not yet spread to the medial area of the thighs. The penis and scrotum are near adult size. A deeper voice is becoming permanent.

Stage 5 for boys is difficult to pinpoint. At this time, the spurt of growth in height ends—usually between 17 and 20 years. There is facial hair on the chin and the upper lip. Pubic hair extends to the medial of the thigh and there is adult distribution of armpit hair and a further increase in muscular strength.

The timing of puberty makes an important difference in ultimate body size in a way that may seem paradoxical at first; the earlier the onset of puberty, the smaller the adult size, and vice versa. Growth in height depends on endochondral bone growth at the epiphyseal plates of the long bones, and the impact of sex hormones on endochondral bone growth is twofold. First, the sex hormones stimulate the cartilage to grow faster, and this is a major factor in the adolescent growth spurt. However, the sex hormones also cause an increase in the rate of skeletal maturation, which for the long bones is the rate at which cartilage is transformed into bone. The acceleration in maturation is even greater than the acceleration in growth. Thus, during the rapid growth of adolescence, the cartilage is used up faster than it is replaced. Toward the end of adolescence, the last of the cartilage is transformed into bone, and the epiphyseal plates close. At that point, of course, growth potential is lost and growth in height stops.

This early cessation of growth after early sexual maturation is particularly prominent in girls. It is responsible for much of the difference in adult size between males and females. Girls mature earlier on average and finish their growth much sooner. Boys are not bigger than girls until they grow for a longer time in adolescence. The difference arises because there is slow but steady growth before the growth spurt, and so when the growth spurt occurs, for those who mature late, it takes off from a higher plateau. The epiphyseal plates close more slowly in males than in females, and therefore the cutoff in growth that accompanies the attainment of sexual maturity is also more complete in girls.

The timing of puberty seems to be affected by both genetic and environmental influences. There are early- and late-maturing families, and individuals in some racial and ethnic groups mature earlier than others. As Fig. 4.4 shows, Dutch boys are about 5 cm (2 inches) taller and 7 kg (15 lb) heavier than their American counterparts at age 10, and it is likely that both heredity and environment play a role in producing that considerable difference. In girls, it appears that the onset of menstruation requires the development of a certain amount of body fat. In girls of a slender body type, the onset of menstruation can be delayed until this level is reached. Athletic girls with low body fat often are slow to begin their menstrual periods, and highly trained female athletes whose body fat levels are quite low may stop menstruating, apparently in response to the low body fat levels.

Seasonal and cultural factors also can affect the overall rate of physical growth. For example, everything else being equal, growth tends to be faster in spring and summer than in fall and winter, and city children tend to mature faster than rural ones, especially in developing countries. Such effects presumably are mediated via the hypothalamus and

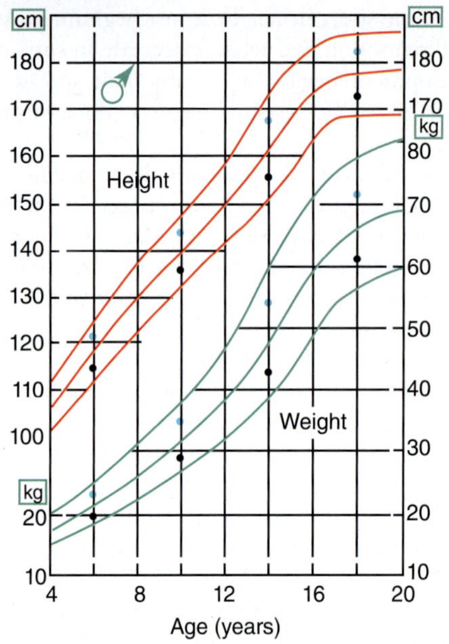

• **Fig. 4.4** Height and weight curves for boys in the United States, showing means ± 2 standard deviations. Note the dots on the graphs at ages 6, 10, 14, and 18. The upper blue dots show median height and weight for boys in the Netherlands; the lower black ones show median height and weight for boys in the United States. Note that at all ages the Dutch boys are larger and heavier than their US counterparts; at age 10 the height and weight differences are nearly 5 cm (2 inches) and 7 kg (15 lb). This is a dramatic illustration of how growth is affected by racial, ethnic, national, and other variables.

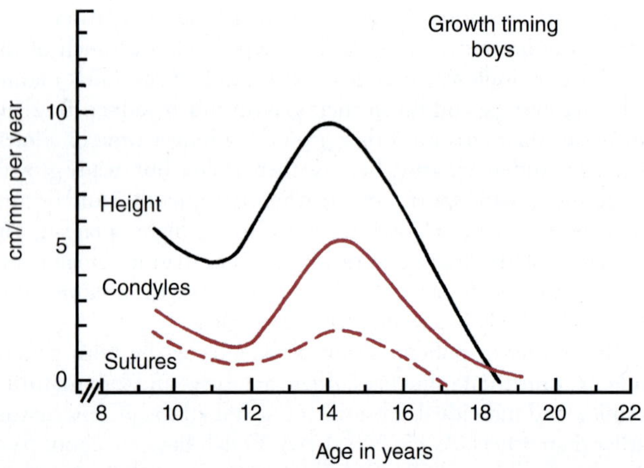

• **Fig. 4.5** On average, the adolescent spurt in growth of the jaws occurs at about the same time as the spurt in height, but it must be remembered that there is considerable individual variation. (Data from the Burlington Growth Study; redrawn from Woodside DG. In: Salzmann JA, ed. *Orthodontics in Daily Practice*. JB Lippincott; 1974.)

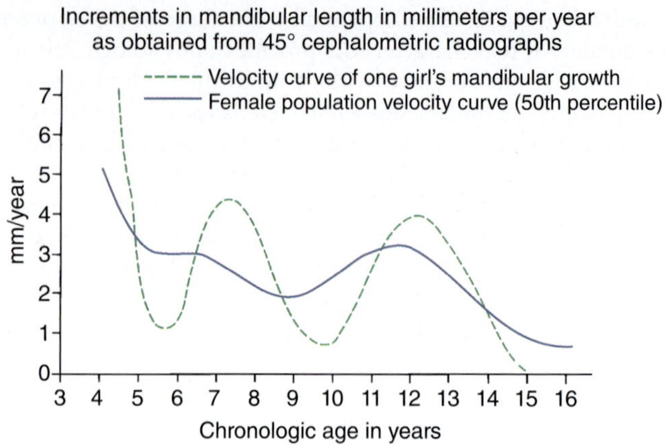

• **Fig. 4.6** Longitudinal data for increase in length of the mandible in one girl, taken from the Burlington growth study in Canada, demonstrates an acceleration of growth at about 8 years of age (juvenile acceleration) that is about equal in intensity to the pubertal acceleration between ages 11 and 14. Changes of this type in the pattern of growth for individuals tend to be smoothed out when cross-sectional or group average data are studied. (From Woodside DG. In: Salzmann JA, ed. *Orthodontics in Daily Practice*. JB Lippincott; 1974.)

indicate that the rate of secretion of gonadotropin-releasing factors can be influenced by external stimuli and epigenetic factors.

In the description given earlier, the stages of adolescent development were correlated with growth in height. Fortunately, the growth of the jaws usually correlates with the physiologic events of puberty in about the same way as growth in height (Fig. 4.5). There is an adolescent growth spurt in the length of the mandible, though not nearly as dramatic a spurt as that in body height, and a modest although discernible increase in growth at the sutures of the maxilla. The cephalocaudal gradient of growth, which is part of the normal pattern, is dramatically evident at puberty. More growth occurs in the lower extremity than in the upper, and within the face, more growth takes place in the lower jaw than in the upper. This produces an acceleration in mandibular growth relative to the growth of the maxilla and results in the differential jaw growth referred to previously. The maturing face becomes less convex as the mandible and chin become more prominent because of differential jaw growth.

Although jaw growth follows the curve for general body growth, the correlation is not perfect. Longitudinal data from studies of craniofacial growth indicate that a significant number of individuals, especially among girls, have a "juvenile acceleration" in jaw growth that occurs 1 to 2 years before the adolescent growth spurt (Fig. 4.6).[4] This juvenile acceleration can equal or even exceed the jaw growth that accompanies secondary sexual maturation. In boys, if a juvenile spurt occurs, it is nearly always less intense than the growth acceleration at puberty.

This tendency for a clinically useful acceleration in jaw growth to precede the adolescent spurt, particularly in girls, is a major reason for careful assessment of physiologic age in planning orthodontic treatment. If treatment is delayed too long, the opportunity to use the growth spurt is missed. In early-maturing girls the adolescent growth spurt often precedes the final transition of the dentition, so by the time the second premolars and second molars erupt, physical growth is all but complete. The presence of a juvenile growth spurt in girls accentuates this tendency for significant acceleration of jaw growth in the mixed dentition. For many girls, if they are to receive orthodontic treatment while they are growing rapidly, the treatment must begin during the mixed dentition rather than after all succedaneous teeth have erupted.

In slow-maturing boys, on the other hand, the dentition can be relatively complete while a considerable amount of physical growth remains. In the timing of orthodontic treatment, clinicians tend to treat girls too late and boys too soon, forgetting the considerable disparity in the rate of physiologic maturation.

Growth Patterns in the Dentofacial Complex

Dimensional Changes

Growth of the Nasomaxillary Complex

As we have noted in the preceding chapters, growth of the nasomaxillary area is produced by two basic mechanisms: (1) passive displacement, created by growth in the cranial base that pushes the maxilla forward, and (2) active growth of the maxillary structures and nose (Fig. 4.7). Because the push from behind decreases greatly as the cranial base synchondroses close at about age 7, most of the growth after that time (i.e., during the time period when most orthodontic treatment is done) is due to active growth at the maxillary sutures and modeling surfaces.

The effect of surface modeling must be taken into account when active growth of the maxilla is considered. Surface changes can either be added to or subtracted from growth at the sutures by surface apposition or resorption, respectively. In fact, the maxilla grows downward and forward as bone is added in the tuberosity area posteriorly and at the posterior and superior sutures, but the anterior surfaces of the bone are resorbing at the same time (Fig. 4.8). For this reason, the distance that the body of the maxilla and the maxillary teeth are carried downward and forward during growth is greater by about 25% than the forward movement of the anterior surface of the maxilla. This amount of surface modeling, which conceals the extent of relocation of the jaws, is even more prominent when the rotation of the maxilla during growth is considered (see the following sections).

The nasal structures undergo the same passive displacement as the rest of the maxilla. However, the nose grows more rapidly than the rest of the face, particularly during the adolescent growth spurt. Nasal growth is produced in part by an increase in the size of the cartilaginous nasal septum. In addition, the proliferation of the lateral cartilages alters the shape of the nose and contributes to an increase in overall size. On average, nasal dimensions increase at a rate about 25% greater than the growth of the maxilla during adolescence (Fig. 4.9), but the growth of the nose is extremely variable among racial or ethnic groups and quite variable within those groups. There are no fixed proportions for nose size except the more prominent the nose, the more prominent the jaws and lips need to be to produce reasonable facial balance.

Mandibular Growth

Growth of the mandible continues at a relatively steady rate before puberty. On average, as Table 4.1 shows, ramus height increases 1 to 2 mm per year and body length increases 2 to 3 mm per year. These cross-sectional data tend to smooth out the juvenile and pubertal growth spurts, which do occur in the growth of the mandible (see previous discussion).

One feature of mandibular growth is an accentuation of the prominence of the chin. At one time it was thought that this occurred primarily by the addition of bone to the chin, but that is incorrect. Although small amounts of bone are added, the change in the contour of the chin itself occurs largely because the area just above the chin, between it and the base of the alveolar process, is a resorptive area. The increase in chin prominence with maturity results from a combination of forward translation of the chin as a part of the overall growth pattern of the mandible and resorption above the chin that alters the bony contours.

An important source of variability in how much the chin grows forward is the extent of growth changes at the glenoid fossa. If

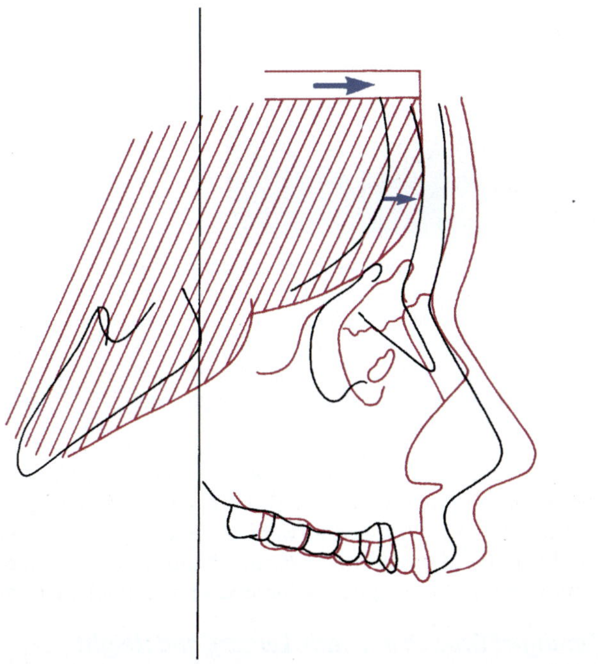

• **Fig. 4.7** Diagrammatic representation of a major mechanism for growth of the maxilla: Structures of the nasomaxillary complex are displaced forward as the cranial base lengthens and the anterior lobes of the brain grow in size. (Redrawn from Enlow DH, Hans MG. *Essentials of Facial Growth*. WB Saunders; 1996.)

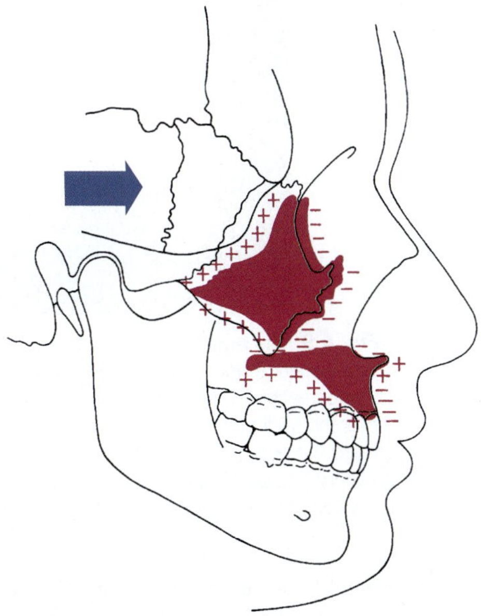

• **Fig. 4.8** As the maxilla is translated downward and forward, bone is added at the sutures and in the tuberosity area posteriorly, but at the same time, surface modeling removes bone from the anterior surfaces (except for a small area at the anterior nasal spine). For this reason, the amount of forward movement of anterior surfaces is less than the amount of displacement. In the roof of the mouth, however, surface modeling adds bone, whereas bone is resorbed from the floor of the nose. The total downward movement of the palatal vault, therefore, is greater than the amount of displacement. (Redrawn from Enlow DH, Hans MG. *Essentials of Facial Growth*. WB Saunders; 1996.)

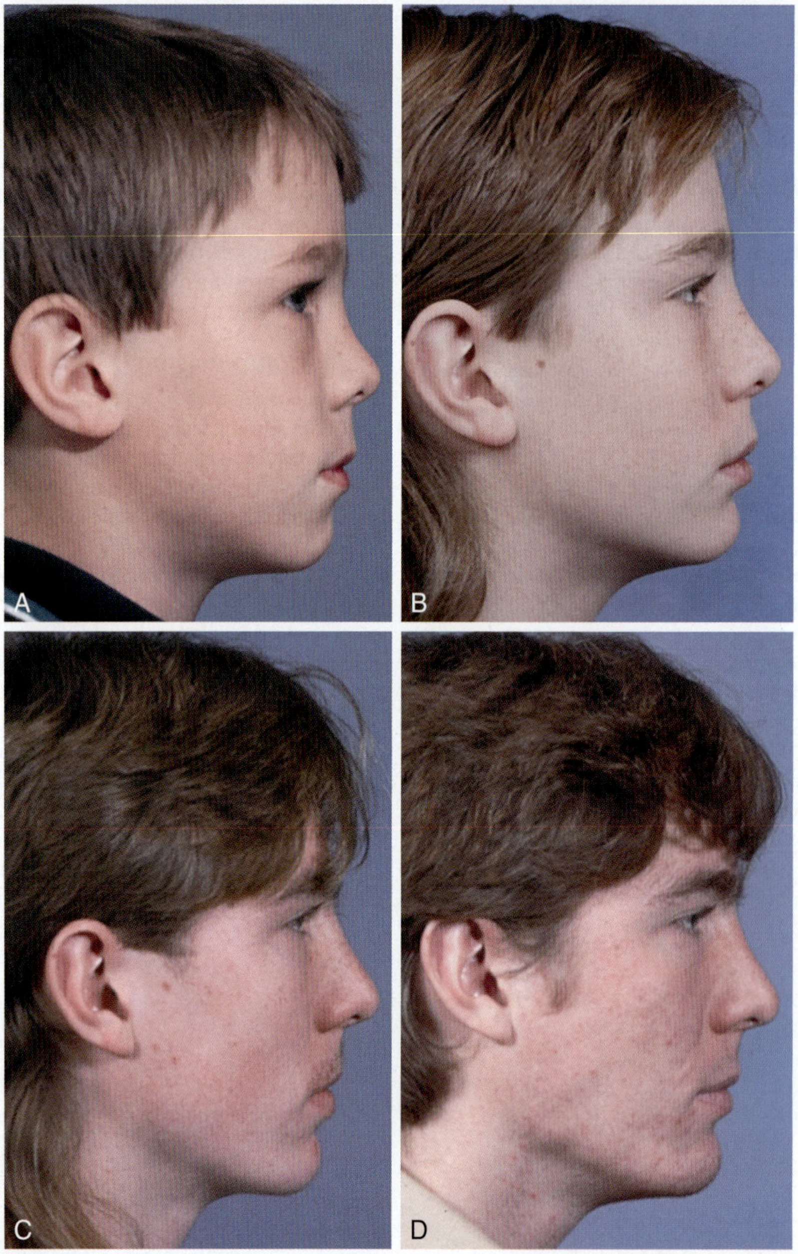

• **Fig. 4.9** The nose is small relative to the jaws before adolescence, then grows much more than the jaws in adolescence and continues to grow after forward growth of the maxilla and mandible has all but stopped. This decreases the apparent prominence of the jaws relative to the midface. In the same boy: (A) age 7 years, 0 months, well prior to adolescence; (B) age 12 years, 8 months, early adolescence; (C) age 15 years, 8 months, toward the end of the adolescent growth spurt, when forward jaw growth is nearly complete but the nose is still growing; (D) age 18 years, 8 months, late adolescence. Note the amount of forward nose growth but largely vertical growth of the jaws beyond age 15 years, 8 months.

the area of the temporal bone to which the mandible is attached moved forward relative to the cranial base during growth, this would translate the mandible forward in the same way that cranial base growth translates the maxilla. However, this rarely happens. Usually the attachment point moves straight down so that there is no anteroposterior displacement of the mandible, but occasionally it moves posteriorly, thus subtracting from rather than augmenting the forward projection of the chin.[5] In both the patients shown in Fig. 4.10, for instance, there was an approximate 7 mm increase in the length of the mandible during orthodontic treatment around the time of puberty. In one of the patients, the temporomandibular joint (TMJ) did not relocate during growth and the chin was projected forward at 7 mm. In the other patient, the TMJ moved posteriorly, resulting in only a small forward projection of the chin despite the increase in mandibular length.

Timing of Growth in Width, Length, and Height

For the three planes of space in both the maxilla and mandible, there is a general sequence in which growth is "completed" (i.e., declines to the very slow rate that characterizes normal adults). Growth in width is completed first, then growth in length, and finally growth in height.

TABLE 4.1 Mandibular Length Changes

Age (years)	Body Length Increase (mm) (Gonion-Pogonion) Male	Female	Ramus Height Increase (mm) (Condylion-Gonion) Male	Female
7	2.8	1.7	0.8	1.2
8	1.7	2.5	1.4	1.4
9	1.9	1.1	1.5	0.3
10	2.0	2.5	1.2	0.7
11	2.2	1.7	1.8	0.9
12	1.3	0.8	1.4	2.2
13	2.0	1.8	2.2	0.5
14	2.5	1.1	2.2	1.7
15	1.6	1.1	1.1	2.3
16	2.3	1.0	3.4	1.6

Data from Riolo ML, et al. *An Atlas of Craniofacial Growth*. University of Michigan Center for Human Growth and Development; 1974.

Growth in the width of both jaws, including the width of the dental arches, tends to be completed before the adolescent growth spurt and is affected minimally if at all by adolescent growth changes (Fig. 4.11). For instance, intercanine width is more likely to decrease than increase after age 12.[6] However, there is a partial exception to this rule. As the jaws grow in length posteriorly, they also grow wider. For the maxilla, this affects primarily the width across the second molars and, if they are able to erupt, the third molars as well. For the mandible, both molar and bicondylar widths show small increases until the end of growth in length. Anterior width dimensions of the mandible stabilize earlier.

Growth in length and height of both jaws continues through the period of puberty. In girls, the maxilla grows slowly downward and forward to age 14 to 15 on average (more accurately, by 2 to 3 years after first menstruation). For males, the maxilla also grows downward and forward.[7] Forward growth of the mandible is greater in males than in females.

In both sexes, growth in vertical height of the face continues longer than growth in length, with the late vertical growth occurring primarily in the maxilla in females and more in the mandible in males.[8] Increases in facial height and concomitant eruption of teeth continue throughout life, but the decline to the adult level (which for vertical growth is surprisingly large [see the following section]) often does not occur until the early 20s in boys and somewhat earlier in girls.

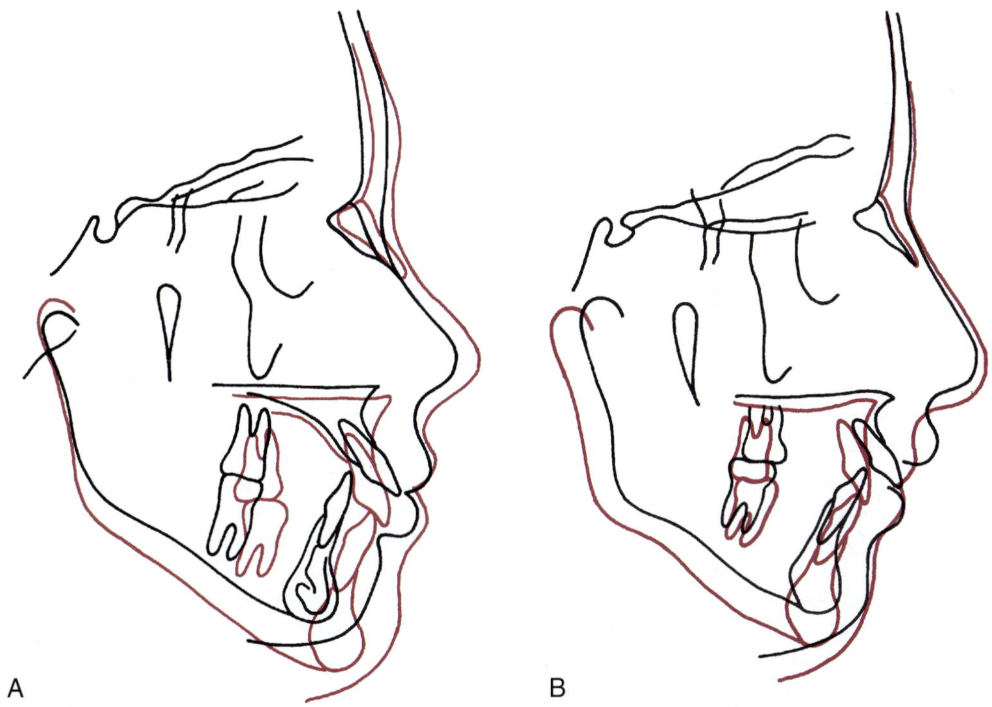

• **Fig. 4.10** Cephalometric tracings showing growth in two patients during the orthodontic correction of moderate class II malocclusion (superimposed on sphenoethmoid triad in cranial base). (A) Changes from age 11 years, 10 months to age 14 years, 11 months. In this patient, approximately 7 mm of mandibular growth was expressed entirely as forward movement of the chin, whereas the area of the temporomandibular joint remained in the same anteroposterior position relative to the cranial base. (B) Changes in another patient from age 11 years, 8 months to age 15 years, 0 months. This patient also had approximately 7 mm of mandibular growth, but the temporomandibular joint area moved downward and backward relative to the cranial base, so much of the growth was not expressed as forward movement of the chin. (Courtesy Dr. V. Kokich.)

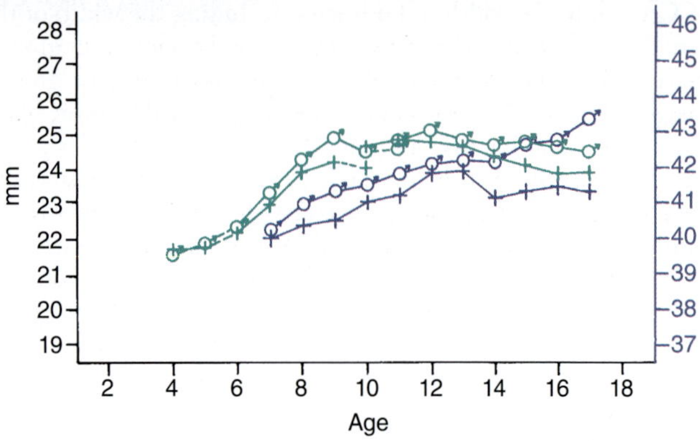

• **Fig. 4.11** Average changes in mandibular canine and molar widths in both sexes during growth. Molar widths are shown in blue, and canine widths are in green. (From Moyers RE, et al. *Standards of Human Occlusal Development*. University of Michigan Center for Human Growth and Development; 1976.)

TABLE 4.2 Terminology: Rotational Changes of the Jaws

Condition	Proffit et al. Contemporary Orthodontics
Posterior growth greater than anterior	Forward rotation (–)
Anterior growth greater than posterior	Backward rotation (+)
Rotation of mandibular plane relative to cranial base	Total rotation (approximately Internal - external rotation)
Rotation of mandibular core relative to cranial base (including rotation at the condyle)	Internal rotation
Rotation of mandibular plane relative to core of mandible	External rotation

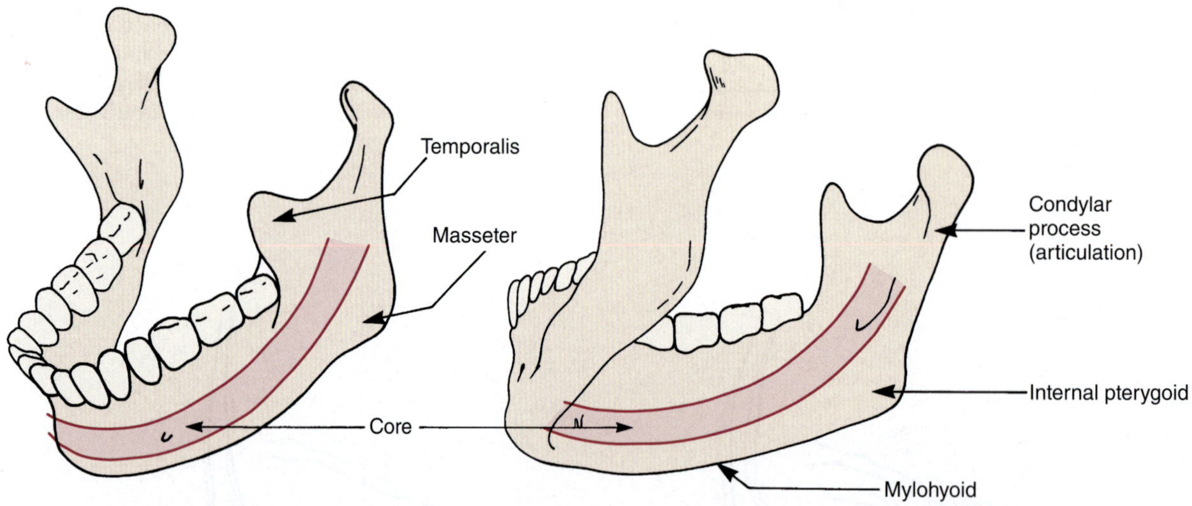

• **Fig. 4.12** The mandible can be visualized as consisting of a core of bone surrounding the inferior alveolar neurovascular bundle and a series of functional processes: the alveolar process, serving the function of mastication; the muscular processes, serving as muscle attachments; and the condylar process, serving to articulate the bone with the rest of the skull.

Rotation of Jaws During Growth

Implant Studies of Jaw Rotation

Until longitudinal studies of growth using metallic implants in the jaws were carried out in the 1960s, primarily by Björk and coworkers in Copenhagen (see Chapter 2), the extent to which both the maxilla and mandible rotate during growth was not appreciated. The reason is that the rotation that occurs in the core of each jaw, called *internal rotation,* tends to be masked by surface changes and alterations in the rate of tooth eruption. The surface changes produce *external rotation.* Obviously, the overall change in the orientation of each jaw, as judged by the palatal plane and mandibular plane, results from a combination of internal and external rotation.

The terminology for describing these rotational changes is itself confusing. The descriptive terms used here are an effort to simplify and clarify a complex and difficult subject (Table 4.2) and are not the terms originally used by Bjork[9] or his successors.[10] It is easier to visualize the internal and external rotation of the jaws by considering the mandible first. The core of the mandible is the bone that surrounds the inferior alveolar nerve. The rest of the mandible consists of several functional processes (Fig. 4.12). These are the alveolar process (bone supporting the teeth and providing for mastication), the muscular processes (the bone to which the muscles of mastication attach), and the condylar process, the function in this case being the articulation of the jaw with the skull.

Let us start with the *total rotation* of the mandible. That is the mandibular plane relative to the cranial base and what you essentially see when you look at a person over time or on an overall cephalometric superimposition registered on, for example, the S-N line (Fig. 4.13). Over time from childhood to adulthood, this would average −2 to −4 degrees of forward rotation.

Now we will look at the *internal* or core rotation of the mandible. This rotation can be determined by observing the core (or stable implants) rotation relative to the cranial base (S-N line) (Fig. 4.14). From childhood to adulthood the core of the mandible rotates forward an average of −10 to −15 degrees.[11] Less (−7 degrees)

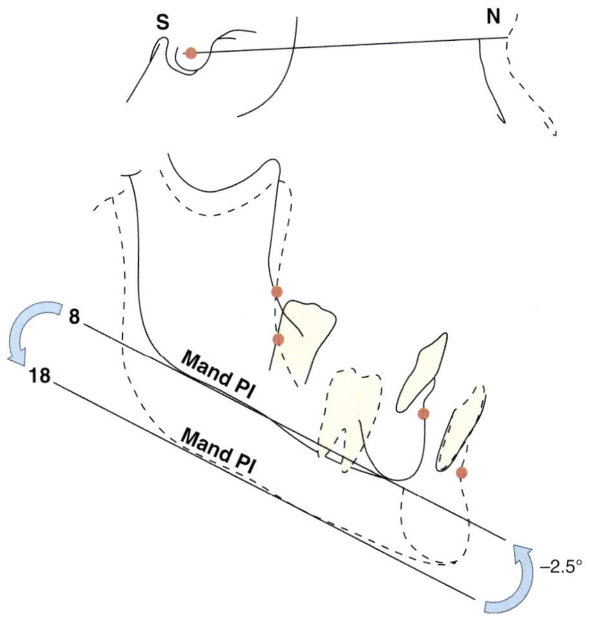

• **Fig. 4.13** Total rotation of the mandible is determined by the change in the mandibular plane relative to the cranial base (S-N). Bolton Standards of Developmental Growth at ages 8 and 18 were superimposed on the cranial base. Note the counterclockwise or negative rotation of the mandibular plane, which is common. The red dots indicate where stable implant markers are placed. (Redrawn using templates from Broadbent Sr H, Broadbent Jr H, Golden W. *Bolton Standards of Dentofacial Developmental Growth*. CV Mosby; 1975.)

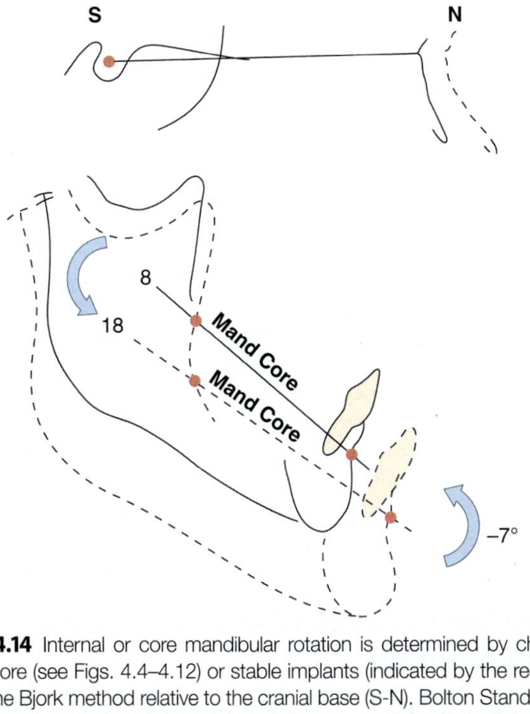

• **Fig. 4.14** Internal or core mandibular rotation is determined by changes in the core (see Figs. 4.4–4.12) or stable implants (indicated by the red dots) using the Bjork method relative to the cranial base (S-N). Bolton Standards of Developmental Growth at ages 8 and 18 were superimposed. Note the counterclockwise or negative rotation (−7 degrees) of the mandibular core during this time period. This change also includes any rotation around the condyle. (Redrawn using templates from Broadbent Sr H, Broadbent Jr H, Golden W. *Bolton Standards of Dentofacial Developmental Growth*. CV Mosby; 1975.)

is observed in Fig. 4.14 because this is only a 10-year time period, but the forward rotation tendency is seen. Internal rotation also reflects rotation forward or backward around the condyle because

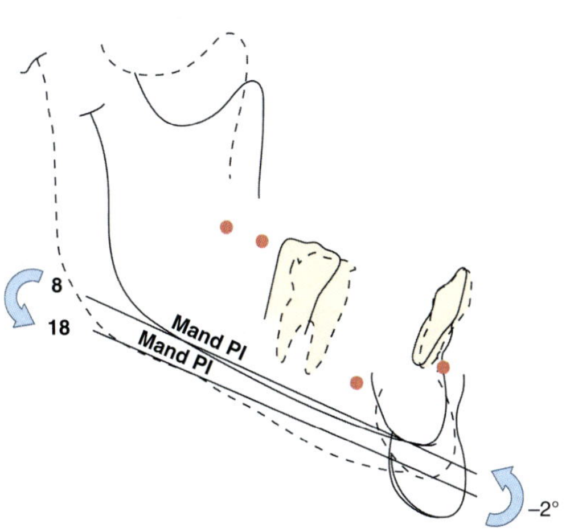

• **Fig. 4.15** The external mandibular rotation is determined by superimposing on the mandibular core or stable implants (indicated by the red dots) and observing the changes in the mandibular plane. The Bolton Standards of Developmental Growth at ages 8 and 18 used here show little mandibular plane change (−2 degrees) or anterior rotation. Usually there is a positive or backward eternal rotation due to modeling. (Redrawn using superimposed templates from Broadbent Sr H, Broadbent Jr H, Golden W. *Bolton Standards of Dentofacial Developmental Growth*. CV Mosby; 1975.)

the core's orientation to the cranial base can change in this way too. The pattern of vertical facial development, discussed in more detail later, is strongly related to the rotation of both jaws.

Finally, there is external rotation of the mandible. If implants are placed in areas of stable bone (the core), away from the functional processes, it can be observed that the core of the mandible rotates during growth in a way that would tend to decrease the mandibular plane angle (i.e., up anteriorly and down posteriorly). The eternal rotation (Fig. 4.15) would be the opposite (down in the anterior and up in the posterior) so the internal and external rotations (surface modeling) generally offset each other to some extent and reduce the total observed rotation that is a net more modest anterior rotation (Fig. 4.13). This means that the posterior part of the lower border of the mandible must be an area of resorption, whereas the anterior aspect of the lower border is unchanged or undergoes slight apposition (Fig. 4.16).

It is less easy to divide the maxilla into a core of bone and a series of functional processes. The alveolar process is certainly a functional process in the classic sense, but there are no areas of muscle attachment analogous to those of the mandible. The parts of the bone surrounding the air passages serve the function of respiration, and the form-function relationships involved are poorly understood. If implants are placed above the maxillary alveolar process, however, one can observe a core of the maxilla that undergoes a small and variable degree of rotation, forward or backward (Fig. 4.17).[12] This internal rotation is analogous to the rotation within the body of the mandible.

At the same time that internal rotation of the maxilla is occurring, there also are varying degrees of modeling of the palate with nasal surface resorption and palatal surface deposition. Similar variations in the amount of eruption of the incisors and molars occur. These changes amount to an external rotation. For most patients, the external rotation is opposite in direction and equal in magnitude to the internal rotation so that the two rotations cancel and the net change in jaw orientation (as evaluated by the palatal plane) is zero (see Fig. 3.19). Until the implant studies were done, rotation of the maxilla during normal growth had not been suspected.

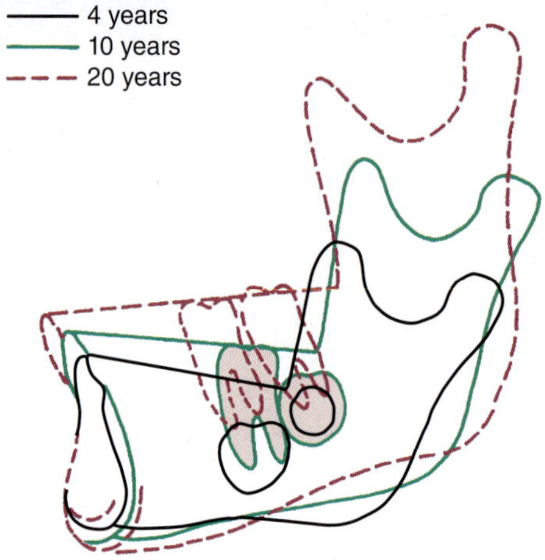

• **Fig. 4.16** Superimposition on implants for an individual with a normal pattern of growth, showing surface changes in the mandible from ages 4 to 20 years. For this patient, there was a 19-degree internal rotation but only a 3-degree change in the mandibular plane angle. Note how the dramatic modeling (external positive rotation) compensates for and conceals the extent of the internal rotation. Note that Figs. 4.16–4.19 and 4.21 are facing the left and others are not. That is a common convention in European countries where these data were derived. (From Björk A, Skieller V. Normal and abnormal growth of the mandible: a synthesis of longitudinal cephalometric implant studies over a period of 25 years. *Eur J Orthod*. 1983;5:1–46.)

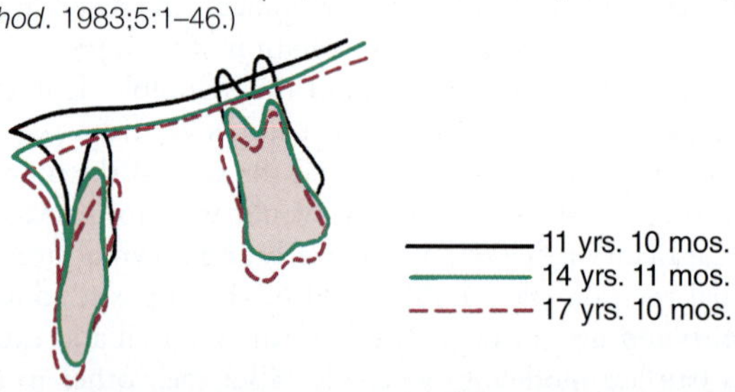

• **Fig. 4.17** Superimposition on implants in the maxilla reveals that this patient experienced a small amount of backward internal rotation of the maxilla (i.e., down anteriorly). A small amount of forward rotation is the more usual pattern, but backward rotation occurs frequently. (From Björk A, Skieller V. Facial development and tooth eruption: an implant study at the age of puberty. *Am J Orthod*. 1972;62:339.)

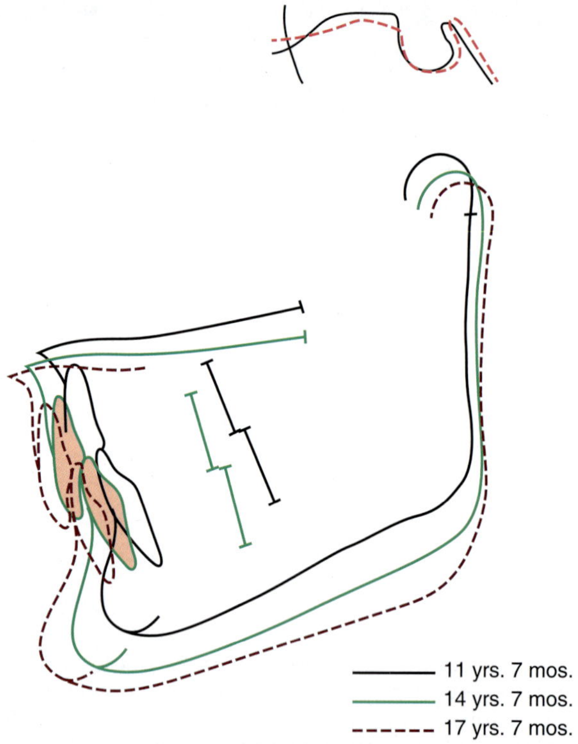

• **Fig. 4.18** Cranial base superimposition shows the characteristic pattern of forward mandibular rotation and a decrease in the mandibular plane angle in an individual with a short face or short-face tendency. As the mandible rotates upward and forward, anterior movement of the incisors is impeded and the bite deepens, creating a deep bite malocclusion that usually includes crowded incisors. (From Björk A, Skieller V. Facial development and tooth eruption: an implant study at the age of puberty. *Am J Orthod*. 1972;62:339.)

Although both internal and external rotation occur in everyone, variations from the average pattern are common. Greater or lesser degrees of both internal and external rotation often occur, altering the extent to which external changes compensate for the upward growth of the mandible when superimposed on the mandibular core implants.[13] You also see the anterior inferior deposition and posterior inferior (near the mandibular angle) resorption. The overall result is a downward and forward movement of the chin point.

Individuals of the short-face type, who are characterized by short anterior lower face height, have more a forward rotation of the mandible during growth, resulting from both an increase in the normal internal rotation and a decrease in external compensation. The condylar growth direction when superimposing on the mandibular core is upward and forward. The result is a more horizontal palatal plane, a low mandibular plane angle, and a smaller gonial angle (Fig. 4.18). A deep bite malocclusion and crowded incisors usually accompany this type of rotation (discussed later).

In long-face individuals, who have excessive lower anterior face height, the palatal plane may rotate down posteriorly creating an incline to the palatal plane, and the mandibular condyle shows an upward and backward growth direction when superimposed on the core implants. Overall, the mandible moves with a downward and backward rotation, with an increase in the mandibular plane angle (Fig. 4.19). The normal deposition under the symphysis and resorption at the posterior of the mandibular plane amplify the presentation. The mandibular changes result primarily from a lack of the normal forward internal rotation or even a backward internal rotation. This type of rotation is associated with anterior open bite malocclusion and mandibular deficiency (because the chin rotates back as well as down). Backward rotation of the mandible also occurs in patients with abnormalities or pathologic changes affecting the TMJs. In these individuals, growth at the condyle is restricted. Backward rotation of the mandible occurred in the core of the mandible.[14]

Interaction Between Jaw Rotation and Tooth Eruption

As discussed in Chapter 3, the growth of the mandible away from the maxilla creates a space into which the teeth erupt. The rotational pattern of jaw growth obviously influences the magnitude of tooth eruption. To a surprising extent, it can also influence the direction of eruption and the ultimate anteroposterior position of the incisor teeth.

The path of eruption of the maxillary teeth is downward and somewhat forward (see Fig. 4.17). In normal growth, the maxilla usually rotates a few degrees forward but frequently rotates slightly

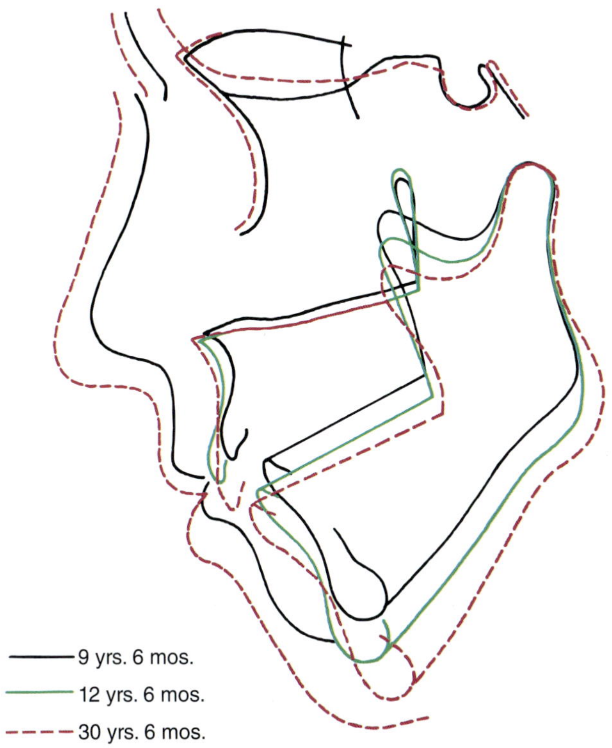

• **Fig. 4.19** Cranial base superimposition showing the pattern of jaw rotation in an individual with the long-face pattern of growth. These patients do not have the normal amount of forward internal rotation and may even have backward internal rotation. As the mandible rotates backward, anterior face height increases, there is a tendency toward anterior open bite, and the incisors are thrust forward relative to the mandible. (From Björk A, Skieller V. Normal and abnormal growth of the mandible:a synthesis of longitudinal cephalometric implant studies over a period of 25 years. *Eur J Orthod*. 1983;5:1–46.)

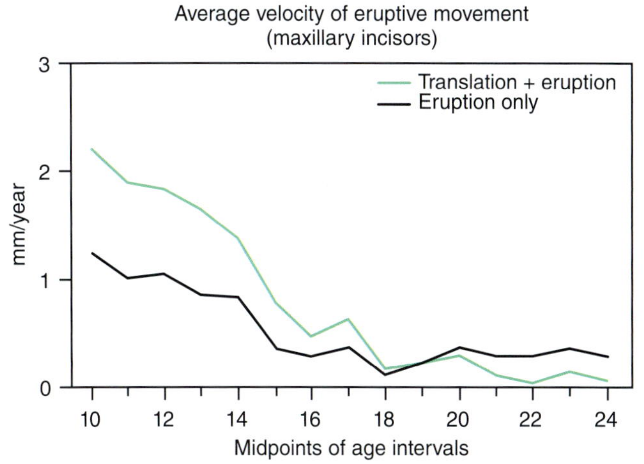

• **Fig. 4.20** The average velocity of continued eruption (movement of the incisors relative to implants in the maxilla) and translocation (movement away from the cranial base) of maxillary incisors in Danish girls, from a mixed longitudinal sample. Note that movement of the teeth away from the cranial base is due to a combination of eruption and translocation as the jaw grows and that small changes due to eruption continue after growth has essentially stopped. (Redrawn from Solow B, Iseri H. Maxillary growth revisited: an update based on recent implant studies. In: Davidovitch Z, Norton LA, eds. *Biological Mechanisms of Tooth Movement and Craniofacial Adaptation*. Harvard Society for Advancement of Orthodontics; 1996.)

backward. Forward rotation tends to tip the incisors forward, increasing their prominence, whereas backward rotation directs the anterior teeth more posteriorly, relatively uprighting them and decreasing their prominence. Movement of the teeth relative to the cranial base obviously could be produced by a combination of *translocation* as the tooth moved along with the jaw in which it was embedded, and true *eruption*, movement of the tooth within its jaw. As Fig. 4.20 shows, translocation contributes about half the total maxillary tooth movement during adolescent growth; the rest is due to eruptive movement of the teeth.

The eruption path of mandibular teeth is upward and somewhat forward, especially in long-face patients. The normal internal rotation of the mandible carries the jaw upward in front. This rotation alters the eruption path of the incisors, tending to direct them more posteriorly than would otherwise have been the case (Fig. 4.21). Note the upward and backward condylar change.

In short-face patients, because the internal jaw rotation tends to upright the incisors, the molars migrate further mesially during growth than do the incisors, and this migration is reflected in the decrease in arch length that normally occurs (Fig. 4.18). Because the forward internal rotation of the mandible is greater than that of the maxilla, it is not surprising that the normal decrease in mandibular arch length is somewhat greater than the decrease in maxillary arch length. Note the upward and forward condylar change.

This explanation for the decrease in arch length that normally occurs in both jaws is different from the 20th-century interpretation that emphasized forward migration of the molar teeth. The modern view places relatively greater importance on the lingual movement of the incisors and relatively less importance on the

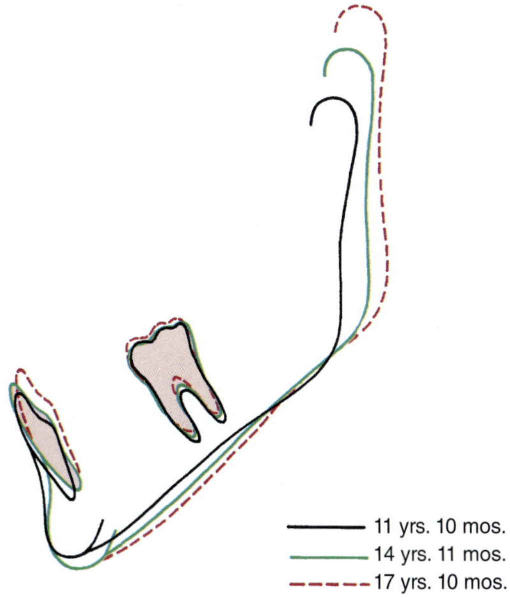

• **Fig. 4.21** Superimposition on mandibular implants shows the lingual positioning of the mandibular incisors relative to the mandible that often accompanies forward rotation during growth and late growth. (From Björk A, Skieller V. Facial development and tooth eruption: an implant study at the age of puberty. *Am J Orthod*. 1972;62:339.)

forward movement of molars. In fact, the same implant studies that revealed the internal jaw rotation also confirmed that changes in the anteroposterior position of the incisor teeth are a major influence on arch length changes.

Given this relationship between jaw rotation and incisor position, it is not surprising that both the vertical and the anteroposterior positions of the incisors are affected in short-face and long-face individuals. When excessive rotation occurs in the short-face type of development, the incisors tend to be carried into an overlapping position even if they erupt very little. This is why there is a strong tendency for deep bite malocclusion in short-face individuals. The rotation also progressively uprights the incisors, displacing them lingually and causing a tendency toward crowding. In the long-face growth pattern, on the other hand, an anterior open bite will develop as anterior face height increases unless the incisors erupt for an extreme distance. The rotation of the jaws also carries the incisors forward, creating dental protrusion.

This interaction between tooth eruption and jaw rotation explains a number of previously puzzling aspects of tooth positioning in patients who have vertical facial disproportions and is a key to understanding the growth pattern in affected individuals.

Maturational and Aging Changes

Maturational changes affect both the hard and soft tissues of the face and jaws as slow growth continues in adult life, with changes in jaw relationships and greater long-term changes in the soft tissues. There are important aging effects on the teeth, their supporting structures, and dental occlusion itself.

Facial Growth in Adults

Although some anthropologists in the 1930s reported small amounts of growth continuing into middle age, it was generally assumed until the late 20th century that growth of the facial skeleton ceased in the late teens or early 20s. In the early 1980s Behrents[15] succeeded in recalling over 100 individuals who had participated in the Bolton growth study in Cleveland in the 1930s and late 1940s, more than 40 years previously. Only a few had ever had orthodontic treatment. While they were participants in the study, the growth of these individuals was carefully evaluated and recorded using both measurements and serial cephalometric films. The magnification in the radiographs was known precisely, and it was possible to obtain new radiographs more than four decades later with known magnification so precise measurements of facial dimensions could be made.

The results were surprising but unequivocal: facial growth had continued during adult life (Fig. 4.22). There was an increase in essentially all the facial dimensions, but both the size and shape of the craniofacial complex altered with time. Vertical changes in adult life were more prominent than anteroposterior changes, so the alterations observed in the adult facial skeleton seem to be a continuation of the pattern seen during maturation. In a point of particular interest, an apparent deceleration of growth in females in the late teens was followed by a resumption of growth during the 20s. It appears that a female's first pregnancy often produces some growth in their jaws. Although the magnitude of the adult growth changes, as assessed in millimeters per year, was quite small, the cumulative effect over decades was surprisingly large.

The data also revealed that rotation of both jaws continued into adult life, in concert with the vertical changes and eruption of teeth. Because implants were not used in these patients, it was not possible to precisely differentiate internal from external rotation, but it seems likely that both internal rotation and surface changes did continue. In general, males showed more anterior-directed change and females showed a more vertically directed change. Males had a net rotation of the jaws in a forward direction, slightly decreasing the mandibular plane angle, whereas females had a tendency toward backward rotation, with an increase in the mandibular plane angle. In both groups, compensatory changes were noted in the dentition, so occlusal relationships were largely maintained. In summary, female skeletal landmarks moved downward and posteriorly, while male landmarks moved more downward and anteriorly.

Both a history of orthodontic treatment and loss of multiple teeth had an impact on facial morphology in these adults and on the pattern of change. In the smaller group of patients who had undergone orthodontic treatment many years previously, Behrents noted that the pattern of growth associated with the

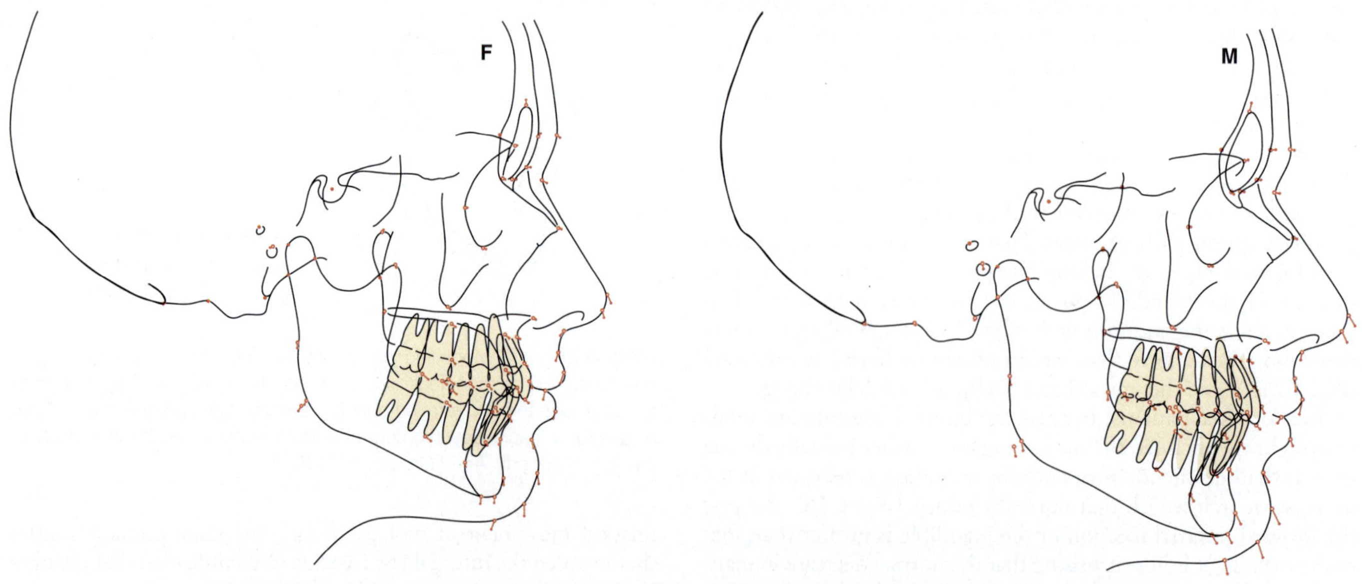

• **Fig. 4.22** Composites of (F) female and (M) male cephalograms who were recalled at approximately 40 years following participation in the Bolton Study. There is a surprising magnitude of skeletal and dental change over this time with an apparent contrast between the sexes. Females tended to have more vertical and backward components of change and males more vertical and forward changes. (From Behrents RG. Growth of the aging craniofacial skeleton. Monograph 17, *Craniofacial Growth Series*. Center for Human Growth and Development, University of Michigan; 1985.)

original malocclusion continued to express itself in adult life. This finding is consistent with previous observations of growth in the late teens but also indicates how a gradual worsening of occlusal relationships could occur in some patients long after the completion of orthodontic treatment. It is interesting that in long-face patients who have surgery to decrease face height by moving the maxilla up (Chapter 22), what looks like a recurrence of the previous growth pattern occurs in some patients long after growth should have stopped.[16]

In the light of Behrents's findings, it seems clear that viewing facial growth as a process that ends in the late teens or early 20s is not correct. It is correct, however, to view the growth process as one that declines to a basal level after the attainment of sexual maturity, continues to show a cephalocaudal gradient (i.e., more mandibular than maxillary changes in adult life), and affects the three planes of space differently. Not only is growth in width the first to drop to adult levels, usually reaching essential completion by the onset of puberty, but width changes thereafter are quite low.[17]

Anteroposterior growth continues at a noticeable rate for a longer period, declining to basal levels only after puberty, with small but noticeable changes continuing throughout adult life. Vertical growth, which had previously been observed to continue well after puberty in both males and females, continues at a modest level far into adult life. Although most of the skeletal change occurs between adolescence and mid-adulthood,[18] skeletal growth comes much closer to being a process that continues throughout life than most observers had previously suspected.

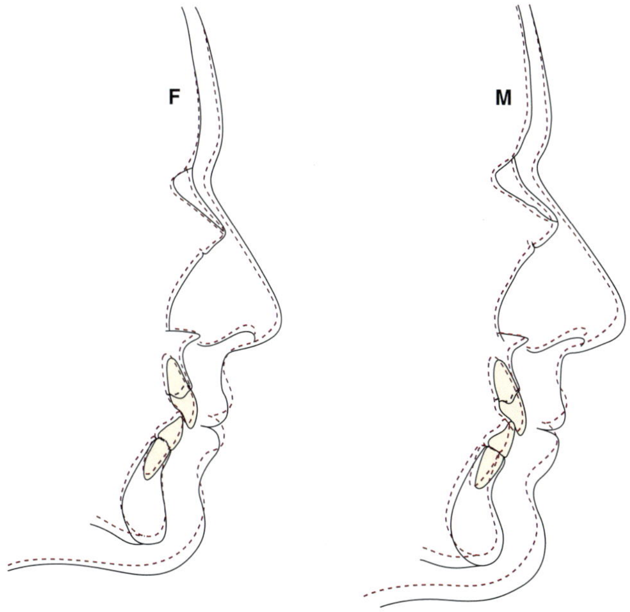

• **Fig. 4.23** These soft tissue profiles of females (*F*) and males (*M*) show changes from 40 years of adulthood. Note the growth of the nose and lowering of the nasal tip (greater in males), flattening of the lips and lengthening of the upper lip (greater in females) and soft tissue accumulations at the chin (greater in males). (From Behrents RG. Growth of the aging craniofacial skeleton. Monograph 17, *Craniofacial Growth Series*. Center for Human Growth and Development, University of Michigan; 1985.)

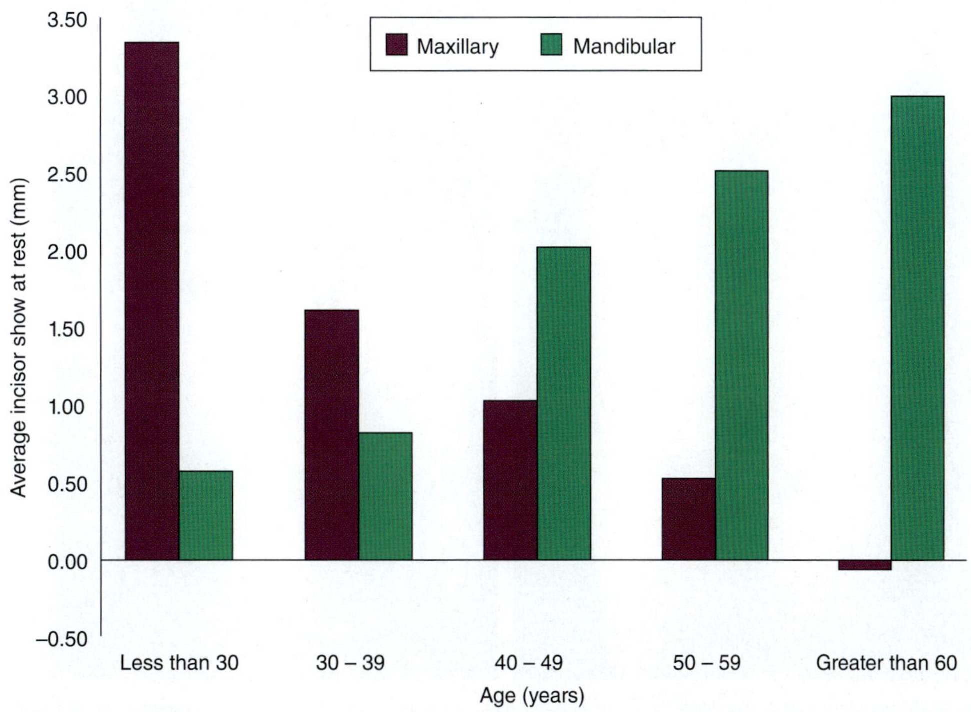

• **Fig. 4.24** Incisor display at rest as a function of age. With aging, both males and females show less of their upper incisors and more of their lower incisors, so display of upper incisors is a youthful characteristic. (Drawn from data: Vig RG, Brundo GC. The kinetics of anterior tooth display. *J Prosthet Dent*. 1978;39:502–504.)

Changes in Facial Soft Tissues

An important concept is that changes in facial soft tissues not only continue with aging, but they are also larger in magnitude than changes in the hard tissues of the face and jaws (Fig. 4.23).

The changes involved an elongation of the nose, which often became significantly longer during adult life and an augmentation of the soft tissue chin.

The soft tissue nose and chin changes are of significance for orthodontic treatment planning, particularly in the case of orthognathic surgery. Projection of the nose and chin will continue with growth from prepubescence into skeletal maturity. In males, a peak in nasal growth occurs around 13 to 14 years of age, continuing up to 16 to 18 years and beyond.[19] Females show a steadier increase in nose growth over time. With growth, the soft tissue profile will become more convex as the nose grows in a downward and forward direction at a greater degree than other soft tissues of the face. The nose can also have a small vertical component with a more acute nasal tip[20]; however, this translates to a clinically insignificant change in the nasolabial angle. Development of the bony chin is largely attributed to the stable lower symphyseal border near pogonion relative to the anterior aspect of the mandibular near the B point that is undergoing modeling resorption. The prominence of the chin can also result from the posterior placement of the mandibular incisors relative to the chin.[21] Soft tissue thickness at pogonion has been shown to average 2.4 mm in males and 1.5 mm in females with the anterior growth of the chin directly related to the growth of the body of the mandible. [22]

The change of greatest significance for orthodontists is that the lips and the other soft tissues of the face sag downward. There is a flattening and lengthening of the upper lip that is greater in females with aging. The result is a decrease in exposure of the upper incisors and an increase in exposure of the lower incisors, both at rest (Fig. 4.24) and on smile (Figs. 4.25 and 4.26). With aging, the lips also become progressively thinner, with less vermilion display (Fig. 4.27). A recent study of individuals followed longitudinally in the Michigan Growth Study revealed that in Americans of European descent, the upper lip lengthened by an average of 3.2 mm and thinned 3.6 mm between adolescence and mid-adulthood. This continued until late adulthood, with a further average mean lengthening and thinning of 1.4 mm. [18]

Because exposure of all the upper incisors and a small amount of gingiva on the smile is both youthful appearing and esthetic, it is important to remember in orthodontic treatment that the vertical relationship of the lip to the teeth will change after adolescence. With age the philtrum length will increase, peaking in the mid-20s for both males and females. The vertical length of the philtrum increases due to differential lip growth contributing to a flattening of the upper lip and further decrease of incisor display on smile.[23,24] Therefore leaving the upper incisors somewhat more exposed than the ideal adult relationship is necessary in the treatment of an adolescent if this relationship is to be ideal later in life (Figs. 4.28–4.30). Knowledge of soft tissue changes during aging is important in planning modern orthodontic treatment, and this is discussed further in Chapter 6.

Changes in Alignment and Occlusion

The alveolar bone bends during heavy mastication, allowing the teeth to move relative to one another (see Chapter 8 for more details). With a coarse diet, not only did occlusal wear reduce the

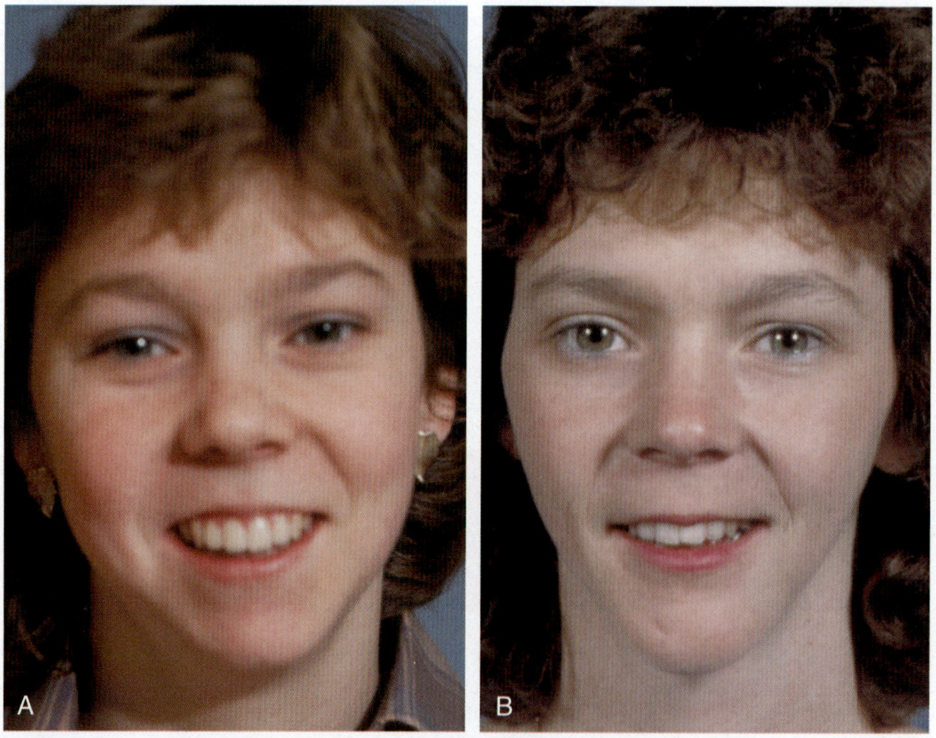

• **Fig. 4.25** Maxillary incisor exposure on smile at age 15 (A) and age 25 (B). An important characteristic of facial aging is the downward movement of the lips relative to the teeth, so that the maxillary incisors have progressively decreased exposure over time after adolescent growth is completed. (From Proffit WR, White RP, Sarver DM. *Contemporary Treatment of Dentofacial Deformity*. Mosby; 2003.)

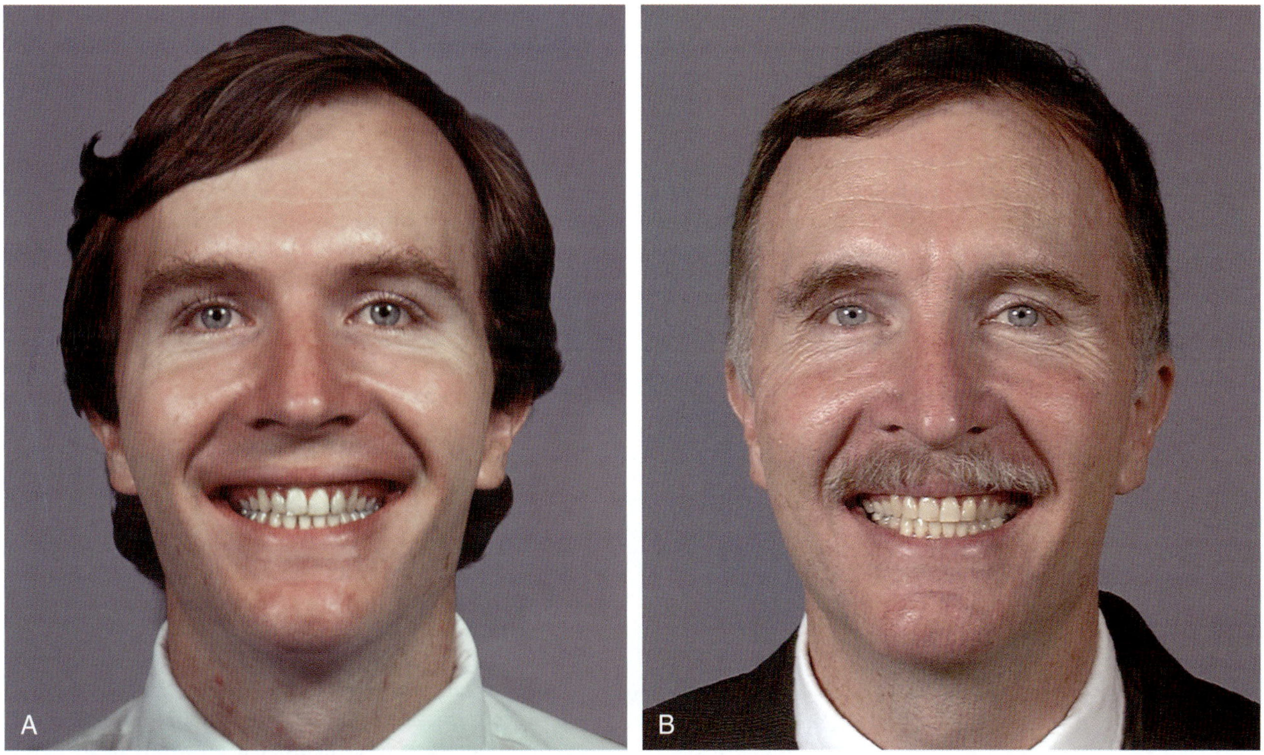

• **Fig. 4.26** Incisor exposure on smile at the completion of orthodontic treatment at age 30 (A) and 20 years later, at age 50 (B). Note that downward movement of the facial soft tissues continues, so the lower incisors are seen more prominently with increasing age.

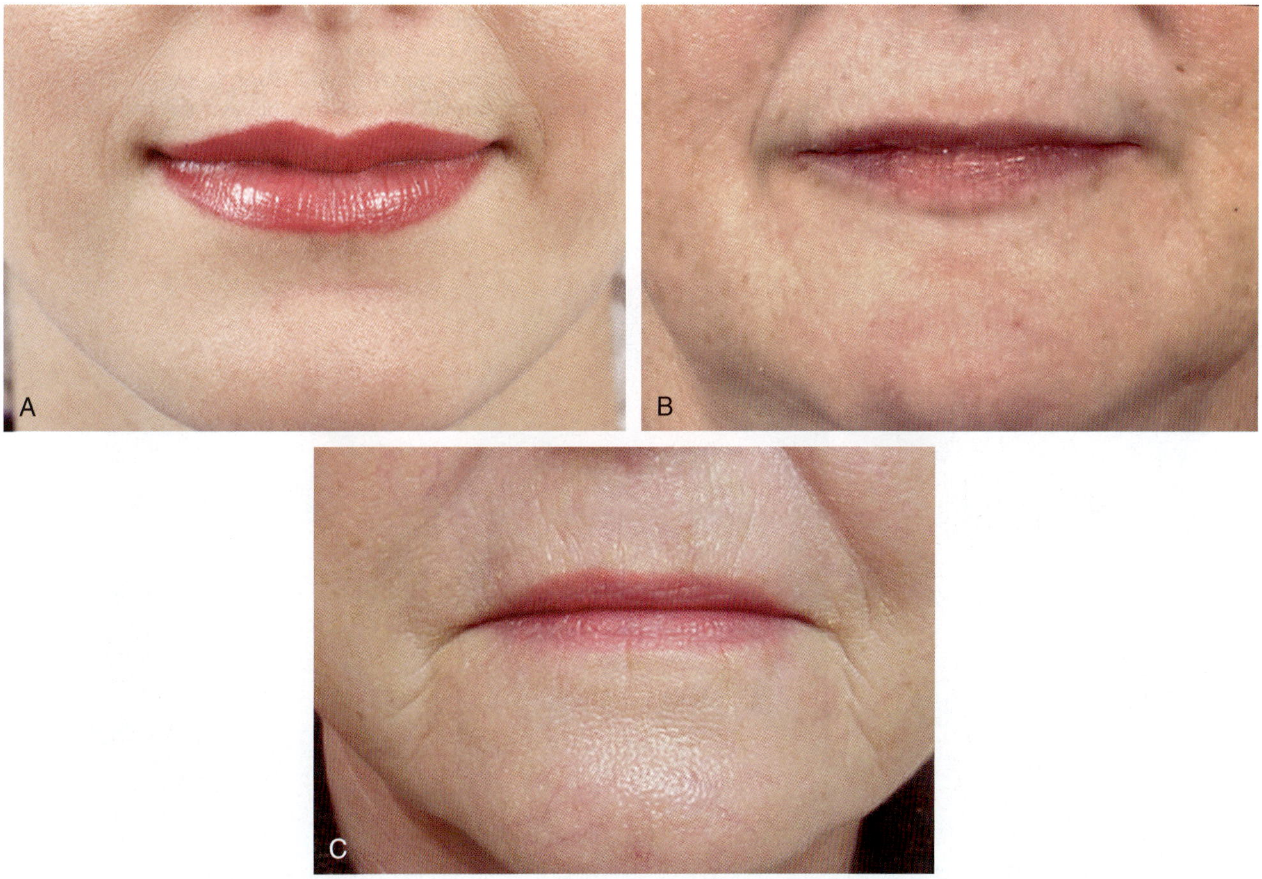

• **Fig. 4.27** A decrease in the fullness of the lips is an obvious sign of aging. (A) Age 20, (B) age 40, (C) age 70.

height of the crowns, but also the width of teeth was reduced as interproximal wear occurred. When this type of interproximal wear occurs, spaces do not open between the posterior teeth, although some spacing may develop anteriorly. Instead, the permanent molars migrate mesially, keeping the contacts reasonably tight even as the contact points are worn off and the mesiodistal width of each tooth decreases. The result in many early native populations was a reduction in arch circumference of 10 mm or more after completion of the permanent dentition at adolescence.

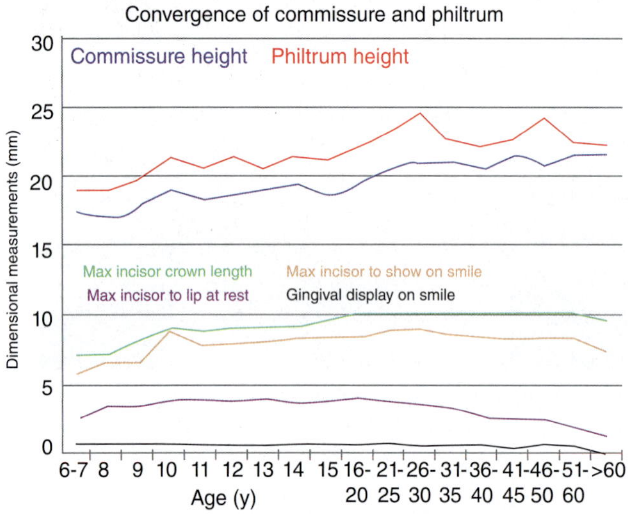

• **Fig. 4.28** This graph compiles many features of lip changes and incisor display. Note that the lip growth changes occur due to an increase in philtrim height that peaks in the mid-20s and an increase in commissure height. As expected, maxillary incisor crown length changes little after 16 years of age, due to reduced passive eruption. Maxillary incisor shown on smile begins to decrease in the mid-20s as does the maxillary incisor to the lip at rest. Gingival display on smile decreases most noticeably after 50 years of age.

In modern populations, there is a strong tendency for crowding of the mandibular incisor teeth to develop in the late teens and early 20s, no matter how well aligned the teeth were initially. Mild crowding of the lower incisors tends to develop if the teeth were initially well aligned, or initially mild crowding becomes worse. These changes appear as early as age 17 to 18 in some individuals and as late as the mid-20s in others. Three major theories to account for this crowding have been proposed.

1. *Lack of "normal attrition" in the modern diet.* As noted in Chapter 1, native populations tend to have a much smaller prevalence of malocclusion than contemporary populations. If a shortening of arch length and mesial migration of the permanent molars is a natural phenomenon, it would seem reasonable that crowding would develop unless the amount of tooth structure was reduced during the final stages of growth. Raymond Begg, a pioneer Australian orthodontist, noted in his studies of the Australian aborigines that malocclusion is uncommon but large amounts of interproximal and occlusal attrition occurred (Fig. 4.31).[25] He concluded that in modern populations the teeth became crowded when attrition did not occur with soft diets, and advocated widespread extraction of premolar teeth to provide the equivalent of the attrition he saw in aborigines. More recent observations have shown that when Australian aborigines change to a modern diet, as they did during the 20th century, occlusal and interproximal wear all but disappear. Nevertheless, late crowding rarely develops,[26] although periodontal disease does become a major problem. It has been observed in other population groups that late crowding may develop even after premolars have been extracted and arch length has been reduced by modern orthodontic treatment. Thus the Begg theory, although superficially attractive, does not explain late crowding.[27]
2. *Pressure from third molars.* Late crowding develops at about the time the third molars should erupt. In most individuals, these teeth are hopelessly impacted because the jaw length did not increase enough to accommodate them via backward modeling of the ramus (Fig. 4.32). It has seemed entirely logical to

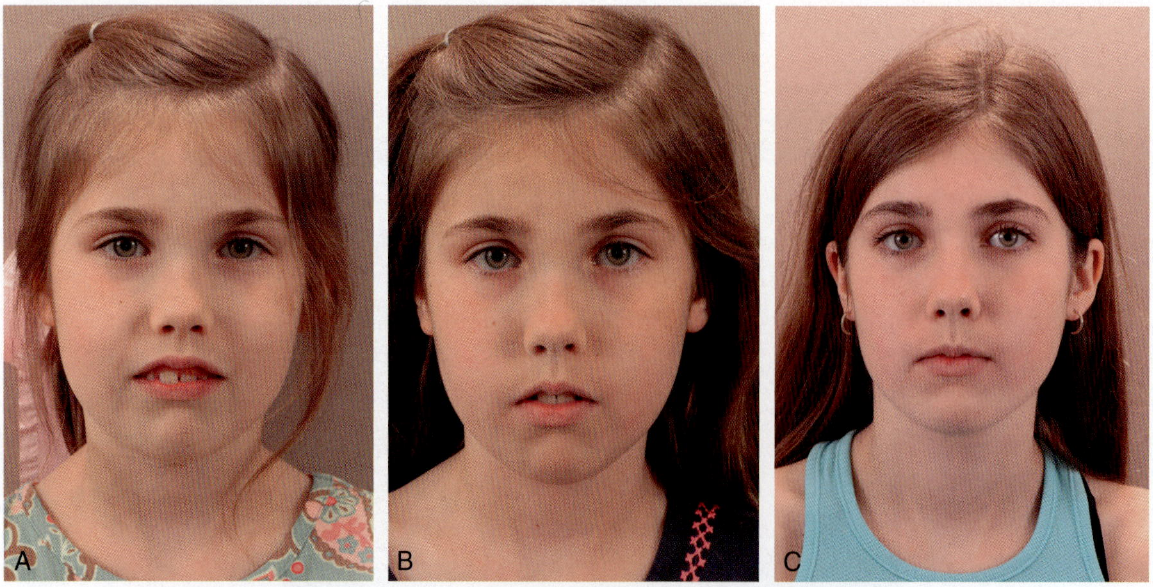

• **Fig. 4.29** This child illustrates the changes in lip competence due to soft tissue growth without treatment at (A) age 8, (B) age 10, and (C) age 14. Notably there are philtrim and commissure height changes that reach equality.

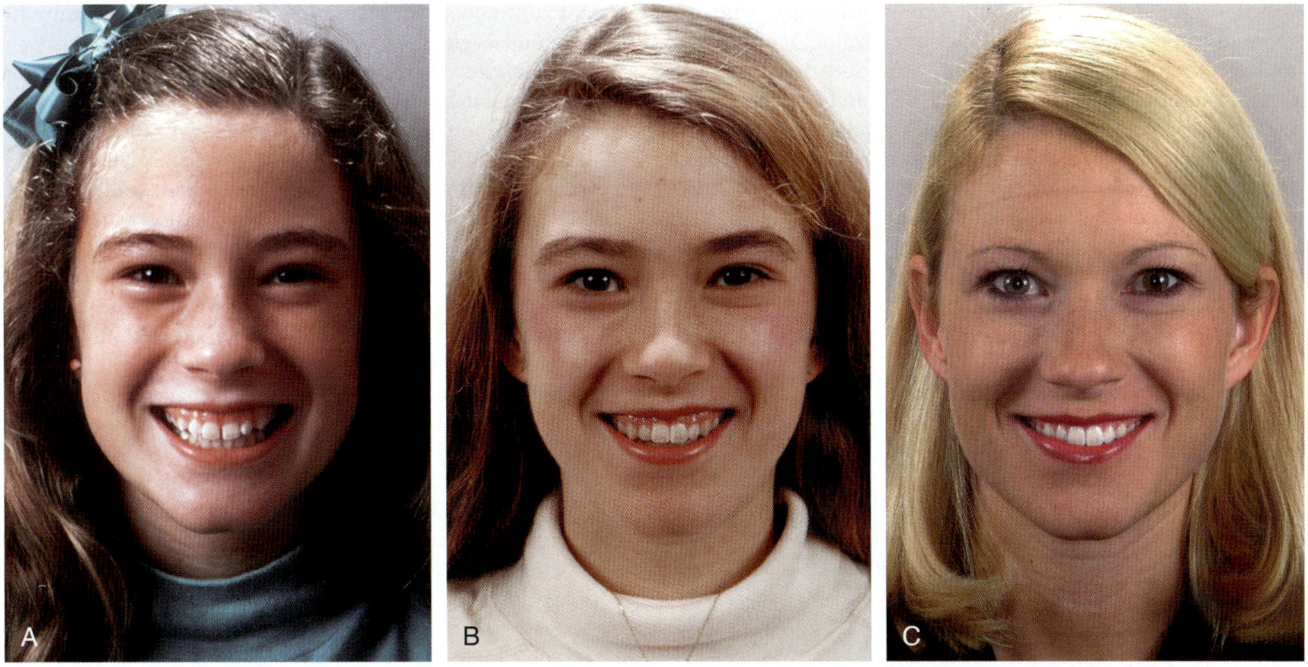

• **Fig. 4.30** The lip to tooth changes due to lip lengthening are even more apparent on smiling. Because lip height increases and the facial soft tissues move downward relative to the teeth with increasing age, what looks like excessive exposure of teeth and gingiva on smile at age 12 (A) appears to be less excessive at age 14 (B), and has totally disappeared at age 24 (C). The patient received no treatment between ages 12 and 24.

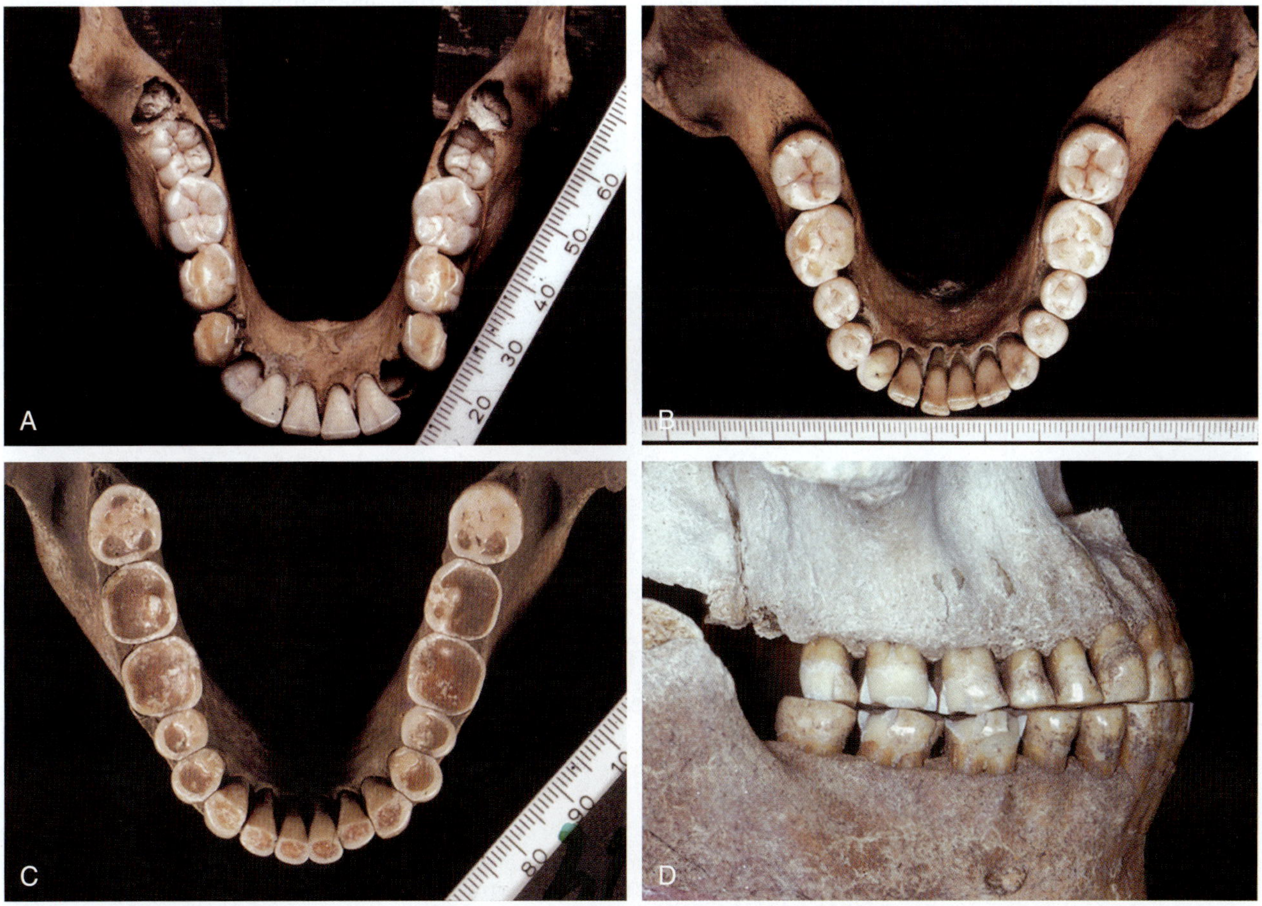

• **Fig. 4.31** Australian aboriginal mandibles of a child approximately at dental age 8 (A), an adolescent at approximately dental age 14 (B), and an adult of indeterminate age (C and D). Note the increasing attrition of the teeth in the younger specimens and the severe attrition of the adult's teeth, with interproximal, as well as occlusal, wear. Arch length in this population shortened by 1 cm or more after adolescence because of the extensive interproximal wear. (Specimens from the Begg Collection, University of Adelaide, Adelaide, Australia. Courtesy Professor W. Sampson.)

dentists and patients that pressure from third molars with no room to erupt is the cause of late incisor crowding. It is difficult to detect such a force, however, even with modern instrumentation that should have found it if it exists.[28] In fact, late crowding of lower incisors can and often does develop in individuals whose lower third molars are congenitally missing. There is some evidence that incisor crowding may be lessened by early removal of second molars, which presumably would relieve pressure from third molars, or management of the leeway space

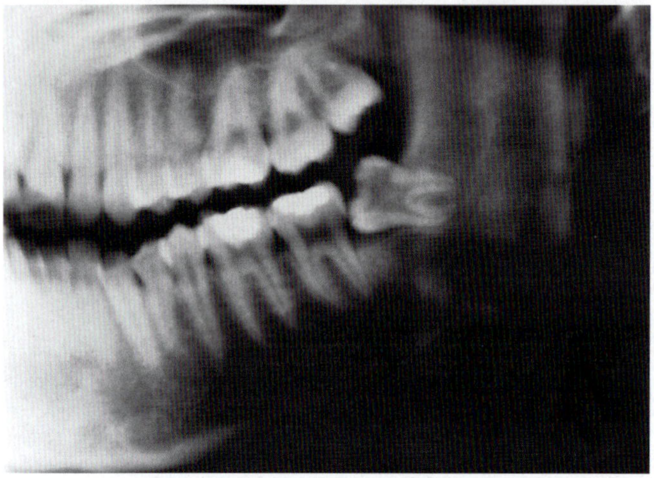

• **Fig. 4.32** It seems reasonable that a horizontally impacted third molar would provide pressure against the dental arch, but it is highly unlikely that there is enough pressure from this source to cause the crowding of mandibular incisors that often develops in the late teens.

to accommodate the transitional crowding, but pressure from third molars clearly is not the total explanation either.[29]

3. *Late mandibular growth.* Because of the cephalocaudal gradient of growth discussed in Chapter 2, the mandible can and does grow more in the late teens than the maxilla. Is it possible that late mandibular growth somehow causes late mandibular incisor crowding? If so, how? Björk's implant studies have provided an understanding of why late crowding occurs and how it indeed relates to the growth pattern of the jaw.

The position of the dentition relative to the maxilla and mandible is influenced by the pattern of growth of the jaws, a concept explored in some detail in previous sections. When the mandible grows forward relative to the maxilla, as it usually does in the late teens, the mandibular incisor teeth tend to be displaced lingually, particularly if forward rotation is also present (as it would be in short-face individuals). This can be seen most clearly when the mandibular growth is excessive (Fig. 4.33), but a milder version of the same uprighting occurs in almost everyone.

In patients with a tight anterior occlusion before late mandibular growth occurs, the contact relationship of the lower incisors with the upper incisors must change if the mandible grows forward. In that circumstance, one of three things must happen: (1) The mandible is displaced distally, accompanied by a distortion of TMJ function and displacement of the articular disc; (2) the upper incisors flare forward, opening space between these teeth; or (3) the lower incisors displace distally and become crowded.

All three of these phenomena have been reported. The second response, flaring and spacing of the maxillary incisors, is rarely seen. Posterior displacement of a "trapped mandible" can happen

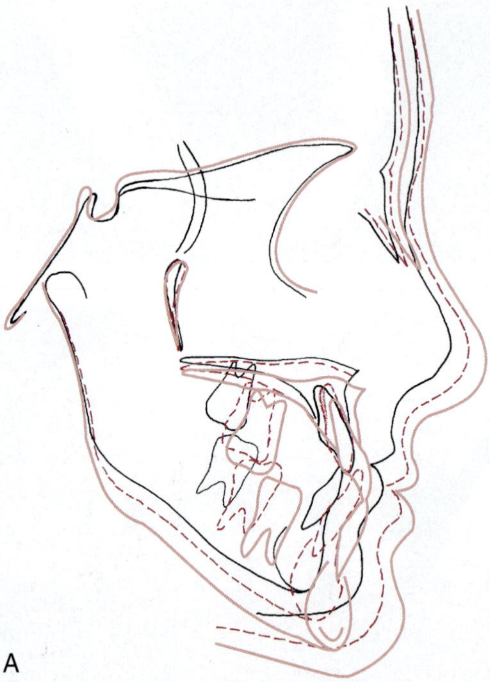

A

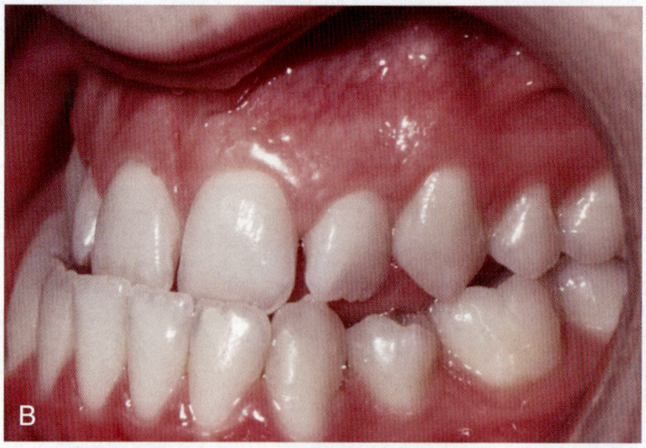

B

• **Fig. 4.33** In this patient with a prolonged class III growth pattern of excessive mandibular growth (A), the lower incisors were increasingly tipped lingually as the mandible grew forward and were noticeably retroclined (B) by the end of adolescent growth. This is a more obvious demonstration of what often happens under normal circumstances, when a small amount of late mandibular growth occurs in the late teens after maxillary growth stops. Late mandibular growth is a major cause of the mandibular incisor crowding that frequently develops at that time.

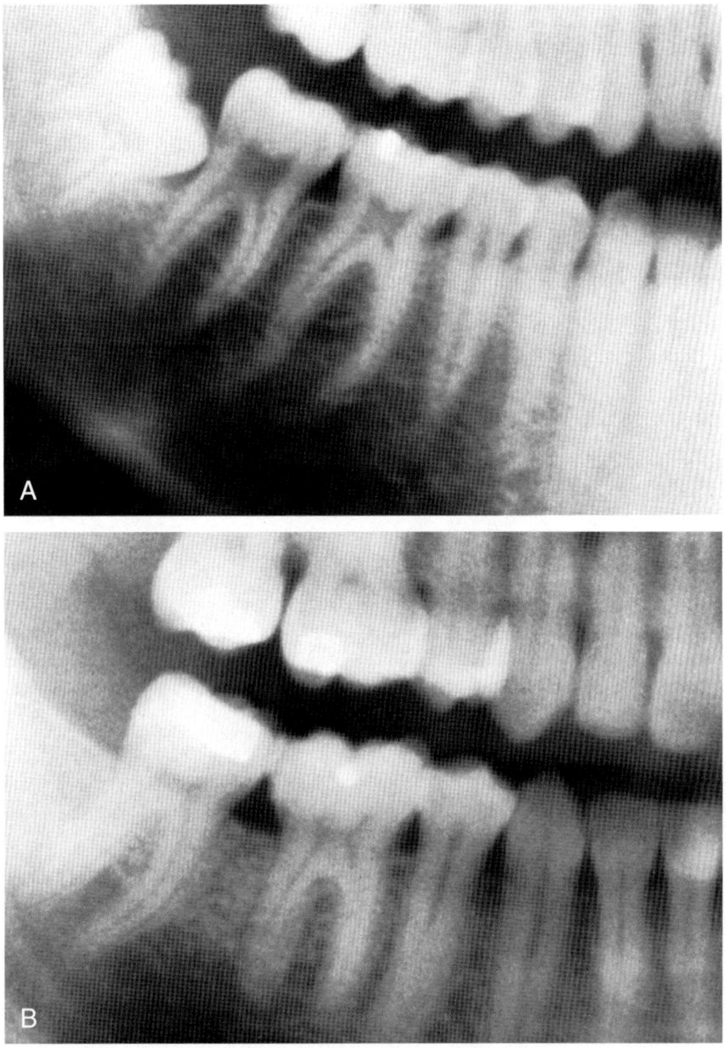

• **Fig. 4.34** The size of the pulp chambers of permanent teeth decreases during adolescence, then continues to fill in more slowly for the rest of adult life. (A) Age 16, (B) age 26.

and may occasionally be related to myofascial pain and dysfunction, but despite the claims of some occlusion theorists, this too seems to be quite rare. Distal displacement of the lower incisors, with concomitant crowding and a decrease in the lower intercanine distance, is the usual response. It is not even necessary for the incisors to be in occlusal contact for late crowding to develop. This also occurs commonly in individuals who have an anterior open bite and backward, not forward, rotation of the mandible (see Fig. 4.21). In this situation, the rotation of the mandible carries the dentition forward, thrusting the incisors against the lip. This creates light but lasting pressure on the lip, which tends to reposition the protruding incisors somewhat lingually, reducing the arch length and causing crowding.

The current concept is that late incisor crowding almost always develops as the mandibular incisors (and perhaps the entire mandibular dentition) move distally relative to the body of the mandible late in mandibular growth. This sheds some light on the possible role of the third molars in determining whether crowding will occur and how severe it will be. If space were available at the distal end of the mandibular arch, it might be possible for all the mandibular teeth to shift slightly distally, allowing the lower incisors to move upright without becoming crowded. However, impacted third molars at the distal end of the lower arch would prevent the posterior teeth from shifting distally, and if differential mandibular growth occurred, their presence might guarantee that crowding would develop. In this case, the lower third molars could be the "last straw" in a chain of events that led to late incisor crowding. As noted previously, however, late incisor crowding occurs in individuals with no third molars at all, so the presence of these teeth is not the critical variable. Instead, the extent of late mandibular growth is. The more your mandible grows after another growth has essentially stopped, the greater the chance your lower incisors will become crowded, and this is true in both those who have undergone orthodontic treatment and those who have not.[30]

Aging Changes in Teeth and Supporting Structures

At the time a permanent tooth erupts, the pulp chamber is relatively large. As time passes, additional dentin slowly deposits on the inside of the tooth so that the pulp chamber gradually becomes smaller with increasing age (Fig. 4.34). This process continues relatively rapidly until the late teens, at which time the pulp

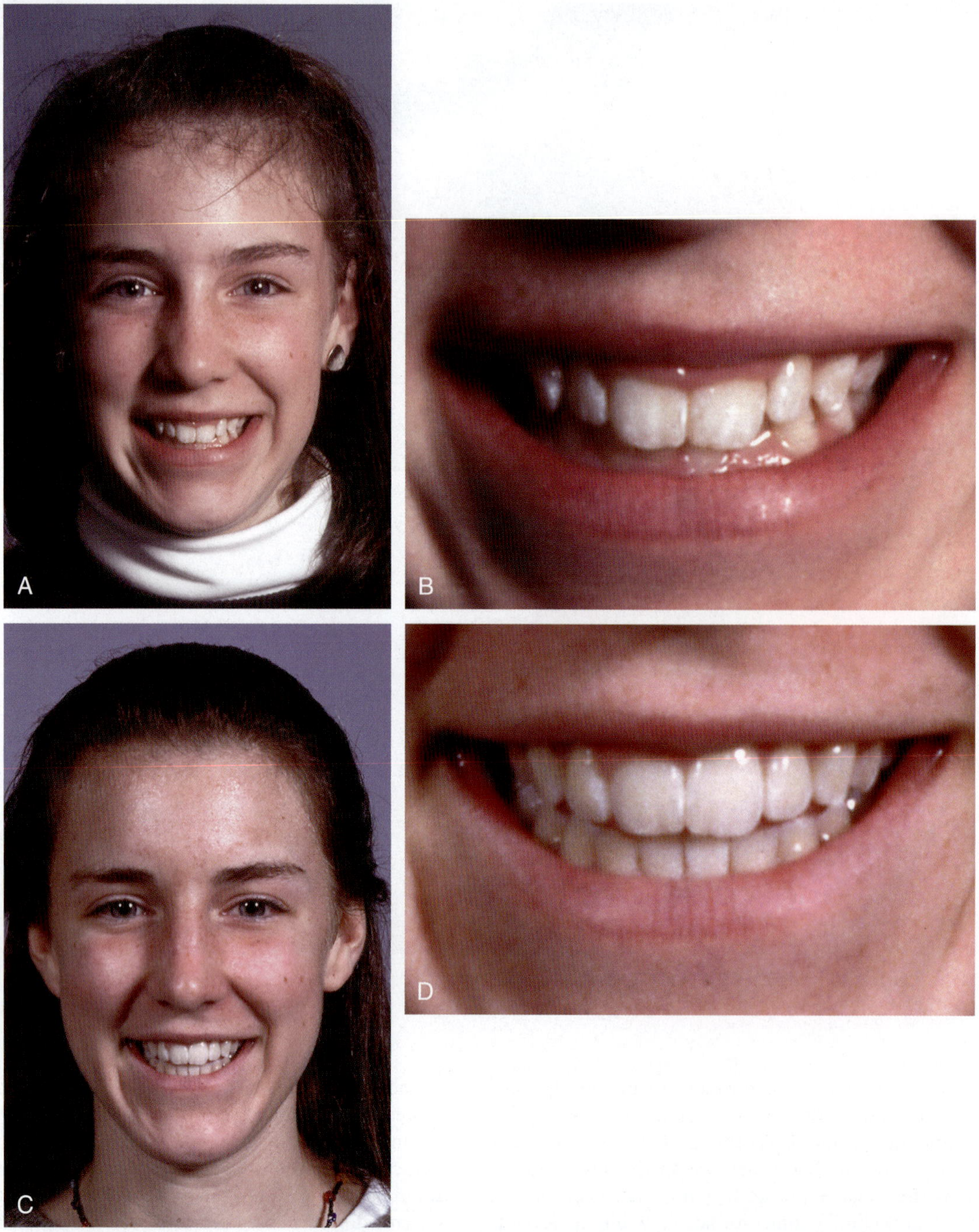

• **Fig. 4.35** The increasing crown height of permanent teeth during adolescence was once thought to result from a downward migration of the gingival attachment but now is recognized to occur mostly from tooth eruption in response to vertical growth. (A and B) Age 10, and (C and D) age 16.

chamber of a typical permanent tooth is about half the size that it was at the time of the initial eruption. Because of the relatively large pulp chambers of young permanent teeth, complex restorative procedures are more likely to result in mechanical exposures in adolescents than in adults. Additional dentin continues to be produced at a slower rate throughout life, so in old age the pulp chambers of some permanent teeth are all but obliterated.

Maturation also brings about greater exposure of the tooth outside its investing soft tissues. At the time a permanent first molar erupts, the gingival attachment is high on the crown. Typically, the gingival attachment is still well above the cementoenamel junction when any permanent tooth comes into full occlusion, and during the next few years, more and more of the crown is exposed. This relative apical movement of the attachment (in normal circumstances) results more from vertical growth of the jaws and the accompanying eruption of the teeth than from downward migration of the gingival attachment. As we have noted previously, vertical growth of the jaws and an increase in face height continue after transverse and anteroposterior growth have been completed. By the time the jaws all but stop growing vertically in the late teens, the gingival attachment is usually near the cementoenamel junction. In the absence of inflammation, mechanical abrasion, or pathologic changes, the gingival attachment should remain at about the same level almost indefinitely. However, many individuals experience some pathology of the gingiva or periodontium as they age, and so further recession of the gingiva is common.

At one time, it was thought that "passive eruption" (defined as an actual gingival migration of the attachment without any eruption of the tooth) occurred. It now appears that if the gingival tissues are entirely healthy, this sort of downward migration of the soft tissue attachment does not occur. What was once thought to be apical migration of the gingiva during the teens is in fact active eruption, compensating for the vertical jaw growth still occurring at that time (Fig. 4.35).

Both occlusal and interproximal wear, often to a severe degree, occurred in native people eating an extremely coarse diet. The elimination of most coarse particles from modern diets has also largely eliminated wear of this type. With a few exceptions (tobacco chewing is one), wearing facets on the teeth now indicates bruxism, not what the individual has been eating.

References

1. Manotas MC, González DM, Céspedes C, Forero C, Rojas Moreno AP. Genetic and epigenetic control of puberty. *Sex Dev.* 2022;16(1):1–10.
2. Shim YS, Lee HS, Hwang JS. Genetic factors in precocious puberty. *Clin Exp Pediatr.* 2022;65(4):172–181. https://doi.org/10.3345/cep.2021.00521.
3. Marshall WA, Tanner JM. Puberty. In: Falkner F, Tanner JM, eds. *Human Growth*. Vol 2. 2nd ed. Plenum Publishing; 1986.
4. Anderson DL, Thompson GW, Popovich F. Interrelationship of dental maturity, skeletal maturity, height and weight from age 4 to 14 years. *Growth.* 1975;39:453–462.
5. Agronin KJ, Kokich VG. Displacement of the glenoid fossa: a cephalometric evaluation of growth during treatment. *Am J Orthod Dentofac Orthop.* 1987;91:42–48.
6. Bishara SE, Jakobsen JR, Treder J, et al. Arch width changes from 6 weeks to 45 years of age. *Am J Orthod Dentofac Orthop.* 1997;111:401–409.
7. Solow B, Iseri H. Maxillary growth revisited: an update based on recent implant studies. In: Davidovitch Z, Norton LA, eds. *Biological Mechanisms of Tooth Movement and Craniofacial Adaptation.* Harvard Society for Advancement of Orthodontics; 1996.
8. Behrents RG. *Growth in the aging craniofacial skeleton. Craniofacial Growth series, Monograph 17.* Center for Human Growth and Development, University of Michigan; 1985.
9. Björk A. The use of metallic implants in the study of facial growth in children: method and application. *Am J Phys Anthropol.* 1968;29:243–254.
10. Solow B, Houston WJ. Mandibular rotations: concept and terminology. *Eur J Orthod.* 1988;10:177–179.
11. Björk A, Skieller V. Normal and abnormal growth of the mandible: a synthesis of longitudinal cephalometric implant studies over a period of 25 years. *Eur J Orthod.* 1983;5:1–46.
12. Björk A, Skieller V. Postnatal growth and development of the maxillary complex. In: McNamara JA, ed. *Factors Affecting Growth of the Midface.* University of Michigan Center for Human Growth and Development; 1976.
13. Houston WJ. Mandibular growth rotations—their mechanisms and importance. *Eur J Orthod.* 1988;110:369–373.
14. Björk A, Skieller V. Contrasting mandibular growth and facial development in long face syndrome, juvenile rheumatoid arthritis and mandibulofacial dysostosis. *J Craniofac Genet Dev Biol.* 1985;1(suppl):127–138.
15. Behrents RG. *A Treatise on the Continuum of Growth in the Aging Craniofacial Skeleton.* University of Michigan Center for Human Growth and Development; 1984.
16. Proffit WR, Phillips C, Turvey TA. Stability following superior repositioning of the maxilla. *Am J Orthod.* 1987;92:151–163.
17. Harris EF. A longitudinal study of arch size and form in untreated adults. *Am J Orthod Dentofac Orthop.* 1997;111:419–427.
18. Pecora NG, Beccetti T, McNamara Jr. JA. The aging craniofacial complex: a longitudinal cephalometric study from late adolescence to late adulthood. *Am J Orthod Dentofac Orthop.* 2008;134:496–506.
19. Subtelny JD. A longitudinal study of soft tissue facial structures and their profile characteristics, defined in relation to underlying skeletal structures. *Am J Orthod.* 1959;45(7):481–507.
20. Bergman RT, Waschak J, Borzabadi-Farahani A, Murphy NC. Longitudinal study of cephalometric soft tissue profile traits between the ages of 6 and 18 years. *Angle Orthod.* 2014;84(1):48–55.
21. Marshall SD, Low LE, Holton NE, et al. Chin development as a result of differential jaw growth. *Am J Orthod Dentofac Orthop.* 2011;139(4):456–464.
22. Nanda RS, Meng H, Kapila S, Goorhuis J. Growth changes in the soft tissue facial profile. *Angle Orthod.* 1990;60(3):177–190. Fall.
23. Dickens ST, Sarver DM, Proffit WR. Changes in frontal soft tissue dimensions of the lower face by age and gender. *World J Orthod.* 2002;3:313–332.
24. Sarver DM. *Dentofacial Esthetics: From Macro to Micro.* Quintessence Publishing Co, Inc; 2020.
25. Begg PR. Stone age man's dentition. *Am J Orthod.* 1954;40:298–312. 373–383, 462–475, 517–531.
26. Brown T, Townsend GC, Pinkerton SK, Rogers JR. *Teeth, Time and the Tanami: Dental Research at Yuendumu.* Univ. of Adelaide Press; 2011.
27. Corruccini RS. Australian aboriginal tooth succession, interproximal attrition and Begg's theory. *Am J Orthod Dentofac Orthop.* 1990;97:349–357.
28. Southard TE, Southard KA, Weeda LW. Mesial force from unerupted third molars. *Am J Orthod Dentofac Orthop.* 1991;99:220–225.
29. Richardson ME. Late lower arch crowding: the aetiology reviewed. *Dent Update.* 2002;29:234–238.
30. Jonsson T, Magnusson TE. Crowding and spacing in the dental arches: long-term development in treated and untreated subjects. *Am J Orthod Dentofac Orthop.* 2010;138:384.e1–384.e7; discussion 384–386.

5

The Etiology of Orthodontic Problems

WILLIAM R. PROFFIT, HENRY W. FIELDS, KAITRIN KRAMER, AND BENJAMIN T. PLISKA

CHAPTER OUTLINE

Malocclusion is a developmental condition. In most instances, malocclusion and craniofacial abnormalities or anomalies are not caused by some pathologic process, but dysregulation or deviation from normal development. These deviations from normal can be characterized as mild, moderate, or severe. Dysmorphology, a field pioneered by geneticist David W. Smith in the 1960s, focused on "the study of, or the general subject of abnormal tissue form." Since then, a number of technological advances have revolutionized and advanced our understanding of modern genetics. When discussing craniofacial anomalies, it is important to define terminology as it relates to normal development and how different terms have changed over time. The term malformation and deformation are commonly used to describe craniofacial anomalies. Malformation is defined as a congenital morphologic anomaly due to an alteration in primary development of a body part or an organ. This is generally thought of as intrinsic changes in molecular and cellular signaling pathways governing development due to mutations caused by teratogens or prenatal exposures, or a combination of the two. Deformation is the altered shape or position of a body part due to mechanical forces that distorts the structure. This can result in asymmetric formation of the final body part.

Occasionally, a specific cause of a dentofacial problem is apparent—for example, a mandibular deficiency secondary to a childhood fracture of the jaw, which would lead to deformation of the mandible, or the characteristic malocclusion that accompanies some genetic syndromes, which with rare exceptions would be a malformation. These problems most often result from a complex interaction among multiple factors that influence growth and development, thereby making it impossible to describe a single specific etiologic factor (Fig. 5.1).

Here, we should clarify several additional terms. A hereditary disorder can be passed from generation to generation and is genetic in nature, due to mutations in the genetic code. Congenital disorders are present at birth and may be inherited or may be caused by de novo mutations. Many craniofacial anomalies can be attributed to a single gene mutation, chromosomal changes, or prenatal exposure to certain environments or drugs. There are three stages of fetal development prior to birth: germinal 0 to 2 weeks, embryonic 3 to 8 weeks, and 9 weeks—birth is the fetal period. Problems that occur in the germinal period are largely due to a failure of implantation in the wall of the uterus, which occurs in approximately 60% of natural conceptions. Most problems impacting craniofacial development occur in the embryonic period of 3 to 8 weeks gestation.

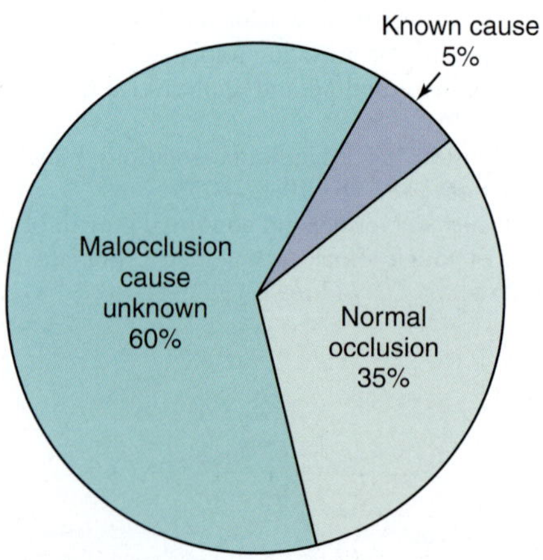

• **Fig. 5.1** From a broad perspective, only about one-third of the US population has normal occlusion, whereas two-thirds have some degree of malocclusion. In the malocclusion group, only a small minority (not more than 5%) have problems attributable to a specific known cause; the remainder are the result of a complex and poorly understood combination of inherited and environmental influences.

TABLE 5.1 Teratogens Affecting Dentofacial Development

Teratogens	Effect
Aminopterin	Anencephaly
Aspirin	Cleft lip and palate
Cigarette smoke (hypoxia)	Cleft lip and palate
Cytomegalovirus	Microcephaly, hydrocephaly, microphthalmia
Dilantin	Cleft lip and palate
Ethyl alcohol	Central midface deficiency
6-Mercaptopurine	Cleft palate
13-*cis* Retinoic acid (Accutane)	Similar to craniofacial microsomia and Treacher Collins syndrome
Rubella virus	Microphthalmia, cataracts, deafness
Thalidomide	Malformations similar to craniofacial microsomia, Treacher Collins syndrome
Toxoplasma	Microcephaly, hydrocephaly, microphthalmia
X-radiation	Microcephaly
Valium	Similar to craniofacial microsomia and Treacher Collins syndrome
Vitamin D excess	Premature suture closure
Zika virus	Microcephaly, brain damage

Although it is difficult to know the precise cause of most malocclusions, we do know in general what the possibilities are, and these must be considered when orthodontic problems are being evaluated. In this chapter we examine etiologic factors for malocclusion under three major headings: known specific causes, hereditary (genetic) influences, and environmental influences. The chapter concludes with a perspective on the interaction of hereditary and environmental influences in the development of the major types of malocclusions.

Specific Causes of Malocclusion

Note here that although the causes of these problems are known, they make up a small percentage of etiologies of malocclusion. The known causes are genetic or environmental or a combination. We will focus our discussion on common craniofacial anomalies by incidence with a direct impact on the dentofacial complex in this section. This includes cleft lip and/or palate, Treacher Collins, craniosynostosis, hemifacial microsomia, microcephaly, and microtia.

Disturbances in Embryologic Development

Defects in embryologic development usually result in death of the embryo. As many as 20% of early pregnancies are lost spontaneously because of lethal embryologic defects, often so early that the mother is not even aware of conception. Although most defects in embryos are of genetic origin, effects from the environment are also important. Chemical and other agents capable of producing embryologic defects if given at the critical time are called *teratogens*. Most drugs do not either interfere with normal development or at high doses kill the embryo without producing defects and therefore are not teratogenic. Teratogens typically cause specific fetal abnormalities. Teratogens known to produce craniofacial problems are listed in Table 5.1, with Zika virus (which causes microcephaly) being the most recent addition.

Fig. 5.2 provides an overview of a succession of stages in human embryonic craniofacial development as it occurs during weeks 3 to 8 after fertilization. Over this short period, morphologic characteristics change from a disklike shape of approximately 0.5 mm in diameter (Fig. 5.2A) to an approximately 25-mm-long (crown to rump), distinctly human form (Fig. 5.2L). This change in form is characterized by formation of the neural plate (developing central nervous system), elevation of its lateral margins to form the neural tube, and subsequent neural tube closure, which occurs in the fourth week of embryonic development. Neural tube formation and closure are accompanied by ventral and lateral folding (differential growth) that results in formation of the foregut (Fig. 5.2D); lengthening and bending of the heart tube (heart development); the appearance of the primitive oral cavity (stomodeum); and formation of the tissues that will contribute to the jaws (maxillary prominence and first arch), nose, and ears. For more detailed description of normal craniofacial embryogenesis, the reader is referred to embryology texts and websites.

Genetic and environmental insults (in this context, *insult* means anything that could have an adverse impact on normal development) can affect the developing face and jaws throughout the embryonic period. It usually is the case that an insult affected growth well before a specific abnormality occurred. With the help of information gained from animal research studies, some abnormalities can be traced to effects that occur during narrow time windows. An example of a phenotype that arises in the third week of development is the characteristic facies of fetal alcohol syndrome (FAS; Fig. 5.3). This is due to deficiencies of midline tissue of the developing brain (neural plate) and is typically caused by exposure to very high maternal ethanol levels. Although such blood levels can be reached only in extreme intoxication in chronic alcoholics, the resulting facial deformity and developmental delay occur frequently enough to be implicated in many cases of midface deficiency.[1] In these children, the delay in dental development matches the skeletal delay.[2]

Many craniofacial defects are related to neural crest cell abnormalities or neurocristopathies. Neurocristopathies are disorders characterized by the abnormal migration, expression, differentiation, or cell death of neural crest cells in embryonic development. Neural crest cell migration away from the cranial neural folds occurs in the latter part of the third and the early part of the fourth week (Fig. 5.4), and this is a time of vulnerability to teratogens. Neural crest cells make up practically all of the mesenchyme (loose connective tissue) of the face and differentiate into much of its skeletal and connective tissue, including the bones of the jaw and the teeth.

The importance of neural crest cell populations and the possibility of drug-induced cell death and/or impairment of their migration have been demonstrated clearly by experience. In the 1960s and 1970s, exposure to thalidomide caused major congenital defects, including facial anomalies in thousands of children. In the 1980s, severe facial malformations related to the anti-acne drug isotretinoin (Accutane) were reported. The similarities in the defects make it likely that both drugs adversely

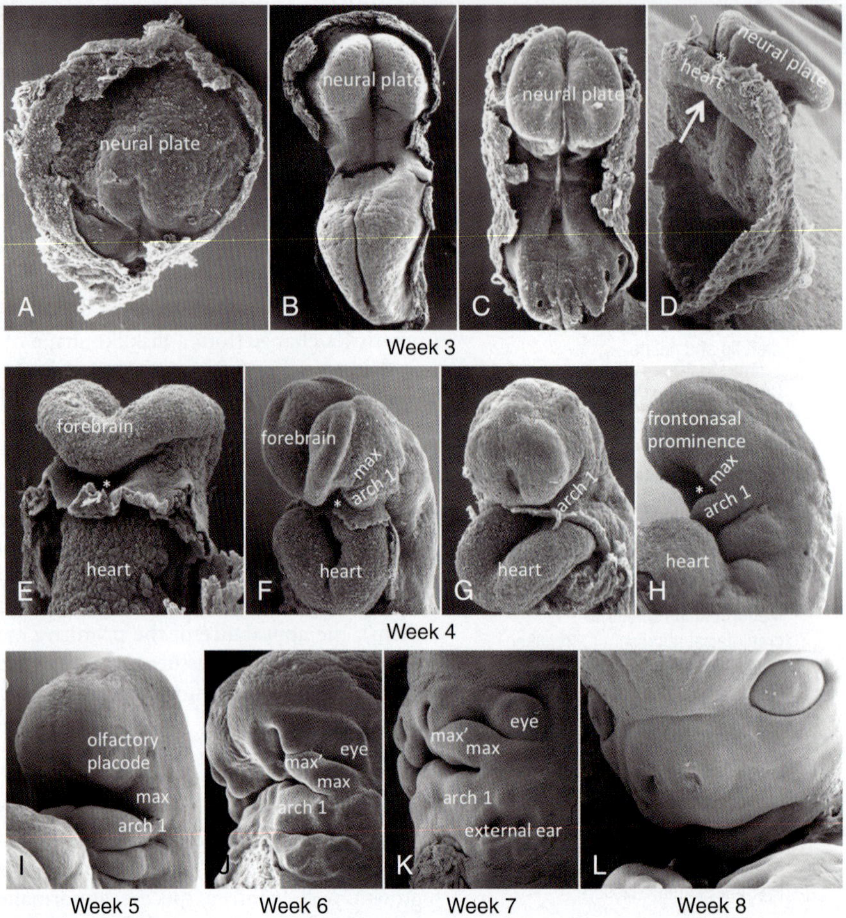

• **Fig. 5.2** This sequence of scanning electron micrographs illustrates a succession of stages of human embryonic development that occur during the third to eighth weeks after fertilization. Views shown in A to C are of the dorsal side of the embryos; D–L are ventrolateral views. Approximate postfertilization ages for each of the embryos are as follows: 17 days (A); 19 days (B); 21 days (C); 21 days (D); 23 days (E); 24 days (F); 25 days (G); 26 days (H); 32 days (I); 41 days (J); 43 days (K); 52 days (L). Notable from the earliest stage shown is the neural plate, which by the end of the fourth week has become the closed neural tube, the most rostral part of which becomes the forebrain. Tissue surrounding the forebrain of a late fourth-week and fifth-week embryo is termed the *frontonasal prominence* (growth center). This structure, along with the first pharyngeal arch and maxillary prominence (*max*, including its most medial and rostral component, *max'*), form the perimeter of the developing oral cavity (*, stomodeum). Distinction among many of the individual facial prominences (growth centers) becomes less apparent with time, and by the end of the embryonic period, the face appears distinctly human. The arrow in D indicates the foregut. (A–I, K, and L, Courtesy Dr. K. Sulik. Reprinted from Hinrichsen JK. The early development of morphology and patterns of the face in the human embryo. *Adv Anat Embryol Cell Biol*. 1985;98:1–79.)

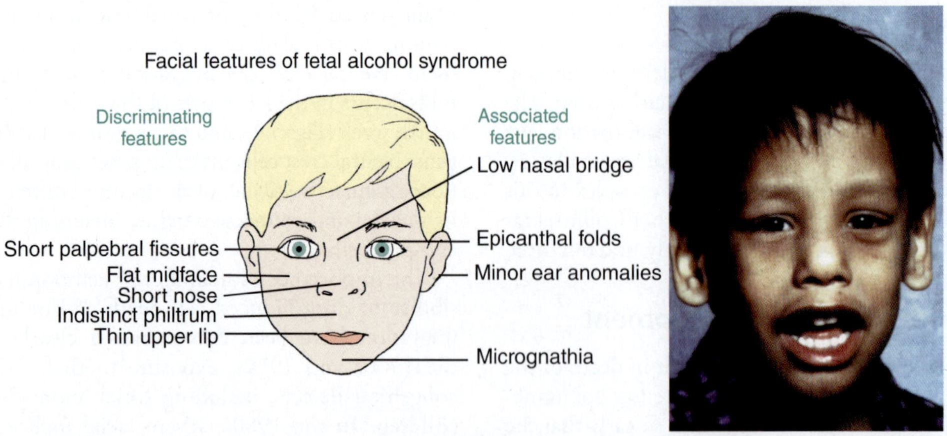

• **Fig. 5.3** The characteristic facial appearance of fetal alcohol syndrome, caused by exposure to very high blood alcohol levels during the first trimester of pregnancy.

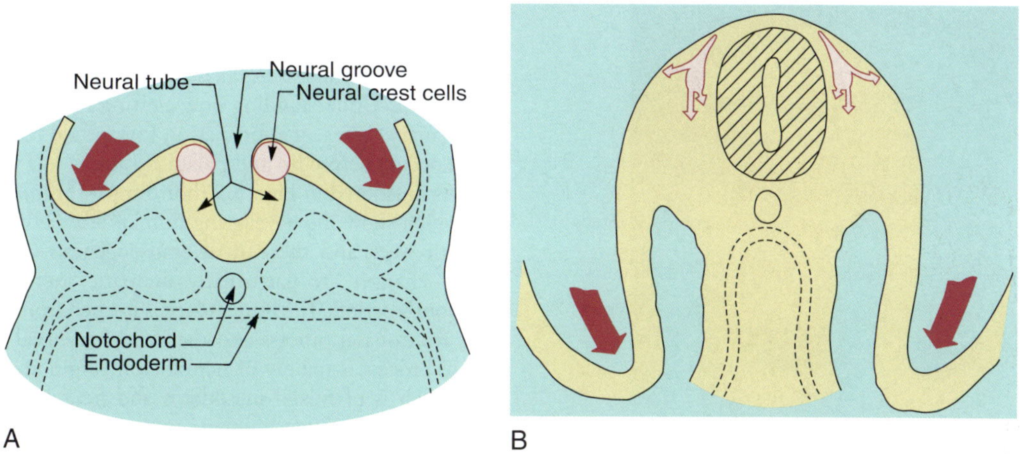

• **Fig. 5.4** Diagrammatic lateral sections of embryos at 20 and 24 days, showing formation of the neural folds, neural groove, and neural crest. (A) At 20 days, neural crest cells *(pink)* can be identified at the lips of the deepening neural groove, forerunner of the central nervous system. (B) At 24 days, the neural crest cells have separated from the neural tube and are beginning their extensive migration beneath the surface ectoderm. The migration is so extensive and the role of these neural crest cells is so important in formation of structures of the head and face that they can almost be considered a fourth primary germ layer. Later stages in the migration can be seen in Fig. 5.2EH.

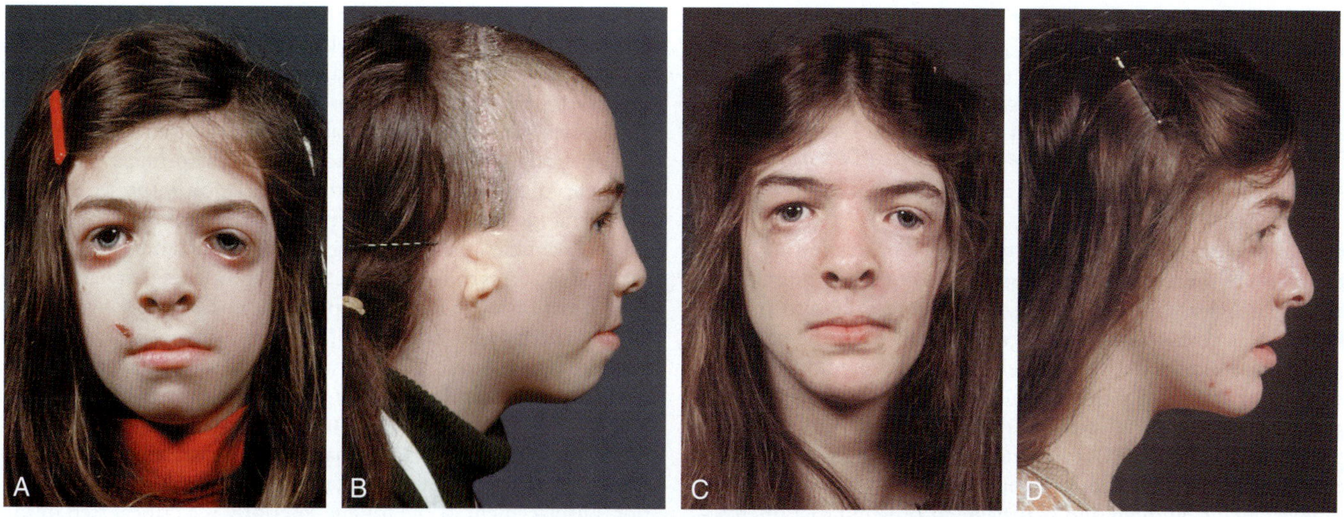

• **Fig. 5.5** In the Treacher Collins syndrome (also called *mandibulofacial dysostosis*), a generalized lack of mesenchymal tissue in the lateral part of the face is the major cause of the characteristic facial appearance. Note the underdevelopment of the lateral orbital and zygomatic areas. The ears also may be affected. Patient at age 12 before (A) and immediately after (B) surgical treatment to advance the midface. Note this patient's ear deformity, which usually is concealed by hair. (C and D) Age 16. Note the change in the lateral orbital margins.

affect neural crest cell migration. Importantly, the time of insult associated with these defects is before the mother knows she is pregnant. From 2010 to the present, Zika virus has caused thousands of cases of microcephaly due to impaired development of the brain. Exposure to Zika virus at any stage of pregnancy, not just during embryogenesis, may impair brain development. The diminished brain growth leads to both microcephaly and severe neurologic deficits. Microcephaly is defined as a small circumference of the head secondary to cessation of brain growth or lack of brain development. There are a number of teratogens described above that are associated with microcephaly as well as associated chromosomal abnormalities and syndromes such Trisomy 21.

In addition to drug-induced neural crest defects, genetic alterations also can adversely affect this cell population and produce craniofacial abnormalities. An example is Treacher Collins syndrome (Fig. 5.5), which is characterized by reduced levels of mesenchymal tissue, especially in the lateral aspects of the face caused by defects in neural crest migration and differentiation. Treacher Collins syndrome is a rare form of mandibulofacial dysostosis contributing to malar and mandibular hypoplasia and now is known to be due to mutations in the *TCOF1, POLR1C and POLR1D* genes.[3] Malformations very similar to this syndrome may result from teratogenic effects on embryos at stages present in the fourth week.[4]

Craniofacial microsomia (often called *hemifacial microsomia*) is characterized by deficient development usually on one side of the

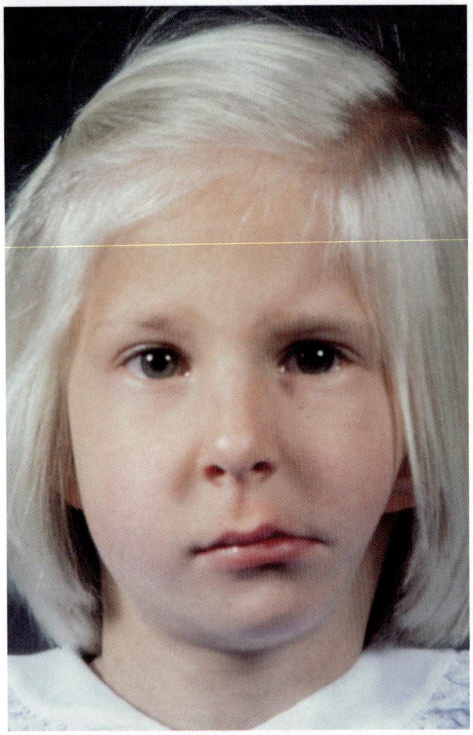

• **Fig. 5.6** In craniofacial microsomia, both the external ear and the mandibular ramus are deficient or absent on the affected side. In this patient with a relatively mild problem, note the use of the hairstyle to conceal the ear and short ramus on the affected left side. (From Proffit WR, White RP, Sarver DM. *Contemporary Treatment of Dentofacial Deformity*. Mosby; 2003.)

face. Typically, the external ear is malformed or missing and both the ramus of the mandible and associated soft tissues (muscle, fascia) are deficient or missing (Fig. 5.6). Some cases also include hearing loss. Facial asymmetry is always seen (thus the common name), and cranial as well as facial structures are affected. The etiology of craniofacial microsomia has been extensively studied, and model systems indicate that the major cause is insult to cell populations (including but not limited to neural crest cells) that are required for proper development of the first pharyngeal (mandibular) arch.[5] Findings and management of hemifacial microsomia will be discussed in more detail in Chapter 7.

In addition to their importance for development of the face, neural crest cells migrate through the lower (pharyngeal) arches and play a major role in formation of the heart and great vessels. This is the basis for the common cooccurrence of craniofacial abnormalities and heart defects such as tetralogy of Fallot.

Orofacial clefts are the most common congenital defects outside of chromosomal defects, second only to heart defects in the entire spectrum of congenital deformities.[6] This includes cleft lip with or without cleft palate and cleft palate only. The primary cause of cleft lip and palate among most infants is unknown. The etiology is thought to be a combination of genetic and environment factors. Smoking (and passive smoking),[7] alcohol use, and certain medication exposure in utero have been shown to increase risk of clefting in babies.[8] Roughly, 30% of cases are associated with a syndrome, while the remaining 70% are of unknown origin. About 1 in 700 babies is born with a cleft palate and 1 in 1600 babies are born with a cleft lip and palate (CLP) in the United States. For dentists and orthodontists, understanding how orofacial clefts arise is important because children with a CLP will require extensive dental and orthodontic rehabilitation. Interestingly, children with cleft lip often only have atypical changes to the dentition but require less extensive intervention compared to children with CLP. Understanding how clefting impacts embryogenesis in humans requires an appreciation for normal facial morphogenesis as it occurs before lip and palate closure.

As illustrated in Figs. 5.2 (bottom row of images) and 5.7, both of which show the developing human face between the end of the fourth week and the end of embryogenesis (eighth week), facial form changes are particularly dramatic over this approximately 1-month period. The human face is formed from two main sources: the frontonasal process and the first pharyngeal arch. The frontonasal process is mainly of neural crest origin and the first pharyngeal arch is of mixed mesoderm and neural crest origin. During the fifth week of development an ectodermal thickening called the nasal placode develops on the frontonasal process. The lateral and medial nasal processes develop lateral and medial to the nasal placode respectively. The nasal placode will eventually give rise to the specialized olfactory epithelium involved in the sense of smell. The first pharyngeal arch gives rise to the maxillary processes which later gives rise to the palatal processes and gives rise to the mandibular processes which makes up the bulk of the first pharyngeal arch. The medial nasal process contributes to the formation of the philtrum of the upper lip. The paired maxillary processes develop and form the lateral aspect of the upper lip before fusion with the medial nasal process. The lower lip is formed by the mandibular process.

The primary palate is formed from a fusion of the medial nasal processes. The primary palate is anterior to the incisive foramen and houses the central and lateral incisors. There have been reports of a dual origin of the lateral incisor from the primary palate and secondary palate contributing to the variation in presentation of the lateral incisor seen in children with clefting.[9]

The secondary palate is formed from bilateral outgrowth of the maxillary process called palatine shelves/processes that occurs after the formation of the primary palate at about 7 to 8 weeks gestation. The palatine shelves initially grow downward and lateral to the tongue. Around 7 to 8 weeks of development the shelves elevate and fuse with each other and the primary palate above the tongue. Fig. 5.8 shows the closure of the palate in mouse embryos (which are very similar to humans at that stage of development) from a frontal view. The secondary palate closes anterior to posterior. Displacement of the tongue inferiorly is a critical step in this process as syndromes that affect mandibular growth such as Pierre Robin Sequence can contribute to cleft palate given the abnormal tongue position during development. Fig. 5.9 shows human embryos at the end of the embryonic period and in the early fetal period. As you can see in Fig. 5.9A, the secondary palatal shelves initially are widely separated. Elevation of the shelves above the tongue is required for midline union. In Fig. 5.9B, note the elevation and (Fig. 5.9C) initial contact of the palatal shelves, which is followed by completion of their midline union (Fig. 5.9D).

The fusion of these distinct developmental processes and embryologic boundaries are tightly regulated and occur at very specific time points. Any deviation from the highly programmed sequence will contribute to the formation of an orofacial cleft at that boundary. For example, a lack of fusion of the medial nasal process and the maxillary process on one side will contribute to a unilateral cleft lip or on both sides a bilateral cleft lip. Lack of fusion of the primary palate with the palatine shelves derived from the maxillary process will contribute to clefting to the alveolus and palate. Typical lip clefts may be unilateral, bilateral, complete, or incomplete (Fig. 5.10).

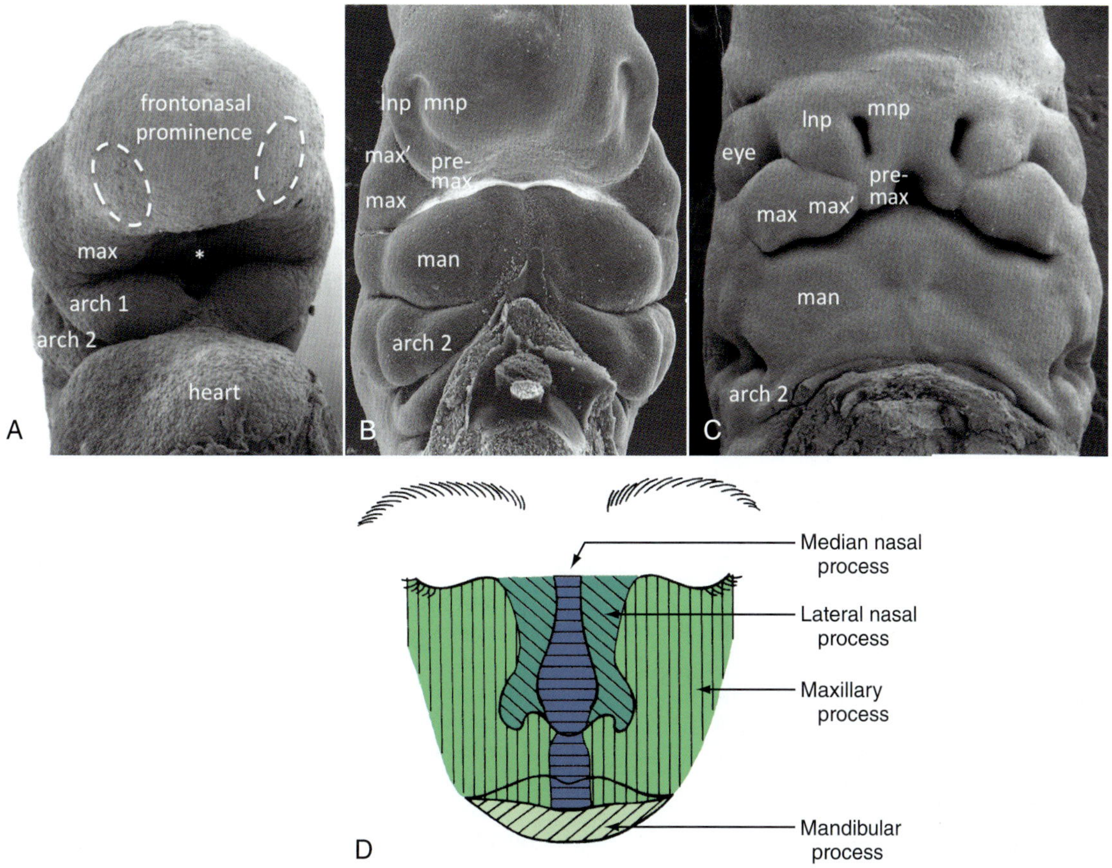

• **Fig. 5.7** Frontal views of human embryos in the fourth (A), sixth (B), and seventh (C) weeks after fertilization. At the stage shown in (A) (fourth week), the olfactory placodes *(dashed circles)* are visible on the surface of the frontonasal prominence, the tissue that envelopes the forebrain. By the middle of the sixth week (B), growth centers that surround the nasal pits and are termed the *medial (mnp)* and *lateral (lnp) nasal prominences* are evident, as are a premaxillary *(premax)* segment, two components of the maxillary region (*max* and *max′*) and the mandibular *(man)* portion of the first pharyngeal arch. These growth centers are also discernable in the early seventh week (43 days) in human embryos (C). *, Stomodeum (primitive oral cavity). (D) Schematic representation of the contribution of the embryonic facial processes to the structures of the adult face. The central part of the nose and the philtrum of the lip are derived from the medial nasal process. The lateral nasal process forms the outer parts of the nose, and the maxillary process forms the bulk of the upper lip and the cheeks. (Courtesy Dr. K. Sulik.)

In addition to cleft lip and cleft palate, other orofacial facial clefts occur that result from the failure of facial prominences to properly form or unite (Figs. 5.7).[10] Orofacial clefts are often named and numbered for the structures (soft tissue and hard tissue) affected.[11] Examples include macrostomia, a defect at the junction of the maxillary and mandibular processes that may result from a growth deficiency and abnormal fusion in either or both processes leading to an enlargement of the mouth at the oral commissure.[12]

Another major group of craniofacial malformations involves craniosynostosis, or early fusion of the fibrous sutures that facilitate the expansion of the craniofacial complex to accommodate the growing brain. Craniosynostosis involves craniofacial abnormalities that become evident in the fetal period.[13] The incidence is 1/2200 births and 25% are syndromic. Syndromic craniosynostosis is generally associated with mutations in certain genes, such as *FGFR2*, *FGFR3*, *FGFR1*, and *TWIST1*, and can involve multiple sutures.[14] Early suture closure leads to characteristic distortions of the skull, depending on the location of the early fusion. Surgical release of the prematurely fused areas is often needed to maintain normal head shape and facial proportions.[15] The ideal time for surgery to release fused cranial sutures is (with a few exceptions) between 3 and 9 months of age.

Helmet therapy, to help reshape the head with gentle pressure, may be used in conjunction with surgery in single suture craniosynostosis, typically sagittal craniosynostosis. Depending on the severity of craniosynostosis and the impact on the forehead and the orbital rim, a fronto-orbital advancement may also be planned to reshape the forehead and improve eye position.[16]

Crouzon syndrome is one of the most frequently occurring member of the group of synostosis syndromes that affect the face.[17] Crouzon syndrome is caused by a mutation in fibroblast growth factor receptors 2 and 3 on chromosome 10 and is characterized by premature fusion of the coronal sutures and underdevelopment of the midface and eyes, which seem to protrude from their sockets (Fig. 5.11). The characteristic protrusion of the eyes is largely an illusion: the eyes appear to bulge outward because of the midface hypoplasia. Intracranial pressure can increase when cranial sutures fuse prematurely. For these children, surgery to release the sutures coupled with distraction osteogenesis to advance the orbits is often necessary.[15] Additionally, children with midface hypoplasia can be at an increased risk for sleep disordered breathing including obstructive sleep apnea contributing to a need for early surgical intervention.[18]

Ear anomalies are often accompanied by other craniofacial anomalies and are most likely a result of interrupted or incomplete neural crest cell migration and apoptosis that result in the absence, or malformation of the external ear at birth. Malformation of the external ear is called microtia. Often the middle and internal ear components can be affected as well, contributing to some degree of hearing loss.[19,20] The causes of ear anomalies are multifactorial in nature including syndromes, gene mutations, and environmental factors. There are several syndromes associated with microtia in addition to isolated cases. Most commonly, there are varying levels of microtia associated with hemifacial microsomia as previously discussed in this chapter.

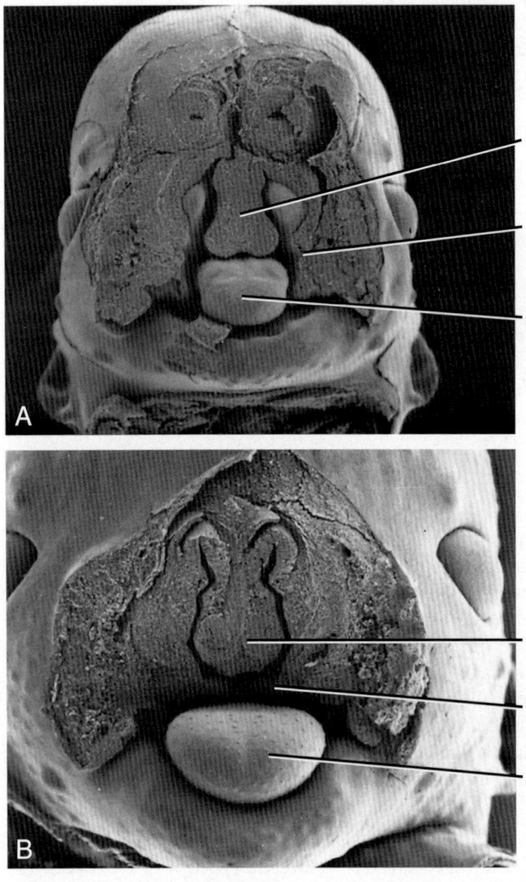

• **Fig. 5.8** Scanning electron micrographs of mouse sectioned in the frontal plane. (A) Before elevation of the palatal shelves. (B) Immediately after depression of the tongue and elevation of the shelves.

Jaw anomalies can be genetic and part of syndromes, but many are environmental and fall into the next category of disturbances in the fetal and perinatal period. Typically, these are described as a small upper or lower jaw, large lower jaw, and jaw positions contributing to anterior open bite, vertical maxillary excess, asymmetry, and occlusal cants. Jaw anomalies are often managed by a multidisciplinary team and this is discussed further in Chapter 22.

Growth Disturbances in the Fetal and Perinatal Period

Fetal Molding and Birth Injuries

Injuries that occur at or during birth can contribute to craniofacial changes. These include intrauterine molding and trauma related to fetal position, intrauterine environment, and traumatic use of instrumentation during birth.

Intrauterine Molding

Pressure against the developing face prenatally can lead to distortion of rapidly growing areas. Strictly speaking, this is not a birth injury, but because the effects are noted at birth, it is considered in that category. On rare occasions, an arm is pressed across the face in utero, resulting in severe maxillary deficiency at birth (Fig. 5.12).

Occasionally, a fetus' head is flexed tightly against the chest in utero, preventing the mandible from growing forward normally. This can be related to a decreased volume of amniotic fluid, which can occur for any of several reasons. The result can lead to a small mandible, posterior positioned tongue, and obstructed airway at birth and is one of the theories behind the characteristic small mandible found in Pierre Robin Sequence (PRS). PRS is not a syndrome that has a defined cause; instead, it is sequence of multiple phenotypes that are related: mandibular hypoplasia, glossoptosis, and upper airway obstruction. PRS is also frequently associated with a cleft palate because the restriction on displacement of the mandible forces the tongue upward and prevents normal closure of the palatal shelves. There are several chromosomal and genetic mutations that have been found to be associated with PRS.[21] About 60% of PRS is associated with a syndrome, the most common being Stickler syndrome.[22] The reduced volume of the oral cavity can lead to respiratory difficulty at birth, and it may be necessary to perform a tracheostomy so the infant can breathe. Early mandibular

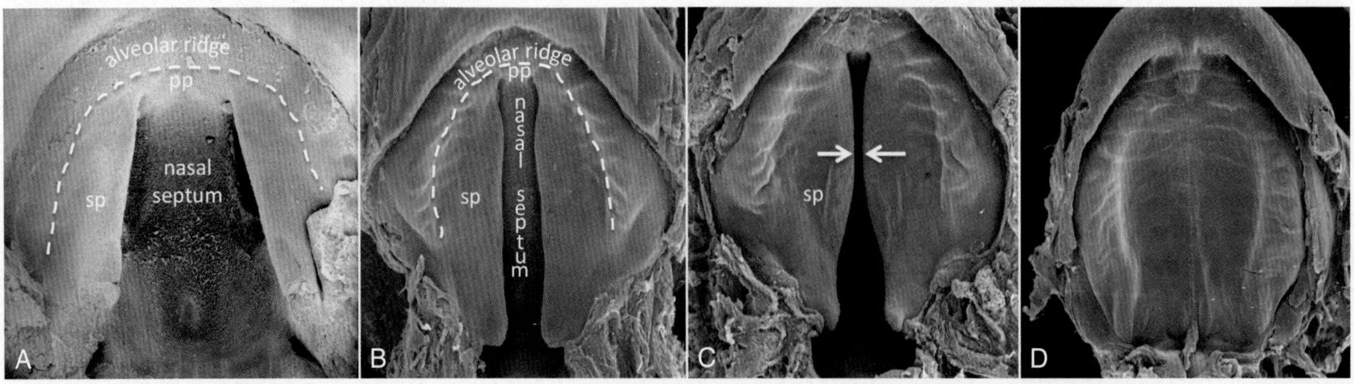

• **Fig. 5.9** The closing human palate in human embryos (A) at the end of the embryonic period (55 days) and (B) in the ninth week, which is the beginning of the fetal period (B to D). Arrows indicate approximate first site of secondary palatal fusion. *pp*, Primary palate; *sp*, secondary palatal shelf. (Courtesy Dr. K. Sulik.)

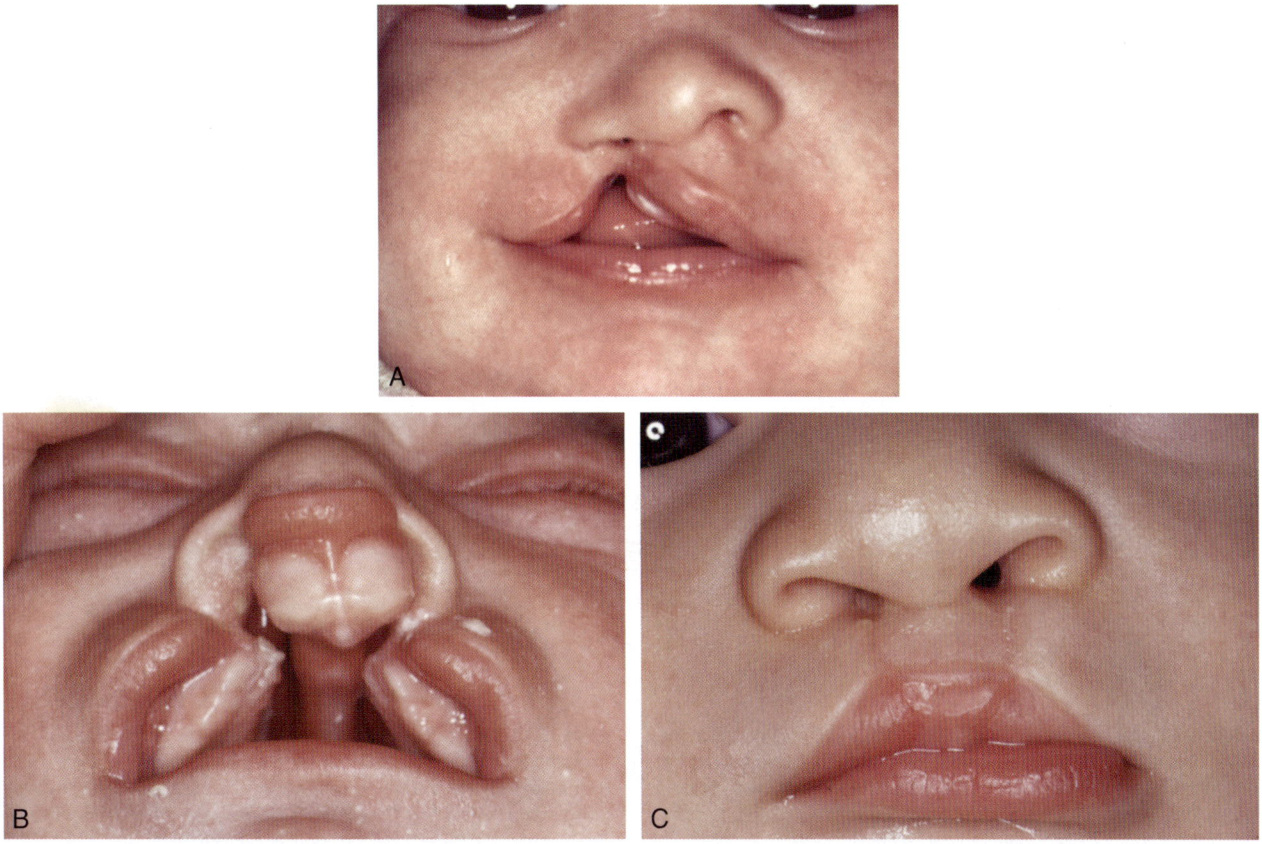

• **Fig. 5.10** Typical human clefts of the lip and palate. (A) Unilateral incomplete cleft lip in an infant. Note that the cleft is not in the midline but lateral to the midline and that there is an intact band of tissue beneath the nostril. (B) Bilateral complete cleft lip and palate in an infant. The separation of the premaxilla from the remainder of the maxilla is shown clearly. (C) Same child after lip repair.

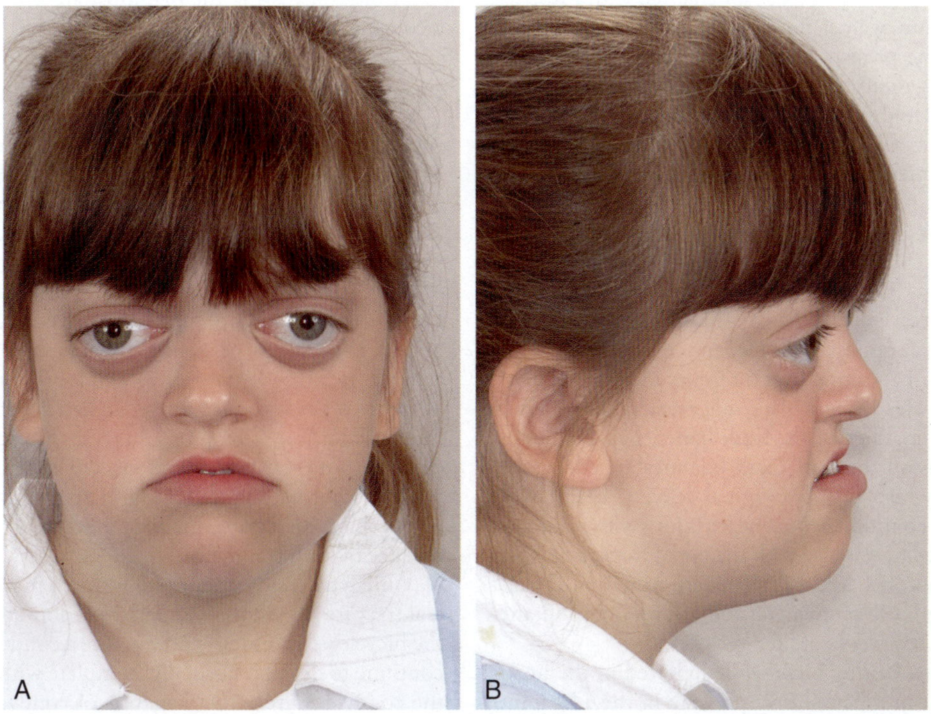

• **Fig. 5.11** (A and B) Facial appearance in Crouzon syndrome of moderate severity, at age 8 years, 8 months. Note the wide separation of the eyes (hypertelorism) and deficiency of the midfacial structures, both of which are characteristic of this syndrome. Because of premature suture fusion along the walls of the orbit, forward development of the midface is retarded, which produces the apparent protrusion of the eyes.

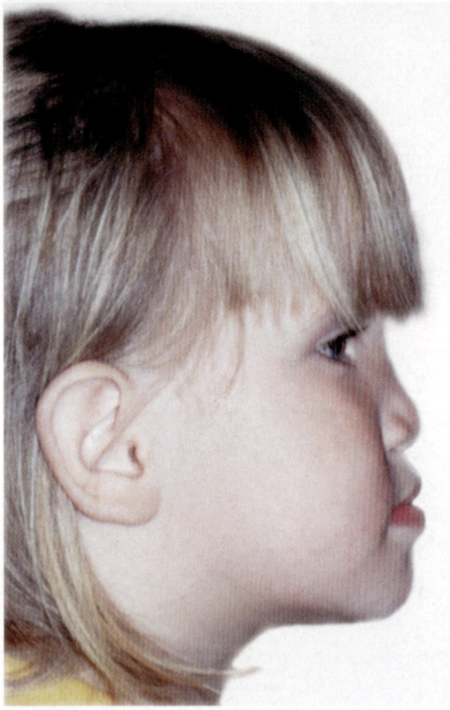

• **Fig. 5.12** Midface deficiency in a 3-year-old child is still apparent, although much improved from the severe deficiency that was present at birth because of intrauterine molding. Before birth, one arm was pressed across her face. (From Proffit WR, White RP, Sarver DM. *Contemporary Treatment of Dentofacial Deformity*. Mosby; 2003.)

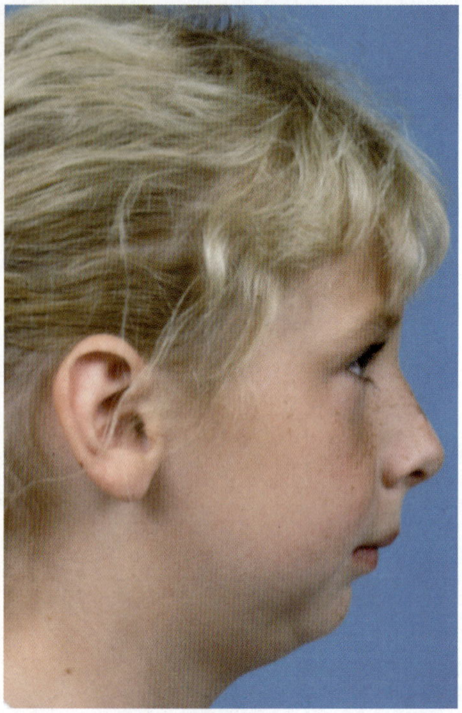

• **Fig. 5.13** This girl was diagnosed at birth as having the Pierre Robin sequence, which results in a very small mandible, airway obstruction, and cleft palate. Some children with this condition have enough postnatal mandibular growth to largely correct the jaw deficiency, but the majority do not. At age 9, her mandibular deficiency persists. (From Proffit WR, White RP, Sarver DM. *Contemporary Treatment of Dentofacial Deformity*. Mosby; 2003.)

advancement via distraction osteogenesis has been used recently in these severely affected infants to bring the tongue forward and provide more space for an airway so that the tracheostomy can be closed. A tongue-lip adhesion is another surgical management for airway to open the oropharyngeal space for children with PRS.

Because the pressure against the face that caused the growth problem would not be present after birth, there is the possibility of normal growth thereafter and perhaps eventually a complete recovery. Some children with PRS at birth do have favorable mandibular growth in childhood, most likely when the original problem was environmental mechanical growth restriction, but a smaller than normal mandible typically persists (Fig. 5.13), and catch-up growth during adolescence does not occur.[23]

Birth Trauma

Birth trauma refers to several clinical conditions that arise because of injury during birth as opposed to a recognized syndrome with a genetic cause. The most common sites for injury include the head, neck, and shoulders. Head traumas include extracranial or intracranial hemorrhage, fractures of the skull bones, ocular injuries, and superficial lesions on the skin. Skull fractures are commonly a result of improperly instrumented vaginal delivery. Facial nerve (CN VII) is the most common cranial nerve injury with traumatic birth. It is often caused by damage with the use of forceps or when the infant face is compressed against the maternal sacrum. If facial nerve injury occurs, it is often unilateral and will resolve spontaneously within the first few weeks of life.[24]

Mandibular factures during birth while reported in the literature, are rare. At least in theory, heavy pressure in the TM joints could cause internal hemorrhage, loss of tissue, and a subsequent underdevelopment of the mandible. At one time this was a common explanation for mandibular deficiency. The contemporary understanding that the condylar cartilage is not critical for proper growth of the mandible indicates that we cannot blame underdevelopment of the mandible on birth injuries. Children with deformities involving the mandible are much more likely to have a congenital syndrome.

Progressive Deformities in Childhood

A progressive deformity is one that steadily becomes worse, which, of course, indicates early treatment. These problems, fortunately, arise much less frequently than the severe but stable deformities that comprise most of the jaw problems encountered in children.

Childhood Fractures of the Jaws

In the frequent falls and impacts of childhood, the condylar neck of the mandible is particularly vulnerable, and fractures of this area are relatively common in children. Fortunately, the condylar process tends to regenerate well after early fractures. The best human data (see Chapter 2) suggest that about 80% to 85% of children with early fractures of the mandibular condylar process have normal mandibular growth afterward and therefore do not develop malocclusions that they would not have had in the absence of such trauma.

Unilateral condylar fracture is much more frequent than bilateral fractures. It seems to be relatively common for a child to crash the bicycle, chip a tooth and fracture a condyle, cry a bit, and then continue to develop normally, complete with total regeneration of the condyle. Often, the diagnosis of condylar fracture was never made. When a problem does arise following condylar fracture, it is usually asymmetric growth deficiency, with the injured side (or, in bilateral fractures, the more severely injured side) lagging

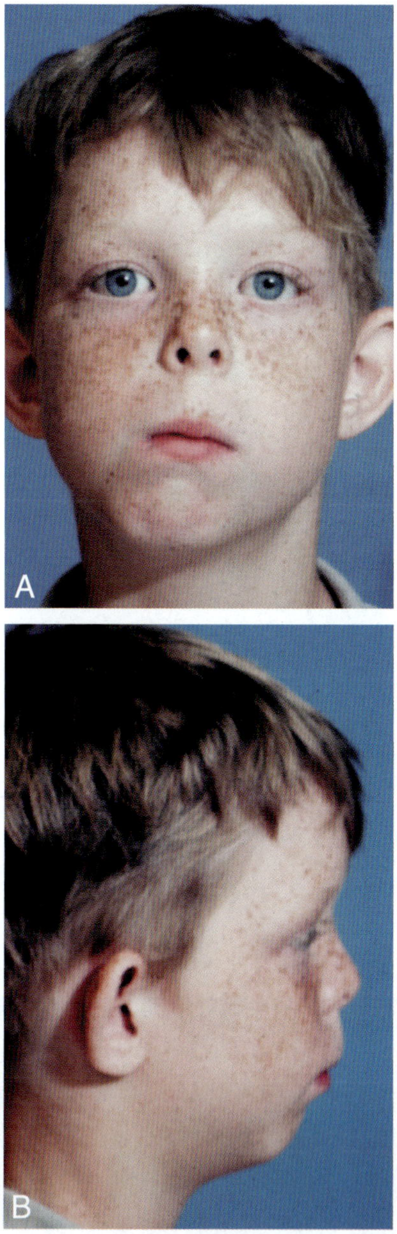

• **Fig. 5.14** (A) This frontal image shows mandibular asymmetry in an 8-year-old boy caused by deficient growth on the affected side after fracture of the right condylar process, probably at age 2. For this patient, growth was normal despite the complete loss of the mandibular condyle until age 6, when an attachment of the condylar process to the underside of the zygomatic arch on the injured side began to restrict growth; then facial asymmetry developed rapidly. (B) This profile view shows considerable mandibular deficiency as well from the restricted growth. (From Proffit WR, White RP, Sarver DM. *Contemporary Treatment of Dentofacial Deformity*. Mosby; 2003.)

(Fig. 5.14). After such an injury, if there is enough scarring around the temperomandibular (TM) joint to restrict translation of the condyle, the normal soft tissues cannot pull the mandible forward on that side as much as the rest of the growing face, and subsequent growth will be restricted.

This concept is highly relevant to the management of condylar fractures in children. It suggests, and clinical experience confirms, that there would be little if any advantage from surgical open reduction of a condylar fracture in a child. The additional scarring produced by surgery could make things worse. The best therapy, therefore, is conservative management at the time of injury and early mobilization of the jaw to minimize any restriction on movement. If deficient growth is observed, however, early treatment is needed (see Chapter 14).

Although an old condylar fracture is the most likely cause of asymmetric mandibular deficiency in a child, other destructive processes that involve the TM joint, such as rheumatoid arthritis (Fig. 5.15), or a congenital absence of tissue as in craniofacial microsomia also can produce this problem. Therefore it is always important for dentists and orthodontists to look for any asymmetry during a clinical exam and also ask about a history of trauma.

Muscle Dysfunction

The facial muscles can affect jaw growth in two ways. First, the formation of bone at the point of muscle attachments depends on the activity of the muscle; second, the musculature is an important part of the total soft tissue matrix whose growth normally carries the jaws downward and forward. Loss of part of the musculature is most likely to result from damage to the motor nerve (muscle atrophies when its motor nerve supply is lost). The result would be underdevelopment of that part of the face, with a deficiency of both soft and hard tissues (Fig. 5.16).

Excessive muscle contraction can restrict growth in much the same way as scarring after an injury. This effect is seen most clearly in torticollis, a twisting of the head caused by excessive tonic contraction of the neck muscles on one side (primarily the sternocleidomastoid) (Fig. 5.17). The result is a facial asymmetry because of growth restriction on the affected side, which can be quite severe and persist until older ages unless the contracted neck muscles are surgically detached at an early age.[25] Oftentimes, less severe cases of torticollis, if caught early, can be treated with Botox injections, neck braces, and/or physical therapy. Conversely, a major decrease in tonic muscle activity (as in muscular dystrophy (genetically influenced), some forms of cerebral palsy (genetic and environmentally influenced), and various muscle weakness syndromes) allows the mandible to drop downward away from the rest of the facial skeleton. The result is increased anterior face height, distortion of facial proportions and mandibular form, excessive eruption of the posterior teeth, narrowing of the maxillary arch, and anterior open bite (Fig. 5.18).[26]

Disturbances Arising in Adolescence or Early Adult Life

Occasionally, unilateral excessive growth of the mandible occurs in individuals who seem metabolically normal. Why this occurs is entirely unknown. It is most likely in girls between the ages of 15 and 20 but may occur as early as age 8 or as late as the early 30s in either sex. The condition was formerly called *condylar hyperplasia*, and proliferation of the condylar cartilage is a prominent aspect; however, because the body of the mandible also is affected (Fig. 5.19), *hemimandibular hypertrophy* now is considered a more accurate descriptive term.[27] The excessive growth may stop spontaneously, but in severe cases removal of the affected condyle and reconstruction of the area are necessary.

In acromegaly, which is caused by an anterior pituitary tumor that secretes excessive amounts of growth hormone, excessive growth of the mandible may occur, creating a skeletal Class III malocclusion in adult life (Fig. 5.20). Often (but not always the mandible is unaffected while the hands and/or feet grow), mandibular growth accelerates again to the levels seen in the adolescent growth spurt, years after adolescent growth was completed.[28] The condylar cartilage proliferates, but it is difficult to be sure whether

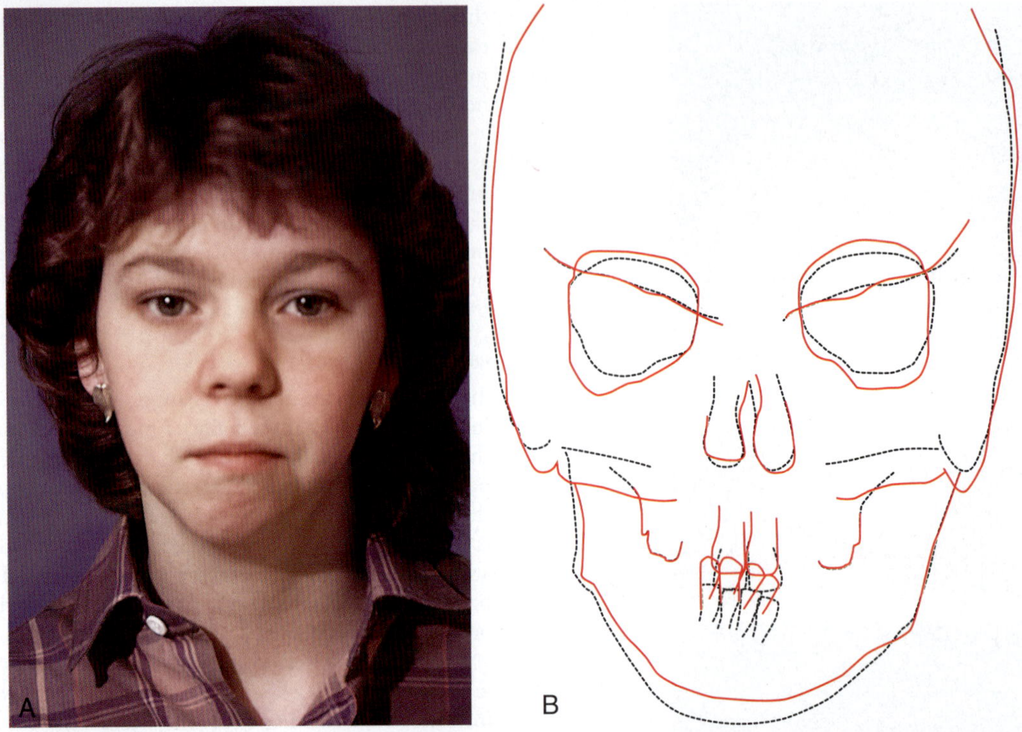

• **Fig. 5.15** Rheumatoid arthritis is an uncommon cause of facial asymmetry, but in the polyarticular form of the disease (multiple joints affected), the temporomandibular joints (TMJs) often are involved, and asymmetry may develop as one side is affected more than the other. (A) Facial appearance at age 12, 2 years after the diagnosis of polyarticular rheumatoid arthritis. (B) Superimposition tracing at ages 11 years, 8 months *(red)* and 13 years, 3 months *(black)*. With a decrease in ramus height on the right side over this period, the mandible rotated down and back. By age 24 the condylar processes on both sides had resorbed almost completely.

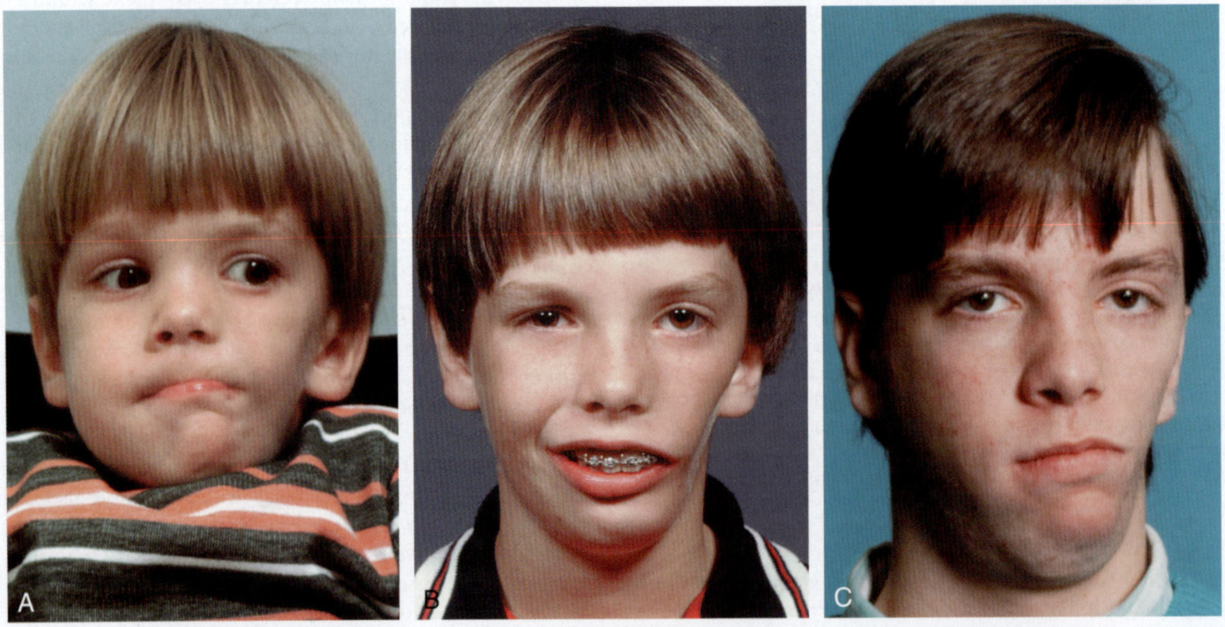

• **Fig. 5.16** Facial asymmetry in a boy whose masseter muscle was largely missing on the left side. The muscle is an important part of the total soft tissue matrix; in its absence growth of the mandible in the affected area also is deficient. (A) Age 4. (B) Age 11. (C) Age 17, after surgery to advance the mandible more on the left than the right side. The soft tissue deficiency from the missing musculature on the left side still is evident.

this is the cause of the mandibular growth or merely accompanies it. Although the excessive growth stops when the tumor is removed or irradiated, the skeletal deformity persists and orthognathic surgery to reposition the mandible is likely to be necessary (see Chapter 22).

Disturbances of Dental Development

Many disturbances of dental development are contributors to malocclusion, and these conditions (such as drift of permanent teeth after early loss of primary teeth) are discussed in Chapter 11. Dental problems that are related to larger congenital, genetic or environmental causes are discussed in the following sections.

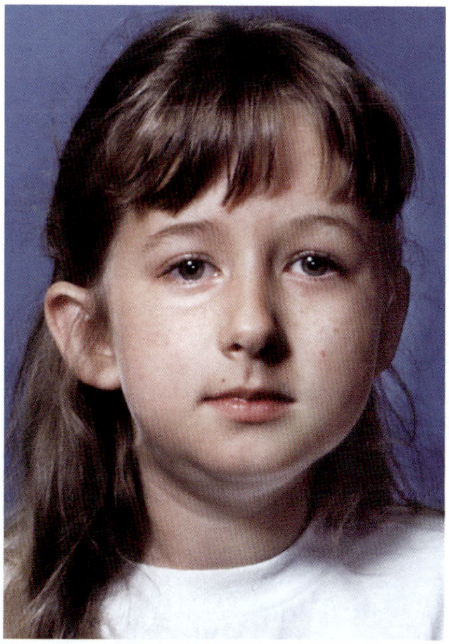

• **Fig. 5.17** Facial asymmetry in a 6-year-old girl with torticollis. Excessive muscle contraction can restrict growth in a way analogous to scarring after an injury. Despite surgical release of the contracted neck muscles at age 1, moderate facial asymmetry developed in this patient, and a second surgical release of the right sternocleidomastoid muscle was performed at age 7. Note that the asymmetry reflects deficient growth of the entire right side of the face, not just the mandible.

Congenitally Missing Teeth

A genetic basis has been established for most instances of congenitally missing teeth (more formally called *tooth agenesis*), and some form of tooth agenesis appears as a phenotype in more than 150 syndromes, but it must be kept in mind that there are both syndromic and nonsyndromic variants. Congenital absence of teeth results from disturbances during the initial stages of formation of a tooth: initiation and proliferation. *Anodontia*, the total absence of teeth, is the extreme form. The term *oligodontia* refers to congenital absence of greater than six, but not all teeth, whereas the rarely used term *hypodontia* implies the absence of only a few teeth. Because the primary tooth buds give rise to the permanent tooth buds, there will be no permanent tooth if its primary predecessor is missing. It is possible, however, for the primary teeth to be present and for some or all the permanent teeth to be absent.

Anodontia and oligodontia are usually associated with a syndrome, *ectodermal dysplasia*, which has a genetic basis. Individuals with ectodermal dysplasia have thin, sparse hair and an absence of sweat glands in addition to their characteristically missing teeth (Fig. 5.21). Occasionally, oligodontia occurs in a patient with no apparent systemic problem or congenital syndrome. In these children, it was once thought that there was a random pattern to the missing teeth, but as more data become available, patterns and an associated syndrome are increasingly being recognized.

Anodontia and oligodontia are rare, but hypodontia is a relatively common finding. It appears that a polygenic multifactorial model of etiology is the best explanation of the cause. As a general rule, if only one or a few teeth are missing, the absent tooth will be the most distal tooth of any given type. If a molar tooth is congenitally missing, it is almost always the third molar; if an incisor is missing, it is nearly always the lateral; if a premolar is missing, it almost always is the second rather than the first. Rarely is a canine the only missing tooth.

Malformed and Supernumerary Teeth

Abnormalities in tooth size and shape result from disturbances during the morphodifferentiation stage of development, perhaps with some carryover from the histodifferentiation stage. The most common abnormality is a variation in size, particularly of maxillary lateral incisors (Fig. 5.22) and mandibular or maxillary second premolars. About 5% of the total population have a significant "tooth size discrepancy" because of disproportionate sizes of the upper and lower teeth. Unless the teeth are matched for size,

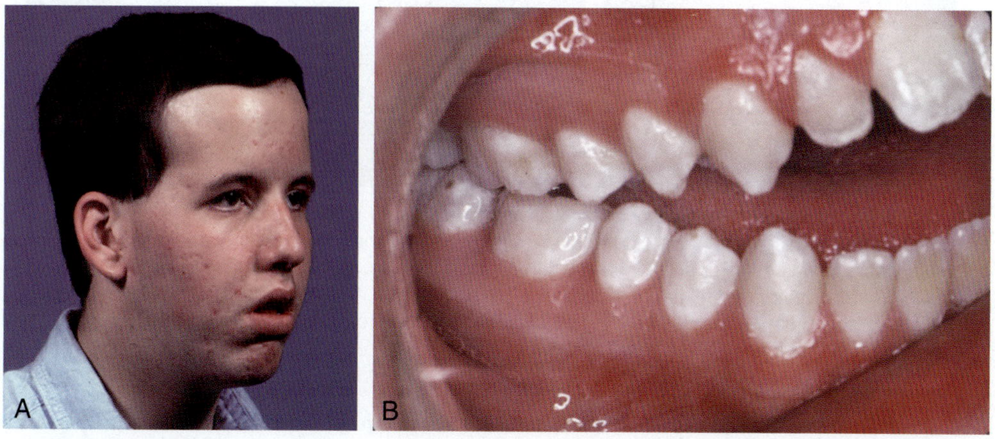

• **Fig. 5.18** (A) Lengthening of the lower face typically occurs in patients with muscle weakness syndromes, as in this 15-year-old boy with muscular dystrophy. (B) Anterior open bite, as in this patient, usually (but not always) accompanies excessive face height in patients with muscular weakness.

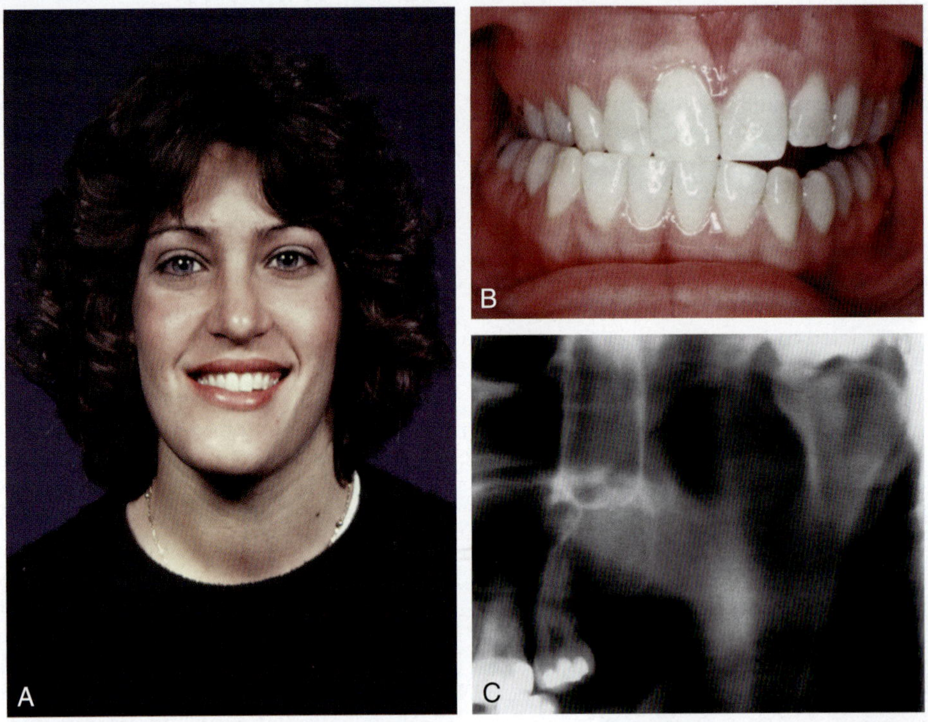

• Fig. 5.19 (A) Facial asymmetry in this 21-year-old female developed gradually in her late teens because of excessive growth of the mandible on the left side, after orthodontic treatment for dental crowding during which there was no sign of jaw asymmetry. (B) The dental occlusion shows an open bite on the affected left side, reflecting the vertical component of the excessive growth. (C) Note the grossly enlarged mandibular condyle on the patient's left side. Why this type of excessive but histologically normal growth occurs and why it is seen predominantly in females is unknown.

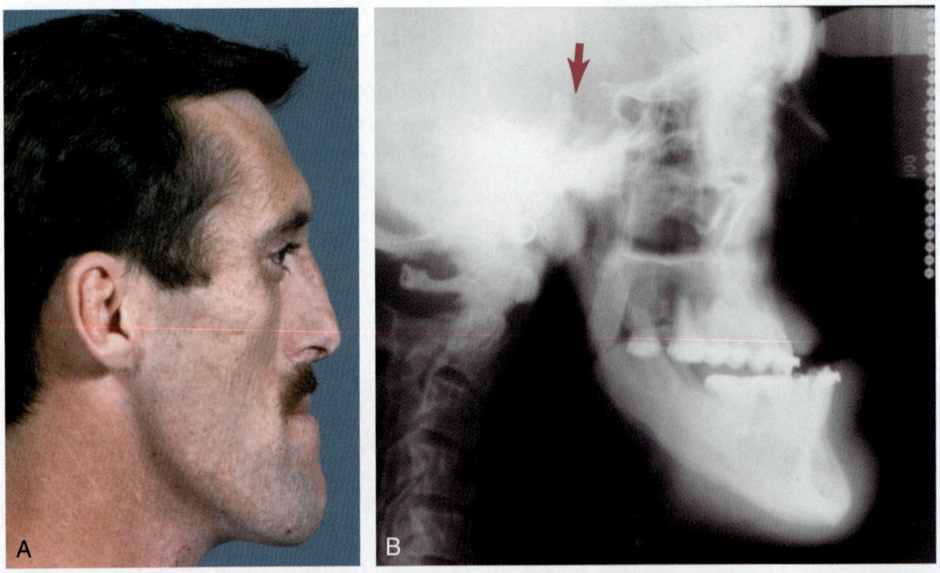

• Fig. 5.20 Profile view (A) and cephalometric radiograph (B) of a 32-year-old male with acromegaly, which had been diagnosed 3 years previously when he had gone to a dentist because his lower jaw was moving forward. After irradiation of the anterior pituitary area, growth hormone levels dropped and mandibular growth ceased. Note the enlargement of sella turcica and loss of bony definition of its bony outline, reflecting the secretory tumor in that location *(arrow)*. (From Proffit WR, White RP, Sarver DM. *Contemporary Treatment of Dentofacial Deformity*. Mosby; 2003.)

normal occlusion is impossible. As might be expected, the most variable teeth, the maxillary lateral incisors, are the major culprits.

Supernumerary or extra teeth also result from disturbances during the initiation and proliferation stages of dental development and, like tooth agenesis, can occur as part of a larger disease process or syndrome or as an idiopathic finding. The most common supernumerary tooth appears in the maxillary midline and is called a *mesiodens*. Supernumerary lateral incisors also occur; extra

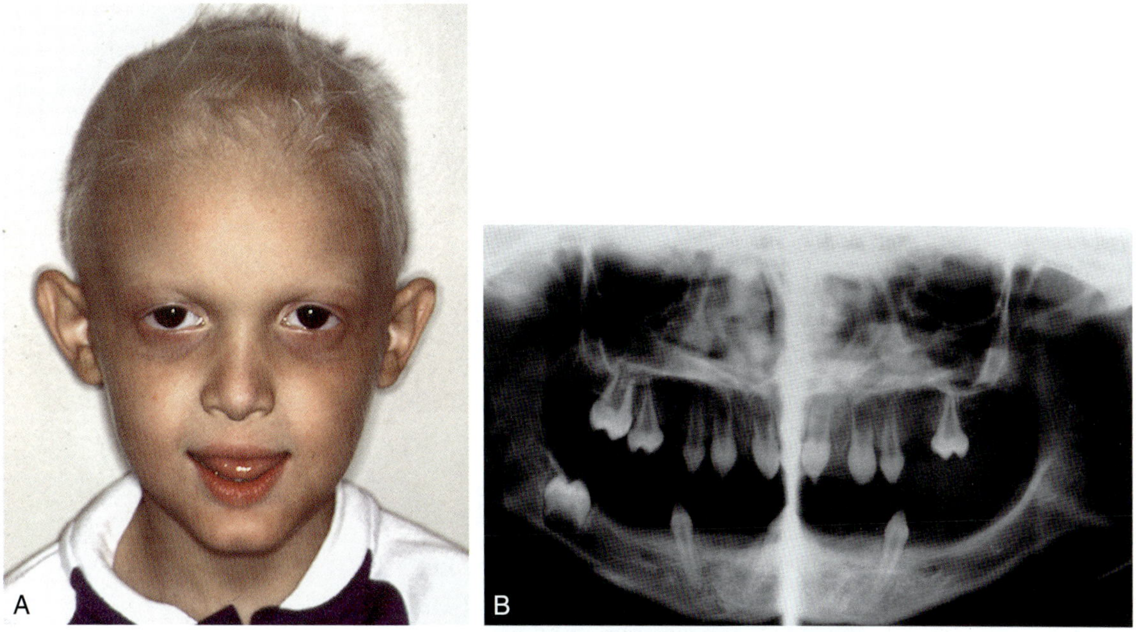

• **Fig. 5.21** (A) A child with ectodermal dysplasia, in addition to the characteristic thin and light-colored hair, is likely to have an overclosed appearance because of lack of development of the alveolar processes. (B) Panoramic radiograph of the same boy, showing the multiple missing teeth. When this many teeth are congenitally missing, ectodermal dysplasia is the most likely cause.

premolars occasionally appear; and a few patients have fourth, in addition to third, molars. The presence of an extra tooth obviously has great potential to disrupt normal occlusal development (Fig. 5.23), and early intervention to remove it is usually required to obtain reasonable alignment and occlusal relationships. Multiple supernumerary teeth are most often seen in the congenital syndrome of cleidocranial dysplasia (see Fig. 3.15), which is characterized by missing clavicles (collar bones), many supernumeraries, and failure of the succedaneous teeth to erupt.

Traumatic Displacement of Teeth

Almost all children fall and hit their teeth during their formative years. When trauma to a primary tooth displaces the permanent tooth bud underlying it, there are two possible results. First, if the trauma occurs while the crown of the permanent tooth is forming, enamel formation will be disturbed and there will be a defect in the crown of the permanent tooth.

Second, if the trauma occurs after the crown is complete, the crown may be displaced relative to the root. Root formation may stop, leaving a permanently shortened root. More frequently, root formation continues, but the remaining portion of the root then forms at an angle to the traumatically displaced crown (Fig. 5.24). This distortion of root form is called *dilaceration.* If it is severe enough, it is almost impossible for the crown to assume its proper position, which might require the root to extend out through the alveolar bone. For this reason, it may be necessary to extract a severely dilacerated tooth or perform a partial root amputation.

Teeth that are displaced laterally by trauma and mobile can be digitally repositioned as soon as possible (see Chapter 12). If the tooth is consolidated in the new position after the accident, it usually can be moved back orthodontically to its original position if it interferes with the patient's occlusion. If there is no occlusal interference, after healing, orthodontics (at a minimum of 3 months) or surgery may be necessary to reposition the tooth, but ankylosis may make this impossible for tooth movement or difficult even with surgery.

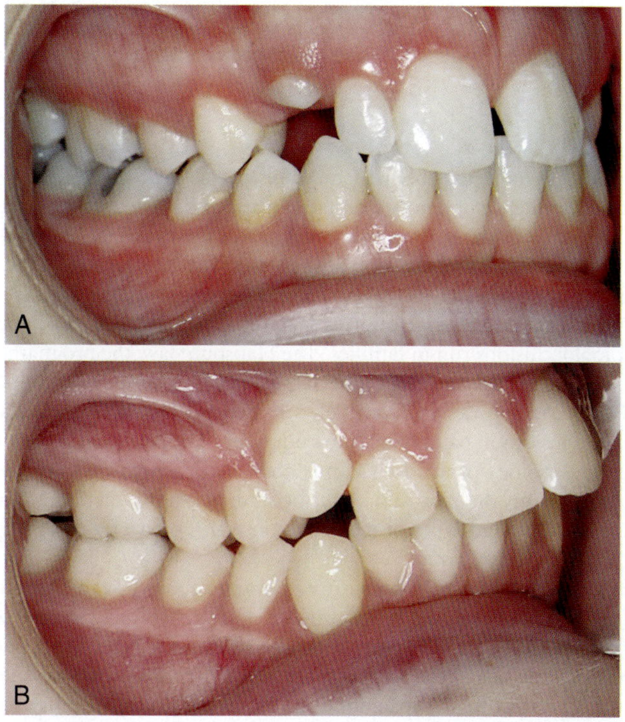

• **Fig. 5.22** Disproportionately small (A) or large (B) maxillary lateral incisors are relatively common. This creates a tooth-size discrepancy that makes normal alignment and occlusion almost impossible. It is easier to build up small laterals than reduce the size of large ones, because dentin is likely to be exposed interproximally after more than 1–2 mm in width reduction.

Genetic Influences

Here we are discussing the genetic impact on skeletal and dental malocclusion features, not individual dental features mentioned earlier

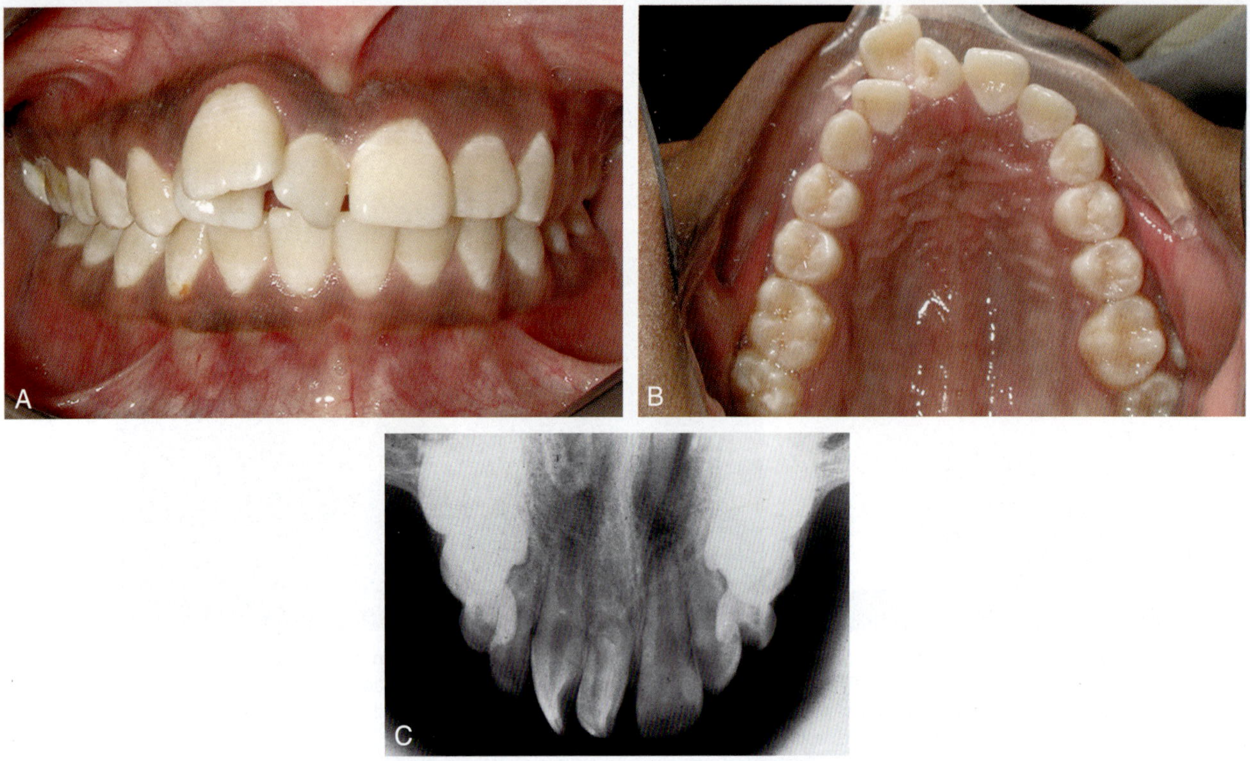

• **Fig. 5.23** (A–C) The maxillary anterior area and often the midline is the most common location for a supernumerary tooth, often called a *mesiodens* because of its location. It can be of almost any shape. The supernumerary tooth may block the eruption of one or both central incisors or, as in this girl, may cause the central incisors to be separated and the right lateral incisor right lateral incisor to be displaced as well.

under specific causes of congenital missing or malformed teeth. A strong influence of heredity on facial features is obvious at a glance: it is easy to recognize familial tendencies in the tilt of the nose, the shape of the jaw, and the look of the smile. The similarity of human faces among relatives—past and present—makes the genetic basis of human craniofacial development even more apparent. Certain types of malocclusions run in families. The Hapsburg jaw, the prognathic mandible of this European royal family, is the best-known example (Fig. 5.25), but dentists routinely see repeated instances of similar malocclusions in parents and their offspring. The pertinent question for the etiology of malocclusion is not whether there are inherited influences on the jaws and teeth, because obviously there are, but whether different types of malocclusions can be directly caused by inherited characteristics.[29]

For much of the 20th century, thoughts about how malocclusion could be produced by inherited characteristics focused on two major possibilities. The first would be an inherited disproportion between the size of the teeth and the size of the jaws, which would produce crowding or spacing. The second would be an inherited disproportion between the size and/or shape of the upper and lower jaws, which would cause improper occlusal relationships. The more independently these characteristics are determined, the more likely that disproportions could be inherited. Could a child inherit relatively large teeth but a jaw too small to accommodate them, for instance, or a large upper jaw and a small lower one? That would be quite possible if jaw and tooth sizes were inherited independently, but if dentofacial characteristics tended to be linked, an inherited mismatch of this type would be unlikely.

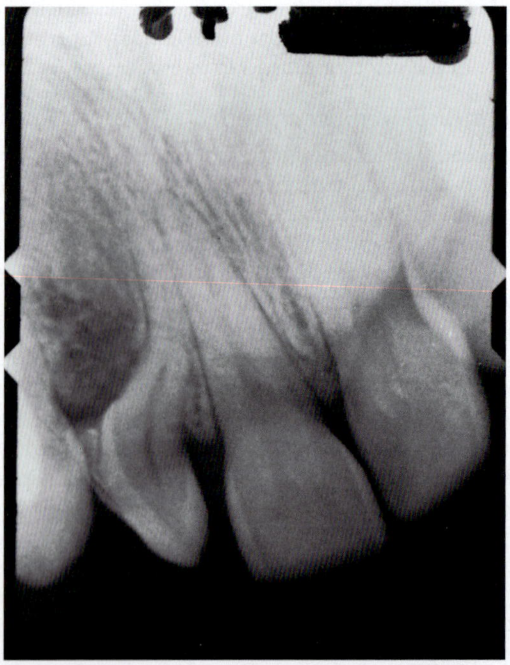

• **Fig. 5.24** Distortion of the root (termed *dilaceration*) of this lateral incisor resulted from trauma at an earlier age that displaced the crown relative to the forming root. This is a more severe dilaceration than what is usually observed (see Fig. 3.17), but even in this child the tooth erupted—dilaceration does not necessarily prevent eruption.

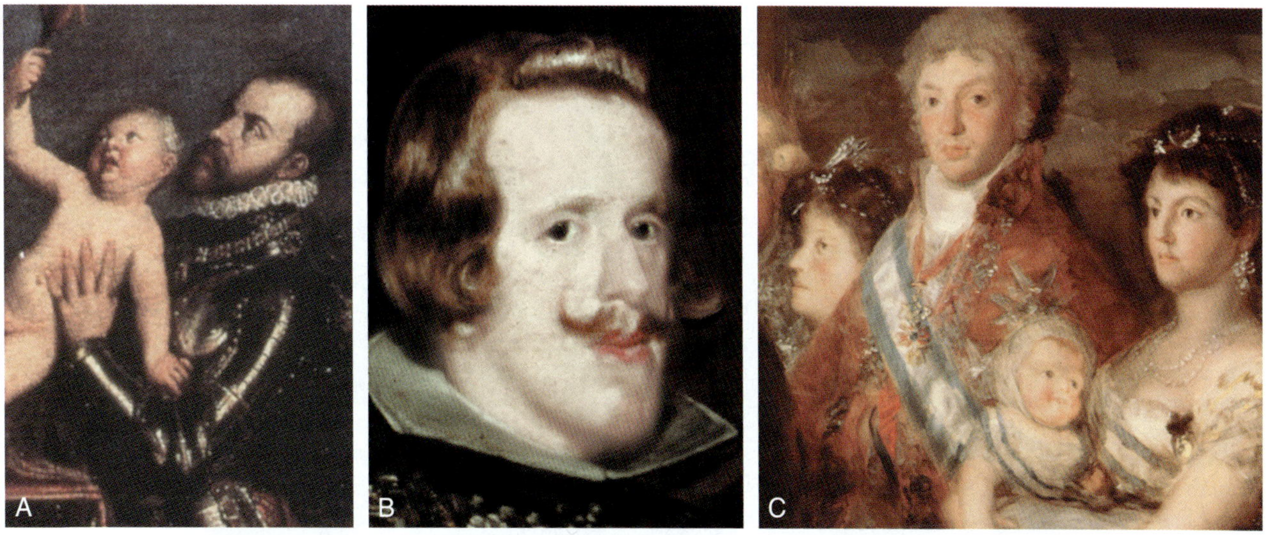

• **Fig. 5.25** Mandibular prognathism in the Hapsburg family became known as the Hapsburg jaw because it recurred over multiple generations in European royalty and was recorded in many portraits. (A) Phillip II and Prince Ferdinand, 1575 (Titian). (B) Phillip IV, 1638 (Velasquez). (C) Charles IV and family, 1800 (Goya). In (C), note the strong lower jaw in baby, father, and grandmother but not in the mother.

Primitive human populations in which malocclusion is less frequent than in modern groups are characterized by genetic isolation and uniformity. If everyone in a group carried the same genetic information for tooth size and jaw size, there would be no possibility of a child inheriting discordant characteristics. In the absence of processed food, one would expect strong selection pressure for traits that produced good masticatory function. Genes that introduced disturbances into the masticatory system would tend to be eliminated from the population (unless they conferred some other advantage). The result should be exactly what is seen in native populations: individuals in whom tooth size-jaw size discrepancies are infrequent and groups in which everyone tends to have the same jaw relationship (not necessarily one that produces ideal dental occlusion). Different human groups have developed impressive variations in facial proportions and jaw relationships. What happens, then, when there is breeding between originally distinct and various human population groups?

One of the characteristics of civilization is the collection of large groups of people into urban centers, where the opportunities for mating outside one's own small population group are greatly magnified. If inherited disproportions of the functional components of the face and jaws were frequent, one would predict that modern urban populations would have a high prevalence of malocclusion and a great variety of orthodontic problems. The United States, reflecting its role as a "genetic melting pot," should have one of the world's highest rates of malocclusion, which it does. In the 1930s and 1940s, as knowledge of the new science of genetics developed, it was tempting to conclude that the great increase in breeding outside of one's native group that occurred as human populations grew and became more mobile was the major explanation for the increase in malocclusion in recent centuries.

This view of malocclusion as primarily a genetic problem was greatly strengthened by breeding experiments with animals carried out in the 1930s. By far the most influential individual in this regard was Professor Stockard, who methodically crossbred dogs and recorded the interesting effects on body structure.[30] Present-day dogs, of course, come in a tremendous variety of breeds and sizes. What would happen if one crossed a Boston terrier with a collie? Might the offspring have the collie's long, pointed lower jaw and the terrier's diminutive upper jaw? Could unusual crowding or spacing result because the teeth of one breed were combined in the offspring with the jaw of the other? Stockard's experiments indicated that dramatic malocclusions did occur in his crossbred dogs, more from jaw discrepancies than from tooth size-jaw size imbalances, and he published pointed comparisons with human malocclusions (Fig. 5.26). These experiments seemed to confirm that independent inheritance of facial characteristics could be a major cause of malocclusion and that the rapid increase in malocclusion accompanying urbanization was probably the result of genetic diversity through crossbreeding of these dogs.

These dog experiments turned out to be misleading, however, because many breeds of small dogs carry the gene for achondroplasia. Animals or humans affected by this condition have deficient growth of cartilage. The result is extremely short extremities and an underdeveloped midface. The dachshund is the classic achondroplastic dog, but most terriers and bulldogs also carry this gene. Achondroplasia is an autosomal dominant trait. Like many dominant genes, the gene for achondroplasia shows variable expressivity, meaning simply that the trait will be expressed more dramatically in some individuals than in others. Most of the unusual malocclusions produced in Stockard's breeding experiments can be explained by the extent to which achondroplasia was expressed in that animal, not based on inherited jaw size.

When discussing humans, achondroplasia is rare, but it does occur and produces the expected changes (Fig. 5.27). In addition to short limbs, the cranial base does not lengthen normally because of the deficient growth at the synchondroses, the maxilla is not translated forward to the normal extent, and a relative midface deficiency occurs. In a number of relatively rare genetic syndromes such as achondroplasia, influences on the form of the face, jaws, and teeth can be discerned, but those cause only a fraction of 1% of orthodontic problems.

A careful examination of the results of genetic diversity in human populations also casts doubt on the hypothesis that independently inherited tooth and jaw characteristics are a major cause of malocclusion. The best data are from investigations carried out in Hawaii by Chung et al.[31] Before its discovery by the European explorers of the 18th century, Hawaii had a homogeneous Polynesian population. Large-scale migration to the islands from Europe, China, and Japan, as well as the arrival of smaller numbers of other racial and ethnic

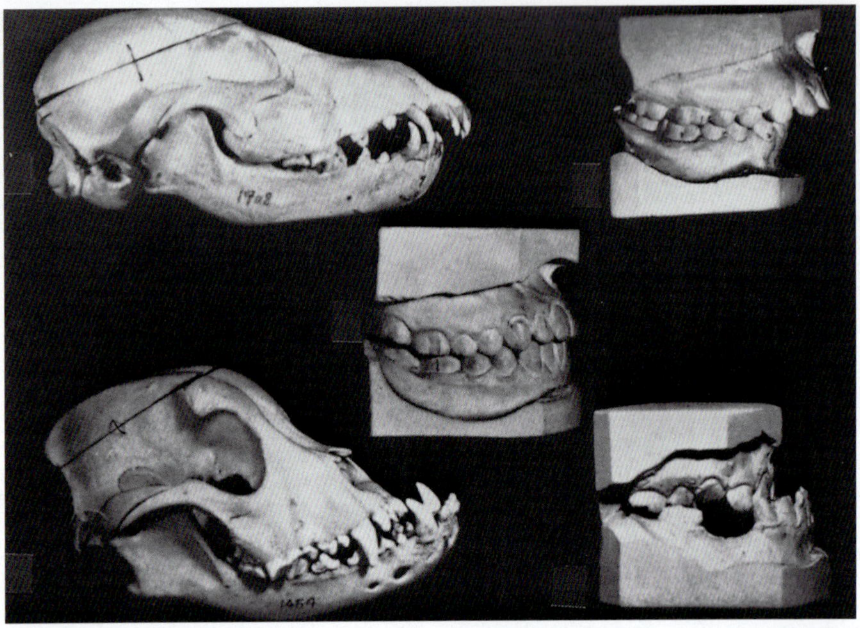

• **Fig. 5.26** In breeding experiments with dogs in the 1930s, Professor Stockard demonstrated that severe malocclusions could be developed by crossing morphologically different breeds. His analogy to human malocclusion was a powerful influence in the rejection of the prevailing belief of the 1920s that improper jaw function caused malocclusion. (From Stockard CR, Johnson AL. *Genetic and Endocrinic Basis for Differences in Form and Behavior*. The Wistar Institute of Anatomy and Biology; 1941.)

groups, resulted in an exceptionally heterogeneous modern population. Tooth size, jaw size, and jaw proportions were all rather different for the Polynesian, Asian, and European contributors to the Hawaiian melting pot. Therefore, if tooth and jaw characteristics were inherited independently, a high prevalence of severe malocclusion would be expected in this population.

The prevalence and types of malocclusion in the current Hawaiian population, although greater than the prevalence of malocclusion in the original population, do not support this concept. The effects of interracial crosses appear to be more additive than multiplicative. For example, about 10% of the Chinese who migrated to Hawaii had Class III malocclusion, whereas about 10% of the Polynesians had crowded teeth. The offspring of this cross seem to have about a 10% prevalence of each characteristic, but there is no evidence of dramatic facial deformities. In other words, if malocclusion or a tendency to malocclusion is inherited, the mechanism is not the independent inheritance of discrete morphologic characteristics such as tooth and jaw sizes.

The classic way to determine to what extent a characteristic is determined by inheritance is to compare monozygotic (identical) with dizygotic (fraternal) twins. Monozygotic twins occur because of the early division of a fertilized egg, so each individual has the same chromosomal DNA and the two are genetically identical. Any differences between them should be solely the result of environmental influences. Twins also occur when two eggs are released at the same time and are fertilized by different spermatozoa. These dizygotic twins are not more similar to ordinary siblings except that they have shared the same intrauterine and family environment. Through the comparison of identical twins, fraternal twins, and ordinary siblings, the proportion of the variability in that characteristic that is due to heredity can be estimated.

Studies of this type are limited in several ways. Not only is it difficult to obtain the twin pairs for study, but also it can be difficult to establish zygosity and confirm that the environments were in fact the same for both members of a twin pair. Nevertheless, well-done twin studies are the best way to evaluate heritability. Using twins with siblings as controls, Hughes et al. reported that the hereditary component for variations in spacing and tooth position within the dental arches was 69% to 89%. It was 53% for overbite, but only 28% for overjet (which therefore appears to have a greater environmental component than crowding/spacing or overbite).[32] Corruccini et al.

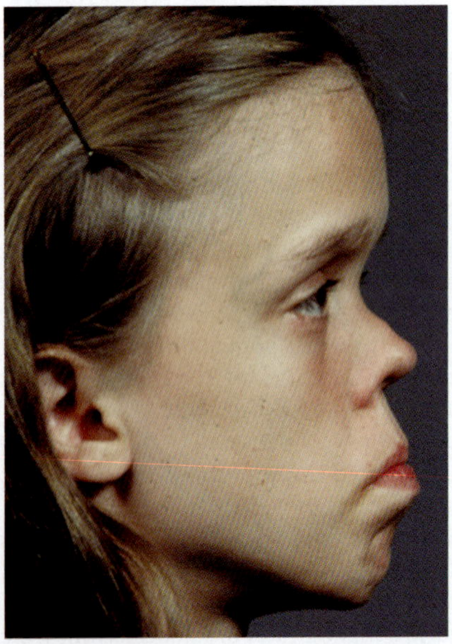

• **Fig. 5.27** In this 14-year-old girl with moderately severe achondroplasia, note the deficient midface, particularly at the bridge of the nose. This results from decreased growth of cartilage in the cranial base, with a resulting lack of forward translation of the maxilla. (From Proffit WR, White RP, Sarver DM. *Contemporary Treatment of Dentofacial Deformity*. Mosby; 2003.)

have argued that with appropriate corrections for unsuspected environmental differences within twin pairs, the heritability for some dental characteristics such as overjet is almost zero.[33]

The other classic method of estimating the influence of heredity is to study family members, observing similarities and differences between mother and child, father and child, and sibling pairs. From an examination of longitudinal cephalometric radiographs and dental casts of siblings who participated in the Bolton-Brush growth study, Harris and Johnson concluded that the heritability of craniofacial (skeletal) characteristics was relatively high but that of dental (occlusal) characteristics was low.[34] For skeletal characteristics, the heritability estimates increased with increasing age; for dental characteristics, the heritability estimates decreased, indicating an increasing environmental contribution to the dental variation. These findings were confirmed and extended in a follow-up study of heritability in Icelandic families.[35] To the extent that the facial skeleton determines the characteristics of a malocclusion, therefore, a hereditary component is likely to be present. When parent-child correlations are used to assist in predicting facial growth, errors are reduced, which in itself strongly indicates the hereditary influence on these dimensions.[36] Purely dental variation, however, seems to be much more environmentally determined.

As was noted in European royal families (see Fig. 5.25), the influence of inherited tendencies is particularly strong for mandibular prognathism. In a recent study of 55 families in Brazil with more than 2000 individuals, the heritability of mandibular prognathism was estimated to be 0.316. The majority of the pedigrees suggested autosomal dominant inheritance with incomplete penetration, and the investigators concluded that there is a major gene that influences the expression of mandibular prognathism.[37] This does not mean that a single gene is responsible, and efforts during the last decade to identify a major gene related to prognathism have not been successful. It is apparent that what we call Class III malocclusion, or even the subcategory mandibular prognathism, really is a group of different phenotypes, and identifying these phenotypes and determining their heritability is a necessary step toward unraveling the genetics of Class III problems.[38]

The long-face pattern of facial deformity seems to be the second most likely type of jaw anomaly to run in families. In general, similar malocclusions are likely to be seen in siblings, especially if the malocclusion is severe, perhaps because their genetically influenced facial types and growth patterns lead to similar responses to environmental factors. Knowing the type of growth associated with different genetic patterns could help greatly with both the type and timing of orthodontic and surgical treatment.

The extent to which other types of malocclusion are related to genetic influences is less clear, despite the recent advances in understanding the genetic basis of tooth agenesis and eruption failure. If dental variations that contribute to malocclusion are not tightly linked to gene expression, a condition such as open bite could be largely due to external influences—for example, sucking habits or tongue posture. Let us now examine the role of the environment in the etiology of malocclusion.

Environmental Influences

Environmental influences during growth and development of the face, jaws, and teeth consist largely of pressures and forces related to physiologic activity. A relationship between anatomic form and physiologic function is apparent in all animals. Over evolutionary time, adaptations in the jaws and dental apparatus are prominent in the fossil record. Form-function relationships at this level are controlled genetically and, although important for a general understanding of the human condition, have little to do with any individual's deviation from the current norm.

On the other hand, there is every reason to suspect that form-function relationships during the lifetime of an individual may be significant in the development of malocclusion and dentofacial malformations. Although the changes in body form are minimal, an individual who does heavy physical work has both heavier and stronger muscles and a sturdier skeletal system than one who is sedentary. If function could affect the growth of the jaws, altered function would be a major cause of malocclusion, and it would be logical for chewing exercises and other forms of physical therapy to be an important part of orthodontic treatment. If, however, function makes little or no difference in the individual's pattern of development, altering his or her jaw function would have little if any impact, etiologically or therapeutically. Because of its importance in contemporary orthodontics, particular emphasis is placed here on evaluating potential functional contributions to both the development of dentofacial problems and to relapse after treatment.

Equilibrium Considerations

The laws of physics state that an object subjected to unequal forces will be accelerated and thereby will move to a different position in space. It follows that if any object is subjected to a set of forces but remains in the same position, any forces must be in balance or equilibrium. From this perspective, the dentition is obviously in equilibrium because the teeth are subjected to a variety of forces but do not move to a new location under usual circumstances.

The effectiveness of orthodontic treatment is itself a demonstration that forces on the dentition are normally in equilibrium. Teeth normally experience forces from masticatory effort, swallowing, and speaking but do not move. If a tooth is subjected to a continuous force from an orthodontic appliance, it does move, so the force applied by the orthodontist has altered the previous equilibrium. The nature of the forces necessary for tooth movement is discussed in detail in Chapter 8, but at this point, we must briefly preview what is known about force magnitude and force duration in producing changes in tooth position.

A key consideration is that the supporting structures of the dentition (cementum, periodontal ligament [PDL] and alveolar bone) are constructed to withstand heavy forces of short duration such as those from mastication. During mastication, the fluid in the PDL space acts as a shock absorber, so that the soft tissues in

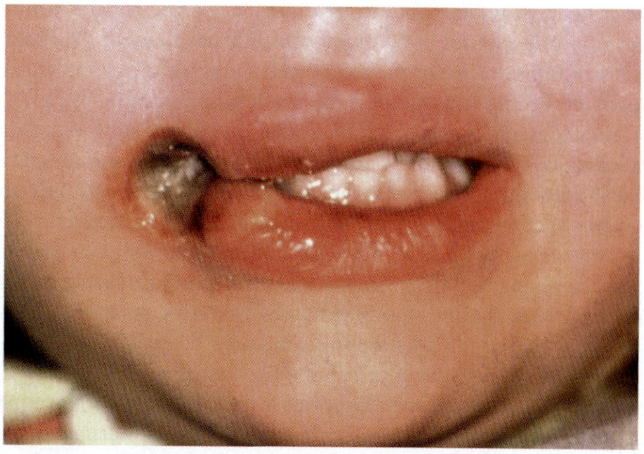

• **Fig. 5.28** Scarring of the corner of the mouth in this child will occur as the burn from biting an electrical cord heals. From equilibrium theory, one would expect a distortion in the form of the dental arch in the region of the contracting scar, and exactly this occurs after an injury of this type.

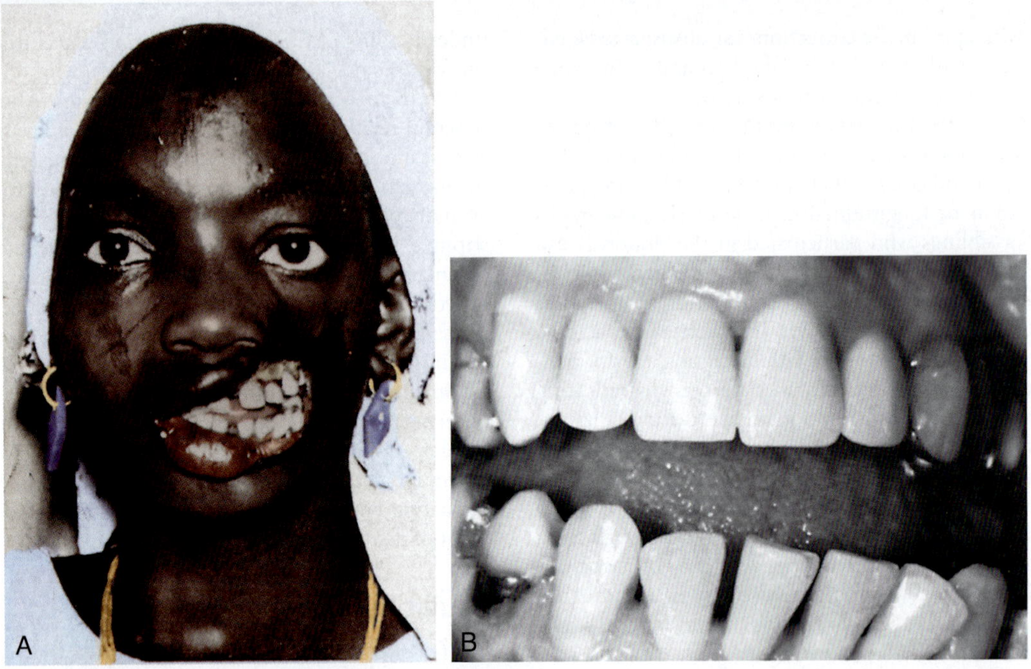

• **Fig. 5.29** (A) In this individual, a large part of the cheek was lost because of a tropical infection. Note the outward splaying of the teeth on the affected side after the restraining force of the cheek was lost. (B) After a paralytic stroke, this patient's tongue rested against the mandibular posterior teeth. Before the stroke, the occlusion was normal; within a few months afterward, an outward splaying of the teeth occurred on the affected side because of the increase in resting tongue pressure. (A, Courtesy Professor J.P. Moss; B Courtesy Dr. T. Wallen.)

the PDL are not compressed, although bending of alveolar bone occurs. Only if pressure is maintained long enough to squeeze out the fluid (a few seconds) is there an impact on the soft tissues. Then, because that begins to hurt, the pressure is released, and the fluid returns before the next chewing stroke. The result is that only light force of long duration (6 hours or so per day) is important in determining whether there is enough of an imbalance of forces to lead to tooth movement, which means that if the balance between long-duration pressure from the tongue versus lip or cheek pressure changes, tooth movement would be expected.

It is easy to demonstrate that this is indeed the case. For example, if an injury to the soft tissue of the lip results in scarring and contracture, the adjacent incisors will be moved lingually as the lip tightens against them (Fig. 5.28). On the other hand, if restraining pressure by the lip or cheek is removed, the teeth move outward in response to unopposed pressure from the tongue (Fig. 5.29A). Pressure from the tongue, whether from an enlargement of the tongue from a tumor or other source or because its posture has changed, will result in labial displacement of the teeth, even though the lips and cheeks are intact, because the equilibrium has been altered (Fig. 5.29B).

These observations make it plain that, in contrast to forces from mastication, light sustained pressures from lips, cheeks, and tongue at rest are important determinants of tooth position. It seems unlikely, however, that the intermittent short-duration pressures created when the tongue and lips contact the teeth during swallowing or speaking would have any significant impact on tooth position. As with masticatory forces, the pressure magnitudes would be great enough to move a tooth, but the duration is inadequate (Table 5.2).

Equilibrium considerations also apply to the skeleton, including the facial skeleton. Skeletal alterations occur all the time in response to functional demands and are magnified under unusual experimental situations. The bony processes to which muscles attach are especially influenced by the muscles and the location of the attachments. The form of the mandible, because it is largely dictated by the shape of its functional processes, is particularly prone to alteration.

TABLE 5.2 Possible Equilibrium Influences: Magnitude and Duration of Force Against the Teeth During Function

Possible Equilibrium Influence	Force Magnitude	Force Duration
Tooth Contacts		
Mastication	Very heavy	Very short
Swallowing	Light	Very short
Soft Tissue Pressures of Lip, Cheek, and Tongue		
Swallowing	Moderate	Short
Speaking	Light	Very short
Resting	Very light	Long
External Pressures		
Habits	Moderate	Variable
Orthodontics	Moderate	Variable
Intrinsic Pressures		
PDL fibers	Light	Long
Gingival fibers	Variable	Long

PDL, Periodontal ligament.

The density of the facial bones, like the rest of the skeleton, increases when heavy work is done and decreases in its absence.

Let us now consider the role of function in the etiology of malocclusion and dentofacial deformity from this perspective.

Masticatory Function

The pressures generated by chewing activity potentially could affect dentofacial development in two ways: (1) greater use of the jaws, with higher and/or more prolonged biting force, could increase the dimensions of the jaws and dental arches, or (2) less use of the jaws might lead to underdeveloped dental arches and crowded and irregular teeth, and the resulting decreased biting force could affect how much the teeth erupt, thereby affecting lower face height and overbite and open bite relationships.

Function and Dental Arch Size

The size and shape of the muscular processes of the jaws reflect muscle size and activity. For example, enlargement of the mandibular gonial angles can be seen in humans with hypertrophy of the mandibular elevator muscles (Fig. 5.30), and changes in the form of the coronoid processes occur in children when temporalis muscle function is altered after injuries. In contrast, the heavy intermittent forces produced during mastication should have little direct effect on tooth positions, so the size of the dental arches would be affected by function only if their bony bases were widened. Maybe the extent of masticatory activity affects the width of the base of the dental arches.

It seems likely that differences in jaw size and facial proportions among various ethnic groups do reflect dietary differences and the accompanying masticatory effort. The characteristic craniofacial morphology of the native population of northern America, which includes broad dental arches, is best explained as an adaptation to the extreme stress they traditionally have placed on jaws and teeth, and changes in craniofacial dimensions from early to modern human civilizations have been related to the accompanying dietary changes.[39] A number of studies by physical anthropologists have indicated that changes in dental occlusion and an increase in malocclusion occur along with transitions from a primitive to a modern diet and lifestyle, to the point that Corruccini has labeled malocclusion a "disease of civilization."[40] In the context of adaptations to changes in diet over even a few generations, it appears that dietary changes probably have played a role in the modern increase in malocclusion. During the development of a

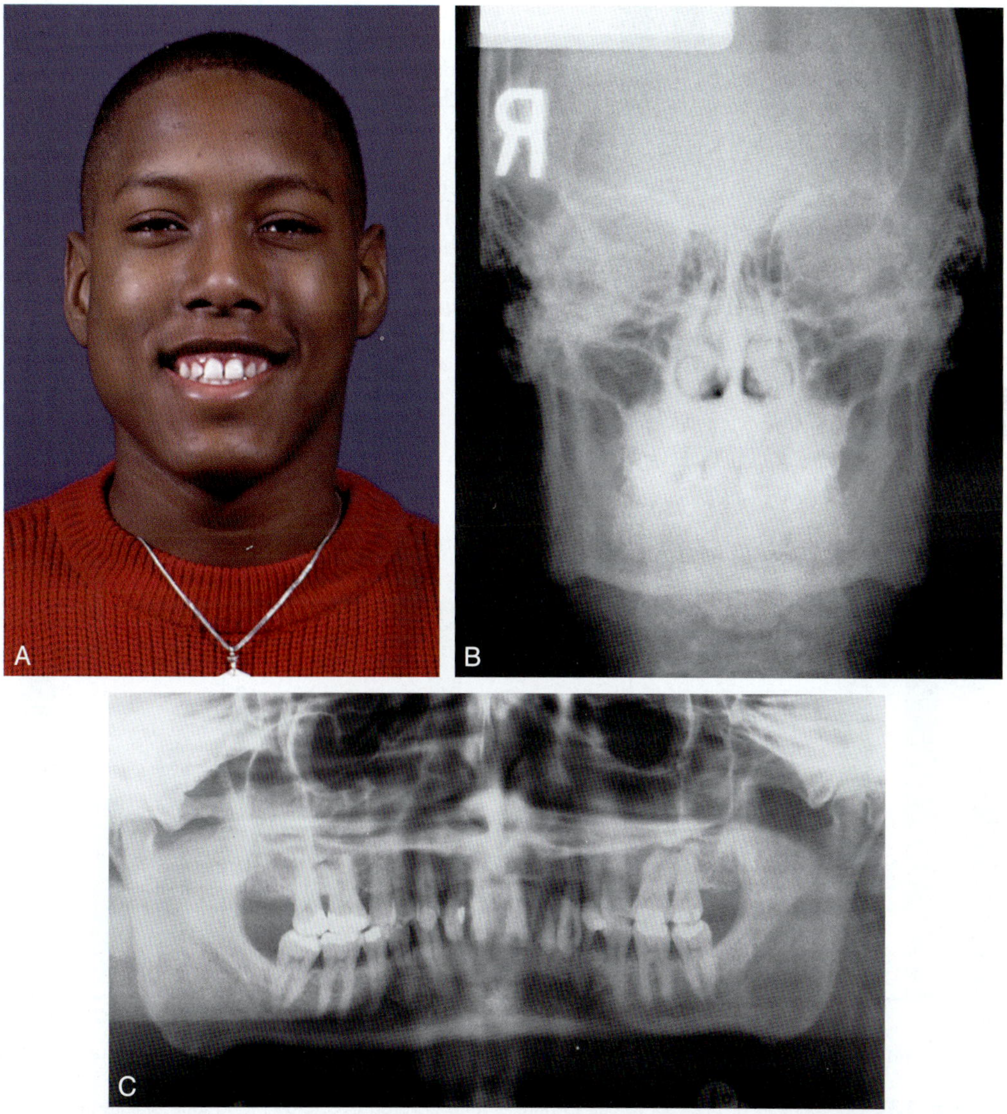

• **Fig. 5.30** Hypertrophy of the masseter muscles leads to excessive bone formation at the angles of the mandible, as would be expected in a bony area that responds to muscle attachment. Note the unusual fullness of the masseteric area, especially on the right side, in the frontal view of the face (A). Bony enlargement at the gonial angles, especially on the right, can be seen in a P-A cephalogram (B) and a panoramic radiograph (C).

single individual, vertical jaw relationships clearly are affected by muscular activity (the effect on tooth eruption is discussed later). Whether masticatory effort influences the size of the dental arches and the amount of space for the teeth is not so clear.

Animal experiments with soft versus hard diets have shown that morphologic changes can occur within a single generation when diet consistency is altered. When a pig, for instance, is raised on a soft rather than a normal diet, there are changes in jaw morphology, in the orientation of the jaws to the rest of the facial skeleton, and in dental arch dimensions.[41] In humans, if dietary consistency affects dental arch size and the amount of space for the teeth as an individual develops, it must do so early in life because dental arch dimensions are established early. Is it possible that a preadolescent child's masticatory effort plays a major role in determining dental arch dimensions? That seems unlikely, but the precise relationship remains unknown.

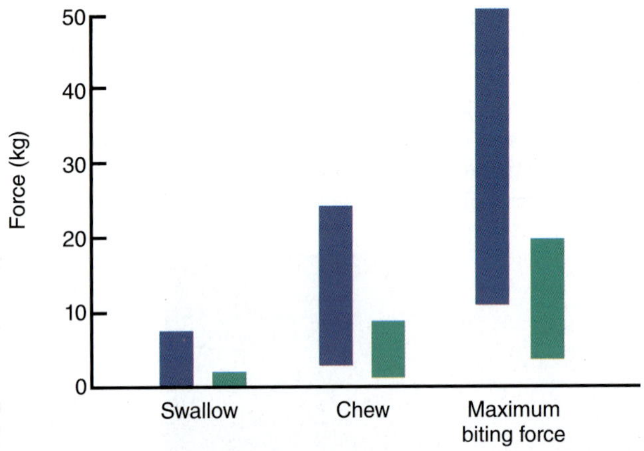

• **Fig. 5.31** Comparison of occlusal force for swallowing, simulated chewing, and maximum effort at 2.5 mm of molar separation in normal-face *(blue)* and long-face *(green)* adults. Note that the normal subjects have much greater occlusal force during swallowing and chewing as well as at maximum effort. The differences are highly significant statistically. (From Proffit WR, Fields HW, Nixon WL. Occlusal forces in normal and long face adults. *J Dent Res*. 1983;62:566–571.)

Biting Force and Eruption

Patients who have excessive overbite or anterior open bite usually have posterior teeth that are infra- or supra-erupted, respectively. It seems reasonable that how much the teeth erupt should be a function of how much force is placed against them during function. Is it possible that differences in muscle strength and therefore in biting force are involved in the etiology of short- and long-face problems?

It was noted some years ago that short-face individuals have higher and long-face persons lower maximum biting forces than those with normal vertical dimensions. The difference between long- and normal-face patients is highly significant statistically for force during occlusal tooth contacts during swallow, simulated chewing, and maximum biting (Fig. 5.31).[42] Such an association between facial morphology and occlusal force does not prove a cause-and-effect relationship. In the rare muscle weakness syndromes discussed earlier, there is a downward and backward rotation of the mandible associated with excessive eruption of the posterior teeth, but this is characteristic of the more usual long-face condition, not just an extension of it. Evidence to document decreased occlusal forces in children who are showing the long-face pattern of growth would strengthen a possible causative relationship.

It is possible to identify a long-face pattern of growth in prepubescent children. Measurement of occlusal forces in this group produces a surprising result: there are no differences between children with long faces and normal faces nor between either group of children and long-face adults.[43] All three groups have forces far below those of normal adults (Fig. 5.32). Therefore it appears that the differences in occlusal force arise at puberty, when the normal

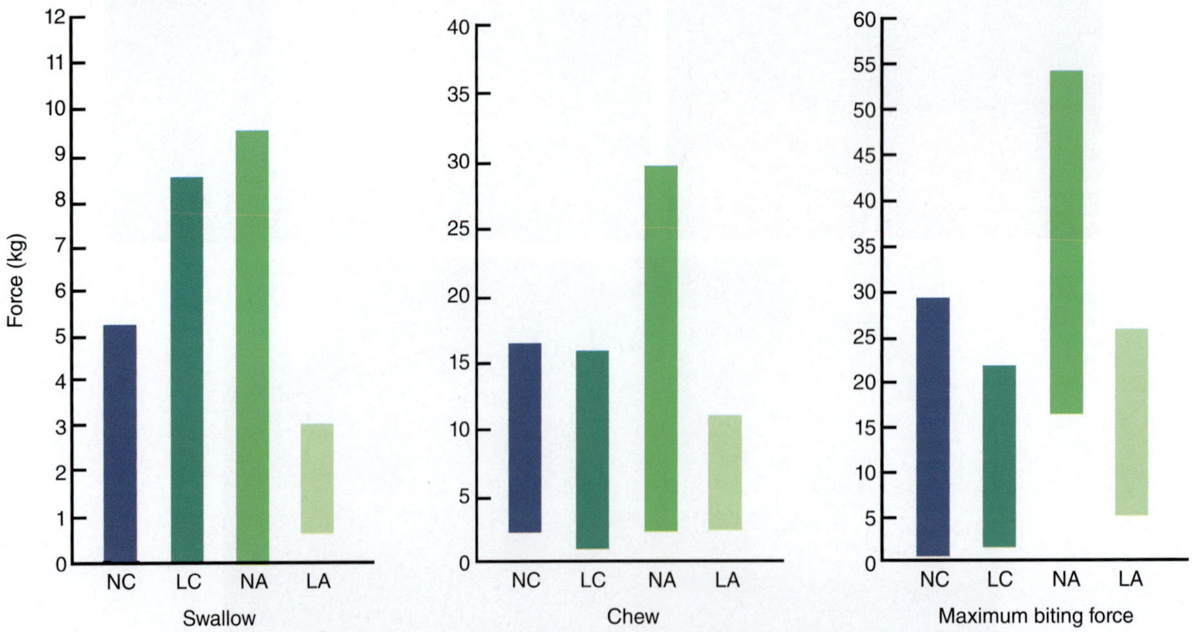

• **Fig. 5.32** Comparison of occlusal forces in normal-face children *(NC, blue)*, long-face children *(LC, aqua)*, normal-face adults *(NA, green)*, and long-face adults *(LA, light green)*. Values for both groups of children and the long-face adults are similar; values for normal adults are significantly higher than for any of the other three groups. The implication is that the differences in occlusal force in adults result from failure of the long-face group to gain strength during adolescence, not to the long condition itself. (From Proffit WR, Fields HW, Nixon WL. Occlusal forces in normal and long face adults. *J Dent Res*. 1983;62:566–571.)

group gains masticatory muscle strength and the long-face group does not. Because the long-face growth pattern can be identified before the differences in occlusal force appear, it seems more likely that the different biting force is an effect rather than a cause.

These findings suggest that the force exerted by the masticatory muscles is not a major environmental factor in controlling tooth eruption and not an etiologic factor for most patients with deep bite or open bite. The effect of muscular dystrophy and related syndromes shows that there can be definite effects on growth if the musculature is abnormal, but in the absence of syndromes of this type, there is no reason to believe that how a patient bites is a major determinant of either dental arch size or vertical dimensions.

Sucking and Other Habits

Almost all normal children engage in non-nutritive sucking of a thumb or pacifier, and as a general rule, sucking habits during the primary dentition years have little if any long-term effect. If these habits persist beyond the time that the permanent teeth begin to erupt, however, malocclusion characterized by flared and spaced maxillary incisors, lingually positioned lower incisors, anterior open bite, and a narrow upper arch is the likely result (Fig. 5.33). The characteristic malocclusion associated with sucking arises from a combination of direct pressure on the teeth and an alteration in the pattern of resting cheek and lip pressures.[44]

When a child places a thumb or finger between the teeth, it is usually positioned at an angle so that it presses lingually against the lower incisors and labially against the upper incisors (Fig. 5.34). There can be considerable variation in which teeth are affected and how much. From equilibrium theory, one would expect that how much the teeth are displaced would correlate better with the number of hours per day of sucking than with the magnitude of the pressure. Children who suck vigorously but intermittently may not displace the incisors much if at all, whereas others, particularly those who sleep with a thumb or finger between the teeth all night, can cause a significant malocclusion.

The anterior open bite associated with thumb-sucking arises by a combination of interference with normal eruption of incisors and excessive eruption of posterior teeth. When a thumb or finger is placed between the anterior teeth, the mandible must be positioned downward to accommodate it. The interposed thumb directly impedes incisor eruption. At the same time, the separation of the jaws alters the vertical equilibrium on the posterior teeth, and as a result, there is more eruption of posterior teeth than might otherwise have occurred. Because of the geometry of the jaws, 1 mm of elongation posteriorly opens the bite about 2 mm anteriorly, so this can be a powerful contributor to the development of anterior open bite (Fig. 5.35).

Although negative pressure is created within the mouth during sucking, there is no reason to believe that this is responsible for the narrowing of the maxillary arch that usually accompanies sucking habits. Instead, arch form is affected by an alteration in the balance between cheek and tongue pressures. If the thumb is placed between the teeth, the tongue must be lowered, which decreases pressure by the tongue against the lingual of upper posterior teeth. At the same time, cheek pressure against these teeth is increased as the buccinator muscle contracts during sucking (Fig. 5.36). Cheek pressures are greatest at the corners of the mouth, and this probably explains why the maxillary arch tends to become V-shaped, with more constriction across the canines than the molars. A child who sucks vigorously is more likely to have a narrow upper arch than one who just places the thumb between the teeth.

Mild displacement of the primary incisor teeth is often noted in a 3- or 4-year-old thumb-sucker, but if sucking stops at this stage, normal lip and cheek pressures soon restore the teeth to their usual positions. If the habit persists after the permanent incisors have begun to erupt, orthodontic treatment may be necessary to overcome the resulting tooth displacements. It is important to realize that transverse constriction of the maxillary arch is the aspect of the malocclusion least likely to correct spontaneously. In many children with a history of thumb-sucking, if the maxillary arch is expanded transversely, both the incisor protrusion and

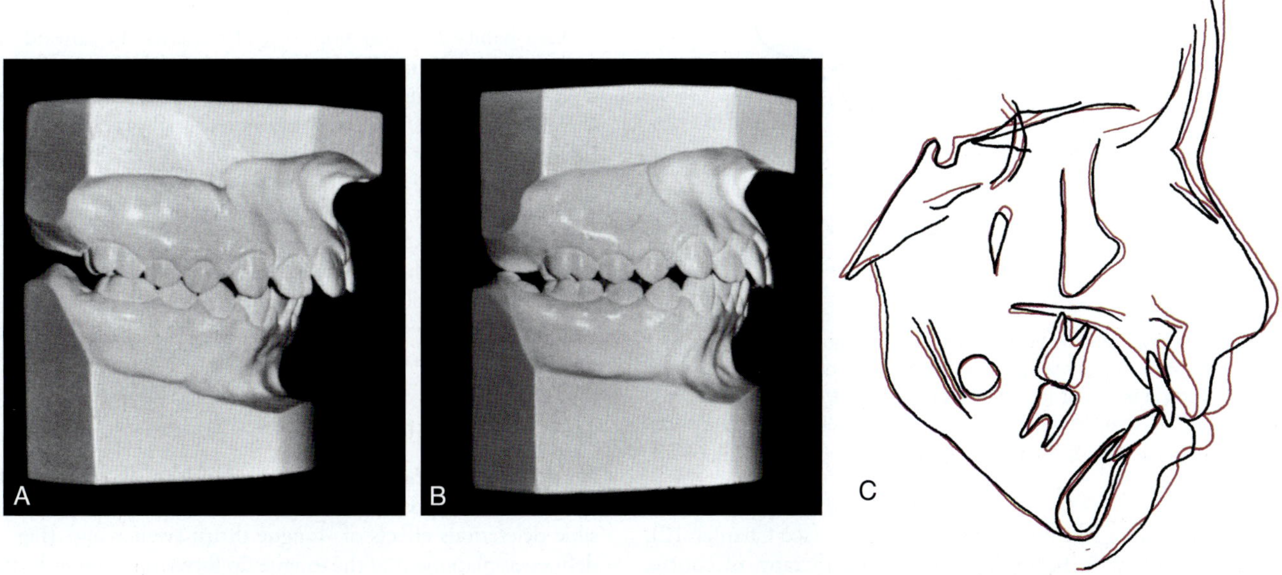

• **Fig. 5.33** In this pair of identical twins, one sucked her thumb up to the time of orthodontic records at age 11 and the other did not. (A) Occlusal relationships in the thumb-sucking girl and (B) her non–thumb-sucking twin. Note the increased overjet and forward displacement of the dentition of the thumb-sucker. (C) Cephalometric tracings of the two girls superimposed on the cranial base of the two girls (Red is the thumb-sucker and black is the non–thumb-sucker). As one would expect with identical twins, the cranial base morphology is nearly identical. Note the forward displacement of the maxillary dentition and anterior alveolus (Points A, the deepest point on the maxilla below ANS (Anterior Nasal Spine), but not at PNS (Posterior Nasal Spine). (Courtesy Dr. T. Wallen.)

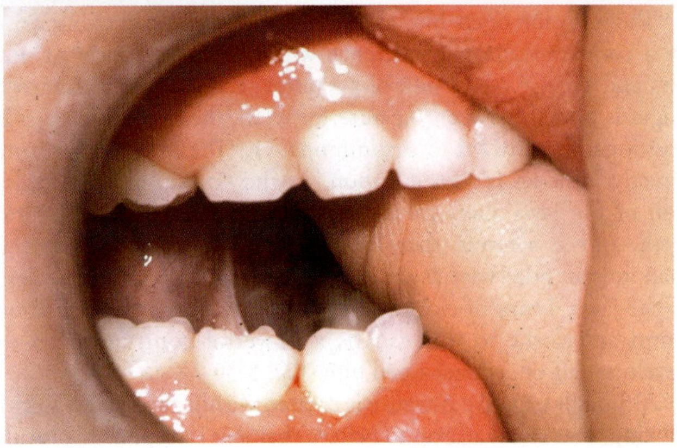

• **Fig. 5.34** A child sucking the thumb usually places it against the roof of the mouth, causing pressure that pushes the lower incisors lingually and the upper incisors labially. In addition, the jaw is positioned downward, providing additional opportunity for posterior teeth to erupt, and cheek pressure is increased while the tongue is lowered vertically away from the maxillary posterior teeth, altering the equilibrium that controls width dimensions. If the thumb is placed on one side instead of in the midline, which is usually the case, the arch and open bite will be asymmetric.

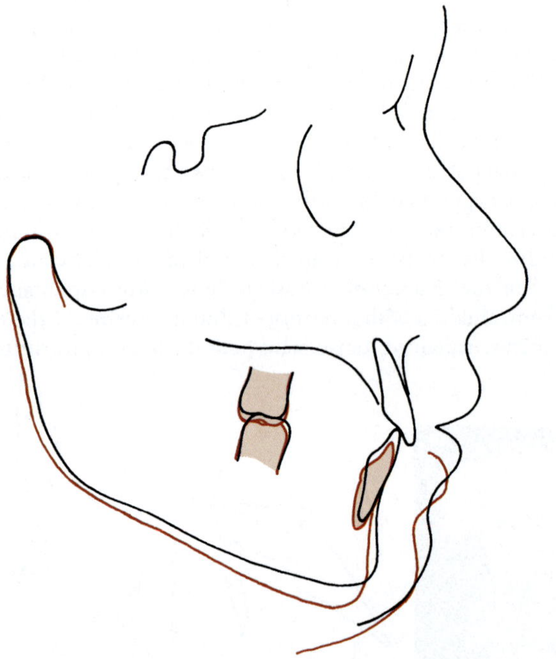

• **Fig. 5.35** Cephalometric tracing showing the effects of posterior eruption on the extent of anterior opening. The only difference between the red and black tracings is that the first molars have been elongated 2 mm in the red tracing. Note that the result is 4 mm of separation of the incisors because of the geometry of the jaw.

anterior open bite will improve spontaneously (see Chapter 12). There is no point in beginning orthodontic therapy, of course, until the habit has stopped.

Whether a habit can serve in the same way as an orthodontic appliance to change the position of the teeth has been the subject of controversy since at least the first century CE, when the philosopher Celsus recommended that a child with a crooked tooth be instructed to apply finger pressure against it to move it to its

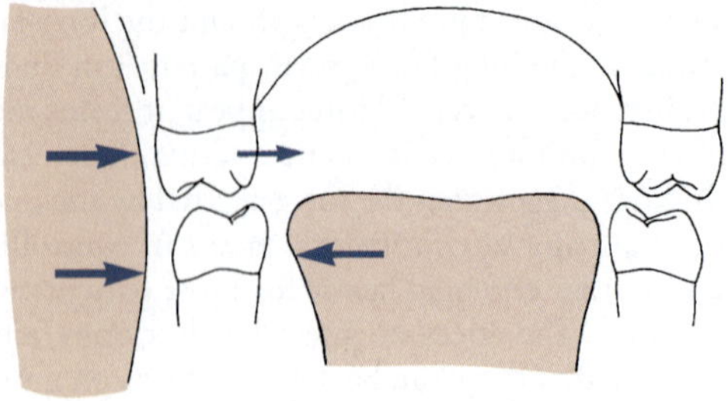

• **Fig. 5.36** Diagrammatic representation of soft tissue pressures in the molar region in a child with a sucking habit. As the tongue is lowered and the cheeks contract during sucking, the pressure balance against the upper teeth is altered, and the upper but not the lower molars are displaced lingually.

proper position. From our present understanding of equilibrium, we would expect that this might work but only if the child kept finger pressure against the tooth for 6 hours or more per day.

This concept also makes it easier to understand how playing a musical instrument might relate to the development of a malocclusion. In the past, many clinicians have suspected that playing a wind instrument could affect the position of the anterior teeth, and some have prescribed musical instruments as part of orthodontic therapy. Playing a clarinet, for instance, might lead to increased overjet because of the way the reeds are placed between the incisors, and this instrument could be considered both a potential cause of a Class II malocclusion and a therapeutic device for treatment of Class III malocclusion. String instruments such as the violin and viola require a specific head and jaw posture that affects tongue versus lip and cheek pressures and could produce asymmetries in arch form. Although the expected types of displacement of teeth are seen in professional musicians,[45,46] even in this group the effects are not dramatic, and little or no effect is observed in most children. It seems quite likely that the duration of tongue and lip pressures associated with playing the instrument is too short to make any difference, except for the most devoted musician.

Can habits affect development of the jaws? In Edward Angle's era, a "sleeping habit" in which the weight of the head rested on the chin was once thought to be a major cause of Class II malocclusion. Facial asymmetries have been attributed to always sleeping on one side of the face or even to "leaning habits," as when an inattentive child leans the side of his or her face against one hand to doze without falling out of the classroom chair. It is not nearly as easy to distort the facial skeleton as these views imply. Sucking habits often exceed the time threshold necessary to produce an effect on the teeth, but even prolonged sucking has little impact on the underlying form of the jaws. On close analysis, most other habits have such a short duration that dental and skeletal effects are unlikely.

Tongue Thrusting

Much attention has been paid at various times to the tongue and tongue habits as possible etiologic factors in malocclusion. The possible deleterious effects of "tongue thrust swallowing" (Fig. 5.37), defined as placement of the tongue tip forward between the incisors during swallowing, still is often thought to be a cause of malocclusion despite the number of studies that have found no such relationship. Let's review what is known now about tongue thrusting as an etiologic factor.

Laboratory studies have indicated that individuals who place the tongue tip forward when they swallow usually do not have

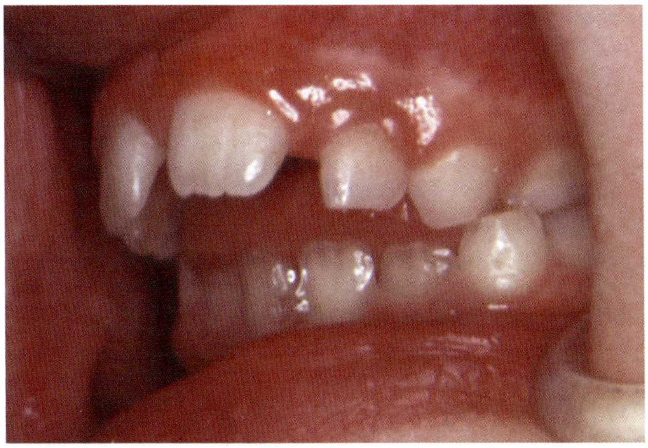

• **Fig. 5.37** The typical appearance of a "tongue thrust swallow" with the lip pulled back. Note the tongue tip between the incisors protruding forward toward contact with the elevated lower lip.

more tongue force against the teeth than those who keep the tongue tip back; in fact, tongue pressure may be lower.[47] The term *tongue thrust* is therefore something of a misnomer because it implies that the tongue is forcefully thrust forward. Swallowing is not a learned behavior but is integrated and controlled physiologically at subconscious levels, so whatever the pattern of swallow, it cannot be considered a habit in the usual sense. It is true, however, that individuals with an anterior open bite malocclusion place the tongue between the anterior teeth when they swallow, whereas those who have a normal incisor relationship usually do not, and it is tempting to blame the open bite on this pattern of tongue activity.

As discussed in detail in Chapter 2, the mature or adult swallow pattern appears in some normal children as early as age 3 but is not present in the majority until about age 6 and is never achieved in 10% to 15% of a typical population. Tongue thrust swallowing in older patients superficially resembles the infantile swallow (described in Chapter 3), and sometimes children or adults who place the tongue between the anterior teeth are spoken of as having a retained infantile swallow. This is clearly incorrect. Only children with brain damage retain a truly infantile swallow in which the posterior part of the tongue has little or no role.

Because coordinated movements of the posterior tongue and elevation of the mandible tend to develop before protrusion of the tongue tip between the incisor teeth disappears, what is called "tongue thrusting" in young children is often a normal transitional stage in swallowing. During the transition from an infantile to a mature swallow, a child can be expected to pass through a stage in which the swallow is characterized by muscular activity to bring the lips together, separation of the posterior teeth, and forward protrusion of the tongue between the teeth. This is also a description of the classic tongue thrust swallow. A delay in the normal swallow transition can be expected when a child has a sucking habit.

When there is an anterior open bite and/or upper incisor protrusion, as often occurs from sucking habits, it is more difficult to seal off the front of the mouth during swallowing to prevent food or liquids from escaping. Bringing the lips together and placing the tongue between the separated anterior teeth is a successful maneuver to close off the front of the mouth and form an anterior seal. In other words, a tongue thrust swallow is a useful physiologic adaptation if you have an open bite, which is why an individual with an open bite usually also has a tongue thrust swallow, but protruding the tongue between the anterior teeth during swallowing is often present in children with good anterior occlusion. After a sucking habit stops, the anterior open bite tends to close spontaneously, but the position of the tongue between the anterior teeth persists for a while as the open bite closes. Until the open bite disappears, an anterior seal by the tongue tip remains necessary.

The modern viewpoint is, in short, that tongue thrust swallowing is seen primarily in two circumstances: in younger children with reasonably normal occlusion, in whom it represents only a transitional stage in normal physiologic maturation; and in individuals of any age with displaced incisors, in whom it is an adaptation to the space between the teeth. The presence of a large overjet (often) and anterior open bite (nearly always) conditions a child or adult to place the tongue between the anterior teeth. A tongue thrust swallow therefore is more likely to be the result of displaced incisors, not the cause. It follows, of course, that correcting the tooth position should cause a change in swallow pattern, and this usually happens. It is neither necessary nor desirable to try to teach the patient to swallow differently before beginning orthodontic treatment.

This is not to say that the tongue has no etiologic role in the development of open bite malocclusion. From equilibrium theory, light but sustained pressure by the tongue against the teeth would be expected to have significant effects. Tongue thrust swallowing simply has too short a duration to have an impact on tooth position. Pressure by the tongue against the teeth during a typical swallow lasts for approximately 1 second. A typical individual swallows about 800 times per day while awake but only a few times per hour while asleep. The total per day therefore is usually under 1000. One thousand seconds of pressure, of course, totals only a few minutes, not nearly enough to affect the equilibrium.

On the other hand, if a patient has a forward resting posture of the tongue, the duration of this light pressure could affect tooth position, vertically or horizontally. Tongue tip protrusion during swallowing is sometimes associated with a forward tongue posture. If the position from which tongue movements start is different from normal, so that the pattern of resting pressures is different, there is likely to be an effect on the teeth, whereas if the postural position is normal, the tongue thrust swallow has no clinical significance.

Perhaps this point can best be put in perspective by comparing the number of children who have an anterior open bite malocclusion with the number of children of the same age reported to have a tongue thrust swallow. As Fig. 5.38 shows, at every age above 6, the number of children reported to have a tongue thrust swallow is about 10 times greater than the number reported to have an anterior open bite. Thus, there is no reason to believe that a tongue thrust swallow always implies an altered rest position and will lead to malocclusion. In a child who has an open bite, tongue posture may be a factor, but the swallow itself is not.

Respiratory Pattern

Respiratory needs are the primary determinant of the posture of the jaws and tongue (and of the head itself, to a lesser extent). Therefore it seems entirely reasonable that an altered respiratory pattern, such as breathing through the mouth rather than the nose, could change the posture of the head, jaw, and tongue. This in turn could alter the equilibrium of pressures on the jaws and teeth and affect both jaw growth and tooth position. To breathe through the mouth, one must lower the mandible and tongue and extend (tip back) the head. If these postural changes were maintained, three effects on growth would be expected: (1) anterior face height would increase, and posterior teeth would super-erupt; (2) unless there was unusual vertical growth of the ramus, the mandible would rotate down and back, opening the bite anteriorly and increasing overjet; and (3) increased pressure from the stretched cheeks might cause a narrower maxillary dental arch.

Exactly this type of malocclusion often is associated with mouth breathing (note its similarity to the pattern also blamed on sucking habits and tongue thrust swallow). The association has been noted for many years: the descriptive term *adenoid facies* has appeared in the English literature for at least a century, and probably longer (Fig. 5.39). Unfortunately, the relationship among mouth breathing, altered posture, and the development of malocclusion is not so clear-cut as the theoretical outcome of shifting to oral respiration might appear at first glance.[48] Recent experimental studies have only partially clarified the situation.

In analyzing this, it is important to understand first that although humans are primarily nasal breathers, everyone breathes partially through the mouth under certain physiologic conditions, the most prominent being an increased need for oxygen during exercise. For the average individual, there is a transition to partial oral breathing when ventilatory exchange rates above 40 to 45 L/min are reached. At maximum effort, 80 or more L/min of air are needed, about half of which is obtained through the mouth. At rest, minimum airflow is 20 to 25 L/min, but heavy mental concentration or even normal conversation leads to increased airflow and a transition to partial mouth breathing.

During resting conditions, greater effort is required to breathe through the nose than through the mouth; the tortuous nasal passages introduce an element of resistance to airflow as they perform their function of warming and humidifying the inspired air. The increased work for nasal respiration is physiologically acceptable up to a point, and indeed respiration is most efficient with modest resistance present in the system. If the nose is partially obstructed, the work associated with nasal breathing increases, and at a certain level of resistance to nasal airflow, the individual switches to partial mouth breathing. This crossover point varies among individuals but is usually reached at resistance levels of about 3.5 to 4 cm H_2O/L per s.[49] The swelling of the nasal mucosa accompanying a

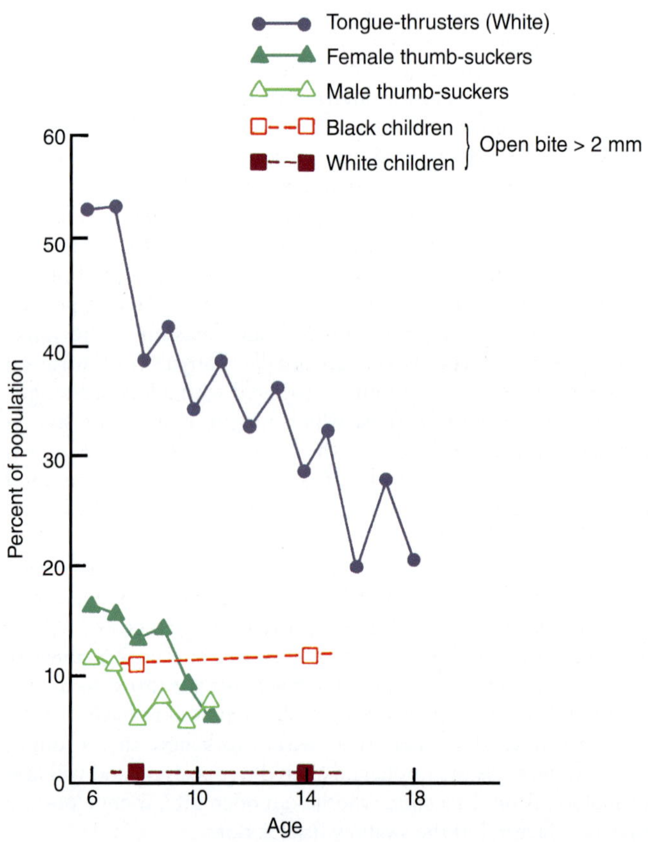

• **Fig. 5.38** Prevalence of anterior open bite, thumb-sucking, and tongue thrust swallowing as a function of age. Open bite occurs much more frequently in blacks than in whites. Note that the prevalence of anterior open bite at any age is only a small fraction of the prevalence of tongue thrust swallowing and is also less than the prevalence of thumb-sucking. (Data from Fletcher SG, Casteel RL, Bradley DP. Tongue-thrust swallow, speech articulation, and age. *J Speech Hear Disord*. 1961;26:201–208; Kelly JE, Harvey CR. An assessment of the occlusion of the teeth of youths 12-17 years. DHEW Pub No [HRA] 76–1644; Vital and health statistics. Series 11, Data from the national health survey; no.162. National Center for Health Statistics; 1977:77–144. https://staging-stacks.cdc.gov/view/cdc/12684.)

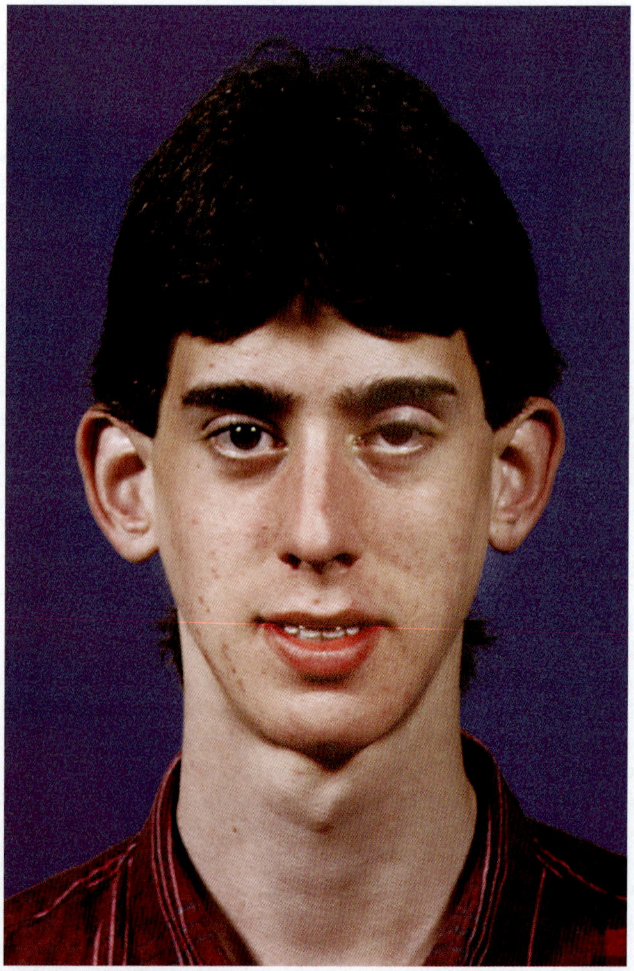

• **Fig. 5.39** The classic adenoid facies, characterized by narrow width dimensions, protruding teeth, and lips separated at rest, has often been attributed to mouth breathing because of enlarged adenoids. Because it is perfectly possible to breathe through the nose with the lips separated, simply by creating an oral seal posteriorly with the soft palate, the facial appearance is not diagnostic of the respiratory mode. On careful study, many patients with this facial type are found not to be obligatory mouth breathers.

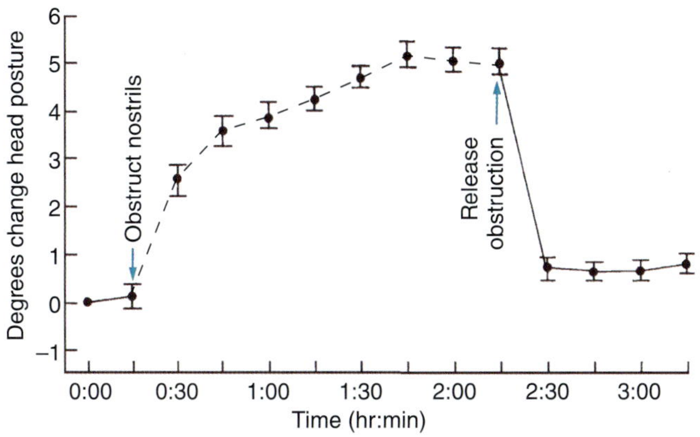

• **Fig. 5.40** Data from an experiment with dental students, showing the immediate change in head posture when the nostrils are totally blocked: The head tips back about 5 degrees, increasing the separation of the jaws. When the obstruction is relieved, head posture returns to its original position. (From Vig PS, Showfety KJ, Phillips C. Experimental manipulation of head posture. *Am J Orthod*. 1980;77:258–268.)

common cold occasionally converts all of us to mouth breathing at rest by this mechanism.

Chronic respiratory obstruction can be produced by prolonged inflammation of the nasal mucosa associated with allergies or chronic infection. It can also be produced by mechanical obstruction anywhere within the nasorespiratory system, from the nares to the posterior nasal choanae. Under normal conditions, the size of the nostril is the limiting factor in nasal airflow. The pharyngeal tonsils or adenoids normally are large in children, and partial obstruction from this source may contribute to mouth breathing in children. Individuals who have had chronic nasal obstruction may continue to breathe partially through the mouth even after the obstruction has been relieved. In this sense, mouth breathing can sometimes be considered a habit.

If respiration influenced the jaws and teeth, it should do so by causing a change in posture that secondarily altered long-duration pressures from the soft tissues. Experiments with human subjects have shown that a change in posture does accompany nasal obstruction. For instance, when the nose is completely blocked, usually there is an immediate change of about 5 degrees in the craniovertebral angle (Fig. 5.40). The jaws move apart, as much by elevation of the maxilla, because the head tips back, as by depression of the mandible. When the nasal obstruction is removed, the original posture immediately returns.

Harvold's classic experiments with growing monkeys showed that totally obstructing the nostrils for a prolonged period in this species leads to the development of malocclusion, but not the type commonly associated with mouth breathing in humans.[50] Instead, the monkeys tend to develop some degree of mandibular prognathism, although their response shows considerable variety. In the evaluation of these experiments, it must be kept in mind that mouth breathing of any extent is completely unnatural for monkeys, who will die if their nasal passages are obstructed abruptly. For these experiments to be carried out, it was necessary to gradually obstruct their noses, giving the animals a chance to learn how to survive as mouth breathers. The variety of responses in the monkeys suggests that the type of malocclusion is determined by the individual animal's pattern of adaptation.

Total nasal obstruction is extremely rare in humans. There are only a few well-documented cases of facial growth in children with long-term total nasal obstruction, but it appears that under these circumstances the growth pattern is altered in the way one would predict (Fig. 5.41). Because total nasal obstruction in humans is so rare, the important clinical question is whether partial nasal obstruction, of the type that occurs occasionally for a short time in everyone and chronically in some children, can lead to malocclusion; more precisely, how close to total obstruction does partial obstruction have to come before it is clinically significant?

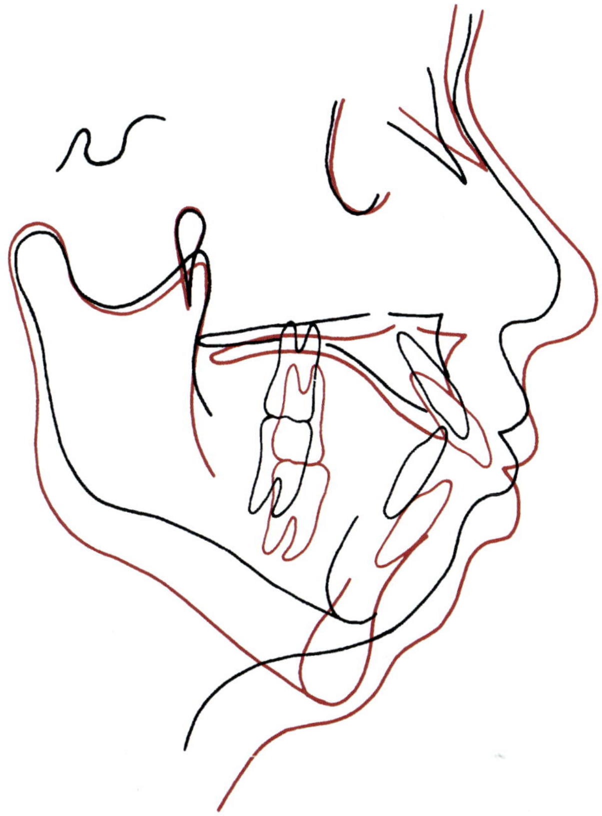

• **Fig. 5.41** Cephalometric superimposition showing the effect of total nasal obstruction produced by a pharyngeal flap operation (for cleft palate speech) that sealed off the nose posteriorly. From age 12 *(black)* to 16 *(red)*, the mandible rotated downward and backward as the patient experienced considerable growth. (Redrawn from McNamara JA. Influence of respiratory pattern on craniofacial growth. *Angle Orthod*. 1981;51:269–300.)

The question is difficult to answer, primarily because it is difficult to know what the pattern of respiration really is at any given time in humans. Observers tend to equate lip separation at rest with mouth breathing (see Fig. 5.39), but this is simply not correct. It is perfectly possible for an individual to breathe through the nose while the lips are apart. To do this, the individual only needs to seal off the mouth by placing the tongue against the palate. Because some lip separation at rest (lip incompetence) is normal in children, many children who appear to be mouth breathers may not be.

Simple clinical tests for mouth breathing can also be misleading. The highly vascular nasal mucosa undergoes cycles of engorgement with blood and shrinkage. The cycles alternate between the two nostrils: When one is clear, the other is usually somewhat obstructed. For this reason, clinical tests to determine whether the patient can breathe freely through both nostrils nearly always show that one is at least partially blocked. One partially obstructed nostril should not be interpreted as a problem with normal nasal breathing.

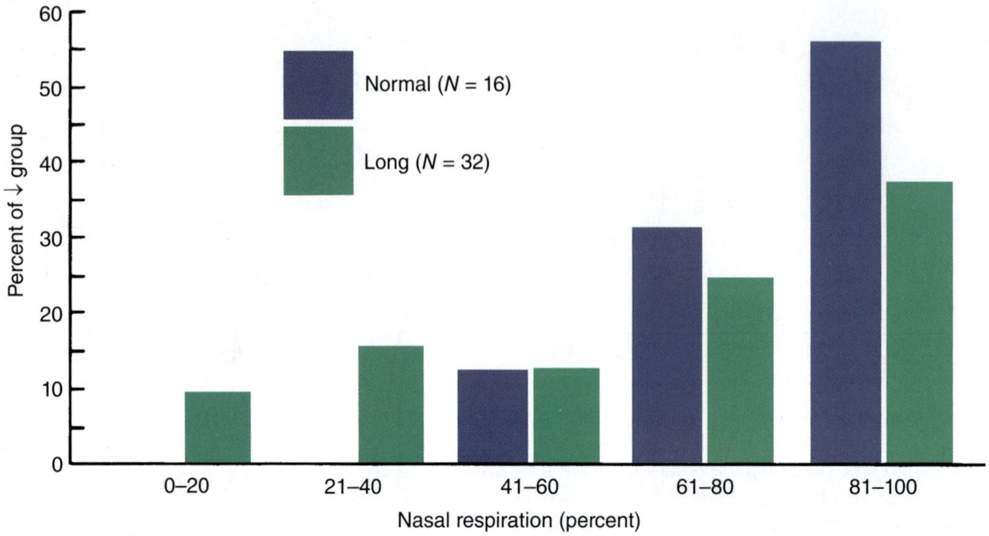

• **Fig. 5.42** Comparison of the percentage of nasal respiration in long-face versus normal-face adolescents. About one-third of the long-face group have less than 50% nasal respiration, whereas none of the normal-face group have such a low nasal percentage, but most of the long-face group are predominantly nasal breathers. The data suggest that impaired nasal respiration may contribute to the development of the long-face condition but is not the sole or even the major cause. (Data redrawn from Fields HW, Warren DW, Black K, Phillips C. Relationship between vertical dentofacial morphology and respiration in adolescents. *Am J Orthod Dentofac Orthop*. 1991;99:147–154.)

The only reliable way to quantify the extent of mouth breathing is to establish how much of the total airflow goes through the nose and how much through the mouth, which requires special instrumentation to simultaneously measure nasal and oral airflow. This allows the percentage of nasal or oral respiration (nasal/oral ratio) to be calculated for the length of time the subject can tolerate being continuously monitored. It seems obvious that a certain percentage of oral respiration maintained for a certain percentage of the time should be the definition of significant mouth breathing, but despite years of effort such a definition has not been produced.

The best experimental data for the relationship between malocclusion and mouth breathing were derived from studies of the nasal/oral ratio in normal versus long-face children.[51] The relationship is not nearly as clear-cut as theory might predict. It is useful to represent the data as in Fig. 5.42, which shows that both normal and long-face children are likely to be predominantly nasal breathers under laboratory conditions. A minority of the long-face children had less than 40% nasal breathing, but none of the normal children had such low nasal percentages. When adult long-face patients are examined, the findings are similar: the number with evidence of nasal obstruction is increased in comparison to a normal population, but the majority are not mouth breathers in the sense of predominantly oral respiration.

It seems reasonable to presume that children who require adenoidectomy and/or tonsillectomy for medical purposes, or those diagnosed as having chronic nasal allergies, would have some degree of nasal obstruction. Although the differences between normal children and those in the allergy or adenoidectomy groups were statistically significant and undoubtedly real, they were not large. Face height on the average was about 3 mm greater in the adenoidectomy group.[52]

Studies of Swedish children who underwent adenoidectomy showed that on the average, children in the adenoidectomy group had a significantly longer anterior face height than control children (Fig. 5.43). They also had a tendency toward maxillary

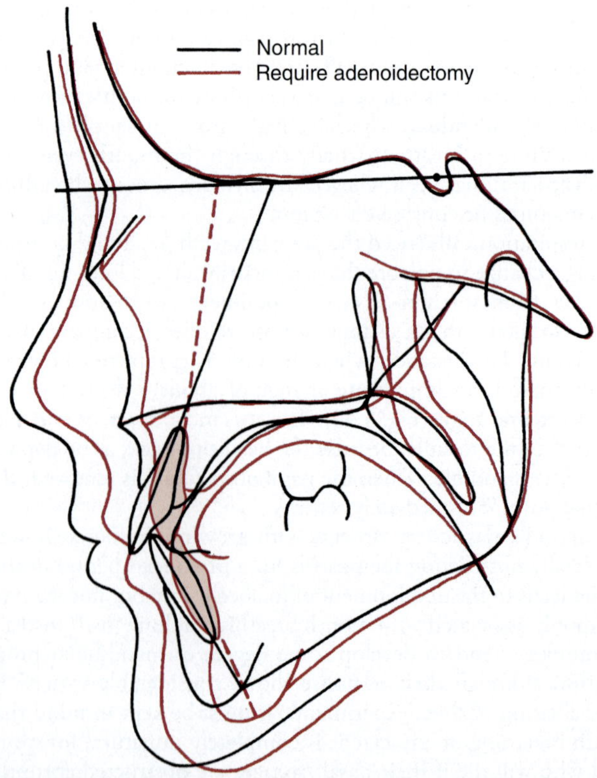

• **Fig. 5.43** Composite (mean) cephalometric tracings for a group of Swedish children requiring adenoidectomy for medical purposes, compared with a group of normal controls. The adenoidectomy group had statistically significantly greater anterior face height and steeper mandibular plane angles than the controls, but the differences were quantitatively not large. The tracing is oriented with the nose to the left, as it is done routinely in Europe, because it was originally published that way. (From Linder-Aronson S. Adenoids: their effect on mode of breathing and nasal airflow and their relationship to characteristics of the facial skeleton and dentition. *Acta Otolaryngol Scand*. 1970;[suppl]:265.)

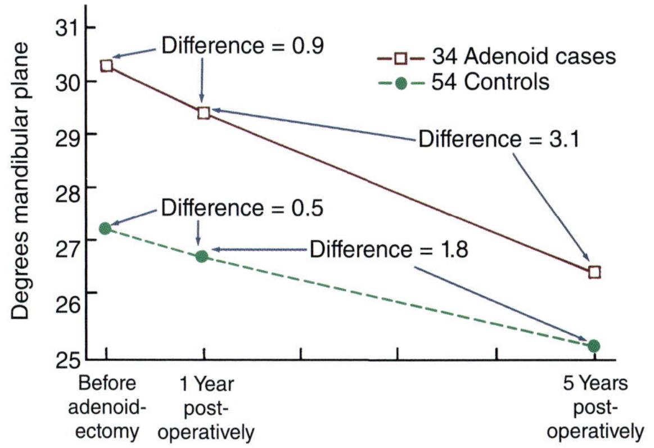

• **Fig. 5.44** Comparison of mandibular plane angles in a group of post-adenoidectomy children compared with normal controls. Note that the differences existing at the time of adenoidectomy decreased in size but did not totally disappear. (From Linder-Aronson S. Effects of adenoidectomy on the dentition and facial skeleton over a period of five years. In: Cook JT, ed. *Transactions of the Third International Orthodontic Congress*. Mosby; 1975:85–100.)

constriction and more upright incisors.[53] Furthermore, when children in the adenoidectomy group were followed after surgery they tended to return toward the mean of the control group, although the differences persisted (Fig. 5.44). It is frequently overlooked that this change occurred in only roughly half of the original sample. When changes did occur they were small and with wide amounts of individual variation leading to the inference that change in mandibular posture as a response to nasopharyngeal obstruction may only actually occur in a subset of affected patients. Similar differences from normal control groups were seen in other groups requiring adenoidectomy and/or tonsillectomy.[54]

It appears therefore that research to this point on respiration has established two opposing principles, leaving a large gray area between them: (1) total nasal obstruction is highly likely to alter the pattern of growth and lead to malocclusion in experimental animals and humans, and individuals with a high percentage of oral respiration are overrepresented in the long-face population; but (2) the majority of individuals with the long-face pattern of deformity have no evidence of nasal obstruction and must therefore have some other etiologic factor as the principal cause. Perhaps the alterations in posture associated with partial nasal obstruction and moderate increases in the percentage of oral respiration are not great enough by themselves to create a severe malocclusion. Mouth breathing, in short, may contribute to the development of orthodontic problems but is difficult to indict as a frequent etiologic agent.

Obstructive Sleep Apnea

It is interesting to consider the other side of this relationship: can malocclusion sometimes cause respiratory obstruction? Obstructive sleep apnea (OSA) has been recognized recently as a more frequent problem than had been appreciated,[55] having a prevalence rate of up to 5% in the general pediatric population and estimated to be present in 9%–38% of adults.[56] The peak prevalence of OSA in children occurs around the ages of 6–7. This is coincident with the increased adenotonsillar growth that reaches its maximum size in relation to the surrounding upper airway anatomy.

OSA is characterized by repeated episodes of partial or complete collapse of the upper airway during sleep followed by arousal to open the airway. This leads to drops in blood oxygen levels, fragmented sleep and daytime sleepiness as well as cardiopulmonary disease, stroke, arthritis, depression and diabetes.[57] This leads to functional problems of lost work time and auto accidents. While all patients with OSA have some anatomical deficiency, it is a common misconception that this always refers to a deficiency in size of the airway or the surrounding skeletal framework such as mandibular or maxillary hypoplasia. The simple fact that airway collapse occurs during sleep and not while a patient is awake serves to highlight the neuromuscular influence on airway function.

Historically, a retrusive mandible with an increased mandibular plane angle and maxillary constriction have been associated with OSA in children. This has been based on small, retrospective studies with subjective reporting of obstructive sleep apnea.

More recently, systematic reviews and meta-analysis of the cephalometric measurements or dental characteristics of children with objectively diagnosed OSA using sleep studies have failed to find a strong relationship between morphology and the disease. The most frequently reported cephalometric differences between children with OSA and healthy controls are in the cephalometric angles SNB and mandibular plane, however these differences are in the order of only a few degrees and relatively small when compared to the ranges observed in the general population.[58] Similarly, smaller intermolar widths (approximately 2 mm) may have little clinical relevance.[59] It would seem that there is perhaps a subset of children with OSA who have a significant alteration to their facial form, however most children with OSA will appear within normal limits.

OSA is unlikely to be a dominant influence in facial growth in at least the majority of patients. The reciprocal is also likely true—outside of syndromic levels of altered craniofacial form, the genetically determined size of the jaws will impact breathing function of some but not most patients with OSA.

OSA's etiology, however, is by no means impacted just by orofacial morphology; obesity, age, and gender seem to be important. The orthodontist's role in treatment of sleep apnea and current recommendations for types of treatment are discussed in Chapter 7.

What is the impact of orthodontic treatment on the airway? It has been proposed that dental extractions for orthodontic purposes may lead to impaired breathing, perhaps from the overly simplistic notion that a reduction in arch length will cause the tongue to take on a posterior position in the oral cavity and lead to increased airway collapsibility. It is misleading to assume that extractions will always lead to a reduced arch length because the indications for extractions and subsequent tooth movement during orthodontic treatment can vary significantly from patient to patient (extractions can be indicated for various levels of crowding, protrusion, or open bite). A recent systematic review and meta-analysis[60] concluded that there is no strong evidence to support the concept that premolar extractions for bimaxillary protrusion or crowded, in growing or adult patients reduce either pharyngeal airway volume or minimal cross-sectional area.

It is important to note however that a change in airway dimensions does not necessary provide any meaningful data on airway function. However, a very large population-based study has helped clarify the relationship between extractions and obstructive sleep apnea. Researchers took advantage of a large patient database from an insurance company that provide both dental and medical care to patients in Minnesota.[61] From the dental records, nearly 2800 adult patients with four missing premolars were recruited and matched based on BMI, age, and gender to an equal number of patients with a full permanent dentition. The medical records of these two groups were then analyzed to determine if the patients with four extracted teeth had a greater prevalence of OSA or associated OSA treatment. Final comparison demonstrated no difference between the two groups and that roughly 10% of both had been diagnosed with OSA, which interestingly is in line with commonly reported prevalence rates of OSA in the general US population.

Is it possible that the retraction force applied to the maxillary arch and transmitted to the maxilla by orthodontic headgear causes negative changes to the upper airway? Classic implant studies have demonstrated that there is little long-term effect on the innate direction or pattern of growth of the face by treatment with headgear. Although there are measurable changes to the maxilla during or immediately following treatment with headgear, these effects on the facial skeleton are temporary and do not impart significant long-term changes on the size or position of the upper or lower jaws.[62]

Further, studies examining the effects of headgear treatment on the upper airway dimensions with cephalometric analysis have reported no negative changes,[63,64] and that neither treatment in the early or late mixed dentition had any adverse effects on upper airway dimensions.[65] In a small study of 10 children who were selected because of preexisting sleep apnea conditions, Pirilä-Parkkinen[66] examined the impact of orthodontic treatment with headgear on children with existing OSA which may cause their conditions to be exacerbated. Importantly, the blood oxygen levels during sleep were not affected while headgear was worn, but rather they had a great number of sleep disturbances.

It is often overlooked that the long-term skeletal effects of headgear compared to functional appliance treatment of class II malocclusions are remarkably similar. Godt and colleagues[67] compared effects on airway space between children treated with headgear and mandibular advancing appliances. They concluded that upper airway changes did not vary significantly between patients treated with either the headgear or functional appliance, supporting the idea that headgear does not significantly affect airway.

There is a substantial body of evidence demonstrating that the long-term skeletal changes from orthodontic treatment with headgear are rather minimal with significant dentoalveolar change being the major contributor to correction of the malocclusion. Long-term effects are at the level of the teeth, and not the actual upper or lower jaw bones. Therefore it is unreasonable to expect any significant effect on airway dimensions from headgear treatment.

Etiology in Contemporary Perspective

Part of the philosophy of the early orthodontists was their belief in the perfectibility of man. Edward Angle and his contemporaries, influenced by the romanticized view of native peoples commonly held in the late 19th and early 20th centuries, took for granted that malocclusion was a disease of civilization and blamed it on improper function of the jaws under modern conditions. Changing jaw function to produce proper growth and improve facial proportions was an important goal of treatment, which unfortunately proved difficult to achieve.

Classic (mendelian) genetics developed rapidly in the first part of the 20th century, and a different view of malocclusion gradually replaced the earlier one. This new view was that malocclusion is primarily the result of inherited dentofacial proportions, which might be altered somewhat by developmental variations, trauma, or altered function, but which are basically established at conception. If that were true, the possibilities for orthodontic treatment also would be rather limited. The orthodontist's role would be to adapt the dentition to the existing facial structures, with little hope of producing underlying changes.

In the 1980s there was a strong swing back toward the earlier view, as the failure of heredity to explain most variation in occlusion and jaw proportions was appreciated and as the new theories of growth control indicated how environmental influences could operate by altering posture. The earlier concept that jaw function is related to the development of malocclusion was revived and strengthened, both by the evidence against simple inheritance and by a more optimistic view of the extent to which the human skeleton can be altered. Clinical applications, some already recognized as unfortunate, reflected extreme optimism about arch expansion and growth modification.

As the 21st century moves ahead, a more balanced view seems to be emerging. Contemporary research has refuted the simplistic picture of malocclusion as resulting from independent inheritance of dental and facial characteristics, but the research findings consistently have shown also that there are no simple explanations for malocclusion in terms of oral function. Mouth breathing, tongue thrusting, soft diet, sleeping posture—none of these can be regarded as the sole or even the major reason for most malocclusions. Along the same lines, it is fair to say that the research has not yet clarified the precise role of heredity as an etiologic agent for malocclusion. The relatively high heritability of craniofacial dimensions and the relatively low heritability of dental arch variations now have been established, but exactly how this relates to the etiologic process of malocclusions that have both skeletal and dental components remains unknown. Conclusions about the etiology of most orthodontic problems are difficult because several interacting factors probably played a role. At least, at this point we are more aware of how much we really do not yet know about the etiology of orthodontic problems.

References

1. Suttie M, Faroud T, Wetherill L, et al. Facial dysmorphism across the fetal alcohol spectrum. *Pediatrics*. 2013;131:e779–e788.
2. Naidoo S, Norval G, Swanevelder S, et al. Foetal alcohol syndrome: a dental and skeletal age analysis of patients and controls. *Eur J Orthod*. 2006;28:247–253.
3. Sanchez E, Laplace-Builhé B, Mau-Them FT, et al. *POLR1B* and neural crest cell anomalies in Treacher Collins syndrome type 4. *Genet Med*. 2020;22:547–556.
4. Sulik KK, Johnston MC, Smiley SJ, et al. Mandibulofacial dysostosis (Treacher Collins syndrome): a new proposal for its pathogenesis. *Am J Med Genet*. 1987;27:359–372.
5. Brandstetter KA, Patel KG. Craniofacial microstomia. *Facial Plast Surg Clin North Am*. 2016;24:495–515.
6. Centers for Disease Control and Prevention. Improved national prevalence estimates for 18 selected major birth defects—United States, 1999-2001. *MMWR Morb Mortal Wkly Rep*. 2006; Jan 6;54(51):1301–1305.
7. Li Z, Liu J, Ye R, et al. Maternal passive smoking and risk of cleft lip with or without cleft palate. *Epidemiology*. 2010;21:240–242.
8. Centers for Disease Control and Prevention. *Facts About Cleft Lip and Cleft Palate*. https://www.cdc.gov/ncbddd/birthdefects/cleftlip.html
9. Garib DG, Rosar JP, Sathler R, Ozawa TO. Dual embryonic origin of maxillary lateral incisors: clinical implications in patients with cleft lip and palate. *Dental Press J Orthod*. 2015; Oct;20(5):118–125.
10. Tessier P. Anatomical classification of facial, craniofacial and laterofacial clefts. *J Maxillofac Surg*. 1976;4:69–92.

11. Sulik KK. Orofacial embryogenesis: a framework for understanding clefting sites. 3rd ed.. In: Fonseca RJ, Marciani RD, Turvey TA, eds. *Oral and Maxillofacial Surgery*. Vol. 3 Elsevier; 2017. [chap 27].
12. Ewings EL, Carstens MH. Neuroembryology and functional anatomy of craniofacial clefts. *Indian J Plast Surg*. 2009 Oct;42 Suppl (Suppl):S19–34. https://doi.org/10.4103/0970-0358.57184. PMID: 19884675; PMCID: PMC2825068.
13. Utria AF, Mundlinger GS, Bellamy JJ, et al. The importance of timing in optimizing cranial vault remodeling in syndromic craniosynostosis. *Plast Reconstr Surg*. 2015;135:1077–1084.
14. Ko JM. Genetic syndromes associated with craniosynostosis. *J Korean Neurosurg Soc*. 2016 May;59(3):187–191.
15. Helman SN, Badhey A, Kadakia S, Myers E. Revisiting Crouzon syndrome: reviewing the background and management of a multifaceted disease. *Oral Maxillofac Surg*. 2014;18:373–379.
16. Sawh-Martinez R, Steinbacher DM. Syndromic craniosynostosis. *Clin Plast Surg*. 2019 Apr;46(2):141–155. https://doi.org/10.1016/j.cps.2018.11.009. PMID: 30851747.
17. Mathijssen IM. Guideline for care of patients with the diagnoses of craniosynostosis: working group on craniosynostosis. *J Craniofac Surg*. 2015 Sep;26(6):1735–1807. https://doi.org/10.1097/SCS.000000 0000002016. PMID: 26355968; PMCID: PMC4568904.
18. Tan HL, Kheirandish-Gozal L, Abel F, Gozal D. Craniofacial syndromes and sleep-related breathing disorders. *Sleep Med Rev*. 2016 Jun;27:74–88.
19. Bartel-Friedrich S, Wulke C. Classification and diagnosis of ear malformations. *GMS Curr Top Otorhinolaryngol Head Neck Surg*. 2007;6:Doc05. Epub 2008 Mar 14. PMID: 22073081; PMCID: PMC3199848.
20. Chen X, Zhang R. Microtia epigenetics: an overview of review and new viewpoint. *Medicine (Baltimore)*. 2019;98(41):e17468.
21. Gangopadhyay N, Mendonca DA, Woo AS. Pierre robin sequence. *Semin Plast Surg*. 2012;26(2):76–82.
22. Karempelis P, Hagen M, Morrell N, Roby BB. Associated syndromes in patients with Pierre Robin Sequence. *Int J Pediatr Otorhinolaryngol*. 2020;131:10984.
23. Suri S, Ross RB, Tompson BD. Craniofacial morphology and adolescent facial growth in Pierre Robin sequence. *Am J Orthod Dentofacial Orthop*. 2010;137:763–774.
24. Collins KA, Popek E. Birth injury: birth asphyxia and birth trauma. *Acad Forensic Pathol*. 2018;8(4):788–864.
25. Yu CC, Wong FH, Lo LJ, et al. Craniofacial deformity in patients with uncorrected congenital muscular torticollis: an assessment from three-dimensional computed tomography imaging. *Plast Reconstr Surg*. 2004;113:24–33.
26. Kiliaridis S, Katsaros C. The effects of myotonic dystrophy and Duchenne muscular dystrophy on the orofacial muscles and dentofacial morphology. *Acta Odontol Scand*. 1998;56:369–374.
27. Obwegeser HL. *Mandibular Growth Anomalies*. Springer-Verlag; 2000.
28. Fleseriu M, Delashaw JB Jr, Cook DM. Acromegaly: a review of current medical therapy and new drugs on the horizon. *Neurosurg Focus*. 2010;29:E15.
29. Carlson DS. Evolving concepts of heredity and genetics in orthodontics. *Am J Orthod Dentofacial Orthop*. 2015;148:922–938.
30. Stockard CR, Johnson AL. *Genetic and Endocrinic Basis for Differences in Form and Behavior*. The Wistar Institute of Anatomy and Biology; 1941.
31. Chung CS, Niswander JD, Runck DW, et al. Genetic and epidemiologic studies of oral characteristics in Hawaii's schoolchildren. II. Malocclusion. *Am J Hum Genet*. 1971;23:471–495.
32. Hughes T, Thomas C, Richards L, et al. A study of occlusal variation in the primary dentition of Australian twins and singletons. *Arch Oral Biol*. 2001;46:857–864.
33. Corruccini RS, Sharma K, Potter RH. Comparative genetic variance and heritability of dental occlusal variables in U.S. and northwest Indian twins. *Am J Phys Anthropol*. 1986;70:293–299.
34. Harris EF, Johnson MG. Heritability of craniometric and occlusal variables: a longitudinal sib analysis. *Am J Orthod Dentofacial Orthop*. 1991;99:258–268.
35. Johannsdottir B, Thorarinsson F, Thordarson A, et al. Heritability of craniofacial characteristics between parents and offspring estimated from lateral cephalograms. *Am J Orthod Dentofacial Orthop*. 2005;127:200–207.
36. Suzuki A, Takahama Y. Parental data used to predict growth of craniofacial form. *Am J Orthod Dentofacial Orthop*. 1991;99:107–121.
37. Cruz RM, Krieger H, Ferreira R, et al. Major gene and multifactorial inheritance of mandibular prognathism. *Am J Med Genet A*. 2008;146:71–77.
38. Moreno-Uribe LM, Howe SC, Kummel C, et al. Phenotypic diversity in white adults with moderate to severe Class II malocclusions. *Am J Orthod Dentofacial Orthop*. 2014;145:305–316.
39. Larsen CS. *Bioarchaeology: Interpreting Behavior From the Human Skeleton*. Cambridge University Press; 1997.
40. Corruccini RS. Anthropological aspects of orofacial and occlusal variations and anomalies. In: Kelly MA, Larsen CS, eds. *Advances in Dental Anthropology*. Wiley-Liss; 1991.
41. Ciochon RL, Nisbett RA, Corruccini RS. Dietary consistency and craniofacial development related to masticatory function in minipigs. *J Craniofac Genet Dev Biol*. 1997;17:96–102.
42. Proffit WR, Fields HW, Nixon WL. Occlusal forces in normal and long face adults. *J Dent Res*. 1983;62:566–571.
43. Proffit WR, Fields HW. Occlusal forces in normal and long face children. *J Dent Res*. 1983;62:571–574.
44. Dogrammaci EJ, Rossi-Fedele G. Establishing the association between non-nutritive sucking behavior and malocclusions. *J Am Dent Assn*. 2016;147:926–936.
45. Grammatopoulos E, White AP, Dhopatkar A. Effects of playing a wind instrument on the occlusion. *Am J Orthod Dentofacial Orthop*. 2012;141:138–145.
46. Kovero O, Kononen M, Pirinen S. The effect of professional violin and viola playing on the bony facial structures. *Eur J Orthod*. 1997;19:39–45.
47. Proffit WR. Lingual pressure patterns in the transition from tongue thrust to adult swallowing. *Arch Oral Biol*. 1972;17:555–563.
48. Vig KW. Nasal obstruction and facial growth: the strength of evidence for clinical assumptions. *Am J Orthod Dentofacial Orthop*. 1998;113:603–611.
49. Warren DW, Mayo R, Zajac DJ, et al. Dyspnea following experimentally induced increased nasal airway resistance. *Cleft Palate Craniofac J*. 1996;33:231–235.
50. Harvold EP, Tomer BS, Vargervik K, et al. Primate experiments on oral respiration. *Am J Orthod*. 1981;79:359–372.
51. Fields HW, Warren DW, Black K, Phillips C. Relationship between vertical dentofacial morphology and respiration in adolescents. *Am J Orthod Dentofacial Orthop*. 1991;99:147–154.
52. Mahony D, Karsten A, Linder-Aronson S. Effects of adenoidectomy and changed mode of breathing on incisor and molar dentoalveolar heights and anterior face heights. *Aust Orthod J*. 2004 Nov;20(2):93–98.
53. Linder-Aronson S. Adenoids: their effect on mode of breathing and nasal airflow and their relationship to characteristics of the facial skeleton and dentition. *Acta Otolaryngol Scand*. 1970;265:1–132.
54. Woodside DG, Linder-Aronson S, Lundstrom A, et al. Mandibular and maxillary growth after changed mode of breathing. *Am J Orthod Dentofacial Orthop*. 1991;100:1–18.
55. Kim KB. How has our interest in the airway changed over 100 years? *Am J Orthod Dentofacial Orthop*. 2015;148:740–747.
56. Senaratna Cv, Perret JL, Lodge CJ, et al. Prevalence of obstructive sleep apnea in the general population: a systematic review. *Sleep Medicine Reviews*. 2017;34:70–81.
57. Centers for Disease Control and Prevention. Sleep: Health benefits of sleep. https://www.cdc.gov/sleep/about_sleep/chronic_disease.html.

58. Fagundes NCF, GianoniCapenakas S, Heo G, FloresMir C. Craniofacial features in children with obstructive sleep apnea: a systematic review and metaanalysis. *J Clin Sleep Med.* 2022;18:1865–1875.
59. Liu Y, et al. The dental and craniofacial characteristics among children with obstructive sleep apnoea: a systematic review and meta-analysis. *Eur J Orthod.* 2023;45:346–355.
60. Orabi N, Flores-Mir C, Elshebiny T, Elkordy S, Palomo JM. Pharyngeal airway dimensional changes after orthodontic treatment with premolar extractions: a systematic review with meta-analysis. *Am J Orthod Dentofacial Orthop.* 2021;160(4): 503–515.
61. Larsen AJ, Rindal DB, Hatch JP, Kane S, Asche SE, Carvalho C, Rugh J. Evidence supports no relationship between obstructive sleep apnea and premolar extraction: an electronic health records review. *J Clin Sleep Med.* 2015;11(12):1443–1448.
62. Melsen B. Effects of cervical anchorage during and after treatment: an implant study. *Am J Orthod.* 1978;73(5):526–540.
63. Hänggi MP, Teuscher UM, Roos M, Peltomäki TA. Long-term changes in pharyngeal airway dimensions following activator-headgear and fixed appliance treatment. *Eur J Orthod.* 2008;30(6):598–605.
64. Kirjavainen M, Kirjavainen T. Upper airway dimensions in Class II malocclusion: effects of headgear treatment. *Angle Orthod.* 2007;77(6):1046–1053.
65. Julku J, Pirilä-Parkkinen K, Pirttiniemi P. Airway and hard tissue dimensions in children treated with early and later timed cervical headgear-a randomized controlled trial. *Eur J Orthod.* 2018;40(3):285–295.
66. Pirilä-Parkkinen K, Pirttiniemi P, Nieminen P, Löppönen H, Tolonen U, Uotila R, Huggare J. Cervical headgear therapy as a factor in obstructive sleep apnea syndrome. *Pediatr Dent.* 1999;21(1):39–45.
67. Godt A, Koos B, Hagen H, Göz G. Changes in upper airway width associated with Class II treatments (headgear vs activator) and different growth patterns. *Angle Orthod.* 2011;81(3):440–446.

SECTION 2

Diagnosis and Treatment Planning

The process of orthodontic diagnosis and treatment planning fits very well with the contemporary problem-oriented approach to health care more generally. Diagnosis in orthodontics, as in other disciplines of dentistry and medicine, requires the collection of an adequate database of information about the patient and the distillation from that database of a comprehensive but clearly stated list of the patient's problems and positive attributes. It is important to recognize that both the patient's perceptions and the doctor's observations are needed in formulating the problem list. Both pathologic and developmental problems may be present. If so, pathologic problems should be separated from the developmental ones so they can receive priority for treatment because pathologic conditions must be under control before treatment of developmental problems begins. The diagnostic process is outlined in detail in Chapter 6.

The next step is to determine the treatment goals. Where are you and the patient going? What do you want to achieve based on the problem list and the positive attributes? This is somewhat scientific and somewhat art and wisdom. The problems will have various priorities, so you need to pick carefully what you can and should address as goals. Some problems will be more difficult to solve—that is included here, too.

Then, the task of treatment planning is to synthesize the possible solutions to these specific goals (often there are several possibilities) into a specific treatment strategy that would provide maximum benefit for this particular patient. Carrying out diagnosis and treatment planning in a series of logical steps, which are outlined in an overview of the entire process in Figures 6-86 and 7-1 is recommended.

Keep in mind that diagnosis and treatment planning, although part of the same process, are different procedures with fundamentally different goals. In the development of a diagnostic database and formulation of a problem list, the goal is truth—the facts about the patient's situation and problems. At that stage there is no room for opinion or judgment. Instead, a factual appraisal of the situation is required. On the other hand, the treatment planning (setting goals and noting possible solutions) is not scientific truth, but wisdom—the plan that a wise and prudent clinician would follow to maximize benefit for the patient.

The first two steps shown in the figure constitute diagnosis:

1. Development of an adequate diagnostic database.
2. Formulation of a problem list by classifying the recognized problems by five characteristics and note the positive attributes.

Treatment planning requires judgment by the clinician as the classified problems are prioritized and treatment goals are determined. Then, alternative possible solutions are evaluated. For this reason, treatment planning inevitably is something of an art form. The first step in treatment planning is to put the problems in a priority order, based on what is important to the patient (chief complaint) and the severity and complexity of treatment. Could patients with the same problem list appropriately end up with different treatment goals? *Yes*, because treatment goals that are prioritized differently usually will produce different plans.

Once a patient's orthodontic treatment problems and goals have been identified and prioritized, four issues must be faced in determining the optimal treatment plan: (1) the timing of treatment, (2) the complexity of the treatment that would be required, (3) the predictability of success with a given treatment approach, and (4) reviewing the proposed plan with the patient's (and parents') goals and desires again. These issues are considered briefly in the next paragraphs.

Timing

Orthodontic treatment can be carried out at any time during a patient's life and can be aimed at a specific problem or can be comprehensive. Usually, treatment is comprehensive (i.e., with a goal of the best possible occlusion, facial esthetics, and stability) and is undertaken in adolescence, as the last permanent teeth are erupting. There are good reasons for this choice. At this point, for most patients there is sufficient growth remaining to potentially improve jaw relationships, and all permanent teeth, including the second molars, can be controlled and placed in a more or less final position. From a psychosocial point of view, patients in this age group often are reaching the point of self-motivation for treatment, which is evident in their improved ability to cooperate during appointments and in appliance and oral hygiene care. A reasonably short course of treatment in early adolescence, as opposed to two stages of early and later treatment, fits well within the cooperative potential of patients and families.

Even though not all patients respond well to treatment during adolescence, treatment at this time remains the gold standard against which other approaches must be measured. For a child with obvious malocclusion, does it really make sense to start treatment early in the preadolescent years? Obviously, timing will depend on the specific problems. Issues in the timing of treatment are reviewed in detail in Chapters 7, 11, 12, 13, and 14.

Treatment Complexity

The complexity of the treatment that would be required affects treatment planning, especially in the context of who should do the treatment. In orthodontics, as in all areas of dentistry, it makes sense that the less complex cases would be selected for treatment in general or family practice, whereas the more complex cases would be referred to a specialist. The only difference in orthodontics is that traditionally the family practitioner has referred a larger number of orthodontic cases. In family practice, an important issue is how you rationally select patients for treatment or referral. Chapter 11 discusses separating children most appropriate for treatment in family practice from those more likely to require complex treatment. A similar discussion for adults is included in Chapter 20.

Predictability and Success With Treatment Methods

If alternative methods of treatment are available, as usually is the case, which one should be chosen? Data gradually are accumulating to allow choices to be based on evidence of outcomes rather than the frequently unsubstantiated claims of advocates and anecdotal case reports. The use of outcomes data as a basis for deciding what the best treatment approach might be is emphasized in Chapter 7.

Patient Interaction in Planning

Finally, but most important, treatment planning must be an interactive process. No longer can the doctor decide, in a paternalistic way, what is best for a patient. Both ethically and practically, patients must be involved in the decision-making process. Ethically, patients have the right to control what happens to them in treatment—treatment is something done *for* them, not *to* them. Practically, the patient's compliance is likely to be a critical issue in success or failure, and there is little reason to select a mode of treatment that the patient would not support. Informed consent, in its modern form, requires involving the patient in the treatment planning process. This is emphasized in the procedure for presenting treatment recommendations to patients in Chapter 7.

The logical sequence for treatment planning, with these issues in mind, is as follows:

1. Prioritization of the items on the orthodontic problem list and include positive attributes to maintain.
2. List the treatment goals so that the most important goals receive the highest priority for treatment.
3. Consideration of possible solutions to each problem and goal, with each evaluated for the moment as if it were the only one the patient had.
4. Evaluation of the interactions among possible solutions to the individual problems.
5. Consideration the synergy of solutions, compromises, benefits to the patient versus risks and costs.
6. Determination of a final treatment plan, with input from the patient and parent, and selection of the specific therapeutic approach (appliance design, mechanotherapy) to be used.

This process culminates in a level of patient-parent understanding of the treatment plan that allows informed consent to treatment. In most instances, after all, orthodontic treatment is elective rather than required. Rarely is there a significant health risk from no treatment, so functional and esthetic benefits must be compared with risks and costs. Interaction with the patient is required to develop the plan in this way.

6

Orthodontic Diagnosis: The Problem-Oriented Approach

DAVID M. SARVER, HENRY W. FIELDS, BENJAMIN T. PLISKA, AND WILLIAM R. PROFFIT

CHAPTER OUTLINE

In diagnosis, whether in orthodontics or other areas of dentistry or medicine, it is important not to concentrate so closely on one aspect of the patient's overall condition that other significant problems are overlooked. In contemporary orthodontics, this is particularly true because patients' concerns and priorities are often critical determinants of treatment plans, and it can be difficult sometimes for the orthodontist not to "rush to judgment" during the initial examination. A natural bias of any specialist (and one does not have to be a dental specialist to already take a very specialized point of view) is to characterize problems in terms of his or her own special interest. This bias must be recognized and consciously resisted.

Diagnosis, in short, must be comprehensive and not focused on only a single aspect of what in many instances can be a complex situation. Orthodontic diagnosis requires a broad overview of the patient's situation and must take into consideration objective findings. It is important not to characterize the dental occlusion while overlooking a jaw discrepancy, soft tissue drape and esthetics, developmental syndrome, systemic disease, periodontal problem, psychosocial problem, or the cultural milieu in which the patient is living.

The problem-oriented approach to diagnosis and treatment planning has been widely advocated in medicine and dentistry as a way to overcome the tendency to concentrate on only one aspect of a patient's problems. The essence of the problem-oriented approach is to develop a comprehensive database of pertinent information so that no problems or positive attributes will be overlooked. This will lead to a problem list that can be prioritized. The prioritized problem list in turn helps establish the goals of treatment. To put it simply, by this exercise we establish any issues to treat and which attributes we want to want to protect. For orthodontic purposes, the database may be thought of as derived from three major sources: (1) interview data from questions (written and oral) of the patient (and parents, if appropriate); (2) clinical examination of the patient; and (3) evaluation of diagnostic records, including dental casts, radiographs, and photographs. Because all possible diagnostic records will not be obtained for all patients, one of the objectives of the clinical examination is to determine what diagnostic records are needed.

At all stages of the diagnostic evaluation, a specialist may seek more detailed information than would a generalist, and this is a major reason for referring a patient to a specialist. The specialist is likely to obtain more extensive and required diagnostic records, some of which may not be readily available to a generalist. In orthodontics, cephalometric radiographs and cone beam computed tomography (CBCT) are examples. Nevertheless, the basic approach is the same for any orthodontic patient and any practitioner. Given a specific problem and the intention to evaluate it and treat it, both the generalist and the specialist should want the same information and records. A competent generalist will follow the same sequence of steps in evaluating a patient as an orthodontist would and will use the same approach in planning treatment if they do the orthodontics. After all, from both legal and ethical perspectives, the same standard of care is required whether the treatment is rendered by a generalist or specialist. With this as background, the diagnostic process can help provide a framework for decisions on whether to refer a patient to a specialist.

Questionnaire and Interview

The goals of the interview process are to establish the patient's chief concern (major reason for seeking consultation and treatment) and to obtain further information about two major areas: (1) medical and dental history; and (2) motivation, expectations, and other social and behavioral factors. In orthodontic specialty practice, it can be quite helpful to send the patient an interview questionnaire to fill out before the first visit to the office (Fig. 6.1). This can be developed for parents and for adult patients. Note its emphasis on learning the extent to which the child, parent, or adult patient is concerned about facial and dental appearance and growth. This can help clarify the parent's or patient's important issues and those of less concern as a starting point. A medical and dental history form, which should be filled out in advance, would accompany it. The medical history form becomes an outline for follow-up questions and discussion because so many parents and patients do not list things they think are of no relevance to orthodontics.

Chief Concern

It is always important to find out why the patient is inquiring about orthodontics. This is an area that must be discovered and ultimately addressed in the treatment plan and treatment for the best success.

Patient Name: Date:

Are you interested in: (Please indicate all that apply)
[ ] Information
[ ] Treatment at this time
[ ] Clarification of previously received or conflicting information

If your child's teeth were to be changed, how would you like them changed?
[ ] Upper teeth Forward/Backward
[ ] Lower teeth Forward/Backward
[ ] Upper teeth up because gums show too much
[ ] Close spaces Upper/Lower
[ ] Straighten crowded teeth Upper/Lower
[ ] Improve the appearance of chipped/cracked/stained/dark/pointed teeth

Do you realize that growth has a strong influence on the success of orthodontic treatment?
Yes _____ No _____

Is it likely that your son or daughter will be an early maturer or late maturer?
Early _____ Late _____

How tall do you think this child will be when growth is completed? ___ ft ___ inches

Are you aware that orthodontic treatment can to some extent alter facial appearance?
Yes _____ No _____

If any features of the face could be changed, what would you like to see:
[ ] Upper lip Forward/Backward
[ ] Lower lip Forward/Backward
[ ] Upper jaw Forward/Backward
[ ] Lower jaw Forward/Backward
[ ] Chin Larger/Smaller
[ ] Nose Larger/Smaller/Different Shape

Would you prefer that facial appearance NOT be discussed in front of your child?
Yes _____ No _____

Is there any significant family history of jaw or teeth problems?

Are you interested in improving the appearance of the teeth at this time even if more treatment will be needed later? Yes _____ No _____

Signature Relationship to Patient

• **Fig. 6.1** Finding out what patients and parents really want can be difficult and is often not revealed by the chief complaint on a past medical history. This type of a supplemental form that really attempts to quantify their desires can help direct the initial interview when filled out in advance. An adult form can be developed, too. (Courtesy Dr. Alan Bloore.)

As we have discussed in some detail in Chapter 1, there are three major reasons for patient concern about the alignment and occlusion of the teeth: impaired dentofacial appearance and a diminished sense of social well-being, impaired function, and impaired oral health. Although more than one of these reasons may often contribute to seeking orthodontic treatment, it is important to establish their relative importance to the patient. The dentist should not assume that appearance is the patient's major concern just because the teeth appear nonesthetic. Nor should the dentist focus on the functional implications of, for instance, a crossbite with a lateral shift without appreciating the patient's concern about what seems to be a trivial space between the maxillary central incisors. For an individual with reasonably normal function and appearance and reasonable psychosocial adaptation, the major reason for seeking treatment may well be a desire to enhance their appearance, thus potentially improving quality of life (QOL). The greater orientation of modern general practice toward cosmetic dentistry increases the chance that a patient may be referred to an orthodontist for comprehensive treatment simply to enhance dental and facial appearance.

When patients inquire about whether they need orthodontic treatment, a series of leading questions should be asked, beginning with, "Do you think you need orthodontic treatment?" If the answer is yes, one might next inquire "What bothers you more about your teeth, your bite or your appearance?" and "What do you want treatment to do for you?" The answer to that and follow-up questions will clarify what is most important to the patient. The dentist or orthodontist may or may not agree with the patient's assessment—that judgment comes later. At this stage, the objective is to find out what is important to the patient.

Medical and Dental History

Orthodontic problems are almost always the culmination of a developmental process, not the result of a pathologic condition. As the discussion in Chapter 5 illustrates, often it is difficult to be certain of the etiology, but it is important to establish the cause of malocclusion if this can be done and at least rule out some of the possible causes—trauma, habits, periodontal disease, growth disturbance, and so on. A careful medical and dental history is needed for orthodontic patients, both to provide a proper background for understanding the patient's overall situation and to evaluate specific concerns. A caution is that many pediatric health histories are not valid as reported by parents or guardians, so careful questioning and clarification is important.[1]

The outline of an appropriate medical and dental history is presented in Fig. 6.2. Many of the items are annotated to explain their implications for an orthodontic patient. Five areas deserve a special comment. First, although most children with a condylar fracture of the mandible recover uneventfully, remember that a

• **Fig. 6.2** (A) A comprehensive form for obtaining the medical and dental history for young orthodontic patients. A separate but similar form is needed for adult patients. Parents need to be told that it is important to report medical conditions and medications because many can affect orthodontic treatment. Updating these forms at least annually is also important as a follow-up. The considerations below explain the basis of some of the questions posed in this medical history form.

Has your child been hospitalized, received general anesthesia, or had emergency department visits: This helps establish a history of serious health problems, anesthetic complications and trauma.

Are your child's immunizations up to date: In the instance of oral-facial trauma, the DPT status is critical. Soft tissue injury is increased with appliances in place; Immunization status also provides an opportunity to discuss HPV vaccination for children 11–12, but possibly starting at age 9. The impact is on prevention of cervical cancer and oropharyngeal cancer. Alerting parents and referring them to their primary care provider or pediatrician is an important step.

Does your child have allergies: This helps identify allergies to all types of allergens. One must also consider latex used in dental treatment gloves and elastics and Nickel found in orthodontic appliances. These sensitivities appear to be increasing in the population.

Heart issues: Some patients need antibiotic coverage during banding and debanding procedures.

Blood/infectious disease: With modern infection control procedures, these patients can be treated normally, but the treatment may need to be modified.

Cancer: This will help determine whether treatments using radiation, chemotherapy, and glucocorticoids altered dental development, jaw growth, somatic growth, or bone density, depending on the site of the lesion and the treatment type and timing. Bisphosphonates are used to treat the effects of some cancer and bone treatments that slow bone resorption while at the same time inhibiting tooth movement, so that orthodontic treatment is limited.

Tonsil/adenoid/sinus problems: This can help with evaluation of respiratory problems, sleep apnea and tooth sensitivity.

Snoring or interupted breathing: This can be indicative of sleep apnea. At the least, a Pediatric Sleep Questionnaire (discussed in this chapter) should be used to screen these patients.

Radiation: Radiation therapy to the jaws can greatly alter local dental and skeletal development. The risk of osteoradionecrosis is also elevated in these patients depending on the radiation dosage and the type of treatment under consideration.

Growth problems: Some children with growth problems may be treated with growth hormones, which can have implications for growth modification treatment timing. In some cancer patients, growth hormones can be part of the postradiation treatment regimen. This, too, can affect treatment timing.

Attention-deficit disorders: These patients can be treated with numerous drugs. The effect on growth of some of these medications is unclear. Behavior management may need to be reconsidered due to issues with focus and the ability to act independently. Some hyperactive behavior may be confused with sleep apnea signs.

Autism: The extent of these spectrum disorders can vary greatly and the behavior of the child can range from great focus to sensory overload. Exploring the types of approaches each child finds helpful can greatly enhance the treatment experience and success.

Bone or joint/arthritis: This may relate to mandibular growth and development and the types of medications that can control the disease, such as glucocorticoids that can cause bone density problems as a related issue.

Rapid growth and parents/siblings growth: This helps establish growth status and timing.

MEDICAL HISTORY
(Child/Adolescent)

PATIENT NAME: ______________________________ DATE: ________________

BIRTH DATE: __________

Name of your child's physician: __________________ Office Phone: ____________

Address of your child's physician: ________________ Date of last exam: __________

1. Is your child in good health? .... Yes No Don't know
2. Does your child have a health problem? .... Yes No Don't know
   If yes, explain: ____________________
3. Has your child ever been hospitalized, had general anesthesia, or emergency room visits? .... Yes No Don't know
   If yes, explain: ____________________
4. Are your child's immunizations up to date? .... Yes No Don't know
5. Does your child have allergies to medications (drugs), medical products (latex), or the environment (dust, mites, pollen, mold)? .... Yes No Don't know
   If yes, please list: ____________________
6. List past medications taken by child: ____________________
7. List daily medications child is now taking: ____________________
8. Has your child ever had or been treated by a physician for:

Check one for each condition

Yes	No	?		Yes	No	?	
			a. Problems at birth				p. Cancer
			b. Heart murmur				q. Cerebral palsy
			c. Heart disease				r. Seizures
			d. Rheumatic fever				s. Asthma
			e. Anemia				t. Cleft lip/palate
			f. Sickle cell anemia				u. Speech or hearing problems
			g. Bleeding/hemophilia				v. Eye problems/contact lenses
			h. Blood transfusion				w. Skin problems/snoring
			i. Hepatitis				x. Tonsil/adenoid/sinus problems
			j. AIDS or HIV+				y. Sleep problems
			k. Tuberculosis				z. Emotional/behavior problems
			l. Liver disease				aa. Radiation therapy
			m. Kidney disease				bb. Growth problems
			n. Diabetes				cc. Attention deficit disorders
			o. Arthritis				dd. Osteoporosis (bisphosphonates)

9. Has your child had any recent rapid growth? ________ If so, how much? ____________
10. Parents: (Father) Ht: _____ Wt: _____ (Mother) Ht: _____ Wt: _____
11. Older brothers and sisters: (1) Ht: ____ Wt: ____ (2) Ht: ____ Wt: ____ (3) Ht: _____ Wt: _____
12. Females: Has menstruation begun? _______ If yes, when? ___________ Pregnant? _______
    Using birth control pills? __________
13. If yes to any above, please explain this or any other problem: ____________________
14. Child's grade in school: ___________ Child's school: ________________
15. Do you consider your child to be (check one): Advanced in learning ___ Progressing normally ___
    Slow learner ___

A

• **Fig. 6.2, cont'd**

DENTAL HISTORY

16. What is your main concern about your child's dental condition? ____________________
17. Has your child been to a dentist before? No Yes If yes, date of last visit: ____________________
18. Regular dentist's name: ____________________
19. Check one for each condition:

Yes	No	?	
			a. Has your child ever had dental x-rays? Date of last x-rays? ____________
			b. Will your child be uncooperative? If yes, explain: ____________
			c. Has your child experienced any complications following dental treatment? If yes, explain: ____________
			d. Has your child had cavities and / or toothaches?
			e. Are your child's teeth sensitive to temperature or food?
			f. Did you or your child ever get instructions in brushing?
			g. Do your child's gums bleed when brushed?
			h. Does your child use fluoride products: rinses, drops, tabs?
			i. Does or has your child had any clicking or pain in the jaw joint?
			j. Does or has your child had any problems opening or closing their mouth?
			k. Has your child inherited any family facial or dental characteristics? If yes, explain: ____________
			l. Has your child ever injured his/her teeth?
			m. Has your child ever injured his/her jaws or face?
			n. Does or did your child use a pacifier?
			o. Does or did your child suck his/her fingers or thumb?

20. Does your child have any other dental problems we should know about? ______ Please explain: ____________________
21. Whom may we thank for referring you to our office? ____________________
22. PERSON COMPLETING THIS FORM: Signature ____________________
Relationship to patient: ____________________

B

• **Fig. 6.2, cont'd** (B) Considerations in understanding the Dental History form:

Main concern: The chief complaint is critical to determine why the patient is seeking care. This must be considered carefully in the planning of the treatment.

X-rays: Reduction in unnecessary radiation is critical to the highest quality care. Many practitioners will request films as part of the examination procedures. Patients seeking second opinions often have already had some records obtained.

Cavities or toothaches: Orthodontic appliances make teeth difficult to clean. This can lead to white spot lesions and cavities as well as soft tissue inflammation and destruction. With poor hygiene the hard tissue can change in weeks. Improving hygiene and using adjuncts to prevent enamel changes may be necessary. Delaying treatment or interruptions in treatment may be indicated.

Bleeding gums: Orthodontic treatment in the face of periodontal disease, either acute or chronic, is contraindicated until the disease stage is either controlled or reversed.

Opening/closing mouth: A previous history of temporomandibular joint (TMJ) problems or treatment merits pretreatment investigation. Limitations or problems with opening, closing, or translation can indicate TMJ problems.

Family facial and dental characteristics: Familial tendency is observed in some skeletal patterns, and missing teeth have a documented genetic component.

Injury to teeth? Dental trauma may have implications during tooth movement because of the increased possibility of pulpal necrosis and root resorption. This also may indicate trauma prevention is indicated. Recommendations are always appropriate for mouth guard protection.

Pacifier/thumb or finger sucking: Habits may explain some aspects of the malocclusion.

Person completeing form: This helps establish the authenticity of the historian.

growth deficit related to an old injury is the most probable cause of true facial asymmetry (Fig. 6.3). It has become apparent in recent years that early fractures of the condyle occur more frequently than was previously thought (see Chapter 5). A mandibular fracture in a child can easily be overlooked in the aftermath of an accident that caused other injuries, so a jaw injury may not have been diagnosed at the time. Although old jaw fractures have particular significance, trauma to the teeth may also affect the development of the occlusion and treatment. Knowing when a traumatic dental injury occurred and the type of injury can help guide your treatment recommendations and should not be overlooked.

Second, it is important to note whether the patient is on long-term medication of any type and, if so, for what purpose. This may reveal systemic disease or metabolic problems that the patient

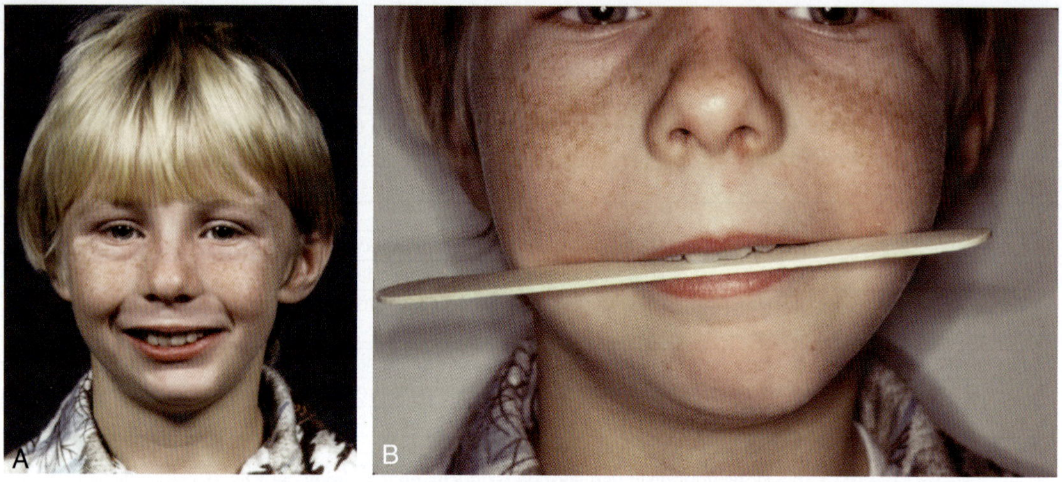

• **Fig. 6.3** (A) Facial asymmetry developed in this boy after fracture of the left mandibular condylar process at age 5 because scarring in the fracture area prevented normal translation of the mandible on that side during growth. See Chapter 2. (B) Note the cant to the occlusal plane and the resulting roll deformity illustrated in more detail in Figs. 6.88, 6.90 and 6.92. This develops as failure of the mandible to grow vertically on the affected side restricts eruption of both maxillary and mandibular teeth. Trauma is the most frequent cause of asymmetry of this type.

did not report in any other way. Chronic medical problems in adults or children do not contraindicate orthodontic treatment if the medical problem is under control, but special precautions may be necessary if orthodontic treatment is to be carried out. For example, orthodontic treatment would be possible in a patient with controlled diabetes, but would require especially careful monitoring because the periodontal breakdown that could accompany loss of control might be accentuated by orthodontic forces (see Chapter 8). It is in the best interest of the orthodontist to engage the patient's primary care provider, who is managing these patients, in treatment planning to ensure no contraindications are overlooked.

Third, many children and adults now survive serious illness and seek orthodontic treatment afterward. Cancer chemotherapy and radiation therapy aimed at head and neck tissues can result in morphologic impacts such as short roots or missing teeth (see Fig. 12.7). In adults being treated for arthritis or osteoporosis, and now increasingly also in children with acute and chronic disease are treated with drugs (such as glucocorticoids) that can be toxic to bone. High doses of resorption-inhibiting agents such as bisphosphonates often are used to counteract the side effects. This impedes orthodontic tooth movement and may increase the chance of complications (see Chapter 8). It is necessary to ask specifically about these medications because parents or patients sometimes do not mention things they think are not related to orthodontic treatment.

Fourth, children, adolescents and adults should be screened for sleep disordered breathing issues. Screening will reduce undiagnosed and untreated patients. The consequences of untreated OSA are significant and can dramatically impact quality of life, neurocognitive development and cardiovascular health. Obstructive sleep apnea has a prevalence rate of up to 5% in the general pediatric population and estimated to be present in 9%–38% of adults.[2] These patients can be expected in a typical general or orthodontic practice.

The peak prevalence of OSA in children occurs around the ages of 4–7, when the increased adenotonsillar growth reaches its maximum size in relation to the surrounding upper airway anatomy. Common symptoms reported by parents include snoring, restless sleep or daytime hyperactivity. Other symptoms during sleep can include gasping, sweaty sleep, frequent awakenings, extended neck positions and bedwetting. Daytime symptoms of negative behaviors of aggression, impulsivity and hyperactivity can be seen. Impaired learning and poor school performance are also noted.

Screening for OSA in children should be based on symptomology and not any particular dentofacial morphology (see Chapter 5). As stated previously, the relationship between OSA and dentofacial morphology has been generally overestimated by the dental profession. Most children with OSA will appear relatively normal in terms of their orthodontic characteristics. In terms of risk factors, the most obvious morphologic characteristics of OSA in children are obesity, hypertrophic tonsils, and adenoids.

Due to its implications for health, screening for OSA should be performed for all patients and this can be most easily done by adding specific questions to the medical history form asking for a history of snoring and witnessed apneas or gasping during sleep. Any positive answers should be followed up with further questions related to the common signs and symptoms of OSA

The most reliable questionnaire for screening for OSA in children is the Pediatric Sleep Questionnaire (PSQ) (Fig. 6.4). The PSQ consists of 22 "yes/no/I don't know" questions relating to daytime and sleep behavior and quality of life that are completed by the parent or care-giver. If greater than one-third of the questions are answered, "yes," then this is suggestive of high risk for a pediatric sleep-related breathing disorder.[3] When applied to an orthodontic-seeking population, based on responses to the PSQ roughly 7% of children will be deemed to be of high risk of having OSA.[4]

Pediatric Sleep Questionnaire

	While sleeping, does your child...	Yes	No	DK
A1	... snore more than half the time?			
A2	... always snore?			
A3	... snore loudly?			
A4	... have 'heavy' or loud breathing?			
A5	... have trouble breathing. or struggle to breathe?			
	Have you ever?	**Yes**	**No**	**DK**
A6	... seen your child stop breathing during the night?			
	Does you child?	**Yes**	**No**	**DK**
A7	... tend to breathe through the mouth during the day?			
A8	... have a dry mouth on waking up in the mornig?			
A9	... occasionally wet the bed?			
	Does you child?	**Yes**	**No**	**DK**
A10	... wake up feeling unrefreshed in the morning?			
A11	... have a problem with sleepiness during the day?			
A12	... Has a teached or other supervisor commented that your child appears sleepy during the day			
A13	... Is it hard to wake your child up in the morning?			
A14	... Does your child wake up with headaches in the morning?			
A15	... Did your child stop growing at a normal rate at any time since birth?			
A16	... Is your child overweight?			
	This child often...	**Yes**	**No**	**DK**
A17	... does not seem to listen when spoken to directly			
A18	... has difficulty organizing tasks and activities			
A19	... is easily distracted by extraneous stimuli			
A20	... fidgets with hands or feet or squirms in seat			
A21	... is on the 'go' or often acts as of 'driven by a motor'			
A22	... interrupts or intrudes on others (e.g. butts into converstions or games)			

The caregiver answers Yes; No; DK= Don't Know
Yes =1; No =0; DK not counted
Scores are averaged.
>0.33 is consistent with OSA
Sensitivity = 0.85 Specificity = 0.87

Chervin, RD et al., Pediatric Sleep Questionnaire (PSQ), Sleep Medicine 2000; 21-32

• **Fig. 6.4** The Pediatric Sleep Questionnaire (*PSQ*) is an excellent way to screen children and adolescents for the risk of sleep apnea. The 22 questions are answered Yes, No or Don't Know (*DK*). Scoring and interpretation are noted on the form. The diagnostic reliability of this questionnaire is very good.

In adults, snoring and daytime sleepiness are the most commonly reported symptoms. The STOP-Bang questionnaire (Fig. 6.5), consisting of four subjective yes/no questions (STOP: **S**noring, **T**iredness, **O**bserved apnea, and high blood **P**ressure) and four demographics items (Bang: **B**MI, **a**ge, **n**eck circumference, **g**ender), has demonstrated high sensitivity and specificity to detect adult patients with severe OSA.[5]

Patients suspected of OSA based on their medical history or results of an administered questionnaire should be referred to their family physician, otolaryngologist, or sleep medicine specialist for definitive diagnosis and management. The gold standard for diagnosis of OSA is a polysomnogram, an overnight study that monitors physiologic information including electroencephalography, pulse oximetry, oronasal airflow, abdominal and chest wall movements, and carbon dioxide partial pressure during sleep.

One common metric from a sleep study is the Apnea-Hypopnea Index (AHI) that is used to describe disease severity by the combined number of apnea (complete obstruction of air movement) and hypopnea (partial obstruction) events per hour. In children <1 event per hour is normal. In adults, less than 5 events per hour is normal (an AHI of 5–15 is mild OSA, 15–30 is moderate, and >30 is severe). The lowest blood oxygen saturation level reached and percentage of sleep time with oxygen saturation below defined thresholds are important adjunctive measures of OSA severity.

Finally, there are a number of questions and examination findings that can reveal oral hygiene issues that make the patient susceptible to white spot lesions. These lesions can proceed rapidly in the presence of poor hygiene and appliances. White spot lesions in orthodontic patients have an incidence of nearly 46% and a prevalence in orthodontic patients of 68%. The lesions are the result a demineralized surface and a subsurface lesion, which, if untreated will lead to caries. The white and opaque lesions appear at the margins of the appliances and the gingival margins during

STOP-Bang questionnaire

Please answer the following question by checking "yes" or "no" for each one.

	Yes	No
Snoring (Do you snore loudly?)	☐	☐
Tiredness (Do you often feel tired, fatigued, or sleepy during the daytime?)	☐	☐
Observed Apnea (Has anyone observed that you stop breathing, or choke or gasp during sleep?)	☐	☐
High Blood **P**ressure (Do you or are you being treated for high blood pressure?)	☐	☐
BMI (Is your body mass index more than 35 kg per m²?)	☐	☐
Age (Are you older than 50 years?)	☐	☐
Neck Circumference (Is your neck circumference greater than 40 cm [15.75 inches]?)	☐	☐
Gender (Are you male?)	☐	☐

Score 1 point for each positive response.

Scoring interpretation: 0 to 2 = low risk, 3 or 4= intermediate risk, ≥5 = high risk.

• **Fig. 6.5** The STOP-Bang questionnaire is an excellent way to screen adults for the risk of sleep apnea based on clinical features of sleep apnea. Scoring and interpretation of results are noted on the form. The sensitivity (the test's ability to positively identify patients with the disease) was 90%, 94%, and 96% to detect any OSA (AHI ≥5), moderate-to-severe OSA (AHI ≥15), and severe OSA (AHI ≥30), respectively. The corresponding Negative Predictive Validity (NPV the percentage of times a negative test indicates the true absence of disease) was 46%, 75%, and 90%.[5] (University Health Network, Toronto, Ontario, Canada (www.stopbang.ca/osa/screening/php). Used with permission from Sauk Prairie Healthcare.)

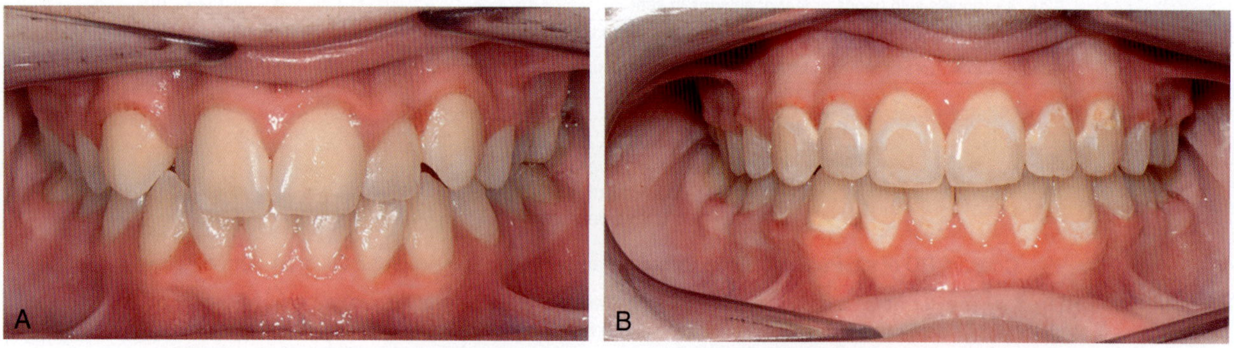

• **Fig. 6.6** White spot lesions. (A) There are no enamel decalcifications (white spot lesions) noted pretreatment, but the plaque accumulations and gingival inflammation are significant findings that oral hygiene will need to improve or the patient will be at increased risk of post treatment lesions. (B) The presence of post treatment white spot lesions along the margins of the previous appliances and the gingival margins. (Courtesy Dr. Samantha Marks.)

treatment (Fig. 6.6), especially the maxillary anterior teeth. Most agree the lesions are more prevalent and severe in males, more frequent in adolescents than adults and accompany longer treatment. If patients are compliant, fluoride toothpaste and mouth rinses can reduce the incidence of lesions. There is some evidence that a spontaneous reduction in the severity of the lesions occurs during the year following appliance removal due to either abrasion of the effected enamel and/or remineralization.[6] Treatments that appear to be the most highly rated include self-assembling (SAP) P_{11}-4 in combination with fluoride varnish (FV) and resin infiltration (RI).[7] The SAP +FV is applied to isolated and clean dry enamel. The RI method involves isolated, cleaned, etched enamel, which is air and chemically dried. The lesion is then infiltrated with a low viscosity resin and light cured.

Social and Behavioral Evaluation

The dynamics of social and behavioral development are discussed in Chapter 2. Some medical or psychological conditions can preclude successful orthodontic treatment due to the underlying problems of the ability to understand treatment, control attention and motor activity or avoid undue focus on and stimulation of the appliances (also discussed in Chapter 2).

Clinical social and behavioral evaluation should explore several related areas beyond these larger underlying problems: the patient's motivation for treatment, what he or she expects as a result of treatment, and how cooperative the patient is likely to be. Information from the preliminary form that the parent filled out in advance of the initial appointment (see Fig. 6.1) can be somewhat helpful in evaluating this.

Motivation for seeking treatment can be classified as external or internal. External motivation is supplied by pressure from another individual or external pressure, as with a reluctant child who is being brought for orthodontic treatment by a determined parent, or with an adult who is seeking alignment of incisor teeth because their new significant other wants the teeth to look better. Internal motivation, on the other hand, comes from within the individual and is based on their own assessment of the situation and desire for treatment. Even quite young children can encounter difficulties in their interaction with others because of their dental and facial appearance. Other children with apparently similar malocclusions do not perceive a problem. Older patients usually are aware of functional problems related to their malocclusion and so are likely to have some component of internal motivation.

Although now some preadolescent children express a desire to have "braces" because many of their peers are having early treatment, it is rare to find strong motivation in that age group. To them, orthodontics is usually something they have to do because a parent requires it. Self-motivation for treatment often does not develop until adolescence. Nevertheless, even in preadolescents, it is important for a patient to have a component of internal motivation. Cooperation is likely to be much better if the patient genuinely wants treatment for himself or herself, rather than just putting up with it to please a parent. Children or adults who feel that the treatment is being done *for* them will be much more receptive patients than those who view the treatment as something being done *to* them.

What the patient expects from treatment is very much related to the type of motivation and should be explored carefully with adults, especially those with primarily cosmetic problems. It is one thing to undertake to correct spacing between the maxillary incisors to improve a patient's appearance and dental function, and something else to do this because the patient has unrealistic expectations of improved esthetics or that they will experience greater social or professional success. If esthetics are the issue and considerable changes can be made with substantial esthetic improvements, there is a reasonable chance for success. If the patient is focused on small esthetic issues that are beyond what laypersons perceive at usual social or professional interaction distances (usually approximately 2 ft), problems can likely arise. Although correcting those problems may be relatively easy, maintaining the correction and satisfaction may be difficult if social or professional problems continue after treatment, as is possible. Then orthodontic treatment may become a focus for resentment.

Cooperation is more likely to be a problem with a child than an adult. Two factors are important in determining this: (1) the extent to which the child sees the treatment as a benefit, as opposed to something else he or she is required to undergo; and (2) the degree of parental control or parenting style. The best cooperation with treatment will most probably be achieved with authoritative (not authoritarian) parents who will be demanding but responsive to their children. Resentful and rebellious adolescents, or those who do as they wish with little parental concern or involvement, are especially likely to become a problem in treatment. It is important to take the time to understand what the patient perceives his or her problems to be and, if necessary, to help the patient appreciate the reality of the situation (see the final section of Chapter 2). They also must understand their role in helping fix the problem and things associated with the treatment process such as food choices and oral hygiene. If a patient is cooperative and avoids appliance breakage and has good oral hygiene, the teeth can be straightened with appliances. But, unless the patient is willing to wear extraoral (headgear or face mask) or intraoral (elastics) adjuncts to treatment, the teeth will not fit together. Having either crooked teeth or teeth that do not fit properly can be considered a treatment failure and should be clearly explained prior to treatment.

Any patient who is under the legal age (which varies among states and countries but most often is 18) cannot legally consent to treatment. The bioethical standard is that he or she should at least assent to treatment. With child or adolescent patients of any age, ask "If your parents and I think that you would benefit from orthodontic treatment, are you willing to help with that?" Treating an unwilling child, even if the parents force an apparent assent, is rarely good judgment.

Clinical Evaluation

There are two goals of the orthodontic clinical examination to (1) evaluate and document statural and facial growth, oral health, dental relationships, jaw function, facial proportions, jaw relationships, and smile characteristics and (2) decide which diagnostic records are required.

Statural and Sexual Maturation Evaluation

The patient's physical growth status should be determined. This is important for several reasons, not the least of which is the gradient of facial growth discussed in Chapters 2 through 4. Rapid growth during the adolescent growth spurt can facilitate orthodontic treatment, but any attempt at growth modification will surely fail in a child who is beyond the peak of the adolescent growth spurt.

Generally speaking, facial growth occurs when statural growth occurs, but not precisely. For normal youths who are approaching puberty, several questions usually provide the necessary information about where the child is on the growth curve: How rapidly has the child grown recently? Have clothes sizes changed recently?

If a child is being followed for referral to an orthodontist at the optimum time or by an orthodontist for observation of growth before beginning treatment, height changes can provide insight into the patient's overall growth status and mandibular growth status, given that statural growth and mandibular growth are generally related (see Fig. 2.4 for current height and weight growth charts). In many instances, height-weight records and the child's progress on growth charts can be obtained from the pediatrician.

If an orthodontist is obtaining height records for patients, they should use a reliable method of measurement. The stadiometer, a wall-mounted ruler with a sliding horizontal height-measuring arm that rests against the top of the child's head, should be used. This method is preferred because it provides stable and accurate measures when the patient is reliably and appropriately positioned. The child's head, shoulders, back, and hips should be at or near the wall. This includes measuring the child without footwear of any type and with the hairstyle mass reduced to a minimum so the horizontal arm touches the top of the head. Done without attention to these details, more than 50% of measures are inaccurate.

It appears that radiographic estimates of mandibular growth, based on hand wrist and cervical vertebrae methods (reviewed later in this chapter and Chapter 3), provide little additional benefit to growth estimates beyond statural measures and chronologic age and are less invasive and radiologically burdensome.[8]

The attainment of recognizable secondary sexual characteristics for girls and boys and the correlation between stages of sexual maturation and facial growth are discussed in Chapter 4 (see Fig. 4.3) and are summarized in Table 6.1.

TABLE 6.1 Adolescent Growth Stages and Related Secondary Sexual Characteristics (After Tanner)

Girls Total Duration of Adolescent Growth: 3½ Years	
Stage 1	
Prepuberty	No visible changes
Stage 2 (About 12 Months Later)	
Beginning of physical growth in height	Appearance of breast buds, initial pubic hair
Stage 3	
Peak velocity in height	Continued and noticeable breast development, underarm hair, pubic hair spread
Stage 4	
Growth spurt slowing	Onset of menstruation (menarche) breasts fullness continues, thicker pubic hair restricted to triangle
Stage 5	
Reach adult height	Pubic hair extends to thighs
Boys Total Duration of Adolescent Growth: 5 Years	
Stage 1	
Prepuberty	No visible changes
Stage 2	
Beginning of adolescent growth, awkward physically	"Fat spurt" weight gain, testes, and scrotum begin to increase in size and there is pubic hair at the base of the penis
Stage 3	
Height spurt beginning	Redistribution and reduction in fat, pubic hair spread, growth of penis. Wet dreams and voice changes begin
Stage 4	
Peak velocity in height	Facial hair appears on upper lip only, underarm hair appears, muscular growth continues. Scrotum and penis near adult size. Public hair not spread to thighs and a permanent deeper voice
Stage 5	
Growth spurt ending	Facial hair on chin and lip, adult distribution and color of pubic and axillary hair, adult body form

Serial cephalometric radiographs offer the most accurate way to determine whether facial growth has stopped or is continuing, because you are not inferring future facial growth changes, but measuring them.

Oral Health

The health of oral hard and soft tissues must be assessed for potential orthodontic patients as for any other. The general guideline is that before orthodontic treatment begins, any disease or pathologic condition must be under control. This includes medical problems, dental caries or pulpal pathology, and periodontal disease.

It sounds trivial to say that the dentist should not overlook the number of teeth that are present or forming, yet almost every dentist, concentrating on details rather than the big picture, has done just that on some occasions. It is particularly easy to fail to notice a missing or supernumerary lower incisor. At some point in the evaluation, count the teeth either clinically or radiographically to be sure they are all there.

The patient's dental health status should be documented with recording of active caries, decalcification, and incipient lesions. The patient's oral hygiene status should be recorded and documented by clinical photographs (Fig. 6.7). Having appliance therapy will make tooth cleaning more difficult and can lead to destruction of various amounts of the hard (white spot lesions on the teeth) and soft tissues, and for a potential patient with inadequate oral hygiene, pretreatment improvement of oral hygiene should be required.

A systematic way to address caries risk is to use a caries risk assessment form, like the one shown in Fig. 6.8 and endorsed by the American Dental Association. Note, as indicated above, simply having appliances is a moderate risk of caries.

In the periodontal evaluation, there are two major points of interest: indications of active periodontal disease, and potential or actual mucogingival problems. Any orthodontic examination should include gentle probing through the gingival sulci, not so much to establish pocket depths as to detect any areas of bleeding. Bleeding on probing indicates inflammation that may extend into the periodontal ligament, and this must be brought under control before orthodontic treatment is undertaken. Periodontal probing is also useful in detecting stages of altered passive and active eruption.

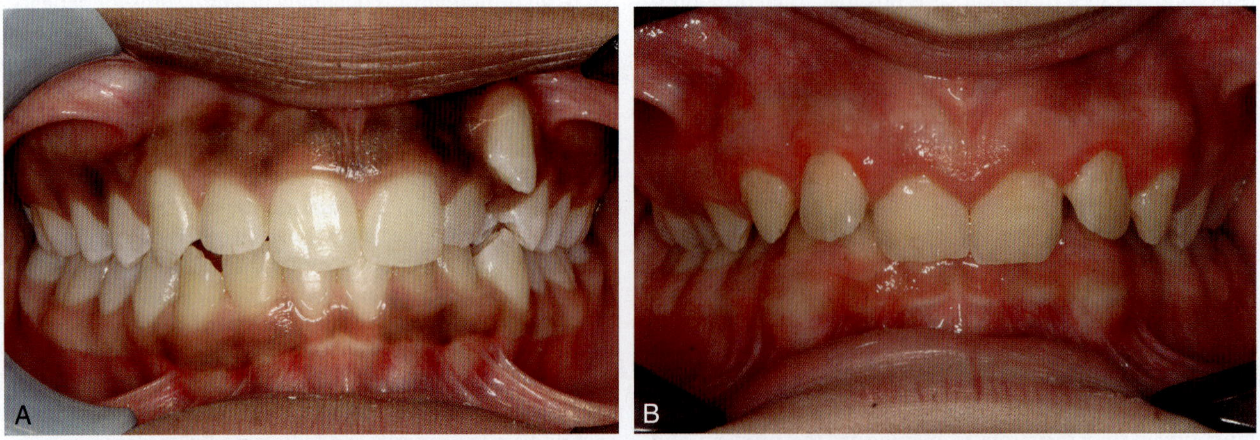

• **Fig. 6.7** Two examples of variations in pretreatment oral hygiene. (A) In spite of considerable localized irregularity, this patient has good oral hygiene with excellent tissue color, crisp gingival margins, and little inflammation. (B) This patient has poor oral hygiene with plaque accumulations, rolled gingival margins, and inflamed marginal tissues. This type of patient should demonstrate improved home care before appliance placement, given the speed with which white spot lesions and soft tissue breakdown can develop.

Caries Risk Assessment Form (Age >6)

Patient Name:				
Birth Date:		Date:		
Age:		Initials:		
		Low Risk	**Moderate Risk**	**High Risk**
	Contributing Conditions	**Check or Circle the conditions that apply**		
I.	Fluoride Exposure **(through drinking water, supplements, professional applications, toothpaste)**	☐ Yes	☐ No	
II.	Sugary Foods or Drinks **(including juice, carbonated or non-carbonated soft drinks, energy drinks, medicinal syrups)**	Primarily at mealtimes ☐		Frequent or prolonged between meal exposures/day ☐
III.	Caries Experience of Mother, Caregiver and/or other Siblings **(for patients ages 6-14)**	No carious lesions in last 24 months ☐	Carious lesions in last 7-23 months ☐	Carious lesions in last 6 months ☐
IV.	Dental Home **: established patient of record, receiving regular dental care in a dental office**	☐ Yes	☐ No	
	General Health Conditions	**Check or Circle the conditions that apply**		
I.	Special Health Care Needs **(developmental, physical, medical or mental disabilities that prevent or limit performance of adequate oral health care by themselves or caregivers)**	☐ No	Yes (over age 14) ☐	Yes (ages 6-14) ☐
II.	Chemo/Radiation Therapy	☐ No		☐ Yes
III.	Eating Disorders	☐ No	☐ Yes	
IV.	Medications that Reduce Salivary Flow	☐ No	☐ Yes	
V.	Drug/Alcohol Abuse	☐ No	☐ Yes	
	Clinical Conditions	**Check or Circle the conditions that apply**		
I.	Cavitated or Non-Cavitated **(incipient)** Carious Lesions or Restorations **(visually or radiographically evident)**	No new carious lesions or restorations in last 36 months ☐	1 or 2 new carious lesions or restorations in last 36 months ☐	3 or more carious lesions or restorations in last 36 months ☐
II.	Teeth Missing Due to Caries in past 36 months	☐ No		☐ Yes
III.	Visible Plaque	☐ No	☐ Yes	
IV.	Unusual Tooth Morphology **that compromises oral hygiene**	☐ No	☐ Yes	
V.	Interproximal Restorations - 1 or more	☐ No	☐ Yes	
VI.	Exposed Root Surfaces **Present**	☐ No	☐ Yes	
VII.	Restorations with Overhangs **and/or** Open Margins; Open Contacts **with Food Impaction**	☐ No	☐ Yes	
VIII.	Dental/Orthodontic Appliances **(fixed or removable)**	☐ No	☐ Yes	
IX.	Severe Dry Mouth (Xerostomia)	☐ No		☐ Yes
	Overall assessment of dental caries risk:	☐ Low	☐ Moderate	☐ High

Patient Instructions:

ADA American Dental Association®
America's leading advocate for oral health

Caries Risk Assessment Form (Age >6)

Circle or check the boxes of the conditions that apply. Low Risk = only conditions in "Low Risk" column present; Moderate Risk = only conditions in "Low" and/or "Moderate Risk" columns present; High Risk = one or more conditions in the "High Risk" column present.

The clinical judgment of the dentist may justify a change of the patient's risk level (increased or decreased) based on review of this form and other pertinent information. For example, missing teeth may not be regarded as high risk for a follow up patient; or other risk factors not listed may be present.

The assessment cannot address every aspect of a patient's health, and should not be used as a replacement for the dentist's inquiry and judgment. Additional or more focused assessment may be appropriate for patients with specific health concerns. As with other forms, this assessment may be only a starting point for evaluating the patient's health status.

This is a tool provided for the use of ADA members. It is based on the opinion of experts who utilized the most up-to-date scientific information available. The ADA plans to periodically update this tool based on: 1) member feedback regarding its usefulness, and; 2) advances in science. ADA member-users are encouraged to share their opinions regarding this tool with the Council on Dental Practice.

• **Fig. 6.8** The Caries Risk Assessment form developed by the ADA can be used as a starting point for evaluation of patient risk. A patient is **Low risk** if all checks are in the Low risk column; **Moderate risk** if checks are in the Low or Moderate category; and **High risk** if one or more checks are in the high risk column. This method should supplement the clinician's clinical judgment. Note that simply placing orthodontic appliances is Moderate risk. (From https://www.ada.org/-/media/project/ada-organization/ada/ada-org/files/resources/public-programs/give-kids-a-smile/gkas_caries_risk_assessment_forms.pdf.)

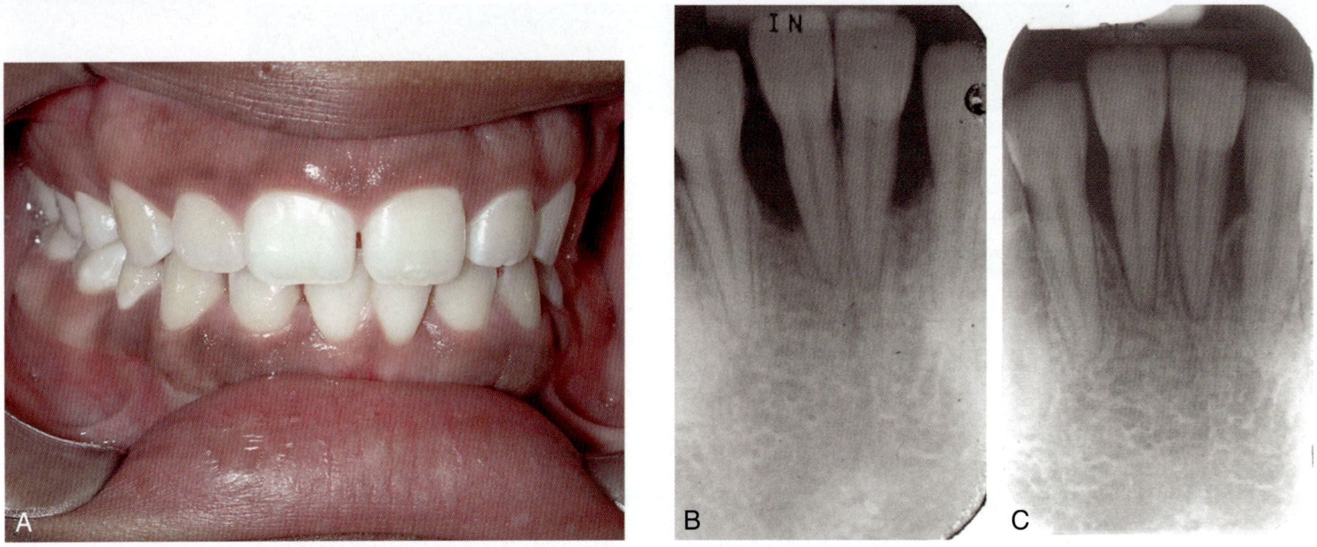

• **Fig. 6.9** Aggressive periodontitis in children and adolescents usually starts with an intensive attack on the supporting tissues around central incisors and/or first molars. (A) Intraoral appearance of a patient who sought orthodontic consultation because of congenitally missing second premolars. (B) Periapical radiograph of the lower central incisor area. (C) Follow-up periapical radiograph of the same incisor area after treatment with antibiotics and curettage and then comprehensive orthodontics. Unless periodontal probing during the orthodontist's clinical examination reveals inflammation and bone loss of this type and a periapical radiograph is obtained, the severe periodontal disease may be overlooked, and if it progresses, loss of the involved teeth is inevitable. If the periodontal problem is brought under control, orthodontic treatment is feasible.

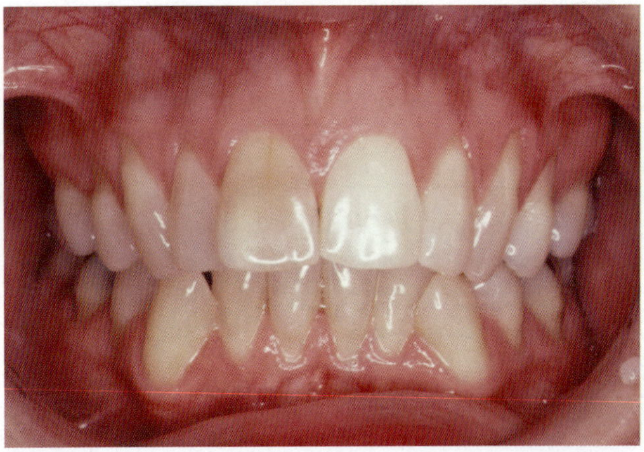

• **Fig. 6.10** In this patient with minimal attached gingiva in the lower incisor region, who has enough crowding that the lower incisors will have to be advanced at least somewhat to align them without extraction, further recession of the gingiva is possible during orthodontic treatment. There is mixed evidence regarding the usefulness of pretreatment and posttreatment soft tissue grafting.

Fortunately, aggressive juvenile periodontitis (Fig. 6.9) occurs rarely, but if it is present, it is critically important to note this before orthodontic treatment begins. Inadequate attached gingiva around crowded incisors may lead to stripping of the gingiva away from the teeth when the teeth are aligned, especially if the dental arch is expanded (Fig. 6.10). The interaction between periodontal and orthodontic treatment for both children and adults is discussed further in Chapter 7.

The developmental status of the patient applies not only to the eruption of teeth and growth of the jaws but also to the quality of the teeth. Teeth with developmental defects of morphology and hard tissue quality are more susceptible to decalcification and decay during treatment, which can become an esthetic issue at the end of treatment. The most common example of this is Molar Incisor Hypomineralization (MIH), which is characterized by clear demarcations between effected and sound enamel and asymmetric involvement of molars and incisors. This problem has been reported in 12%–20% of children. Extraction of a defective tooth rather than a sound one should be considered when extractions are part of the plan (Fig. 6.11). Photographic documentation is also important here, too. Patients and parents soon forget the pretreatment status of their teeth and gums.

Dental Relationships—Intra and Interarch

Certainly documenting the clinical presence or absence of teeth is important to development of the dentition, its stage, timing, and symmetry. Many novice clinicians do not give the clinical dental examination much importance and instead just rely on the records to document the occlusal characteristics. This is a huge mistake, because without the patient or an accurate clinical exam, there is no way to validate the occlusion recorded on the casts or on a cephalometric radiograph. Is there really an anterior or posterior crossbite, a midline discrepancy? Which midline is off? Are the overbite and overjet correct? Or, does the patient have a CR-CO shift?

Documenting these relationships is critical:

- Molar and canine relationships (using Angle classification)

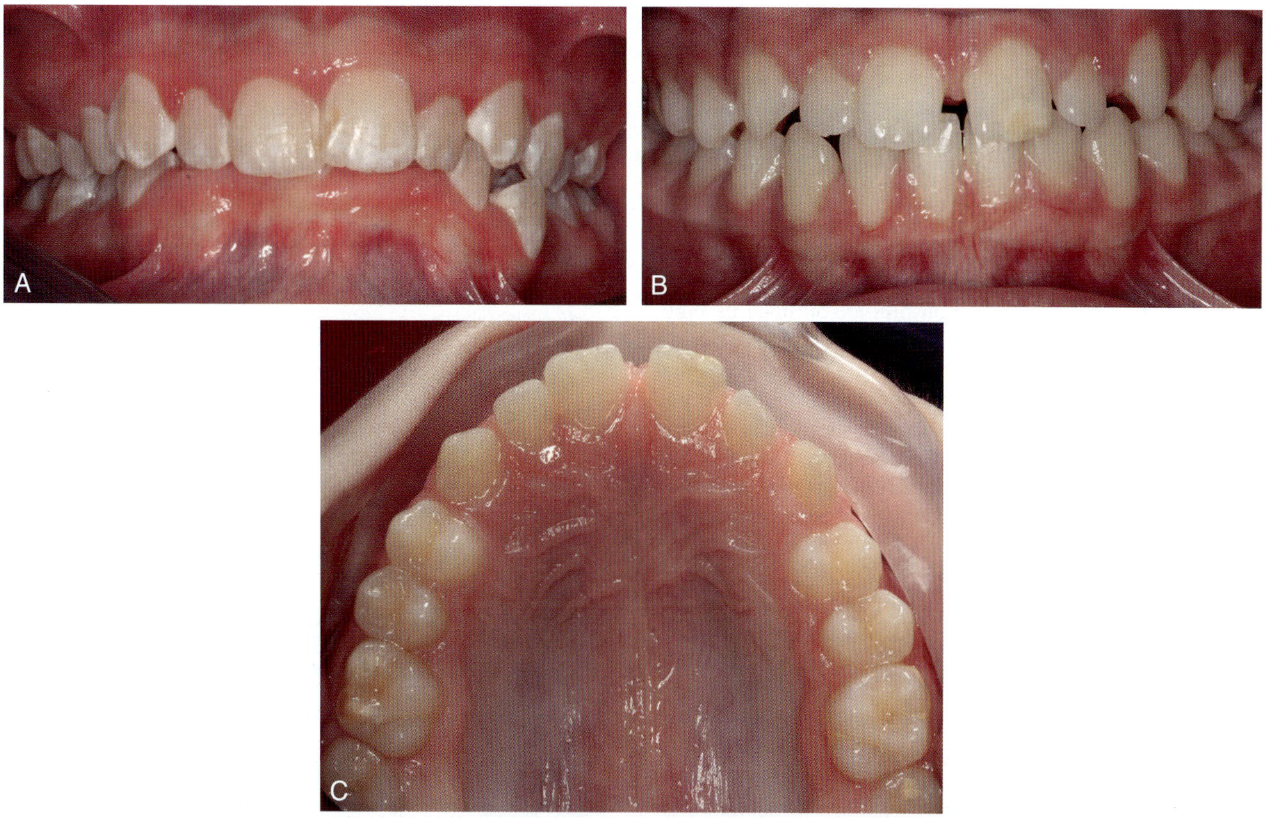

• **Fig. 6.11** Enamel defects of several types can be present on permanent teeth at multiple locations. Differentiating between those with local versus systemic causes can be accomplished by noting whether teeth forming during the same time are affected and the extent of the involvement. (A) This patient most likely has a form of fluorosis given the extent of the involvement and the history. This is distinguished from typical white spot lesions because the involvement is largely incisal and not primarily gingival or outlining previous bracket locations. (B) The maxillary left central incisor has a local hypoplastic incisal defect with discoloration and some defective morphology. If this is the only hypoplastic defect, then it is most likely the result of either trauma to the primary tooth that displaced it into the developing permanent tooth bud, or pulpal degeneration of one or more primary teeth that affected developing permanent teeth. Note also the narrow maxillary lateral incisors. (C) The same patient shown in (B) also has a defect on the permanent maxillary right first molar. This leads to the conclusion the patient has molar incisor hypomineralization. Although the lesions are not severe, they should be monitored for breakdown of the enamel and the need for restoration.

- Overbite (percentage and mm overlap) and overjet (mm)
- Anterior and posterior crossbites (including the teeth involved and buccal or lingual, if posterior)
- CR-CO shifts (amount in mm and direction)
- Midline relationships in CR and CO (mm) (upper to lower and to the facial midline, which is part of the extraoral examination)

Jaw and Occlusal Function

In the evaluation of function, it is important to note in the beginning whether the patient has normal coordination and movements. If not, as in an individual with cerebral palsy or other types of severe neuromuscular disease, normal adaptation to the changes in tooth position produced by orthodontics may not occur, and the equilibrium effects discussed in Chapter 5 may lead to post-treatment relapse. Three aspects of oral function require evaluation: mastication (including but not limited to swallowing), speech, and the presence or absence of temporomandibular joint (TMJ) problems.

Patients with severe malocclusion often have difficulty in normal mastication, not so much in being able to chew their food (although this may take extra effort) but in being able to do so in a socially acceptable manner. These individuals often have learned to avoid certain foods that are hard to incise and chew and may have problems with cheek and lip biting during mastication. If asked, patients report such problems and usually indicate that after orthodontic treatment they can chew better. Unfortunately, there are almost no reasonable diagnostic tests to evaluate masticatory efficiency, so it is difficult to quantify the degree of masticatory handicap and difficult to document functional improvement.

Swallowing is almost never affected by malocclusion. It has been suggested that lip and tongue weakness may indicate problems in normal swallowing, but there is no evidence to support this contention (see Chapter 5). Oral gymnastic tests (such as measuring lip strength or how hard the patient can push with the tongue) therefore add little or nothing to the diagnostic evaluation.

Speech problems can be related to malocclusion, but normal speech is possible in the presence of severe anatomic distortions. Speech difficulties in a child therefore are unlikely to be solved by orthodontic treatment. Specific relationships are outlined in Table 6.2. If a child has a speech problem and the type of malocclusion related to it, a combination of speech therapy and orthodontics may help. It is best to rely on a speech professional for diagnostic input and caution everyone regarding what can be successfully accomplished. If the speech problem is not listed as related to malocclusion, orthodontic treatment may be valuable in its own right but is unlikely to have any impact on speech. It appears that speech can be altered by orthognathic surgery, which will be addressed in Chapter 22.

Jaw function is more than TMJ function, but evaluation of the TMJs is an important aspect of the diagnostic workup. A form for recording routine clinical examination of TMJ function is shown in Box 6.1. As a general guideline, if the mandible moves normally, its function is not severely impaired, and by the same token, restricted movement usually indicates a functional problem.[9] For that reason, the most important indicators of joint function are the amount of maximum opening and the ability of the mandible to translate beyond the hinge movement. Palpating the muscles of mastication and TMJs should be a routine part of any dental examination, and it is important to note any signs of TMJ problems such as joint pain, noise, limitation of opening, or deviation on opening.

Because the articular eminence is not well developed in children, it can be more challenging to find the sort of positive "centric relation" position that can be determined in adults. Nevertheless, it is important to note whether the mandible shifts laterally or anteriorly when a child bites down. Children with an apparent unilateral crossbite often have a bilateral narrowing of the maxillary arch, with a shift to the unilateral crossbite position. This is the most common cause of apparent but not true facial asymmetry. It is vitally important to verify this during the clinical examination or to rule out a shift and confirm a true unilateral crossbite, because treatment of these problems is different.

Similarly, many children and adults with a class II malocclusion and an underlying skeletal class II jaw relationship will habitually position the mandible forward in a "Sunday bite," making the occlusion look better than it really is. Sometimes an apparent class III relationship results from a forward shift to escape incisor interferences in what is really an end-to-end incisor relationship (Fig. 6.12). These patients are said to have pseudo–class III malocclusion.

Other occlusal interferences with functional mandibular movements, although of interest, are less important than they would be if treatment to alter the occlusion were not being contemplated. Balancing interferences, presence or absence of canine protection in lateral excursions, and other such factors take on greater significance if they are still present when the occlusal changes produced by orthodontic treatment are nearing completion.

TABLE 6.2 Speech Difficulties Related to Malocclusion

Speech Sound	Problem	Related Malocclusion
/s/, /z/ (sibilants)	Lisp	Anterior open bite, large gap between incisors
/t/, /d/ (linguoalveolar stops)	Difficulty in production	Irregular incisors, especially lingual position of maxillary incisors
/f/, /v/ (labiodental fricatives)	Distortion	Skeletal class III
th, sh, ch (linguodental fricatives [voiced or voiceless])	Distortion	Anterior open bite

• BOX 6.1 Screening Examination for Jaw Function (Temporomandibular Joint [TMJ])

Jaw function/TMJ complaint now: ☐ **No** ☐ **Yes**

If yes, specify: ______

History of pain: ☐ No ☐ Yes _____ duration

History of sounds: ☐ No ☐ Yes _____ duration

TMJ tenderness to palpation: ☐ No ☐ Yes ☐ Right ☐ Left

Muscle tenderness to palpation: ☐ No ☐ Yes

If yes, where? ______

Range of motion:
Maximum opening _____ mm
Right excursion _____ mm
Left excursion _____ mm
Protrusion _____ mm

Deviations on opening?
Deviations on opening?
R_____ L_____
At what point?_____ mm

Facial and Dental Appearance: The Evolution To Today's Soft-Tissue Paradigm

The soft-tissue paradigm in orthodontic diagnosis actually had its beginnings in the earliest days of orthodontics. Norman Kingsley (1829–1913), an artist/dentist and the most important person in the early development of orthodontics, wrote extensively on the importance of recognizing the artistic form of the face as the start of orthodontic diagnosis in his book *Treatise on Oral Deformities*. Kingsley was followed by Edward H. Angle (1855–1930) who established the Angle classification of malocclusion with its emphasis on

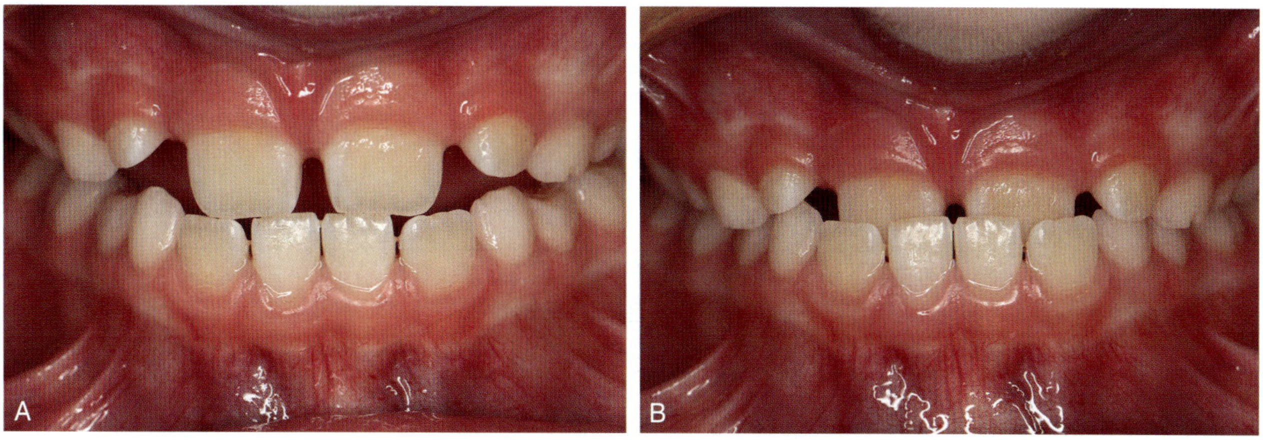

• **Fig. 6.12** Anterior crossbite with a forward mandibular shift. (A) When the anterior teeth contact in centric relation and cause an interference so that a natural continuation to centric occlusion is not possible, (B) the mandible shifts forward so maximum intercuspation of the posterior teeth can be achieved.

occlusion and felt that an ideal occlusion including all the teeth meant ideal facial esthetics. However, the soft tissues of the face were still of importance in the Angle school, to the degree that he incorporated into his curriculum Dr. Edmund Wuerpel, an art professor, who taught the students about Greco-Roman sculpture and facial proportion. Technological advances in orthodontics, primarily the advances in radiographic cephalometry, diverted attention from the clinical facial examination as attention focused on the lateral cephalometric radiograph. The use of cephalometric "analyses" followed, but any cephalometric analysis has an inherent weakness. It is either someone else's idea of ideal, or it is a result of a series of quantitative measurements from a cross-sectional sample resulting in "norms." This focus did not mean that the attention to facial form was entirely lost, but it was focused strongly on the profile and its relationship to the Angle classification of malocclusion.[10–14]

As coordinated surgical and orthodontic treatment continued to evolve in the 1980s, orthodontic diagnosis and treatment planning were greatly influenced by these interdisciplinary experiences. As a consequence, orthodontists now visualize cases in a vastly different way than they did two decades ago. The focus on occlusion began to shift to the face, and now with the involvement in interdisciplinary cosmetic dentistry, that focus includes smiles.

Effect of Background Facial Attractiveness on Perceptions of Dental Esthetics

Although it has been and now is widely recognized that the background facial appearance plays a role in the perception of the appearance of the teeth,[15] it has been difficult to quantify these relationships. The discovery that the length and number of times an individual looks at features of the face is proportional to its importance to them allowed new insights regarding facial and smile esthetics. This concept provides a way to determine how the teeth and the face affect each other in quantitative terms. In recent studies, the movements of the eyes in samples of young adults were tracked while they were looking at images of faces of young adults with different levels of facial attractiveness. The faces were digitally combined with teeth that had different levels of dental attractiveness (quantified using the Aesthetic Component of the Index of Orthodontic Treatment Need [IOTN-AC]—see Fig. 1.25). The frequency and duration of gazes were recorded for both sexes.

In general, the eye tracking for the facial images showed that the most attention was paid to the eyes. These data showed that for attractive and average females, unattractive teeth (high borderline esthetic dental need at IOTN level 7) became a focus for the viewers sooner when the female model had moderate or high background attractiveness than it did for images with unattractive background esthetics.[16] This attention rivaled looking at the eyes. For men, the most attention was directed at the mouth when the males were unattractive or of average attractiveness and the dental esthetics need was severe (esthetic dental need at IOTN level 10). Then it surpassed the eyes.[17]

These studies demonstrated that overall facial attractiveness influences how people look at teeth (smiles) and that they tolerate different levels of dental attractiveness based on this. So, malalignment is more noticeable in average and attractive women and average and unattractive men.

How much of facial attractiveness is determined by the teeth? This was determined quantitatively in a study[18] that examined young adults ratings of attractiveness for other young adults when faces of different attractiveness and different levels of dental attractiveness were combined as in the previous studies. The difference was that the models were rated with lips closed and lips apart during a posed smile. The difference in ratings was the contribution, either positive or negative, of the teeth. There is a clear interaction between the attractiveness of the face and the teeth. Males and females are judged differently (Fig. 6.13).

We also know that people make judgments regarding intelligence and interpersonal temperament for children and young adults based on the appearance of the teeth.[15,18,19] For females there were some positive social ratings that accompanied good dental attractiveness for unattractive and average models. Both benefitted in positive judgments of intelligence with attractive smiles. For attractive females only social class and popularity were improved with attractive teeth. The data show a good deal of overlap between the best and worst dentitions. For males, especially average and attractive ones, the data separated significantly. Attractive teeth showed nearly uniform benefit, including integrity and intelligence, for average attractive males. For attractive males, attractive teeth showed benefits especially for social class, compliance, popularity, and intelligence (Fig. 6.14).

It seems that unattractive teeth affect females, especially attractive females, more than males. Socially and intellectually, attractive

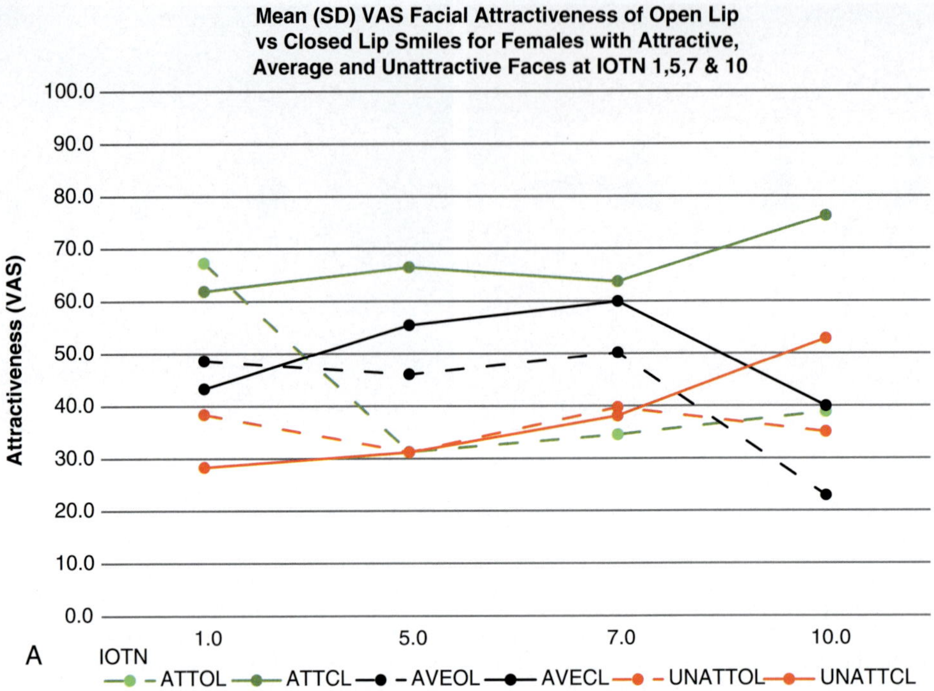

A

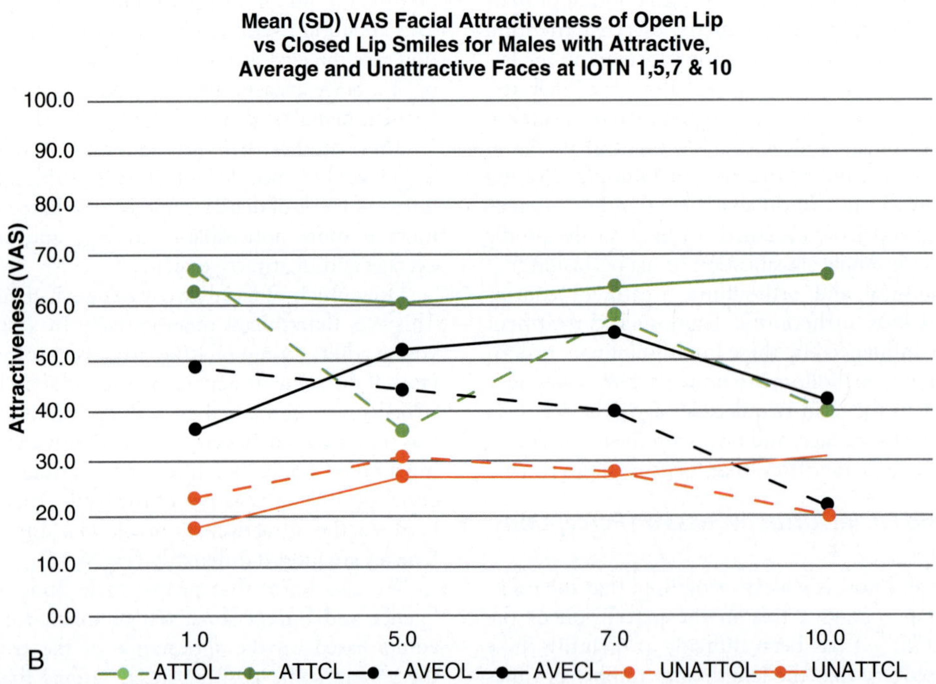

B

• **Fig. 6.13** The effect of open (*OL*) and closed lip (*CL*) smiles for (A) females and (B) males of varying facial and dental attractiveness. (A) When the female models revealed their teeth, all benefitted by near ideal teeth, but unattractive models (*UNATT*) gained about 10% compared to 5% for average (*AVE*) and attractive (*ATT*) females. Essentially "borderline" and "extreme need" dental esthetics, caused a neutral or negative impact. But, for attractive females, there was up to −37% impact. (B) When males revealed near ideal teeth, average (*AVE*) attractive males had a 12% increase in attractiveness with unattractive (*UNATT*) and attractive (*ATT*) males getting approximately 5% improvement. Unattractive males had a gradual decrease in attractiveness as the dental attractiveness decreased. But, average and attractive males had more dramatic decreases reaching −27% for attractive males. Data from Papio MA, Fields, HW, Beck FM, et al. The Role of Dental and Background Facial Attractiveness on Facial Attractiveness and Perceived Integrity, Social and Intellectual Attractiveness. *Am J Orthod Dentofacial Orthop* 2019; 1256:464–74.

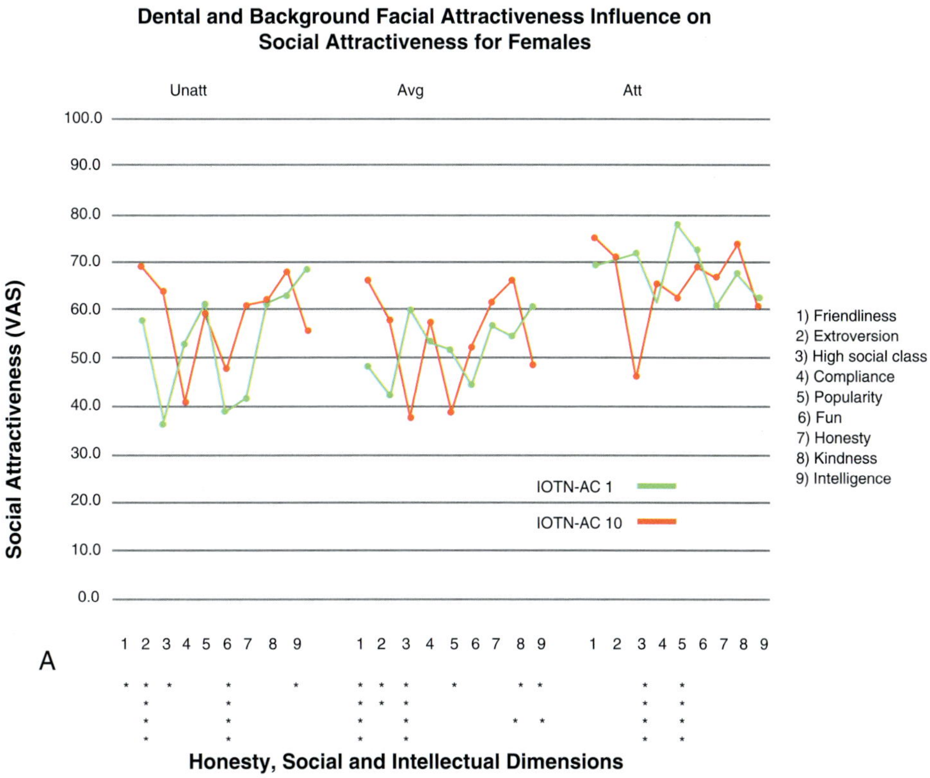

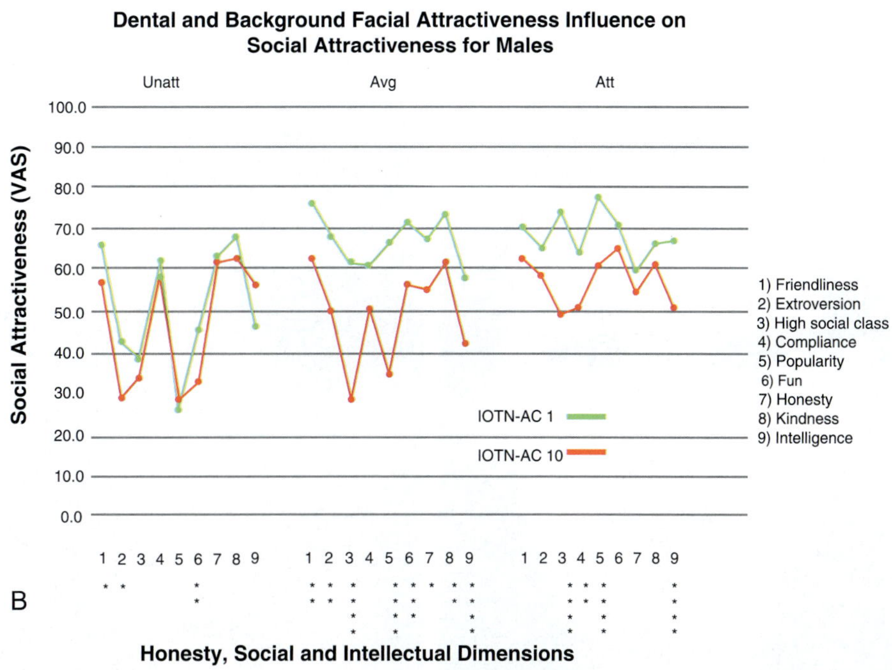

• **Fig. 6.14** Judgments on Social, Integrity, and Intellectual qualities for (A) females and (B) males. (A) For females there were some positive social ratings that accompanied good dental attractiveness for unattractive (*UNATT*) and average (*AVE*) models. Both benefitted in positive judgments of intelligence with attractive smiles. For attractive (*ATT*) females only social class and popularity were improved with attractive teeth. The data show a good deal of overlap between the best and worst dentitions. (B)For males, especially average and attractive ones, the data separated significantly for the attractive and unattractive teeth. Attractive teeth showed nearly uniform benefit, including integrity and intelligence, for average (*AVE*) attractive males. For attractive (*ATT*) males, attractive teeth showed benefits especially for social class, compliance, popularity, and intelligence. The females and males had similar ranges for unattractive and attractive faces, but the average males benefitted more than average females by about 15 percentage points. Data from Papio MA, Fields, HW, Beck FM et al. The Role of Dental and Background Facial Attractiveness on Facial Attractiveness and Perceived Integrity, Social and Intellectual Attractiveness. *Am J Orthod Dentofacial Orthop*. 2019; 1256:464–74.

teeth benefit males more. This information can be helpful when advising patients regarding their need for treatment and helps explain how important it is to assess the facial as well as the dental attractiveness of the patient.

Systematic Examination of Facial and Dental Appearance

A systematic examination of facial and dental appearance should be done in the following three steps:

1. *Facial proportions in all three planes of space (macroesthetics).* Examples of problems that would be noted in this first step would be asymmetry, excessive or deficient face height, mandibular or maxillary deficiency or excess, and so on. In performing this evaluation, keep in mind that both the evolutionary and prenatal development of the face can provide additional insight into the origin and significance of unusual facial morphology.
2. *The dentition in relation to the face (mini-esthetics).* This includes the display of the teeth at rest, during speech, and on smiling. It includes such assessments as smile arc, excessive gingival display, inadequate anterior tooth display, inappropriate gingival heights, and the extent of the buccal corridors (the dark spaces in the corners of the mouth beyond the teeth).
3. *The teeth in relation to one another (microesthetics)* This includes assessment of tooth proportions in height and width, gingival shape and contour, connectors, incisal embrasures, black triangular holes (gingival embrasures), and tooth shade.

Let us evaluate what you are looking for in each step.

Macroesthetics: Facial Proportions

The first step in evaluating facial proportions is to take a good look at the patient, examining him or her for developmental characteristics and a general impression. Humans are very adept at evaluating faces and in fact have a dedicated neural system for that purpose.[20] Even so, with faces as with everything else, looking too quickly at the details carries the risk of missing the big picture. It is a mistake for any dentist to focus on just the teeth after a cursory look at the face. It is a disastrous mistake for an orthodontist not to evaluate the face carefully.

Facial Esthetics Versus Facial Proportions. Because a major reason for orthodontic treatment is to overcome psychosocial difficulties related to facial and dental appearance and enhance social well-being and QOL in doing so, evaluating dental and facial esthetics is an important part of the clinical examination. Judgments regarding dental esthetics are affected by the background attractiveness of the patient's face, so this context is important. Whether a face is considered attractive is greatly affected by cultural and ethnic factors, but whatever the culture, a severely disproportionate face becomes a psychosocial problem. For that reason, it helps to recast the purpose of this part of the clinical evaluation as an evaluation of facial proportions, not esthetics per se. Distorted and asymmetric facial features are a major contributor to facial esthetic problems, whereas proportionate features are generally acceptable even if not beautiful.

Facial Form Analysis. In the next sections you will learn how to examine the face clinically in all dimensions: frontal, anteroposterior, and vertical. Taken together and without using any radiography, this process is called the facial form analysis and is the macroesthetic evaluation (Fig. 6.15). The extraoral soft tissue contours inform us about the position and proportions underlying jaws and teeth. During this exercise, we must take into consideration the maturity of the patient. Expectations change for what is appropriate facial form as maturity changes. In this context, we

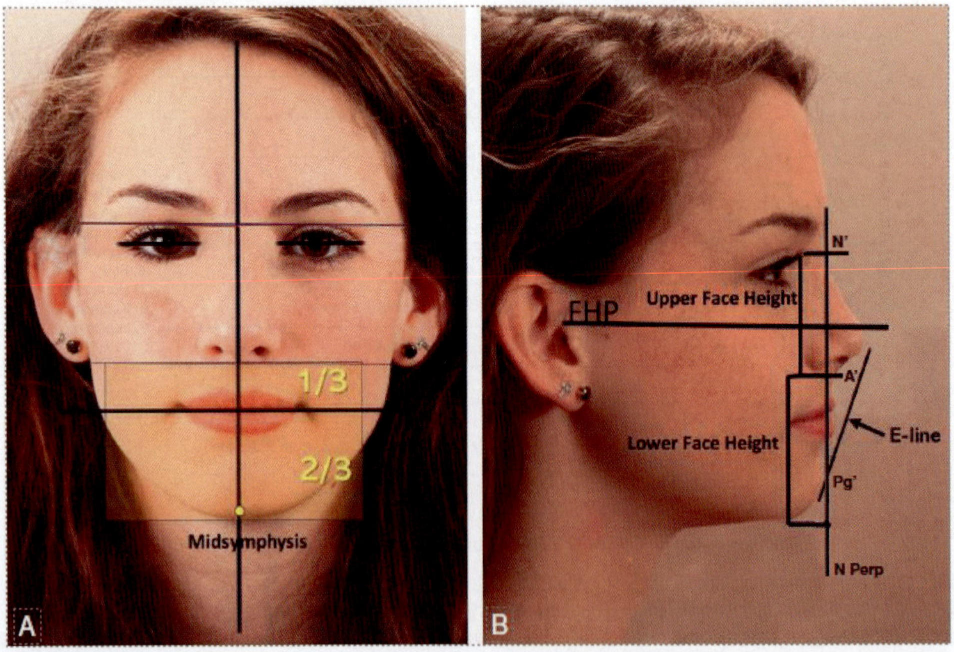

• **Fig. 6.15** These are the hallmarks of the proportional evaluations that are made in Macroesthetic considerations. These also make up a portion of the Facial Form Analysis. (A) The frontal view is used to examine facial symmetry and proportional segments of the lower face. (B) The lateral view displays the vertical facial proportions of the upper and lower face (nearly equal). The Nasion Perpendicular (N Perp, a line perpendicular to the Frankfort Horizontal plane [*FHP*]) is used to judge the position of the maxilla (the base of the nose (A') should be on this line) and mandible (soft tissue pogonion (Pg') should be either on the line or up to 4 mm behind it). Finally, lip protrusion is evaluated relative to the E-line (a line from the tip of the nose to the tip of the chin. Ideally, the lips should lie near the E-line or slightly anterior to it, depending upon the size of the nose and chin.

TABLE 6.3 Checklist for the Facial Form Analysis

Frontal at Rest	Frontal Smile	Frontal Widths	Profile
To Midsagittal Plane • Nasal tip • Maxillary dental midline • Mandibular dental midline • Chin (midsymphysis)	• Maxillary incisor display • Maxillary incisor crown height • Gingival display • Smile arc • Occlusal plane cant?	• Alar base • Nasal tip • Buccal corridor	**Ant/Post Jaw Position** • Maxillary projection • Mandibular projection • Chin projection **Vertical Lower Face** • Lower Face proportion • Mandibular plane
Vertical • Lip separation (lips relaxed) • Lip vermilion display • Maxillary incisor display (lips relaxed) • Lower face proportion • Philtrum length • Commissure height • Chin height			**Nose** • Nasal radix • Nasal dorsum contour • Nasal tip projection • Nasolabial angle **Lip** • Lip protrusion • Labiomental sulcus **Throat Form** • Chin-throat angle • Throat length • Submental contour (fat pad)

must project what the ultimate later adolescent and adult esthetics will be, given the current time point. This is the heart of the clinical extraoral examination.

Dentofacial characteristics that should be noted as part of the facial examination are shown in Table 6.3. This checklist is just that: a list of things that should be noted systematically during the clinical examination that is part of the Facial Form Analysis. As in many other things, if you do not look for it, you will not see it. Precise measurements are not necessary, but deviations from the normal should be considered when the problem list is developed. Computer programs currently in use already allow positive findings from the digital data acquired during the clinical examination to "flow through" to the preliminary problem list.

Frontal Examination. The first step in analyzing facial proportions is to examine the face in frontal view. Low-set ears or eyes that are unusually far apart (hypertelorism) may indicate either the presence of a syndrome or a microform of a craniofacial anomaly. If a syndrome is suspected, the patient's hands should be examined for syndactyly, because there are several dental-digital syndromes. If a syndrome is suspected the patient should be referred to their primary care physician for additional workups such as genetics.

In the frontal view, one looks for bilateral symmetry in the fifths of the face and for proportionality of the widths of the eyes, nose, and mouth (Fig. 6.16). A small degree of bilateral facial asymmetry exists in essentially all normal individuals. This can be appreciated most readily by comparing the real full-face photograph with composites consisting of two right or two left sides (Fig. 6.17). This "normal asymmetry," which usually results from a small size difference between the two sides, should be distinguished from a chin or nose that deviates to one side, which can produce severe disproportion and esthetic problems (see Fig. 6.3).

Before the advent of cephalometric radiography, dentists and orthodontists often used anthropometric measurements (i.e., measurements made directly during the clinical examination) to help establish facial proportions (Fig. 6.18). Although this method was largely replaced by cephalometric analysis for many years, the recent emphasis on soft tissue proportions has brought soft tissue evaluation back into prominence. Farkas's modern

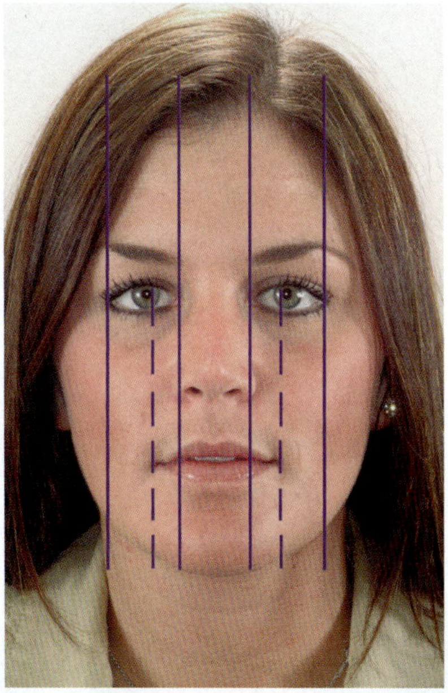

• **Fig. 6.16** Facial proportions and symmetry in the frontal plane. An ideally proportional face can be divided into central, medial, and lateral equal fifths. The separation of the eyes and the width of the eyes, which should be equal, determine the central and medial fifths. The nose and chin should be centered within the central fifth, with the width of the nose the same as or slightly wider than the central fifth. The interpupillary distance *(dashed line)* should equal the width of the mouth.

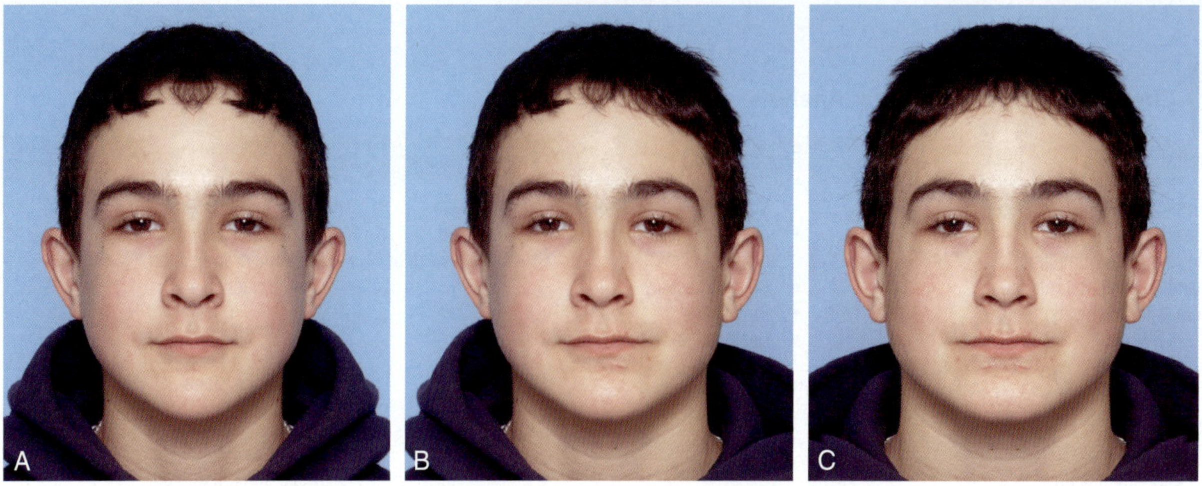

• **Fig. 6.17** Composite photographs are the best way to illustrate normal facial asymmetry. For this boy, whose mild asymmetry rarely would be noticed and is not a problem, the true photograph is in the center (B). On the patient's right, (A) is a composite of the two right sides; on the left, (C) is a composite of the two left sides. This dramatically illustrates the difference in the two sides of a normal face, in which mild asymmetry is the rule rather than the exception. Usually, the right side of the face is a little larger than the left, rather than the reverse as in this individual.

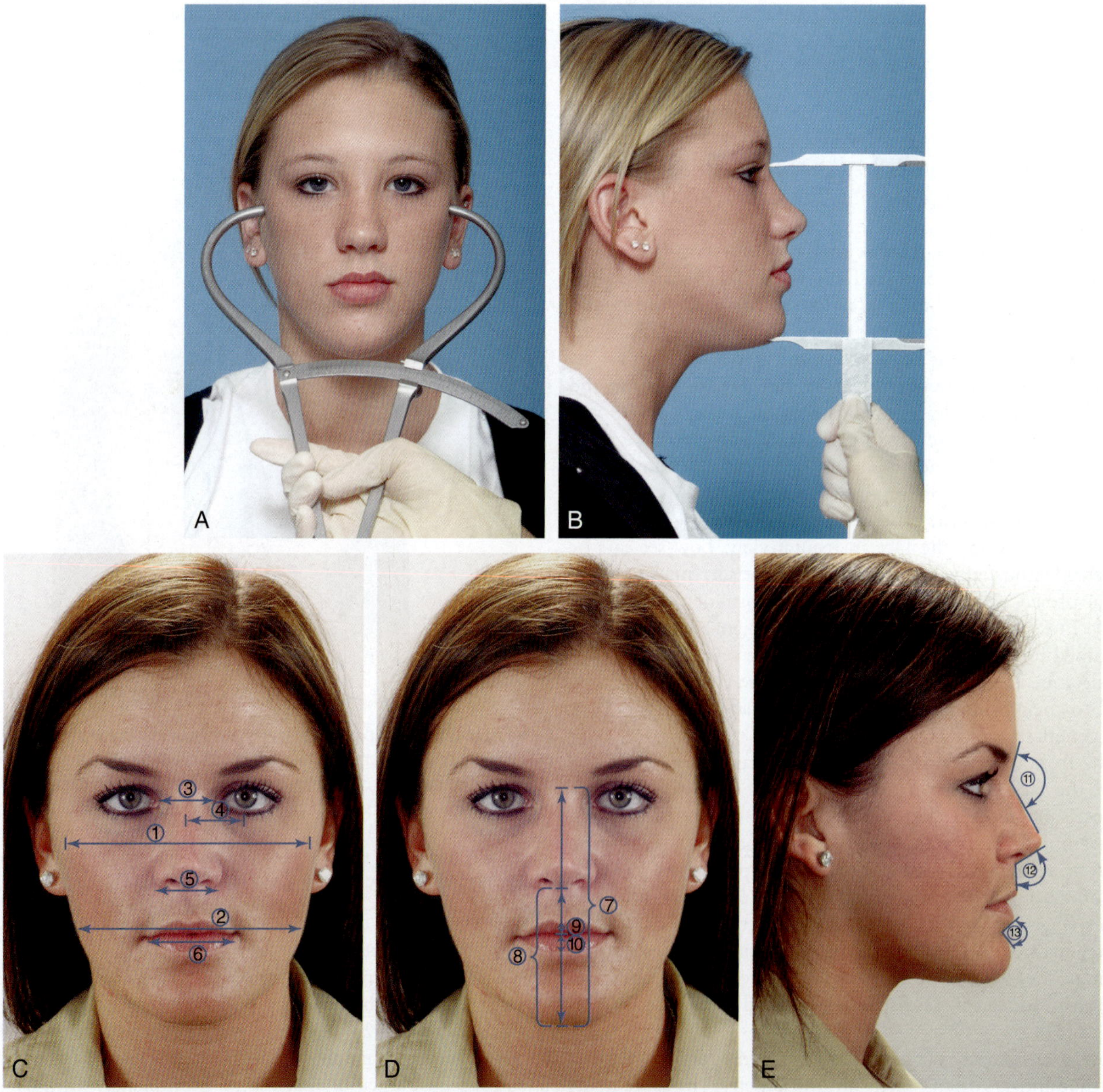

• **Fig. 6.18** Facial measurements for anthropometric analysis are made with either (A) bow calipers or (B) straight calipers. (C–E) Frequently used facial anthropometric measurements; the numbers are keyed to Table 6.3.

studies of Canadians of northern European origin provided the data for Table 6.4.[21]

Note that some of the measurements in Table 6.4 could be made on a cephalometric radiograph, but many could not. When there are questions about facial proportions, it is much better to make the measurements clinically because soft tissue proportions as seen on visual examination determine facial appearance. During the clinical examination, one can record measurements.

TABLE 6.4 Facial Anthropometric Measurements (Young Adults)

Parameter	Male (SD)	Female (SD)
1. Zygomatic width (zy-zy) (mm)	137 (4.3)	130 (5.3)
2. Gonial width (go-go)	97 (5.8)	91 (5.9)
3. Intercanthal distance	33 (2.7)	32 (2.4)
4. Pupil-midfacial distance	33 (2.0)	31 (1.8)
5. Nasal base width	35 (2.6)	31 (1.9)
6. Mouth width	53 (3.3)	50 (3.2)
7. Face height (N-gn)	121 (6.8)	112 (5.2)
8. Lower face height (subnasale-gn)	72 (6.0)	66 (4.5)
9. Upper lip vermilion	8.9 (1.5)	8.4 (1.3)
10. Lower lip vermilion	10.4 (1.9)	9.7 (1.6)
11. Nasofrontal angle (degrees)	131 (8.1)	134 (1.8)
12. Nasolabial angle (degrees)	99 (8.0)	99 (8.7)
13. Labiomental sulcus	Obtuse	Obtuse

Data from Farkas LG. *Anthropometry of the Head and Face in Medicine.* Elsevier Science; 1991. Measurements are illustrated in Fig. 6.18. *SD*, Standard deviation.

The proportional relationship of facial height to width (the facial index) establishes the overall facial type and the basic proportions of the face. It is important to remember that face height cannot be evaluated unless face width is known, and face width is not evaluated when a lateral cephalometric radiograph is analyzed.

Differences in facial types and body types must obviously be taken into account when facial proportions are assessed, and variations from the average ratios can be compatible with good facial esthetics. An important point, however, is to avoid treatment that would change the ratios in the wrong direction—for example, treatment with interarch elastics that could rotate the mandible downward in a patient whose face already is too long for its width.

Finally, the face in frontal view should be examined from the perspective of the vertical facial thirds. The artists of the Renaissance period, primarily da Vinci and Durer, established the proportions for drawing anatomically correct human faces (Fig. 6.19). They concluded that the distance from the hairine to the base of the nose, base of nose to bottom of nose, and bottom of nose to chin should be the same. Farkas's studies show that in modern Whites of European descent, the lower third is very slightly longer. The artists also saw that the lower third has a proportion of one-third above the mouth to two-thirds below, which is still true.

It is important to note the cause of vertical problems such as excessive display of the maxillary gingiva, which is done best by examining the position of lips and teeth relative to the vertical thirds of the face (Fig. 6.20). It also is important to keep in mind that different ethnic and national groups view facial esthetics somewhat differently (there are differences even in countries as closely matched as the United States and Canada) and that both gender and overall facial attractiveness influence how people are perceived. As the examining doctor, you need to notice and evaluate disproportions, even though you know that as treatment is planned, aspects of facial appearance that would be a problem for

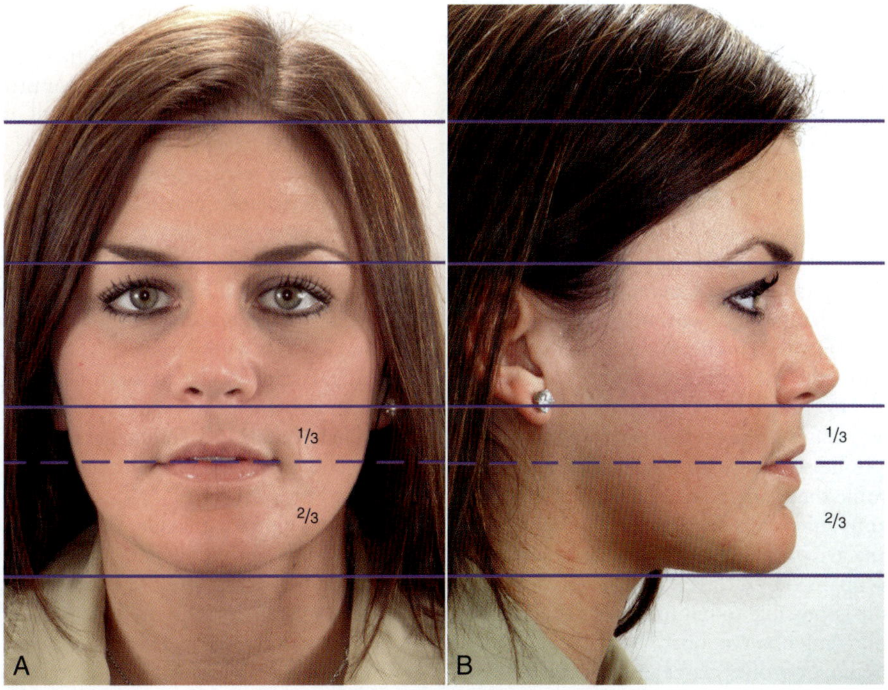

• **Fig. 6.19** Vertical facial proportions in the frontal (A) and lateral (B) views are best evaluated in the context of the facial thirds, which the Renaissance artists noted were equal in height in well-proportioned faces. In modern Whites the lower facial third often is slightly longer than the central third. The lower third also includes thirds: the mouth should be one-third of the way between the base of the nose and the chin.

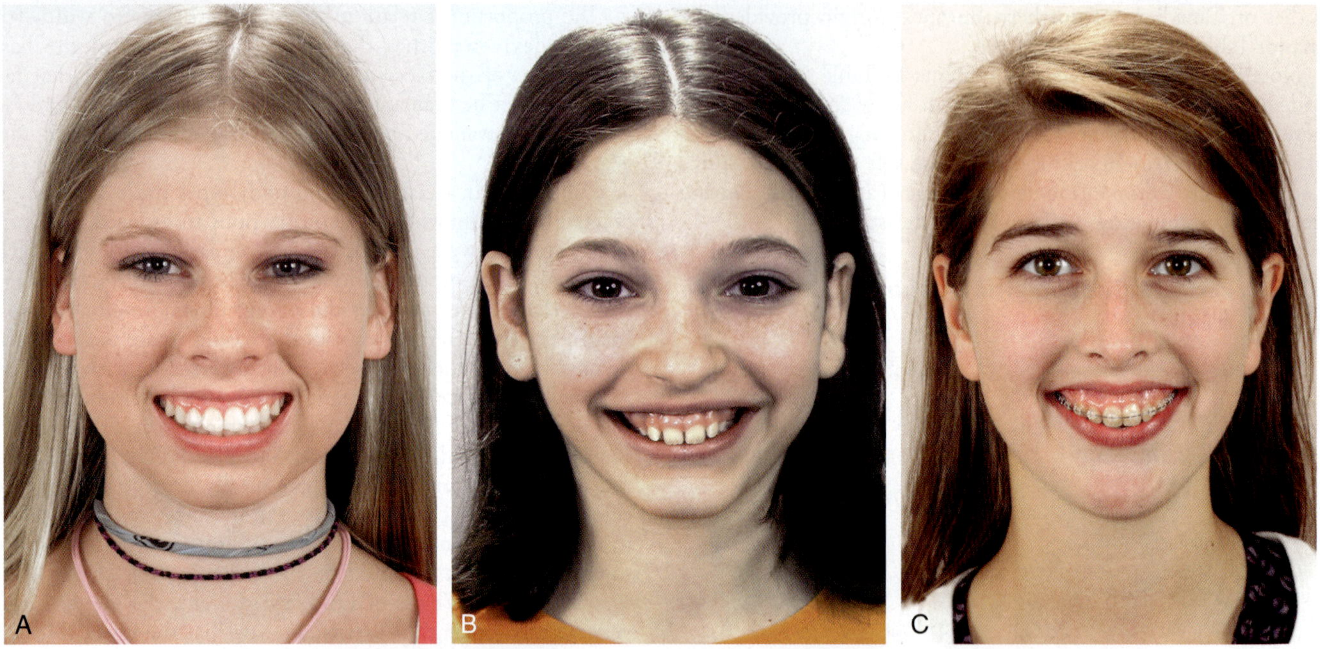

• **Fig. 6.20** The usual cause of excessive display of maxillary gingiva is a long face due to excessive downward growth of the maxilla, which moves the maxilla down below the upper lip and results in a disproportionately long lower third of the face. (A) This should not be confused with display of gingiva in childhood because the gingival recession that accompanies eruption is incomplete, or with (B) gingival display due to a combination of incomplete eruption and a short upper lip. (C) Note that for the patients in (A and C), the lower third of the face is long, whereas for the patient in (B), the lower third is about the same length as the middle third.

some individuals are not a problem for others with a different ethnic background.

Profile Analysis. The three goals of the profile evaluation are approached in four clear and distinct steps, discussed below.

1. *Establishing the overall facial form and if the teeth are consistent with the jaws and are proportionately positioned in the anteroposterior (AP) plane of space.* This step requires placing the patient in the physiologic natural head position (NHP), which is the head position the individual adopts in the absence of other cues. This can be accomplished reliably with the patient either sitting upright or standing and looking at the horizon or a distant object, but not reclining in a dental chair. With the head in this position, note the relationship between two lines, one dropped from the bridge of the nose (soft tissue Nasion or N') to the base of the upper lip (soft tissue A point or A'), and a second one extending from that point downward to the chin (soft tissue Pogonion or Pg') (Fig. 6.21). These line segments ideally should form a nearly straight line, with only a slight inclination in either direction. A large angle between them (>10 degrees or so) indicates either profile convexity (upper jaw prominent relative to chin) or profile concavity (upper jaw behind chin). A marked convex profile therefore indicates a skeletal jaw relationship usually accompanied by a class II dental relationship, whereas a marked concave profile indicates a skeletal jaw relationship usually accompanied by a class III dental relationship. During this process it is possible to confirm the skeletal classification with the following observations:
   - If the patient has a convex profile, class II molars and >5 mm overjet, they have a class II skeletal relationship (extending the dental classification to the skeletal).
   - If the patient has a slightly convex to straight profile, class I molars and 2 to 5 mm of overjet, they have a class I skeletal relationship (extending the dental classification to the skeletal).
   - If they have a concave profile, class III molars and 0 to negative overjet, they have a class III skeletal relationship (extending the dental classification to the skeletal).

   It is the consistency that is confirmational.[22] But, knowing the overall facial form, does not tell us the cause of a problem, if one exists (class II or III). Is the class II due to a protrusive maxilla or a retrusive mandible or both. Similarly, is a class III due to a retrusive maxilla or a protrusive mandible or both.
2. *Determining maxillary and mandibular contributions to skeletal malocclusions.* This step also requires having the patient in the same natural head position as Step 1. Then a line is imagined that connects the external auditory meatus with Orbitale (making this a soft tissue Frankfort Horizontal line) (see Fig. 6.15). Perpendicular to this line and through N' another line is imagined. The position of A' and Pg' relative to this vertical line (called Nasion Perpendicular) tells us the position of the maxilla and mandible to the cranial base (Frankfort Horizontal) and to each other.

   For a normal maxilla, A' should be near (within ±2 mm) of Nasion Perpendicular. If A' is more anterior to Nasion Perpendicular the maxilla is protrusive and if it is posterior to it, the maxilla is retrusive. For a normal mandibular position in a child or adolescent, Pg' should be on or up to 4 mm posterior to Nasion Perpendicular. Pg' anterior to Nasion Perpendicular demonstrates mandibular protrusion, while more than 4 mm posterior to the vertical reference line is mandibular retrusion.

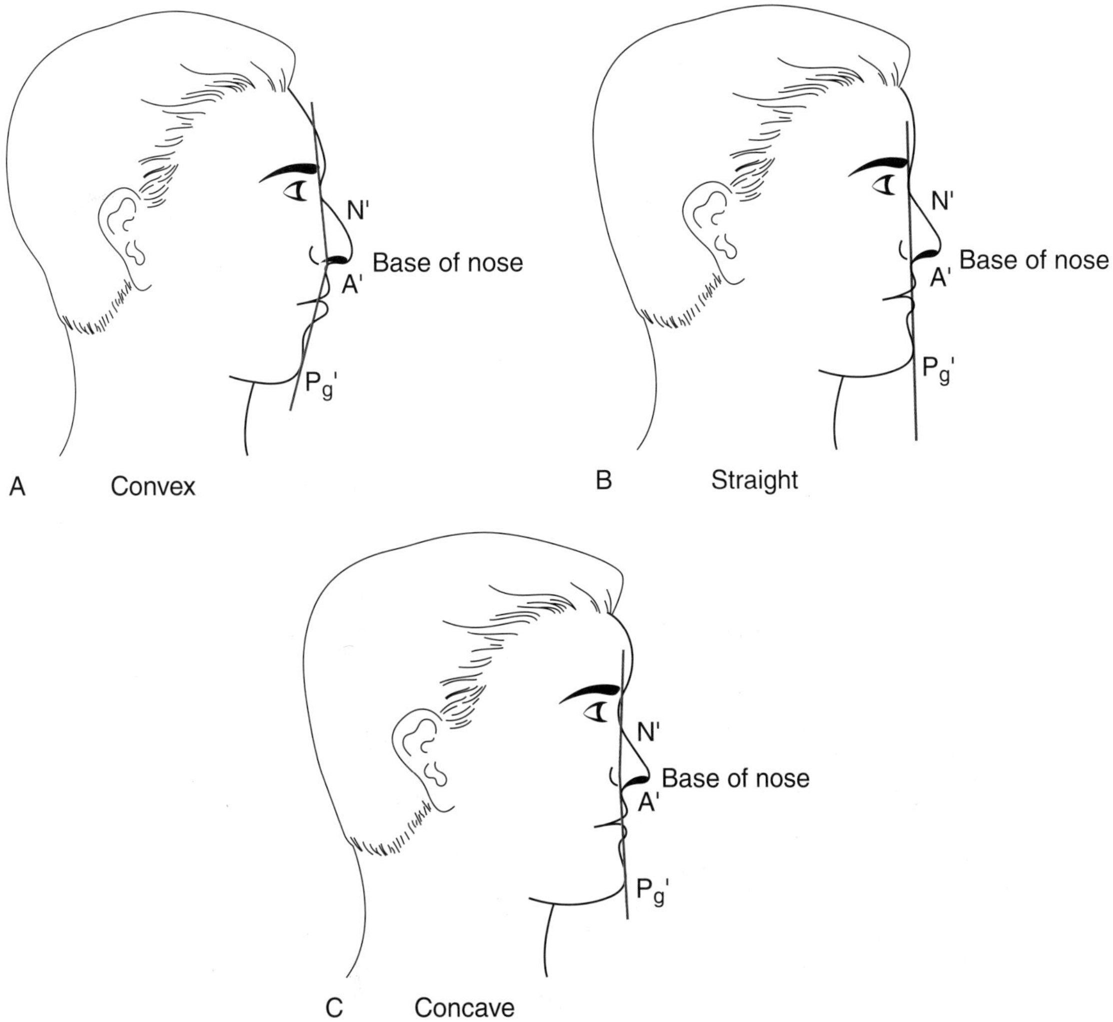

• **Fig. 6.21** Accentuated profile convexity or concavity results from a disproportion in the size of the jaws but does not by itself indicate which jaw is at fault. (A) A convex facial profile indicates a class II jaw relationship, which can result from either a maxilla that projects too far forward or a mandible too far back. (B) A straight or slightly convex profile is normal and usually reflects a normal jaw relationship. (C) A concave profile indicates a class III jaw relationship, which can result from either a maxilla that is too far back or a mandible that protrudes forward.

These positions show the contributions of each jaw to a class II or class III malocclusion (Fig. 6.22).

Not only the prominence of the chin, but also the submental soft tissue contours should be evaluated. Throat form is an important factor in establishing optimal facial esthetics, and poor throat form is a major contributor to esthetic impairment in patients with mandibular deficiency (Fig. 6.23).

3. *Evaluation of lip posture and incisor prominence.* Detecting excessive incisor protrusion (which is relatively common) or retrusion (which is less frequent) is important because of the effect on space within the dental arches. If the incisors protrude, they align themselves on the arc of a larger circle as they lean forward, whereas if the incisors are upright or retrusive, less space is available (Fig. 6.24). In the extreme case, incisor protrusion can produce ideal alignment of the teeth instead of severely crowded incisors, at the expense of lips that protrude and are difficult to bring into function over the protruding teeth. This is *bimaxillary dentoalveolar protrusion*, meaning simply that in both jaws the teeth protrude (Fig. 6.25). Dentists often refer to the condition as just *bimaxillary protrusion*, a simpler term but a misnomer because it is not the jaws, but the teeth that protrude. Physical anthropologists use bimaxillary protrusion to describe faces in which both jaws are prominent relative to the cranium, and the different terminology must be kept in mind when faces are described in the anthropology literature.

Determining how much incisor prominence is too much can be difficult, especially when changes over time in public preference for both lip and chin prominence and ethnic differences are considered. This is simplified by understanding the relationship between lip posture and the position of the incisors. The teeth protrude excessively if (and only if) two conditions are met: (1) The lips are prominent and everted and (2) the lips are separated at rest by more than 3 to 4 mm (which is sometimes termed *lip incompetence*). In other words, excessive protrusion of the incisors is revealed by prominent lips that are separated when they are relaxed, so that the patient

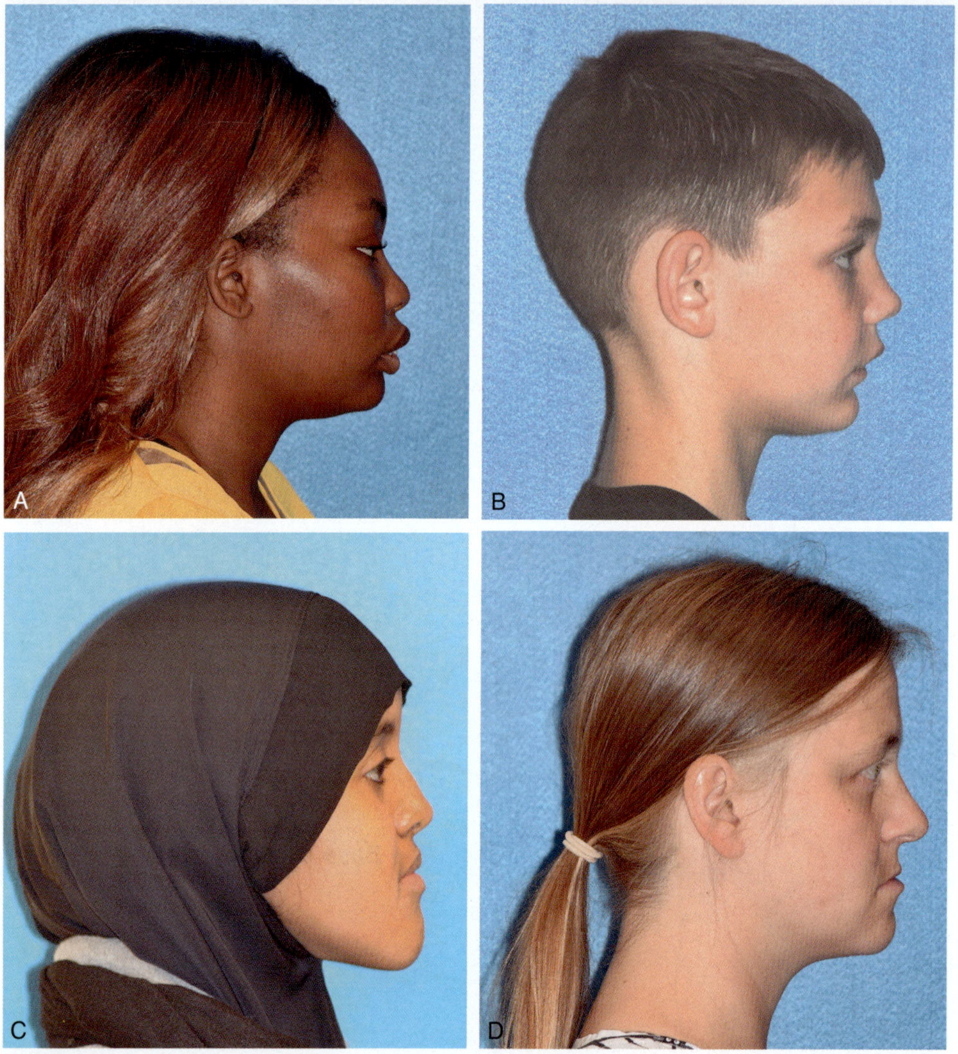

• **Fig. 6.22** These patients demonstrate facial skeletal discrepancies evident on clinical facial form analysis that were also confirmed by cephalometric evaluation. Patients A and B have class II malocclusions for different reasons. A has a protrusive maxilla and B, has a retrusive mandible. Patients C and D have class III malocclusions for different reasons. C has a protrusive mandible and D has a retrusive maxilla.

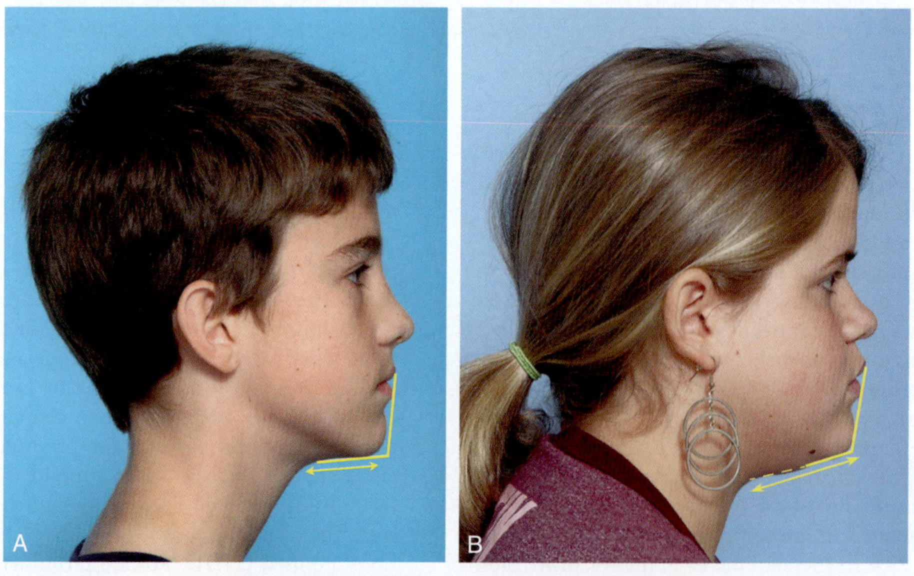

• **Fig. 6.23** Throat form is evaluated in terms of the contour of the submental tissues (straight is better), chin-throat angle (closer to 90 degrees is better), and throat length (longer is better, up to a point). Both submental fat deposition and a low tongue posture contribute to a stepped throat contour, which becomes a "double chin" when extreme. (A) For this boy who has a mild mandibular deficiency, throat contour and the chin-throat angle are good, but throat length is short, as usually is the case when the mandible is short. (B) For this girl with more chin projection, throat contour is affected by submental fat, and the chin-throat angle is somewhat obtuse, but throat length is good.

must strain to bring the lips together over the protruding teeth (see Fig. 6.26). For such a patient, retracting the teeth (possible either through extraction space, existing spacing, or interproximal reduction) tends to improve both lip function and facial esthetics. On the other hand, if the lips are prominent but close over the teeth without strain, the lip posture is largely

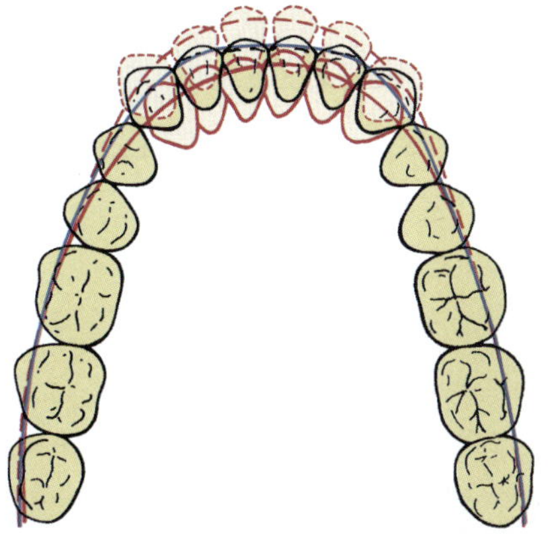

• **Fig. 6.24** If the incisors flare forward, they can align themselves along the arc of a larger circle, which provides more space to accommodate the teeth and alleviates crowding. Conversely, if the incisors move lingually, there is less space, and crowding becomes worse. For this reason, crowding and protrusion of incisors must be considered two aspects of the same thing; how crowded and irregular the incisors are reflects both how much room is available and where the incisors are positioned relative to supporting bone.

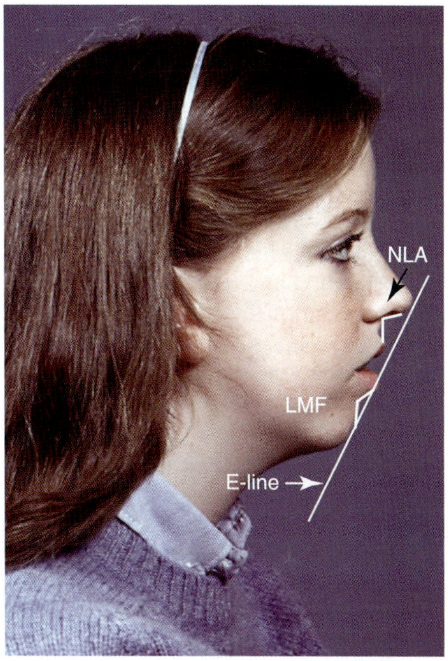

• **Fig. 6.26** Lip prominence is evaluated by observing several relationships while the lips are at rest. Lips that are more than 4 mm apart at rest or when there is lip strain to approximate them are most likely protrusive. The nasal labial angle (*NLA*) should be slightly obtuse and the labiomental fold (LMF) or sulcus should be obtuse. Another guide is the E-line that runs from the tip of the nose to the tip of the chin. Lips several millimeters posterior to this line are retrusive and currently lips can protrude to or slightly anterior to the line and be considered normal. Lips more anterior than that are protrusive.

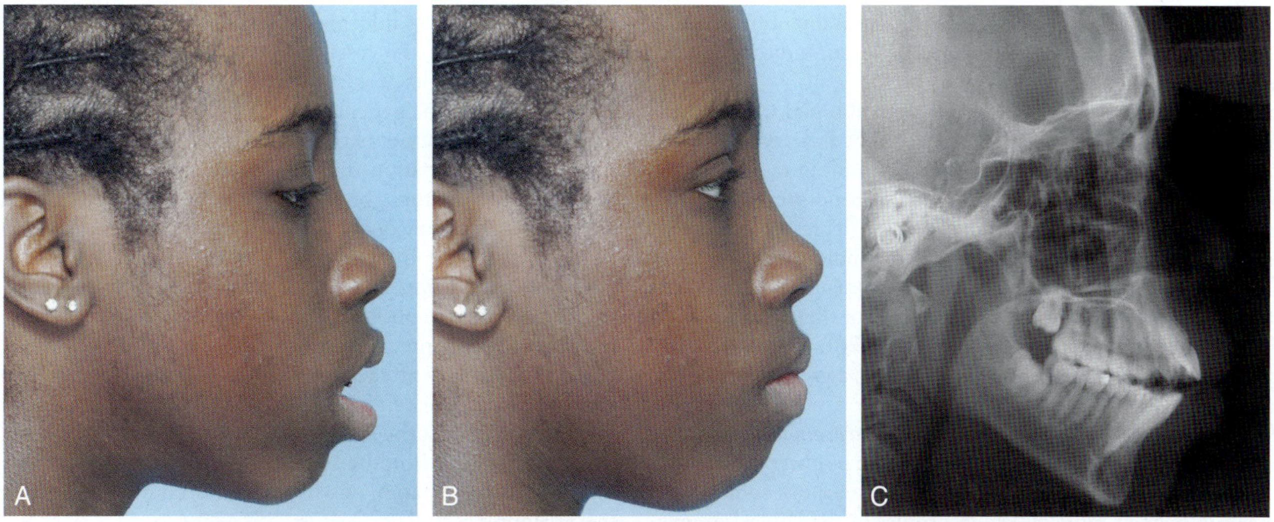

• **Fig. 6.25** Bimaxillary dentoalveolar protrusion is seen in the facial appearance in three ways. (A) Excessive separation of the lips at rest is called *lip incompetence*. The general guideline that holds for all racial groups is that lip separation at rest should be not more than 4 mm. (B) Excessive effort to bring the lips into closure creates lip strain and prominence of lips in the profile view, as shown in both (A) and (B). Remember that all these soft tissue characteristics must be present to make the diagnosis of dental protrusion, not just protruding teeth as seen in a cephalometric radiograph of the same girl. (C) Different racial groups and individuals within those groups have different degrees of lip prominence that are independent of tooth position. As a result, excessive dental protrusion must be a clinical diagnosis. It cannot be made accurately from cephalometric radiographs.

independent of tooth position. For that individual, retracting the incisor teeth would have little effect on lip function or prominence.

Lip prominence is strongly influenced by racial and ethnic characteristics and to a considerable extent also is age dependent (see Chapter 2). Whites of northern European backgrounds often have relatively thin lips, with minimal lip and incisor prominence. Whites of southern European and Middle Eastern origin normally have more lip and incisor prominence than their northern counterparts. Greater degrees of lip and incisor prominence normally occur in individuals of Asian and African descent, so a lip and tooth position normal for Asians or Blacks would be excessively protrusive for most whites. Although multiculturalism demonstrated by multiracial individuals has begun to blur these lines of distinction, more lip prominence now is being recognized as a desired esthetic quality.[23]

Lip posture and incisor prominence should be evaluated by viewing the profile with the patient's lips relaxed. In evaluating lip protrusion, it is important to keep in mind that everything is relative, and the lip relationships with the nose and chin affect the perception of lip fullness. The larger the nose, the more prominent the chin must be to balance it, and the greater the amount of lip prominence that will be esthetically acceptable. It can be helpful to look at lip prominence relative to a line from the tip of the nose to the chin (the E-line of cephalometric analysis), which can be visualized easily on clinical examination (see Figs. 6.15B and 6.26). The lips should be at or 1 to 2 mm anterior to the E-line, but this varies by the age of the patients and gender. If the lips are both prominent and incompetent (separated by more than 3–4 mm), the guideline is that the anterior teeth are excessively protrusive. Is that a problem? It depends on both the patient's perception and the cultural setting, not just on the objective evaluation.

Another helpful guideline is to consider the nasolabial angle, the angle between the ventral surface of the nose and the labial surface of the lip (see Fig. 6.26). A mildly obtuse angle is considered normal. A more acute angle can indicate dental and lip protrusion.

Vertical facial and dental relationships also play a role here. Some patients with short lower face height have everted and protrusive lips because they are overclosed (deep overbite and low mandibular plane angle) and the upper lip presses against the lower lip or because the upper incisor depresses the lower lip, not because the teeth protrude. One indicator of lip protrusion caused by overclosure is the labiomental fold angulation, the angle between the labial surface of the lower lip and the labial surface of the chin (see Fig. 6.26). Under normal conditions this is usually somewhat obtuse; a greatly decreased angle indicates overclosure.

4. *Reevaluation of vertical facial proportions and evaluation of mandibular plane angle.* Vertical proportions can be observed during the full-face examination (see previous section) but sometimes they can be seen more clearly in profile. In the clinical examination, the inclination of the mandibular plane to the true horizontal (or Frankfort Horizontal Plane if the patient is in near natural head position) should be noted. The mandibular plane is visualized readily by placing a finger or mirror handle along the lower border (Fig. 6.27). A steep mandibular plane angle usually accompanies long anterior facial vertical dimensions and a skeletal open bite tendency, whereas a flat mandibular plane angle often correlates with short anterior facial height and deep bite malocclusion. This is also a good time to validate the nearly equal vertical middle and lower facial thirds (see Figs. 6.15B, 6.19B, and 6.27).

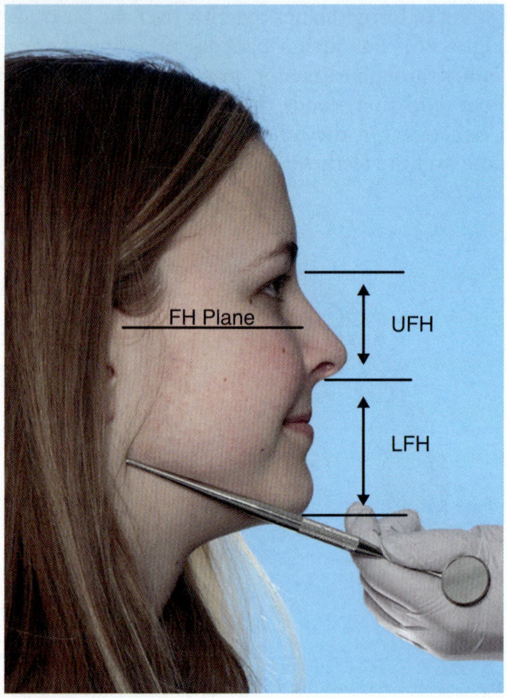

• **Fig. 6.27** The mandibular plane angle can be visualized clinically by placing a mirror handle or other instrument along the border of the mandible. For this patient, the mandibular plane angle is normal, neither too steep nor too flat. The middle and lower thirds of the face are also nearly equivalent.

Facial form analysis carried out this way takes only a couple of minutes but provides information that simply is not present from dental radiographs and casts. Such an evaluation by the primary care practitioner is an essential part of the evaluation of every prospective orthodontic patient.

During the macroesthetic examination, and in other parts of the clinical examination discussed later, it is important to note not only what is wrong, but also what is right. After all, you don't want to damage some of the good attributes of dentofacial appearance while treating the bad ones. For instance, in a patient with a well-supported upper lip and a deficient mandible, you would want to protect the position of the upper lip. Retraction of upper incisors in a patient who does not have a prominent upper lip can damage the dentofacial appearance. A common example is removal of maxillary first premolars in a patient with a deficient mandible to correct the class II malocclusion. While the problem, the malocclusion, is addressed, facial balance is not considered. This is a clear illustration of why it is important to note both positive attributes as well as negative.

Mini-esthetics: Tooth-Lip Relationships and Smile Analysis

Mini-esthetic issues deal with maxillary to mandibular midlines and their angulation, gingival display, transverse occlusal cant, buccal corridors, and smile arc (Fig. 6.28). Evaluation of tooth-lip relationships begins with an examination of symmetry, in which it is particularly important to note the relationship of the dental midline of each arch to the skeletal midline of that jaw (i.e., the

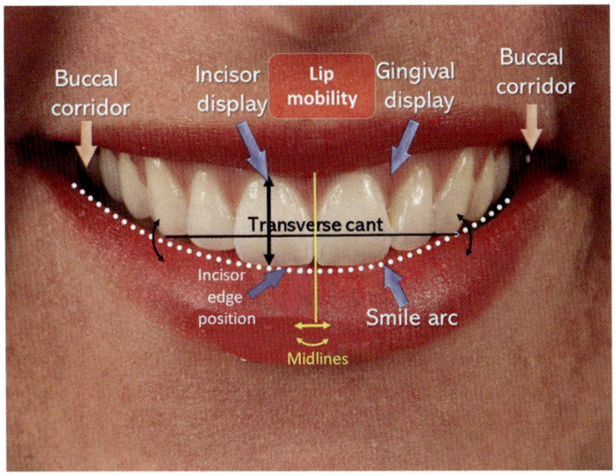

• **Fig. 6.28** Mini-esthetic issues deal with maxillary to mandibular midlines and their angulation, gingival and incisal display, transverse occlusal cant, buccal corridors and smile arc.

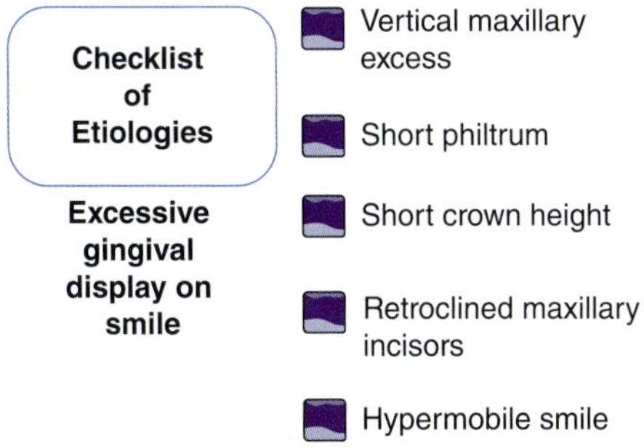

• **Fig. 6.30** Any of the above variables, (1) vertical maxillary excess (long-face syndrome), (2) short upper lip (philtrim), (3) short clinical crown height, (4) retroclined maxillary incisors, and (5) hypermobile smile. alone or in combination, can lead to excessive gingival display.

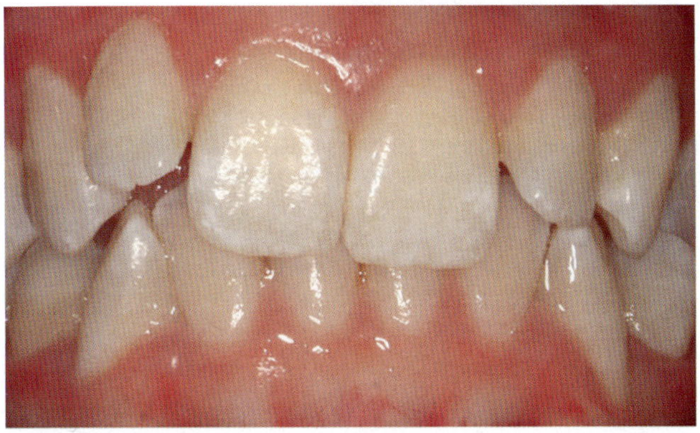

• **Fig. 6.29** These maxillary central incisors are tipped mesiodistally. Laypersons find this objectionable esthetically when the inclination of the mesial proximal surface of an incisor exceeds a 2-mm deviation from where you would expect the normal, slightly angulated, surface to intersect the occlusal plane.

lower incisor midline relative to the midline of the mandible, and the upper incisor midline relative to the midline of the maxilla).

The midlines can be influenced by another feature that draws negative attention to the smile, which is excessive inclination of the upper teeth as they tip toward the left or right (Fig. 6.29). Both dentists and laypersons notice a nonesthetic quality of the smile when this inclination exceeds a 2-mm deviation from the normal, but tolerate a tilt less than that.

These measurements can be obtained only through a direct clinical examination. Dental casts, even if mounted on an articulator, will show the relationship of the midlines to each other but provide no information about the dental-skeletal midlines. This must be recorded during the clinical examination.

A second aspect of dental–soft tissue relationships is the vertical relationship of the teeth to the lips at rest and on smile. During the clinical examination, it is important to note the amount of incisor display both at rest and on smile. For patients with excessive incisor display, (Fig. 6.30) there are five potential etiologies: (1) vertical maxillary excess (long-face syndrome), (2) short upper lip (philtrum), (3) short clinical crown height, (4) retroclined maxillary incisors, and (5) hypermobile smile. In an individual patient a gummy smile may be one of these factors or a combination of several of them. Recording lip height or length at the philtrum and the commissure height (from the base of the nose to a line horizontal line through the commissures) can clarify the source of the problem. Remember, however, that whatever the cause of excessive display, this tends to decrease with advancing age, so what looks like a problem at a younger age may not be as the patient gets older (see Fig. 4.28).

A third important relationship to note is whether an up-down transverse rotation of the dentition is revealed when the patient smiles or the lips are separated at rest (Fig. 6.31) there may be a *transverse cant of the occlusal plane* but is better described as a *transverse roll of the esthetic line of the dentition* (see the section in this chapter on classification by dentofacial traits). Neither dental casts nor a photograph with lip retractors will reveal this. Dentists detect a transverse roll at 1 mm from side to side, whereas laypersons are more forgiving and see it at 2.3 mm (2.8 degrees)—but at that point, it is a problem.[24,25]

Facial attractiveness is defined more by the smile than by soft tissue relationships at rest. For this reason, it is important to analyze the characteristics of the smile and to think about how the dentition relates to the facial soft tissues dynamically, as well as statically. There are two types of smiles: the posed or social smile and the enjoyment smile (also called the *Duchenne smile* in the research literature). The social smile is reasonably reproducible and is the one that is presented to the world routinely. The enjoyment smile varies with the emotion being displayed (for instance, the smile when you are introduced to a new colleague differs from the smile when your team just won the year's most important game). The social smile is the focus of orthodontic diagnosis.

In smile analysis, the oblique view and the frontal and profile views are important. It is important to keep in mind that these features of the smile are viewed differently by patients when the full face is the context (i.e., when they are looking into a large mirror mounted so that they can see their whole face at about 2-ft distance—the normal social distance of interaction), instead of just seeing their lips and teeth (as in a hand-held mirror that shows only part of the face or just the lips and teeth). When patients have complaints about these specific smile components, it is best to have them point out what concerns them while they are looking into a large mirror that lets them see their entire face—just as others will view them in real-life encounters.

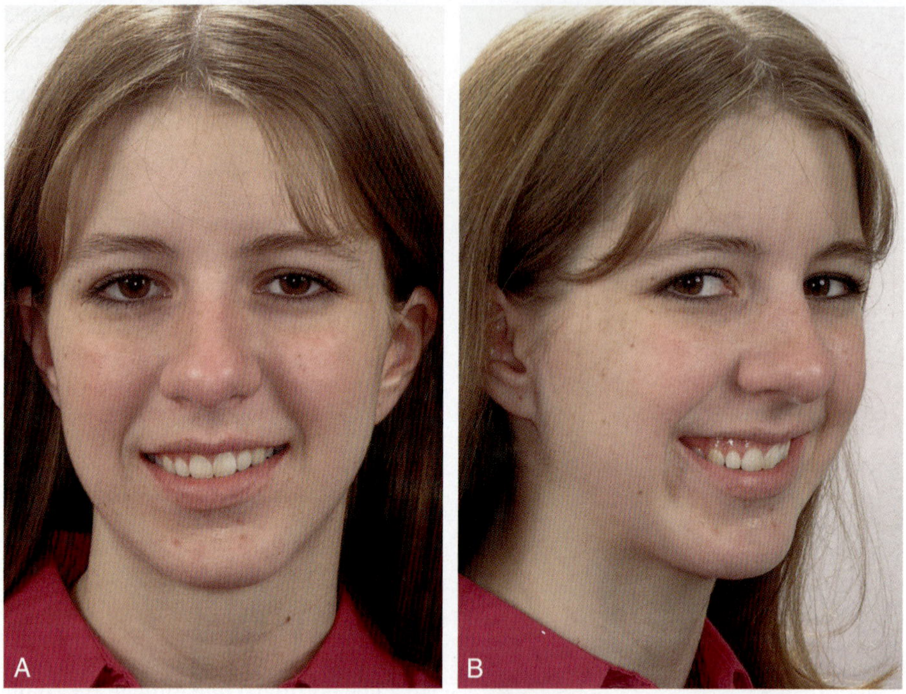

• **Fig. 6.31** A cant to the occlusal plane can be seen in both frontal (A) and oblique (B) views. This is a "roll deformity" that results from the orientation of the jaws and teeth rather than their position (roll is discussed further in the classification section of this chapter, later). It becomes an esthetic problem if it is noticeable, and lay observers do notice a cant of this degree of severity, or, in general, of 2–3 degrees to the horizontal.

TABLE 6.5 Smile Variables

Variable	Ideal	Maximum	Minimum
Variables Best Viewed in Full Face			
Smile arc	Tracks the lower lip	0.6 mm higher at canines	Greater than flat
Buccal corridor (as % black space of intercommissure width)			
Gingival display	2.3 mm tooth coverage	0.8 mm tooth coverage	4.5 mm tooth coverage
Occlusal cant	0	2.8 degrees	
Upper to lower dental midlines	0	3.6 mm	
Variables Viewed Either in Full Face or as Close-up of Lower Face			
Upper dental midline to face	0 mm	3.2 mm	
Upper central to central incisor gingival height discrepancy	0 mm	2.1 mm	
Upper lateral to central incisor gingival height discrepancy	−0.4 mm	0.4 mm	−1.9 mm
Overbite	2 mm	5.4 mm	0.9 mm
Upper central to lateral incisal edge step	1.2 mm	2.0 mm	

Data from Springer NC; Chang C, Fields HW, et al. Smile Esthetics from the Patients' Perspective. *Am J Orthod Dentofac Orthop.* 2011;140:e171–e180.

The following variables need to be considered, when conducting clinical smile assessment (Table 6.5).

1. *Amount of incisor and gingival display.* Using computer-altered photographs, recent research has established a range of acceptability for incisor and gingival display at the central incisors (Fig. 6.32).[25,26] Although some display of gingiva is acceptable and can be both esthetic and youthful appearing, the ideal elevation of the lip on smile for young adults is slightly below the gingival margin with approximately 2 mm of tooth coverage, so that most but not quite all of the upper incisor can be seen. More importantly, the acceptable range of tooth display is from minimal gingival display up to 4 to 5 mm coverage of the incisor crown. Beyond that, the smile appearance is less attractive.

   It also is important to remember that the vertical relationship of the lip to the incisors will change over time, with the amount of incisor exposure decreasing (see Chapter 4).[27] This

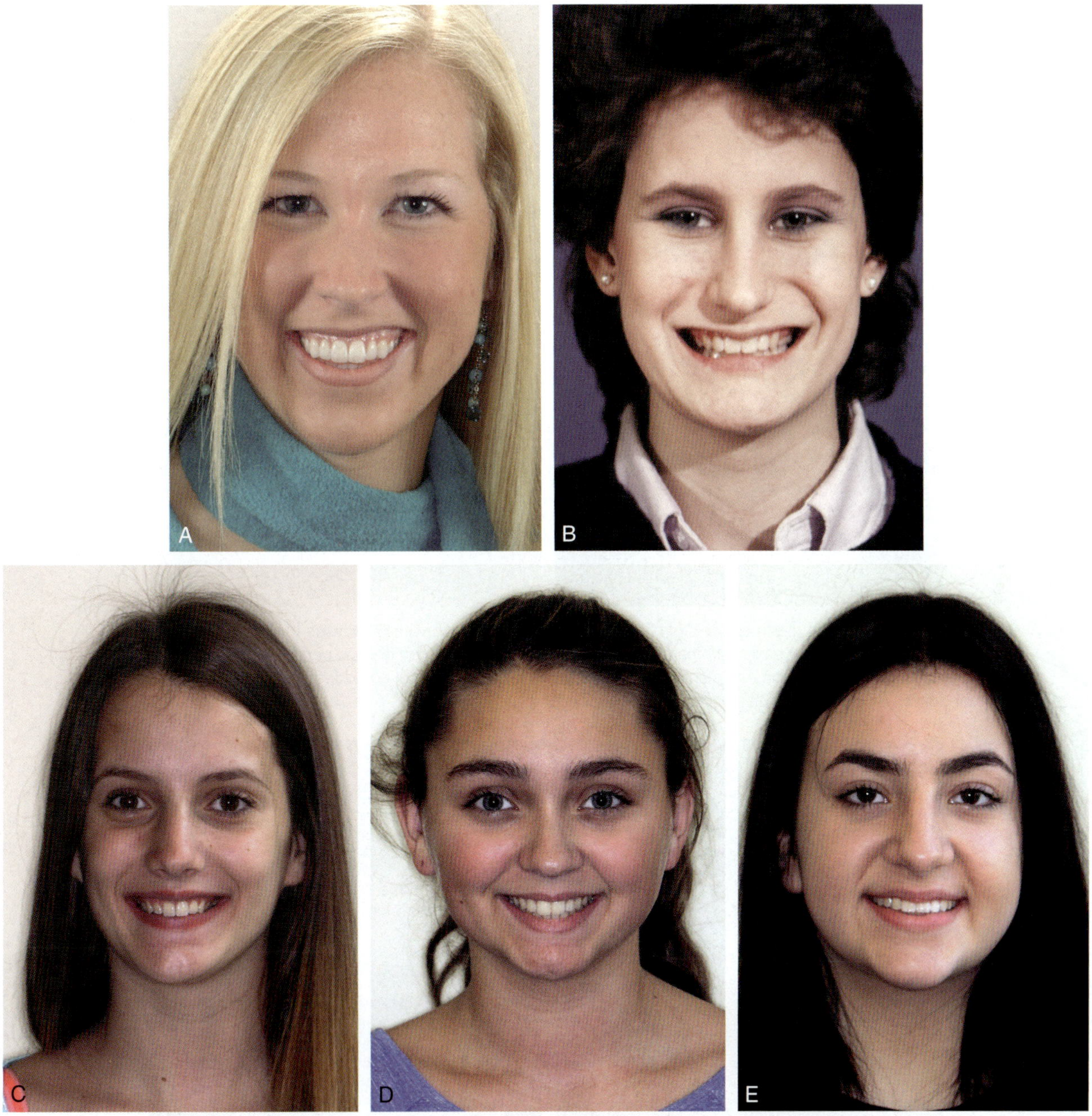

• **Fig. 6.32** (A) Display of all the maxillary incisors and some gingiva on smiling is a youthful and appealing characteristic. (B) No gingival display is less attractive, although it is not considered objectionable at this level by laypersons. (C) There is agreement among laypersons regarding the acceptable range of gingival and tooth display during a posed smile. This girl shows 1–2 mm of gingiva, which is the maximum acceptable amount on a social smile. (D) Overlap by the lip of the cervical margin of the tooth by 1–2 mm is ideal. (E) Tooth coverage by the lip of 4 mm is considered to be the maximum acceptable amount.

makes it even more important to note the vertical tooth-lip relationship during the diagnostic evaluation and to keep it in mind during treatment.

2. *Transverse dimensions of the smile relative to the upper arch.* There are several factors that can contribute to an esthetic balance in these dimensions (Fig. 6.33). Depending on the facial index (i.e., the width of the face relative to its height), a broad smile may be more attractive than a narrow one—but what does that mean exactly? A dimension of interest to prosthodontists, and more recently to orthodontists, is the amount of buccal corridor that is displayed on smile—that is, the distance between the maxillary posterior teeth (especially the premolars) and the inside of the cheek (Figs. 6.28 and 6.34).

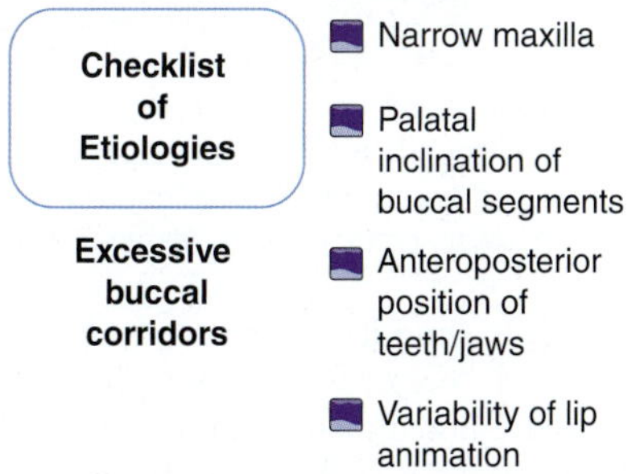

• **Fig. 6.33** The above factors can contribute to differences in the dark space between the posterior teeth and the inside of the cheek known as the buccal corridor. In extreme cases, this can be nonesthetic.

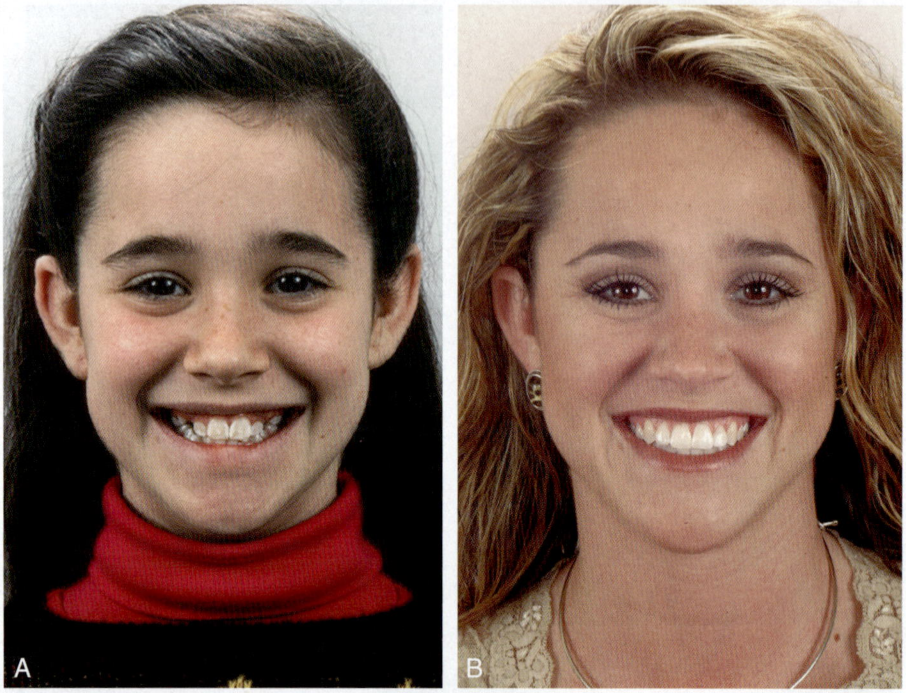

• **Fig. 6.34** (A) Before treatment, this girl had a narrow maxillary arch with quite wide buccal corridors. (B) On 5-year recall, the broader smile (with narrow but not obliterated buccal corridors) is part of the esthetic improvement created by orthodontic treatment. It must be remembered that buccal corridor evaluation is subjective and that during clinical studies it has been shown to be unreliable.

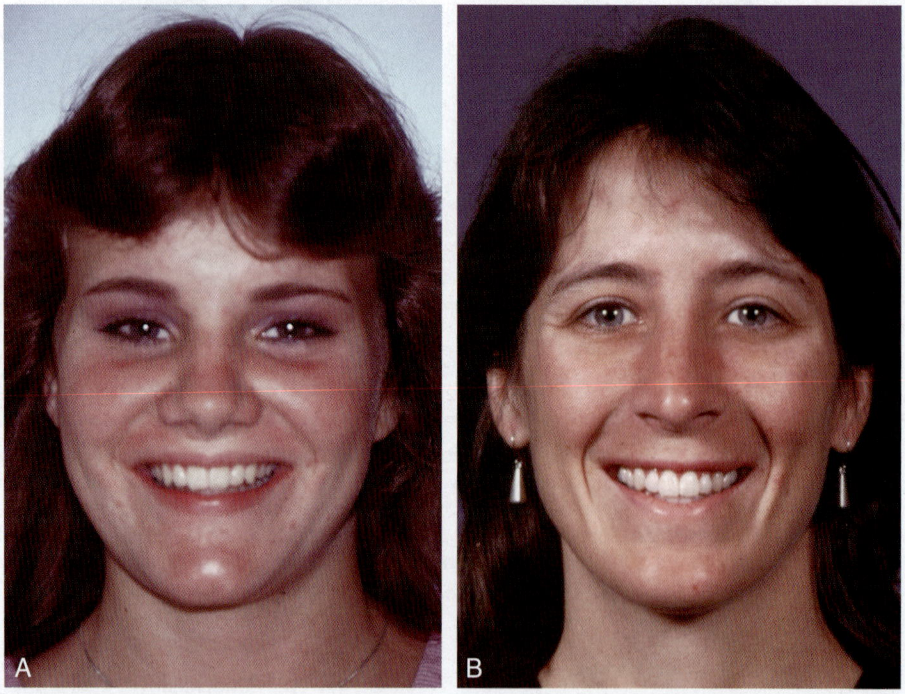

• **Fig. 6.35** The width of the maxillary dental arch, as seen on smile, should be proportional to the width of the midface. (A) A broad smile is appropriate for a face with relatively large width across the zygomatic arches, but a narrower smile (B) is preferred when the face width is narrow. The patient in (B) was appropriately treated with maxillary premolar extraction to prevent overexpansion during treatment.

Prosthodontists consider excessively wide buccal corridors (sometimes called "negative space") to be nonesthetic, and orthodontists have noted that widening the maxillary arch can improve the appearance of the smile if cheek drape is significantly wider than the dental arch. Although minimal buccal corridors are favored by most observers, especially in females, the transverse width of the dental arches can and should be related to the width of the face (Fig. 6.35). Too broad an upper arch, so that there is no buccal corridor, is nonesthetic. The relationship of the cheeks to the posterior teeth on smile is just

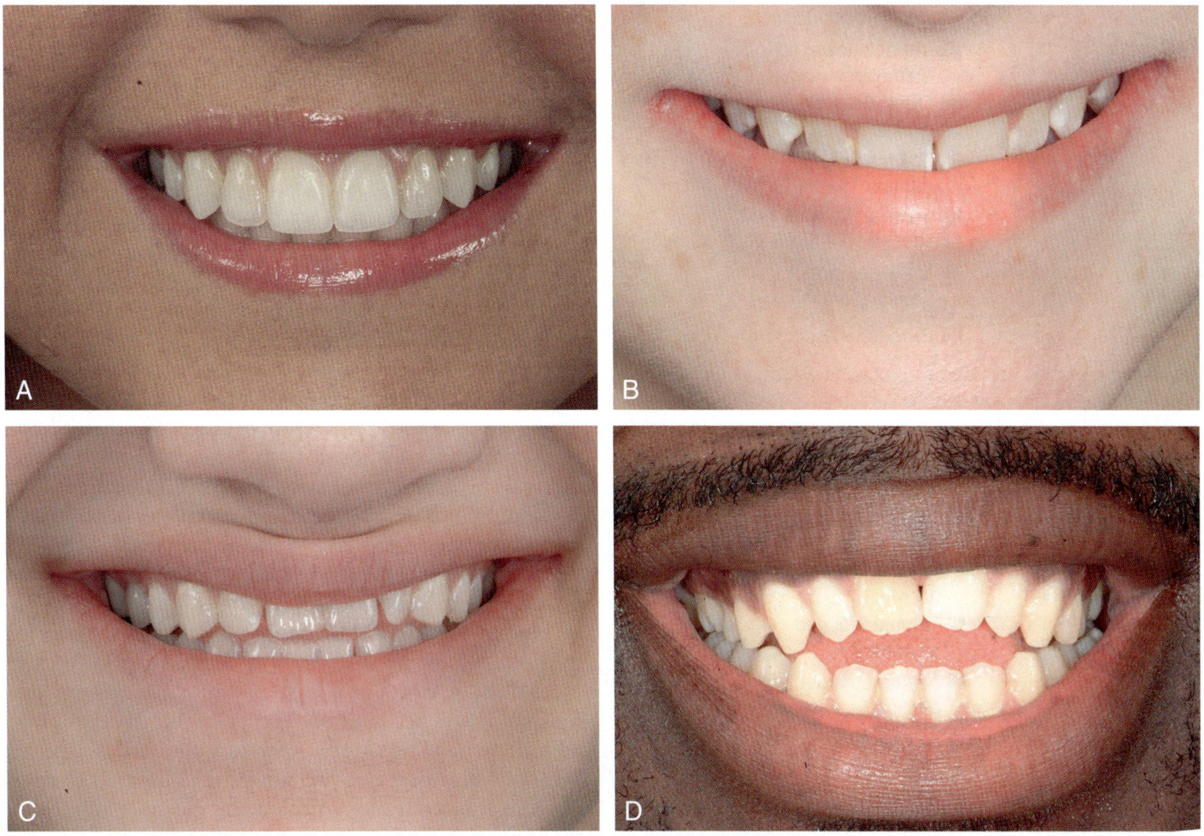

• **Fig. 6.36** There is great variation in smile arcs. (A) The ideal smile arch is defined as one where the contours of the incisal edges of the maxillary anterior teeth track the curvature of the lower lip. If the lip and dental contours match, they are said to be consonant. (B) This excessive smile arch shows none of the lower incisal edge, but the incisal edges of the lateral incisors and canine cusp tips are visible or nearly so. (C) A flat smile arc (nonconsonant) is just that and can pose either or both of two problems: It is less attractive, and it tends to make you look older (because older individuals often have wear of the incisors that tends to flatten the arc of the teeth). The characteristics of the smile arc must be monitored during orthodontic treatment. It is the most important factor in smile esthetics. (D) The reverse smile arc contrasts with the lip line in most cases and is often related to an anterior open bite.

another way of evaluating the width of the dental arches. But, this measure has proven unreliable.

3. *The smile arc*. The smile arc is traditionally defined as the contour of the incisal edges of the maxillary anterior teeth relative to the curvature of the lower lip during a social smile (Fig. 6.36). For best appearance, the contour of the incisal edges of these teeth should parallel the curvature of the lower lip. If the lip and dental contours match, they are said to be consonant. Another way to evaluate the smile arc is to evaluate the entire maxillary occlusal plane based on the oblique view (Fig. 6.37). There are numerous etiologies of an apparent nonconsonant smile arc (Fig. 6.38).

   A flattened (nonconsonant) smile arc can pose either or both of two problems: It is less attractive, and it tends to make you look older (because older individuals often have wear of the incisors that tends to flatten the arc of the teeth). The characteristics of the smile arc must be monitored during orthodontic treatment because it is surprisingly easy to flatten it in the pursuit of other treatment objectives. The data indicate that

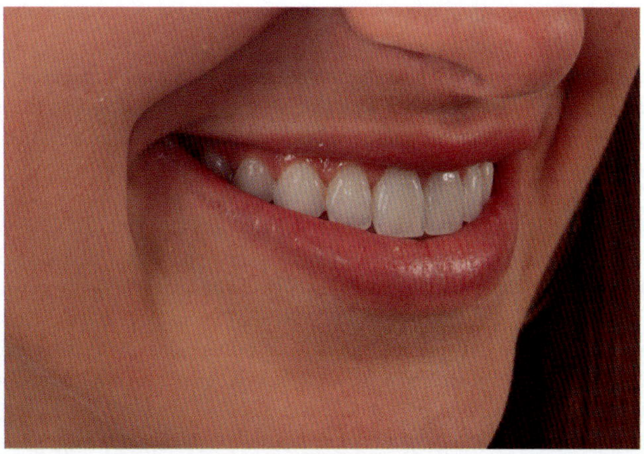

• **Fig. 6.37** Smile arcs can be evaluated from the frontal or oblique view. This oblique view provides good a perspective of the incisors and the canines and premolars so it is possible to evaluate the arc of the entire occlusal plane.

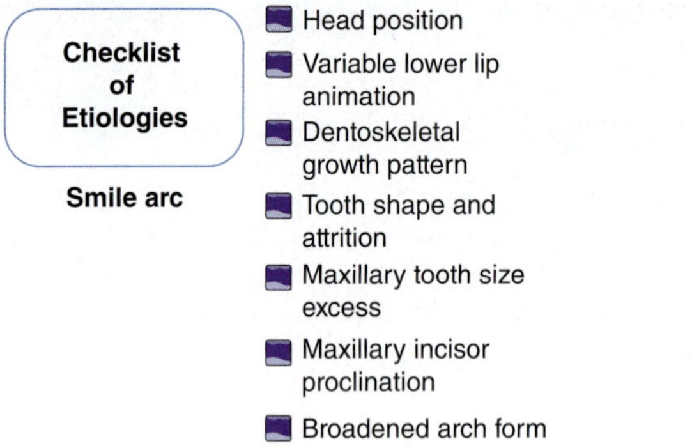

• **Fig. 6.38** These variables can lead to problems with ideal smile arcs. Because this is an interaction between the vertical and transverse dimensions of the lips and the teeth, changes that affect them can lead to imbalance and disproportions. Clearly, it is easier to alter the teeth than the lips.

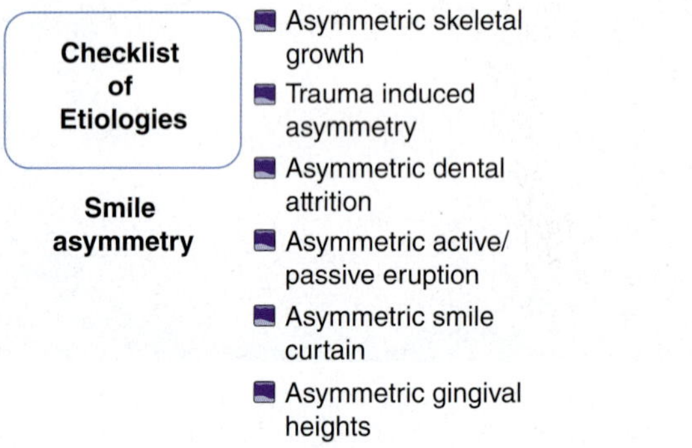

• **Fig. 6.39** The variables listed here can cause smile asymmetry and can be based among gingival, dental, facial soft tissue, or skeletal etiologies.

it is the most important factor in smile esthetics, the only one that by itself can change the rating of a smile from acceptable to nonesthetic, is the smile arc.[28]

4. *Smile asymmetries*

Smile asymmetries can have several causes: asymmetric facial growth or trauma-induced skeletal asymmetry, asymmetric dental attrition, asymmetric active/passive eruption, asymmetric smile curtain, asymmetric smile animation, or asymmetric gingival heights (Figs. 6.39 and 6.40).

Although there are modest differences among nationalities and ethnic groups in their judgment of smile esthetics,[29,30] the acceptable ranges had some commonality for groups that were predominantly of European descent. Similar data for Asian and African groups are beginning to emerge.

Microesthetics: Close-up Dental Appearance

Subtleties in the proportions and shape of the teeth and associated gingival contours have been emphasized in the burgeoning literature on "cosmetic dentistry" in recent years (Fig. 6.41). These factors must be considered in the development of an orthodontic problem list if an optimal esthetic result is to be obtained, and treatment planning to correct them is discussed in Chapter 7 along with the orthodontic aspects of maximally esthetic treatment.

Tooth Proportions. The smile, of course, reveals the maxillary anterior teeth, and two aspects of proportional relationships are important components of their appearance: the tooth widths in relation to one another and the height-width proportions of the individual teeth.

Width Relationships and the "Golden Proportion". The apparent widths of the maxillary anterior teeth on smile, and their actual mesiodistal width, differ because of the curvature of the dental arch such that not all of the lateral incisors and only a portion of the canine crowns can be seen in a frontal view. For best appearance, the apparent width of the lateral incisor (as one would perceive it from a direct frontal examination) should be 62% of the width of the central incisor, the apparent width of the canine should be 62% of that of the lateral incisor, and the apparent width of the first premolar should be 62% of that of the canine (Fig. 6.42). This ratio of recurring 62% proportions appears in a number of other relationships in human anatomy and sometimes is referred to as the "golden proportion." Whether it has any mystical significance or not, it is an excellent guideline when lateral incisors are disproportionately small or (less frequently) large, and the width ratios of the central and lateral are the best way to determine what the posttreatment size of the lateral incisor should be. The same judgment is used when canines are narrowed to replace missing lateral incisors.

Height-Width Relationships. The range in height-width relationships for maxillary central incisors is shown in Fig. 6.43. Note that the width of a visible tooth (i.e., incisors through premolars) should be about 80% of its height. In examining an orthodontic patient, it is important to note both height and width because if disproportions are noted, this allows a determination of which is at fault. If the vertical measurement is short for the width the incisors look nearly square. There are several possible causes: incomplete eruption in a child (active eruption), or periodontal maturation (passive eruption) both of which may correct themself with further development. Loss of crown height from attrition in an older patient may indicate restoration of the missing part of the crown is needed. Excessive gingival height is best treated with crown lengthening. Perhaps an inherent malformation of crown form could suggest a more extensive restoration with facial laminates or a complete crown (see Chapter 20). The disproportion and its probable cause should be included in the patient's problem list to focus attention on doing something about it before orthodontic treatment is completed.

Connectors and Embrasures. These elements, illustrated in Fig. 6.41, also can be of real significance in the appearance of the smile and should be noted as problems if they are incorrect. The connector (also referred to as the interdental contact area) is where adjacent teeth appear to touch and may extend apically or occlusally from the actual contact point. In other words, the actual contact point is likely to be a very small area, and the connector includes both the contact point and the areas above and below that are so close together they look as if they are touching. The normal connector height is greatest between the central incisors and diminishes from the centrals to the posterior teeth, moving apically in a progression from the central incisors to the premolars and molars. The embrasures (the triangular spaces incisal and gingival to the contact) ideally are larger in size than the connectors, and the gingival embrasures are filled by the interdental papillae.

Embrasures: Black Triangles. Short interdental papillae leave an open gingival embrasure above the connectors, and these "black triangles" can detract significantly from the appearance of the teeth on smile, especially when they reach 2 to 3 mm.[31] Black triangles in adults usually arise from loss of gingival tissue related to periodontal disease, but when crowded and rotated maxillary

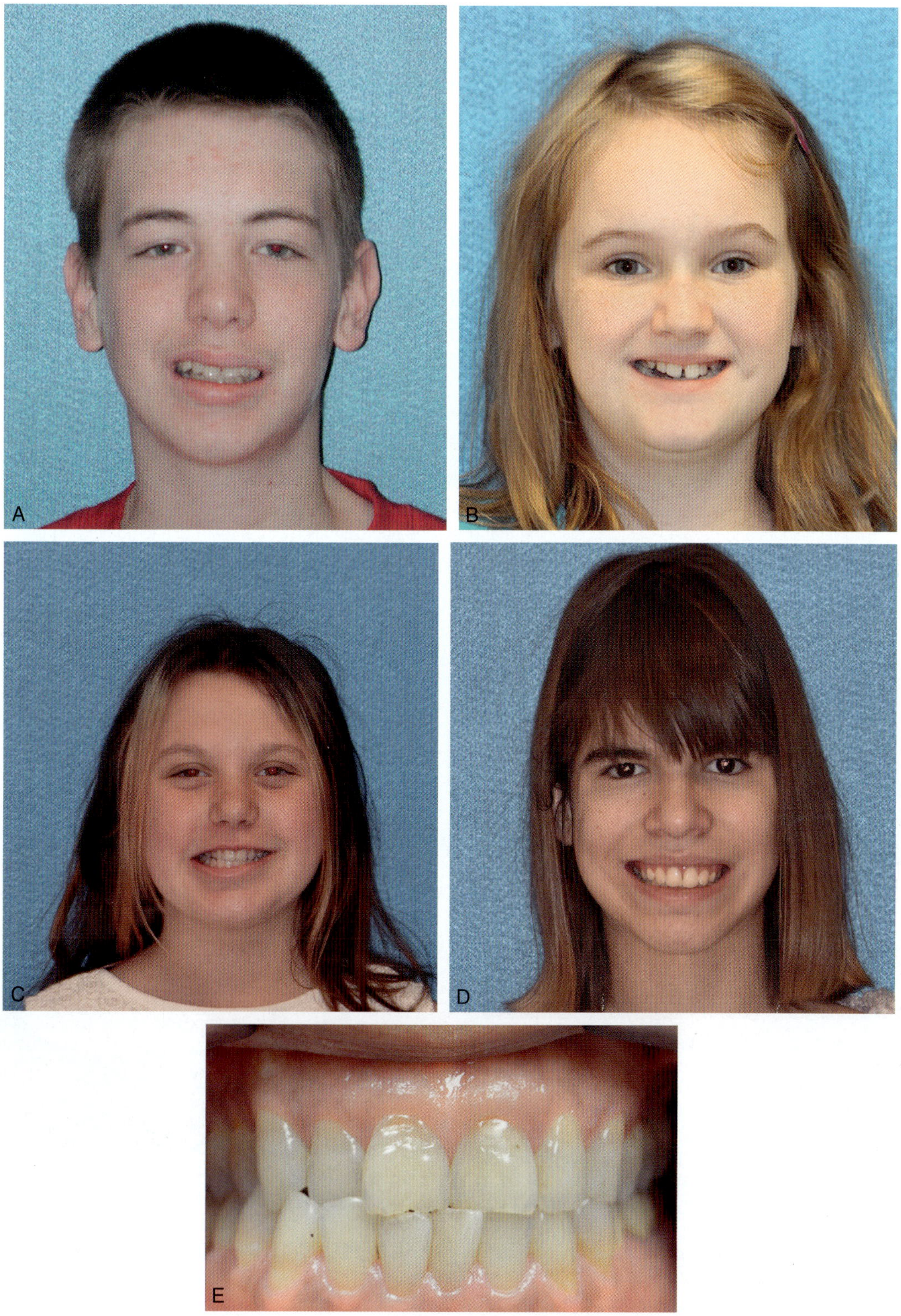

• **Fig. 6.40** The causes of smile asymmetry can include: (A) skeletal asymmetry from developmental problems or trauma, Note the mandible deviates to the right and is accompanied by the asymmetry and an occlusal cant. (B) Asymmetric active eruption is evident in the maxillary right anterior teeth leading to this asymmetric smile. (C) This is an asymmetric smile from asymmetric soft tissue animation. This has not caused dental changes due to the short duration of the animations and little effect on soft tissue equilibrium. (D) The asymmetric smile is due to the more incisal gingival margin levels on the left than the right, in spite of the reasonably level occlusal plane, most likely due to the differences in passive eruption of erupted teeth. (E) The incisal wear of this patient has caused an asymmetry due to the cant of the occlusal plane that is more inferior on the left.

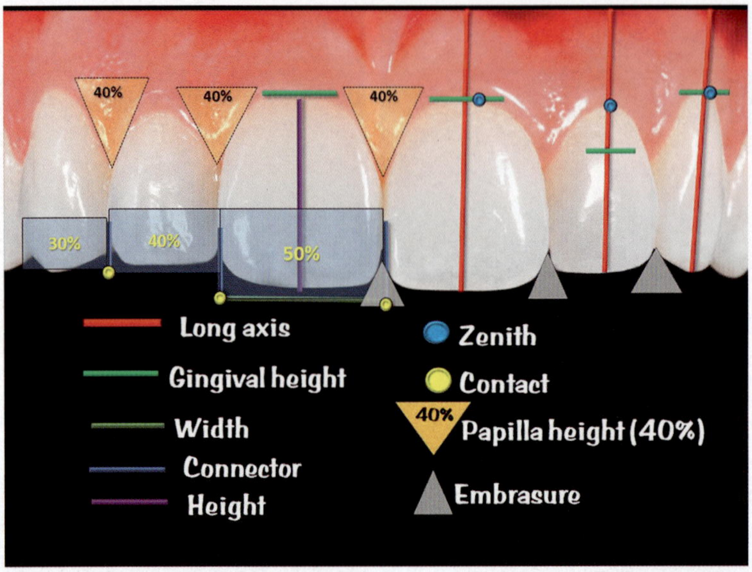

• **Fig. 6.41** This is a summary of the microethetic elements of a smile that deal with the dental proportions, gingival heights and detailed dental positioning that effect the approximation of the teeth to each other and the gingival contours.

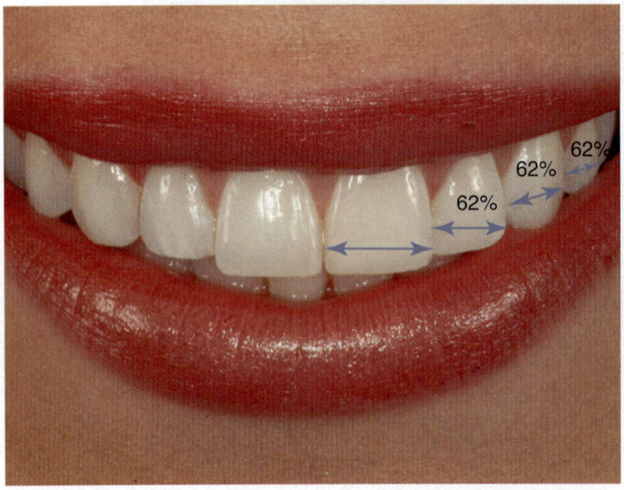

• **Fig. 6.42** Ideal tooth width proportions when viewed from the front are one of many illustrations of the "golden proportion"—1.0 : 0.62 : 0.38 : 0.24, and so on. In this close-up view of attractive teeth on smile, it can be seen that the width of the lateral incisor is 62% of the width of the central incisor; the apparent width of the canine is 62% of the width of the lateral incisor; and the apparent width of the first premolar is 62% of the width of the canine—which is the other way of representing the golden proportion.

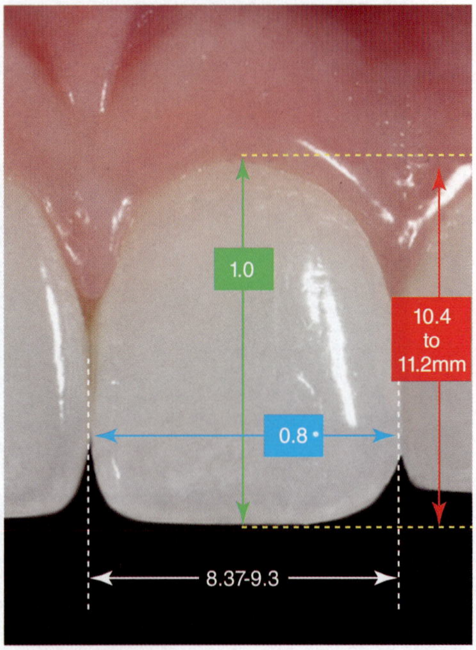

• **Fig. 6.43** (A) Height-width proportions for maxillary central incisors, with the normal range of widths and heights. The width of the tooth should be about 80% of its height. How to manage changes in height-width proportions will depend on multiple mini- and macroesthetic considerations.

incisors are corrected orthodontically in adults, the connector moves incisally and black triangles may appear, especially if severe crowding was present (Fig. 6.44). For that reason, both actual and potential black triangles should be noted during the orthodontic examination, and the patient should be prepared for reshaping of the teeth to minimize this esthetic problem.

Gingival Heights, Shape, Contour, and Color. Proportional gingival heights are needed to produce a normal and attractive dental dimensional gradation (Fig. 6.41). In general, the central incisor has the highest gingival level, the lateral incisor is approximately 1.5 mm lower, and the canine gingival margin again is at the level of the central incisor. Maintaining these gingival relationships becomes particularly important when canines are used to replace missing lateral incisors or when other tooth substitutions are planned. Both laypersons and dentists readily recognize differences of more than 2 mm and unilateral occurrences are distracting.

Gingival shape refers to the curvature of the gingiva at the margin of the tooth. For best appearance, the gingival shape of the maxillary lateral incisors should be a symmetric half-oval or half-circle. The maxillary centrals and canines should exhibit a gingival shape that is more elliptical and oriented distally to the long axis of the tooth (see Fig. 6.41). The gingival zenith (the most apical point of the gingival tissue) should be located distal to the longitudinal

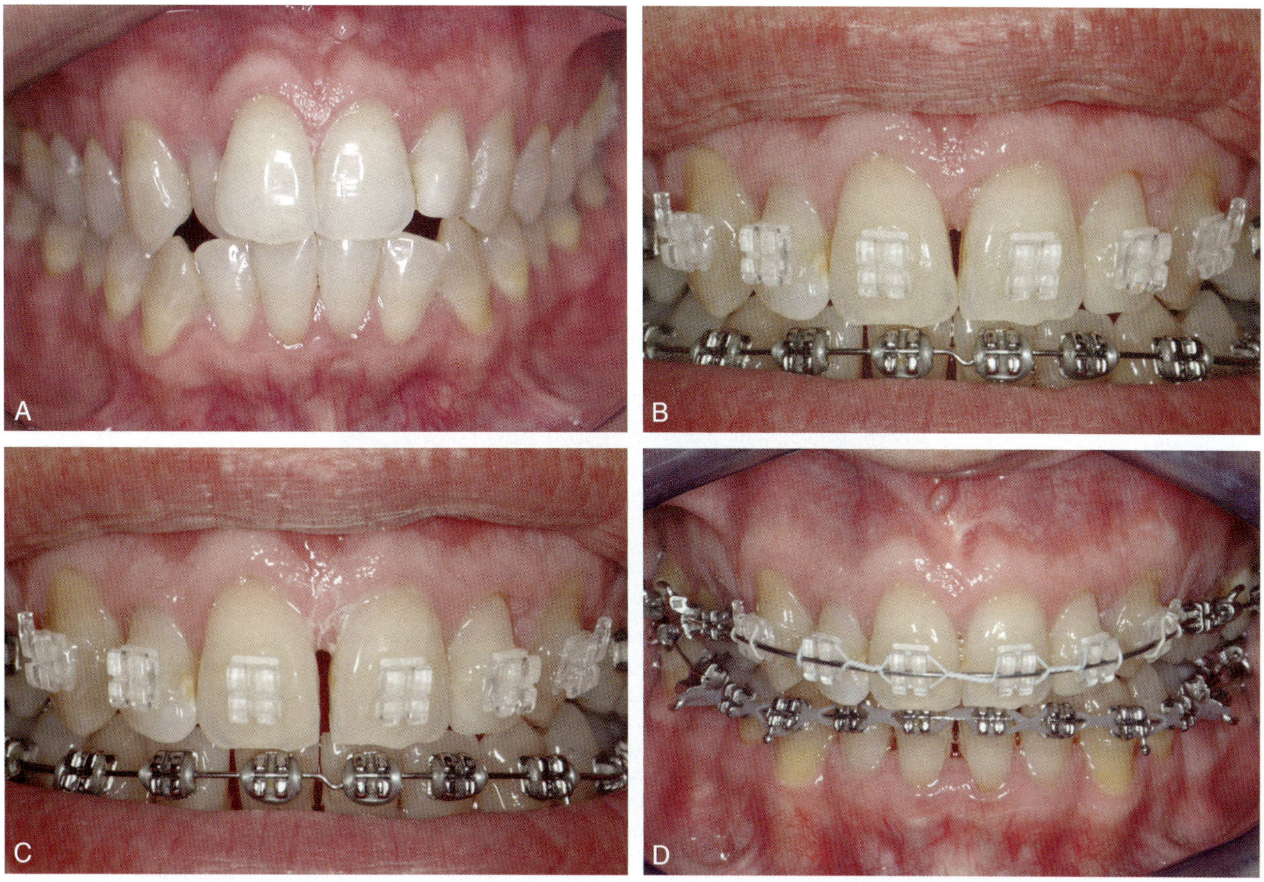

• **Fig. 6.44** (A) Crowded and rotated maxillary incisors at the beginning of orthodontic treatment in an adult. (B) After alignment of the incisors, a black triangle was present between the central incisors. (C) With the orthodontic appliance still in place, the incisors were reshaped so that when the contact point would be moved apically the midline connector would be lengthened. (D) After the space was closed the black triangle was no longer apparent.

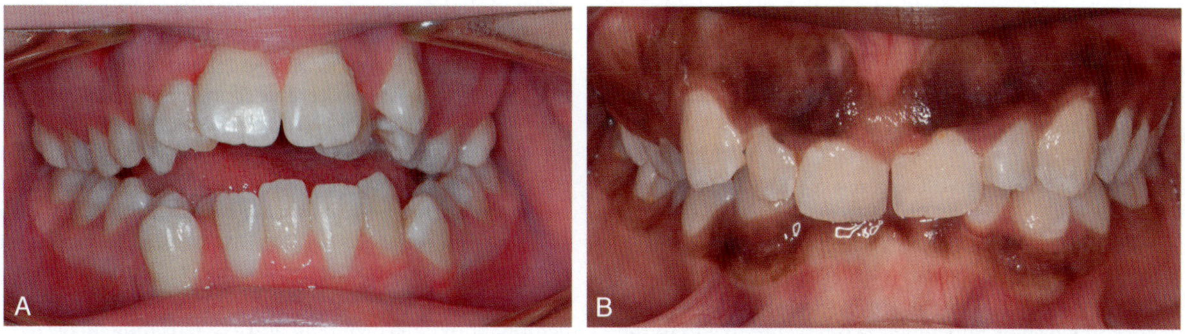

• **Fig. 6.45** (A) Gingival inflammation and (B) patchy pigmentation are considered unattractive. Although inflammation can be generalized or localized, the color change attracts attention. Gingival pigmentations is not uncommon among various ethnic and racial groups. It is the unevenness, like seen in (B) that attracts attention. (Courtesy Dr. Samantha Marks)

axis of the maxillary centrals and canines; the gingival zenith of the maxillary laterals should coincide with their longitudinal axis.

Other than black triangles, variations in gingival color are considered most unattractive, when they are the result of papillary gingival inflammation and patchy pigmentation (Fig. 6.45).

Tooth Shade and Color. The color and shade of the teeth change with increasing age, and many patients perceive this as a problem. The teeth appear lighter and brighter at a younger age and darker and duller as aging progresses (Fig. 6.46). This is related to the formation of secondary dentin as pulp chambers decrease in size and to thinning of the facial enamel, which results in a decrease in its translucency and a greater contribution of the darker underlying dentin to the shade of the tooth. A normal progression of shade change from the midline posteriorly is an important contributor to an attractive and natural-appearing smile. The maxillary central incisors tend to be the brightest in the smile, the lateral incisors less so, and the canines the least bright– known as tonal gradation.[32] The first and second premolars are more closely matched to the lateral incisors. They are lighter and brighter than the canines (see Fig. 6.46C).

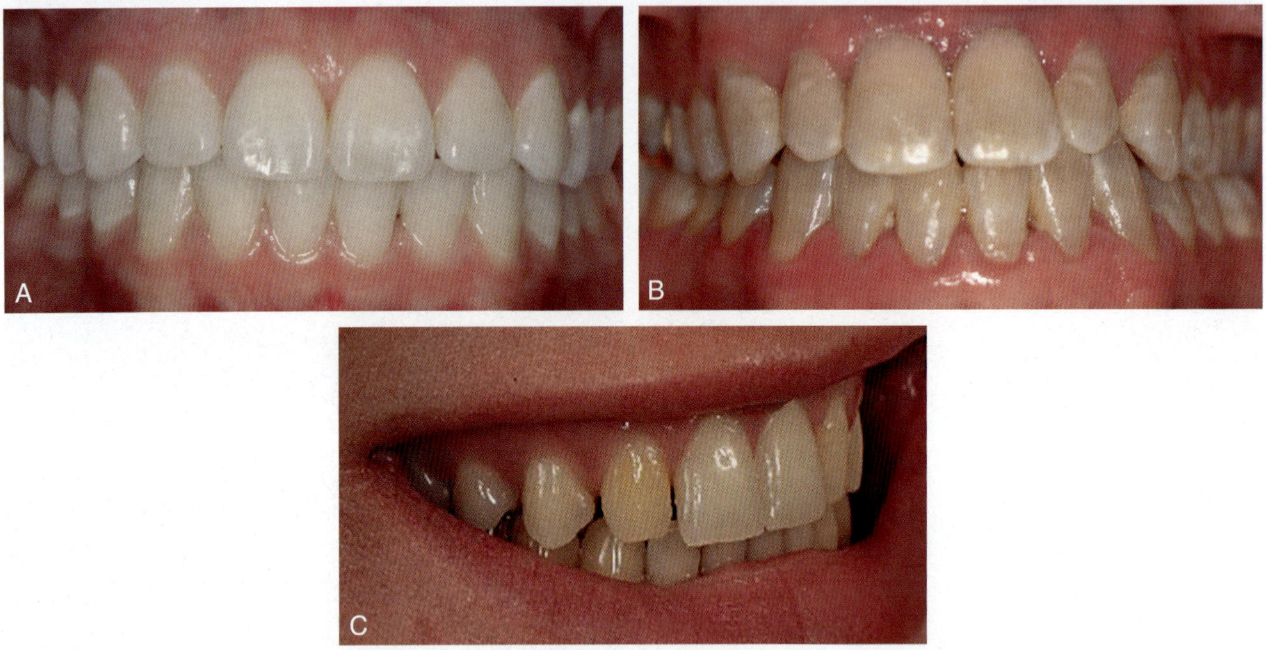

• **Fig. 6.46** (A) The teeth in younger patients show less incisal and occlusal wear and have more ideal shape because they have not been restored. Their color is also lighter even without whitening agents. (B) These teeth belong to an older patient and demonstrate extrinsic staining and likely pulpal obliteration along with more wear, decalcifications, and restoration. (C) Tonal gradation, which is the differing light and darkness of the teeth from the central incisors through the premolars. Note the lighter centrals, darker canines and then lighter premolars.

At present, even young patients are quite likely to be aware of the possibility of bleaching their teeth to provide a more youthful appearance and may benefit from having this done at the end of orthodontic treatment. If color and shade of the teeth are a potential problem, this should be on the orthodontic problem list so that it is included in the final treatment plan if the patient desires it. It is important to recognize that any restorations will not be lightened by bleaching, so they may need to be replaced or modified to match the final color.

Diagnostic Records

Which Diagnostic Records Are Needed?

Which orthodontic records are ideal is not a clear-cut or simple judgment and depends on the problems that exist and the type of treatment anticipated.[33] Orthodontic diagnostic records are taken for two purposes: to document the starting point for treatment (after all, if you do not know where you started, it is hard to tell where you are going or how far you have come), and to add to the information gathered on clinical examination. It is important to remember that the records are supplements to, not replacements for, the clinical examination.

Orthodontic records fall into the same three major categories used for development of the diagnostic database: those for evaluation of the (1) health of the teeth and oral structures, (2) alignment and occlusal relationships of the teeth, and (3) facial and jaw proportions, which include both facial photographs, cephalometric radiographs, and computed tomography (CT) images, if necessary. Digital photography now has replaced film, digital images have done the same for radiographs and digital casts have replaced plaster.

Records for Health of Teeth and Oral Structures

A major purpose of intraoral photographs, which should be obtained routinely for patients undergoing complex orthodontic treatment, is to document the initial condition of the hard and soft tissues. Five standard intraoral photographs are suggested: right, center, and left views with the teeth in occlusion, and maxillary and mandibular occlusal views (Fig. 6.47). Maximum lateral retraction of the cheeks and lips is needed. If there is a special soft tissue problem (for instance, no attached gingiva in the lower anterior or palatal impingement on the maxillary lingual tissue), additional photographs of those area areas are needed.

Current guidelines for growth and development radiographs developed by the American Dental Association (ADA) and the US Department of Health and Human Services for new or recall patients were revised in 2012. A panoramic radiograph is valuable for orthodontic evaluation at most ages beyond the early mixed dentition years. The panoramic image has two significant advantages over a series of intraoral radiographs: It yields a broader view and thus is more likely to show any pathologic lesions and supernumerary or impacted teeth, and the radiation exposure is much lower. It also gives a view of the mandibular condyles, which can be helpful, both in its own right and as a screening image to determine if tomography (CBCT) or magnetic resonance imaging (MRI) of the joint is needed. TMJ symptoms often are due to problems with the intraarticular disc or the ligaments that suspend it, which cannot be seen in radiographs, but can be seen with MRI. Imaging of the TMJ and recommendations for current practice are covered in detail in an overview based on a multisite study.[34]

The panoramic radiograph should be supplemented with periapical or occlusal radiographs only when greater detail is required. In addition, for children and adolescents, periapical views of incisors are indicated if there is evidence or suspicion of root resorption, periodontal disease or previous trauma. Pretreatment radiographs for adults (those over 18 years old) should include a panoramic radiograph, bitewings and periapical radiographs, according to the American Board of Orthodontics. [35] The principle is that periapical or other radiographs to supplement the panoramic radiograph

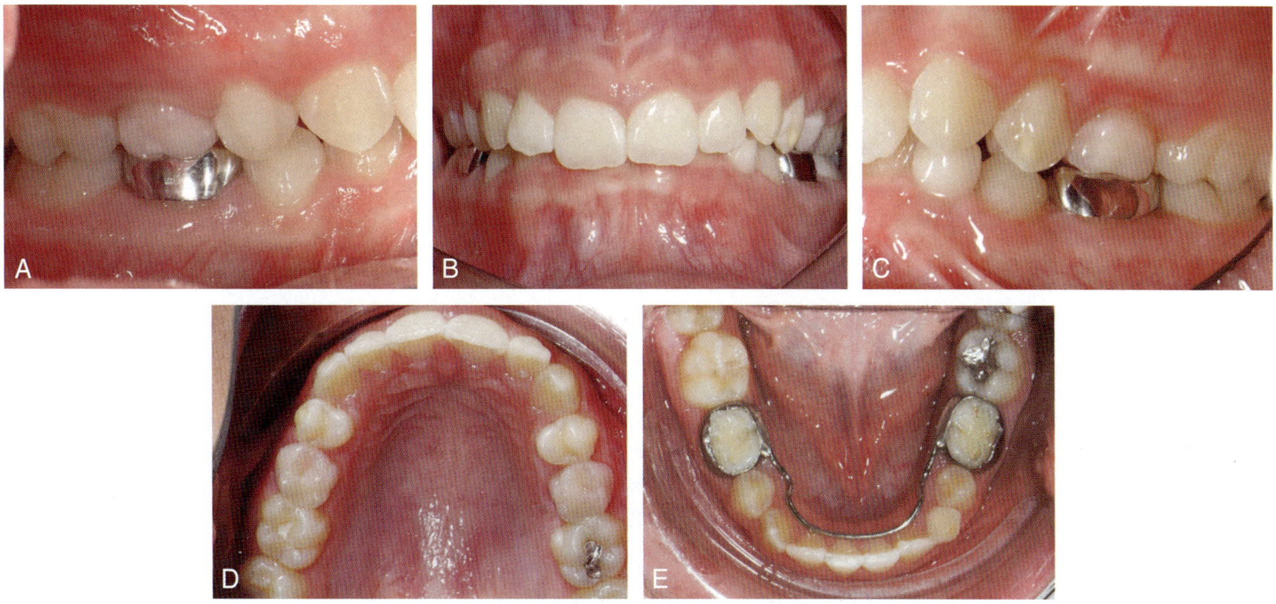

• **Fig. 6.47** (A–E) Patient F.P., age 12 years 3 months, intraoral views before treatment. There is moderate maxillary incisor crowding, with the midline off due to displacement of the maxillary incisors. The maxillary incisors are tipped lingually, there is minimal overjet despite class II buccal segments, and overbite is excessive. A pediatric dentist had placed a lingual arch to maintain alignment of the lower incisors.

are ordered only if there is a specific indication for doing so, in order to keep the amount of radiation to a minimum that is consistent with obtaining the necessary diagnostic information.

A frequent problem that deserves radiographic follow-up is localization of an unerupted maxillary canine that cannot be palpated in the buccal vestibule at dental age 10. Now that CBCT has become widely available, it is the preferred method for localizing canines (Fig. 6.48). Both the position of the impacted tooth and the extent of damage to the roots of other teeth can be evaluated better with true three-dimensional (3D) images. The use of 3D imaging, including its possible replacement of panoramic and cephalometric radiographs, is discussed further in the section of this chapter on analysis of these images.

Dental Records

Evaluation of the occlusion requires two things: impressions for dental casts or digital scanning into computer memory, and a record of the occlusion (either a wax bite or a buccal scan) so that the casts or images can be related to each other. For some, but not all patients, a facebow transfer of the dental casts to an articulator may be needed. The following paragraphs consider this in greater detail.

Physical Versus Virtual Casts

Whether physical plaster or virtual orthodontic diagnostic casts are to be produced, an impression of the teeth that also gives maximum displacement of the lips and cheeks is desired. Being able to visualize the inclination of the teeth, not just the location of the crown, is important. If the impression is not well extended, important diagnostic information may be missing. If the impressions are to be poured in dental stone without great delay, alginate impressions are satisfactory; if virtual models will be produced, a more accurate and stable impression material (such as modified alginate or polysiloxane) should be used. At this point, direct intraoral scanning of the teeth and supporting tissues is the most common method for obtaining virtual casts if there is adequate lip and cheek retraction. Their accuracy has been well established.[36]

At the minimum, a wax bite or polysiloxane record of the patient's usual interdigitation (maximum intercuspation) should be made, and a check should be made to be sure that this does not differ significantly from the initial contact position. An anterior shift of 1 to 2 mm from the retruded position is of little consequence unless it creates a pseudo–class III relationship, but lateral shifts or anterior shifts of greater magnitude should be noted carefully and a bite registration in an approximate centric relation position should be made.

Dental casts for orthodontic purposes were usually trimmed so that the bases were symmetric and then polished. Now that digital images often are used, they still are prepared to look like trimmed and polished casts (Fig. 6.49). There are two reasons for doing this: (1) If the casts are viewed with a symmetric base that is oriented to the midline of the palate, it is much easier to analyze arch form and detect asymmetry within the dental arches; and (2) neatly trimmed and polished casts are more acceptable for presentation to the patient, as will be necessary during any consultation about orthodontic treatment. In specialty practice, virtual casts have the great advantage that they eliminate the need for storage space and can be used for computer-assisted measurements, analyses and fabrication of appliances.

At present the most popular and efficient way to generate accurate digital casts and occlusal relationships is from direct intraoral scans.[37] This also eliminates impressions that are unpleasant for patients, which becomes more important when multiple scans may be needed to obtain data required for a computer-controlled wire-bending robot to fabricate archwires. Application of this technology is discussed in Chapter 10.

Articulator Mounting

Whether it is desirable to mount casts on an adjustable articulator as part of an orthodontic diagnostic evaluation is a matter of continuing debate. There are three reasons for mounting casts on articulators. The first is to record and document any discrepancy between the occlusal relations at the initial contact of the teeth

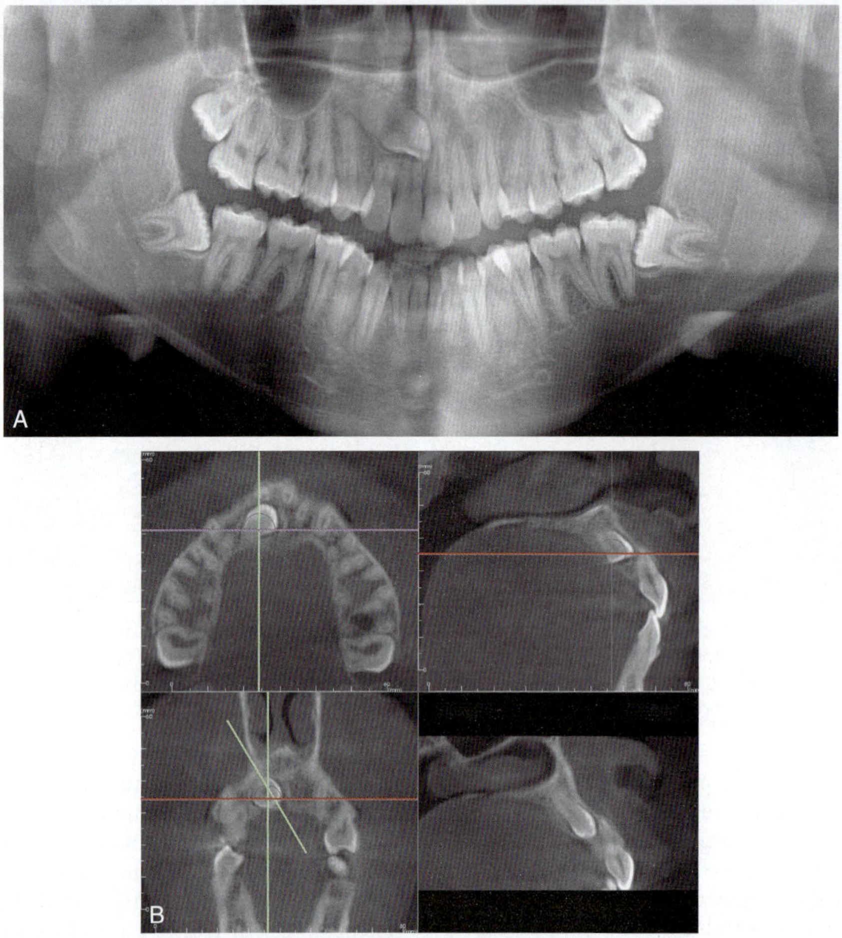

• **Fig. 6.48** (A) An impacted maxillary canine, seen in a panoramic radiograph and (B) in cone beam computed tomography (*CBCT*) sections in various planes of space. (For an overall three-dimensional view of a similar case, see Fig. 6.78). Note that it is impossible to evaluate the extent of root resorption of the lateral and central incisors from the panoramic radiograph, and it is difficult to determine whether the canine is facial or lingual to the incisors. From the CBCT slices, it is apparent that the lateral incisor root has been damaged but the central incisor root is intact, although it is very close to the crown of the canine, and the canine is on the palatal side. This information changes the treatment plan and biomechanics from what it would have been if the panoramic radiograph were supplemented with periapicals that determined the palatal canine position but not the details of its relationship to the other teeth: it will be important for the orthodontist to first move the canine palatally, away from the incisors, before beginning to bring it down toward the occlusal plane. Otherwise, the central incisor root is almost sure to be damaged during the movement of the canine.

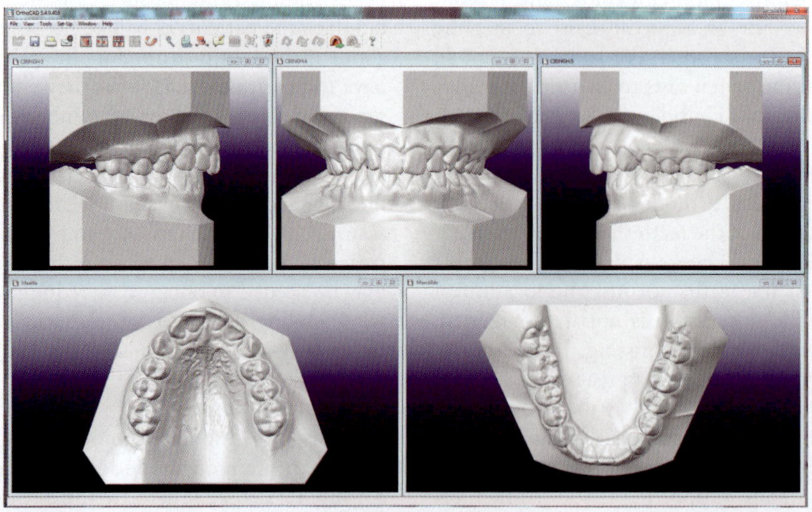

• **Fig. 6.49** Digital casts, which usually are produced from intraoral scans, can be displayed with or without symmetric bases. The advantage of the bases is that they help the observer detect asymmetries within the dental arches. These five views are traditionally available for diagnostic and treatment planning purposes.

and the relations at the patient's full or habitual occlusion. The second is to record the lateral and excursive paths of the mandible, documenting these and making the tooth relationships during excursions more accessible for study. A third, which increasingly is superseded by CBCT images, is to display the orientation of the occlusal plane to the face.

Knowing the centric occlusal relationship when the condyles are positioned "correctly" obviously is important for orthodontic diagnostic purposes if there is a significant difference between it and the usual intercuspation. Unfortunately, there is no current agreement as to what the "correct" centric position is, although the "muscle-guided" position (the most superior position to which a patient can bring the mandible using his or her own musculature) seems most appropriate for orthodontic purposes. It is now generally accepted that in normal individuals this neuromuscular position is anterior to the most retruded condylar position. Lateral shifts or large anterior shifts are not normal and should be recorded. Articulator-mounted casts are one way, but not the only way, to do that.

The second reason for mounting casts—to record the excursive paths—is important when restorative dentistry is being planned because the contours of the replacement or restored teeth must accommodate the path of movement. This is much less important when tooth positions and jaw relationships will change during treatment.

The current consensus is that for preadolescent and early adolescent orthodontic patients (i.e., those who have not completed their adolescent growth spurt), there is little point in an articulator mounting. In these young patients, the contours of the TMJ are not fully developed, so condylar guidance is much less prominent than in adults. The shape of the temporal fossa in an adult reflects function during growth. Thus, until mature canine function is reached and the chewing pattern changes from that of the child to the normal adult (see Chapter 3), completion of the articular eminence and the medial contours of the joint should not be expected. In addition, the relationships between the dentition and the joint that are recorded in articulator mountings change rapidly while skeletal growth is continuing and tend to be only of historic interest after orthodontic treatment.

The situation is different when growth is complete or largely complete. In adults with symptoms of temporomandibular dysfunction (TMD; clicking, limitation of motion, pain), articulator-mounted casts may be useful to document significant discrepancies between habitual and relaxed mandibular positions. These patients often need therapy to reduce muscle spasm and splinting before the articulator mounting is done. An articulator mounting may also be needed to plan orthodontic or surgical treatment of adults with significant cants of the occlusal plane or asymmetries.

It is widely anticipated that virtual articulators will replace physical ones before long; at present they are continuing to evolve (Fig. 6.50). Software used for surgical treatment planning already has produced something like a true virtual articulator. It is possible to virtually relate casts to each other for model surgery and fabrication of bite wafers for surgery. This has proven to be equally as accurate as, if not more accurate than, manual methods.[38] The current limitations include the costs of these systems and the knowledge level to use and apply them. Interestingly, these systems can also include a haptic system that introduces the feel of the articulator and restoration contact for the laboratory technician. To make them more attractive to the orthodontic community, set-up modules can be included.

That does not change the indication for articulator use in orthodontics; physical or virtual, articulators are indicated primarily for adult patients with functional problems, not for children or adolescents.

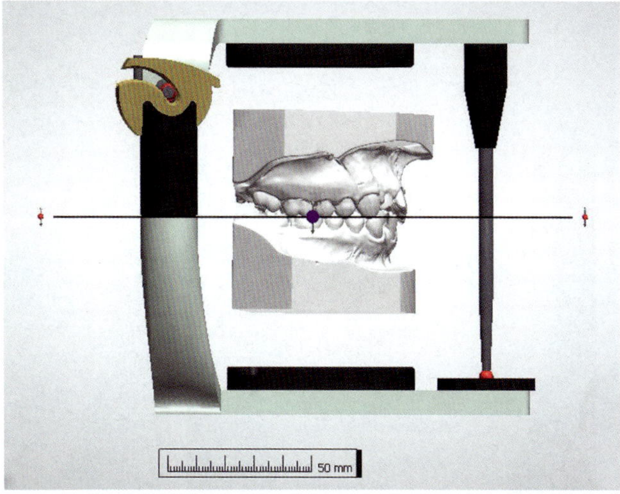

• **Fig. 6.50** The 3 Shape virtual articulator (3Shape A/S, Copenhagen, Denmark) provides for some individualization of the settings for the mounted cast along with various movements and view perspectives. This technology, intended to replace physical articulators, is progressing and has shown reasonable accuracy when used in conjunction with surgical planning and splint construction.

Records for Dentofacial Proportions

For any orthodontic patient, facial and jaw proportions, not just dental occlusal relationships, must be evaluated. This is done best by a careful clinical evaluation of the patient's face (as described previously), and data from the clinical examination are an important part of the diagnostic database, but both a cephalometric radiograph and facial photographs, and sometimes CT images, are needed as records to support the clinical findings.

Radiographs

Like all radiographic records, cephalograms should be taken only when they are indicated. Lateral cephalometric radiographs are the standard for comprehensive orthodontic treatment. They allow analysis of the pretreatment form (positions and relationships) for diagnosis and treatment planning. In 1992 this was estimated to alter treatment in about 20% of cases,[39] and that proportion still is accepted. More important, they provide for evaluation of progress and the posttreatment result when follow-up cephalograms are taken. Treatment changes cannot be understood without cephalometric superimpositions. It is irresponsible to undertake growth modification treatment in a child without a pretreatment lateral cephalometric radiograph, because knowing the timing, direction, and magnitude of the pretreatment growth and subsequent changes due to treatment and growth are critical to success.

The major indication for a frontal (posteroanterior [PA], not AP) cephalometric radiograph was facial asymmetry, and this now is an indication for 3D imaging instead (see the section on analysis of 3D images, later), so PA cephalograms are obsolete. For treatment of minor problems in children or for adjunctive treatment procedures in adults, cephalometric radiographs usually are not required, simply because jaw relationships and incisor positions would not be changed significantly.

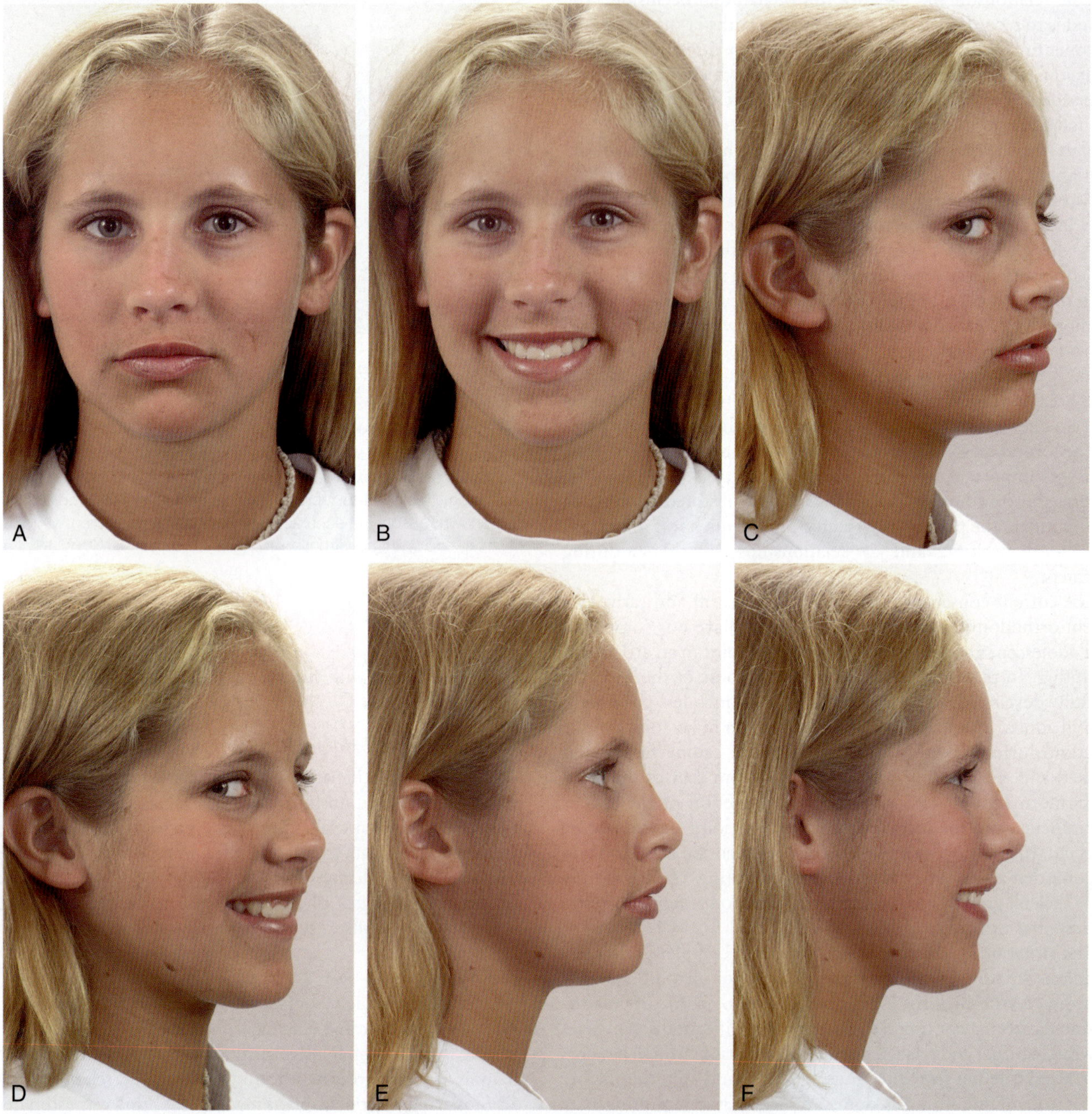

• **Fig. 6.51** (A–F) Patient F.P., age 12 years 3 months, facial views before treatment. Note the mildly short anterior face height, the lack of mandibular projection, and the appearance of the maxillary incisors on smile—very upright with short clinical crowns but minimal gingival display.

Facial Photographs

A series of facial photographs has been a standard part of orthodontic diagnostic records for many years. The minimum set is three photographs, frontal at rest, frontal smile, and profile at rest, but it can be valuable to have a record of tooth-lip relationships in other views. The oblique smiling photo, for instance, provides an excellent view of both vertical tooth-lip relationships and the smile arc. So, a more complete set of facial photographs includes the original three mentioned above and additionally the lateral smiling and oblique resting and smiling (Fig. 6.51). Although 3D photography now is available and has potential as a valuable research tool (see Fig. 2.11), it is little used clinically at this point for orthodontic diagnostic evaluation and requires more development including refinement of the superimposition capabilities.

With the advent of digital records, it is easy now to obtain a short segment of digital video as the patient smiles and turns from a frontal to a profile view. The resulting set of images allows analysis of facial relationships at rest and in function. It is important to keep in mind that images are never a substitute for careful clinical evaluation—they are just a record of what was observed clinically, or what should have been observed and recorded—and the current view of digital video is that the gain in diagnostic information over careful clinical analysis simply is not worth the time and effort to obtain and analyze it.

Diagnostic Records Summary

In summary, minimal diagnostic records for any orthodontic patient consist of data from the clinical examination of dentofacial characteristics, dental casts trimmed to represent the occlusal relationship (or their electronic equivalent), facial and intraoral photographs, and appropriate radiographs for that individual patient. The radiographs are the judgment call in deciding what records are needed.

The guideline for radiography is that you should obtain the images you need, while keeping the radiation dose as low as possible. With that in mind, a panoramic radiograph is needed for almost every patient and may be available from the patient's family dentist (preferably less than 1 year old). Obtaining a lateral cephalogram is sensible unless there is severe enough facial asymmetry to indicate that a full-field CBCT is indicated.

If you have the panoramic radiograph and there is a suspected localized issue, you will best serve the patient in terms of radiation by getting a cephalometric radiograph and a small-field CBCT view, because you will likely need higher resolution of the problem area.

If none of these images are available and you need a panoramic, cephalometric radiograph and a close-up view of a specific localized area, a full-field image can address all these issues, although the panoramic and cephalometric radiographs constructed from CBCT have lower resolution than individual images.

Analysis of Diagnostic Records

Comments on the analysis of intraoral radiographs appear in the previous section on clinical evaluation, along with assessment of intraoral and facial clinical findings that were recorded photographically. In this section, the focus is on four things: (1) dental cast analysis to evaluate symmetry and space excess or deficiency within the dental arches, (2) cephalometric analysis of dentofacial relationships, (3) analysis of 3D CBCT images, and (4) integration of information from all sources into the problem-oriented format that facilitates treatment planning.

Cast Analysis: Symmetry, Space, and Tooth Size

Symmetry

An asymmetric position of an entire arch should be detected in the facial and esthetic examination, but an asymmetry of arch form may be present even if the face looks symmetric. Evaluating dental casts from the occlusal view when the cast bases have been trimmed symmetrically can make it easier to see a distortion of arch form in either physical or virtual casts (see Fig. 6.49).

Asymmetry within the dental arch, but with a symmetric arch form also can occur. This is due either to severe crowding or spacing or to drift of anterior or posterior teeth on one side of the arch, which is sometimes due to premature loss of a primary or permanent tooth followed by movement of both anterior and posterior teeth.

Alignment, Crowding, and Spacing: Space Analysis

It is important to quantify the amount of space available for alignment of the teeth within the dental arches because treatment varies depending on whether the space is adequate, deficient, or excessive. In adolescents and adults the amount of available space and the amount required to align all the teeth can be measured directly from the erupted teeth. If permanent teeth are unerupted after their expected eruption time, contralateral teeth can be measured or periapical radiographs can be exposed so that measurement ratios can be established (see later in this chapter) to establish the true space status in each arch. In the mixed dentition, if clinically significant space problems are discovered before the eruption of all permanent teeth, planned space regaining, expansion or extraction can be planned before the problem is clinically apparent. In the mixed dentition, the true amount of crowding is deceptive, because there often is a difference between the apparent crowding at one point in time and the true ultimate crowding after the transition from the mixed to permanent dentition.

Space analysis, using the dental casts or virtual casts to measure the space available for the teeth and a prediction of the size of unerupted canines and premolars, is required for this purpose and will reveal the true ultimate crowding. The steps in mixed dentition space analysis and the assumptions that underlie it are covered in detail in Chapter 11.

Tooth Size Analysis

For good occlusion, the upper and lower teeth must be proportional in size. If large upper teeth are combined with small lower teeth, as in a denture set-up with mismatched tooth sizes, there is no way to achieve ideal occlusion. Although the natural teeth match very well in most individuals, approximately 5% of the population have some degree of disproportion among the sizes of individual teeth. This is termed *tooth size discrepancy*. Variation in the width of the upper lateral incisors (enlarged, diminutive, or peg shaped) is the most common cause, but variations in the size of premolars or other teeth also may be present. Occasionally, all the upper teeth will be too large or too small to fit properly with the lower teeth or vice versa.

Tooth size analysis, often called *Bolton analysis* after its developer,[40] is carried out by measuring the mesiodistal width of each permanent tooth. A standard table (Table 6.6) is then used to

TABLE 6.6 Tooth Size Relationships

Maxillary Anterior Sum of 3-3	Mandibular Anterior Sum of 3-3	Maxillary Total Sum of 6-6	Mandibular Total Sum of 6-6
40	30.9	86	78.5
41	31.7	88	80.3
42	32.4	90	82.1
43	33.2	92	84.0
44	34.0	94	85.8
45	34.7	96	87.6
46	35.5	98	89.5
47	36.3	100	91.3
48	37.1	102	93.1
49	37.8	104	95.0
50	38.6	106	96.8
51	39.4	108	98.6
52	40.1	110	100.4
53	40.9		
54	41.7		
55	42.5		

From Bolton WA. Disharmony in tooth size and its relation to the analysis and treatment of malocclusion. *Angle Orthod.* 1958;28:113–120.

compare the summed widths of the maxillary to the mandibular anterior teeth (canine to canine) and the total width of all upper to lower teeth (permanent first molar through permanent first molar, excluding second and third molars). One advantage of entering measured individual tooth widths into a computer template during space analysis is that the computer then can quickly provide individual tooth, interarch and intraarch measurements (Fig. 6.52), and the computer can calculate a tooth size analysis (Fig. 6.53).

A quick check for anterior tooth size discrepancy can be done by comparing the size of upper and lower lateral incisors. Unless the upper laterals are wider, a discrepancy almost surely exists. A

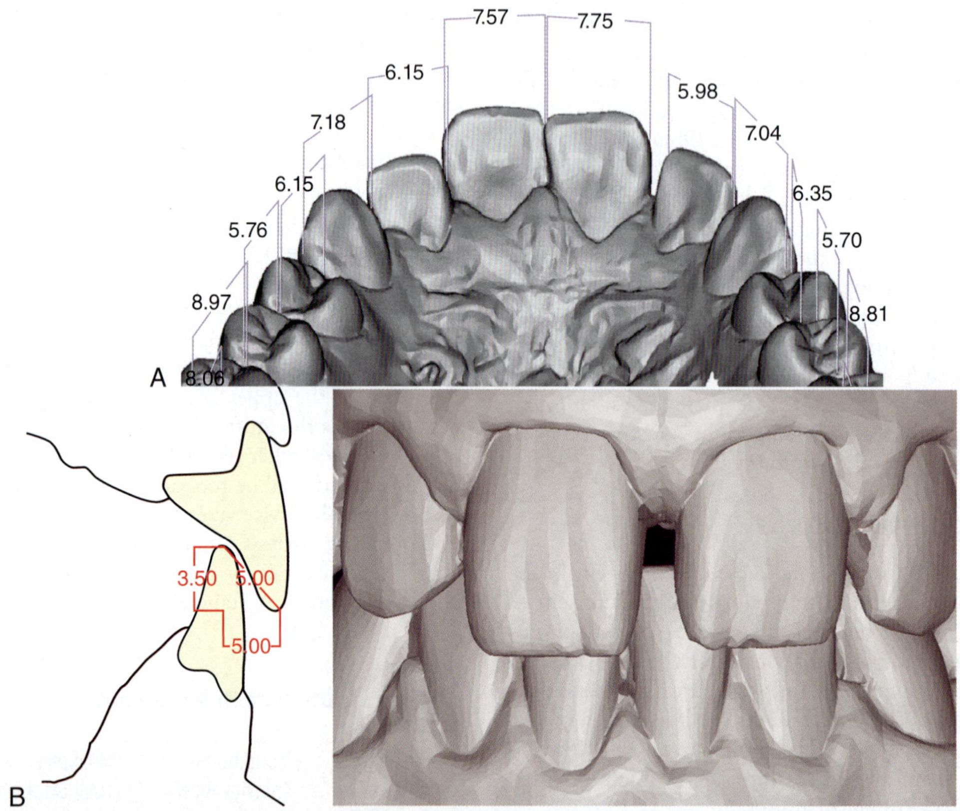

• **Fig. 6.52** (A) Accurate measurements can be achieved from digital casts derived from direct intraoral scans. Usually, virtual casts are related to each other with use of a scan of the buccal interdigitation. (B) It is possible to create sagittal representations of the digital casts and juxtapose them as shown here so that precise measurements can be made.

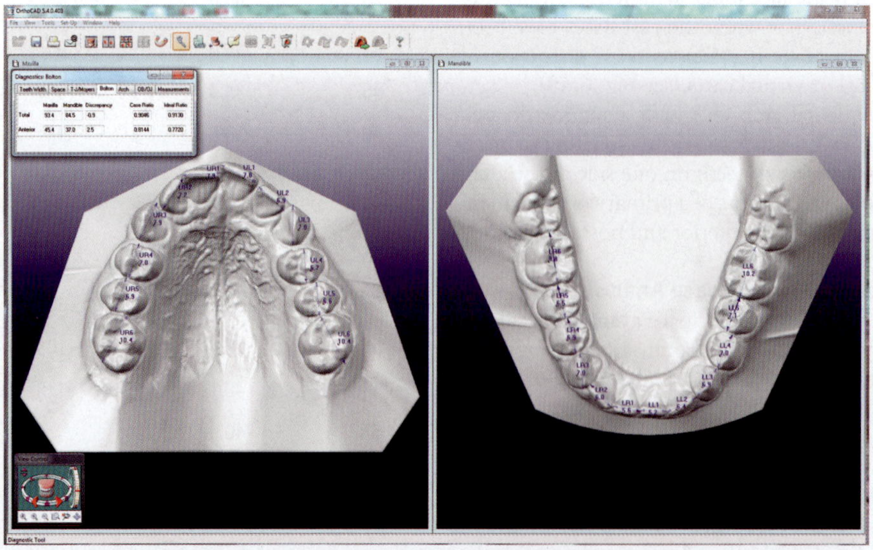

• **Fig. 6.53** Tooth-size analysis (Bolton analysis) also is readily available from digital casts. This requires accurate measurement of the width of each of the teeth, so that the sum of the incisor widths in each arch, and the sum of the widths of all the teeth, can be compared with these sums for the other arch (see Table 6.6).

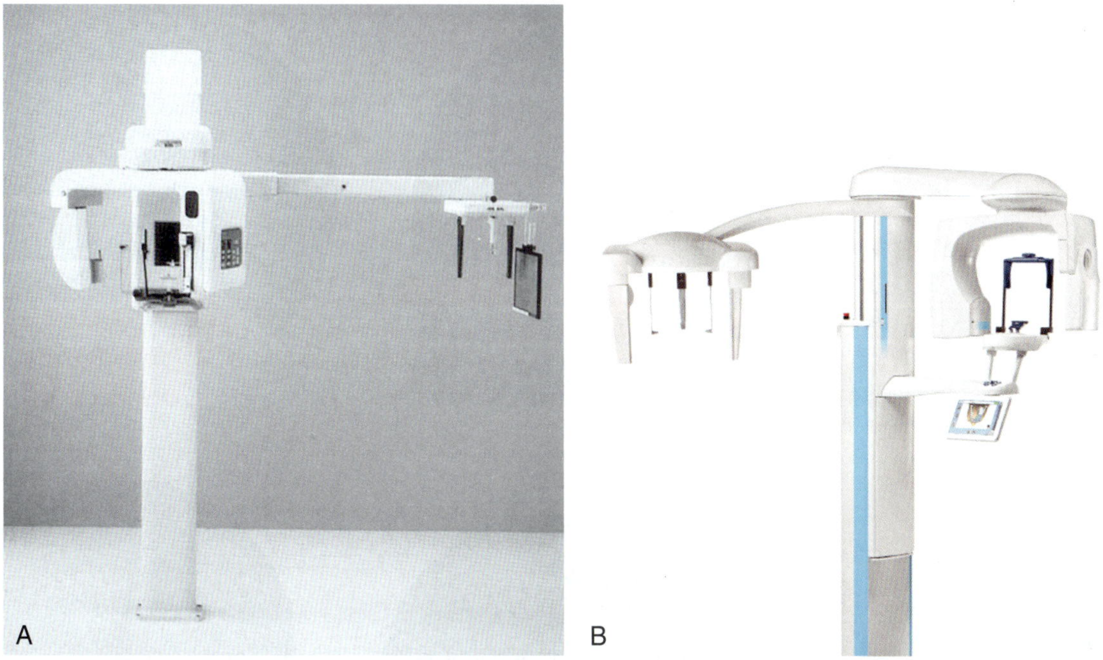

• **Fig. 6.54** (A) A more traditional cephalometric and panoramic machine that was film based. (B) A digital cephalometric, panoramic, and CBCT combination machine. (A, From https://pocketdentistry.com/14-cephalometric-radiography/. B, Courtesy Planmecca USA, Hoffman Estates, IL.)

quick check for posterior tooth size discrepancy is to compare the size of upper and lower second premolars, which should be about equal size. A tooth size discrepancy of less than 1.5 mm is rarely significant, but larger discrepancies create treatment problems in achieving ideal interdigitation, overjet and overbite, and must be included in the orthodontic problem list.

Cephalometric Analysis

Early Cephalometrics: From Research to Clinical Application

The introduction of radiographic cephalometrics in 1934 by Hofrath in Germany and Broadbent in the United States provided both a research and a clinical tool for the study of malocclusion and underlying skeletal disproportions. The original purpose of cephalometrics was research on growth patterns in the craniofacial complex. The machines had specific dimensions so that the magnification was consistent and images overtime could be compared. New digital machines (Fig. 6.54B) that produce less radiation have various magnification among manufacturers, which must be carefully monitored. The concepts of normal development presented in Chapters 2 and 3 were largely derived from such cephalometric studies.

It soon became clear, however, that cephalometric radiographs could be used to evaluate dentofacial proportions and clarify the anatomic basis for a malocclusion. The orthodontist needs to know how the major functional components of the face (cranial base, jaws, teeth) are related to one another (Fig. 6.55). Any malocclusion is the result of an interaction between jaw position and the position the teeth assume as they erupt. The teeth are affected by the jaw relationships (see Chapter 4 for a discussion of dental compensation or adaptation). For this reason, apparently similar malocclusions as evaluated from the dental occlusions may turn out to be quite different when evaluated

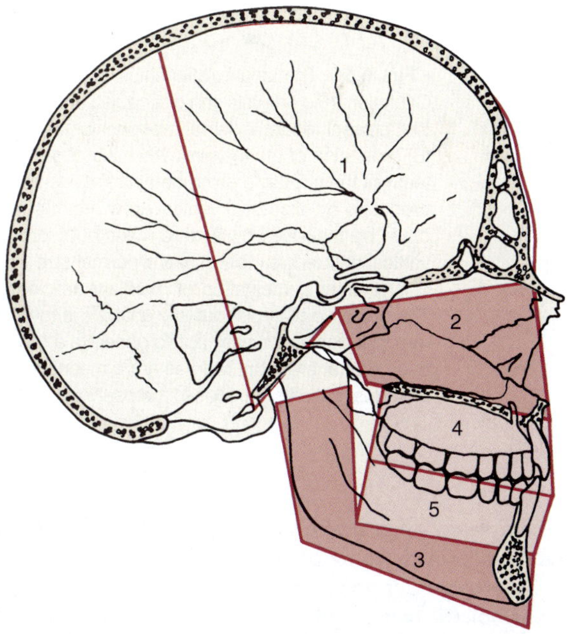

• **Fig. 6.55** The structural components of the face, shown superimposed on the anatomic drawing. The cranium and cranial base *(1)*, the skeletal maxilla and nasomaxillary complex *(2)*, and the skeletal mandible *(3)* are parts of the face that exist whether there is or is not a dentition. The maxillary teeth and alveolar process *(4)* and the mandibular teeth and alveolar process *(5)* are independent functional units, which can be displaced relative to the supporting bone of the maxilla and mandible, respectively. The major goal of cephalometric analysis is to establish the relationship of these components in both the anteroposterior and vertical planes of space.

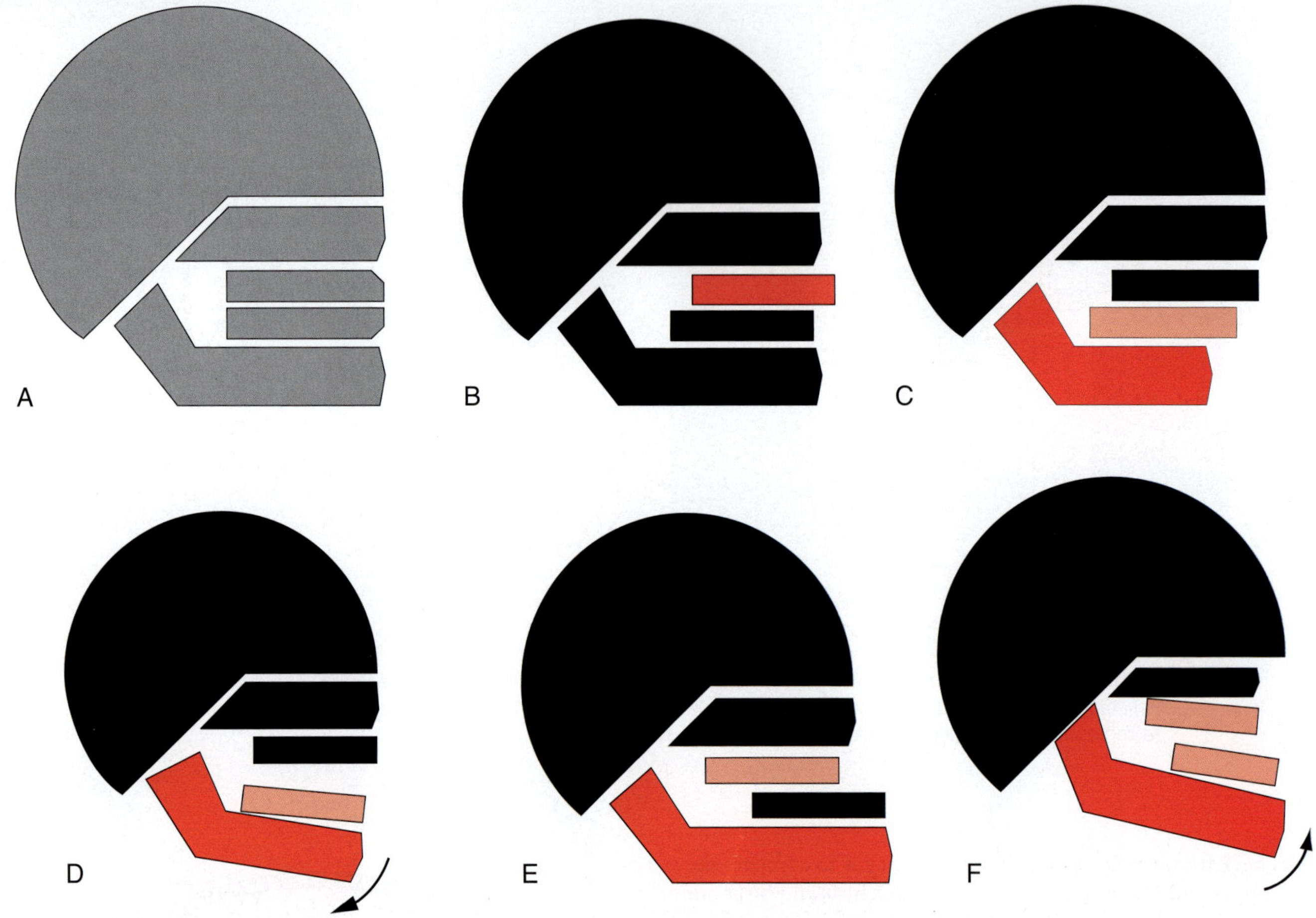

• **Fig. 6.56** The ideal relationships of the facial and dental components can be represented as shown in (A). Cephalometric analysis can distinguish and clarify the differing dental and skeletal contributions to malocclusions that present identical dental relationships. A class II division 1 malocclusion, for example, could be produced by (B) protrusion of the maxillary teeth although the jaw relationship was normal, (C) mandibular deficiency with the teeth of the mandible protruded in relationship to the jaw, (D) downward and backward rotation of the mandible produced by excessive vertical growth of the maxilla, or a number of other possibilities. A class III malocclusion could be produced by (E) true mandibular prognathism with a normal maxilla, (F) maxillary anteroposterior and vertical deficiencies that make a normal-size mandible look prominent because the maxillary vertical deficiency or any other combination of maxillary deficiency and mandibular excess allowed it to rotate up and forward, The objective of cephalometric analysis is to visualize the contribution of skeletal and dental relationships to the malocclusion in this way, not to generate a table of numbers that are estimators of relationships. Measurements and other analytic procedures are a means to the end of understanding dental and skeletal relationships for an individual patient, not ends in themselves.

more completely (Fig. 6.56). Although careful observation of the face can provide some of this information, cephalometric analysis allows greater precision.

Cephalometric radiographs are not taken as a screen for pathologic problems, but the possibility of observing pathologic changes on these radiographs should not be overlooked. Occasionally, previously unsuspected anomalies in the cervical spine (Fig. 6.57) or degenerative changes in the vertebrae are revealed in a cephalometric radiograph. Other pathologic changes in the skull, jaws, or cranial base also can be observed.[41] This becomes particularly important when full-view 3D images of the head are obtained (see later), and examination of such images by a radiologist is needed to be sure that a pathologic condition is not overlooked.

Perhaps the most important clinical use of radiographic cephalometrics is in recognizing and evaluating changes brought about by orthodontic treatment and growth. Superimpositions taken from serial cephalometric radiographs before, during, and after treatment can be superimposed to study changes in jaw and tooth positions retrospectively (see later in this chapter, Fig. 6.73). The observed changes result from a combination of growth and treatment (except in nongrowing adults). It is all but impossible to know what is really occurring during treatment of a growing patient without reviewing cephalometric superimpositions, which is the reason that cephalometric radiographs are required for comprehensive orthodontic treatment of children and adolescents.

For diagnostic purposes, the major use of radiographic cephalometrics is in characterizing the patient's dental and skeletal relationships. In this chapter, we focus on the use of cephalometric analysis to compare a patient to his or her ethnic and racial peers, using population standards. The use of cephalometric predictions

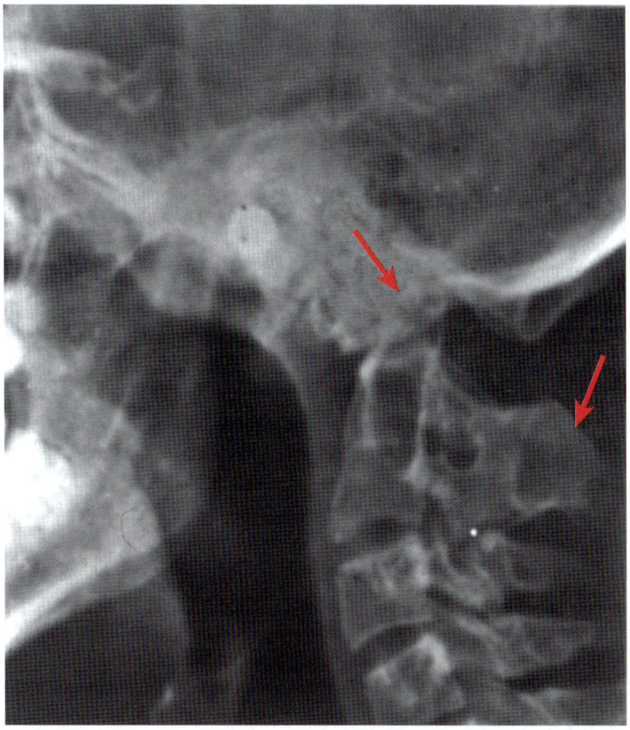

• **Fig. 6.57** Vertebral pathologic characteristics can be observed in cephalometric radiographs and sometimes is discovered by the orthodontist. This patient has fusion of the first and second cervical vertebrae *(left arrow)*, with the odontoid process extending into the margin of foramen magnum *(right arrow)*. This is a potentially life-threatening situation because a blow to the head or extreme positioning of the head could lead to damage to the spinal cord at the foramen level.

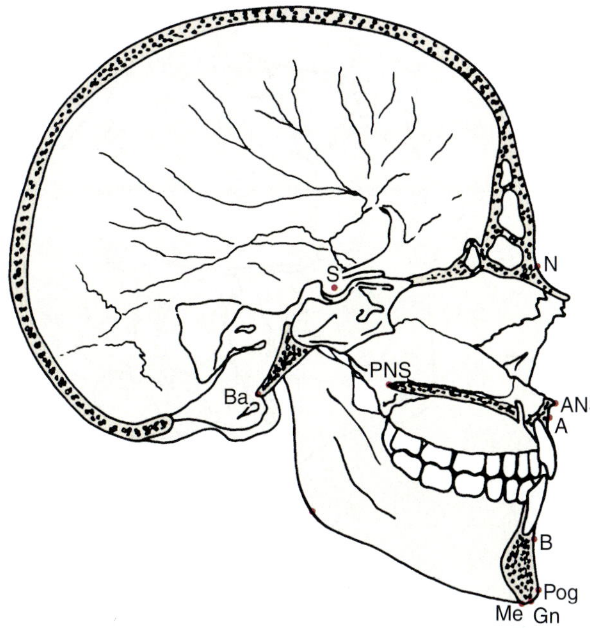

• **Fig. 6.58** Definitions of cephalometric landmarks as they would be seen at the midline in a dissected skull. *A*, The innermost point on the contour of the premaxilla between anterior nasal spine and the incisor tooth; *ANS*, anterior nasal spine, the tip of the anterior nasal spine (sometimes modified as the point on the upper or lower contour of the spine where it is 3 mm thick: see Harvold analysis); *B*, the innermost point on the contour of the mandible between the incisor tooth and the bony chin; *Ba*, basion, the lowest point on the anterior margin of foramen magnum, at the base of the clivus; *Gn*, gnathion, the most inferior *and* anterior point on the mandibular symphysis—that is, the point of the chin; *Me*, menton, the most inferior point on the chin; *N*, nasion, the anterior point of the intersection between the nasal and frontal bones; *PNS*, posterior nasal spine, t the most distal extent of the horizontal process of palatine bone; *Pog*, pogonion, the most anterior point on the contour of the chin; *S*, sella, the midpoint of the cavity of sella turcica. Note that some of these points can vary depending on head position.

to estimate orthodontic and surgical treatment outcomes is covered for children, adolescents, and adults later, in the clinical treatment chapters.

Development of Cephalometric Analysis

Cephalometric analysis is commonly carried out not on the radiograph itself, but on a tracing or digital model that emphasizes the relationship of selected points. In essence, the tracing or model is used to reduce the amount of information on the radiograph to a manageable level. Common cephalometric midline bony landmarks and a typical tracing are shown in Figs. 6.58 and 6.59, respectively.

Cephalometric landmarks are represented as a series of points, which are usually defined as physical locations on the skull or soft tissue (e.g., the junction of the nasal and frontal bones) but often as an extreme point (e.g., the most anterior point on the bony chin), or occasionally as constructed points such as the intersection of two planes (e.g., the intersection of the mandibular plane and a plane along the posterior margin of the ramus for Gonion). The extreme points can change depending on the patient's head position, so it is important that head position be consistent. The *x,y* coordinates of these points are used to enter cephalometric data in a computer-compatible format. Computer analysis now is the usual method in almost all orthodontic offices. An adequate set of points are digitized from the radiograph that represent the cranium, jaws, teeth and soft tissue that allow their respective relationships and sizes to be determined. This set of points is a digital model, which means that 50 to 100 landmark locations should be specified (Fig. 6.60).

The principle of cephalometric analysis, however, is not different when computers are used or when radiographs are evaluated manually. The goal is to determine the skeletal and dental relationships that exist in an individual patient and determine how they contribute to their malocclusion. How do you do that? One way is to compare the patient with a normal reference group, so that differences between the patient's actual dentofacial relationships and those expected for his or her age and racial or ethnic group are revealed. This type of cephalometric analysis was first popularized after World War II in the form of the Downs analysis, developed at the University of Illinois and based on skeletal and facial proportions of a reference group of 25 untreated adolescent whites selected because of their ideal dental occlusions.

From the very beginning, the issue of how to establish the normal reference standards was difficult. It seems obvious that patients with severe cranial disproportions should be excluded from a normal sample. Because normal occlusion is not the usual finding in a randomly selected population group, one must make a further choice in establishing the reference group, either excluding individuals with obvious craniofacial deformities while including most malocclusions, or excluding essentially all those

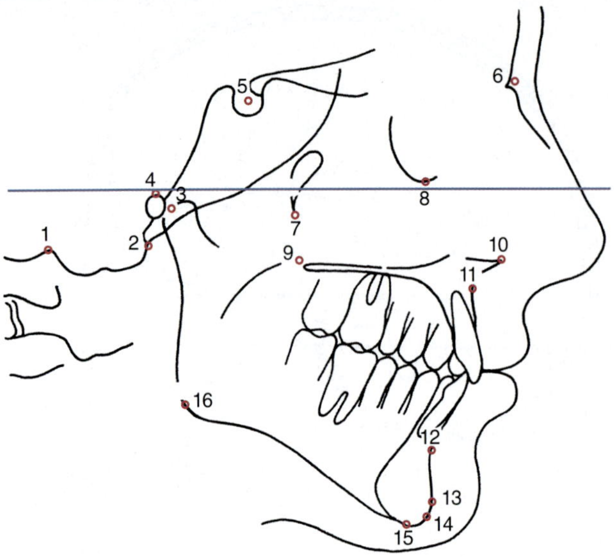

• **Fig. 6.59** Definitions of cephalometric landmarks (as seen in a lateral cephalometric tracing). *1, Bo*, Bolton point, the highest point in the upward curvature of the retrocondylar fossa of the occipital bone; *2, Ba*, basion, the lowest point on the anterior margin of the foramen magnum, at the base of the clivus; *3, Co, condylion*, post posterior and superior point on the mandibular condyle; *4, Po*, porion, the midpoint of the upper contour of the external auditory canal (anatomic porion), or the midpoint of the upper contour of the metal ear rod of the cephalometer (machine porion); *5, S*, sella, the midpoint of the cavity of sella turcica; *6, N*, nasion, the point where the outer surface of the frontal bone and the superior surface of the nasal bone intersect *7, Ptm*, pterygomaxillary fissure, the point at the base of the fissure where the anterior and posterior walls meet; *8, Or*, orbitale, the lowest point on the inferior margin of the orbit; *9, PNS*, the most distal extent of the horizontal process of palatine bone; *10, ANS*, anterior nasal spine, the tip of the anterior nasal spine (sometimes modified as the point on the upper or lower contour of the spine where it is 3mm thick; see Harvold analysis); *11, point A*, the innermost point on the contour of the premaxilla between anterior nasal spine and the incisor tooth; *12, point B*, the innermost point on the contour of the mandible between the incisor tooth and the bony chin; *13, Pog*, pogonion, the most anterior point on the contour of the chin; *14, Gn, gnathion*. the most anterior and inferior point on the chin; 15 *Me*, menton, the most inferior point on the mandibular symphysis—that is, the bottom of the chin; *16, Go*, gonion, the midpoint of the contour connecting the ramus and body of the mandible.

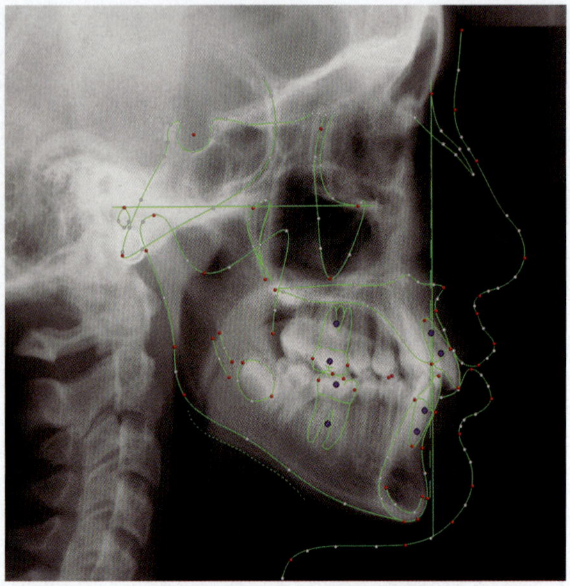

• **Fig. 6.60** A standard lateral digitization model for a current cephalometric analysis and prediction program (Dolphin Imaging, Patterson Dental, St. Paul, MN). Similar digital models, which usually can be customized to provide specific points that the clinician wants, are used in all current programs.

with malocclusion to obtain an ideal sample. In the beginning, the latter approach was chosen. Comparisons were made only with patients with excellent occlusion and facial proportions, as in the 25 individuals chosen for the Downs standards. Perhaps the extreme of selectivity in establishing a reference standard was exemplified by Steiner, whose original ideal measurements were reputedly based on one Hollywood starlet. Although the story is apocryphal, if it is true, Dr. Steiner had a very good eye because recalculation of his original values based on averages from much larger samples produced only minor changes.

The standards developed for the Downs, Steiner, and Wits analyses are still useful but have largely been replaced by newer standards based on less rigidly selected groups. A major database for contemporary analysis is the Michigan growth study, carried out in Ann Arbor and involving a typical group of children, including those with mild and moderate malocclusions.[42] Other major sources are the Burlington (Ontario) growth study,[43] the Bolton study in Cleveland,[44] and numerous specific samples collected in university projects to develop standards for specific racial and ethnic groups that are included in texts on cephalometrics.[45]

Remember, the goal of cephalometric analysis is to evaluate the relationships, both horizontally and vertically (2D), of the five major functional components of the face (see Figs. 6.55 and 6.56): the cranium and cranial base, the skeletal maxilla (described as the portions of the maxilla that would remain if there were no teeth and alveolar processes), the skeletal mandible (similarly defined), the maxillary dentition and alveolar process, and the mandibular dentition and alveolar process. In this sense, any cephalometric analysis is a procedure designed to yield a description of the relationships among these functional units.

There are two basic ways to approach this goal. One is the approach chosen originally in the Downs analysis and followed by most workers in the field since that time. This approach uses selected linear and angular measurements based on a set of selected points to establish the appropriate comparisons. The other is to express the normative data graphically rather than as a series of measurements and to compare the patient's dentofacial form directly with the graphic reference (usually called a *template*). Then any differences can be observed without making measurements

Both approaches are employed in contemporary cephalometric analysis. In the sections following, contemporary measurement approaches are discussed first, and then cephalometric analysis via direct comparison with a reference template is presented.

Measurement Analysis

Choice of a Horizontal (Cranial) Reference Line. In any technique for cephalometric analysis, it is necessary to establish a reference area or reference line. The same problem was faced in the craniometric studies of the 19th century. By the late 1800s, skeletal remains of humans had been found at many locations and were under extensive study. An international congress of anatomists and physical anthropologists was held in Frankfort, Germany, in 1882, with the choice of a horizontal reference line

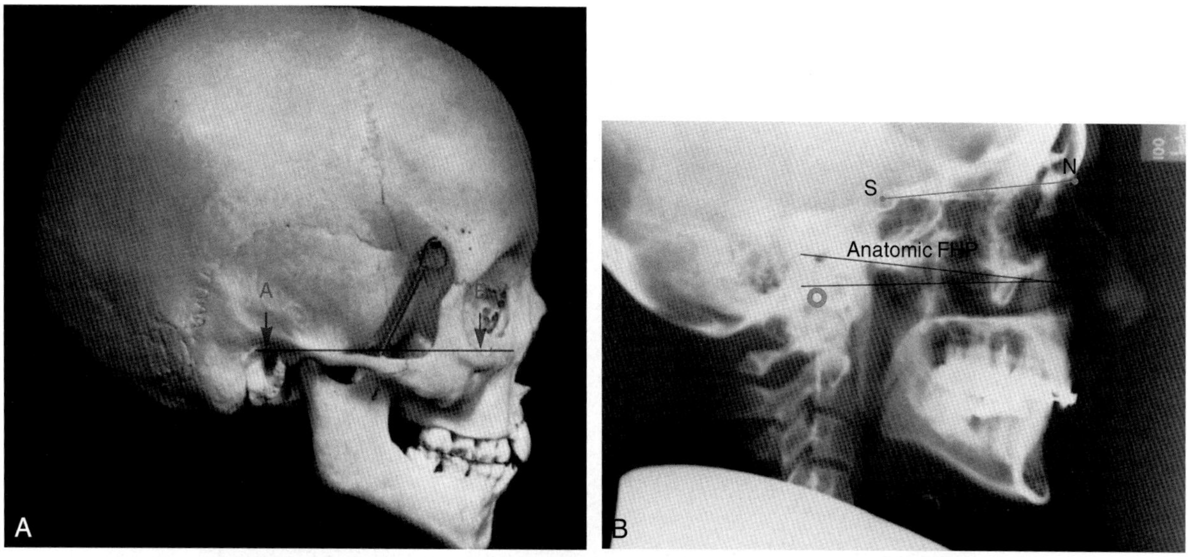

• **Fig. 6.61** (A) The Frankfort plane as originally described for orientation of dried skulls. This plane extends from the upper border of the external auditory canal *(A)* (porion) anteriorly to the upper border of the lower orbital rim *(B)* (orbitale). (B) Use of "machine porion," the upper surface of the ear rod of the cephalometric headholder, can give a different Frankfort plane than use of "anatomic porion," the upper surface of the shadow of the bony auditory canal. Both porion and orbitale, the landmarks for the Frankfort plane, are difficult to locate accurately on cephalometric films, making it a relatively unreliable reference for cephalometric analysis. Another approach to defining the cranial base is to use the points S (sella) and N (nasion) with a reference plane drawn between them. The points are visible and reliable to locate. On average the S-N line is inclined 6–7 degrees upward anteriorly from the anatomic Frankfort Plane.

for orientation of skulls being an important item on the agenda. At the conference, the Frankfort plane, extending from the upper rim of the external auditory meatus (porion) to the inferior border of the orbital rim (orbitale), was adopted as the best representation of the natural orientation of the skull (Fig. 6.61), because it was often parallel to the true horizontal when people were standing in a relaxed position. This Frankfort plane was employed for orientation of the patient from the beginning of cephalometrics and remains commonly used for analysis.

In cephalometric use, however, the Frankfort plane has two difficulties. The first is that both its anterior and posterior landmarks, particularly porion, can be difficult to locate reliably on a cephalometric radiograph. A radiopaque marker is placed on the rod that extends into the external auditory meatus as part of the cephalometric head positioning device, and the location of this marker, referred to as "machine porion," is often used to locate porion. The shadow of the auditory canal can be seen on cephalometric radiographs, usually located slightly above and posterior to machine porion. The upper edge of this canal can also be used to establish "anatomic porion," which gives a slightly different (occasionally, quite different) Frankfort plane (Fig. 6.61B).

An alternative horizontal reference line, easily and reliably detected on cephalometric radiographs, is the line from sella turcica to the junction between the nasal and frontal bones (N)—the line (S-N) (see Fig. 6.61B). In the average individual, the S-N plane is oriented at 6 to 7 degrees upward anteriorly to the Frankfort plane. Another way to obtain a Frankfort line is simply to draw it at a specific inclination to S-N, usually 6 degrees. However, although this increases reliability and reproducibility, it decreases accuracy.

The second problem with the Frankfort plane is more fundamental. It was chosen as the best anatomic indicator of the true or physiologic horizontal line. Everyone orients their head in a characteristic position, which is established physiologically, not anatomically. As the anatomists of a century ago deduced, for most patients the true horizontal line closely approximates the Frankfort plane. Some individuals, however, show significant differences, up to 10 degrees.

For the skulls they examined, the anatomists had no choice but to use an anatomic indicator of the true horizontal. For living patients, however, it is possible to use a "true horizontal" line, established physiologically rather than anatomically, as the horizontal reference plane (Fig. 6.62). This approach requires taking cephalometric radiographs with the patient in natural head position (NHP, i.e., with the patient holding the head level as determined by the patient's own internal physiologic mechanism). This position is obtained when relaxed individuals look at a distant object or into their own eyes in a mirror and incline their heads up and down in increasingly smaller movements until they feel comfortably positioned. NHP can be reproduced within 1 or 2 degrees.[46]

In contemporary usage, cephalometric radiographs should be taken in NHP, so that the physiologic true horizontal plane is established. Although NHP is not as precisely reproducible as orienting the head to the Frankfort plane, the potential errors from lower reproducibility are smaller than those from inaccurate head orientation. The inclination of SN to the true horizontal plane (or to the Frankfort plane if true horizontal plane is not known) should always be noted. If the inclination of S-N differs significantly from 6 degrees, any measurements based on S-N should be corrected by this difference.

Steiner Analysis. Developed and promoted by Cecil Steiner in the 1950s, the Steiner analysis can be considered the first of the modern cephalometric analyses for two reasons: It displayed measurements in a way that emphasized not just the individual measurements but their interrelationship in a pattern, and it offered specific guides for use of cephalometric measurements in treatment planning.[47] Elements of it remain useful today.

In a sense, the Steiner analysis was based on evaluating the compensations necessary to compensate for the difference between

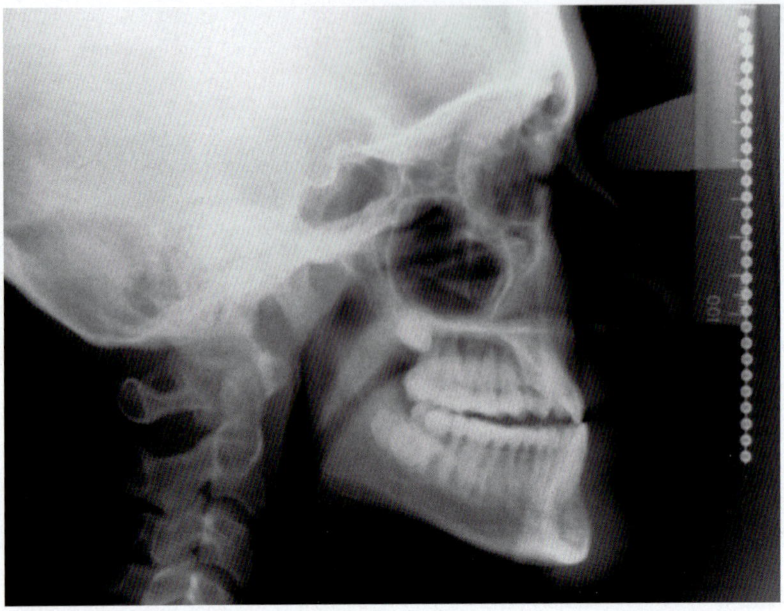

• **Fig. 6.62** If the cephalometric radiograph is taken with the patient in natural head position (NHP), a line perpendicular to the true vertical (shown by the image of the freely suspended chain that is seen on the edge of the film) is the true (physiologic) horizontal line. NHP is preferred in modern cephalometrics to anatomic head positioning.

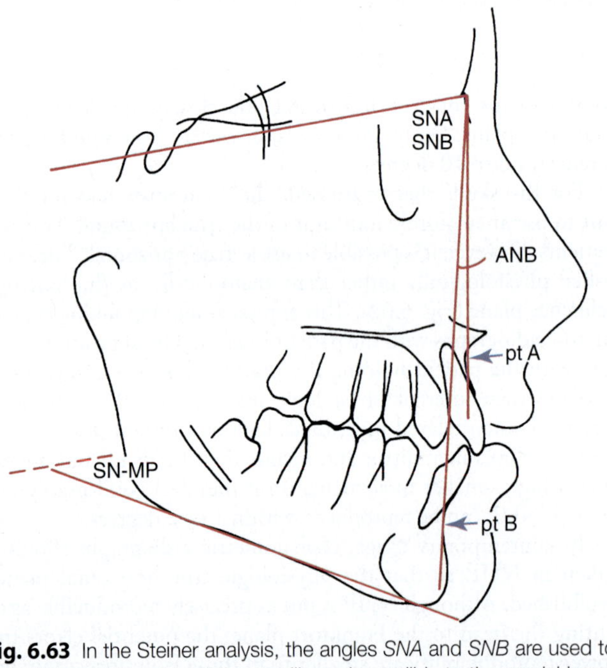

• **Fig. 6.63** In the Steiner analysis, the angles *SNA* and *SNB* are used to establish the relationship of the maxilla and mandible to the cranial base; the *ANB angle* shows the difference between the maxilla and mandible; the *SN-MP* (mandibular plane) angle is used to establish the vertical position of the mandible.

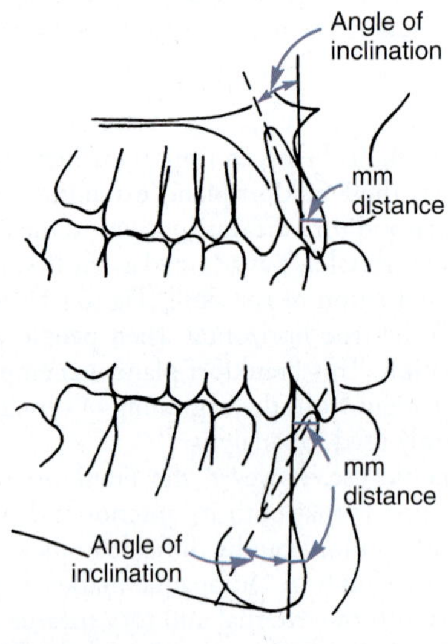

• **Fig. 6.64** In the Steiner analysis, the relationship of the upper incisor to the NA line is used to establish the position of the maxillary dentition relative to the maxilla. Both the millimeter distance that the labial surface of the incisor is in front of the line and the inclination of the long axis of the incisor to the line are measured. The position of the lower incisor relative to the mandible is established by similar measurements to the line NB. In addition, the prominence of the chin is established by measuring the millimeter distance from the NB line to pogonion, the most prominent point on the bony chin. Remember, these angles and distances can be affected by the protrusion and retrusion of the maxilla and mandible relative to the nasion.

SNA and SNB (angles advocated by Riedel),[48] which indicates the magnitude of the anteroposterior skeletal jaw discrepancy (Fig. 6.63). To Steiner, this difference (the ANB angle) was the measurement of real interest. One can argue, as he did, that which jaw was at fault is of mostly theoretical interest—what really matters is the magnitude of the discrepancy between the jaws that must be overcome in treatment, and this is what the ANB angle measures. In today's world, this is a myopic viewpoint. We now have methods to affect each jaw's position during treatment (orthodontically or surgically) that make the origin of the orthodontic problem more meaningful in diagnostic and treatment planning terms.

Steiner then measured the angular and millimeter relationship of the upper incisor to the NA line and the lower incisor and the chin to the NB line, thus establishing the relative protrusion of the dentition (Fig. 6.64). The millimeter distance establishes how prominent the incisor is relative to its supporting bone (protrusion or retrusion), and the inclination (proclined or retroclined) indicates whether the tooth has been tipped to its position or

TABLE 6.7 Cephalometric Values for Selected Groups (All Values in Degrees Except as Indicated)

	American White	American Black	Chinese (Taiwan)	Israeli	Japanese
SNA	82	85	82	82	81
SNB	80	81	78	79	77
ANB	2	4	4	3	4
1-NA	4mm	7mm	5mm	5mm	6mm
	22	23	24	24	24
Ī – NB	4mm	10mm	6mm	6mm	8mm
	25	34	29	27	31
1 to	131	119	124	126	120
GoGn-SN	32	32	35	32	34
Ī – MnPl	93	100	93	93	96
Ī – FH	62	51	57	57	57
Y-axis	61	63	61	61	62

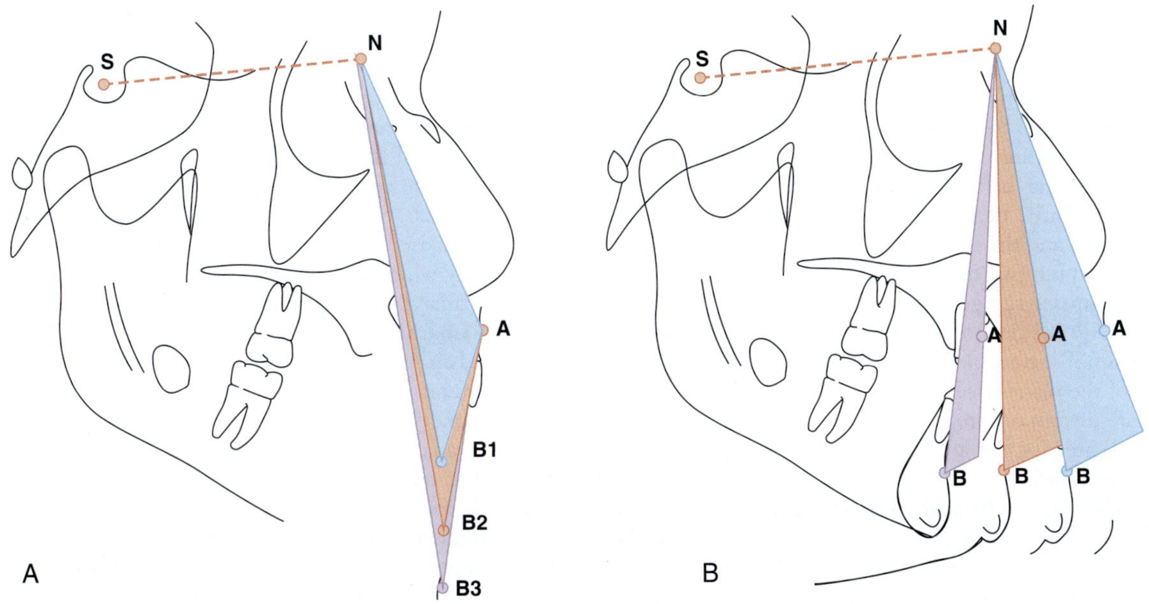

• **Fig. 6.65** There are two issues with interpreting the ANB angle that need to be recognized. (A) First, as the lower face height increases and when A point and B point are in the same anteroposterior position relative to each other, the ANB angle increases (and vice versa). Note for all three B points 1, 2, 3 relative to A, as the face is longer, the angle is larger from blue to red to purple. (B) Second, When A and B points have the same anteroposterior relationship to each other, it can be interpreted differently using ANB because the amount of protrusion or retrusion of those points to N can either increase or decrease, respectively, the apparent difference between them. Note the blue, red, and purple angles diminishing as the position of A and B points become more retrusive.

has moved there bodily. The prominence of the chin (pogonion) compared with the prominence of the lower incisor establishes the balance between them: The more prominent the chin, the more prominent the incisor can be, and vice versa. This important relationship is often referred to as the *Holdaway ratio*. Another important measurement included in the Steiner analysis is the inclination of the mandibular plane to S-N, which was its only indicator of the vertical proportions of the face (see Fig. 6.63). Tabulated standard values for five racial groups are given in Table 6.7.

There were significant problems with the Steiner analysis, however, that led to its replacement. First, its reliance on ANB was problematic. The ANB angle is influenced by two factors other than the AP difference in jaw position. One is the vertical height of the face. Vertical face height problems most often occur below the palatal plane, so the vertical difference between A point and B point commonly distort the ANB angle. Practically, as the distance between A point and B point increases, so does the ANB angle, even when the anteroposterior difference between the points does not change (Fig. 6.65A).

The second problem with ANB is that as the jaws become more protrusive relative to nasion, the ANB angle increases, even though their position relative to each other does not change. When they become more retrusive, the effect is the opposite (Fig. 6.65B). This causes exaggeration or minimization of the data. The validity of these criticisms led to the use of different indicators of jaw discrepancy in the later analyses presented in the following sections.

It should not be overlooked that relying on tooth movement alone to correct skeletal malocclusion, particularly as the skeletal discrepancies become large, is not necessarily the best approach to orthodontic treatment. It is usually better to correct skeletal discrepancies at their source than only to attempt to achieve a solely dental compromise or camouflage. It is fair to say that the Steiner compromises reflect the prevailing attitude of Steiner's era, that the effects of orthodontic treatment are almost entirely limited to the alveolar process.

Sassouni Analysis. The Sassouni analysis was the first to emphasize vertical, as well as horizontal, relationships and the interaction between vertical and horizontal proportions.[49] Sassouni pointed out that the horizontal anatomic planes—the inclination of the anterior cranial base, palatal plane, occlusal plane, and mandibular plane—tend to converge toward a single point in well-proportioned faces. The inclination of these planes to each other reflects the vertical proportionality of the face (Fig. 6.66A).

If the planes intersect relatively close to the face and diverge quickly as they pass anteriorly, the facial proportions are long anteriorly and short posteriorly, which predisposes the individual to an open bite malocclusion. Sassouni coined the term *skeletal open bite* for this anatomic relationship. If the planes are nearly parallel so that they converge far behind the face and diverge only slowly as they pass anteriorly, there is a skeletal predisposition toward anterior deep bite, and the condition is termed *skeletal deep bite.*

In addition, an unusual inclination of one of the planes stands out because it misses the general area of intersection. Sassouni evaluated the AP position of the face and dentition by noting the relationship of various points to arcs drawn from the area of intersection of the planes (see Fig. 6.66). Unfortunately, as a face becomes more disproportionate, it is more and more difficult to establish the center for the arc, and the AP evaluation becomes more and more arbitrary.

Although the total arcial analysis described by Sassouni is no longer widely used, his analysis of vertical facial proportions has become an integral part of the overall analysis of a patient.

Harvold and Wits Analyses. Both the Harvold[50] and Wits[51] analyses are aimed solely at describing the severity or degree of jaw disharmony. Harvold, using data derived from the Burlington growth study, developed standards for the "unit length" of the maxilla and mandible referenced to age and sex norms. The maxillary unit length is measured from the posterior wall of the glenoid fossa to the lower border of the anterior nasal spine where it is vertically 3 mm thick; the mandibular unit length is measured from the same point to the most anterior point of the chin (Fig. 6.67). These unit lengths attempted to quantify the size of the respective jaws. The difference between the maxillary and mandibular unit lengths (mandible-maxilla) provides an indication of the size discrepancy between the jaws. Smaller differences indicate more class II relationships and larger ones, more class III relationships. In analyzing the difference between maxillary and mandibular unit lengths, it must be kept in mind that the shorter the vertical distance between the maxilla and mandible, the more anteriorly the chin will be placed for any given unit difference, and vice versa. Harvold did quantify the lower face height to account for this factor. The positions of the teeth have no influence on the Harvold figures (Table 6.8).

The Wits analysis was conceived primarily as a way to overcome the limitations of ANB as an indicator of jaw discrepancy. It is based on a projection of points A and B to the functional occlusal plane, along which the linear difference between these points is measured (Fig. 6.68A) If the AP position of the jaws is normal, the projections from points A and B will intersect the occlusal plane at very nearly the same point. The magnitude of a discrepancy in the class II direction can be estimated by how many millimeters the point A projection is anterior to the point B projection, and vice versa for class III.

The Wits analysis, in contrast to the Harvold analysis, is influenced by the teeth both horizontally and vertically. Horizontally, because points A and B are somewhat influenced by the prominence of the dentition. Vertically, because the occlusal plane is determined by the vertical position of the teeth. There is a skeletal vertical influence. If A and B points are in identically anteroposterior positions for two patients, but the lower face is longer in one, that patient will appear to have more mandibular protrusion when A and B points are projected to the occlusal plane (see Fig. 6.68A). The Wits analysis uses the functional occlusal plane, drawn along the maximum intercuspation of the posterior teeth, that is, from the permanent first molar intercuspation point to the first premolar or primary first molar intercuspation point. This is not the traditional Downs analysis occlusal plane influenced by the vertical position of the incisors. Downs used the molar intercuspation point and an anterior point that bisects the overbite or open bite. So, if the occlusal plane rotates and points A and B do not change, the skeletal malocclusion will change (see Fig. 6.68B). This approach fails to distinguish skeletal discrepancies from problems caused by displacement of the dentition, and it does not specify which jaw is at fault if there is a skeletal problem. If the Wits analysis is used, these limitations must be kept in mind.

McNamara Analysis. The McNamara analysis, originally published in 1984,[52] combines elements of previous approaches (Ricketts and Harvold) with original measurements to attempt a more precise definition of jaw and tooth positions. In this method, both the anatomic Frankfort plane and the basion–nasion line are used as reference planes. The AP position of the maxilla and mandible are evaluated with regard to their position relative to the "nasion perpendicular," a vertical line extending downward from nasion perpendicular to the Frankfort plane (Fig. 6.69). The maxilla should be on or slightly ahead of this line, the mandible slightly behind. The second step in the procedure is a comparison of maxillary and mandibular length, using condylion, instead of the fossa. The mandible is positioned in space with the lower anterior face height (ANS–menton). The upper incisor is related to the maxilla with a line through point A perpendicular to the Frankfort plane, similar to but slightly different from Steiner's relationship of the incisor to the N-A line. The lower incisor is related as in the Ricketts analysis, primarily by using the A-pogonion line.

The McNamara analysis has two major strengths. First, it relates the jaws via the nasion perpendicular, in essence projecting the difference in AP position of the jaws to an approximation of the true vertical line. (Using a true vertical line, perpendicular to the true horizontal rather than anatomic Frankfort, would be better yet; the major reason for not doing so in constructing the analysis is that the cephalometric radiographs from which the normative data were derived were not taken in NHP.) This means that AP differences in jaw relationships are measured along the dimension (nearly true horizontal) in which they are visualized by both

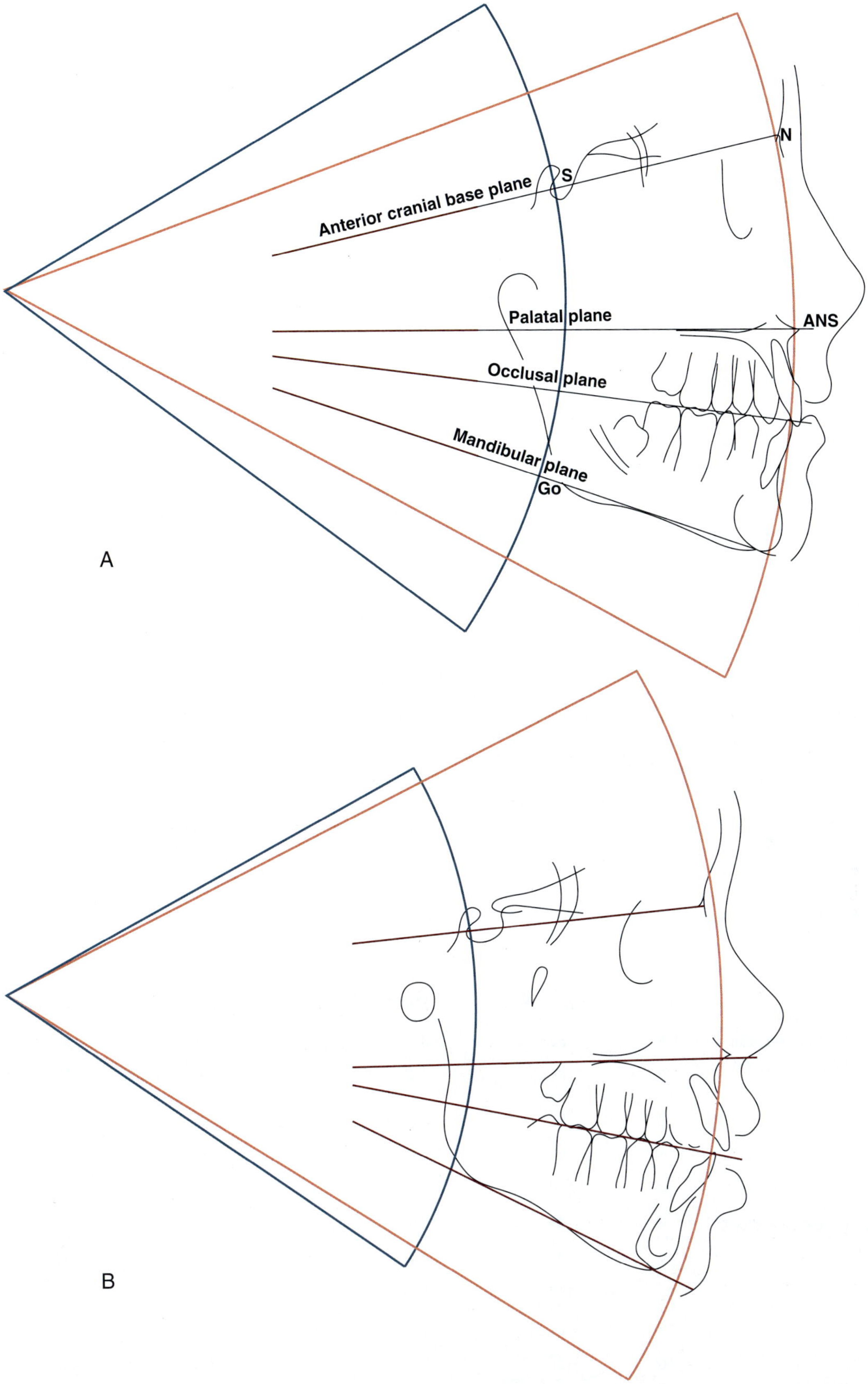

• Fig. 6.66 Sassouni contributed the idea that if a series of anteroposterior planes (anterior cranial base [S-N], palatal, functional occlusal, and mandibular) are drawn, they will project toward a common meeting point in a well-proportioned face, and that if this is not the case, the orientation of the individual planes will make it easy to visualize the disproportion. The anterior arc (*orange*) passes through N, ANS, and Pg, while the posterior arc (*blue*) passes through S and Go. (A) For this patient with a reasonably normal face and normal occlusion, the horizontal planes converge toward a common point not far behind the tracing, and vertical proportions are well within the range of normal. The arcs are good as well. (B) Inspection of the horizontal planes for this patient makes it clear that the palatal plane is rotated downward posteriorly and the mandible rotated downward anteriorly. These rotations of the jaws contribute to an open bite tendency, so the skeletal pattern revealed here is often referred to as "skeletal open bite." The arcs are reasonably good.

the patient and the diagnostician. Second, the normative data are based on the Michigan, Burlington, and Bolton samples.

Template Analysis. In the early years of cephalometric analysis, it was recognized that representing the norm in graphic form might make it easier to recognize a pattern of relationships. The "Moorrees mesh," which was developed in the 1960s and updated more recently, presents the patient's disproportions as the distortion of a grid. In recent years, direct comparison of patients with templates derived from the various growth studies has become a reliable method of analysis, with two major advantages: Compensatory skeletal and dental deviations within an individual can be observed directly, and changes in dimensions and angles with changing ages can be evaluated by using age-appropriate templates.

Any individual cephalometric tracing easily can be represented as a series of coordinate points on an *(x,y)* grid, which is what is done when a radiograph is digitized for computer analysis. But cephalometric data from any group also could be represented graphically by calculating the average coordinates of each landmark point, then connecting the points. The resulting average or composite tracing often is referred to as a *template*.

Templates of this type have been prepared by using the data from the major growth studies, showing changes in the face and jaws with age. At present, templates exist in two forms: *schematic* (Michigan, Burlington) and *anatomically complete* (Broadbent-Bolton, Alabama). The schematic templates show the changing position of selected landmarks with age on a single template. The anatomically complete templates, a different one for each age, are particularly convenient for direct visual comparison of a patient with the reference group while accounting for age. The Bolton templates, which are readily available (Department of Orthodontics, Case-Western Reserve School of Dentistry, Cleveland, Ohio), are most often used for template analysis.

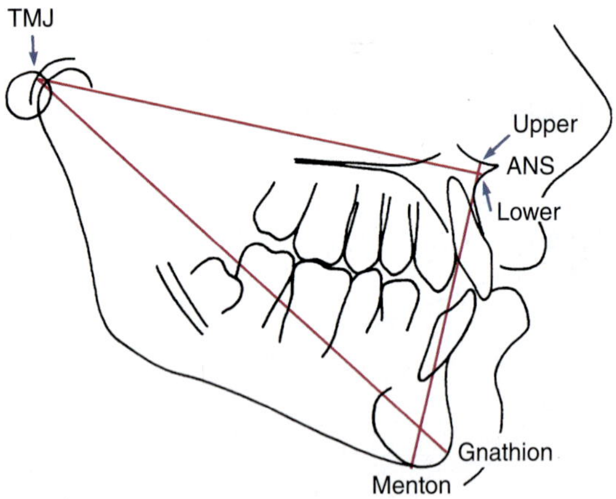

• **Fig. 6.67** Measurements used in the Harvold analysis. Maxillary length is measured from the temporomandibular joint *(TMJ)*, the posterior wall of the glenoid fossa, to lower anterior nasal spine *(ANS)*, defined as the point on the lower shadow of the ANS where the projecting spine is 3 mm thick. Mandibular length is measured from TMJ to the gnathion, the most anterior and inferior point on the chin in the *lateral* views. Lower face height is measured from the upper ANS, the similar point on the upper contour of the spine where it is 3 mm thick, to menton.

Template Analysis Techniques

Superimposition on anatomic templates using a pretreatment cephalometric tracing can give you a graphic impression of the differences between your patient and a developmentally similar male or female. In a template analysis the first step is to pick the correct template from the set of age and sex-different ones that

TABLE 6.8 Harvold Standard Values (Millimeters)

		MALE		FEMALE	
	Age	Mean Value	Standard Deviation	Mean Value	Standard Deviation
Maxillary length (temporomandibular joint to anterior nasal spine) (see Fig. 6.67)	6	82	3.2	80	3.0
	9	87	3.4	85	3.4
	12	92	3.7	90	4.1
	14	96	4.5	92	3.7
	16	100	4.2	93	3.5
Mandibular length (temporomandibular joint to pogonion)	6	99	3.9	97	3.6
	9	107	4.4	105	3.9
	12	114	4.9	113	5.2
	14	121	6.1	117	3.6
	16	127	5.3	119	4.4
Lower face height (ANS-Me)	6	59	3.6	57	3.2
	9	62	4.3	60	3.6
	12	64	4.6	62	4.4
	14	68	5.2	64	4.4
	16	71	5.7	65	4.7

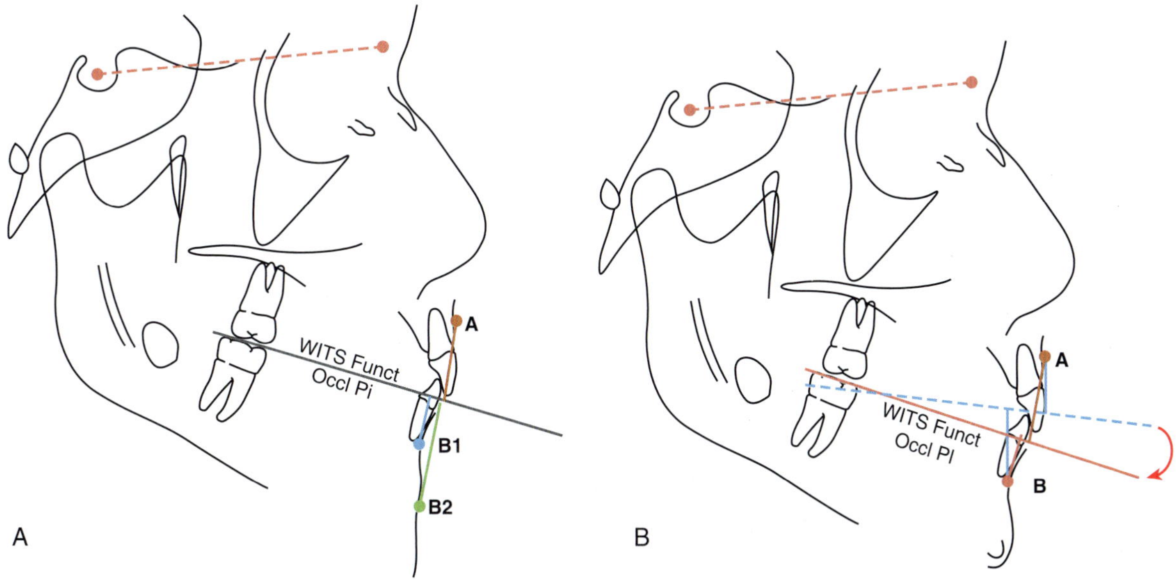

• **Fig. 6.68** There are known geometric idiosyncrasies with the WITS analysis. (A) The WITS analysis uses the functional occlusal plane determined by the intercuspationi of the posterior teeth. Points A and B are projected perpendicular to the occlusal plane. Normally B point in at or 1 mm anterior to A point. If it more anterior to A point it indicates a class III skeletal relationship and posterior to A point indicates a class II skeletal relationship. Points A and B1 demonstrate a class II relationship. Note that when there is a longer lower face height as with B2, although the anteroposterior relationship is the same, the relationship is class I. (B) It is also true that when the functional occlusal plane changes its angulation, that can be interpreted as a skeletal change, even when there was none. The blue occlusal plane and the projections from A and B points show a significant class II relationship, but simply tipping the occlusal plane down anteriorly, leads to an impression the skeletal relationships are nearly class I without true skeletal change.

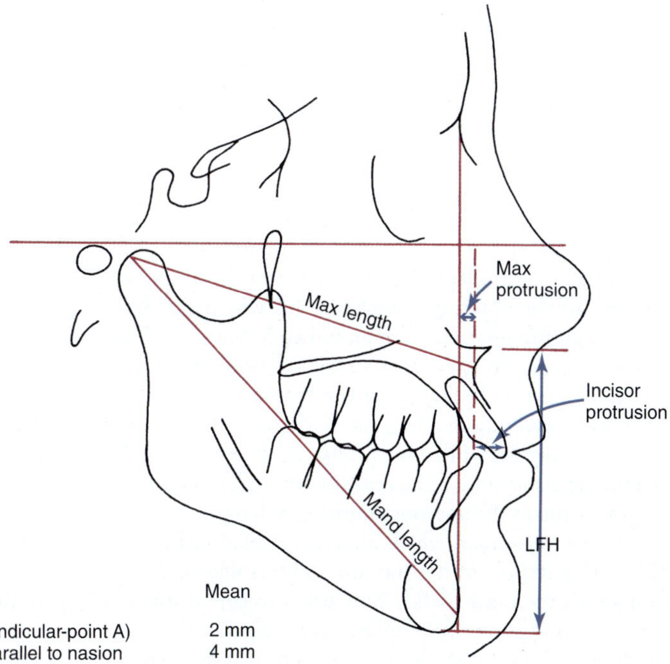

Measurements	Mean
Maxillary protrusion (mm distance from nasion perpendicular-point A)	2 mm
Maxillary incisor protrusion (mm distance from line parallel to nasion perpendicular to labial surface of incisor)	4 mm
Maxillary length } Mandibular length } Lower face height (LFH) }	As in Harvold analysis

• **Fig. 6.69** Measurements used in the McNamara analysis for a mixed dentition patient: *maxillary protrusion* (millimeter distance from nasion [N] perpendicular–point A), mean is 0 mm; *maxillary incisor protrusion* (millimeter distance from line parallel to N perpendicular to labial surface of incisor), mean is 4–6 mm; *mandibular protrusion* (millimeter distance from N perpendicular to Pg; mean is –6 to –8 mm); *maxillary length* and *mandibular length*, both measured from Co and in the lateral view, with means of approximately 86 and 106 mm, respectively; *lower face height* (*LFH*, measured from ANS to Me; mean is 60 mm). Some of these are subtle differences from the Harvold analysis but make it a different analysis.

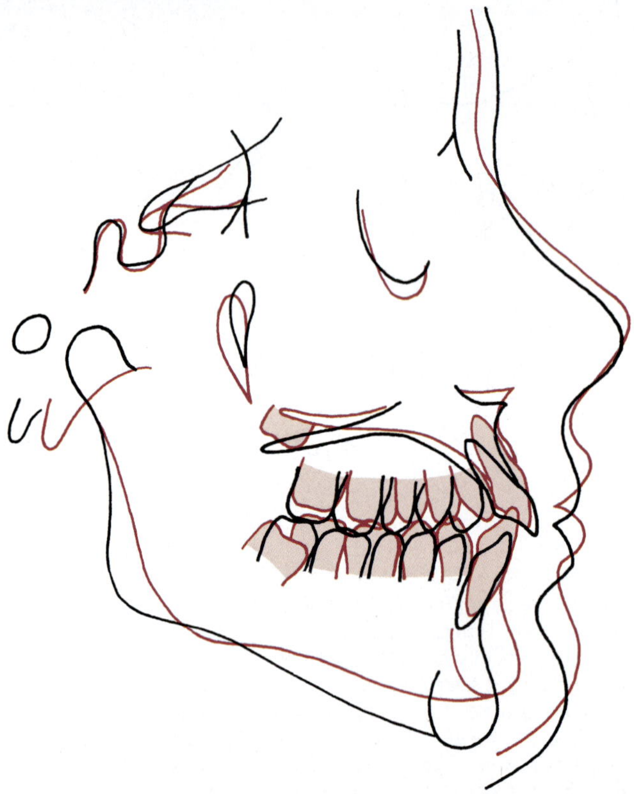

• **Fig. 6.70** Cranial base superimposition of the standard Bolton template for age 14 *(red)* on the tracing of a 13-year-old boy. The age 14 template was chosen because it matches cranial base length. Note that from a comparison of the template with this patient, the considerable increase in the lower face height and downward rotation of the mandible can be seen clearly. It also is apparent that the patient's maxilla is rotated down posteriorly. This comparison of a patient's tracing to a template is a direct approach toward describing the relationship of functional facial units.

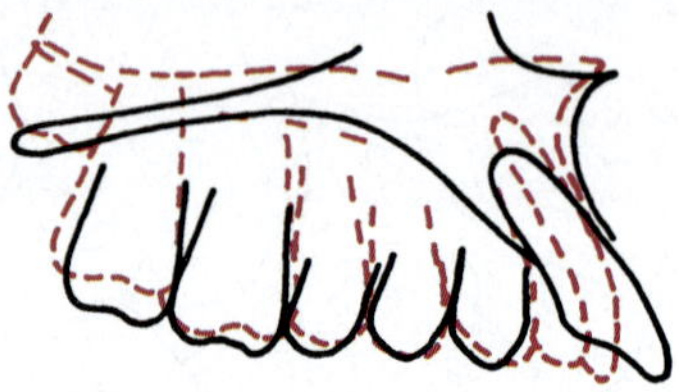

• **Fig. 6.71** Superimposition of the Bolton template on the maxilla (primarily on the anterior palatal contour) of the patient shown in Fig. 6.66. This superimposition clearly reveals the forward protrusion of the maxillary incisors relative to the maxilla but also shows that the vertical relationship of the maxillary teeth to the maxilla for this patient is nearly ideal.

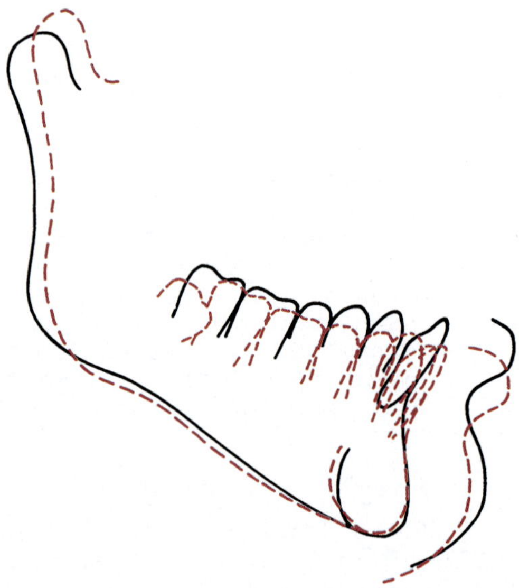

• **Fig. 6.72** Superimposition of the Bolton template on the mandible of the patient in Fig. 6.66. This superimposition indicates that the patient's mandible is longer than the ideal, but the ramus is shorter and inclined posteriorly. All the mandibular teeth have erupted more than normal, especially the incisors.

represent the reference data. Two things must be kept in mind: (1) the patient's physical size and (2) his or her developmental age. The best plan usually is to select the reference template initially so that the length of the anterior cranial base (of which the SN distance is a good approximation) is approximately the same for the patient and the template, and then to consider developmental age, moving forward or backward in the template age if the patient is developmentally quite advanced or retarded. In almost all instances, correcting for differences between developmental and chronologic age also leads to the selection of a template that more nearly approximates the anterior cranial base length.

1. *Cranial base superimposition*, which allows the relationship of the maxilla and mandible to the cranium to be evaluated (Fig. 6.70). In general, the most useful approach is to superimpose on the SN line, registering the template over the patient's tracing at the nasion rather than the sella if there is a difference in cranial base length. (For growth prediction with templates, it is important to use the posterior superimposition points described with the prediction method. For analysis, registering SN at N is usually preferable.)

   To judge the changes relative to the cranial base, the AP and vertical position of maxilla and mandible can be observed and described. It is important at this stage to look not at the position of the teeth, key observations are the position of the landmarks that indicate the skeletal units (i.e., anterior nasal spine and point A for the anterior maxilla, posterior nasal spine for the posterior maxilla; point B, pogonion and gnathion for the anterior mandible, and gonion for the posterior mandible). The object is to evaluate the position of the skeletal units. For the template analysis evaluate how the patient's jaw positions differ from the norm. Compensations within the individual's skeletal pattern are observed directly.
2. *Maxillary superimposition*. The second superimposition is on the maximum contour of the palate to evaluate the relationship of the maxillary dentition to the maxilla (Fig. 6.71. Again, it is important to evaluate the position of the teeth both vertically and anteroposteriorly. The template analysis makes it easy to see whether the teeth are displaced vertically, which is information often not obtained in measurement analysis techniques.
3. *Mandibular superimposition*. The third superimposition is on the symphysis of the mandible along the lower border, to evaluate the relationship of the mandibular dentition to the mandible. Fig. 6.72). If the shadow of the mandibular canal is shown on the templates, a more accurate orientation can be obtained by registering along this rather than the lower border posteriorly. Both the vertical and the AP positions of the anterior and posterior teeth should be noted.

Template analysis in this fashion quickly provides an overall impression of the way in which the patient's dentofacial structures are related. Sometimes the reason for making measurements, which is to gain an overall understanding of the pattern of the patient's facial relationships, is overlooked in a focus on acquiring the numbers themselves. Comparing the patient's features with a template is an excellent way to overcome this hazard and be sure that one does not miss the forest while observing the trees.

Template analysis often is thought of as somehow less scientific than making a series of measurements, but really that is not so. Remember that the template contains exactly the same information as a table of measurements from the same data bases. The information is just expressed in a different way. The difference is that with the template method, there is greater emphasis on the clinician's individual assessment of whatever about the patient may be abnormal, and a corresponding de-emphasis of specific criteria.

Templates easily can be used with computer analysis as well. The technique would be to store the templates in computer memory, then pull up the appropriate template for comparison to the patient's digitized tracing, and use the computer to make the series of superimpositions. The clinician, looking at the superimpositions, should be stimulated to make his own assessment of interactions among the various components of the face.

Serial Cephalometric Superimposition Techniques

Serial superimpositions are designed to detect growth and treatment changes. Although there are numerous superimposition variations that can give different impressions of changes, it is best to use a method that has a sound biologic basis and a result that coincides with our understanding of facial growth. With these acknowledgments, we will discuss the method currently adapted by the American Board of Orthodontics.[53–56]

The three separate superimpositions described here provide a comprehensive 2D analysis of facial growth. Superimpositions of two or more tracings are helpful when observing continued growth in a class III patient with mandibular prognathism. In that case, you will wait to treat when growth is completed with either surgical or traditional orthodontics. Another application is when a patient is in treatment, and you are trying to judge the effect of treatment.

Cranial Base Serial Superimposition Technique

This documents maxillary and mandibular skeletal changes in direction and amount and overall facial height changes relative to the cranial base. No interpretation of maxillary or mandibular dental changes are appropriate. Specifically, the tracings are registered on the anterior wall of sella turcica and use the superior plane of the sphenoid bone and continue on to the cribriform plate (Fig. 6.73A). All of these points are considered reasonably stable after 6 years of age. For anteroposterior orientation, the anterior wall of sella turcica and a line bisecting the greater wings of the sphenoid bone are useful. For vertical orientation, the intersection of the anterior wall of sella turcica and the anterior clinoid processes and the plane of the sphenoid bone and the cribiform plate serve well. The final positioning is a best fit. As a simplified alternative, some clinicians use the S-N line and register at S.

Maxillary Serial Superimposition Technique

This is just a superimposition of the maxilla and removes maxillary position change and adjusts for modeling changes, so changes in tooth position, both vertically and anteroposteriorly relative to the maxilla, are obvious. The method is to superimpose on the anterior side of the zygomatic process between the key ridge and orbital (Fig. 6.73B). This provides primary anteroposterior orientation. For vertical orientation, use the floor of the orbit and the nasal floor. Here it is critical to account for modeling changes—apposition at the floor of the orbit and resorption at the floor of the nose. The vertical distance is divided 3/5 in favor of orbital apposition and 2/5 for nasal floor resorption.

Mandibular Serial Cephalometric Superimposition

This superimposition provides information on the movement of the mandibular teeth relative to the mandible and the length and direction of condylar growth. The method is to register on the anterior surface of the bony chin contour below pogonion, the inner aspect of the posterior and inferior symphysis and the mandibular nerve canals (see Fig. 6.73C). Additionally, the lower surface of the crypt of the developing third molar (if present) before root development is included secondarily. The chin contour and posterior symphysis provide anteroposterior orientation and the inferior aspect of the symphysis and the alveolar nerve canal (and possibly the third molar crypt) provide vertical orientation.

Cervical Vertebral Maturation Staging From Cephalometric Radiographs

Another approach to evaluating facial growth status is to get an estimate of how much mandibular growth remains, which would be especially important for a child with a skeletal class II problem who would benefit from orthodontic treatment to modify growth, if that is possible. This has been attempted by using the stage of development of the cervical vertebrae as seen in a cephalometric radiograph to determine the timing and status of mandibular growth[57]. Studies using a diagnostic testing model that evaluates sensitivity, specificity and positive and negative predictive validity of a given diagnostic test have had limited success in validating this method[58,59] (see Fig. 3.12 and Chapter 3 and earlier in this chapter for more details). Additionally, the stage of vertebral development is not useful in establishing whether jaw growth has subsided to adult levels in a teenager with mandibular prognathism.

The stage of dental development should *not* be used to estimate the stage of jaw growth. As we emphasized earlier (see Fig. 3.13), dental development correlates less well with skeletal growth than almost any other developmental index.

Hand-wrist radiographs are an alternative method for evaluating skeletal maturity, but these also are not an accurate way to determine when growth is completed.[60] Serial cephalometric radiographs offer the most accurate way to determine whether facial growth has stopped or is continuing, because you are not inferring future facial growth changes, but measuring them.

Cephalometric Methodology in a Digital Age

Today, with digital images, it is still important to follow a sequence of steps in cephalometric analysis to ensure that the conclusions reached are defensible:

1. Look carefully at the overall image for pathologic issues. The most likely indication of pathologic conditions will take the form of radiolucencies or opacities in unexpected places or to a bigger extent than expected. Sometimes it is the shape or size of a structure, such as the sella turcica or a condyle, that signals a problem. Remember, about one cephalometric radiograph in a thousand will show significant pathologic problems—so in a practice with the current average of 250 to 300 new patients per year, you should expect to see such problems once in 3 to 4 years.
2. Look for head positioning errors or indications of facial asymmetry. The ear rods should be concentric (unless the image was deliberately taken using only one ear rod because of clinically observed asymmetry). If the right and left structures in the

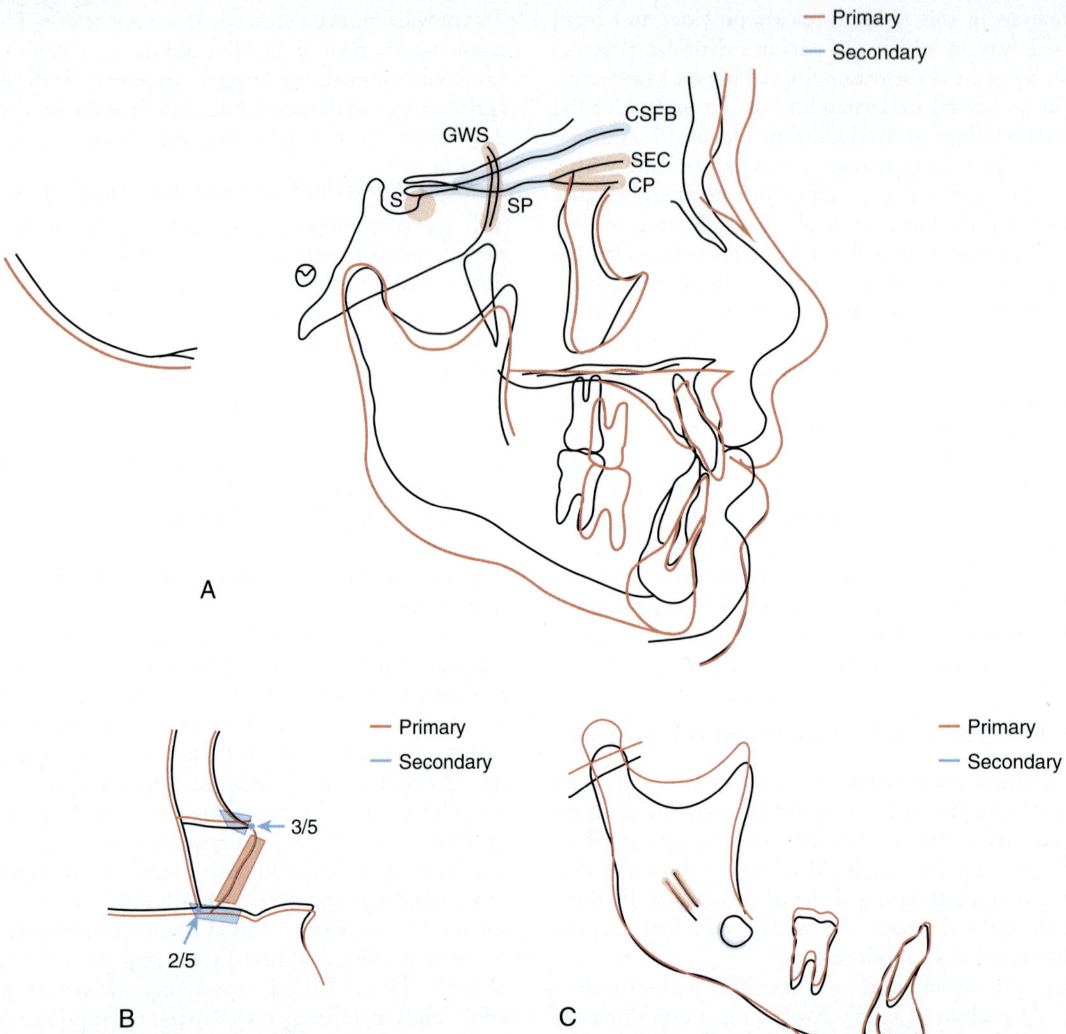

• **Fig. 6.73** Serial cephalometric superimposition techniques can provide information regarding growth and treatment changes. Here we review the anatomic areas of registration for each superimposition. (A) The cranial base superimposition demonstrates changes in the position of the jaws to the cranial base and each other. Primary registration is on the anterior wall of sella turcica, the spheno-ethmoid plane and the greater wings of the sphenoid. Secondary registration is on the roof of the orbit. (B) The maxillary superimposition shows changes of the teeth to the maxilla. The primary anteroposterior registration is along the anterior surface of the zygomatic bone with vertical registration on the floor of the orbit and the floor of the nose. The apposition on the floor of the orbit and the resorption on the floor of the nose should be divided 3/5 to 2/5, respectively. (C) The mandibular superimposition demonstrates mandibular tooth movement relative to the mandible and amount and direction of condylar growth. Primary registration is on the inner aspect of the symphasis, the anterior symphasis below Pg and the inferior alveolar nerve canal. The lower surface of the developing third molar crypt prior to root formation provides further orientation.[53] (From American Board of Orthodontics. Superimpositions. https://ntiiiby.americanboardortho.com/orthodontists/become-certified/clinical-exam/mail-in-cre-submission-procedure/case-record-preparation/superimpositions/.)

upper part of the image (e.g., orbits, key ridges, greater wings of the sphenoid) are evenly spaced and those in the lower part are not (or vice versa), that usually indicates skeletal asymmetry. If all are evenly spaced, but to a greater or lesser extent than is normal, it usually indicates a positioning problem.

3. Check the landmark points. Contemporary cephalometric points are either manually or AI identified. This is a point identification exercise whose integrity depends upon a reliable and valid method. If it is not, the method collapses. Because all the points in the template are digitized, go back and check them for accuracy. Reevaluate particularly critical points such as A, B, PG, Me, Co, Or, N, Go, and Po and the occlusal plane. Errors in locating them can dramatically alter your measurements and impression of the patient's problem.
4. Beware of the common geometric issues that can affect interpretation of result of cephalometric measures. These have been alluded to earlier and have been captured in Figs. 6.65 and 6.68. Protrusion or retrusion of the maxilla and mandible can fool the practitioner. More maxillary and mandibular protrusion increases anteroposterior differences; less decreases it for the same differences. This same protrusion must be factored into evaluation of incisors as well. Vertical differences also can cause interpretation problems. Increased or decreased lower face height magnifies or decreases skeletal anteroposterior differences.

5. Make certain that extremal points are truly extremal. Cast true vertical and horizontal reference lines so that the depth or prominence of A, B Pog, and Me are valid.
6. Look for consistency in similar types of measures. AP measures hopefully tell consistent stories, as should vertical measures. If not, then be certain they are not being affected by commonly known shortcomings of the individual measures such as differences created by maxillary and mandibular protrusion relative to the cranial base or aberrant face height.
7. Look for facial proportionality or lack of it. This can be a key issue. For example, if the lower face is long and the mandibular plane angle is high, but the patient is large and the upper and lower face heights are proportional, this is less of a problem than it would be in a patient with disproportionate face heights and an open bite. This method of moving from the small details to the bigger picture and making certain you can explain what you see, and any inconsistencies will serve you well. It is not just the numbers, but what they mean. And remember—superimposing a normal template can help in determining exactly what's different about your patient.

Three-Dimensional Imaging in Modern Orthodontics

Axial CT and its improved version, spiral CT, have been available for over 40 years now and quickly came to be widely used in medical applications. Neither form of CT was used to generate typical orthodontic diagnostic records because of their considerable cost and the relatively large radiation dose, which is quite acceptable for major medical problems, but not for most elective treatment including orthodontics.

The advent of CBCT for views of the head and face in the early 21st century changed this because the cost of the equipment (and therefore the cost of obtaining the images) is significantly less than for medical CT, and the radiation dose also is greatly reduced. At this point, CBCT is being widely used in orthodontics. There is a consensus that it provides new information that could improve the treatment plan in certain situations, and enough enthusiasm to lead some orthodontists to advocate use of CBCT on all orthodontic patients, replacing panoramic, cephalometric, and occlusal radiographs, as well as tomograms of the TMJ. There is a significant radiation dose increase in doing this, however (Table 6.9).

Does the additional information from CBCT translate into better treatment plans and improved treatment outcomes? Answering that question requires an understanding of the critical variables in use of CBCT, and then careful examination of its applications in orthodontic diagnosis and treatment planning. Let us start with the basic concepts in 3D imaging.

Basic Concepts

A CBCT scan is derived from a cone-shaped X-ray beam that is directed through the patient's head, and information is captured on a flat two-dimensional (2D) area detector as a series of slices as the X-ray beam rotates totally or partially around the subject and moves vertically as it does so. Each slice contains hundreds of thousands of voxels, the 3D equivalent of pixels in a digital camera. A darker grayscale intensity of a voxel reflects that more radiation reached it.

Two types of image resolution are important: contrast resolution, the ability to distinguish between tissues of different densities (which is somewhat limited because CBCT images have low soft

TABLE 6.9 Communicating Radiation Risks to Patients: Effective Doses and Cancer Risks From Dentomaxillofacial Radiologic Imaging

Examination	Effective Dose (mSv)[a]	Equivalent Background Radiation[b]	Estimated Cancer Risk[c]	RELATIVE RADIATION LEVELS[D]	
				Adult	Child
Bitewings, 4 images Cephalometric	0.005	<1 day	1 in 4 million	☢	☢
Los Angeles to New York City, 5-hour air travel	0.015	~1.5 days			
Panoramic, direct digital	0.02	~2 days	1 in a million	☢	☢
Full-mouth x-rays, digital sensor with rectangular collimation	0.03	~3 days	1 in 600,000	☢	☢☢
Los Angeles to Osaka, 15-hour air travel	0.045	~5 days			
CBCT, limited FOV	0.05	~6 days	1 in 400,000	☢	☢☢
Full-mouth x-rays, storage phosphor with round collimation CBCT, both jaws Chest radiograph	0.1	~ 12 days	1 in 200,000	☢☢	☢☢
Los Angeles to Singapore, round trip, 33-hour air travel	0.1	~ 12 days			
CBCT, both jaws with cranium	0.15	~ 2 weeks	1 in 130,000	☢☢	☢☢
Mammogram	0.4	~ 7 weeks	1 in 50,000	☢☢	☢☢☢
Multidetector computed tomography, maxillofacial	0.8	~ 14 weeks	1 in 25,000	☢☢☢	☢☢☢
Multidetector computed tomography, chest	7.0	~ 2 years	1 in 3,000	☢☢☢	☢☢☢☢

[a]Median effective doses of typical imaging protocols collated from multiple published studies.
[b]Equivalent background radiation is based on the average annual US background exposure of 3.1 mSv.
[c]Cancer risk estimated at 5.5%/Sv as per ICRP publication No. 103.
[d]Relative radiation levels. From American College of Radiology, ACR Appropriateness Criteria, www.acr.org/-/media/ACR/Files/Appropriateness-Criteria/ RadiationDoseAssessmentIntro.pdf.
From Mallya SM. Effective and safe use of X-rays: understanding the risks for practical decision-making. *J. Calif. Dent. Assoc.* 2021;49(5):301–309.

tissue contrast), and spatial resolution, the ability to distinguish between separate structures that are positioned very close together. Smaller voxel size provides better spatial resolution. Because voxels are cubes, the resolution is the same for the three planes of space.

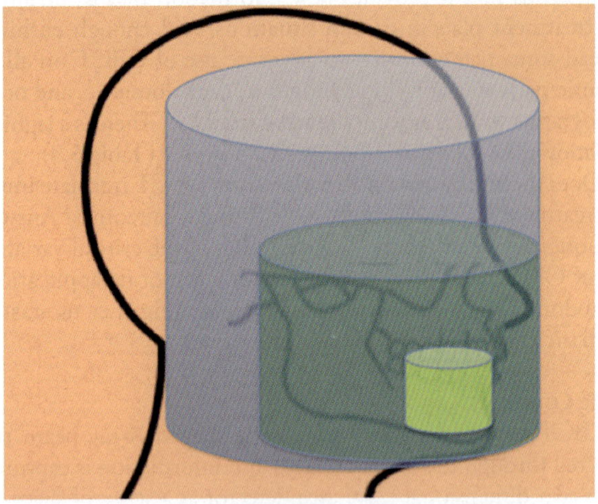

• **Fig. 6.74** Different fields of view provide different areas of coverage of the head and different levels of radiation. Use of the smallest one that will yield the critical information is most important.

The amount of radiation exposure is determined by three things: the resolution needed for adequate diagnostic accuracy—the greater the resolution that is needed, the larger the resolution dose; the voxel size—the smaller the voxels, the greater the amount of radiation; and the field of view (FOV), which reflects the size of the irradiated area—the larger the FOV, the greater the radiation dose (Fig. 6.74). The radiation can be reduced by accepting the lower resolution that comes with larger voxels and using the smallest FOV that would be compatible with an adequate diagnosis. A recent addition to CBCT imaging is a "quick scan" feature, which minimizes radiation exposure but is adequate only for dental anomalies and impacted teeth in a small area, not evaluation of, say, resorption caused by an ectopic tooth. This does bring the radiation down to the equivalent of two digital radiographs, which is the minimum that would be needed with 2D radiography.

Orthodontic Applications of Cone Beam Computed Tomography

The ability to view structures from all three planes of space without any superimposition and geometric distortions is the key advantage of CBCT over conventional images (Fig. 6.75). Synthetic cephalometric and panoramic images also can be produced (Fig. 6.76). The key disadvantage, of course, is the increased radiation exposure, and the simplest way to balance this risk against the

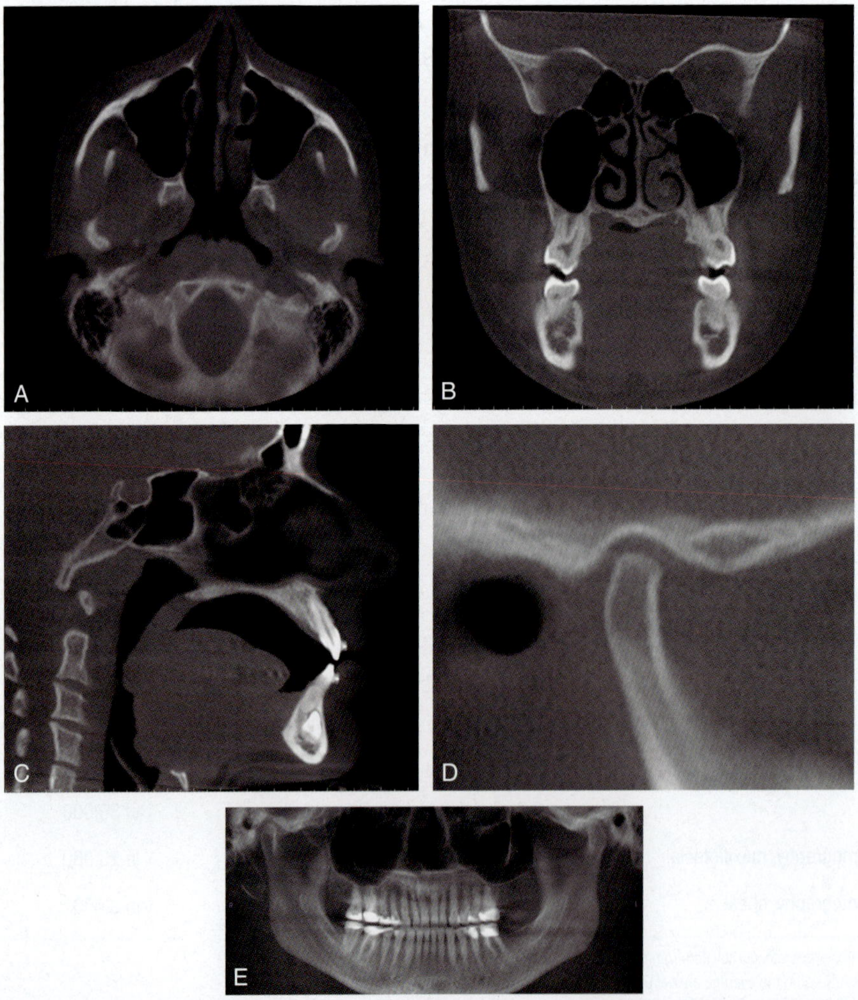

• **Fig. 6.75** Selection of cone beam computed tomography (*CBCT*) images demonstrating the ability to provide all three planes of space: (A) axial; (B) coronal; (C) sagittal for examination of the entire head with a large field of view (*FOV*). In addition, (D) the bony temporomandibular joint area can be imaged with a smaller FOV or extracted from a large FOV. (E) A synthetic panoramic radiograph can also be extracted.

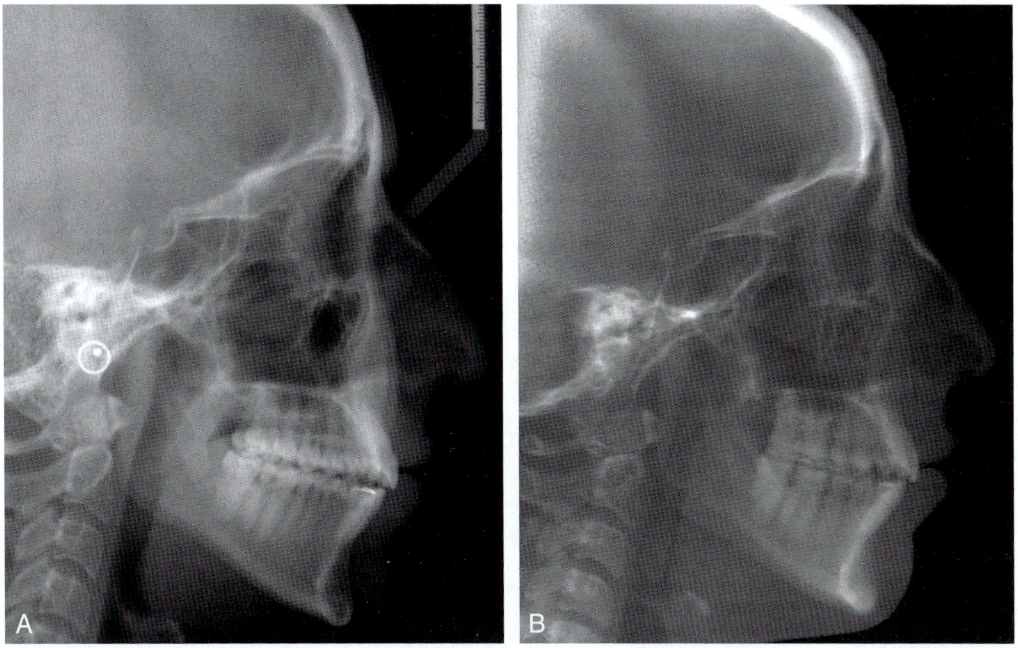

• **Fig. 6.76** Comparison of (A) standard cephalometric radiograph and (B) "synthetic ceph" created from a thick slice of cone beam computed tomography (*CBCT*) data from the same individual. They are similar in a number of ways, and studies have shown that the same measures on both are equal, but they do not look exactly alike.

benefits is to follow the rule that CBCT is indicated when it is the only way to get the necessary information for appropriate treatment. Five situations in which enough data now exist to support use of CBCT for orthodontic patients are as follows:

- Ectopically erupting or impacted teeth (especially maxillary canines, but other teeth as well) requiring surgical exposure and orthodontic tooth movement to bring them into the mouth. Or, ectopically erupting teeth that are suspected of causing resorption of adjacent teeth or those in the eruption path. Supernumerary teeth may also require 3D imaging to determine their location, potential for eruption problems involving other teeth and timing and difficulty of extraction.
- Severe facial asymmetry, especially asymmetries involving roll and yaw (see later section)
- Syndromes, congenital deformities, and sequelae of facial trauma
- Dental fractures and transplantation
- Hard tissue problems in the TMJ

Let us consider these uses in the order of their frequency as CBCT applications.

Ectopically Erupting or Impacted Teeth. In evaluating ectopically erupting or impacted teeth (including supernumeraries), CBCT provides four types of information that can significantly change the treatment plan that would have resulted from 2D radiographs: (1) presence or absence of teeth or supernumeraries (Fig. 6.77); (2) the position of the teeth relative to one another (Fig. 6.78); (3) clear demonstration of the extent of damage (resorption) to the roots of adjacent permanent teeth (Fig. 6.79); and (4) definition of the path along which an unerupted tooth should be moved so that the tooth can be brought into the mouth efficiently and with the least further damage to adjacent teeth (Fig. 6.80).[61] This allows adjustments such as bringing an impacted canine facially or lingually before beginning to bring it toward the occlusal plane, to avoid the remaining root of a damaged lateral incisor, and makes it possible for the surgeon and orthodontist to plan and apply the best treatment. For instance, the orthodontist may need to alter the anchorage appliance to include transpalatal arches with multiple attachment points so the direction of traction to the impacted canine is optimal. The

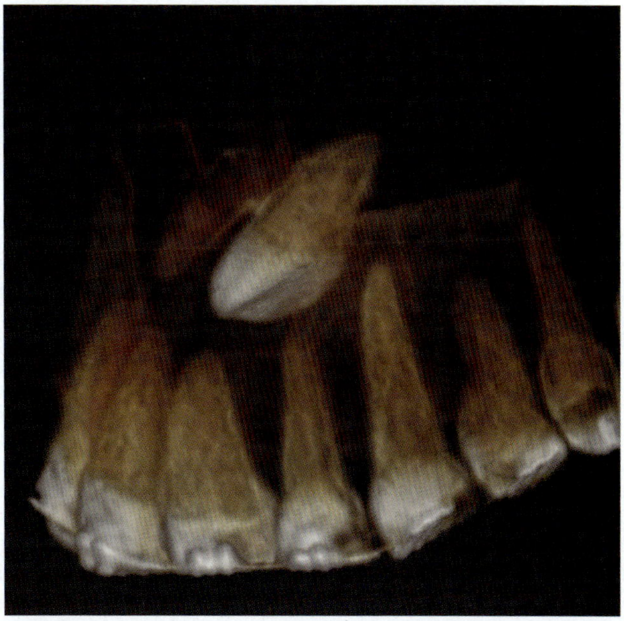

• **Fig. 6.77** Cone beam computed tomography (*CBCT*) images can provide added value in detecting the presence or absence of ectopic, impacted, or supernumerary teeth, as in the image. The number of supernumerary teeth is also easier to determine on a CBCT image.

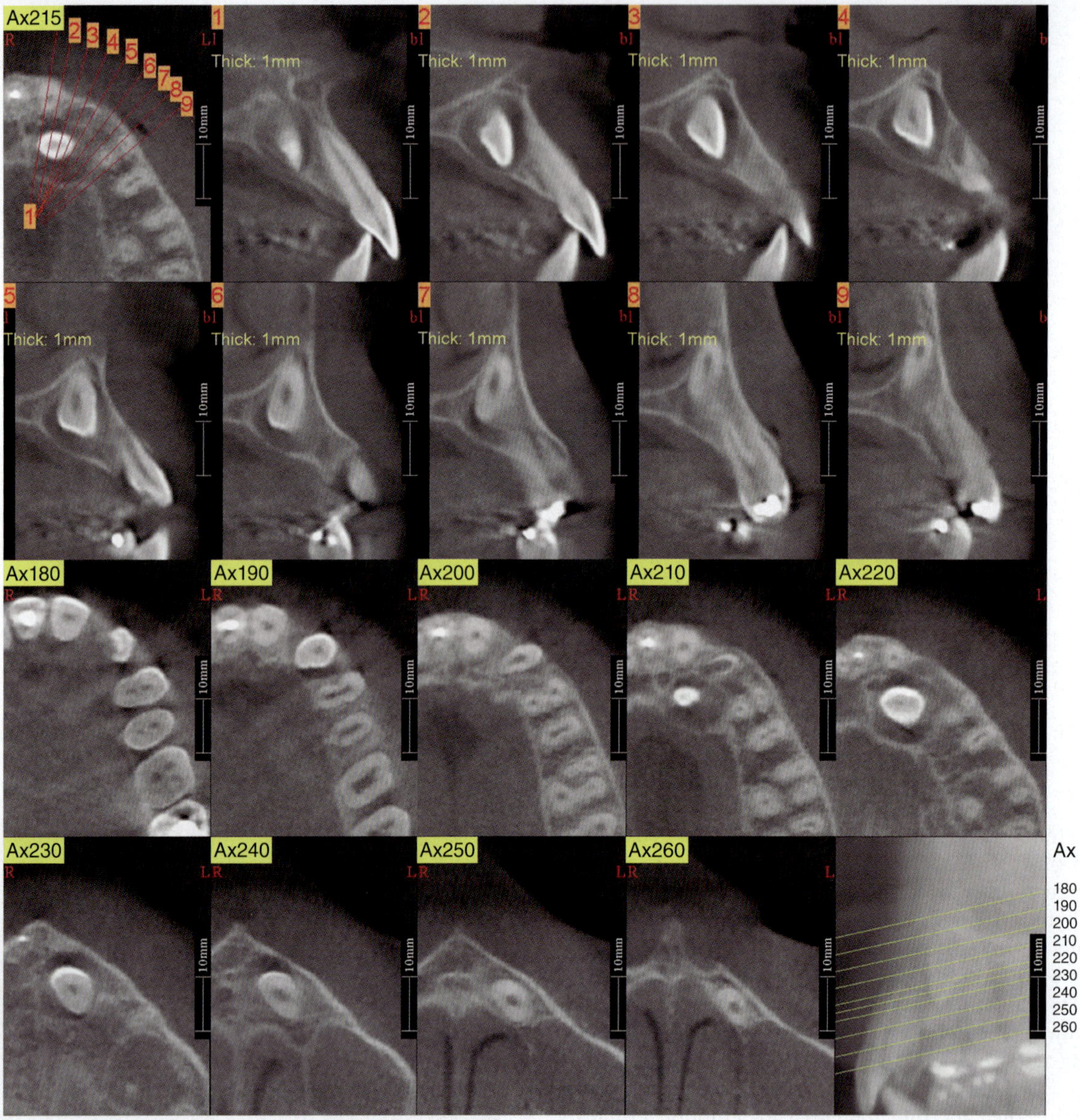

• **Fig. 6.78** The position of unerupted teeth relative to one another is best detected on a cone beam computed tomography (*CBCT*) image. This series of images shows the crown of an impacted canine, moving along the upper dental arch *(top two rows)* and from the occlusal plane upward *(lower two rows)*. The relationship of the impacted tooth to both the bone around it and the other teeth can be seen in detail at each level.

surgeon can place an attachment on the tooth at the most favorable location for biomechanical advantage in moving it, and if a bone anchor is needed for anchorage, the 3D image facilitates placing it for best advantage.

Facial Asymmetry and Complex Orthognathic Surgery. Until CBCT became readily available, the major indication for a frontal cephalometric radiograph was facial asymmetry. Even with the addition of this image to the standard panoramic and lateral cephalometric views, evaluating asymmetry required extrapolation among the three images and was qualitative, not quantitative. With these three radiographs of a patient with an asymmetric mandible, one could see in the lateral cephalometric view that the ramus and mandibular body are longer on one side, in the panoramic view that the ramus is longer on one side primarily because the condylar neck is longer, and in the frontal cephalometric view that the chin is off to one side—but the magnitude of the difference could be only approximated. With the multiple images and FOVs available from CBCT images (Fig. 6.81), the primary source of the asymmetry can be identified in a way that allows treatment to be targeted to it.

The same considerations apply to diagnosis and planning for complex orthognathic surgery, when simultaneous maxillary, mandibular, chin, and alveolar surgery may be necessary. For these patients, 3D imaging provides more precise diagnostic evaluation, but it is even more valuable in planning the surgical cuts and making splints for intermediate and final jaw positions (see Chapter 22). Although facial asymmetry is not the major component of many of these patients' problems, about 40% of all orthognathic surgery patients are asymmetric, and asymmetry is part of the problem for most of the complex cases.

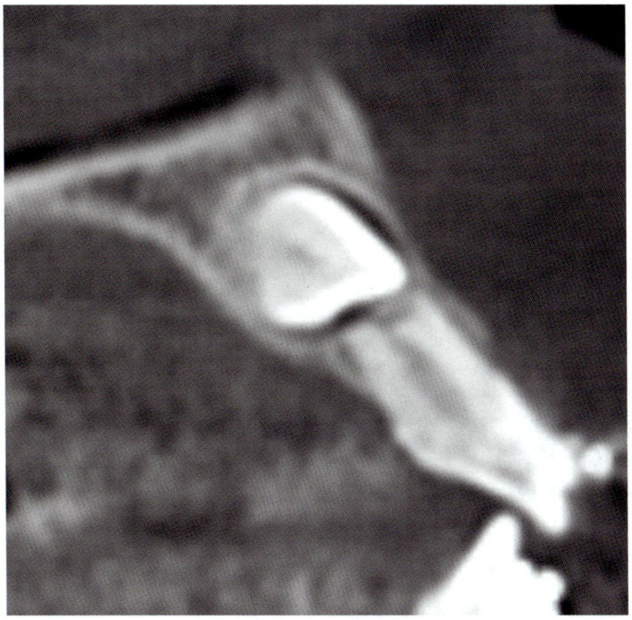

• **Fig. 6.79** The amount of damage (resorption) caused by a migrating and erupting impacted tooth is clearly demonstrated on this cone beam computed tomography (*CBCT*) image. This can lead to fully informed decisions as to extraction or retention of the damaged tooth, and as to the direction of moving the impacted tooth to minimize further damage to the damaged tooth if it is to be retained.

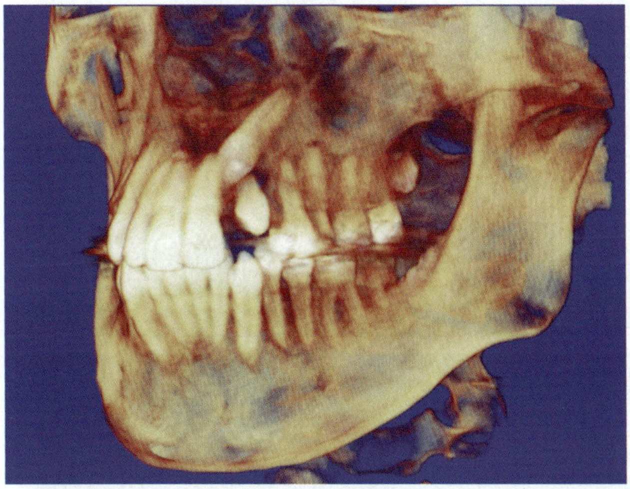

• **Fig. 6.80** An impacted canine can be seen on this medium-field-of-view cone beam computed tomography (*CBCT*) image. By rotating the image, different relationships of the teeth can be viewed. This type of image can help in planning the biomechanics necessary to move the impacted canine into occlusion.

It is possible to produce a precisely dimensioned stereolithographic model of an asymmetric facial skeleton from CT data (Fig. 6.82), so that the orthodontist and surgeon can see it in the 3D world rather than as a series of images on a computer screen. A stereolithographic model allows more precise surgical planning, including the ability to shape fixation plates in advance and determine exactly how fixation screws are to be placed. This technology is discussed in more detail in Chapter 22.

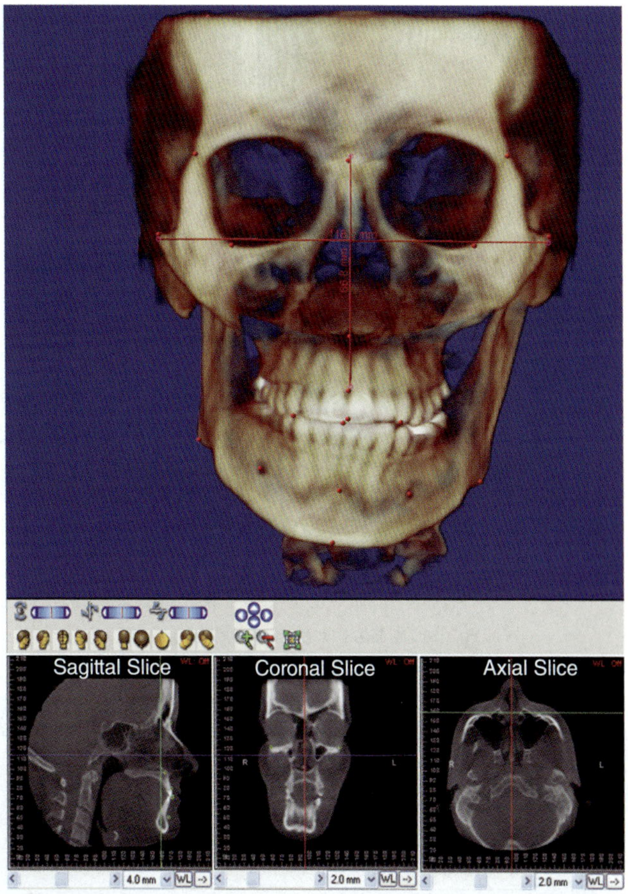

• **Fig. 6.81** Large-field cone beam computed tomography (*CBCT*) and the axial, coronal, and sagittal slices are useful in confirming the presence of clinically detected skeletal asymmetry. By measuring distances on the different views, the source of the problem can be identified and more readily addressed.

Congenital Deformities, Syndromes, and Facial Trauma. In a sense, because asymmetry usually is a major component of their problem list, patients with a syndrome or who have experienced trauma also present the same diagnostic problems as asymmetry for other reasons—quantitative measurements rather than qualitative approximations are required. A major difference is that treatment at younger ages is likely to be required. For instance, for the alveolar graft surgery that patients with cleft lip and palate need at age 7 to 9, CBCT provides valuable information such as the size of the alveolar defect and the precise location of any impacted or supernumerary teeth and allows for both linear and volumetric measurements (Fig. 6.83). For orthodontists, cleft lip and palate is the major condition that goes in the congenital deformity group. Treatment planning for them and other special circumstances is discussed at the end of the treatment planning chapter (see Chapter 7), and appropriate use of CBCT is included there. Although orthodontists are needed as part of the team that manages such patients, their diagnostic evaluation and treatment is largely beyond the scope of this book, and the reader is referred to texts that focus on management of these cases.[62,63]

Dental Trauma and Transplantation. In cases of dental trauma, usually affecting the anterior teeth, the extent of fractures that are cervical and root related are often not appreciated with clinical or 2D radiographic examinations. Tooth mobility may

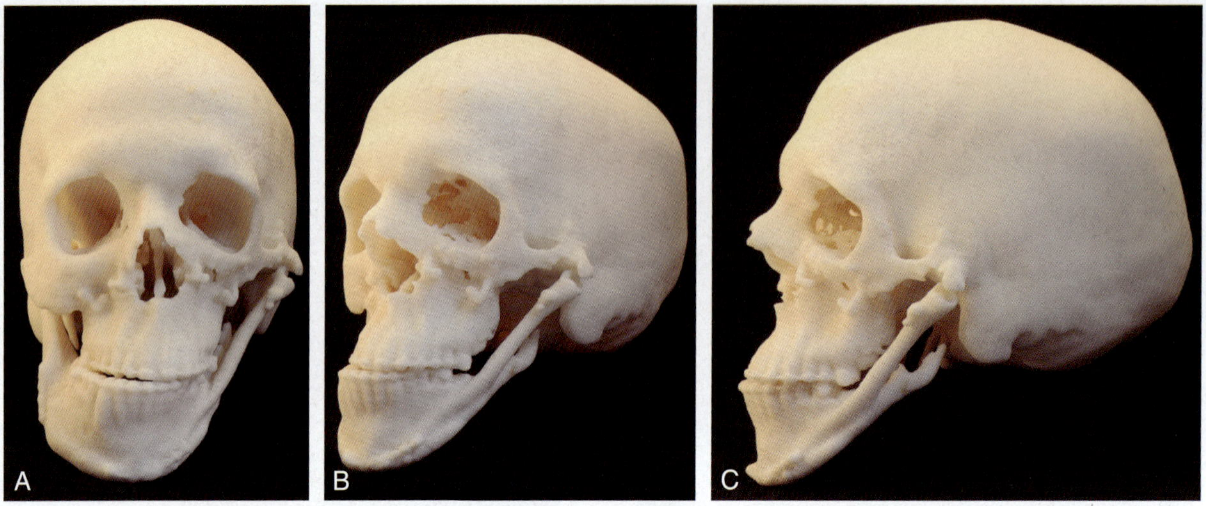

• **Fig. 6.82** (A–C) Stereolithographic model of the head of a patient with grade 3 (severe) hemifacial microsomia, in which the ramus of the mandible is completely missing on the affected left side. Having undergone a previous surgery in which a rib graft was placed to connect the body of the mandible on the left side to a point of articulation with the skull, at this time she required additional surgery to improve function and gain better symmetry. A model like this is an essential part of planning complex surgical treatment. (Courtesy Dr. T.A. Turvey.)

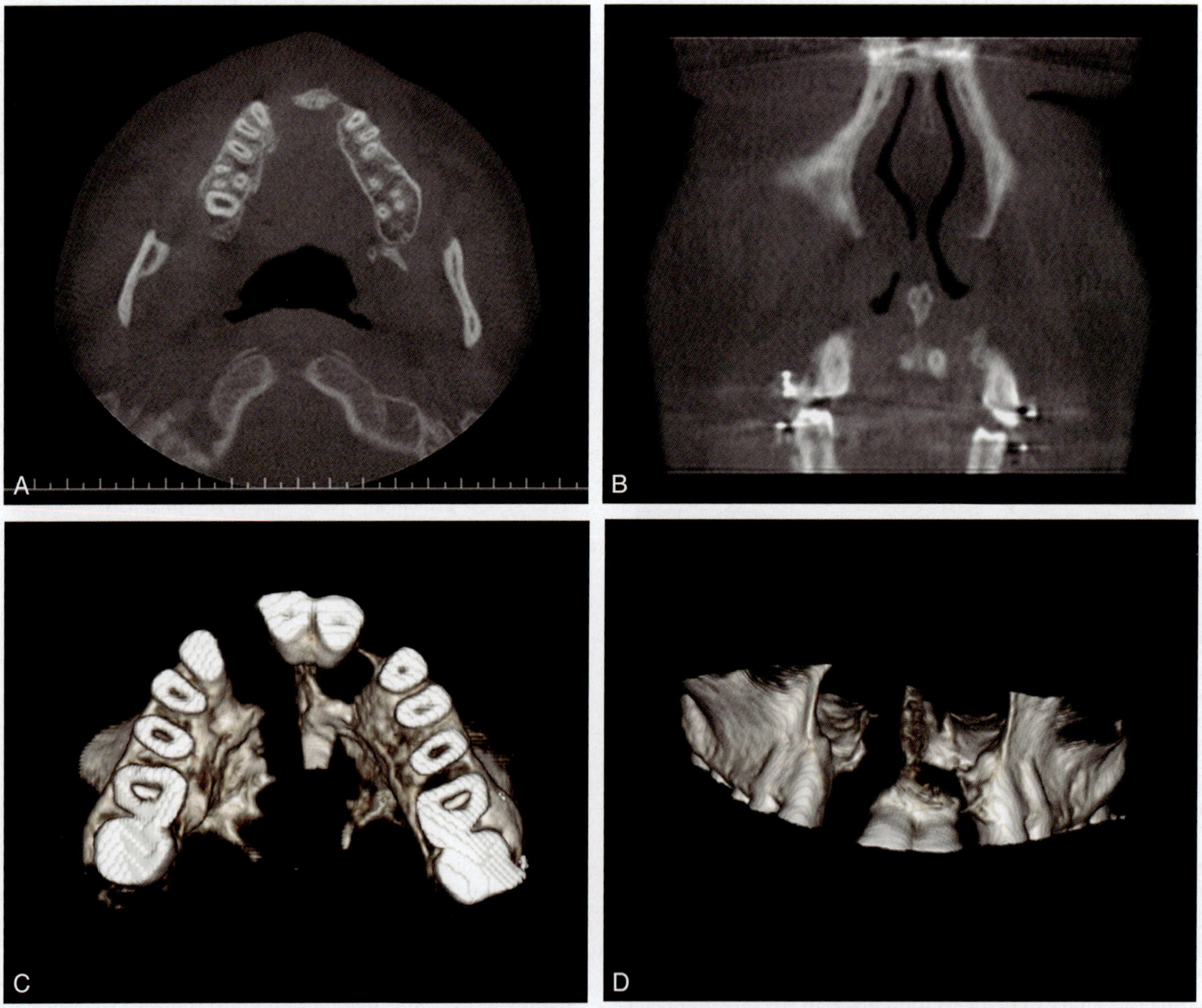

• **Fig. 6.83** In patients with cleft lip and palate, (A–D) the cone beam computed tomography (*CBCT*) images can be extremely useful in determining the location and extent of the clefting, the location of teeth relative to the cleft, and the location and timing of an alveolar bone graft so that erupting teeth near the cleft site can bring new bone with them.

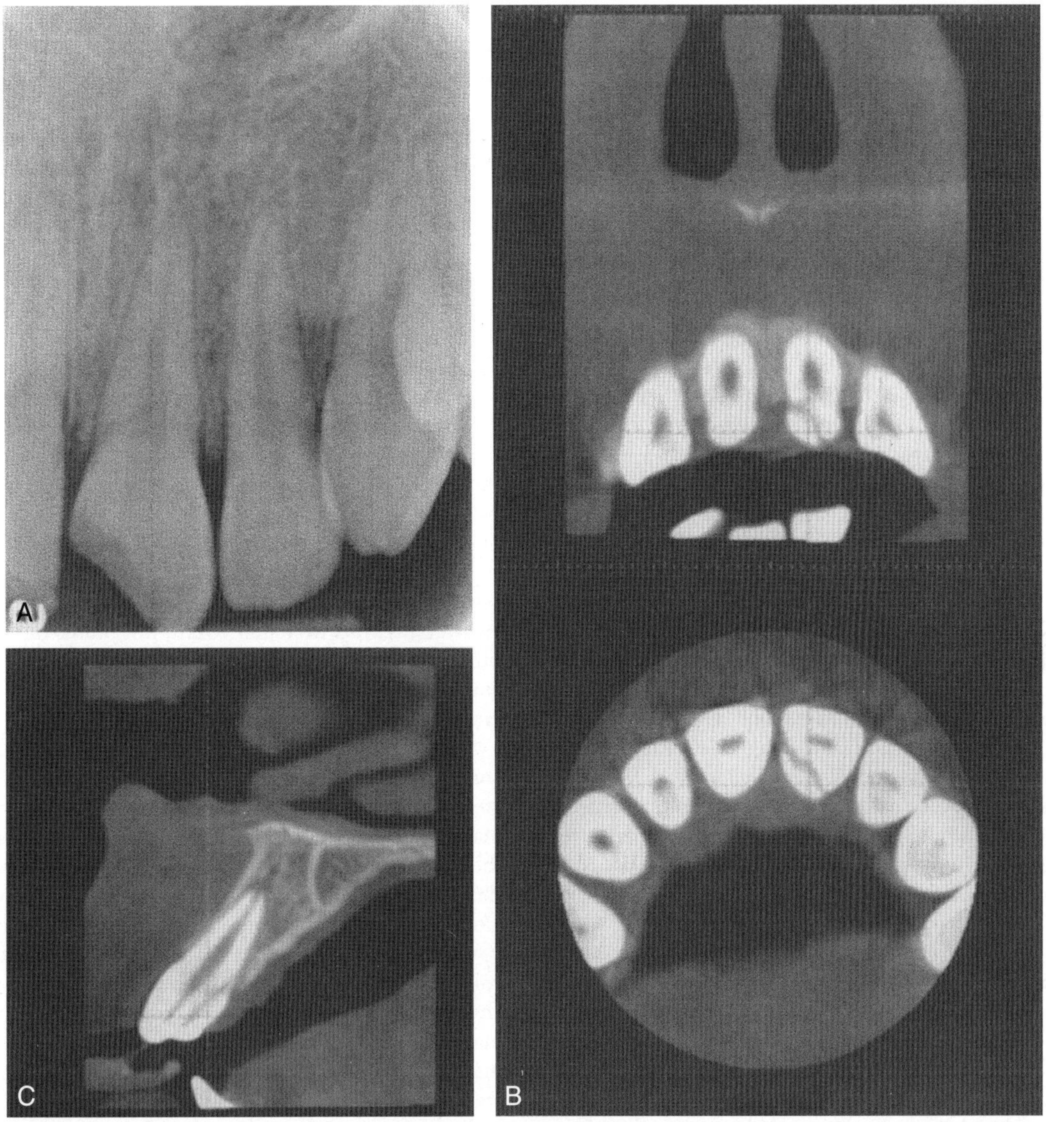

• **Fig. 6.84** (A) A periapical image of a traumatic dental injury showing the mesioincisal fracture. (B) Small filed cone beam computed tomography coronal (above) and axial (below) images showing the shear crown fracture on the lingual surface of the incisor. (C) Small field sagittal view shows the fracture on the lingual surface extending down the root surface. This will be a more challenging treatment.

suggest a more extensive fracture. It may be necessary, given the clinical presentation and existing radiographs, to obtain a small field dental CBCT to examine specific groups of teeth for a full fracture assessment (Fig. 6.84).

Another creative use of CBCT imaging is to use stereolithographic printing to fabricate a model of a tooth that is planned to be transplanted. At the time of the transplantation, the site is prepared by "fitting" the analogue to the receptor site before harvesting the actual donor tooth. With this method, there is little manipulation of the donor tooth and less chance of injury to the tooth or supporting periodontal tissues before the actual final surgical steps. Because intact periodontal ligament structures are critical to transplant success, this approach should improve the outcomes. Tooth transplantation is discussed in more detail in Chapter 12.

Hard Tissue Aspects of Temporomandibular Joint Problems. Distortion or malformation of TMJ hard tissues is relatively infrequent, but certainly can be a component of TMD, and if the mandibular condyle or the adjacent hard tissues are abnormal, CBCT can be a valuable aspect of their evaluation. It is important to keep in mind, however, that the soft tissues in the joint are more likely to be involved in TMD than the hard tissues—and if that is the case, MRI would be the appropriate diagnostic imaging, not CBCT. These issues are discussed in Chapter 20.

Diagnostic Scope of Cone Beam Computed Tomography Imaging

Pathologic Issues

There are two important considerations for detection of pathologic conditions in radiographs taken for orthodontic diagnosis. First, orthodontic diagnosis is appropriately focused on developmental problems, but just as an orthodontist should pick up pathologic problems on cephalometric and panoramic radiographs (which they have been taught to do in typical specialty training), pathologic changes on CBCT images also should be detected. Is the orthodontist responsible for doing so? Should a maxillofacial radiologist with training in evaluation of CBCT images review the images created at the orthodontist's request? The answer to both questions is *yes*—either the orthodontist develops the expertise needed to detect unexpected pathologic features, or they must get an expert evaluation for that purpose.

Is it an advantage or a disadvantage that large-field CBCT images offer the possibility of diagnosing conditions in this FOV that would not have been diagnosed this early without the 3D imaging? This leads to the same discussion as with other diagnostic procedures that are not focused on a specific condition or indication for their use. For some patients, the discovery of an unexpected lesion would lead to further diagnostic evaluation and perhaps more successful treatment than would have occurred with later discovery. For others, the same discovery and further diagnostic evaluation may lead to treatment that really was not needed but exposed the patient to unfortunate side effects. That is the situation with CBCT of the head: Along with the possibility of diagnosis of unsuspected pathologic conditions, there is also the risk of overtreatment of things that would never have become a problem—and that risk may be greater than the benefit. It is not yet clear what the risk-benefit ratio for detection of lesions outside the scope of orthodontic treatment is, but the risk of overdiagnosis and overtreatment is real.

As use of CBCT in orthodontics increases, as it seems clear that it will, the specific indications for using it should be kept in mind. Orthodontic specialty training will need, at the least, a focus on competency of interpretation for small-field images of the maxilla and mandible, but it seems likely that full-field images will require the expertise of a radiologist. This should be a sensible way to manage the risk of overdiagnosis or underdiagnosis for the patient and liability for the orthodontist.

The usefulness of CBCT in diagnosis of sleep apnea (little or none) and its role in planning for placement of mini-implants for skeletal anchorage (useful in special situations only) are discussed in more detail in the special section on these conditions at the end of Chapter 7.

Evaluation of Growth and Treatment Changes

A major use of lateral cephalometrics, in many ways its most important use, is evaluation of the changes produced by growth and/or treatment. This was the purpose for which cephalometrics was developed originally. Careful clinical examination usually can produce a comprehensive problem list that cephalometric radiographs confirm, but the most skilled clinicians cannot evaluate changes over time without superimposed cephalometric tracings. In essence, we have used tracings to discard much of the information on a cephalometric radiograph so that when we superimpose the tracings, we can see more clearly the changes in which we are really interested.

Extending this method to sequential 3D images is problematic. One possibility is to create a "synthetic ceph" from the CBCT images, which is comparable enough to conventional cephalograms to be used clinically (see Fig. 6.76),[64] and doing cephalometric analysis as it has been done for the last 50 years. But the major reason for CBCT imaging in the first place was to go beyond such a limited view that discards too much of the information. In addition, the landmarks that are used with lateral cephalograms are not reliable as the FOV is rotated away from the AP plane of space. Efforts to define landmarks for 3D superimposition are finding some success at present, but at best using them for superimposition provides a rather limited view of the changes occurring in a patient.

In cephalometric analysis, cranial base superimposition is on the sella turcica, sphenoid and cribiform plane, and the ethmoid triad, or oriented along the SN line. Rather than superimposing on landmarks, a more successful method for 3D images is to superimpose on the cranial base structure, using a voxel-based system. Although this method continues to use stable anatomic areas, it attempts to match voxels, not points or surfaces. This has proven to be more effective than landmark based systems for the cranial base[65] and voxel-based superimposition on the mandibular symphysis has been introduced.[66]

This magnifies the problem of too much information for easy comprehension. Changes at thousands of points now can be evaluated, but thousands of measurements are orders of magnitude too many. The solution is to display changes as color maps, showing the change at the thousands of points by the intensity of color and the direction of change by the color itself, as seen in Fig. 6.85.[67] Color maps are not recommended for precise quantification.

In the earlier growth and development chapters, the use of color maps generated from 3D superimpositions to show growth changes already has been introduced. Now you are seeing color maps showing changes produced by treatment and will encounter more of these later in this book and in the future orthodontic literature. Using color maps to evaluate change, of course, forces the orthodontist away from the old cephalometric "numbers game" of decisions based on specific measurements, and toward looking at the overall pattern of change.

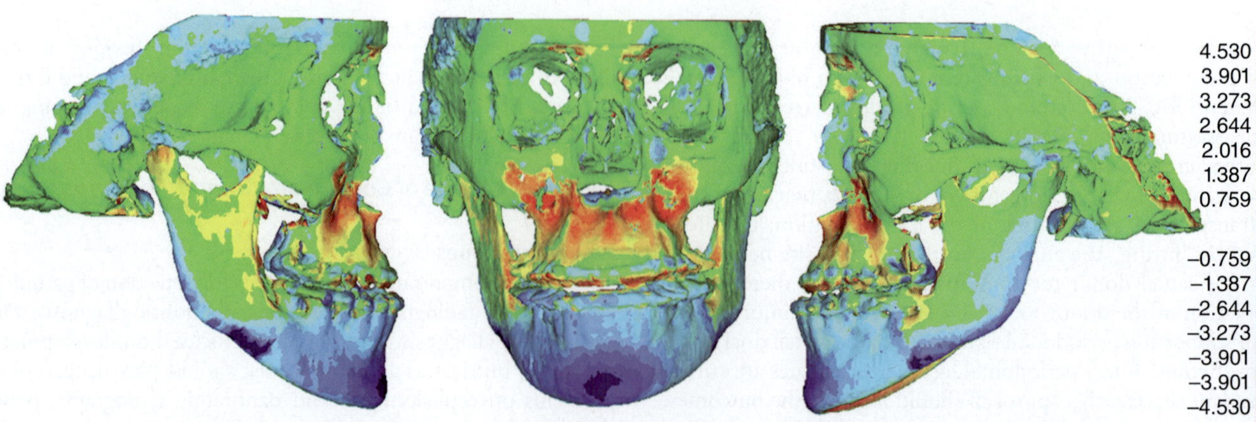

• **Fig. 6.85** Color map representing changes between preoperative and postoperative findings in a patient who underwent both maxillary advancement and asymmetric mandibular setback to correct class III malocclusion. The green color indicates little or no change; the gradient of red and blue colors displays the amount and direction of change. Red indicates forward movement toward the viewer in the center image; the more intense the red, the greater the movement, with 4.5 mm being the maximum on the scale displayed on the right side. Blue indicates backward movement away from the viewer in the center image, with the darkest blue indicating 4.5 mm.

One of the early problems with this method was that the difference between surface points on two images was determined by pairing of the closest points on the two images and not the same points on the two images. For instance, this was a problem when vertical changes also occurred, and dissimilar points came close to one another because of the new orientation. For this reason, early images created with this technology may have given us the wrong impressions. Newer algorithms are attempting to use comparable points for better analyses. This methodology will continue to evolve.

As we have already pointed out, the human brain is an analog computer, and to really understand digital information, you have to do a mental digital-to-analog conversion. Color maps make that much easier.

OSA Radiographic Airway Evaluation

The obstruction of the airway is a complex interaction of collapsibility, ventilatory control, and compensation mechanisms. Perhaps unfortunately, CBCT imaging has not proven useful in screening for the presence of OSA or predicting treatment response to the use of mandibular advancing appliances. This lack of utility stems from inherent limitations in the technique as quantification of the airway volume or cross-sectional area has poor reliability between different examiners.[68] Reliability is weakened as there is some subjectivity to the process of segmentation of the airway from the surrounding soft tissues using contemporary software, or that the airway has been divided into vertical portions that are not always similarly defined. Additionally, multiple landmarks and dimensions have been offered as keys to diagnostic validity. Patients are imaged in different postural positions (sitting or reclined). It also has been observed that there is a significant level of variance, often in the range of what has been previously attributed to a treatment effect in other studies, in volumetric measurements from repeat scans of the same patient, despite controlling for head posture and tongue position.[69]

More recent studies exploring differences in CBCT-imaged airway between patients with OSA and healthy matched controls failed to find differences in volume in specific regions or in the minimal cross-sectional area of the airway beyond those attributed to differences in adenoid and tonsil size.[70] As these tissues can be easily assessed clinically or with traditional radiography, CBCT data is does not provide any additional useful information.

There are large variations in airway dimensions between the sleep and awake states, which are amplified in patients with OSA. It is theorized that differences in airway dynamics between patients with OSA and healthy controls may be due to decreased tonic airway stiffness or decreased inspiratory activity of airway dilator muscles during sleep.[71]

CBCT assessment of the airway in adults has also been investigated as a means to predict treatment response to mandibular advancing oral appliances. These studies have shown that there are no differences in 3D skeletal or airway morphology in responders and non-responders to oral appliance therapy[72] and that changes in airway volume had no relation to the change in function of breathing during sleep from oral appliance treatment.[73]

The research has led to the conclusion that there is relatively poor correlation between the static image of the upper airway of an awake patient captured by CBCT, and how that airway functions during sleep.

Orthodontic Classification

Classification has traditionally been an important tool in diagnosis and treatment planning. An ideal classification of orthodontic conditions would summarize the diagnostic data and imply the treatment plan. In our concept of diagnosis, classification can be viewed as the (orderly) reduction of the database to a list of the patient's problems and positive attributes that are to be maintained (Fig. 6.86).

Development of Classification Systems

The first useful orthodontic classification, still important now, was Angle's classification of malocclusion into classes I, II, and III. The basis of the Angle classification was the relationship of the first molar teeth and the alignment (or lack of it) of the teeth relative to the line of occlusion. Angle's classification thus created the following four groups:

Normal occlusion	Normal (class I) molar relationship, teeth on line of occlusion
Class I malocclusion	Normal (class I) molar relationship, teeth crowded, rotated, and so on
Class II malocclusion	Lower molar distal to upper molar, relationship of other teeth to line of occlusion not specified
Class III malocclusion	Lower molar mesial to upper molar, relationship of other teeth to line of occlusion not specified

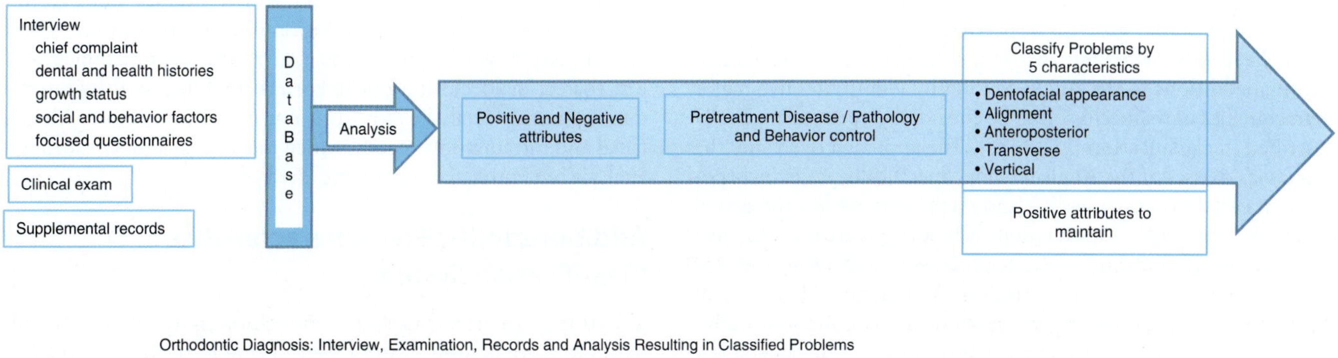

• **Fig. 6.86** Conceptually, classification can be viewed as an orderly way to derive a list of the patient's problems from the database.

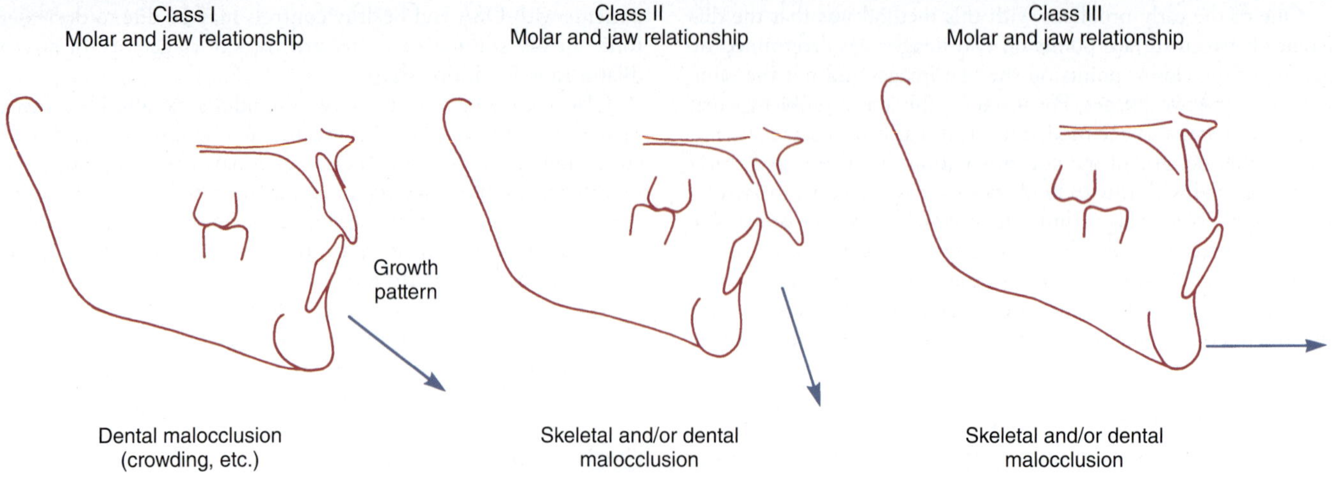

• **Fig. 6.87** The Angle classification has come to describe four different things that can be seen on clinical examination, dental casts, and/or cephalograms: the type of malocclusion, the molar relationship, the jaw relationship, and the pattern of growth, as shown here diagrammatically. Although the jaw relationship and growth pattern correlate with the molar relationship, the correlations are far from perfect. It is not unusual to observe a class I molar relationship in a patient with a class II jaw relationship or to find that an individual with a class I molar and jaw relationship grows in a class III pattern, which ultimately will produce a class III malocclusion.

The Angle system was a tremendous step forward, not only because it provided an orderly way to classify malocclusion but also because for the first time it provided a simple definition of normal occlusion and thereby a way to distinguish normal occlusion from malocclusion.

Almost immediately, it was recognized that the Angle classification was not complete because it did not include important characteristics of the patient's problem. The deficiencies in the original Angle system led to a series of informal additions at an early stage. A series of subdivisions of class I was proposed by Martin Dewey, initially Angle's protégé but later his rival. Gradually, Angle's classification numbers were extended to refer to four distinct but related characteristics: the classification of malocclusion, as in the original plan; the molar relationship; the skeletal jaw relationship; and the pattern of growth (Fig. 6.87). Thus a class II jaw relationship meant the mandible was positioned distally relative to the maxilla. This was usually found in connection with a class II molar relationship but occasionally could be present with a class I molar relationship. Similarly, a class II growth pattern was defined as a downward and backward growth direction of the mandible, which would tend to create and maintain class II jaw and molar relationships. Class I and class III growth patterns show balanced and disproportionate forward mandibular growth, respectively.

In the 1960s Ackerman and Proffit formalized the system of informal additions to the Angle method by identifying five major characteristics of malocclusion to be considered and systematically described in classification (Fig. 6.88). The approach overcame the major weaknesses of the Angle scheme. Specifically, it (1) incorporated an evaluation of crowding and asymmetry within the dental arches and included an evaluation of incisor protrusion, (2) recognized the relationship between protrusion and crowding, (3) included the transverse and vertical, as well as the AP, planes of space (coronal, axial and sagittal planes, in anatomic and radiologic terms), and (4) incorporated information about skeletal jaw proportions at the appropriate point, that is, in the description of relationships in each of the planes of space. Experience has confirmed that a minimum of five characteristics must be considered in a complete diagnostic evaluation.

Although the elements of the Ackerman-Proffit scheme now are often not combined exactly as originally proposed, classification by five major characteristics is now widely used. Like other aspects of orthodontic diagnosis, classification is affected by the major changes that have occurred recently such as the development of 3D imaging and other advances in orthodontic technology. The most important change, however, is the greater emphasis now on evaluating facial soft tissue proportions and the relationship of the dentition to the lips and cheeks, on smile and at rest.

Recent revision of the classification scheme has focused on broadening it to incorporate these new aspects of orthodontic diagnosis. Fifty years ago, most orthodontists viewed their role as correcting malocclusion by straightening teeth. At present, the goal of treatment takes into account facial and dental appearance, as well as the relationships of the teeth. Today, evaluation of dentofacial appearance includes full-face evaluation, consideration of anterior tooth display at rest and during smile, and assessment of soft tissues in the oblique (three-quarters) view, as well as in frontal and profile views. Little has changed regarding the description of crowding or spacing within the dental arches, but a clearer understanding of the line of occlusion in relationship to the goals of treatment now is required. The goal of treatment no longer is to just correct malocclusion but to correct it while also bringing the dentition and facial skeleton into normal relationships with the facial and intraoral soft tissues, which means that a more thorough analysis of dentofacial traits is required.

Additions to the Five-Characteristics Classification System

Two things particularly help this more thorough analysis: (1) evaluating the orientation of the *esthetic line of the dentition*, which is related to but different from Angle's functional line of occlusion, and (2) supplementing the traditional 3D description of facial and

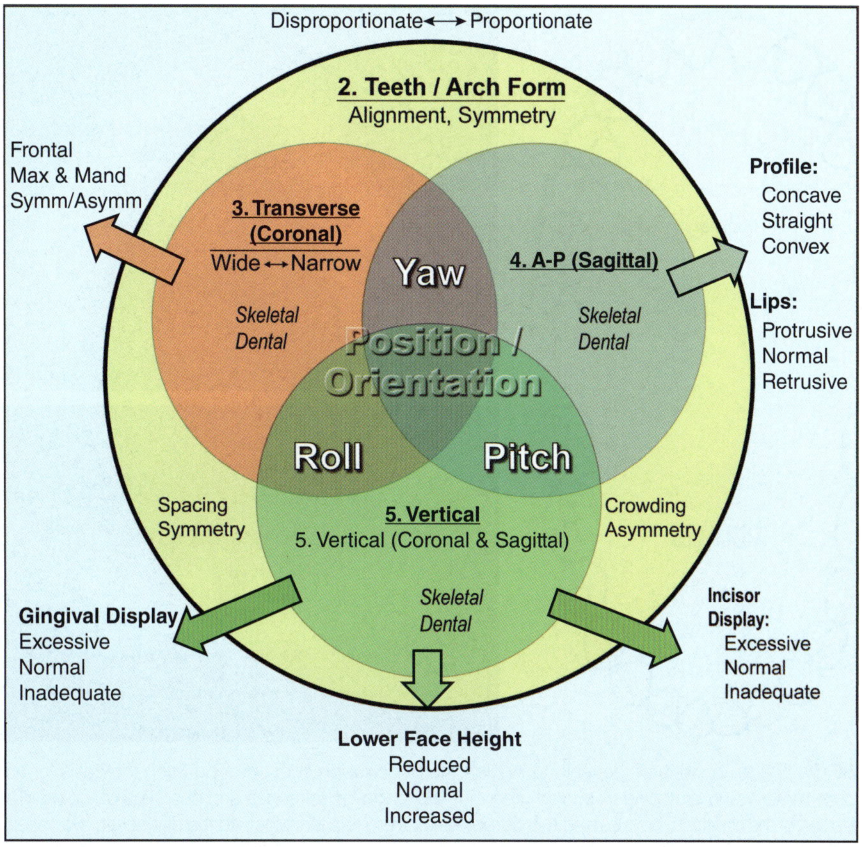

• **Fig. 6.88** Ackerman and Proffit represented the five major characteristics of malocclusion via a Venn diagram. The sequential description of the major characteristics, not their graphic representation, is the key to this classification system, but the interaction of the tooth and jaw relationships with facial appearance must be kept in mind. Note that for each characteristic, the items to be evaluated are listed within the box or circle, with a spectrum of potential problems within that area represented by opposing terms (spacing ↔ crowding, symmetry ↔ asymmetry). The items to be evaluated for dentofacial appearance appear as a backdrop to the dental issues but are related to the dimension they are related to by arrows. The circle for each plane of space (and anatomic plane) represents not only the position but also the orientation of jaws and teeth in that plane of space, and the overlaps between the circles representing the three planes of space are labeled for the orientation problem (Yaw, Roll and Pitch) that this interaction could represent.

dental relationships with rotational characteristics around each plane of space. These factors will be considered in turn.

1. *Esthetic line of the dentition.* For over a century, Angle's line of occlusion has been used to characterize the positions of the teeth within the dental arch and as a reference for assessing arch form and arch symmetry. Angle's concept was that if the buccal occlusal line of the mandibular dental arch was coincident with the central fossae line of the maxillary dental arch and the teeth were well aligned, ideal occlusion would result. The line of occlusion is hidden from view when the maxillary and mandibular teeth are in contact.

   In modern analysis, another curved line characterizing the appearance of the dentition is important, the one that is seen when evaluating anterior tooth display (Fig. 6.89). This line, the esthetic line of the dentition, follows the facial edges of the maxillary anterior and posterior teeth. The orientation of this line, like the orientation of the head and jaws, is best described when the rotational axes of pitch, roll, and yaw are considered in addition to transverse, AP, and vertical planes of space.

2. *Pitch, roll, and yaw in systematic description.* A key aspect of our previous classification system was its incorporation of systematic analysis of skeletal and dental relationships in all three planes of space, so that deviations in any direction would be incorporated into the patient's problem list. A complete description, however, requires consideration of both translation (forward-backward, up-down, right-left) in 3D space and rotation about three perpendicular axes (pitch, roll, and yaw) (Fig. 6.90.[74] This is exactly analogous to what would be necessary to describe the position of an airplane in space. The introduction of rotational axes into systematic description of dentofacial traits significantly improves the precision of the description and thereby facilitates development of the problem list.

Evaluating pitch, roll, and yaw of the esthetic line of the dentition is particularly useful in determining the relationship of the teeth to the soft tissues that frame their display. From this perspective, an excessive upward-downward rotation of the dentition relative to the lips and cheeks would be noted as pitch (up or down, in front or back) (Fig. 6.91). Pitch of the dentition relative to the facial soft tissues must be evaluated on clinical examination. Pitch of the jaws and teeth relative to each other and to the facial skeleton also can and should be noted clinically, but this

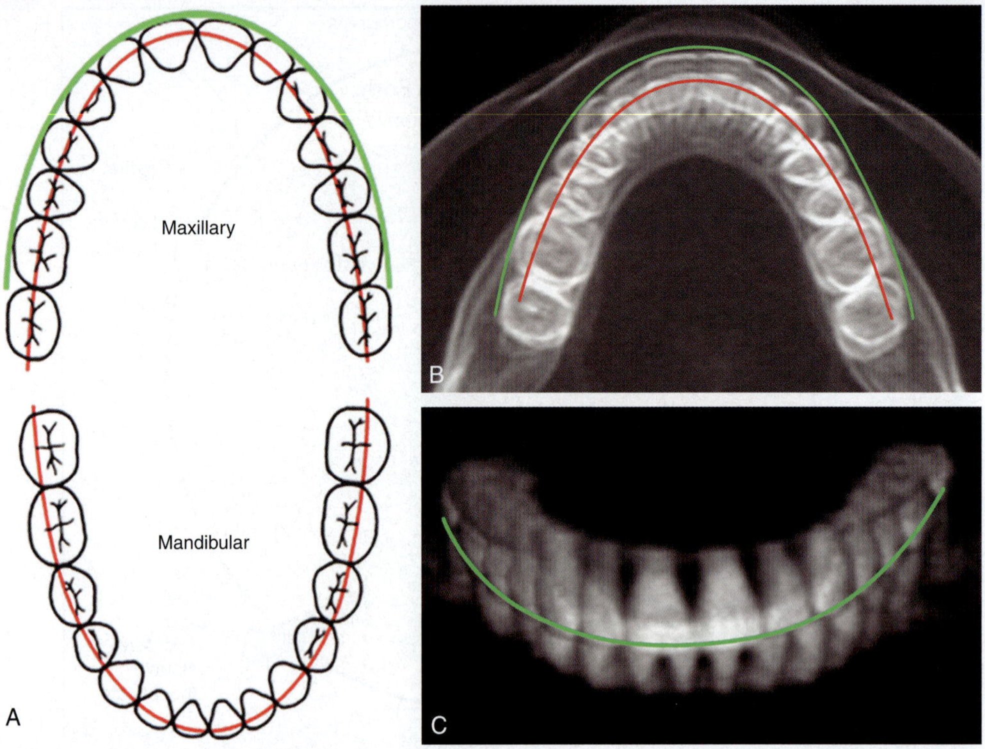

• **Fig. 6.89** (A) The relationship of the teeth to Angle's line of occlusion *(red)* has long been the basis for analysis of dental arch symmetry and crowding. A curved green line along the incisal edges and cusp tips of the maxillary teeth, the esthetic line of the dentition, now is used to incorporate tooth-lip relationships into the diagnostic evaluation of tooth positions. (B) In vivo submental-vertex cone beam computed tomography (CBCT) view of an individual with normal occlusion showing the maxillary dentition superimposed on the mandibular dentition as it is in life. For this individual, the teeth are aligned and positioned so that the line of occlusion is almost ideally placed for both arches. If a patient has an asymmetry characterized by rotation of the maxilla, mandible, or dentition (any or all of the aforementioned) around the vertical axis, it can be detected in this radiographic projection. The esthetic line of the dentition *(green)* also can be seen in this projection, drawn as it was in (A). (C) A cross-sectional "block" of a CBCT image can be manipulated on the computer screen around all three rotational axes. This is simply a different perspective of the image shown in (B), in which the esthetic line of the dentition is shown in its relationship to the incisal edges and cusp tips of the upper teeth.

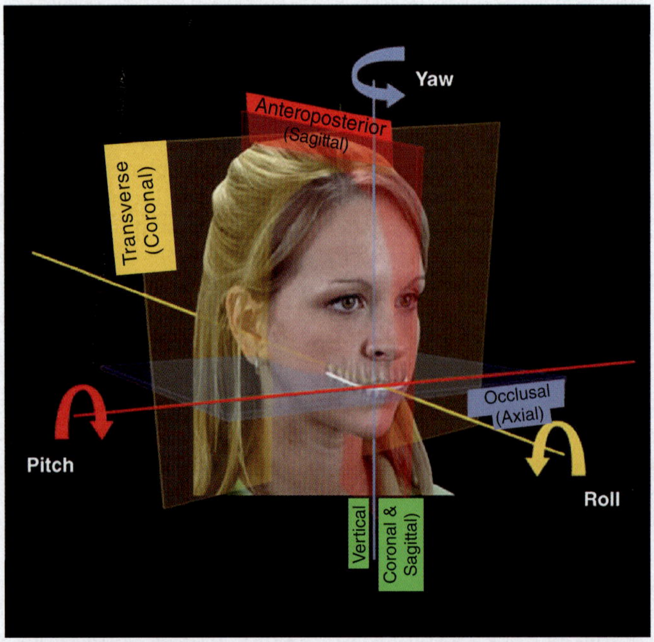

• **Fig. 6.90** In addition to relationships in the transverse (coronal), anteroposterior (sagittal), vertical (coronal and sagittal), and occlusal (axial) planes of space used in traditional analysis, rotations around axes perpendicular to these planes also must be evaluated. These rotations are pitch, viewed as up-down deviations around the antero-posterior axis; roll, viewed as up-down deviations around the transverse axis; and yaw, viewed as left-right deviations around the vertical axis. The rotations should be evaluated for the jaws and for the esthetic line of the dentition.

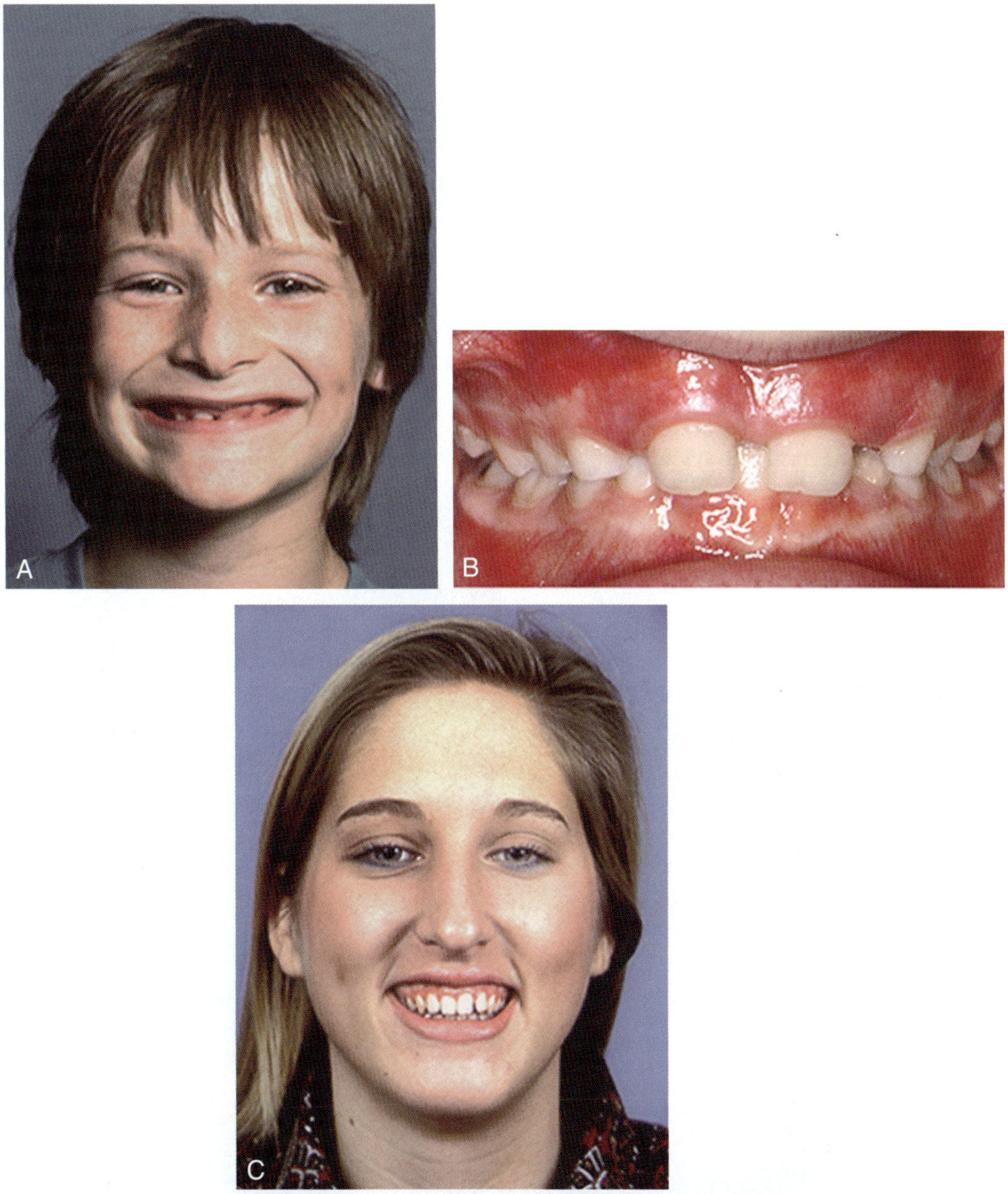

• **Fig. 6.91** The vertical relationship of the teeth to the lips and cheeks during growth or treatment can be conveniently described as downward or upward translation with no pitch deviation, which is rare, or as pitch upward or downward anteriorly and upward or downward posteriorly. The comparison is of the esthetic line of the dentition to the intercommissure line. (A) and (B) downward pitch of the anterior teeth, so that the lower lip almost completely covers the esthetic line of the dentition on smile. Anterior deep bite usually accompanies a pitch of this type. (C) for this girl, who does not have anterior open bite despite her long-face skeletal pattern, the entire dentition is translated down, but a downward pitch posteriorly can be observed clinically. Note that the esthetic line of the dentition tilts down posteriorly relative to the intercommissure line and that there is greater exposure of gingiva posteriorly than anteriorly.

can be confirmed from the cephalometric radiograph in the final classification step, where pitch is revealed as the orientation of the palatal, occlusal, and mandibular planes relative to the true horizontal (see Fig. 6.66).

Roll, which is analogous to the banking of an airplane, is described as rotation up or down on one side or the other. On clinical examination, it is important to relate the coronal or transverse orientation of the dentition (the esthetic line) to both the facial soft tissues and the facial skeleton. The relationship to the facial soft tissues is evaluated clinically with the intercommissure line as a reference. Neither dental casts nor a photograph using an occlusal plane marker (Fox plane) will reveal this. It is seen with the lips relaxed and more clearly on smile, in both frontal and oblique views (Fig. 6.92; also see Fig. 6.3). The relationship to the facial skeleton is viewed relative to the interocular line. The use of a Fox plane to mark a cant of the occlusal plane may make it easier to visualize how the dentition relates to the interocular line, but with this device in place it is impossible to see how the teeth relate to the intercommissure line.

Rotation of the jaw or dentition to one side or the other, around a vertical axis, produces a skeletal or dental midline discrepancy

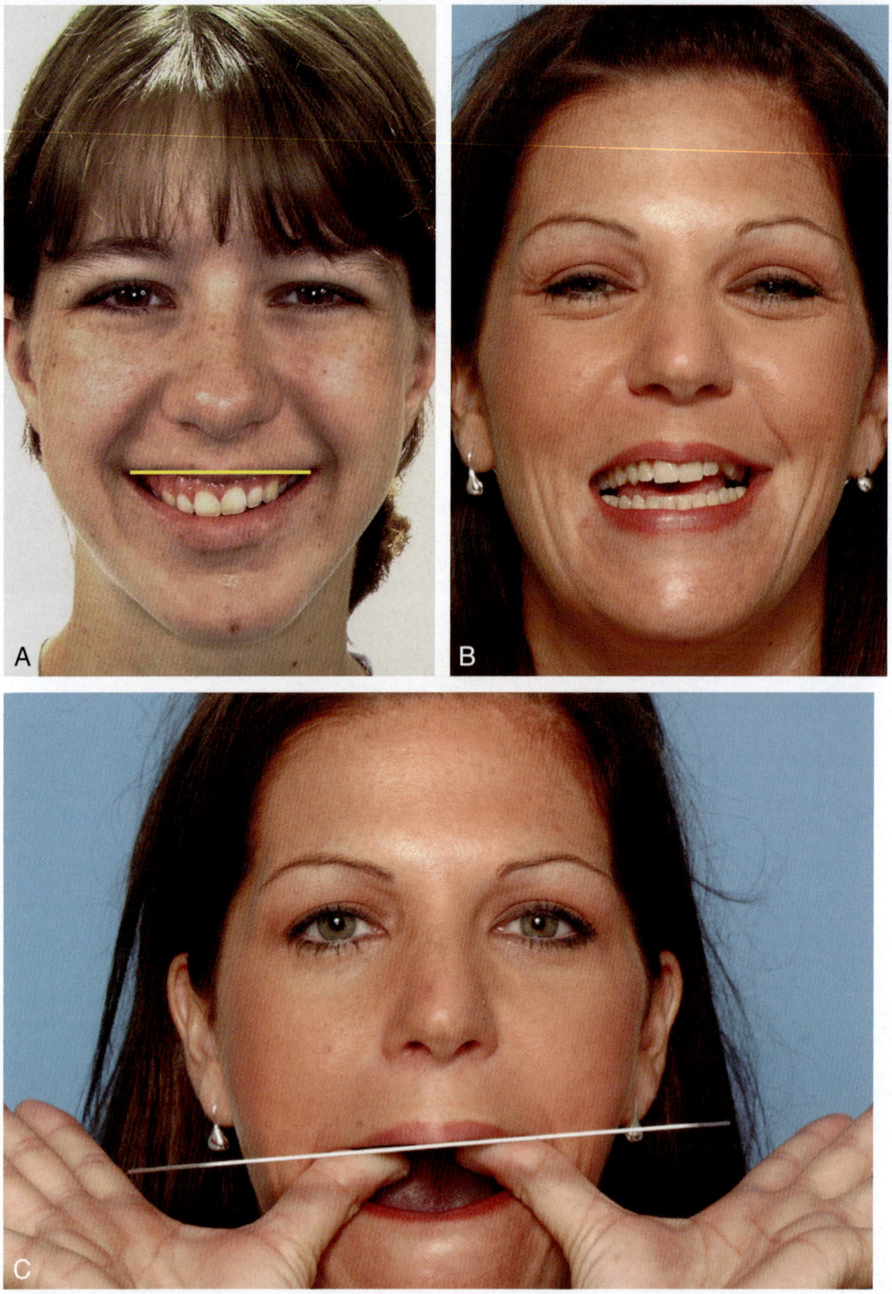

• **Fig. 6.92** *Roll* describes the vertical position of the teeth when this is different on the right and left sides. (A) This image shows a downward roll of the dentition on the right side relative to the intercommissure line *(yellow)*. Note that the maxillary incisors tilt to the left. The chin deviates to the left, reflecting asymmetric mandibular growth with lengthening of the mandibular body and ramus on the right side. The vertical position of the gonial angles can be confirmed by palpation. In this case there is a skeletal component to the roll. (B) Roll of the dentition down on the right side and slightly up on the left, relative to the intercommissure line. There is no transverse displacement of the chin, but the entire right side of the face is larger; note that the interocular line rolls opposite to the esthetic line of the dentition. (C) A Fox plane device demonstrates the orientation of the occlusal plane relative to the interocular line, but the relationship of the teeth to the intercommissure line cannot be observed while one is using it.

that is best described as yaw (Fig. 6.93). Yaw of the dentition relative to the jaw, or yaw of the mandible or maxilla that takes the dentition with it, may be present. The effect of yaw, in addition to dental and/or skeletal midline deviations, typically is a unilateral class II or class III molar relationship. Extreme yaw is associated with asymmetric posterior crossbites, buccal on one side and lingual on the other. Yaw has been left out of all previous classifications, but characterizing transverse asymmetries in this way makes it easier to accurately describe the relationships.

Dental midline deviations can be just a reflection of displaced incisors because of crowding. This should be differentiated from a yaw discrepancy in which the whole dental arch is

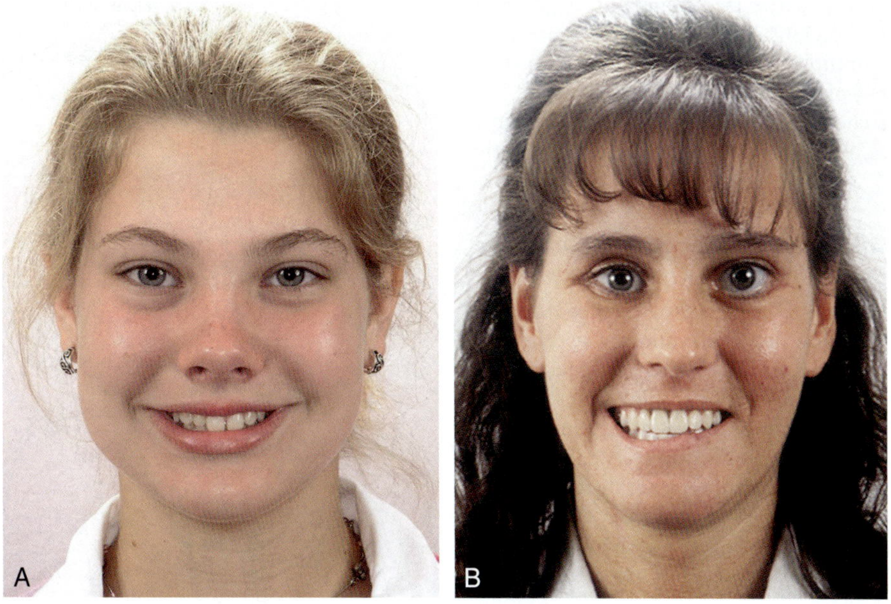

• **Fig. 6.93** (A) Yaw of the maxillary dentition to the left side is apparent in this girl, who also has slight yaw of the mandible in the same direction. Note that the yaw of the esthetic line of the dentition is greater than the yaw of the chin. In her clinical examination, it will be important to evaluate the relationship of the midline of the mandibular dentition to the chin. A compensatory yaw of the mandibular teeth back toward the skeletal midline often is present in patients with this type of asymmetry. (B) Severe yaw of the maxillary dentition to the right in this woman, who has almost no yaw of the mandible. Note that she also has more elevation of the right commissure on smile, so relative to the intercommissure line, she has a downward roll of the dentition on the right. This should be noted in the clinical examination because it will be important to determine whether she considers it a problem.

rotated off to one side. If a true yaw discrepancy is present, the next question is whether the jaw itself is deviated, or whether the dentition deviates relative to the jaw. A yaw deviation of the maxilla is possible but rare; an asymmetry of the mandible that often includes yaw is present in 40% of patients with deficient or excessive mandibular growth,[75] and in these patients the dentition is likely to be deviated in a compensatory direction relative to the jaw. All of this can be detected with a careful clinical examination—and must be because it may not be seen clearly in typical diagnostic records.

Despite these additions to the diagnostic evaluation, dentofacial traits still can be adequately delineated by five major characteristics. The additional items that now must be included in diagnostic evaluation and classification are shown in Box 6.2. Examining the five major characteristics in sequence provides a convenient way of organizing the diagnostic information to be sure that no important points are overlooked.

• BOX 6.2 Classification by the Five Characteristics of Dentofacial Traits

Dentofacial Appearance (Includes Multiple Planes)

Frontal, lateral, oblique, and vertical facial proportions; symmetry; anterior tooth and gingival display; orientation of the esthetic line of occlusion and cant; profile with lip protrusion

Alignment

Crowding or spacing, arch form, symmetry, orientation of the functional line of occlusion

Anteroposterior

Angle classification, skeletal and dental; dental and skeletal protrusion/retrusion; anterior crossbite; overjet

Transverse

Posterior crossbites, skeletal and dental; midlines

Vertical

Bite depth, skeletal and dental;

Classification by the Characteristics of Malocclusion

Step 1: Evaluation of Facial Proportions and Esthetics (Coronal and Sagittal or Transverse and Anteroposterior)

Step 1 is carried out during the initial clinical examination, while facial asymmetry, AP and vertical facial proportions, and lip protrusion /retrusion, lip-tooth relationships and gingival display (at rest and on smile) are evaluated. This also includes evaluating whether a cant to the dentition exists (a roll up or down one or both sides of the occlusal plane). This can only be evaluated relative to the face.

This evaluation has been covered earlier in this chapter in the context of macro- and mini-esthetic considerations. Incorporation of the data into the classification scheme, using axes of rotation in addition to the traditional three planes of space, is described in the previous section. The results are summarized as the positive findings (problems) and negative findings (positive attributes) from this part of the examination. The clinical findings can be checked against the facial photographs and lateral cephalometric radiograph, which should confirm the clinical judgment.

Step 2: Evaluation of Alignment and Symmetry Within the Dental Arches (Axial Plane)

Step 2 is carried out by examining the dental arches from the occlusal (axial) view, evaluating first the symmetry within each dental arch and second the amount of crowding or spacing present. Space analysis quantifies crowding or spacing, but these figures must be interpreted in the light of other findings in the total evaluation of the patient. A major point is the presence or absence of excessive incisor protrusion, which cannot be evaluated without knowledge of lip separation at rest. For that reason, the dentofacial relationships noted in the initial clinical examination must be considered immediately along with the relationship of the teeth to the line of occlusion.

Step 3: Evaluation of the Transverse Plane of Space (the Coronal and Axial dimensions of the Transverse Plane)

At this stage, the casts are brought into occlusion and the occlusal relationships are examined, beginning with the transverse (posterior crossbite) plane of space. The objectives are to accurately describe the occlusion and to distinguish between skeletal and dental contributions to malocclusion. Now the evaluation is primarily of the dental casts (midline deviations to each other and to the facial midline) and radiographs, but it must be kept in mind that both roll and yaw of the jaws (asymmetry) and dentition affect dentofacial transverse relationships. These factors should have been noted in Step 1 of classification and can be confirmed in this step.

Posterior crossbite is described in terms of the position of the upper molars (Fig. 6.94). Thus, a bilateral maxillary lingual (or palatal) crossbite means that the upper molars are lingual to their normal position on both sides, whereas a unilateral mandibular buccal crossbite would mean that the mandibular molars are buccally positioned on one side. This terminology specifies which teeth (maxillary or mandibular) are displaced from their normal position.

It is also important to evaluate the underlying skeletal relationships to answer the question, "Why does this crossbite exist?" in the sense of the location of the anatomic abnormality. If a bilateral maxillary palatal crossbite exists, for instance, is the basic problem that the maxilla itself is narrow, thus providing a skeletal basis for the crossbite, or is it that the dental arch has been narrowed although the skeletal width is correct?

The width of the maxillary skeletal base can be seen by the width of the palatal vault on the casts. If the base of the palatal vault is wide, but the dentoalveolar processes lean inward, the crossbite is dental in the sense that it is caused by a distortion of the dental arch. If the palatal vault is narrow and the maxillary teeth lean outward but nevertheless are in crossbite, the problem is skeletal in that it basically results from the narrow width of the maxilla. Just as there are dental compensations for skeletal deformity in the AP and vertical planes of space, the teeth can compensate for transverse skeletal problems, tipping facially or lingually if the skeletal base is narrow or wide respectively.

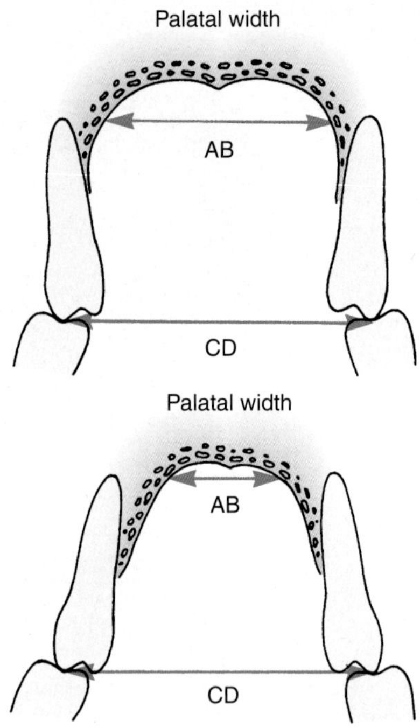

• **Fig. 6.94** Posterior crossbite can be either *dental*, as in a patient with adequate palatal width (i.e., distance *AB* approximately equals distance *CD*), or *skeletal* because of inadequate palatal width (i.e., distance *CD* is considerably larger than distance *AB*). Because it shows the palate, you can see both dental and skeletal width on a maxillary cast.

Transverse displacement of the lower molars on the mandible is rare, so the question of whether the mandibular arch is too wide can be used both to answer the question of whether the mandible or maxilla is at fault in a posterior crossbite and to implicate skeletal mandibular development if the answer is positive. Tabulated data for normal molar and canine widths are shown in Table 6.10. If there is a crossbite and measurements across the arch show that the mandible is wide while the maxillary arch is normal, a skeletal mandibular discrepancy is probably present.

Step 4: Evaluation of the Anteroposterior Plane of Space (the Sagittal and Axial dimensions of the A-P Plane)

Examining the dental casts in occlusion will reveal any AP problems in the buccal occlusion or in the anterior relationships. The Angle classification, in its extended form, describes this well.

It is important to ask whether an end-to-end, class II or class III buccal segment relationship, or excessive overjet or reverse overjet of the incisors, is caused by a jaw (skeletal) discrepancy, displaced teeth on well-proportioned jaws (dental class II or III), or a combination of skeletal and dental displacement. Deficient or excessive jaw growth almost always produces an occlusal discrepancy as well, but if the jaw discrepancy is the cause, the problem should be described as a *skeletal* class II or class III. The terminology simply means that the skeletal or jaw relationship is the cause of the class II dental occlusion. The distinction between dental and skeletal is important because the treatment for a skeletal class II relationship in a child or adult will be different from treatment for a dental class II problem. Cephalometric analysis is needed to be precise about the nature of the problem. The object is to accurately evaluate the underlying anatomic basis of the malocclusion (Fig. 6.95).

TABLE 6.10 Arch Width Measurement

	MALE			FEMALE		
Age	Canine	First Premolar	First Molar	Canine	First Premolar	First Molar
Maxillary Arch						
6	27.5[a]	32.3[a]	41.9	26.9[a]	31.7[a]	41.3
8	29.7[a]	33.7[a]	43.1	29.1[a]	33.0[a]	42.4
10	30.5[a]	34.4[a]	44.5	29.8[a]	33.6[a]	43.5
12	32.5	35.7	45.3	31.5	35.1	44.6
14	32.5	36.0	45.9	31.3	34.9	44.3
16	32.3	36.6	46.6	31.4	35.2	45.0
18	32.3	36.7	46.7	31.2	34.6	43.9
Mandibular Arch						
6	23.3[a]	28.7[a]	40.2	22.2[a]	28.4[a]	40.0
8	24.3[a]	29.7[a]	40.9	24.0[a]	29.5[a]	40.3
10	24.6[a]	30.2[a]	41.5	24.1[a]	29.7[a]	41.0
12	25.1	32.5	42.1	24.8	31.6	41.8
14	24.8	32.3	42.1	24.4	31.0	41.1
16	24.7	32.3	42.8	23.9	31.0	41.5
18	24.8	32.8	43.0	23.1	30.8	41.7

[a]Primary predecessor.
All measurements: millimeter distance between centers of teeth.
Data from Moyers RE, et al. *Standards of Human Occlusal Development.* In: Monograph 5, Craniofacial Growth Series. University of Michigan, Center for Human Growth and Development; 1976.

Occasionally the molar occlusion is class II on one side and class I on the other. Angle called this a *class II subdivision,* right or left, depending on which was the class II side. In modern classification, the subdivision label rarely is useful because it does not describe the real problem. The asymmetric molar relationship reflects either an asymmetry within one or both the dental arches (typically due to loss of space when one primary second molar was lost prematurely) or a yaw discrepancy of the jaw or dentition. These must be distinguished and should already have been addressed in the first or second steps in the classification procedure.

The sagittal plane also is where dental issues like protrusion/retrusion and proclination/retroclination of the incisors are evaluated. Anterior crossbite is a sagittal problem as well.

Step 5: Evaluation of the Vertical Plane (or Vertical Dimensions of the Sagittal and Coronal Planes of Space)

With the casts in occlusion, vertical problems can be described as anterior open bite (failure of the incisor teeth to overlap), anterior deep bite (excessive overlap of the anterior teeth), or posterior open bite (failure of the posterior teeth to occlude, unilaterally or bilaterally). As with all aspects of malocclusion, it is important to ask, "Why does the open bite (or other problem) exist?" Because vertical problems, particularly anterior open bite, can result from environmental causes or habits, the "why" in this instance has two important components: At what anatomic location is the discrepancy, and can a cause be identified?

It is obvious that if the posterior teeth erupt a normal amount, but the anterior teeth do not, there will be a pitch discrepancy of the line of occlusion and the esthetic line of the dentition. This would result in two related problems: an anterior open bite and less than the normal display of the maxillary anterior teeth. Upward pitch anteriorly of the maxillary dentition is possible but rarely is the major reason for an anterior open bite. Instead, anterior open bite patients usually have at least some excessive eruption of maxillary posterior teeth. If the anterior teeth erupt a normal amount but the posterior teeth erupt too much, anterior open bite is inevitable. In this case, the relationship of the anterior teeth to the lips would be normal, and there would be excessive display of the posterior teeth. The line of occlusion and the esthetic line of the dentition then would be pitched down posteriorly.

This leads to an important but sometimes difficult concept: a patient with a *skeletal* open bite will usually have an anterior bite malocclusion that is characterized by excessive eruption of posterior teeth, downward rotation of the mandible and maxilla, and normal (or even excessive) eruption of anterior teeth (Fig. 6.96). This facial and dental pattern is often referred to as the "long-face syndrome," and some patients with this problem do not have an anterior open bite.

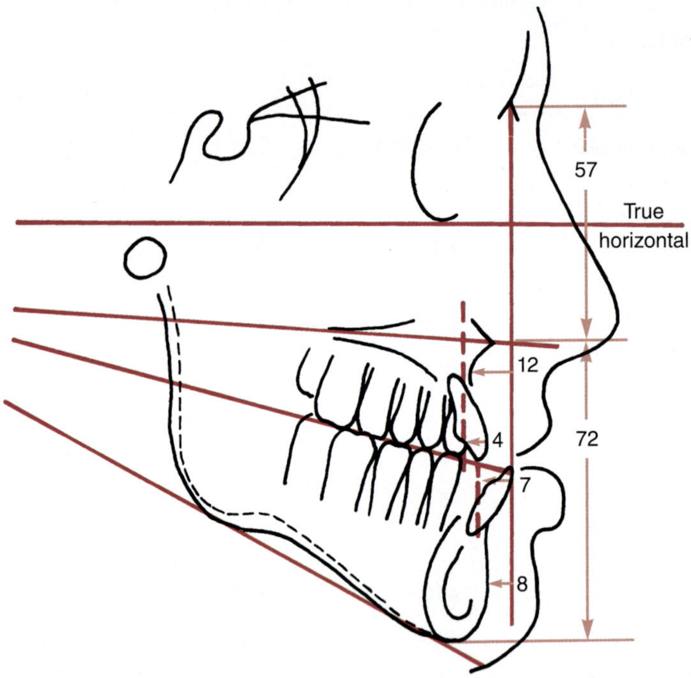

• **Fig. 6.95** Cephalometric analysis combining elements of the measurement approaches presented earlier. A description in words of this patient's problems would be that the maxilla is quite deficient relative to the mandible and the cranial base, but the maxillary teeth are reasonably well related to the maxilla. The mandible is fairly well related in the anteroposterior plane of space to the cranial base, but the mandibular teeth protrude relative to the mandible. Vertical proportions are good. A summary of this type, not a table of measurements, is needed for adequate diagnosis.

The reverse is true in a short-face, skeletal deep bite relationship (Fig. 6.97). In that circumstance, one would expect to see a normal amount of eruption of incisor teeth but rotation of both jaws in the opposite direction and insufficient eruption of the posterior teeth. The skeletal component is revealed by the rotation of the jaws, reflected in the palatal and mandibular plane angles. If the angle between the mandibular and palatal planes is low, there is a skeletal deep bite tendency (i.e., a jaw relationship that predisposes to an anterior deep bite, regardless of whether one is present). Similarly, if the mandibular-palatal angle is high, there is a skeletal open bite tendency.

It is important to remember that if the mandibular plane angle is unusually flat or steep, correcting an accompanying deep bite or open bite may require an alteration in the vertical position of posterior teeth so that the mandible can rotate to a more normal inclination. Cephalometric analysis is required for evaluation of patients with skeletal vertical problems, again with the goal of accurately describing skeletal and dental relationships. As the tracings in this chapter illustrate, most measurement analyses do a much better job of identifying AP than vertical problems.

A careful clinical evaluation of the relationship of the dentition to the soft tissues also is critically important. Open bites and deep bites can result from almost any combination of skeletal and dental components, and the problem is likely to include improper tooth-lip relationships. Careful analysis is required if the approach to treatment is to be esthetic and stable.

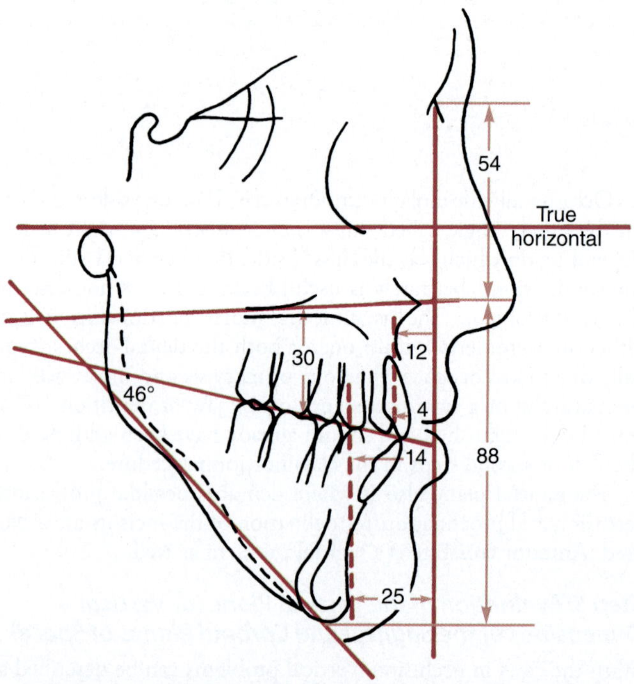

• **Fig. 6.96** Cephalometric analysis for a patient with severe vertical problems. Note that the Sassouni lines clearly indicate the skeletal open bite pattern and that the measurements confirm both long anterior facial dimensions and severe mandibular deficiency related to downward and backward rotation of the mandible. Measurement of the distance from the upper first molar mesial cusp to the palatal plane confirms that excessive eruption of the upper molar has occurred.

Development of a Problem List

If positive findings from a systematic description of the patient are recorded (i.e., if the procedure previously described is used), the

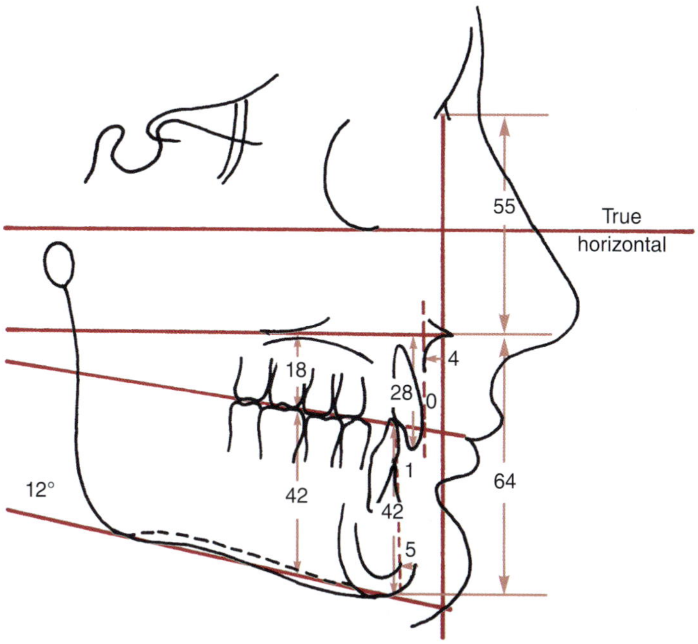

• **Fig. 6.97** Cephalometric analysis of a patient with short anterior vertical dimensions. The measurements show excessive eruption of the lower molar compared with the upper molar and document the distal displacement of the lower incisor relative to the mandible. Note that the Sassouni planes are almost parallel, confirming the skeletal deep bite tendency.

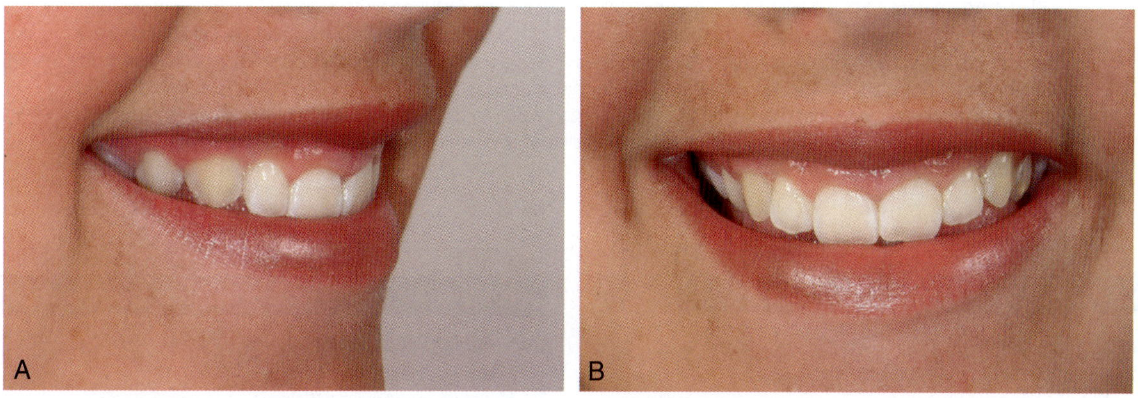

• **Fig. 6.98** (A and B) Patient F.P., age 12 years 3 months. Close-up views of the smile can be a valuable part of the diagnostic records when dental and facial appearance is an important consideration in developing a treatment plan. For this patient, the short clinical crowns coupled with almost no display of the gingiva should be noted in the problem list. Note that the oblique smile view allows an excellent view of these characteristics.

automatic and important result is a list of the patient's problems. The step-by-step procedure is designed to ensure that the important distinctions have been made and that nothing has been overlooked.

The problem list often includes two types of problems: (1) those relating to disease or pathologic processes and (2) those relating to disturbances of development that have created the patient's malocclusion. The set of developmental abnormalities related to malocclusion is the orthodontic problem list. A developmental problem is just that (e.g., moderate mandibular deficiency), not the findings that indicate its presence (e.g., weak chin, increased facial convexity, and increased ANB angle all are findings, not problems).

Having several problems within a major category is not uncommon (maxillary protrusion and maxillary dental retrusion) and would be quite possible. But some subproblems may all be part of crowding or malalignment. When possible, the problems should be indicated quantitatively or at least classified as mild, moderate, or severe (e.g., 5-mm mandibular incisor crowding, severe mandibular skeletal deficiency).

The initial diagnostic records for a patient with a moderate orthodontic problem, whose primary reason for treatment was improvement of her dental and facial appearance, are shown in Figs. 6.47, 6.51, 6.98, and 6.99 and the steps in developing a problem list are illustrated in Boxes 6.3 through 6.5. Similar diagnostic workups for patients with various levels of severity problems are briefly reviewed in Chapters 20 and 22.

With the completion of a problem list and positive attributes, the diagnostic phase of diagnosis and treatment planning is completed, and the more subjective process of treatment planning

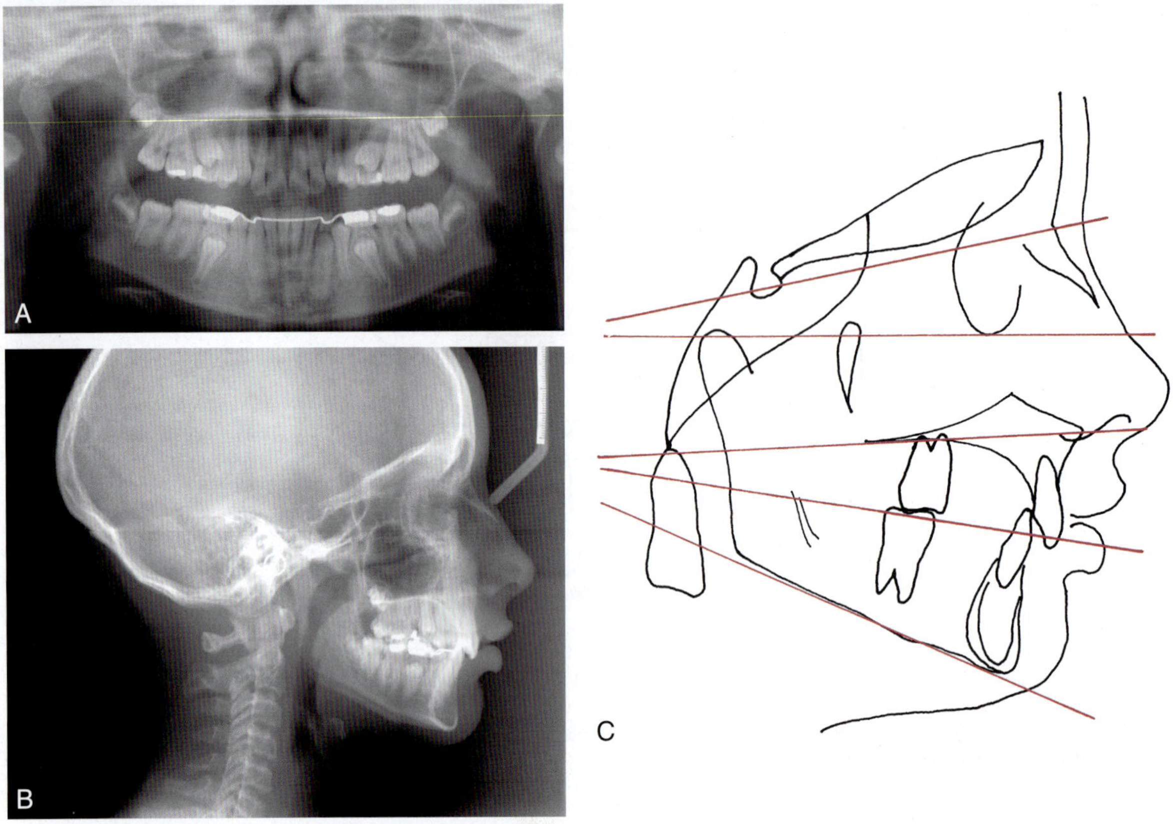

• **Fig. 6.99** Patient F.P., age 12 years 3 months. (A) Panoramic and (B) cephalometric radiographs before treatment. (C) Cephalometric tracing before treatment. To assist in visualization of skeletal and dental relationships, drawing this set of horizontal and vertical reference lines and evaluating relationships relative to the true horizontal line and perpendiculars to it is recommended. Note that mandibular deficiency is the major contributor to her class II malocclusion, and that the deep overbite is primarily due to excessive eruption of the lower incisors. The maxillary incisors are tipped lingually, which is the reason that overjet is not excessive despite the skeletal class II relationship and the class II molar relationship.

• BOX 6.3 Patient F.P.: Interview Data

Chief Concern

"I don't like the way my teeth stick out and look ugly."

Medical, Dental, Social History

- Hemangioma removed from leg at age 4
- No chronic medications
- Regular dental care, no restorations
- Lives with both parents, good progress in school, seems well adjusted without any major social problems

Motivation

- Largely external, mother wants treatment for a problem that she perceives as important
- Patient agrees that she needs treatment, will have to be convinced that this requires her cooperation

Expectation

- General improvement in appearance, seems realistic

Other Pertinent Information

- Older brother treated successfully previously; mother very supportive of orthodontic treatment, father much less so

• BOX 6.4 Patient F.P.: Clinical Examination Data

Dentofacial Proportions

- Mildly short lower third of face
- Moderate mandibular deficiency
- Inadequate display of maxillary incisors
- Maxillary incisors as wide as they are tall: short maxillary incisor crowns
- Moderate facial and dental asymmetry: mild roll down on right and yaw to left are not severe enough to be noticed as a problem
- Mandibular midline left of facial midline

Health of Hard and Soft Tissues

- Hypoplastic area, upper left first premolar
- Mild gingivitis
- Moderate overgrowth of gingiva, anterior maxilla

Jaw Function

- Maximum opening 45 mm
- Normal range of motion
- No joint sounds
- No pain on palpation

• BOX 6.5 Patient F.P.: Analysis of Examination and Diagnostic Records for Classified Problem List (Not Yet Prioritized)[a]

- Pathologic problems
- Mild gingivitis, mild gingival overgrowth
- Hypoplastic area maxillary left premolar

Classified Problems

1. Facial Proportions and Esthetics
    - Deficient chin projection, mandibular deficiency
    - Mildly short lower third of face
    - Maxillary incisors tipped lingually, short crowns
2. Dental Alignment and Symmetry
    - Moderate maxillary incisor crowding
    - Maxillary incisor displaced
3. Transverse Relationships
    - Mandibular dental midline left of facial midline
    - Anteroposterior Relationships
    - Moderate mandibular deficiency
    - Class II buccal segments, minimal overjet
    - Maxillary incisors tipped lingually
4. Vertical Relationships
    - Deep bite, excessive eruption of lower incisors
    - Mildly short face

[a]Using the Ackerman-Proffit classification to generate the initial problem list.

begins. Thorough diagnostic evaluation means that all problems have been identified and characterized at this stage, omitting nothing of significance. The steps in treatment planning (see Fig 7.1) and the outcome of treatment for the patient above are presented at the end of Chapter 7 in Boxes 7.1 through 7.8 and Figs. 7.31 through 7.35.

References

1. Chiao C, Tuncer AH, Jin M, et al. Accuracy of parent-reported health history in a dental setting. *J Am Dent Assoc.* 2022;153(11):1053–1059.
2. Senaratna CV, Perret JL, Lodge CJ, et al. Prevalence of obstructive sleep apnea in the general population: a systematic review. *Sleep Med Rev.* 2017;34:70–81.
3. Chervin RD, Weatherly RA, Garetz SL, et al. Pediatric sleep questionnaire: prediction of sleep apnea and outcomes. *Arch Otolaryngol-Head Neck Surg.* 2007;133:216–222.
4. Rohra AK, Demko CA, Hans MG, et al. Sleep disordered breathing in children seeking orthodontic care. *Am J Orthodont Dento Orthoped.* 2018;154(1):65–71.
5. Nagappa M, Liao P, Wong J, Auckley D, Ramachandran SK, Memtsoudis S, et al. Validation of the STOP-bang questionnaire as a screening tool for obstructive sleep apnea among different populations: a systematic review and meta-analysis. *PLoS ONE.* 2015;10(12):e0143697.
6. Sundararaj D, Venkatachalapathy S, Tandon A, Pereira A. Critical evaluation of incidence and prevalence of white spot lesions during fixed orthodontic appliance treatment: A meta-analysis. *J Int Soc Prev Community Dent.* 2015;5(6):433–439. https://doi.org/10.4103/2231-0762.167719. PMID: 26759794; PMCID: PMC4697225.
7. Xie Z, Yu L, Li S, et al. Comparison of therapies of white spot lesions: a systematic review and network meta-analysis. *BMC Oral Health.* 2023;23:346. https://doi.org/10.1186/s12903-023-03076-x.
8. Mellion Z, Behrents RG, Johnston LE. The pattern of facial skeletal growth and its relationship to various common indexes of maturation. *Am J Orthodont Dentof Orthoped.* 2013;143:845–854.
9. Okeson JP. *Management of Temporomandibular Disorders and Occlusion.* 7th ed. Mosby-Elsevier; 2013.
10. Ackerman JL, Proffit WR, Sarver DM. The emerging soft tissue paradigm in orthodontic diagnosis treatment planning. *Clin Orth Res.* 1999;2:49–52.
11. Sarver DM, Ackerman JL. "About Face-The re-emerging soft tissue paradigm". *Am J Orthod Dentofac Orthoped.* 2000;117:575–576.
12. Sarver DM. Hard tissue analysis-any substance in it anymore? Invited paper in *Oracle. Proceedings of the 39th Indian Orthodontic Conference.* November 2004.
13. Sarver DM. Soft-tissue-based diagnosis and treatment planning. *Clin Impress.* 2005;14(1):21–26.
14. Sarver DM. The interaction of hard tissue, soft tissue, and growth over time, and its impact on orthodontic diagnosis and treatment planning. Invited centennial article. *Am J Orthod Dentofacial Orthop.* 2015;148:380–386.
15. Shaw WC. The influence of children's dentofacial appearance on their social attractiveness as judged by peers and lay adults. *Am J Orthod.* 1981;79:399–415.
16. Richards MR, Fields HW, Beck FM, Firestone AR, Bernhardt-Walther D, Rosenstiel SF, Sacksteder JM. The contribution of dental attractiveness and female facial attractiveness to smile esthetics evaluated by eye tracking. *Am J Orthod Dentofacial Orthop.* 2015;147:472–482.
17. Baker RS, Fields HW, Johnson EK, et al. The contribution of dental attractiveness and male facial attractiveness to smile esthetics evaluated by eye tracking. *Am J Orthod Dentofacial Orthop.* 2018;153:523–533.
18. Papio MA, Fields HW, Beck FM, Firestone AR, Rosenstiel SF. The role of dental and background facial attractiveness on facial attractiveness and perceived integrity, social and intellectual attractiveness. *Am J Orthod Dentofacial Orthop.* 2019;1256:464–474.
19. Shaw WC, Rees MD, Charles CR. The influence of dentofacial appearance on the social attractiveness of young adults. *Am J Orthod.* 1985;87:21–26.
20. Rossion B, Hanseeuw B, Dricot L. Defining face perception areas in the human brain: a large scale factorial fMRI face localizer analysis. *Brain Cogn.* 2012;79:138–157.
21. Farkas LG. *Anthropometry of the Head and Face in Medicine.* Elsevier Science; 1991.
22. Bomeli P, Fields H, Beck M, Vig K, Firestone A, Shanker S. Concordance between dental and skeletal relationships. *J Dent Res.* 2003;82(Special Issue A):1139.
23. Berneburg M, Dietz K, Niederle C, et al. Changes in esthetic standards since 1940. *Am J Orthod Dentofac Orthop.* 2010;137:450.e1–450.e9;discussion 450–451.
24. Kokich VO Jr, Kiyak HA, Shapiro PA. Comparing the perception of dentists and lay people to altered dental esthetics. *J Esthet Dent.* 1999;11:311–324.
25. Springer NC, Chang C, Fields HW, Beck FM, Rosenstiel SF, Firestone AR, Christensen JC. Smile esthetics from the patients' perspective. *Am J Orthod Dentofacial Orthop.* 2011;139:e91–101.
26. Chang C, Springer NC, Fields HW, et al. Smile esthetics from patients' perspective for faces of varying attractiveness. *Am J Orthod Dentofac Orthop.* 2011;140:e171–e180.
27. Dickens ST, Sarver DM, Proffit WR. Changes in frontal soft tissue dimensions of the lower face by age and gender. *World J Orthod.* 2002;3:313–320.
28. Parekh S, Fields HJ, Rosenstiel S, et al. Attractiveness of variations in the smile arc and buccal corridor space as judged by orthodontists and laymen. *Angle Orthod.* 2006;76:612–618.
29. Sharma N, Rosenstiel SR, Fields HW, et al. Layperson's esthetics and smile characterization between Caucasian and Indian populations. *J Prosthetic Dent.* 2012;107:327–335.

30. McLeod C, Fields HW, Hechter F, et al. Esthetics and smile characteristics evaluated by laypersons: a comparison of Canadian and US data. *Angle Orthod*. 2011;81:198–205.
31. Batra P, Daing A, Azam I, Miglani R, Bhardwaj A. Impact of altered gingival characteristics on smile esthetics: Laypersons' perspectives by Q sort methodology. *Am J Orthod Dentofacial Orthop*. 2018;154(1):82–90. e2.
32. Sarver DM, Sinclair P. Master Clinician: David M. Sarver. *J Clin Orthod*. 2021 Mar;55(3):147–158.
33. Rischen RJ, Breuning KH, Bronkhorst EM, Kuijpers-Jagtman AM. Records needed for orthodontic diagnosis and treatment planning: a systematic review. *PLoS ONE*. 2013;8(11):e74186.
34. Hollender AM, Anderson Q, Kartha K, et al. Research diagnostic criteria for temporomandibular disorders (RDC/TMD): development of image analysis criteria and examiner reliability for image analysis. *Oral Surg Oral Med Oral Pathol Oral Radiol Endod*. 2009;107:844–860.
35. American Board of Orthodontics. https://ntiiiby.americanboard-ortho.com/orthodontists/ become-certified/clinical-exam/mail-incre-submission-procedure/case-record-preparation/periodontal-documentation/.
36. Stevens DR, Flores-Mir C, Nebbe B, et al. Validity, reliability, and reproducibility of plaster vs digital study models: comparison of peer assessment rating and Bolton analysis and their constituent measurements. *Am J Orthod Dentofacial Orthop*. 2006;129:794–803.
37. Grauer D, Cevidanes LH, Tyndall D, et al. Registration of orthodontic digital models. In: McNamara JAJr, Hatch N, Kapila SD, eds. *Effective and Efficient Orthodontic Tooth Movement. Monograph 48, Craniofacial Growth Series*. University of Michigan, Department of Orthodontics and Pediatric Dentistry and Center for Human Growth and Development; 2011.
38. Kwon TG, Choi JW, Kyung HM, Park HS. Accuracy of maxillary repositioning in two-jaw surgery with conventional articulator model surgery versus virtual model surgery. *Int J Oral Maxillofac Surg*. 2014:732–738.
39. Atchison KA, Luke LS, White SC. An algorithm for ordering pretreatment orthodontic radiographs. *Am J Orthod Dentofacial Orthop*. 1992;102:29–44.
40. Bolton WA. Disharmony in tooth size and its relation to the analysis and treatment of malocclusion. *Angle Orthod*. 1958;28:113–130.
41. Kantor ML, Norton LA. Normal radiographic anatomy and common anomalies seen in cephalometric films. *Am J Orthod Dentofac Orthop*. 1987;91:414–426.
42. Riolo ML, et al. *An Atlas of Craniofacial Growth, Monograph 2, Craniofacial Growth Series*. University of Michigan, Center for Human Growth and Development; 1974.
43. Popovich F, Thompson GW. Craniofacial templates for orthodontic case analysis. *Am J Orthod*. 1977;71:406–420.
44. Broadbent BH Jr, Broadbent BH Jr, Golden WH. *Bolton Standards of Dentofacial Developmental Growth*. Mosby; 1975.
45. Jacobson A, Jacobson RL. *Radiographic Cephalometry: From Basics to 3-D Imaging*. Quintessence; 2006.
46. Lundstrom A, Lundstrom F, Lebret LM, et al. Natural head position and natural head orientation: basic considerations in cephalometric analysis. *Eur J Orthod*. 1995;17:111–120.
47. Steiner CC. Cephalometries in clinical practice. *Angle Orthod*. 1959;29:8–29.
48. Riedel RA. An analysis of dentofacial relationships. *Am J Orthod*. 1957;43:103–119.
49. Sassouni V. A classification of skeletal facial types. *Am J Orthod*. 1969;55:109–123.
50. Harvold EP. *The Activator in Interceptive Orthodontics*. CV Mosby; 1974.
51. Jacobson A. The "Wits" appraisal of jaw disharmony. *Am J Orthod*. 1975;67:125–131.
52. McNamara JA. A method of cephalometric evaluation. *Am J Orthod*. 1984;86:449–469.
53. American Board of Orthodontics. https://ntiiiby.americanboardortho.com/orthodontists/ become-certified/clinical-exam/mail-in-cre-submission-procedure/case-record-preparation/superimpositions/.
54. Buschang PH, LaPalme L, Tanquay R, Demirjian A. The technical reliability of superimposition on cranial base and mandibular structures. *Eur J Orthod*. 1986;8:152–156.
55. Doppel D, Damon W, Joondeph D, Little R. An investigation of maxillary superimposition techniques using metallic implants. *Am J Orthod Dentofac Orthop*. 1994;105:161–168.
56. Nielsen IL. Maxillary superimposition: a comparison of three methods for cephalometric evaluation of growth and treatment change. *Am J Orthod Dentofac Orthop*. 1989;95:422–431.
57. Baccetti T, Franchi L, McNamara JA Jr. The cervical vertebral maturation (CVM) method for the assessment of optimal treatment timing in dentofacial orthopedics. *Semin Orthod*. 2005;11:119–129.
58. Perinetti G, Primozic J, Sharma B, Cioffi I, Contardo L. Cervical vertebral maturation method and mandibular growth peak: a longitudinal study of diagnostic reliability. *Eur J Orthod*. 2018;40(6):666–672.
59. Morris KM, Fields HW, Beck FM, Kim DG. Diagnostic testing of cervical vertebral maturation staging: an independent assessment. *Am J Orthod Dentofacial Orthop*. 2019;156:626–632.
60. Deicke M, Pancherz H. Is radius-union an indicator for completed facial growth? *Angle Orthod*. 2005;75(3):295–299.
61. Alqerban A, Jacobs R, Fieuws S, Willems G. Comparison of two cone beam computed tomographic systems versus panoramic imaging for localization of impacted maxillary canines and detection of root resorption. *Eur J Orthod*. 2011;33:93–102.
62. Proffit WR, White Jr RP, Sarver DM. *Contemporary Treatment of Dentofacial Deformity*. Mosby; 2003.
63. Hanson J, Hennekam RCM, Allanson JE. *Gorlin's Syndromes of the Head and Neck*. 5th ed. Oxford University Press; 2010.
64. Grauer D, Cevidanes LS, Styner MA, et al. Accuracy and landmark error calculation using CBCT-generated cephalograms. *Angle Orthod*. 2010;80:286–294.
65. Ponce-Garcia C, Ruellas ACd, Cevidanes LHS, et al. Measurement error and reliability of three available 3D superimposition methods in growing patients. *Head Face Med*. 2020;16:1.
66. Koerich L, Weissheimer A, de Menezes LM, Lindauer SJ. Rapid 3D mandibular superimposition for growing patients. *Angle Orthod*. 2017;87:473–479.
67. Cevidanes LH, Bailey LJ, Tucker SF, et al. Three-dimensional cone-beam computed tomography for assessment of mandibular changes after orthognathic surgery. *Am J Orthod Dentofac Orthop*. 2007;131:44–50.
68. Zimmerman JN, Vora SR, Pliska BT. Reliability of upper airway assessment using CBCT. *The European Journal of Orthodontics*. 2019;41(1):101–108.
69. Obelenis Ryan DP, Bianchi J, Ignácio J, et al. Cone-beam computed tomography airway measurements: can we trust them? *Am J Orthodont Dentofac Orthop*. 2019;156(1):53–60.
70. Hsu WC. Evaluation of Upper airway in children with obstructive sleep apnea using cone-beam computed tomography. *Laryngoscope*. 2021;131:680–685.
71. Bitners AC, Sin S, Agrawal S, et al. Effect of sleep on upper airway dynamics in obese adolescents with obstructive sleep apnea syndrome. *Sleep*. 2020:43.
72. Chen H, Aarab G, Lobbezoo F, et al. Differences in three-dimensional craniofacial anatomy between responders and non-responders to mandibular advancement splint treatment in obstructive sleep apnea patients. *Eur J Orthodont*. 2019;41(3):308–315.
73. Marco-Pitarch R, García-Selva M, Plaza-Espín A, et al. Dimensional analysis of the upper airway in obstructive sleep apnoea syndrome patients treated with mandibular advancement device: a bi- and three-dimensional evaluation. *J Oral Rehabil*. 2021;48:927–936.
74. Ackerman J, Proffit WR, Sarver DM, et al. Pitch, roll and yaw: describing the spatial orientation of dentofacial traits. *Am J Orthod Dentofac Orthop*. 2007;131:305–310.
75. Severt TR, Proffit WR. The prevalence of facial asymmetry in the dentofacial deformities population at the University of North Carolina. *Int J Adult Orthod Orthogn Surg*. 1997;12:171–176.

7

Orthodontic Treatment Planning: From Problem List to Specific Plan

HENRY W. FIELDS, DAVID M. SARVER, WILLIAM R. PROFFIT, KAITRIN KRAMER, AND BENJAMIN T. PLISKA

CHAPTER OUTLINE

Treatment Planning Concepts and Goals

Orthodontic diagnosis is complete when a comprehensive list of the patient's problems and positive attributes have been developed and pathologic and developmental problems have been separated. At that point, the objective in treatment planning is to set treatment goals and design the strategy that a wise and prudent clinician, using the best evidence-based information available and their best judgment, would employ to address the problems while maximizing benefit to the patient and minimizing cost and risk.

It is important to view the goals of treatment in that way. Otherwise, an inappropriate emphasis on some aspect of the case is likely, whether the proposed treatment is medical, dental, or just orthodontics. For example, consider a patient with periodontal problems who seeks orthodontics because they are concerned about mildly crowded lower incisors. For that individual, controlling periodontal disease might be more beneficial than aligning teeth that would require permanent retention. This should be emphasized when a treatment plan is discussed with the patient, even though they initially sought only orthodontic treatment. Any treatment plan should be developed, in collaboration with the patient, to do what on balance would be best for that individual.

When a group of dentists and dental specialists meets to plan treatment for a patient with complex problems, questions for the orthodontist often are along the lines of "Could you retract the upper incisors enough to correct the overjet?" or "Could you develop incisal guidance for this patient?" To a question phrased as "Could you …?" the answer often is yes, given an unlimited commitment to treatment. The more appropriate question is not "Could you …?" but "Should you …?" or "Would it be best for the patient to …?" Cost-benefit and risk-benefit analyses (Fig. 7.1) are introduced appropriately when the question is rephrased that way.

A treatment plan in orthodontics, as in any other field, may be less than optimal if it does not take full advantage of the possibilities or if it is too ambitious. There is always a temptation to jump to conclusions and proceed with a superficially obvious plan without considering all the pertinent factors. The treatment planning approach advocated here is specifically designed to avoid both missed opportunities and excessive treatment, while appropriately involving the patient in the planning.

Before we talk in detail about the steps in going from the problem list to the final treatment plan that are outlined in Fig. 7.1, let us examine some important concepts that underlie orthodontic treatment planning more generally.

Major Issues in Planning Treatment

Patient Input

Modern treatment planning must be an interactive process. No longer can the doctor decide, in a paternalistic way, what is best for a patient. Both ethically and practically, patients and parents must be involved in the decision-making process. Ethically, patients have the right to control what happens to them in treatment—treatment should be something done for and with them, not to them. Practically, the patient's compliance is likely to be a critical issue in success or failure, and there is little reason to select a mode of treatment that the patient would not support. We also should emphasize that the doctor has an obligation not to simply follow the patient's instructions when it may lead to an undesirable outcome or side effect. Informed consent, in its modern form, requires involving the patient in the treatment planning process, which results in their understanding of the proposed treatment. This is emphasized in the procedure for presenting treatment recommendations that is provided later.

Predictability and Complexity of Treatment

If alternative methods of treatment are available, as usually is the case, which one should be chosen? Data are continuing to accumulate to allow choices to be based on evidence of outcomes rather than anecdotal reports and the claims of advocates of particular approaches. This chapter, like all the chapters in this book, has been significantly updated with information that was not available when the previous edition was written. How to judge new data and evaluate the quality of evidence for clinical decisions is emphasized in Chapter 1.

The complexity of the proposed treatment affects treatment planning, especially who should do the treatment. The focus of this chapter is on planning comprehensive orthodontic treatment. In orthodontics, as in all areas of dentistry, it makes sense that the less complex cases would be selected for treatment in general practice, and the more complex cases would be referred to a specialist. In general practice, an important issue is how you rationally select patients for treatment or referral. A formal scheme is presented in Chapter 11 for separating child patients most appropriate for orthodontic treatment in general practice from those more likely to require complex treatment, and a similar scheme for adults appears in Chapter 20.

Treatment Possibilities

As further background for planning comprehensive treatment, it is important to consider three controversial aspects of current orthodontic treatment planning: (1) the extent to which arch expansion versus extraction is indicated as a solution for crowding in the dental arches, (2) the extent to which growth modification versus extraction for camouflage or orthognathic surgery should be considered as solutions for skeletal problems, and (3) the extent of the application of Temporary Anchorage Devices (TADs) to retract, protract, expand, extrude or intrude teeth.

Dental Crowding: To Expand or Extract?

Since the beginning of the specialty, orthodontists have debated the limits of expansion of the dental arches and whether the advantages of extraction of some teeth to provide space for the others outweigh the disadvantages. With extraction, the loss of a tooth or teeth is a disadvantage, while avoiding expansion of intercanine dimensions and supporting tissue health are likely an advantage. There may also be positive or negative effects on facial esthetics. But, for any individual patient the decision is a value judgment. It is not only appropriate, but necessary to discuss

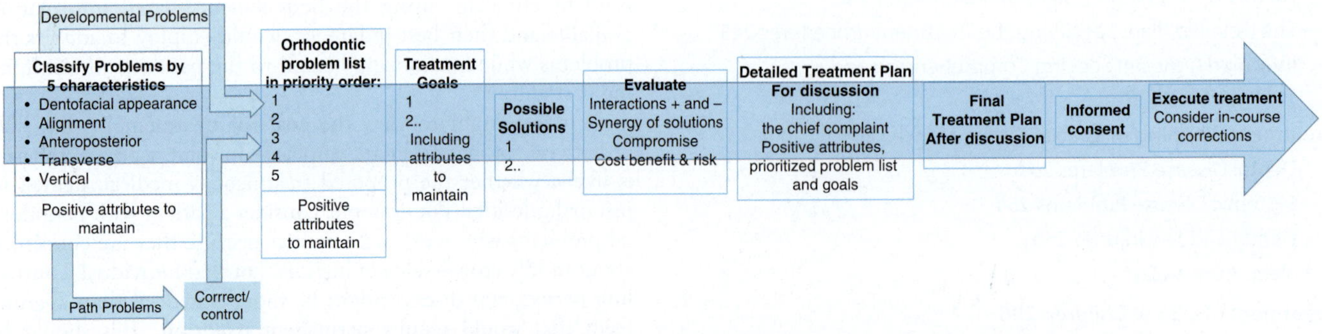

• **Fig. 7.1** The treatment planning sequence. In treatment planning the goal is wisdom, not scientific truth-judgment is required. Interaction with the patient and parent, so that they are involved in the decisions that lead to the final plan and understand cost and risk versus benefit, is the key to informed consent.

the pros and cons with the patient and parent before making the expansion-extraction decision.

In a rational contemporary view, many orthodontic patients can and should be treated without removal of teeth, but some will require extraction to compensate for crowding and/or incisor protrusion that affects facial esthetics. For others, extraction to camouflage a jaw discrepancy will be needed. The number in both groups varies depending on the population being treated. Let's first consider dental crowding and malalignment. In such situations, facial and dental esthetics, posttreatment stability and dental occlusion are the key factors.

Esthetic Considerations

If the major factors in extraction decisions are stability and esthetics, it is worthwhile to review existing data that relate these factors to expansion and extraction. Consider esthetics first. The conceptual relationship between expansion-extraction and esthetics is illustrated in Fig. 7.2. All other things being equal, expansion of the arches moves the patient in the direction of more prominent teeth, but extraction tends to reduce the prominence of the teeth. Facial esthetics can become unacceptable on either the too-protrusive or too-retrusive side.

At what point have the incisors been moved too far forward so that facial appearance is compromised? The answer likely is found in soft tissue, not hard tissue, relationships. Note that this has remarkably little to do with the prominence of the teeth relative to the supporting bone as seen in a profile view. You cannot determine the esthetic limit of expansion from tooth-bone relationships on a cephalometric radiograph.

At what point are the incisors retracted or proclined to the point of adversely affecting facial esthetics? This too depends largely on the soft tissues. The size of the nose and chin has a profound effect on relative lip prominence. For a patient with a large nose and/

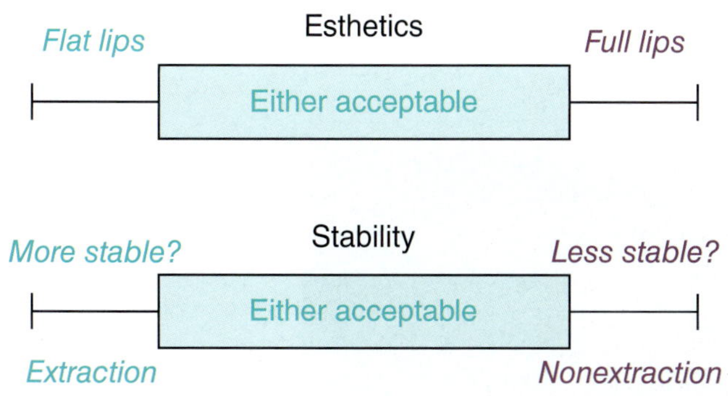

• **Fig. 7.2** Expansion of the dental arches tends to make the teeth more prominent, and extraction makes them less prominent. The choice between extraction and nonextraction (expansion) treatment is a critical esthetic decision for some patients who are toward the extremes of incisor protrusion or retrusion initially. Because there is an acceptable range of protrusion, many can be treated with satisfactory esthetics either way. This is especially true if expansion is managed so as not to produce too much incisor protrusion, or if space closure after extraction is controlled so as not to produce too much incisor retraction. Similarly, expansion tends to make arches less stable, and extraction may favor stability and soft tissue health, but the extraction-nonextraction decision probably is a critical factor in stability largely for patients who are toward the extremes of the protrusion-retrusion distribution. There are no data to show the percentage of patients who could be treated satisfactorily with either extraction or arch expansion versus the number for whom the extraction-nonextraction decision is critical in determining a satisfactory outcome.

or a large chin (either hard or soft tissue chin button), a choice of nonextraction treatment and moving the incisors forward is preferable to extraction treatment and retracting the incisors at least somewhat. When the prominence of the incisors creates excessive lip separation at rest so that the patient must strain to bring the lips together, the teeth are too protrusive and retracting the incisors improves the facial appearance (Fig. 7.3).

The upper incisors are too lingually tipped if the upper lip inclines backward—it should be slightly forward from its base at soft tissue point A (Fig. 7.4A). For best esthetics, the lower lip should be at least as prominent as the chin (Fig. 7.4B). Variations in chin morphology may put the proper incisor-chin relationship beyond the control of orthodontics alone, in which case surgical repositioning of the chin perhaps should be considered (see the sections in this chapter on Class II camouflage and maximizing esthetic changes in treatment, and Chapters 16, 20 and 22).

When similar cases have been treated by either nonextraction or extraction, the resulting esthetics have demonstrated 2 mm fuller lips for the nonextraction patients.[1] In Black patients, extractions produced more lip retrusion and nonextration more protrusion following treatment.[2] In borderline extraction patients the difference in treatment approach was usually approximately a 2 mm difference in lip protrusion.[3] Comparison of patients with comparable malocclusions who were treated either way showed little or no difference. For both frontal and profile appearance, this has been confirmed by more recent studies.[4,5]

Studies completed with similar pretreatment samples or matched borderline extraction samples can be difficult to evaluate because beyond the subtleties of the sample selections, the amount of change in both groups would be related to the amount of crowding and protrusion that was present initially and to the clinician's decision as to how to manage arch expansion or closure of extraction spaces by controlling anchorage.

Stability Considerations

For stable results, using the leeway space to alleviate transitional crowding as described by Gianelly appears to show the most promise.[6–8] But, if crowding is present, how much can arches be expanded? The lower arch is more constrained than the upper, due to the surrounding upper dental arch, but both are constrained by alveolar bone dimension, periodontal tissue support and lip, tongue and cheek pressure. So, its limitations for stable expansion may be somewhat tighter than the upper arch. When treating cases with borderline crowding, those treated with nonextration and extraction on average had similar posttreatment crowding results, but the difference in the follow-up results was affected as much by growth direction and incisor protrusion as by initial crowding.[3]

Current guidelines for the limits of expansion of the lower arch, admittedly based on limited data, are presented in Fig. 7.5. The 2-mm limitation for forward movement of the lower incisors obviously is subject to considerable individual variation but makes sense in light of the observation that lip pressure increases sharply 2 mm out into space usually occupied by the lip (see Chapter 5). If lip pressure is the limiting factor in forward movement, as it probably is, the initial position of the incisors relative to the lip would be a consideration in how much movement could be tolerated. This suggests and clinical observation seems to confirm (again, limited data!) that incisors tipped lingually away from the lip can be moved farther forward than upright incisors. Incisors tipped labially that remain crowded probably represent the equivalent

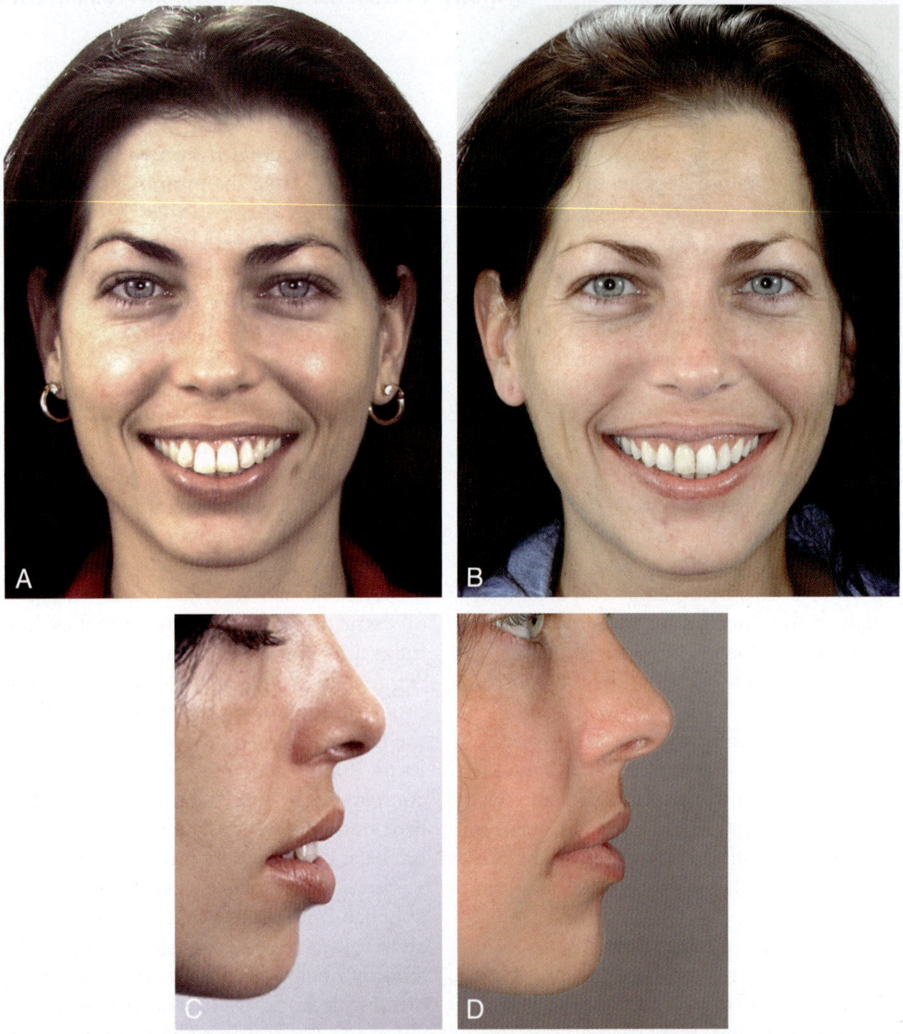

• **Fig. 7.3** In patients with excessive incisor protrusion, retracting the incisors improves facial esthetics. This young woman sought treatment because of dissatisfaction with the appearance of her teeth. After orthodontic treatment with premolar extraction and incisor retraction, dental and facial appearance were significantly improved. (A and B) Appearance on smile before and after treatment. (C and D) Profile before and after treatment. Although the idea goes back to Edward Angle and was revived in the late 20th century, it simply is not true that arch expansion always gives better facial esthetics.

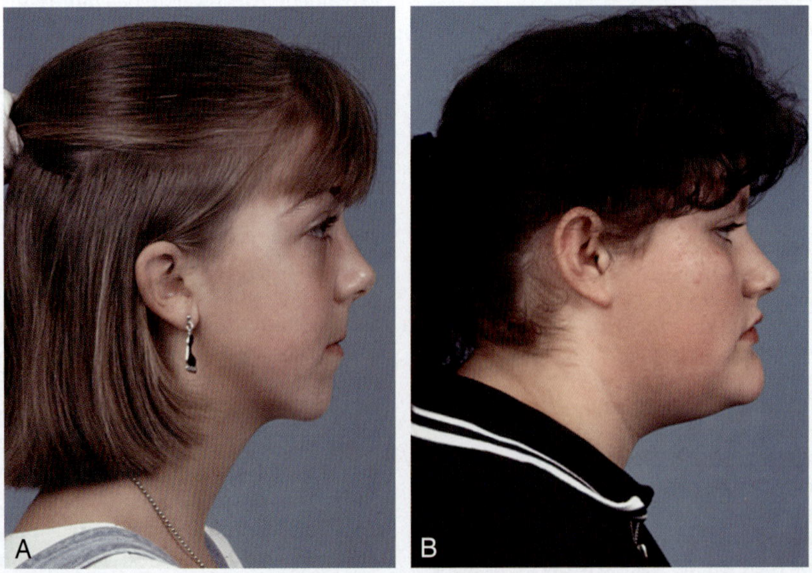

• **Fig. 7.4** (A) An upper lip that inclines backward relative to the true vertical line, which can result from retraction of upper incisors to correct excessive overjet, tends to compromise facial esthetics, as does a poorly defined labiomental sulcus when lip strain is required to bring the lips together. (B) This patient has reasoniable upper lip position, but due to retroclined mandibular incisors, and a prominent chin and dental compensation for a skeletal Class III jaw relationship, there is a poorly defined labiomental sulcus.

of a titrated endpoint in a chemical reaction, in that they have already become as protrusive as the facial soft tissues will allow. Moving them any further forward carries great risk of instability (see Fig. 7.2).

There also is a supporting soft tissue limitation in how far the incisors, especially the lower incisors, can be moved facially. Fenestration of the alveolar bone and stripping of the gingiva become increasingly likely as the incisors are advanced. The amount of attached gingiva is a critical variable. Although correction of gingival stripping after it has occurred is possible (Fig. 7.6), pretreatment consultation with a periodontist is advisable if the gingival attachment is questionable, depending on the amount and direction of planned tooth movement. Placing a gingival graft before orthodontic treatment begins may be the best option for these patients, or rethinking the amount of planned advancement or proclination.

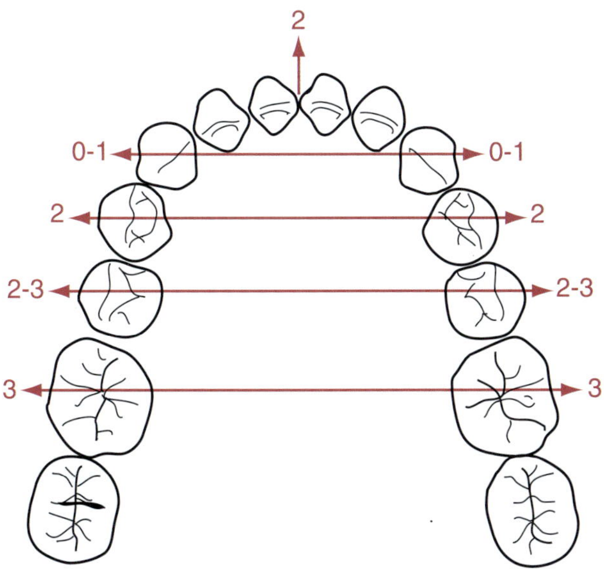

• **Fig. 7.5** Because the lower arch is more constrained, the limits of expansion for stability seem to be tighter for it than the maxillary arch. The available data suggest that moving lower incisors forward more than 2 mm is problematic for stability, probably because lip pressure seems to increase sharply at about that point. A considerable body of data shows that expansion across the canines is not stable, even if the canines are retracted when they are expanded. Expansion across the premolars and molars, in contrast, can be stable if it is not overdone.

As Fig. 7.5 illustrates, there may be more opportunity to expand transversely than anteroposteriorly—but only posterior to the canines. Numerous reports show that transverse expansion across the canines is almost never maintained, especially in the lower arch. In fact, intercanine dimensions typically decrease as patients mature, probably because of lip pressures at the corners of the mouth, whether or not they had orthodontic treatment. Expansion across the premolars and molars is much more likely to be maintained, presumably because of the relatively low cheek pressures.[9]

One approach to arch expansion is to expand the upper arch by opening the midpalatal suture (Fig. 7.7). If the maxillary base is narrow, this is appropriate treatment (see the later discussion of transverse maxillary deficiency). Some clinicians theorize (with no supporting evidence) that generously expanding the upper arch by opening the suture, temporarily creating a buccal crossbite, allows the lower arch then to be expanded more than otherwise would have been possible. If the limiting factor is cheek pressure, it seems unlikely that the method of expansion would make any difference. Excessive expansion carries the risk of fenestration of premolar and molar roots through the alveolar bone. There is an increasing risk of fenestration beyond 3 mm of transverse tooth movement.[10]

Contemporary Extraction Guidelines for Alignment

Contemporary guidelines for orthodontic extraction in Class I crowding cases can be summarized as follows:

- **Less than 4 mm of arch length discrepancy:** Extraction rarely indicated (only if there is severe incisor protrusion or, in a few instances, a severe vertical discrepancy). In some cases this amount of crowding can be managed without arch expansion by slightly reducing the width of selected teeth, being careful

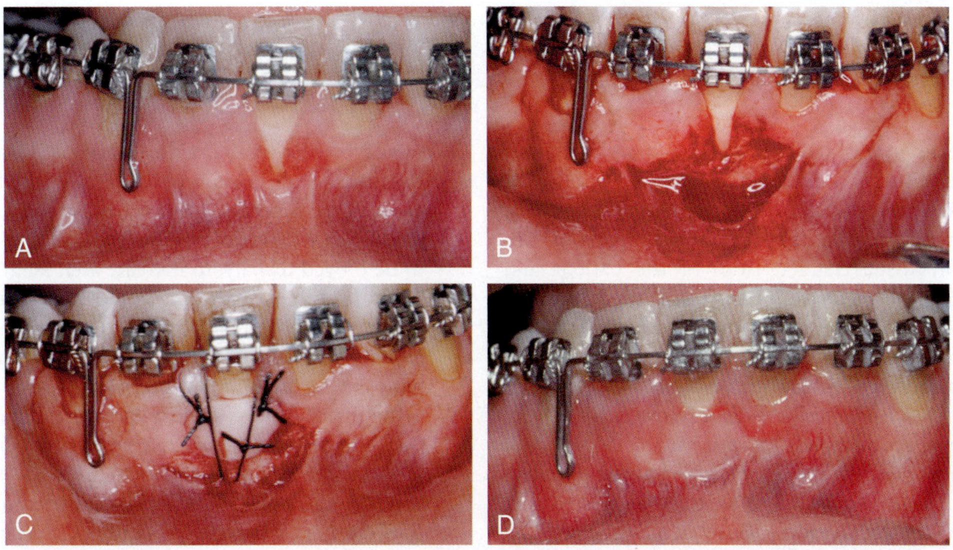

• **Fig. 7.6** (A) Gingival recession beginning to appear in a patient whose crowded lower incisors were aligned with some advancement despite premolar extraction to provide space. (B) Preparation of a bed for a free gingival graft. (C) The graft (tissue taken from the palate) sutured in position. (D) Two weeks later. (Courtesy Dr. J. Moriarty.)

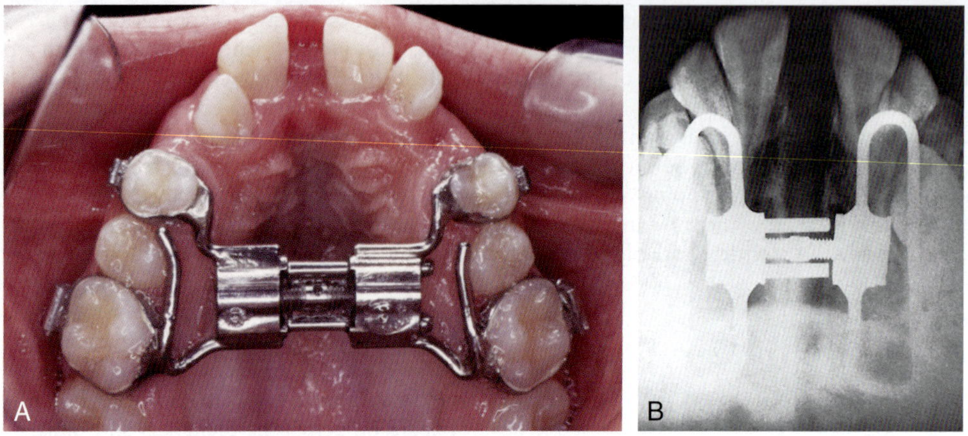

• **Fig. 7.7** Transverse force across the maxilla in children and adolescents can open the midpalatal suture. (A) The expansion force is usually delivered with a jackscrew mechanism fixed to maxillary teeth, as in this Hyrax expander with metal framework and jackscrew, seen at the end of rapid expansion (0.5 mm/day). The maxilla opens as if on a hinge, with its apex at the bridge of the nose. (B) The suture also opens on a hinge anteroposteriorly, separating more anteriorly than posteriorly, as shown in this radiograph of a patient after rapid expansion.

TABLE 7.1 Estimated Space From Various Extractions[a]

Extraction	Relief of Incisor Crowding	INCISOR RETRACTION[b]		POSTERIOR FORWARD[b]	
		Maximum	Minimum	Maximum	Minimum
Central incisor	5	3	2	1	0
Lateral	5	3	2	1	0
Canine	6	5	3	2	0
First premolar	5	5	2	5	2
Second premolar	3	3	0	6	4
First molar	3	2	0	8	6
Second molar	2	1	0	–	–

[a]With typical anchorage management (not skeletal anchorage).
[b]Anteroposterior plane of space in absence of crowding.
Values in millimeters.

to coordinate the amount of reduction in the upper and lower arches (see further discussion in Chapter 16).

- **Arch length discrepancy of 5 to 9 mm:** Nonextraction or extraction treatment possible. The decision depends on both the hard and soft tissue characteristics of the patient and on how the final position of the incisors will be controlled; any of several different teeth could be chosen for extraction. Nonextraction treatment usually requires transverse expansion across the molars and premolars, and inevitably some anterior incisor movement. With anterior incisor movement or leveling of the arches (see Chapter 15) the incisor tipping will also reduce the overbite, which can be a negative side effect in some patients. As early as the 1920s, it was suggested that normal occlusion required a critical width across the maxillary first premolars (Pont's index), and other indices based on arch width have been proposed as predictors of whether extraction is necessary. The modern conclusion is that such indices are not acceptable predictors of whether extraction or expansion would be best for individual patients.[11] This is not surprising, because the key criterion is the amount of lip support from the anterior teeth needed for satisfactory facial appearance. Finally, additional treatment time is required if the posterior teeth are to be moved distally, to increase arch length.
- **Arch length discrepancy of 10 mm or more:** Extraction is almost always required. For these patients, the amount of crowding virtually equals the amount of tooth mass being removed (extracting two premolars), and there would be little or no effect on lip support and facial appearance. The extraction choice is four-first premolars or perhaps upper first premolars and mandibular lateral incisors (which may provide better long-term stability). Second premolar or molar extraction rarely is satisfactory because it does not provide enough space near crowded anterior teeth or options to correct midline discrepancies (Table 7.1). If attempted, mini-implants would nearly always be needed to make this approach work without incisor proclination. Another option available to the clinician

is surgically facilitated orthodontic treatment which includes a soft tissue flap and synthetic bone augmentation material.

Dental Protrusion Plus Crowding

The presence of protrusion in addition to crowding, of course, complicates the extraction decision. Retracting the incisors to reduce lip prominence requires space within the dental arch. The effect is to increase the amount of arch length discrepancy, with about 2 mm of additional space in the arch (1 mm on each side) required for 1 mm of retraction of the central incisors. With that adjustment, the guidelines described earlier can be applied. To say it differently, if there is 6 mm of crowding in both arches and normal overjet, and the incisors need to be moved back 3 mm to correct lip protrusion and incompetence, 12 mm of space in the dental arch would be needed.

As a general rule, the lips will move about two-thirds of the distance that the incisors are retracted (i.e., 3 mm of incisor retraction will reduce lip protrusion by 2 mm). But there is a great deal of individual variation. This set of patients with protrusion and crowding are challenging and anchorage control following extractions is critical. Again, possibly even mini-implants may be needed to reinforce the anchorage.

A final set of guidelines could be as follows:

- The more you can expand without moving the incisors forward or increasing intercanine width, the more patients you can treat satisfactorily (from the perspective of both esthetics and stability) without extraction.
- The more you can close extraction spaces without over-retracting the incisors, the more patients you can treat satisfactorily (again, and especially from the perspective of esthetics) with extraction.
- For oral health, excessive expansion increases the risk of mucogingival problems.
- For masticatory function, expansion or extraction makes no difference.

Guidelines for extraction to camouflage jaw discrepancies are presented later, in the discussion of that approach to skeletal problems.

Skeletal Problems: Macro-esthetic Considerations

The important question in planning treatment for skeletal problems is whether orthodontic treatment, either by compensatory tooth movement and frequently extraction (camouflage) or growth modification, can bring the patient close enough to normal with acceptable facial esthetics, Alternatively, a combination of orthodontics and surgery would be required. This can be best answered by following up on the diagnostic information from the macro-esthetics part of the clinical examination and considering the possibilities for correcting facial disproportions. There are three possibilities: (1) orthodontic camouflage, (2) orthognathic and/or plastic surgery, and (3) for growing patients only, orthodontic growth modification.

Orthodontic Camouflage

If you can make facial disproportion disappear (or at least reduce it to the point that it is no longer a problem for the patient) without changing the jaw proportions that underlie it, you have solved the patient's problem satisfactorily by camouflaging it. In this sense, the success of camouflage treatment is in the eye of the beholder. Is the facial appearance satisfactory with camouflage, or is a greater change from surgery needed to overcome the perception of deformity? In borderline situations, only the patient and family or friends can answer this question. It is not the doctor's decision.

As we have noted already, orthodontic camouflage of mandibular deficiency by retracting the upper incisors tends to be more successful in a northern European-derived population, in which most people have a convex profile with little or no chin projection. Camouflage of mandibular excess by retracting the lower incisors is rarely indicated in patients of European or African descent but can be effective in patients of Asian descent, who often have prominence of the lower lip more because of protruding incisors than a large mandible. In these situations and with other jaw discrepancies, it still is up to the patient to decide whether tooth movement alone would be successful treatment. Computer predictions using pretreatment facial images can help with these decisions (Fig. 7.8).

Surgery

Computer image predictions of the outcome of orthodontics alone or of orthognathic surgery are also an important tool to help the patient and parents or family understand the likely facial or profile effect of alternative treatments (Fig. 7.8). Because surgery and camouflage are both most common when little or no growth remains, the uncertainty of growth prediction is removed, and the predictions are accurate enough for clinical use. Data from a randomized clinical trial showed that surgery patients appreciate the improved communication that the computer predictions made possible and, compared with those who did not see their predictions before surgery, are more likely to be satisfied with the outcome of treatment.[12] Letting the patients see their prediction images now is a routine part of surgical planning (see Chapter 22).

For everyone, advancing age is indicated by increased facial wrinkles, looser skin in the cheeks and throat because of loss of tissue in the deeper layers of the skin, a decrease of facial bony support in the midface and decreased fullness of the lips. Until recently, face lift surgery approached these problems primarily by pulling the skin tighter. The emphasis now in improving facial appearance in adults is on "filling up the bag"—adding volume rather than decreasing it.

One of the advantages of mandibular advancement surgery, and to a lesser extent of maxillary advancement as well, is that it does add volume and makes adults look younger by doing so (Fig. 7.9). Genioplasty, the most frequently used adjunct to orthodontics, also enhances facial appearance by adding volume to the lower face. In addition it improves the stability of the lower incisors and decreases the chance of gingival stripping by adding bone in front of protruding lower incisors,[13] and so is not just a cosmetic procedure.

Orthognathic procedures that decrease volume (mandibular setback and superior repositioning of the maxilla are the best examples) do improve facial proportions but can make the patient look older because of the effects on the skin. For that reason, almost all surgical Class III treatment now includes some maxillary advancement, which often is combined with mandibular setback in prognathic patients. The goal is to correct the jaw discrepancy without making the patient look prematurely older. Maxillary advancement or minimal mandibular setback also reduces the potential for sleep disordered breathing.

For some patients, maximizing the improvement of esthetics requires facial plastic surgery in addition to orthodontics or

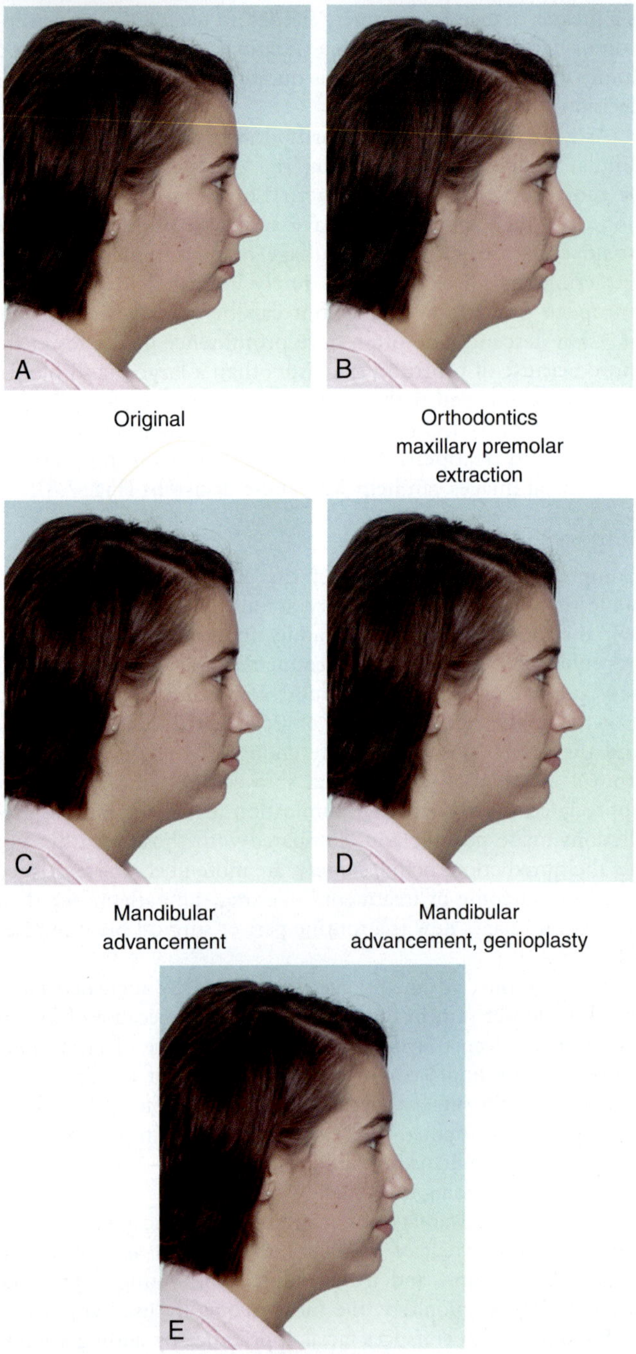

• **Fig. 7.8** Presenting a computer-generated simulation of the posttreatment profile can greatly help patients understand the differences among alternative treatment approaches. For this patient, the pretreatment profile (A) is shown alongside the probable profile outcomes for orthodontic camouflage of a skeletal Class II problem with retraction of the anterior teeth into first premolar extraction spaces (B), versus mandibular advancement to correct the jaw relationship (C), mandibular advancement supplemented with genioplasty (D) and rhinoplasty (E). Although showing patients these simulations heighten their esthetic awareness, it does not seem to create unrealistic expectations.

orthognathic surgery (Fig. 7.10). Rhinoplasty is particularly effective when the nose is deviated to one side, has a prominent dorsal hump, or has a bulbous or distorted tip. Deficient facial areas, such as the paranasal deficiency, that often are seen in patients with maxillary deficiency, can be improved by placing grafts or alloplastic implants subperiosteally.

The interactions of orthodontists and surgeons in the treatment of patients who need orthognathic and facial plastic surgery are discussed in Chapter 22.

Growth Modification

If possible, the best way to correct a jaw discrepancy would be to get the patient to grow out of it. Because the pattern of facial growth is established early in life and rarely changes significantly, this is unlikely without treatment. To some extent, however, jaw growth in all three dimensions can be modified, with a combination of restraint of excessive growth, stimulation of favorable growth and redirection of growth. The attitudes of orthodontists to this have varied greatly over time, with back-and-forth enthusiasm and pessimism about making significant changes in jaw relationships. Most recently, great optimism in the late 20th century has been tempered by better outcomes data.

Modern growth modification is discussed in detail in Chapters 13 and 14, in the context of how much change can be accomplished in each dimension. There is an interesting contrast in success compared with camouflage; greater growth modification is possible in Class III than in Class II patients—just the reverse of the possibilities for camouflage.

As a note of context here, we need to consider all three options for facial change: growth modification, camouflage and orthognathic surgery. You will see in the later chapters that growth modification is a modest enterprise and either as a result of the appliance design and its side effects or the need to create a better occlusion, growth modification treatment always includes some form of camouflage. Camouflage is camouflage and allows clinicians to make acceptable occlusions fit with acceptable facial esthetics and skeletal structures. Orthognathic surgery treatment, in its ideal form, decompensates the teeth to normal and then includes skeletal changes via surgery to near normal for an improved facial esthetic and occlusal result. Data suggests that the first stage of orthognathic surgery treatment, decompensation of the teeth is not fully realized, which limits the ideal surgical change.[14,15] This results in an improved, but not ideal, result that includes dental compensation. All types of orthodontic care that attempts to modify the skeletal relationships or accommodate them, regardless of approach, include camouflage.

Mini-implant (TAD) Augmented Treatment

Another, more contemporary controversy is beginning to take shape. In its most dramatic form, some have argued that the place for orthognathic surgery is dwindling because so much more can now be accomplished with mini-implants than was previously possible with either orthodontics, growth modification or camouflage. This brings us back to consideration of the question previously posed: "Can" or "should" we use a particular treatment option?

Certainly mini-implants have provided new options for anchorage related to space opening, closing, dental protraction and retraction. They have been used successfully for intrusion of anterior and posterior teeth. These same treatments can improve soft tissue profiles and vertical facial relationships. Certainly, the potential for nonsurgical palatal expansion now can extend into

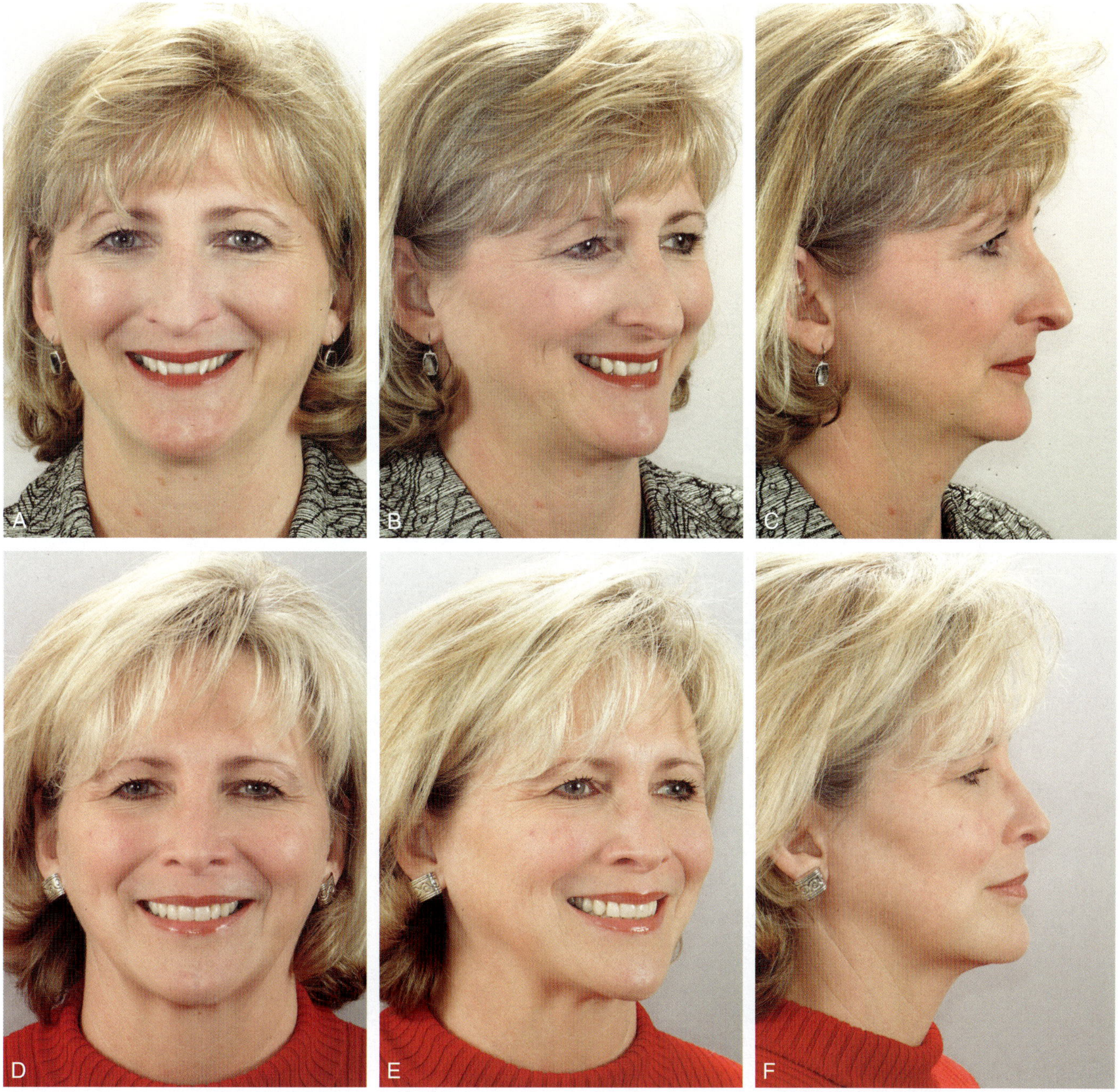

• **Fig. 7.9** Surgical mandibular advancement tightens the skin around the mandible, decreasing wrinkles around and beneath the chin, which tends to make the patient look younger. (A–C) Patient at age 48, before treatment that involved proclining the maxillary central incisors to produce overjet, then advancing the mandible; (D–F) at age 51, 1 year after completion of treatment.

adulthood. Growth modification to address maxillary retrusion can be enhanced with mini-implants (TADs) and boneplates (Figs. 7.11–7.13). Often these treatments can reduce costs and risks.

The limitations, it seems, are the length of treatment, amount of change needed, stability and the number of problems addressed. Differentiating between intruding one or two teeth, versus multitooth segments needs to be considered carefully. And, is it really in the patient's best interest to distalize the whole maxillary dentition to avoid premolar extraction when the nonextraction lower arch will determine the upper incisor position in either case? How important is it to be able to proclaim the treatment was done either nonsurgically or nonextration?

Orthognathic surgery usually addresses multiple problems and planes of space at one time point with an established record of stability/instability. The database for making mini-implant decisions will grow, but it should not be driven by a desire to provide a proof of concept rather than better patient care. These envelopes of successful mini-implant treatment remain to be established (see Chapter 22).

Mini-Esthetic Considerations: Improving the Smile Framework

The primary goal of mini-esthetic treatment is to enhance the smile by correcting the relationship of the teeth to the surrounding

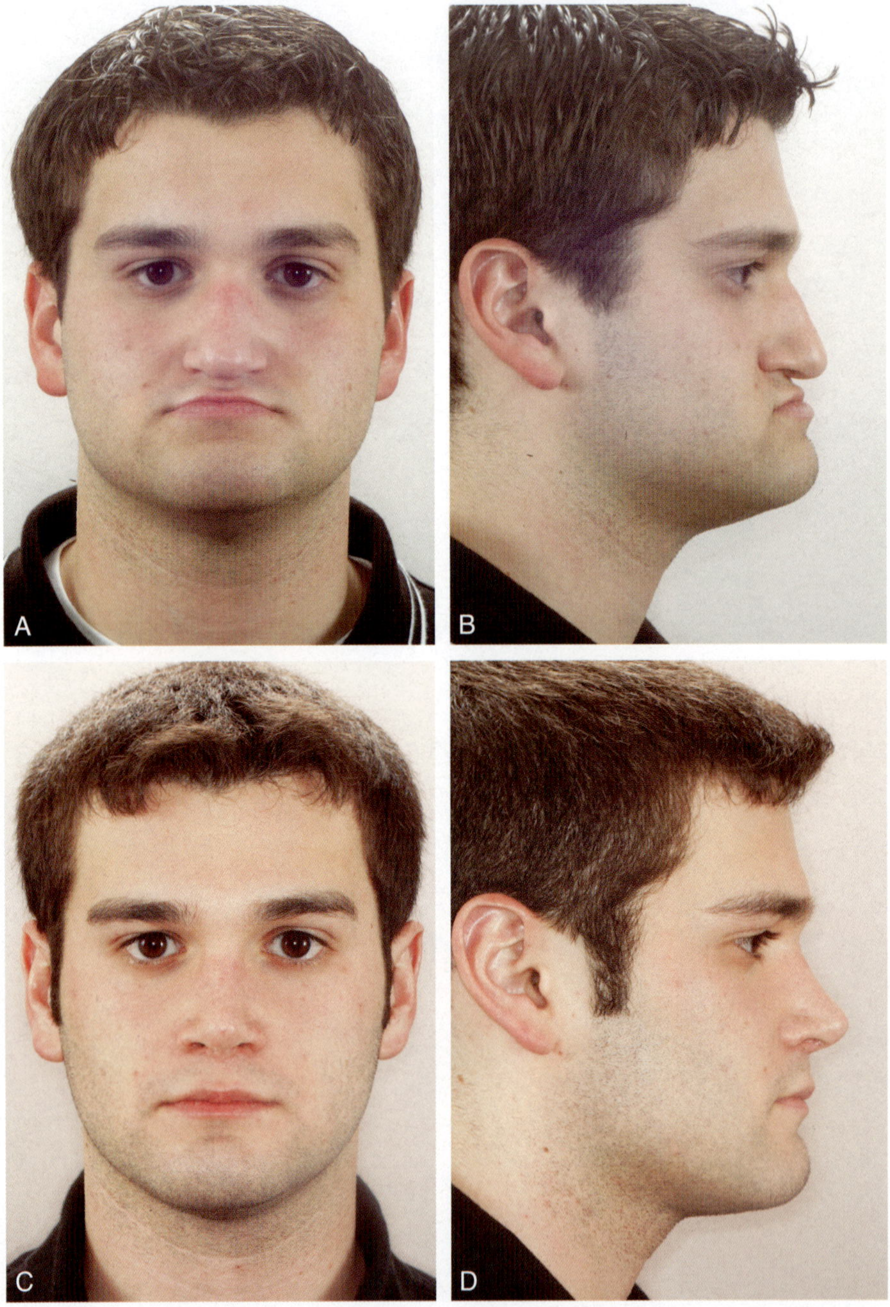

• **Fig. 7.10** It is quite possible to combine rhinoplasty with orthognathic surgery, and correcting a nasal deformity can be a significant adjunct to the improved appearance after contemporary maxillofacial surgery. (A and B) Frontal and profile photographs before treatment. Note that this man's skeletal Class III problem was largely maxillary deficiency and that there was abnormal anatomy of the nasal bridge, a widened nasal base, and an enlarged and bulbous nasal tip. (C and D) Frontal and profile photographs after maxillary advancement and rhinoplasty. The improvement in the nose nicely complements the better projection of the maxilla.

soft tissues on smiling. In the development of the problem list, the examination focuses on three aspects of the smile: the vertical relationship of the lips to the teeth, the transverse dimensions of the smile, and the smile arc. This section considers the possibilities for problems of this type.

It is important to display most of the crowns of the maxillary anterior teeth in a social smile, and the general guideline is that there should be at least 75% display of the central incisor.[16] The amount of display is a function of the age of the patient, with a peak before adolescence of an average display of 85%, little change up to about the late 20's and then a gradual decrease as aging lowers the lips across the anterior teeth (see Fig. 4.24). Exposure of all the crown and some gingiva is both esthetically acceptable and youthful appearing (see Figs. 2.33, 2.34, and 6.31 and Table 6.5). Obviously, the goal in treatment should be to position the teeth relative to the upper lip so that they are displayed on smile within these guidelines. In applying the guidelines, it should be kept in mind that tooth display is greater in females and that minor excess

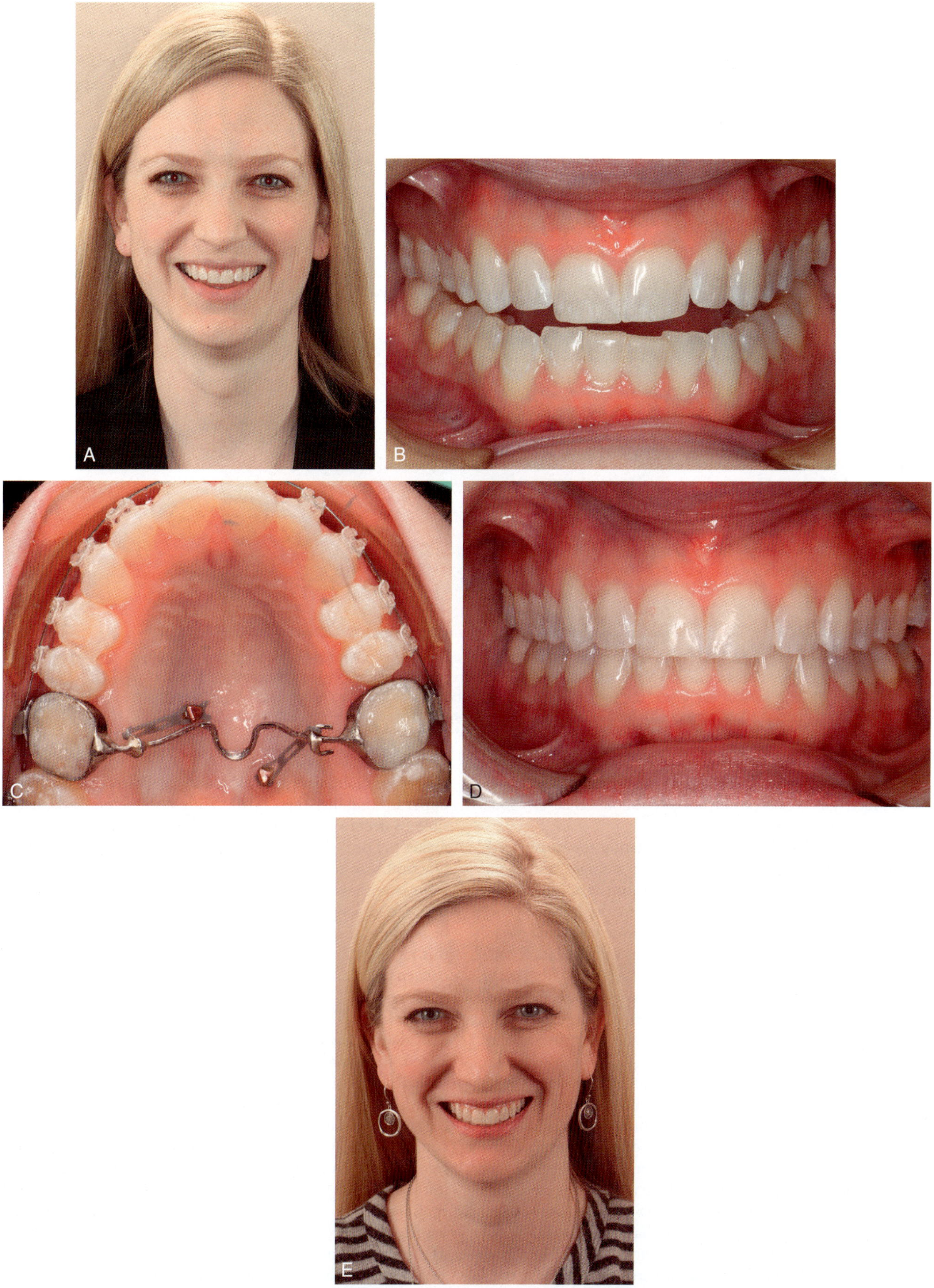

• **Fig. 7.11** TADs used for posterior intrusion and reduction of an anterior openbite. (A) This adult female was concerned about her irregular teeth and (B) her anterior openbite. TAD posterior intrusion was initiated after initial alignment using palatal TADs and alastic chain traction to TPA. (C) Posttreatment facial esthetics are good and (D) anterior overbite is established. To obtain the total anterior bite closure of 5 mm (2 mm openbite and 3 mm posttreatment overbite), approximately 2.5 mm or posterior stable intrusion was accomplished.

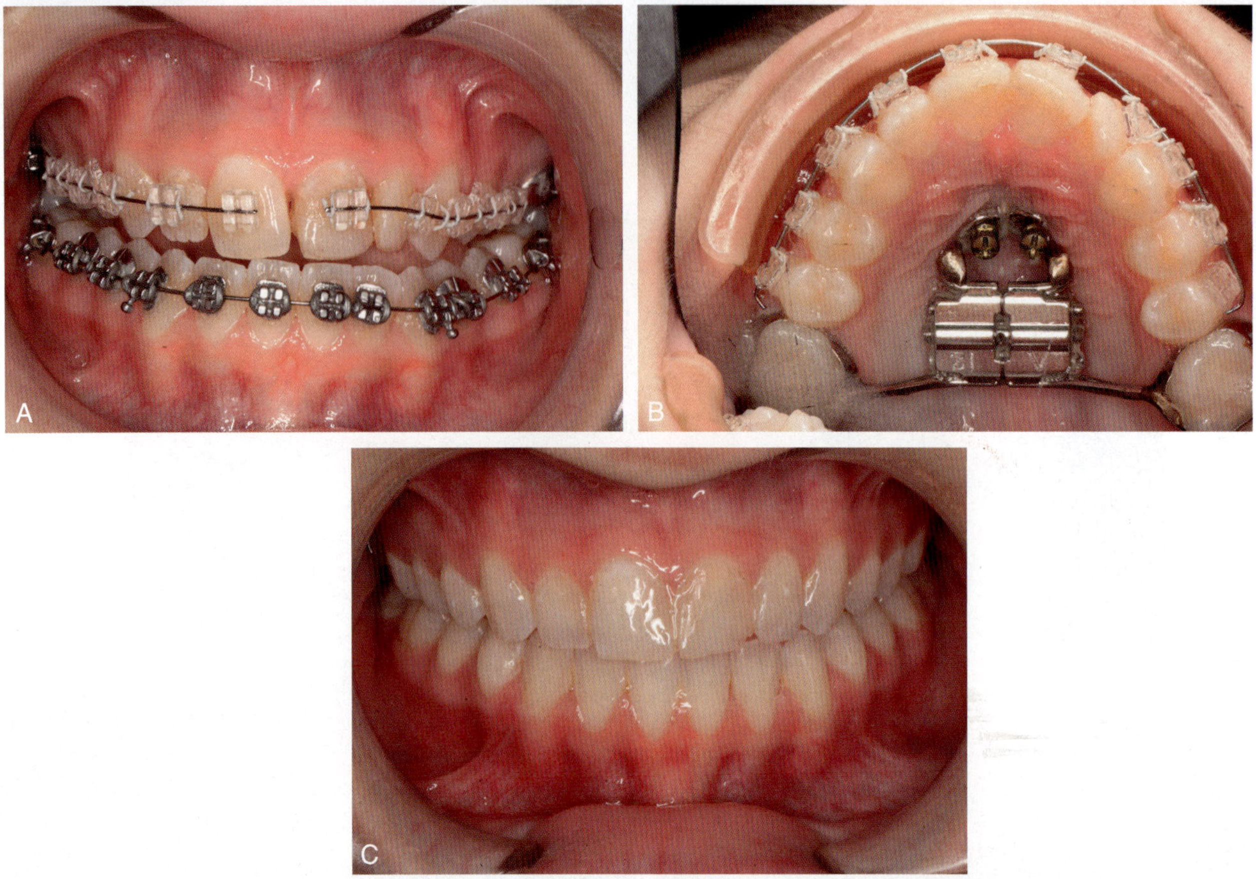

• **Fig. 7.12** TADs used for posterior expansion in an adult. (A) the patient in treatment during early alignment displaying anterior and posterior openbite due to transverse maxillary constriction and interferences. (B) Posterior expansion using midpalatal TADs attached to the maxillary first molars. (C) Posttreatment occlusion with adequate overbite and buccal overjet with the maxillary constriction resolved.

gingival display will usually self-correct with age.[17] What looks like too much gingival exposure in early adolescence can look almost perfect a few years later.

If the tooth display is inadequate, elongating the upper teeth improves the smile, makes the patient look younger, and is the obvious plan. There are several possible treatment approaches to accomplish this, which would be selected on the basis of other aspects of the patient's problems. In orthodontic treatment alone, extrusive mechanics with archwires, judicious use of Class II elastics to take advantage of their tendency to rotate the occlusal plane down anteriorly, and anterior vertical elastics could be considered. Rotating the maxilla down in front as it is advanced surgically can improve smile esthetics, especially in patients with maxillary deficiency (Fig. 7.14).

As noted in Chapter 6, there are five potential etiologies for a gummy smile: (1) vertical maxillary excess (long-face syndrome), (2) short philtrum upper lip, (3) short clinical crown height, (4) retroclined maxillary incisors, and (5) hypermobile smile. In an individual patient, a gummy smile may be one of these factors or a combination of several of them. There are now six treatment approaches to excessive gingival display: (1) intrusion of the maxillary incisors using segmented arch mechanics (Figs. 7.25), (2) intrusion of maxillary incisors using temporary skeletal anchorage (see Figs. 7.13), (3) orthognathic surgery to move the maxilla up (see Chapter 22), (4) vestibuloplasty alone or combined with maxillary orthognathic surgery to lengthen the philtrim area and reduce lip mobility (Figs. 7.15), and (5) Botox therapy to reduce upper lip mobility (Fig. 7.16). With all these methods, it is possible to overdo intrusion of the anterior teeth, which, of course, makes the smile less attractive and the patient look older. Another practical way to improve excess gingival display that can result from overgrowth of the gingiva is (6) recontouring the gingiva with crown lengthening to gain normal crown heights. This can be accomplished with experience using laser surgery (see later in this chapter Case FP) which makes this much easier and more convenient than previously.

Transverse Dimensions of the Smile. "She [or he] has a broad, welcoming smile" often is used as a compliment. Exactly what does that mean? In patients whose arch forms are narrow or collapsed, the smile may also appear narrow, which is less appealing esthetically. In the diagnostic examination of the smile framework, the width of the buccal corridors was noted (Fig. 7.17). Transverse expansion of the maxillary arch, which decreases buccal corridor width, improves the appearance of the smile *if* the buccal corridor width was excessive before treatment. Prosthodontists have learned that too wide a denture set-up, so that the buccal corridor is obliterated, is not esthetic. Too much expansion of the natural dentition can produce the same unnatural appearance of the teeth, so transverse expansion is not for everyone.

Should this be done only with dental expansion or by opening the midpalatal suture? That depends on the amount of expansion that is needed to meet the other goals of proper occlusion and

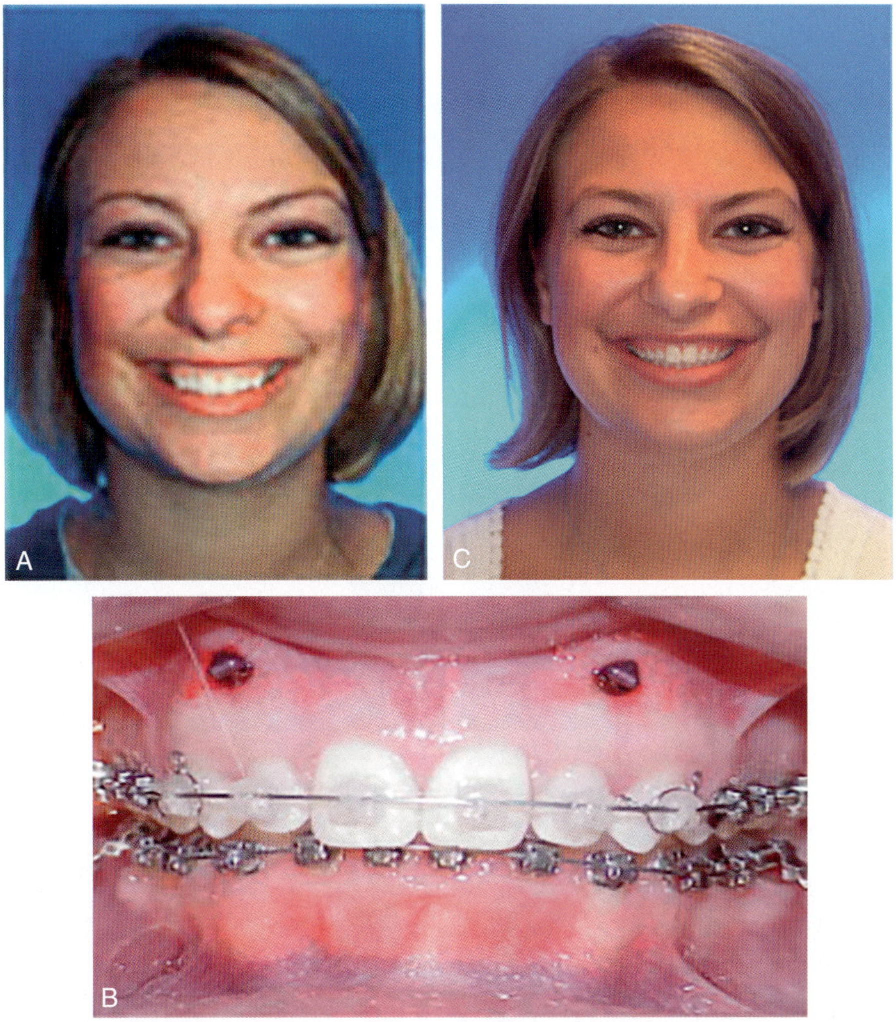

• **Fig. 7.13** (A) An adult with excessive gingival display upon smiling. (B) Dentoalveolar maxillary bilateral anterior TADs used as anchorage with coil springs to intrude the anterior teeth. (C) Posttreatment smile show significant reduction in gingival display to the cervical area of the incisors. (Courtesy Dr. Larry Hutta.)

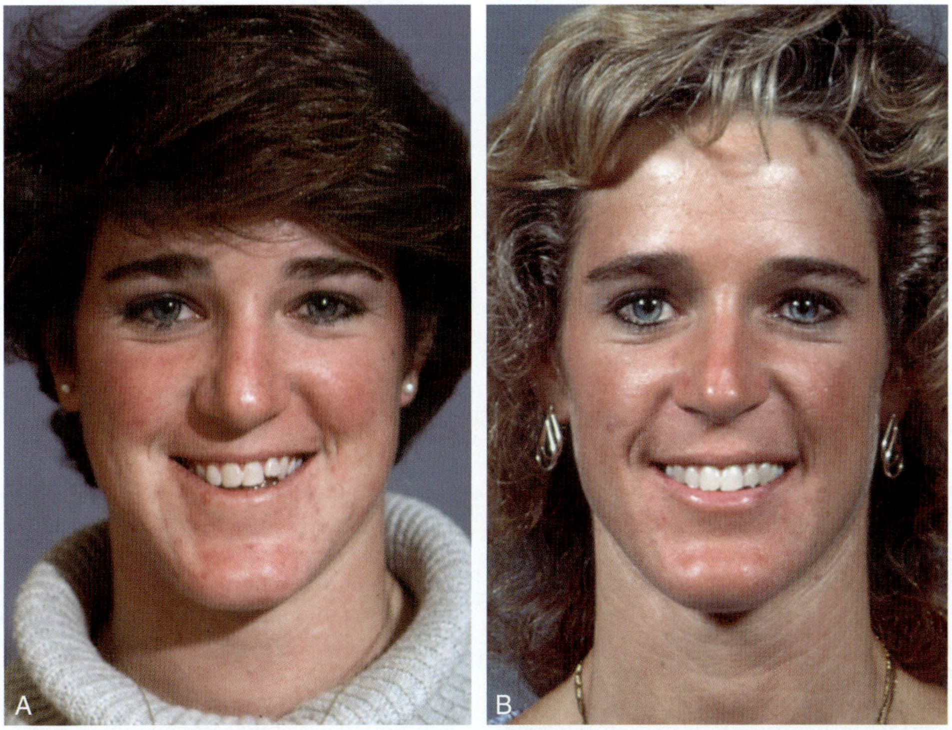

• **Fig. 7.14** Inadequate exposure of the maxillary teeth impairs the appearance of the smile, and increasing incisor display for such a patient improves it. (A) Before treatment, the patient's chief complaint was her facial appearance. Although her problem would traditionally be described as a mild skeletal Class III problem due to maxillary deficiency, the frontal rather than the profile appearance was (appropriately) her major concern. (B) After treatment to bring the maxilla forward and rotate it down anteriorly, to increase incisor display.

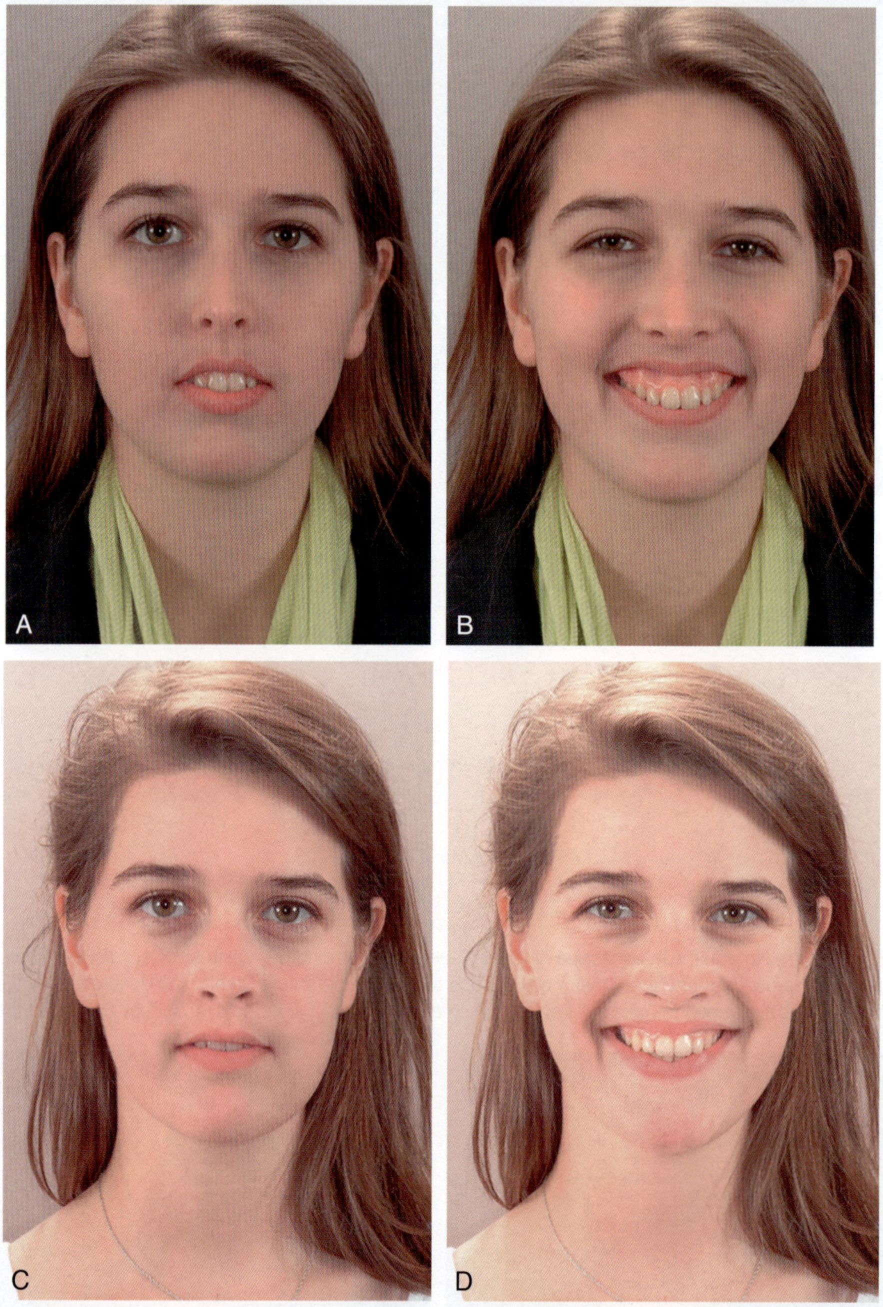

• **Fig. 7.15** (A) This 18-year-old girl demonstrated, At rest, a philtrum length that was significantly shorter than her commissure height. (B) An excessive gingival display on smile (5 mm). (C) The patient 1 year after superior repositioning of the maxilla via Lefort I osteotomy in combination with lengthening of the upper philtrum through a surgical coronal vestibuloplasty. Her final result reflected greatly improved resting lip balance. (D)This image reflects the increase in length of the middle portion of the upper lip, with improved balance with the outer commissures and a significant reduction of gingival display on smile.

long-term stability. An important consideration in widening a narrow arch form, particularly in an adult, is the axial inclination of the buccal segments. Patients in whom the posterior teeth are already flared laterally are not good candidates for dental expansion.

The Smile Arc

Obtaining and maintaining a proper smile arc requires directing the treatment at the real problem (Fig. 7.18). This may mean taking this into account when brackets are placed on the teeth (Fig. 7.19). The traditional guideline for placing brackets has been based on measurements from the incisal edge so that the central incisor bracket is placed at about the middle of the clinical crown, the lateral incisor bracket about 0.5 mm closer to the incisal edge than the central, and the canine about 0.5 mm more apically. The effect is to position the teeth very nicely in relation to one another, as they would be in a denture set-up, without taking into consideration the vertical tooth–lip relationship that the prosthodontist would emphasize. The result may not be compatible at all with the best appearance of the teeth on smile because the smile arc was not considered. Research has suggested that the smile arc is the most

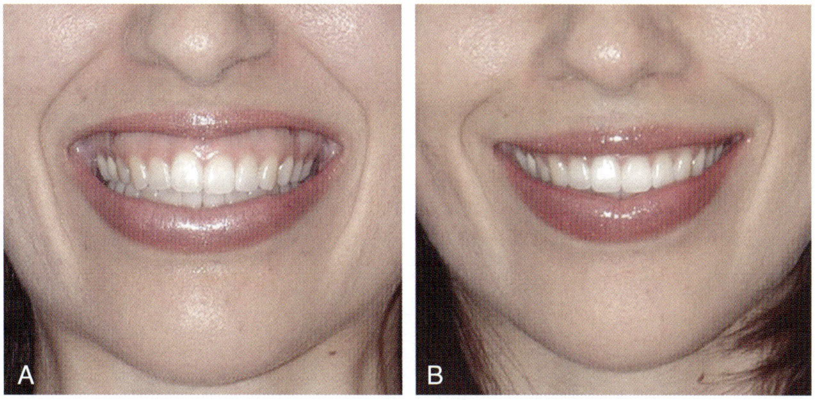

• **Fig. 7.16** (A) Pre and (B) post operative images of a patient with a gummy smile who underwent successful Botox therapy. Some data estimate that with an average preoperative gingival margin to upper lip distance of 5 mm, the gingival exposure can be reduced to approximately 1 mm. The authors estimated 30–32 weeks to return to baseline, but many retreat at 3–4 months. (Polo M. Botulinum toxin type A (Botox) for the neuromuscular correction of excessive gingival display on smiling (gummy smile). *Am J Orthod Dentofac Orthop*. 2008;133:195–203).

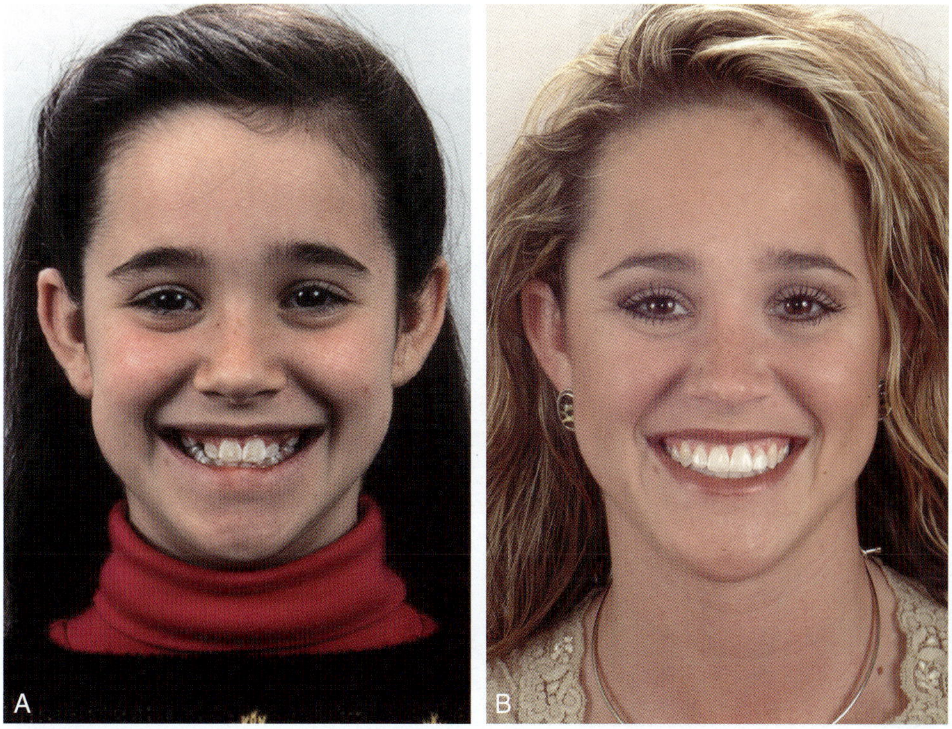

• **Fig. 7.17** For patients with wide buccal corridors, transverse expansion of the maxilla can improve smile esthetics. (A) Age 12, before treatment. (B) Age 15, after orthodontic treatment with widening of the maxillary arch.

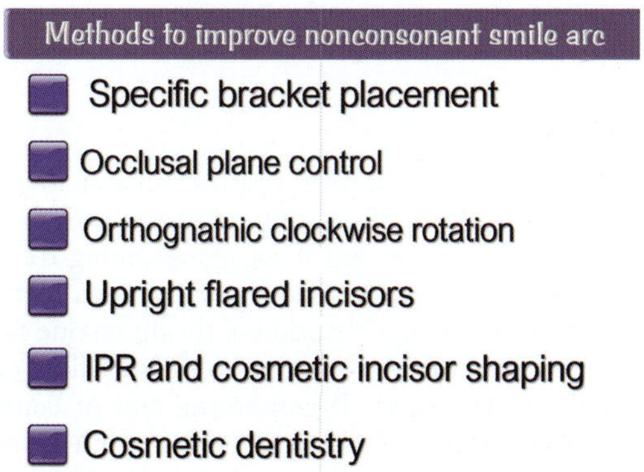

• **Fig. 7.18** These are the elements that can be used to improve the smile arc.

important determinant of the attractiveness of the smile—more important than buccal corridor space, although both play a significant role.[18]

What would you do differently in placing brackets to obtain the best smile arc? The usual problem is that the smile arc is too flat. If that is the case, putting the maxillary central incisor brackets more gingivally would increase the arc of the dentition, bring them closer to the lower lip, and make the smile arc more consonant with the lower lip. If the smile arc were distorted in some other way, placing the brackets to compensate for this by altering tooth positions would be the solution. Of course, if the smile arc had been flattened during treatment, step bends in the

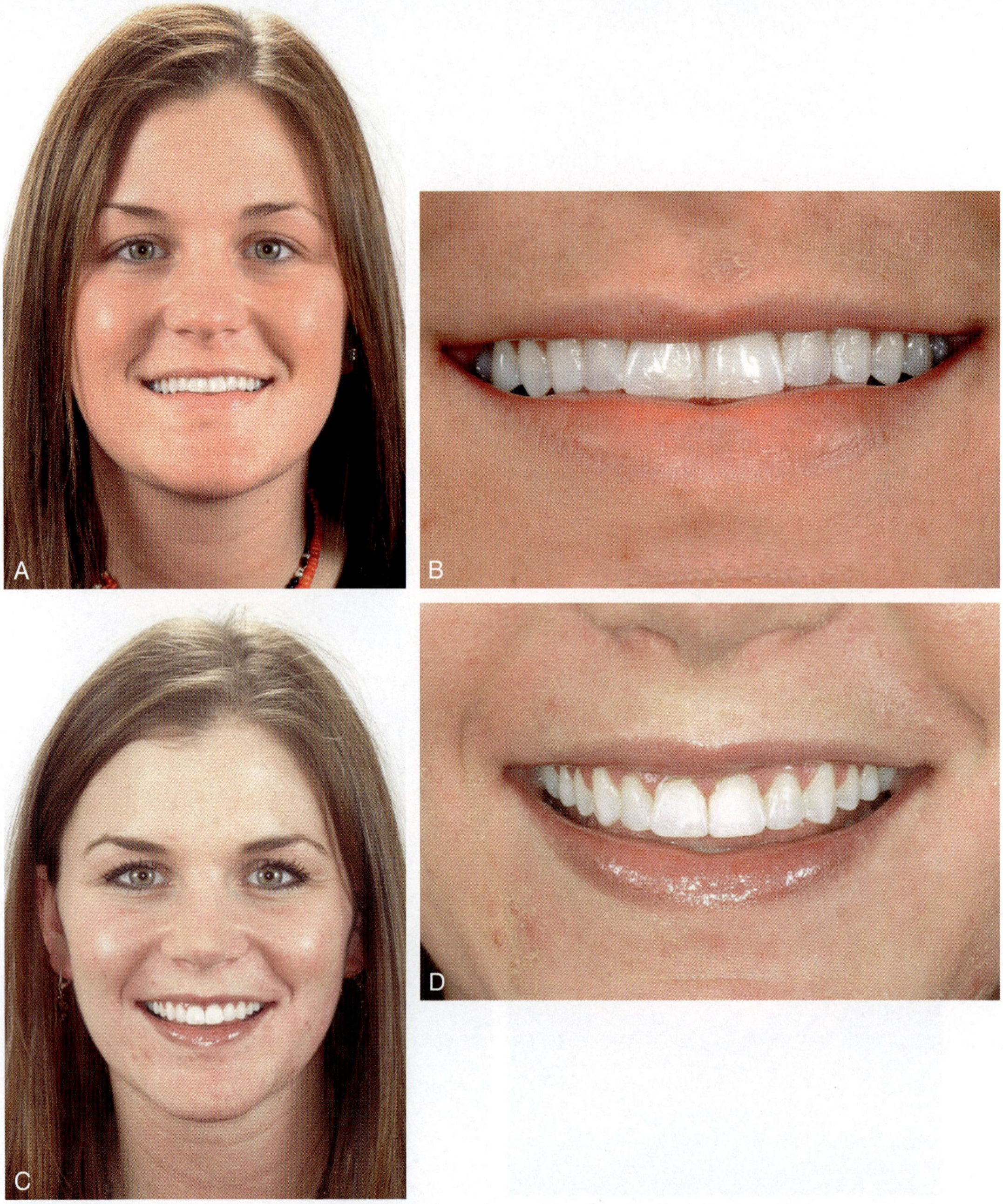

• **Fig. 7.19** The smile arc is the most important single thing in smile esthetics. (A and B) Full-face and close-up views of the smile before treatment. Note the flat smile arc and inadequate display of maxillary incisors. (C and D) One year later, after orthodontic (not orthognathic surgery) treatment. The improvement in facial appearance is largely due to better lip support by the upper teeth that decreased the paranasal folds and attainment of a correct smile arc.

archwire would be an alternative to rebonding brackets to correct it. Repositioning incisors to obtain a better smile arc may be needed in orthognathic surgery patients, as well as in patients who are to receive orthodontic treatment only.

Another solution may be to upright flared incisors that have reduce the smile arc. Simply tipping them lingually to close space or retract after extractions will increase their vertical exposure and provide a more consonant arc (Fig. 7.20) Restorative solutions to smile arc improvement also should be considered. They can include incisor reshaping Fig. 7.21, and cosmetic dentistry (Figs. 7.22 and 7.24).

Smile Symmetry

An asymmetric smile sometimes is a patient's major concern. It is possible that this is due to more eruption of the teeth or different crown heights on one side, and if so, repositioning the teeth or changing the gingival contours should be included in the treatment plan. However, greater elevation of the lip on one side when smiling, gives the appearance of a cant to the maxillary dentition when it really is symmetric. If concerning and of considerable magnitude this condition would need either vestibular surgery or Botox or both to address excessive gingival display.[19] A number of the solutions for excessive and deficient gingival or tooth display

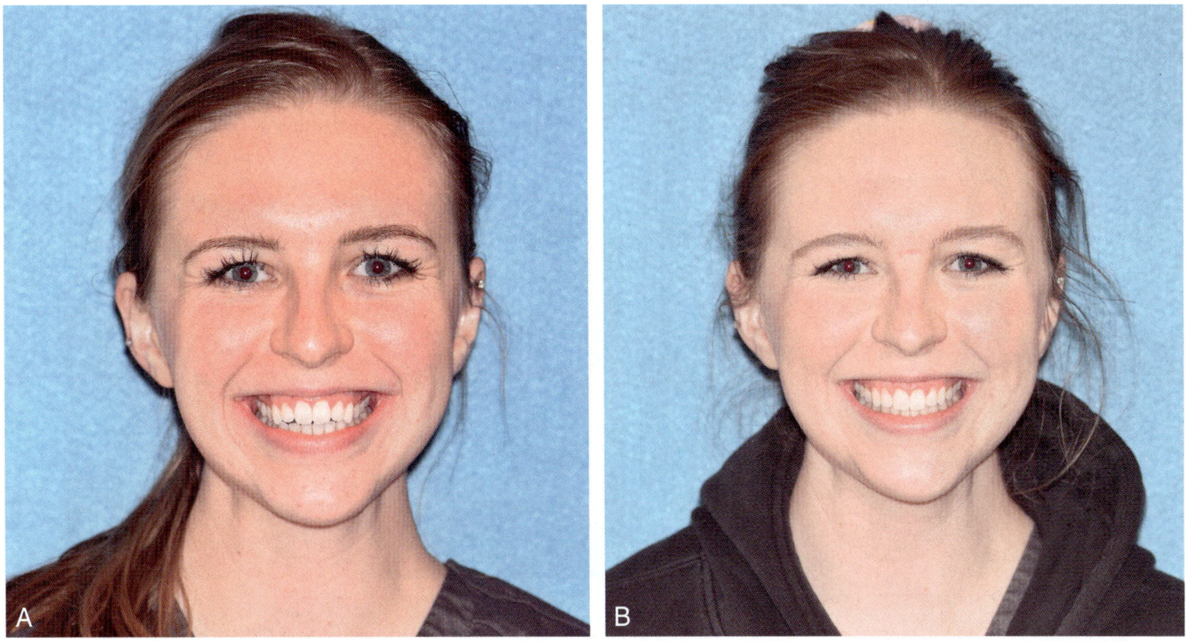

• **Fig. 7.20** (A) This patient has a reverse smile arc that led to a small openbite. (B) Retracting the teeth made the smile arc consonant with the lower lip and reduced the overjet. (Courtesy Dr. Ian Segall.)

are effective treatments for asymmetric smiles and considered previously with smile arc such as gingiva contouring or crown lengthening. If the magnitude of the vertical asymmetry is too great, it may require maxillary and mandibular surgery.

Micro-Esthetic Considerations: Enhancing the Appearance of the Teeth

Treatment plans for problems relating directly to the appearance of the teeth fall into three major categories: (1) reshaping teeth to change tooth proportions; (2) orthodontic preparation for restorations to replace lost tooth structure and correct problems of tooth shade and color; and (3) reshaping of the gingiva.

Reshaping Teeth

Often, it is desirable to do minor reshaping of the incisal edges of anterior teeth to remove mamelons or smooth out irregular edges from minor trauma. Another option is flattening the facial line angle (s) to alter apparent tooth width and alignment. When minor reshaping is planned, it must be considered when brackets are placed, and it may be better to do this before beginning fixed appliance treatment so the clinician can visualize final tooth form and thus proper bracket placement.

Changing Tooth Proportions

Extensive changes in tooth proportions are needed primarily when one tooth is to substitute for another, and the most frequent indication is substituting maxillary canines for congenitally missing maxillary lateral incisors. When a lateral incisor is missing, the treatment alternatives always are closing the space and substituting the canine, or prosthetic replacement of the missing tooth with a single-tooth implant or fixed bridge. The technique for reshaping a canine is illustrated in Fig. 7.23. It requires significant removal of facial, occlusal, interproximal, and lingual enamel. The canine is normally a darker color than the lateral incisor, and removal of facial enamel to get light reflection from the facial surface as it would be from a lateral incisor can further darken the tooth. In some patients, composite buildups or ceramic laminates are needed to obtain good tooth contour and color.

Closing the space and reshaping the canine to look like a lateral incisor can provide an excellent esthetic result, perhaps superior to an implant in the long run. It is important to keep in mind, however, that canine substitution works best when the dental arch was crowded anyway or there was some dental protrusion. It may not be compatible with excellent occlusion and smile esthetics if closing the lateral incisor space would result in significant retraction of the central incisors. In that circumstance, encouraging the permanent canine to erupt into the lateral incisor position, so that alveolar bone is formed in the area of the missing tooth, and then moving the canine distally to open space is the best way to prepare for an eventual implant.[20] The implant should not be placed until vertical growth is essentially complete, in the late teens or early twenties, because late vertical growth will produce an apparent infra-occlusion of the crown on the implant (see Chapter 20 for further discussion of this important point).

Correcting Black Triangles

Decreasing or eliminating spaces between teeth gingival to the contact points, which are unsightly if they are not filled with an interdental papilla, can be accomplished most readily by removing enamel at the contact point so the teeth can be moved closer together (see Fig. 6.44). Moving the contact area apically eliminates much if not all the space. When this is done, however, care is required not to distort the proportional relationships of the teeth to each other, and if possible the progression of connector heights (see later) should be maintained. Clinically, this means that if the central incisors are narrowed, it may be necessary also to slightly narrow the lateral incisors and move their contact area more apically to maintain a good dental appearance.

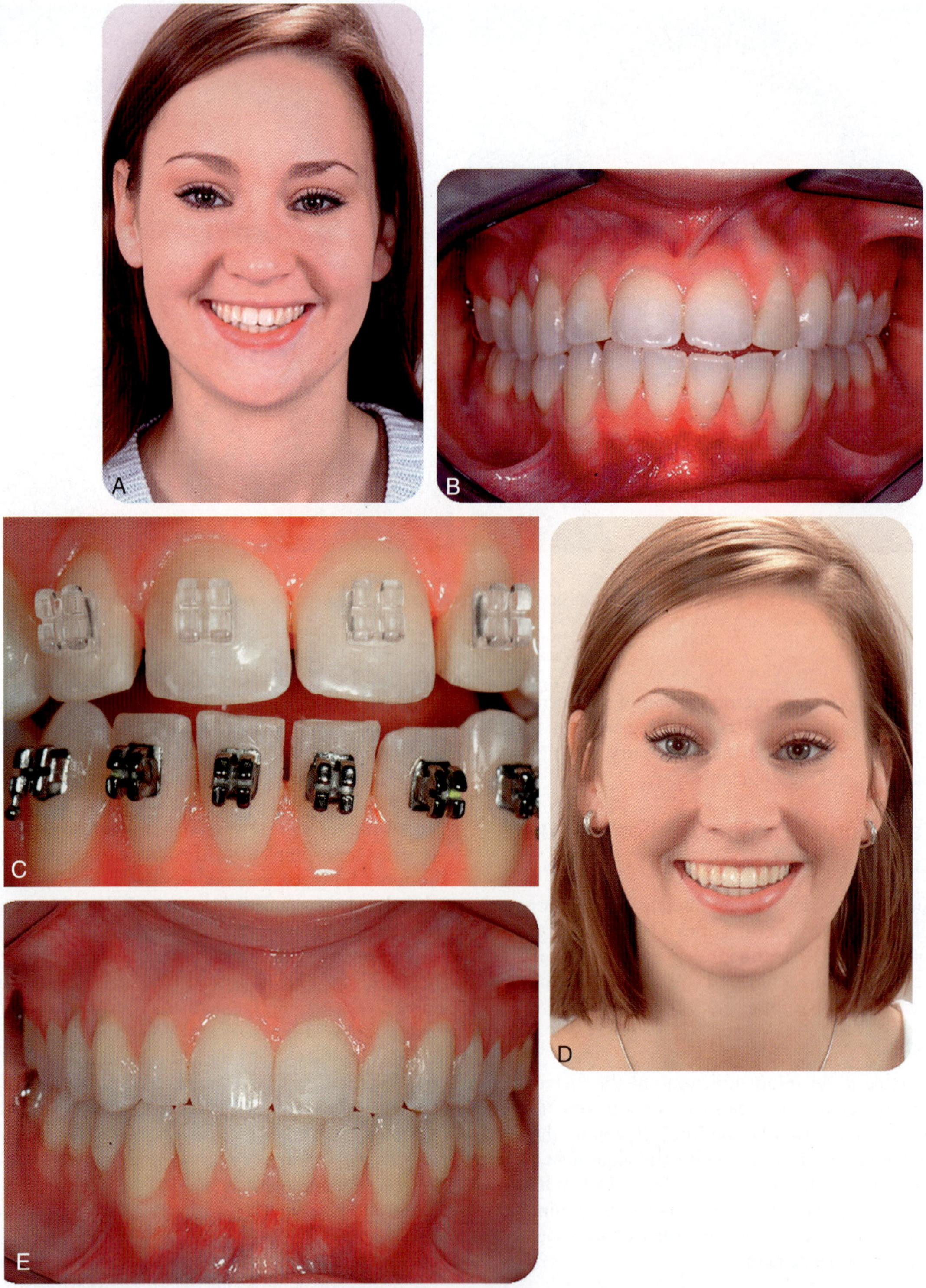

• **Fig. 7.21** Smile arc changes facilitated by incisor reshaping. (A) Pretreatment, the patient had a flat smile arc with the chief complaint of flared, or extreme proclinated maxillary incisors. (B) It was accompanied by incisor irregularity and an anterior openbite. A common method of uprighting anterior teeth is to extract four premolars, but it was felt that her facial appearance would be adversely affected through flattening of the profile and loss of lip support. (C) Miinimal interproximal reshaping changed the tooth proportions and contacts while also allowing retraction. (D) An improved smile with more inferior positioning of the maxillary incisal edges and more superior positioned mandibular incisal edges. (E) Good alignment, overbite and improved smile esthetics.

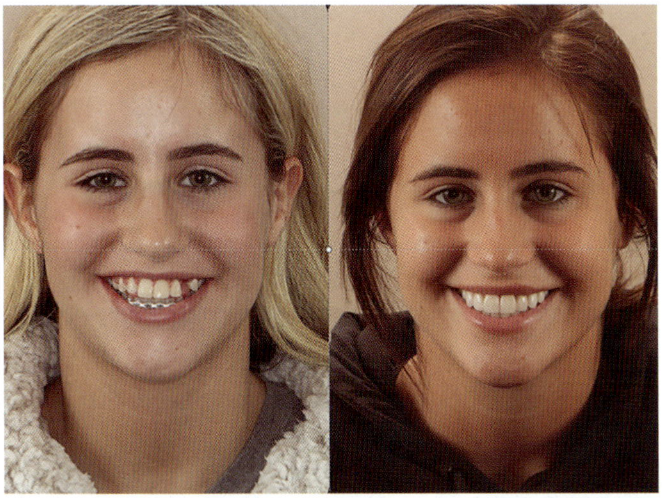

• **Fig. 7.22** (A) Poor maxillary tooth positioning, a flat smile arc and a missing tooth detracted from this patient's smile esthetic. (B) Tooth alignment with veneers provided the tooth proportions, smile arc for improved smile esthetics.

Interaction Between Orthodontist and Restorative Dentist

When the teeth are small or if tooth color or appearance is to be improved by restorative dentistry, during orthodontic treatment it is necessary to position them so that the restorations will bring them to normal size and position. In modern practice, the restorations are either composite buildups or ceramic laminates, laminates being used particularly when it is desirable to change tooth color and shade in addition to the size of the crown (Fig. 7.24).

There are two ways to manage the orthodontic-restorative interaction. The first is to carefully plan where the teeth are to be placed, place a vacuum-formed retainer immediately after the orthodontic appliance is removed that the patient wears full time, and send the patient to the restorative dentist for completion of the treatment. A new retainer is needed as soon as the restorations have been completed. This has two advantages: The restorative work can be scheduled at everyone's convenience after the orthodontic treatment is completed, and any gingival inflammation related to the orthodontic treatment has time to resolve. It also has disadvantages: Excellent patient cooperation is required to maintain the precise spacing needed for the best restorations, so the restorative work may be compromised by tooth movement, and the teeth are nonesthetic until this is accomplished.

An alternative, which is most applicable when composite buildups rather than laminates are planned, is for the orthodontist to deliberately provide slightly more space than the restorative dentist requires to bring the teeth to just the right size, remove the brackets from the teeth to be restored, send the patient immediately to the restorative dentist, replace the brackets the same day after the restorations are completed, and close any residual space before removing the orthodontic appliance (Fig. 7.25). This has the advantage of eliminating compromises in the restorative work, but the disadvantage that careful coordination of the appointments is required and following final appliance removal, resurfacing the restorations may be necessary.

Reshaping Gingival Contours: Applications of a Soft Tissue Laser

Appropriate display of the teeth requires removal of excessive gingiva covering the clinical crown and is enhanced by correcting the gingival contours. Treatment of this type now can be carried out effectively with the use of a diode laser (see Fig. 7.26). A laser of this type, in comparison to the carbon dioxide (CO_2) or erbium:yttrium-aluminum-garnet (Er:YAG) lasers also used now in dentistry, has two primary advantages: (1) It does not cut hard tissue, so there is no risk of damage to the teeth or alveolar bone if it is used for gingival contouring, and (2) it creates a "biologic dressing" because it coagulates, sterilizes, and seals the soft tissue as it is used. There is no bleeding, no other dressing is required, and there is no waiting period for healing.

Use of a soft tissue laser as part of finishing procedures is illustrated and discussed further in Chapter 17.

Planning Comprehensive Orthodontic Treatment

Steps in Planning Comprehensive Treatment

The focus of the rest of this chapter is on comprehensive treatment, in adolescence or later, when the permanent teeth are present at least for the latter part of the treatment period. Planning for mixed dentition treatment to prevent later problems or to keep existing problems from getting worse is covered in Chapter 11, and planning more complex mixed dentition treatment is discussed in Chapter 12. Skeletal growth modification treatments are addressed in Chapters 13 and 14.

Prior to any type of anticipated treatment, orthodontic diagnosis results in a comprehensive list of the patient's problems noted under the appropriate five characteristics of malocclusion (see Fig. 7.1). Of course, there can be several findings under each of the five characteristics. The classification scheme exists to make the treatment planning process work efficiently. Having too many overlapping findings appearing on the problem list only creates confusion. Accompanying the problem list is a list of positive attributes that need to be maintained (see Fig. 7.1).

The goal of treatment is to deal with the problems in a way that creates maximum benefit to the patient—not just to straighten the teeth. Use of a logical sequence of steps on the way from the problem list to the final plan, keeping this goal in mind, is strongly recommended. The sequence of steps is illustrated in Fig. 7.1. Let us now consider this sequence and the logic behind it as we develop the treatment plan for the patient whose diagnostic workup was illustrated in Chapter 6 (see Figs. 6.98–6.99). Her problem list (diagnosis) is repeated in Box 7.1.

Pathologic Versus Developmental Problems

An important principle is that a patient does not have to be in perfect health to have orthodontic treatment, but any problems related to disease and pathology must be under control (i.e., the progression of any acute or chronic conditions must be stopped). For this reason, pathologic problems must be addressed before treatment of orthodontic (developmental) problems can begin. Thus in a treatment sequence, orthodontic treatment must appear after control of systemic disease, periodontal disease, and caries.

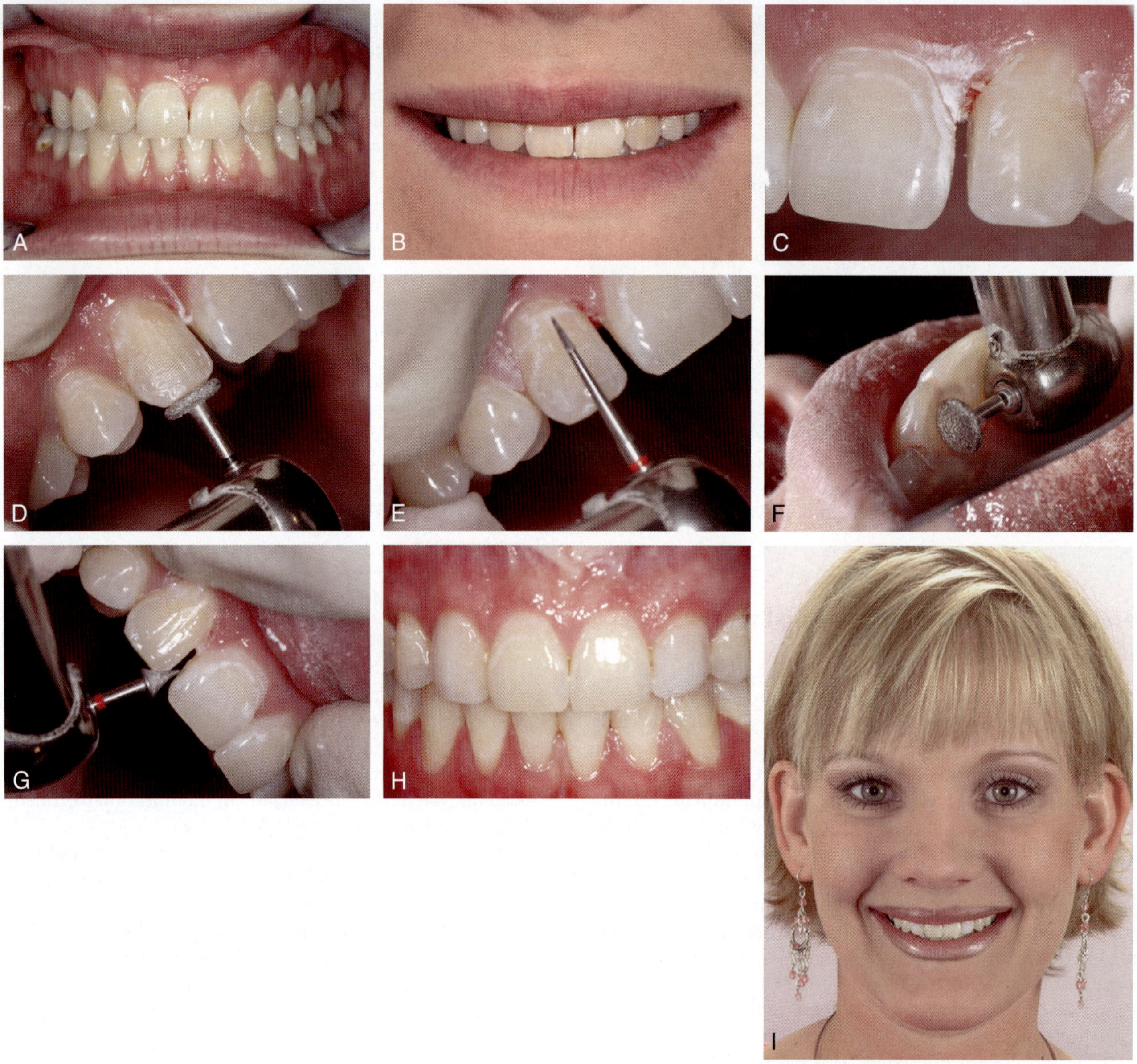

• **Fig. 7.23** To reshape a maxillary canine that is to substitute for a missing maxillary lateral incisor (A and B), the steps in treatment consist of interproximal reduction (C), flattening the tip (D), flattening the facial surface (E), reducing cingulum thickness (F), and rounding the corners of the flattened crown (G). At that point, a lateral bracket can be placed on the canine during orthodontic treatment. If the gingival margin of the canine is visible (which is undesirable when it is to substitute for a lateral incisor), it can be concealed by elongating the tooth and increasing the amount of gingival reduction. Recontouring the gingiva over the first premolar that becomes a substitute for the canine also enhances appearance. In (H), note that the gingival margin of the first premolar has been reshaped (with a diode laser) to make it look more like a canine. (I), Smile at completion of treatment.

The first step in treatment planning is to separate pathologic from developmental (orthodontic) problems (see Fig. 7.1). Even when pathologic problems are mild, as one would expect them to be in the healthy adolescents who are the majority of orthodontic patients, they must not be overlooked in the treatment plan. For a typical patient of that type, the plan for the pathologic problems would include oral hygiene instruction and monitoring gingival health during orthodontic treatment. Other items might be included for specific problems, as in our example patient (Box 7.2). For patients with more complex disease-related problems, the plan often is appropriate referral to another medical or dental clinician before orthodontic treatment begins. For instance, does this patient have sleep disordered breathing as indicated from the screening form, or will the history of bisphosphonate use make substantial tooth movement impossible?

Periodontal health is an important issue, especially for older patients, and interaction with a periodontist often is needed to plan and carry out appropriate orthodontic treatment. Two important points must be kept in mind: (1) orthodontic treatment in the presence of active periodontal disease is likely to accelerate the disease process, so periodontal control is essential before orthodontics begins; but (2) in the absence of active disease, even

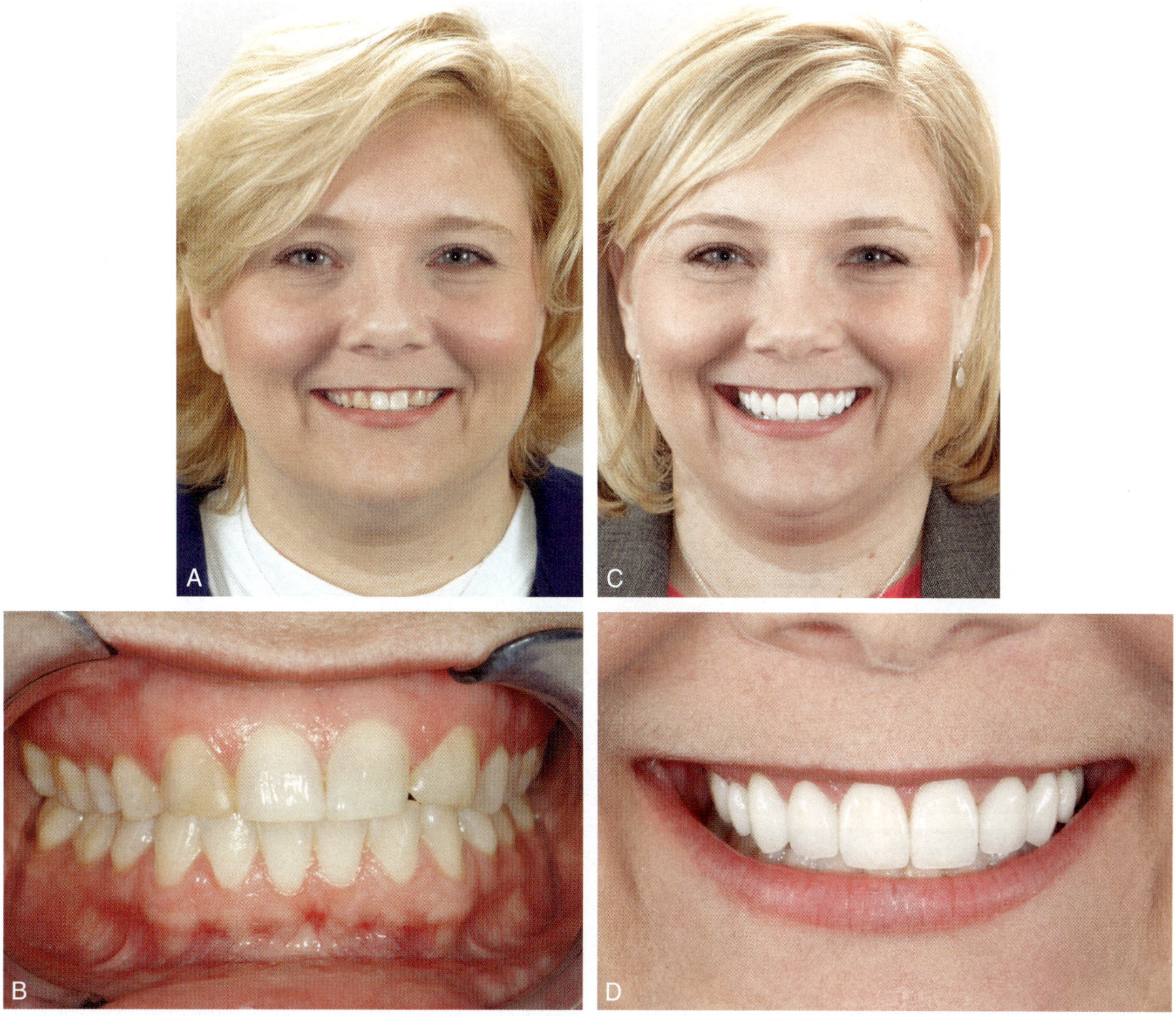

• **Fig. 7.24** Laminate veneers can be used to correct both the color and contour of teeth in canine substitution treatment. (A and B) Pretreatment and posttreatment appearance of teeth on full-face smile and close-up. Note the buildups on canines used after previous treatment to fill in the space of congenitally missing maxillary lateral incisors. (C and D) Appearance after space closure and laminate veneers for the maxillary anterior teeth. Among the things that can be corrected with laminate veneers is the length of the teeth so that there is proper display on smile as seen in the facial photographs.

if significant bone loss has occurred previously, careful orthodontic treatment will not lead to further bone loss and can facilitate other types of dental treatment such as restorative dentistry, prosthodontics, and periodontal surgery.

Behavioral problems also must be considered. Does the patient (of any age) have a nonnutritive sucking problems? Are there concentration or cooperation issues while in the chair? Can the patient tolerate intraoral appliances of any kind? These issues must be considered prior to treatment during frank conversation. This may limit the scope and length of appointments and overall treatment.

Setting Priorities for the Orthodontic Problem List

Putting the patient's orthodontic (developmental) problems in priority order (see Fig. 7.1) is the most important single step in the entire treatment planning process. The problem list should be prioritized. But the issue is, according to what? Certainly, the patient's chief complaint has to be weighed here. The patient's perception of their condition is important in setting these priorities. It is always difficult for the clinician to avoid imposing their own feelings at this stage, and it is not totally inappropriate to reveal them; but ignoring the patient's chief complaint can lead to serious errors in planning treatment. For instance, consider the patient who complains of a protruding chin and who has a Class III malocclusion. If the clinician formulates the problem as Class III malocclusion and concentrates on bringing the teeth into correct occlusion while ignoring the chin, it is not likely that the patient will be happy with the treatment result. The plan did not deal with the patient's problem.

Also, the magnitude of the problem is a factor, e.g., 4 mm of overjet is not as much concern as 9 mm. One can also consider the difficulty of treating a problem. Addressing a mixed dentition

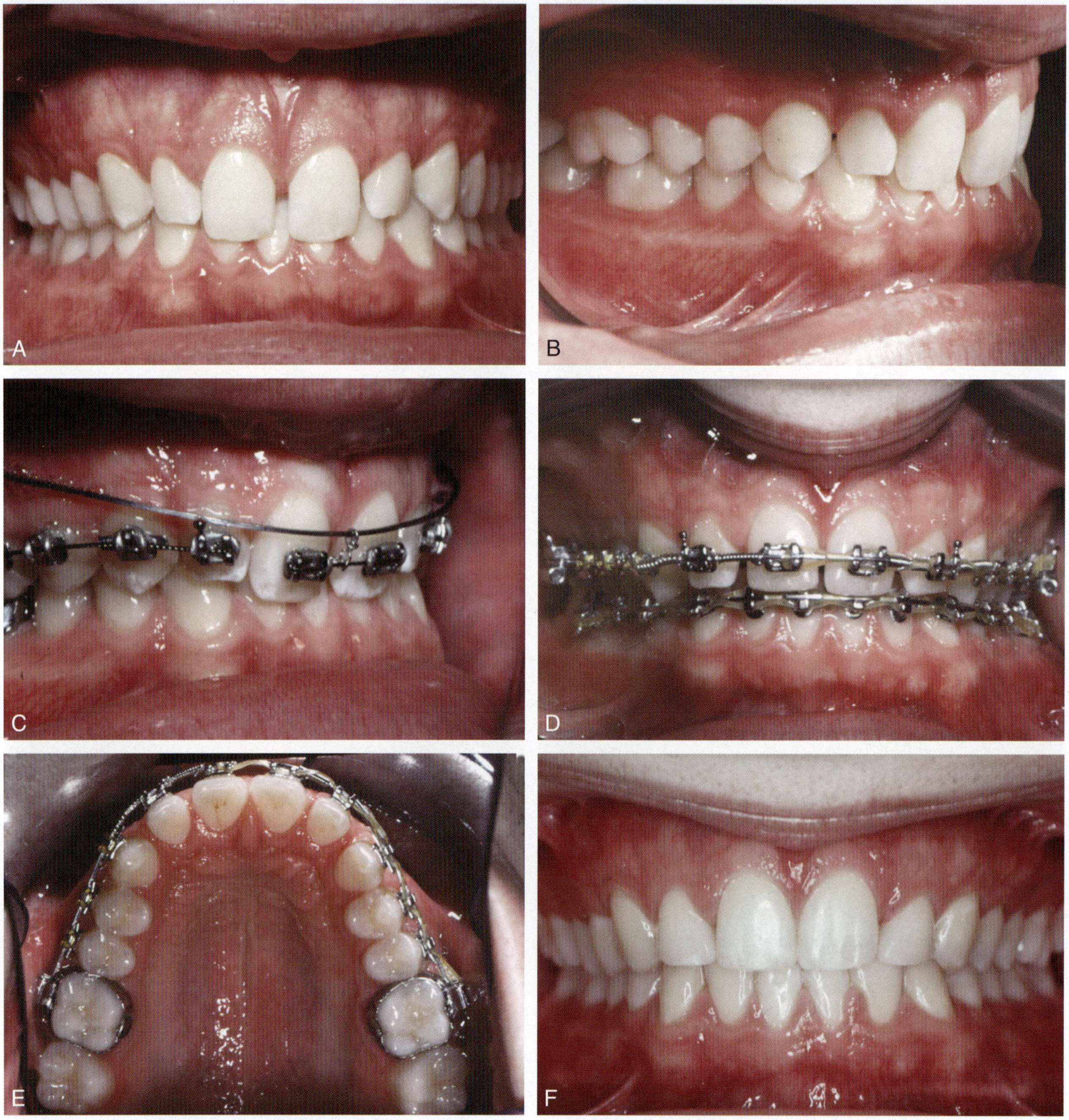

• **Fig. 7.25** (A and B) This patient's complaint was the appearance of his upper incisors. The central incisors were elongated and quite upright; the lateral incisors were small, and the excess space was seen as a maxillary midline diastema. (C) Intrusion archwire to central incisors. (D and E) After intrusion and spacing of the incisors to allow buildups of the lateral incisors. (F) At completion of orthodontic and restorative treatment.

posterior crossbite is easier than one in a nongrowing post-adolescent. Finally, the required sequence of treatment might influence the priority. In the mixed dentition, aligning anterior teeth is a lower priority than addressing the impacted incisor that will prevent space closure. Or, closing maxillary anterior space by retraction cannot be accomplished without first treating the deep overbite, making the vertical problem more important because it is difficult to retract the upper incisors when the lower incisors are in the way. The diagnostic problem list is objective; the prioritized problem list has some subjectivity involved.

All told, the doctor does not have to agree with the patient's initial thoughts as to what is most important. Indeed, often it is necessary to educate the patient about the nature of the problems. But, the importance of various problems must be discussed. It is possible that the patient wants something you cannot provide or will be contrary to their dentofacial welfare or the standard of care. Say, a parent wants their child treated nonextraction and you believe that the crowding and the periodontal condition both point toward an extraction plan. That is the ideal point to suggest a second opinion. You are not compelled to violate the standard

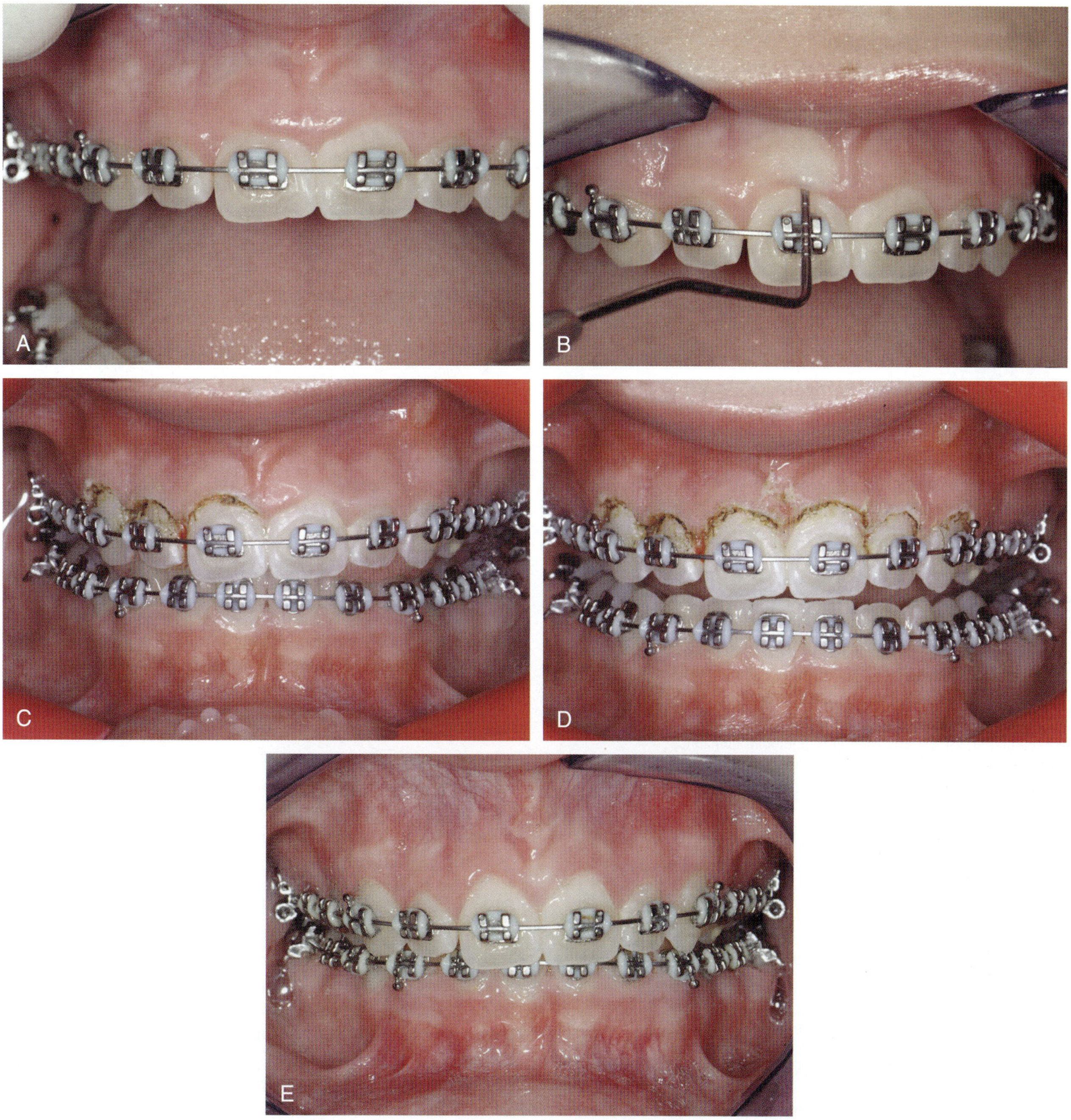

• **Fig. 7.26** For patient F.P., whose diagnostic workup is illustrated in Figs. 6.98–6.99, treatment was deferred until she was entering her adolescent growth spurt. A fixed appliance was placed at age 12 years 5 months, and high-pull headgear was started at age 12 years 10 months. Dentally and skeletally, she responded well to treatment, but the gingival overgrowth of the maxillary incisors worsened rather than improved (A). A diode laser now offers a painless and efficient way to manage problems of this type, and she was scheduled for gingival recontouring at age 13 years 11 months. A periodontal probe was used to establish the depth of the gingival sulcus (B), and the laser was used to recontour the tissue (C, one side done; D, gingival recontouring completed). Because the tissue is ablated (vaporized) and the heat of the laser seals the ablation site, no bleeding occurs and no periodontal dressing is needed. Healing occurs within a few days. (E) The greatly improved tissue contours 4 weeks later.

of care. These approaches to prioritizing problems will facilitate patient and parent interactions that will lead to obtaining true informed consent to treatment—they will understand the focus of the plan and understand the reasoning. The prioritization for our example patient is shown in Box 7.3.

Setting Treatment Goals

Having evaluated the patient's history, their clinical status and their records provides a good basis for the problems and the attributes to maintain. When the problems have been prioritized it is a good point to list the treatment goals. Where are you going??

• BOX 7.1 Patient F.P.: Problem List (Diagnosis)

In the order they appeared in the evaluation sequence including pathologic processes and classified problems

- Mild gingivitis, mild gingival overgrowth
- Hypoplastic area maxillary left premolar
- Mandibular deficiency
- Maxillary incisors tipped lingually, short crowns
- Moderate maxillary incisor crowding
- Mandibular dental midline left of facial midline
- Class II buccal segments, minimal overjet
- Deep bite, excessive eruption of mandibular incisors

• BOX 7.2 Patient F.P.: Pathologic Problems with a plan to address them

- Mild gingivitis
  Hygiene instruction
- Hypoplastic area, upper left first premolar
  Restore at end of orthodontic treatment

• BOX 7.3 Patient F.P.: Prioritized Problem List

Tentative: awaiting parent/patient interaction

- **Alignment and symmetry**
  - Malaligned and nonesthetic maxillary incisors
- **Anteroposterior and Dentofacial Proportions**
  - Skeletal Class II, excess overjet—mandibular deficiency
- **Vertical**
  - Anterior deep bite—excessive eruption of mandibular incisor
- **Transverse**
  - Midline discrepancy—mandibular to left

As an example, you will align the maxillary incisors, reduce the mandibular deficiency, reduce the deep overbite bite and correct the mandibular midline. And, you will maintain the smile arc and lip posture. Those can be listed as shown in Box 7.4

Factors in Evaluating Treatment Possibilities

The next step in the planning process is to list the possibilities for treatment of each of the problems, beginning with the highest priority problem. At this stage, each problem is considered individually, and for the moment the possible solutions are examined as if this problem were the only one the patient had. Broad possibilities, not details of treatment procedures, are what is sought at this stage (Box 7.5). The more complex the total situation, the more important it is to be sure no possibilities are overlooked.

As we continue to develop the treatment plan for our illustrative patient, references to aspects of treatment that have not yet been presented in the text are inevitable. The first-time reader is urged to follow the logic rather than concentrate on details that will be discussed more fully in the following chapters.

Possible Solutions

First, let's consider the possible solutions to this patient's most important problem: the unattractive smile and appearance of the maxillary incisors. Correcting this will require alignment of the teeth, but proper anterior tooth relationships cannot be achieved until overjet is reduced and the deep bite is corrected—so the best solution to the first problem can be determined only after the impact of possible solutions to overjet and overbite have been considered.

• BOX 7.4 Patient F.P.: Treatment Goals

Align maxillary incisors
Reduce mandibular deficiency
Reduce anterior deep bite
Correct mandibular midline
Attributes to maintain:
Smile arc
Lip protrusion and competence

• BOX 7.5 Patient F.P.: Possible Solutions

Malaligned and nonesthetic maxillary incisors:
- *Align, lingual root torque, reduce overjet and overbite*
- *Remove excess gingiva?*

Skeletal Class II
Growth modification: Differential forward growth of mandible
- *Headgear?*
- *Herbst appliance?*
- *If unfavorable growth: Orthodontic camouflage? Orthognathic surgery?*

Anterior deep bite
- *Absolute intrusion: If needed, only for lower incisors?*
- *Relative intrusion: Allow lower molar eruption as mandible grows vertically, prevent further lower incisor eruption*

Midline discrepancy—mandibular to left
- *Resolve with Cl II skeletal and dental correction—limited elastic wear*

As we have noted, there are three ways that the Class II jaw relationship and overjet can be treated (Fig. 7.27): (1) differential forward growth of the mandible, which is ideal if it can be achieved; (2) orthodontic camouflage, retracting the maxillary incisors and proclining the mandibular incisors to make the teeth fit even though the jaws do not; or (3) orthognathic surgery to correct the jaw position. Because our patient has not yet reached the adolescent growth spurt, growth modification would be the primary possibility, with camouflage and surgery as possibilities if growth modification does not succeed.

Class II growth modification can be done in several ways, which are discussed in detail in Chapter 14. For this patient, differential forward growth of the mandible while maintaining vertical control of the maxillary posterior teeth and bringing the maxillary incisors facially would increase the display of the maxillary incisors and the prominence of the chin (Fig. 7.28). The two most effective ways to do that would be high-pull headgear or a fixed functional appliance such as the Herbst appliance. The functional appliance would be more likely to move the lower incisors forward, which is undesirable for this patient, so headgear would be preferred if she would agree to wear it.

There also are three ways to correct the anterior overbite (Fig. 7.29): (1) absolute intrusion of the upper and lower incisors, moving their root apices closer to the nose and lower border of the mandible, respectively; (2) relative intrusion of the incisors, keeping them where they are while the mandible grows and the posterior teeth erupt; and (3) extrusion of the posterior teeth, which would

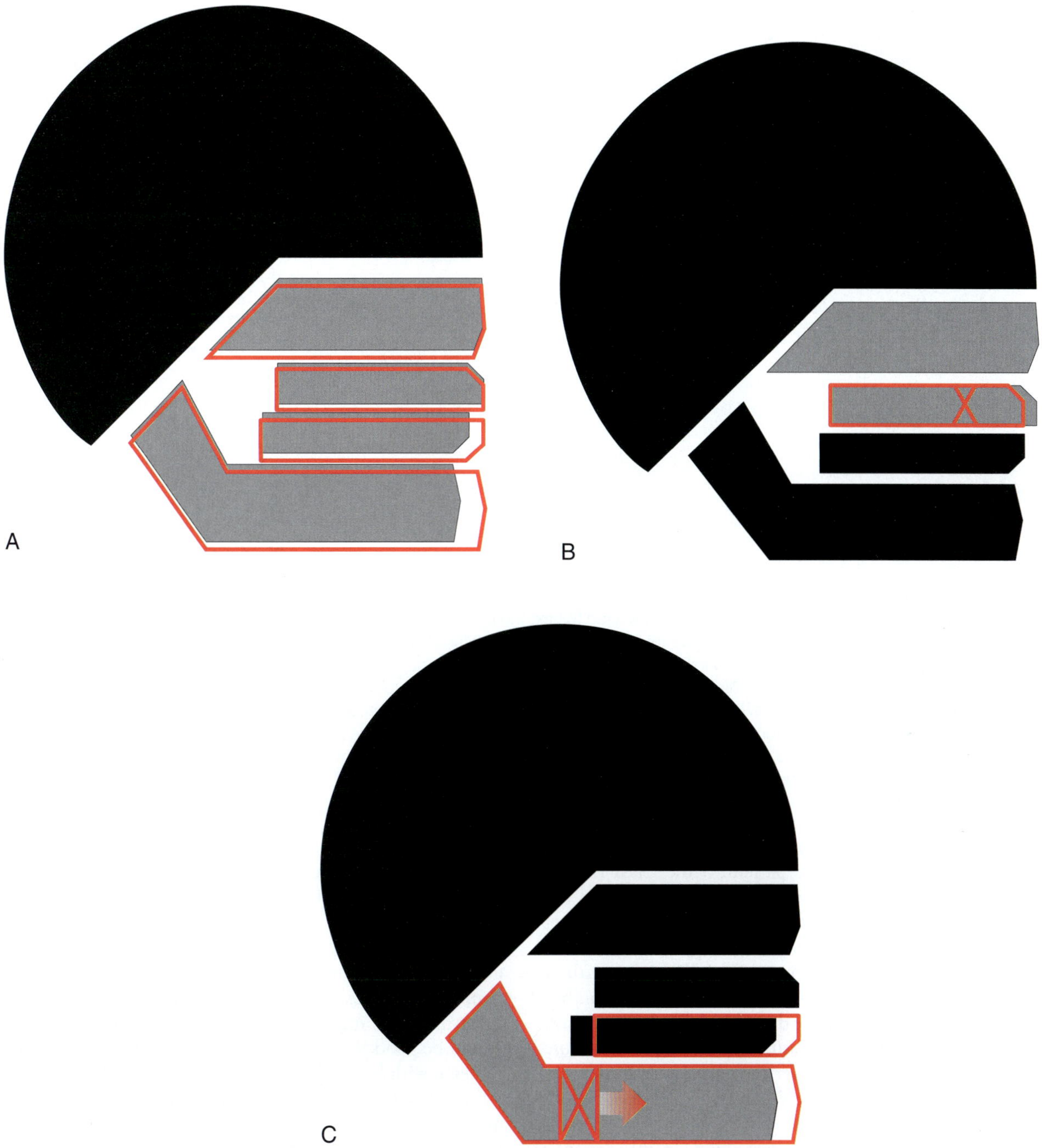

• **Fig. 7.27** The possibilities for correction of a skeletal Class II problem include (A) differential forward growth of the mandible, which is the ideal method if the patient has not yet gone through the adolescent growth spurt; (B) camouflage by retraction of the maxillary incisors after extraction (X), which can be quite successful *if* the other facial features allow it; and (C) orthognathic surgery to move the mandible forward to a normal relationship. In the absence of growth, camouflage and surgery are the only possibilities.

rotate the mandible downward and backward. Relative intrusion of incisors and extrusion of posterior teeth are identical in terms of tooth movement. The difference is whether vertical growth of the ramus compensates for the increase in molar height (i.e., whether the mandibular plane angle is maintained [relative intrusion] or increases as the mandible rotates downward and backward [extrusion]).

In an immature 12-year-old like our example patient, vertical growth can be expected, so relative intrusion would be the preferred approach. It is significant that in the absence of growth, leveling the arches by extrusion of posterior teeth would cause the mandible to rotate downward and backward, accentuating a Class II tendency (Fig. 7.30), which would be highly undesirable for this patient. Controlling the vertical position of the maxillary posterior teeth so that the vertical space between the jaws created by growth could be used largely for elongation of the lower molars would facilitate leveling by relative intrusion. Thus high-pull headgear that appears to be the best approach to a skeletal Class II problem also would facilitate correction of the deep bite, if used along with a fixed appliance to level the lower arch that would elongate the mandibular molars.

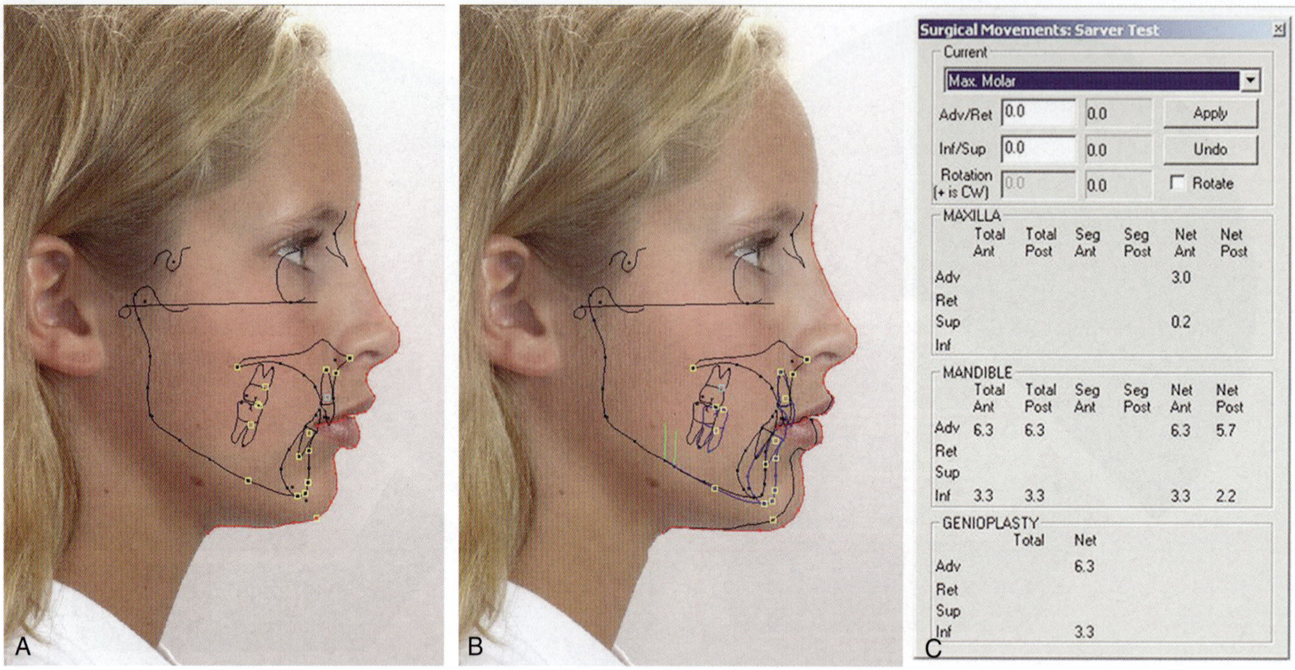

• **Fig. 7.28** Computer predictions of growing patients often are inaccurate because of the difficulty of predicting growth but nevertheless can be used to help the patient and parents understand what is expected to occur. (A) Patient F.P., cephalometric tracing merged with facial profile image, using the Orthotrac imaging system (Carestream Dental LLC, Atlanta, GA). (B) Prediction of treatment with forward growth of the mandible while the maxilla is held in place and the upper incisors are tipped facially and elongated. (C) Computer screen showing the measured amount of change. An adolescent is more likely to cooperate with treatment if he or she understands exactly what is desired and what the benefit would be, and images of changes in your own face are easier to understand than word descriptions, pictures of a different patient, or other generalized educational materials.

Often, the same problem list prioritized differently results in a different treatment plan. For this patient, if the Class II malocclusion was considered the most important problem and the relationship of the upper incisors to the lip and gingiva was not considered important, Class II camouflage might be chosen as the most efficient approach to treatment. Class II elastics, with or without premolar extraction, would correct the malocclusion but might harm rather than enhance the dental and facial appearance.

The objective at this stage of treatment planning is to be sure that no reasonable possibilities are overlooked. It is easy to develop the mindset that "For this problem, we always …." Sometimes an alternative approach would be better but is overlooked unless a conscious effort is made to keep an open mind. In this patient's case, if obtaining proper soft tissue relationships to the upper incisors were not a priority in treatment, she almost surely would not have normal incisor display after treatment, and an optimal result would not be achieved.

Additional factors are pertinent in evaluating treatment possibilities and now must be considered (see Fig. 7.1).

Interaction Among Possible Solutions and Positive Synergy

The interaction among possible solutions to a patient's various problems is much easier to see when the possibilities are listed as previously described. As in the case of the girl in the previous section, it will be clear for nearly every patient that some solutions to a high-priority problem would also solve other problems, but others would not and might even make other things worse.

Consider the opposite situation to our example patient, a patient with an anterior openbite. Often, this problem is due not to decreased eruption of incisors but to excessive eruption of posterior teeth and downward-backward rotation of the mandible. If so, using vertical elastics to elongate the anterior teeth is not a good solution. Treatment should be aimed at depressing the elongated posterior teeth, or preventing them from erupting further while everything else grows (relative intrusion). This would allow the mandible to rotate upward, bringing the incisor teeth together. But if the mandible rotates upward, it also will come forward—which would be good if the patient had a skeletal Class II malocclusion to begin with but bad if the malocclusion was Class I or Class III.

Another important interaction, which also came into play in our illustrative case (Box 7.6), is the relationship between incisor prominence and facial appearance, especially on smile. If the teeth are crowded, is expansion of the arches indicated to gain the space needed to align them? The answer depends on the relationship of the teeth to their soft tissue environment. In developing the treatment plan, it is necessary to plan the final position of the incisors and then determine what is needed to put them in the desired position. Quantifying the extent of the crowding does not tell you what to do about it. You have to look at the effect of the possible treatments on the patient's appearance.

Compromise

In patients with many problems, it may not be possible to solve them all. This type of compromise has nothing to do with the clinician's skill. In some cases, no plan of treatment will solve all of the patient's problems. Then, careful setting of priorities from the problem list is particularly important.

In a broad sense, the major goals of orthodontic treatment are ideal occlusion, ideal facial esthetics, and ideal stability of result.

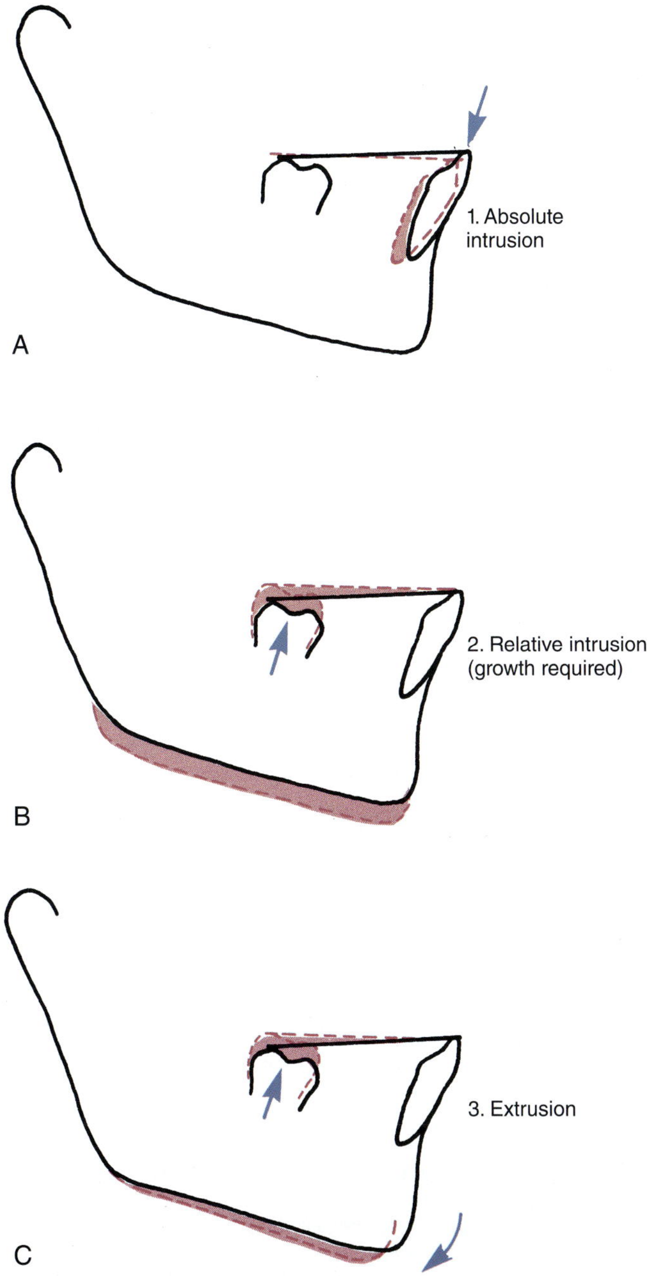

• **Fig. 7.29** There are three possible ways to level out a lower arch with an excessive curve of Spee: *1*, absolute intrusion (A); *2*, relative intrusion (B), achieved by preventing eruption of the incisors while growth provides vertical space into which the posterior teeth erupt; and *3*, elongation of posterior teeth (C), which causes the mandible to rotate downward in the absence of growth. Note that the difference between *2* and *3* is whether the mandible rotates downward and backward, which is determined by whether the mandibular ramus grows longer while the tooth movement is occurring.

Often it is impossible to maximize all three. In fact, attempts to achieve an absolutely ideal dental occlusion, especially if that prohibits extractions, can diminish both facial esthetics and stability after treatment. In the same way, efforts to achieve the most stable result after orthodontic treatment may result in less than optimal occlusion and facial esthetics, and positioning the teeth to produce ideal facial esthetics may detract from occlusion and stability.

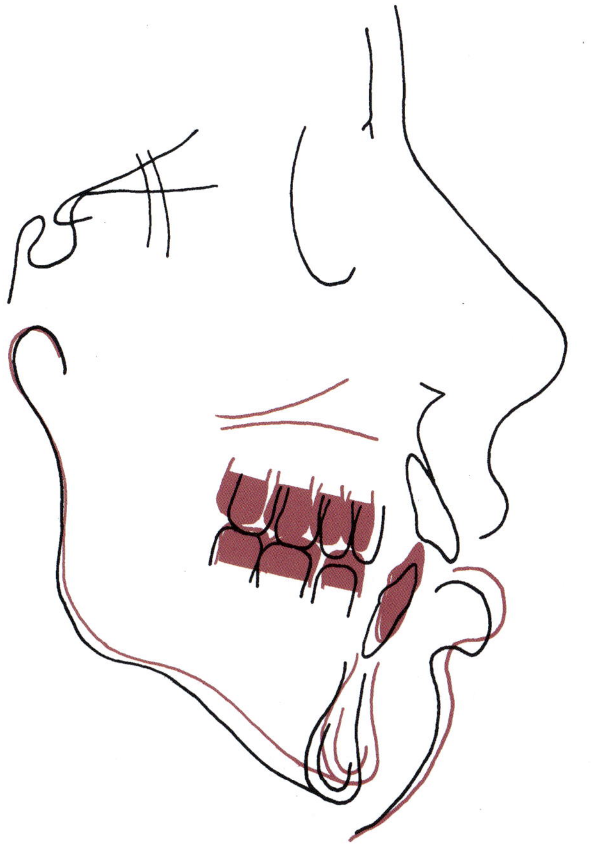

• **Fig. 7.30** There is a strong interaction between the vertical position of the maxilla and both the anteroposterior and vertical positions of the mandible, because the mandible rotates backward as it moves down and forward as it moves up unless vertical growth of the ramus matches downward movement of the maxillary posterior teeth. This superimposition (red = initial, black = progress) shows the effect on chin position of excessive vertical growth of the maxilla and excessive eruption of the maxillary posterior teeth that was not matched by vertical growth of the ramus. This is the classic long-face pattern of growth that makes the Class II jaw relationship worse, but extrusion of maxillary posterior teeth during orthodontic treatment does the same thing. Superior repositioning of the maxilla and/or intrusion of maxillary posterior teeth (see Chapters 20 and 22) would be the key to both reducing face height and correcting the Class II relationship.

• BOX 7.6 Patient F.P.: Interaction of Treatment Possibilities

- Repositioning the maxillary incisors for better appearance will increase overjet and require greater use of the mechanics for Class II correction.
- Extrusive mechanics to correct the deep bite may lead to a more vertical growth direction for the mandible, compromising the Class II correction. Class II elastics could tip occlusal plane clockwise.
- Correcting the deep bite with any intrusion of the maxillary incisors would compromise the smile arc, which is excellent now.

Other Considerations in Planning Treatment

- Patient is immature; growth modification will be more efficient if timed with growth spurt.
- Rotating the maxilla down anteriorly will improve incisor display and smile appearance.

One way to avoid having to face compromises of this type, of course, is to emphasize one of the goals at the expense of the others. In the early 20th century, Edward Angle, the father of modern orthodontics, solved this problem by focusing solely on the occlusion and declaring that facial esthetics and stability would take care of themselves. Unfortunately, they did not. As we have noted, echoes of Angle's position are encountered occasionally even now, particularly among dentists strongly committed to avoiding extraction at all costs.

As important as dental occlusion is, it is not the most important consideration for all patients. Sometimes, ideal occlusion must be compromised, by extraction or other changes within the dental arches, to gain acceptable esthetics and stability. Adjustments in the other goals also may be needed. It is quite possible that placing the teeth for optimal facial esthetics may require permanent retention because they are not stable in that position, or, alternatively, that placing the teeth in a position of maximum stability is likely to make the facial appearance worse, not better.

If various elements of a treatment plan are incompatible, benefit to the patient is greatest if any necessary compromises are made so that the patient understands and agrees that their most important problems are solved, while less important problems are deferred or left untreated. If the major goals of orthodontic treatment cannot be reached, those of greatest importance to that patient should be favored. Doing this successfully requires both judgment and thought on the part of the clinician and input from the patient and parent. For our example patient, would better stability result if the maxillary incisors were retracted to correct the excess overjet be worth the negative impact on her facial appearance? Given her chief complaint, almost certainly not.

Analysis of Benefit Versus Cost and Risk

Practical considerations related to the difficulty of various treatment procedures compared with the benefit to be gained from them also must be considered in evaluating treatment possibilities. The difficulty should be considered in both risk and cost to the patient, with cost calculated not only in money but also in cooperation, discomfort, aggravation, time, and other factors that can be collectively labeled as the "burden of treatment." These must be contrasted to the probable benefit from that procedure.

For instance, for a patient with anterior openbite, jaw surgery to decrease face height has greater cost and risk than elastics to elongate the incisors or mini-implants to intrude the posterior teeth, which are two other possibilities for correcting the bite relationship. But if the simpler and less risky procedures would provide little real benefit to the patient, but jaw surgery would provide considerable benefit, the cost- and risk-benefit analyses might still favor the more difficult procedure. "Is it worth it?" is a question that must be answered not only from the point of view of what is involved, but also in terms of the benefit to the patient.

Special Considerations

At this stage, it is important to consider any pertinent special considerations about the individual patient. Should the treatment time be minimized because of possible exacerbation of periodontal disease? Should treatment options be left open as long as possible because of uncertainty of the pattern of growth? Should visible orthodontic appliances be avoided because of the patient's vanity, even if it makes treatment more difficult? Or even impossible? Such questions must be addressed from the perspective of the individual patient. Rational answers can be obtained only when the treatment possibilities and other important factors influencing the treatment plan have been considered.

For our example patient, interactions, thoughts about necessary compromises, and other considerations (which in her case are quite minor) are shown in Box 7.6. The information now has been assembled. Only at this point are treatment possibilities ready to be discussed with the patient and parents (Box 7.7).

• BOX 7.7 Patient F.P: Outline of Case Presentation

During the treatment presentation, it is appropriate to involve the patient and parents in the treatment decisions, which is necessary to obtain informed consent. The points to be discussed (in this sequence) are as follows:

General and Oral Health

- Two minor problems with oral health:
  - *Mild gingivitis: Better oral hygiene is required to prevent damage to the teeth and periodontal structures during orthodontic treatment.*
  - *Hypoplastic area in first premolar: May require restoration in the future, no treatment needed now.*

Orthodontic Problems

- Appearance of upper incisors: Tipped back and not aligned properly, which partially conceals their relative protrusion.
- Lower jaw has not grown forward properly
- Overbite: Lower front teeth have erupted too much, into the palate
- Midlines are not coincident.

Most Important Problem (But not always the one treated first due to sequencing of the treatment discussed earlier)

- Upper incisor position and crowding (do you agree?)
  - Alignment of teeth and correction of bite
    - *Requires braces on all the teeth.*

Correction of Other Problems

- *Deficient mandible*
  - Restrain downward and forward growth of the upper jaw
    - *Requires favorable growth and cooperation.*
- *Deep bite*
  - Managing lower tooth eruption
    - *Requires favorable growth and braces on the teeth*
- Lower midline correction
  - Moving some lower teeth more than others
    - *May require cooperation wearing elastics*

Benefits From Treatment

- Improved facial and dental appearance
  - *For an adult patient, this is when to show computer image predictions.*
- More normal jaw movements and teeth that fit together well

Risks of Treatment (For All Patieints)

- Discomfort after appliance adjustment
- Decalcification and gingival enlargement and inflammation if hygiene is inadequate
- Root resorption, especially maxillary incisors
- Future need to wear retainers
- Any other pertinent items (that are important to **this** patient) The patient may need an impacted tooth removed or uncovered. Other teeth may need to be extracted. Orthognathic surgery may be necessary or a future possibility.
  - *A signed form acknowledging this discussion is strongly recommended.*

Treatment Schedule, Costs, and So On

- Included with the presentation of the final treatment plan (see Box 7.7).
- Schedule and costs will vary in individual practices.

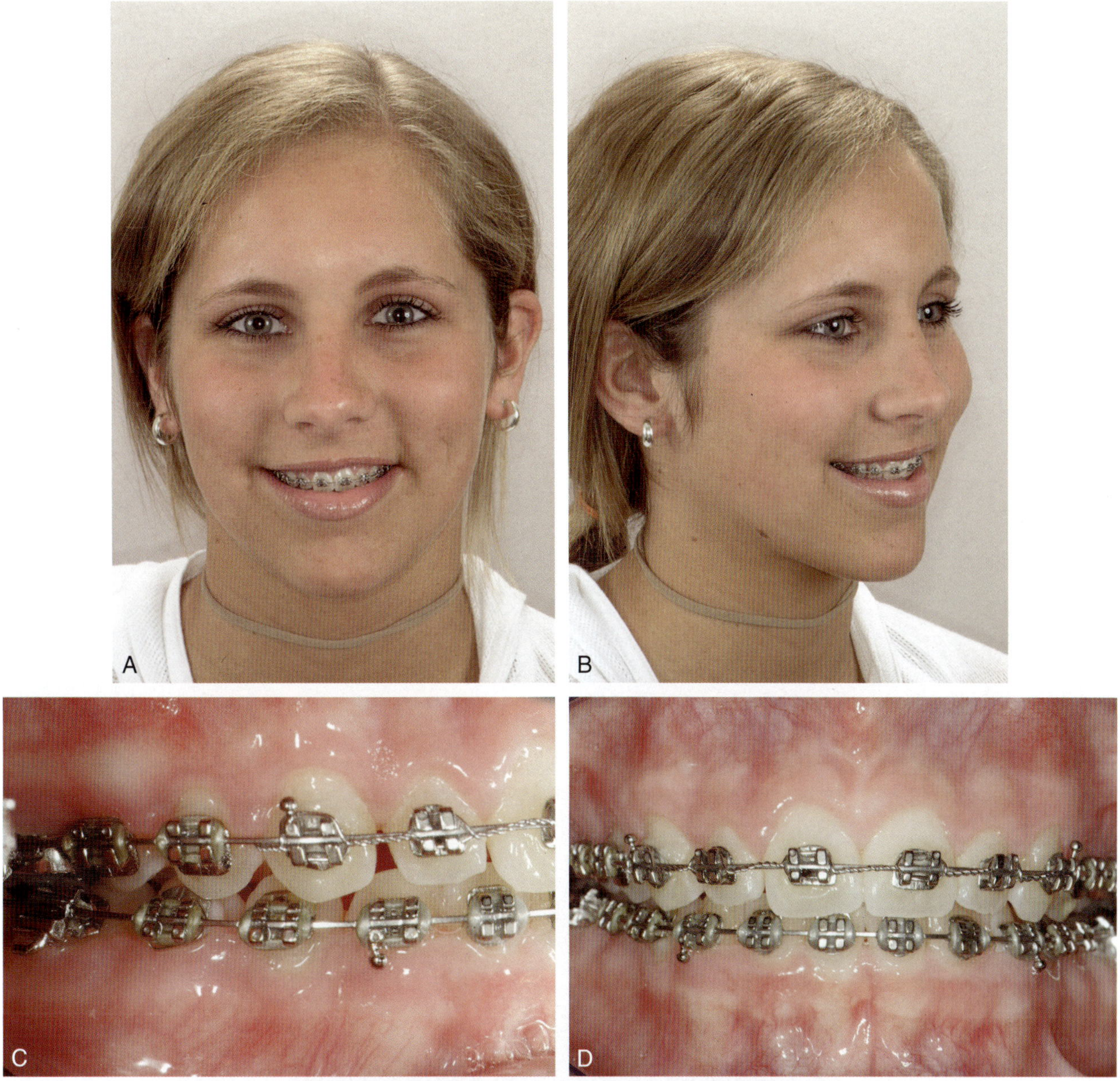

• **Fig. 7.31** For patient F.P., fixed appliance treatment and high-pull headgear were continued following the gingival surgery, with an effort to align and place lingual root torque on the maxillary incisors for better display on smile while maintaining the overbite correction. (A and B) Progress records at age 14-5 showed good incisor display; and (C and D) a nearly corrected malocclusion.

The Detailed Plan: Specifying the Treatment Procedures

At this point, the patient and/ or parent should be presented with their chief complaint and your prioritized problem list, positive attributes and treatment goals. Their affirmation should be obtained so that you know you are heading in the right direction. Discussion of any concerns may require reordering of the problem list and goals. Next, the reasonable treatment possibilities should be discussed to determine which direction you will be heading, together. The pros and cons of each direction is essential for the patient and/ or parent to understand, as are the limitations of each direction. Now you have jointly determined the final plan (Fig. 7.8). Note that for this patient, the conceptual plan leads directly to the therapy plan, which usually is the case. For any patient, the selected treatment procedures must meet two criteria: *effectiveness* in producing the desired result and *efficiency* in doing so without wasting either doctor or patient time or money. Progress, completion and 6- and 13-year follow-ups of this case are shown in Fig. 7.31–Fig. 7.35.

There are good facial esthetics and dental esthetics. The post-treatment stability also appears to be good.

For a relatively simple treatment plan, the associated treatment procedures are also reasonably simple or at least straightforward. Nevertheless, choices must be made and clearly specified in the treatment plan. For example, if the plan is to expand a narrow maxillary arch, it would be possible to do this with an expansion lingual arch, an expansion labial arch, or a banded or bonded

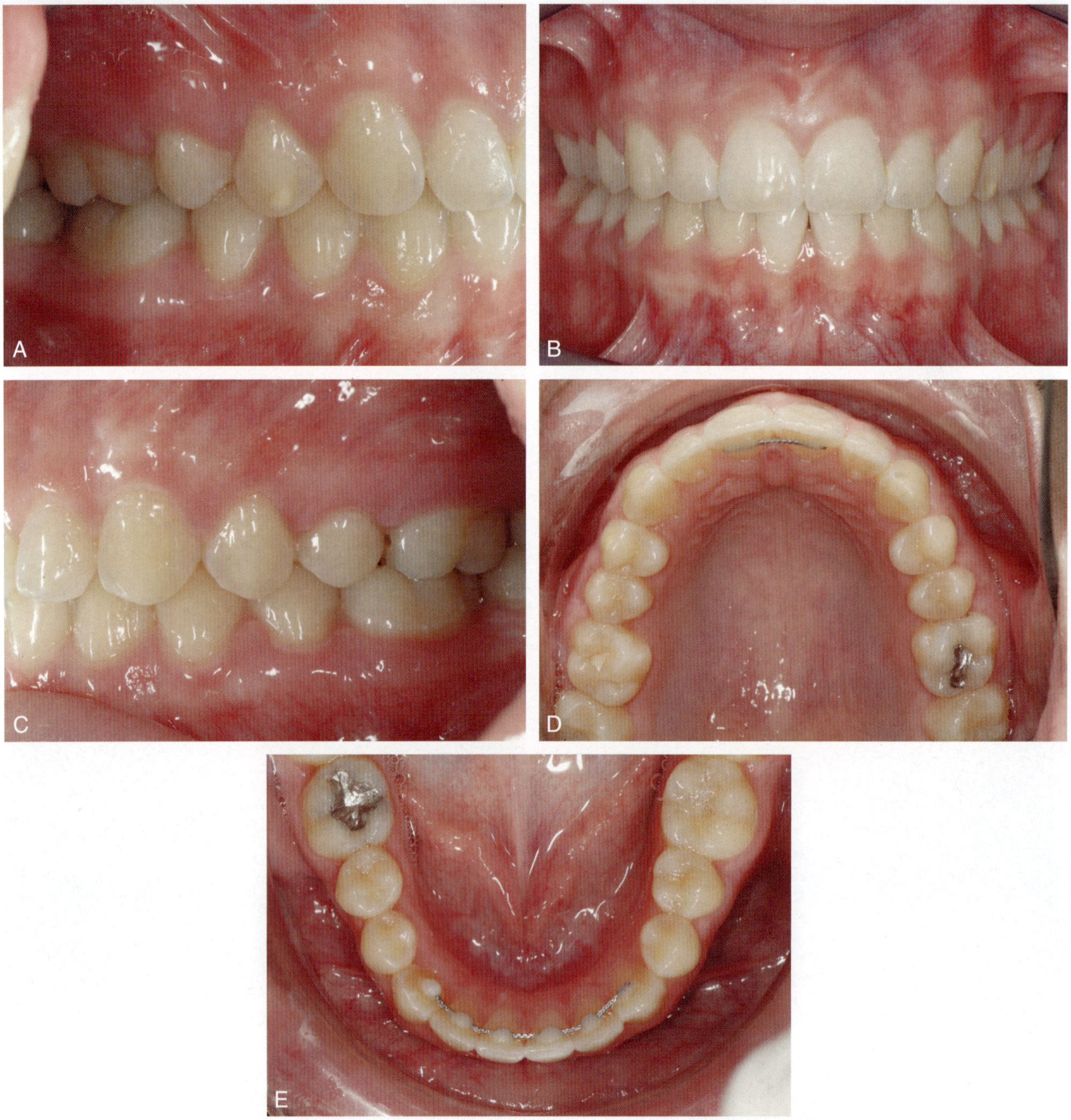

• **Fig. 7.32** Patient F.P. The orthodontic appliance was removed at age 14 years 9 months, 23 months after treatment began. The intraoral views and panoramic radiograph (A to F) show excellent alignment and occlusion, with normal gingival contours. Note (D) the bonded maxillary retainer to maintain the rotation correction and space closure for the maxillary central incisors and (E) the bonded canine-to-canine retainer for the lower arch. In the close-up smile images (G and H), note the consonant smile arc and improved maxillary incisor display.

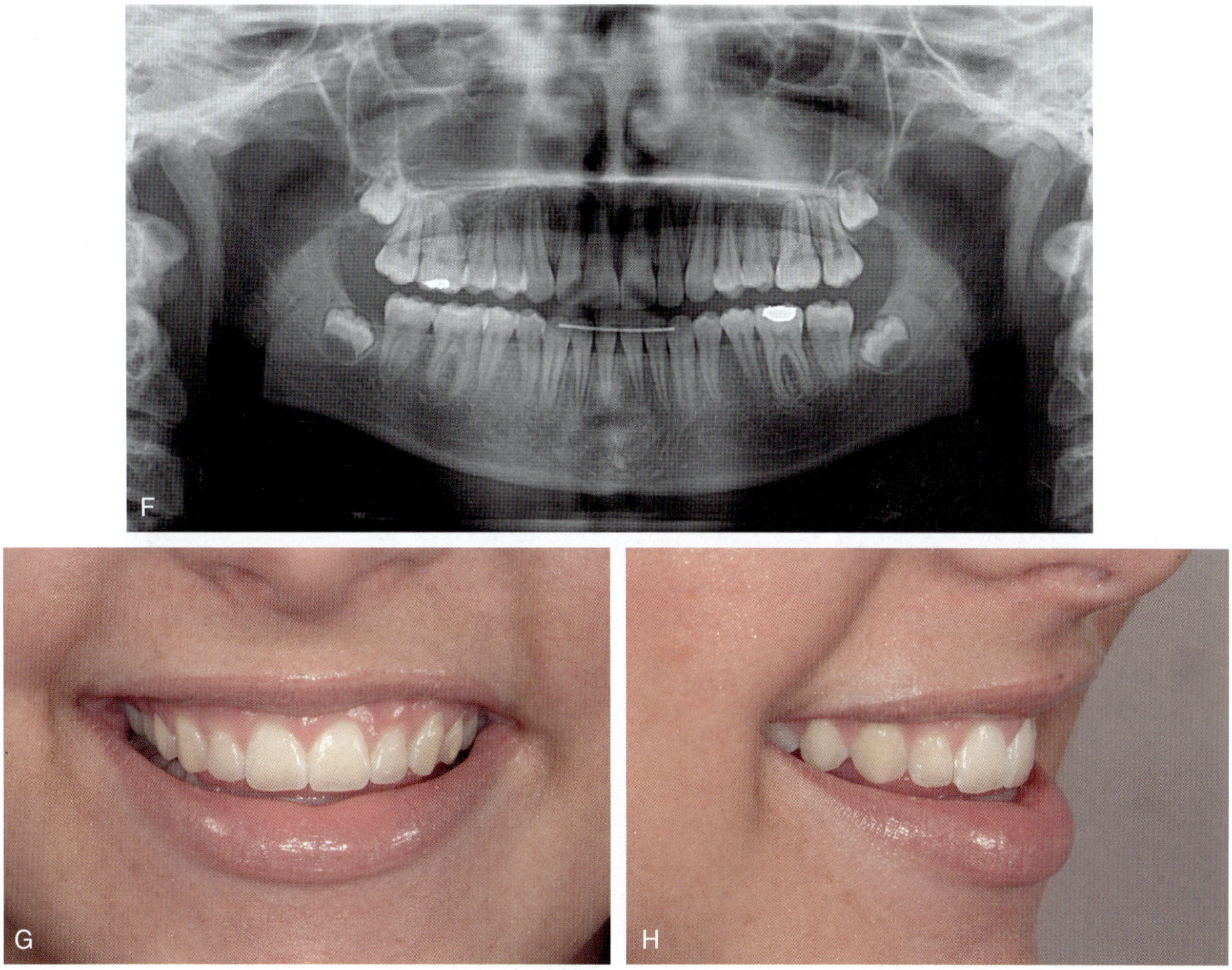

• **Fig. 7.32, cont'd**

maxillary palatal expander. The treatment plan must specify which, and the effectiveness and efficiency of the various possibilities must be considered. There is a time and a place for everything, and this last step is the place for the practical considerations of which treatment method and what orthodontic therapy to use.

The most serious errors in orthodontic treatment planning are those that result from first thinking of which appliance to use, not what the appliance is supposed to accomplish. The treatment mechanics should not be allowed to determine the treatment result. It is an error to establish the treatment mechanics before establishing the broader goal of treatment. The treatment procedures should be manipulated to produce the desired result, not the other way around.

As careful as the original treatment plan was established, there are situations during treatment that require adjustments in the treatment plan during treatment. These can occur due to cooperation from the patient or unexpected occurrences during treatment like problems with closing space, occlusal cants developing, open or deep bites that develop or fail to resolve or unexpected soft tissue responses. Clearly, the best direction of treatment is a straight line from initiation to completion. That rarely happens to a greater or lesser extent. Successful, experienced clinicians make the fewest and smallest and effective in-course corrections from the initial treatment plan (the straight line) to the successful completion. Sage clinicians are always thinking what problems certain treatment conditions and biomechanics can cause them and what they can do to counteract them. That awareness is critical to timely and successful treatment.

Informed Consent: Seeking Comprehension and Understanding

Not so long ago, it was taken for granted that the doctor should analyze the patient's situation and prescribe what they determined to be the best treatment—with little or no regard for whether that treatment was what the patient desired. This is best described as a paternalistic or maternalistic approach to patient care: the doctor, as a father or mother figure, knows best and makes the decisions.

At present, this approach is not defensible, ethically or legally. From an ethical perspective, patients have the right to determine what is done to them in treatment, and increasingly they demand that right. It is unethical not to inform patients of the alternatives, including the likely outcome of no treatment, that are possible in their case. This approach really addresses risk management.

The modern doctrine of informed consent has made the ethical imperative a legal one as well. Legally, the doctor now is liable for problems arising from failure to fully inform the patient about the treatment that is to be performed. Informed consent is not obtained from just a discussion of the risks of treatment. Patients must be informed what their problems are, what the treatment

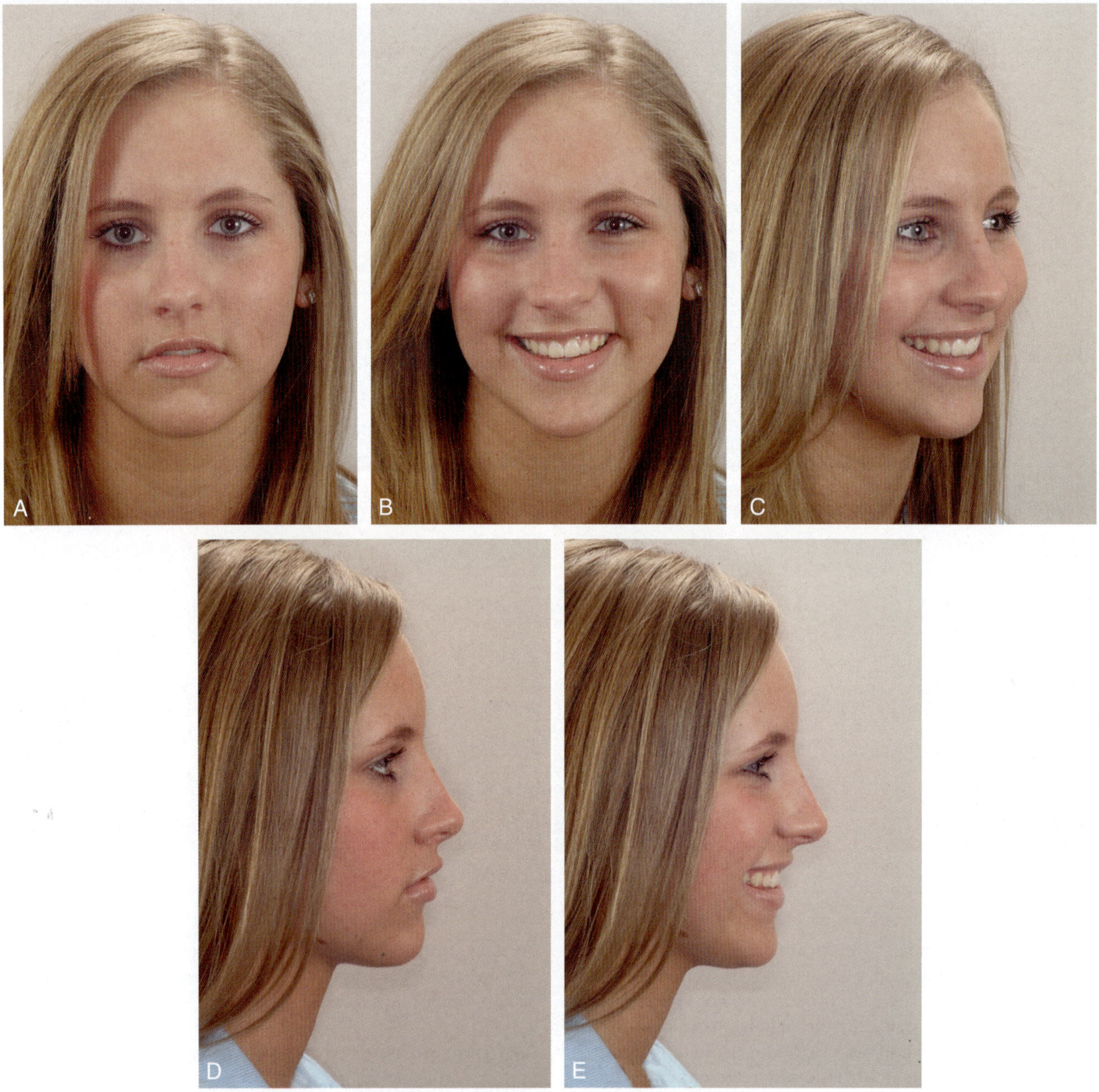

• **Fig. 7.33** Patient F.P. (A) to (C) The posttreatment frontal and 45 degree facial appearance. (D and E) Posttreatment lateral facial appearance. (F) The posttreatment cephalometric radiograph and (G) a cephalometric superimposition showing changes during treatment. In the overall superimposition tracing, note the lack of change in the maxillary position relative to the cranial base and the downward and forward mandibular change.

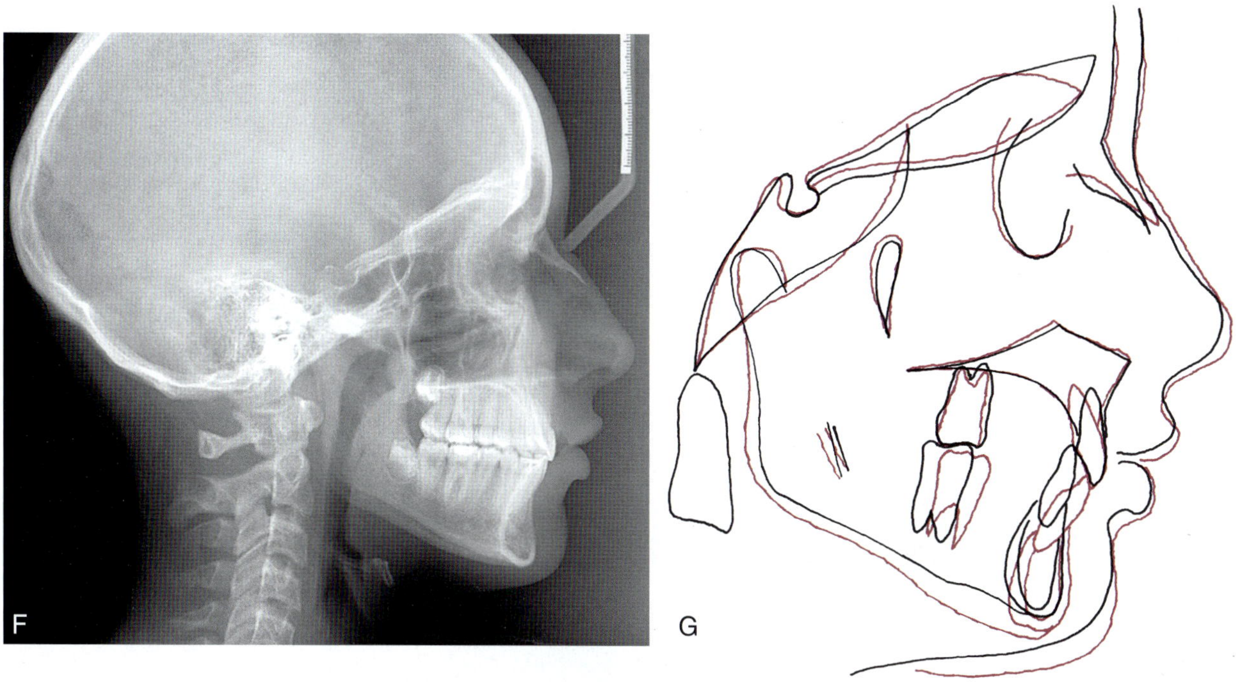

• **Fig. 7.33, cont'd**

alternatives are, and what the possible outcomes of treatment or no treatment are likely to be, in a way they can understand. Simply providing a brochure, video, or written consent form that uses complex language often does not lead the patient to really comprehend the treatment and its consequences.

Having a signed informed consent form is essentially meaningless. All the patient needs to say is that they "...did not understand." Those three words can invalidate any written form. This is often the case because the forms use dental jargon, are too dense with lots of small type and images that are attractive but not informative. This is known as poor processability. Using long, multisyllable word, long sentences and complicated terms leads to poor readability and can be quantified.[21,22] People can understand 7 point, on average, in one presentation.[23] Often case presentations and informed consent documents cover 10 to 20 points.

Similar items should be grouped together and the most important items should be either first or last, so they are remembered.[24] These documents should aim for 7 to 8th grade reading levels.[25] Unfortunately over half of US adults have functional reading levels below that benchmark[26]. This makes true understanding difficult in some situations.

An effective method to insure that patients understand is to ask the patient and parent to tell you what you just told them in your case presentation—not to test them, but to make sure you were clear to them. This takes the burden off them. This is known as "teach back" or Check For Understanding (CFU).[27] You can then correct any errors and indicate in your record that you provided the information including the patient's problems, potential treatment solutions, risks and benefits of each plan, alternative treatments, including no treatment, used teach back or CFU with the required corrections to check for understanding and answered all questions. The detail is dictated by what a reasonable person would want to know. Many of the problems with true informed consent is the low level of health literacy in the United States—being able to read, understand, and act on health information in written form. Those who are young, old, did not speak English before entering school, those who have less education, and those who get their health information primarily from radio and television are most likely to not understand informed consent discussions.[28] For them, understanding the risks and limitations of treatment quite possibly is better with a formal audiovisual presentation than even an extensive discussion.[29]

Recent studies have demonstrated that patient recall of information presented to them is enhanced by putting the information in layperson's terminology and by using visual presentation (images on a computer screen) instead of just words. It may be useful to have patients and parents write down what they believe they saw or heard so it can be confirmed or corrected immediately.[30]

The problem-oriented method of diagnosis and treatment planning lends itself very well to the patient involvement that modern treatment planning requires. As noted above, discussion with the patient and parents should begin with an outline of the patient's problems, positive attributes and treatment goals. The patient involvement begins with the prioritization of the problem list. Perhaps the doctor's single most important question in obtaining informed consent is, "Your most important problem, as I see it, is .... Do you agree?" When problems related to informed consent for orthodontic treatment arise, almost always they result from treatment that failed to address what was most important to the patient, or from treatment that focused on what was not an important problem to the patient.

The problem-oriented method also requires examining the possible solutions to the patient's problems, starting with the most important one. This is exactly the way in which a discussion with the patient and parents is structured most effectively (see Box 7.7). Interactions, unavoidable compromises, and practical considerations must be considered by the clinician. The advantages and disadvantages to the possible treatment approaches must be clear. The doctor's role is to clarify this to the best of their ability, involving the patient in the final decision as to the treatment

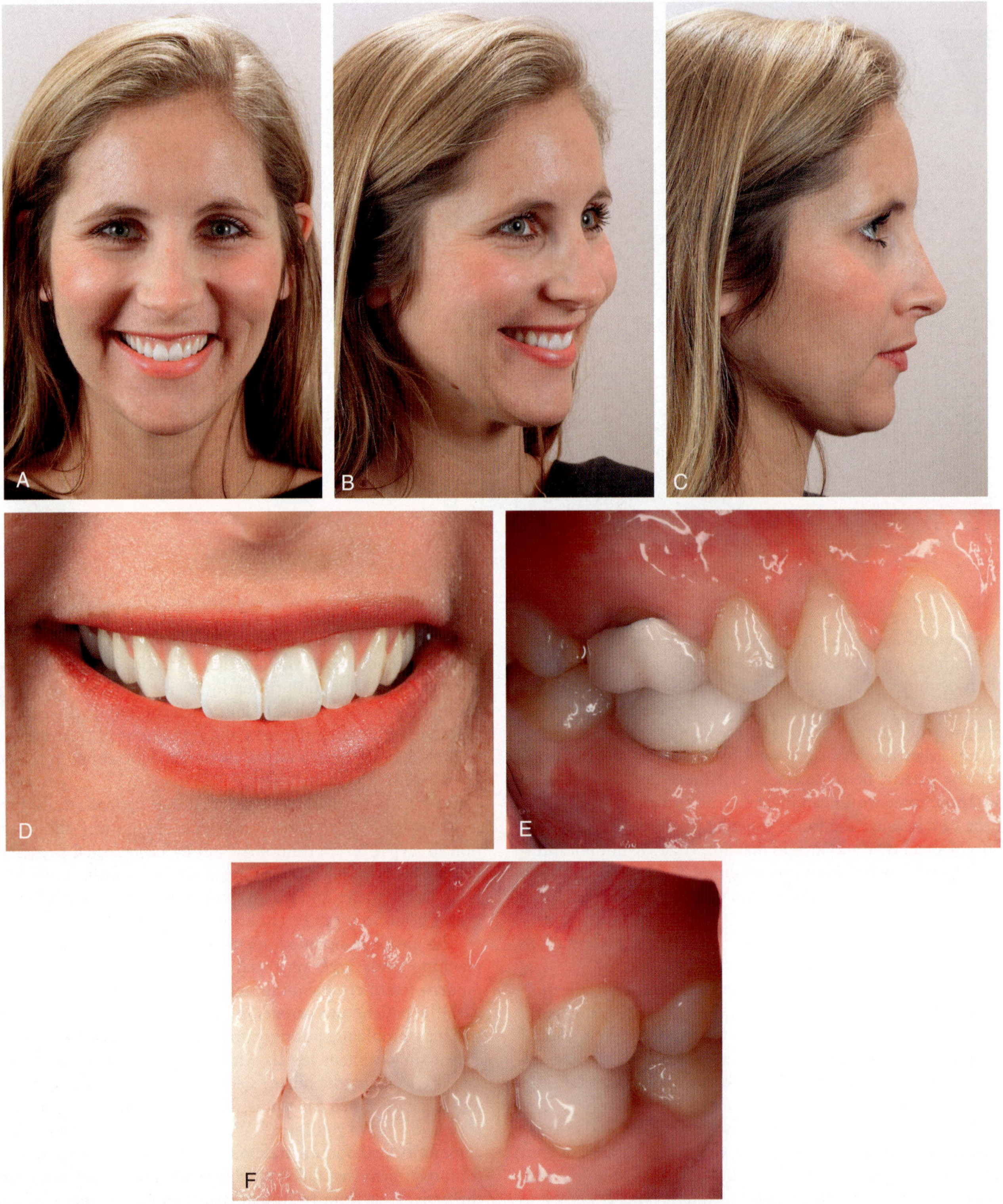

• **Fig. 7.34** Patient F.P., age 21, 6-year follow-up. (A) to (C) Facial photos. (D) Smile arc. (E and F) Dental occlusion. She had almost no growth after completion of treatment, cooperated with wearing retainers at night to age 18, and had a stable result.

approach that will be used. From a practical perspective, involving the patient and parents in decisions about treatment has important advantages. It places the responsibility where it belongs: on a patient who has been led to understand the uncertainties involved. The problems, after all, belong to the patient, not the doctor. For both adults and children, a patient who "owns" the problems and recognizes that this is the case is more likely to be cooperative and oriented toward helping with treatment than one who takes the attitude that it is all up to the doctor.[31]

Several specific situations in orthodontics particularly require interaction between the doctor and the patient and parent while considering the final treatment plan. Every patient should have

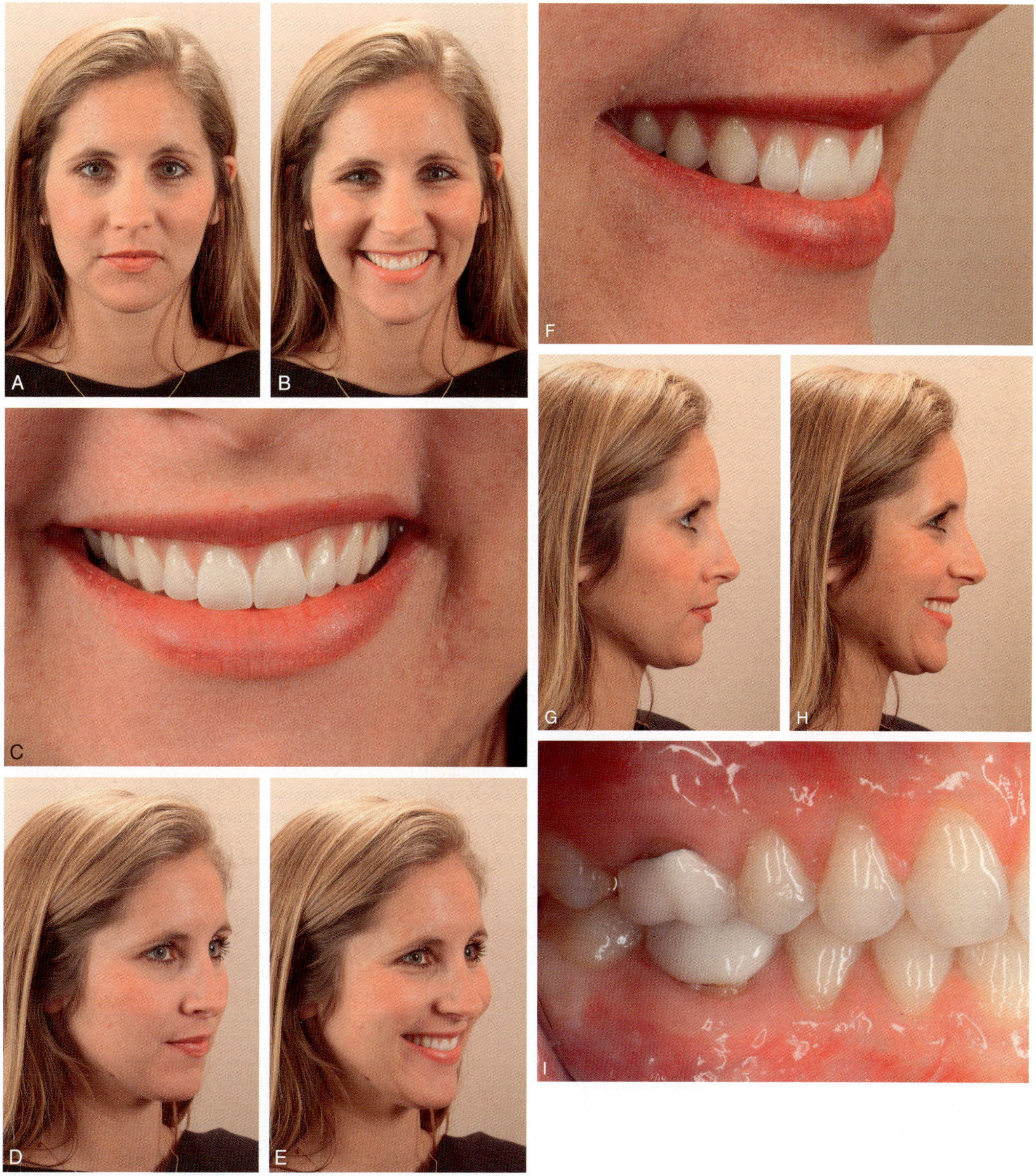

• **Fig 7.35** Patient F.P., age 28, 13-year follow-up. (A–C) Frontal facial photos; (D–F) 45 degree facial smile arc photos; (G and H) Facial profile photos and (I–M) Dental occlusion. Here facial and smiling esthetic dental occlusion are excellent. She continues to have more restorations on her permanent molars and some recession in the premolar areas and lower incisors. Her upper lingual bonded retainer is intact to hold the incisor position and the lower lingual bonded retainer has been removed.

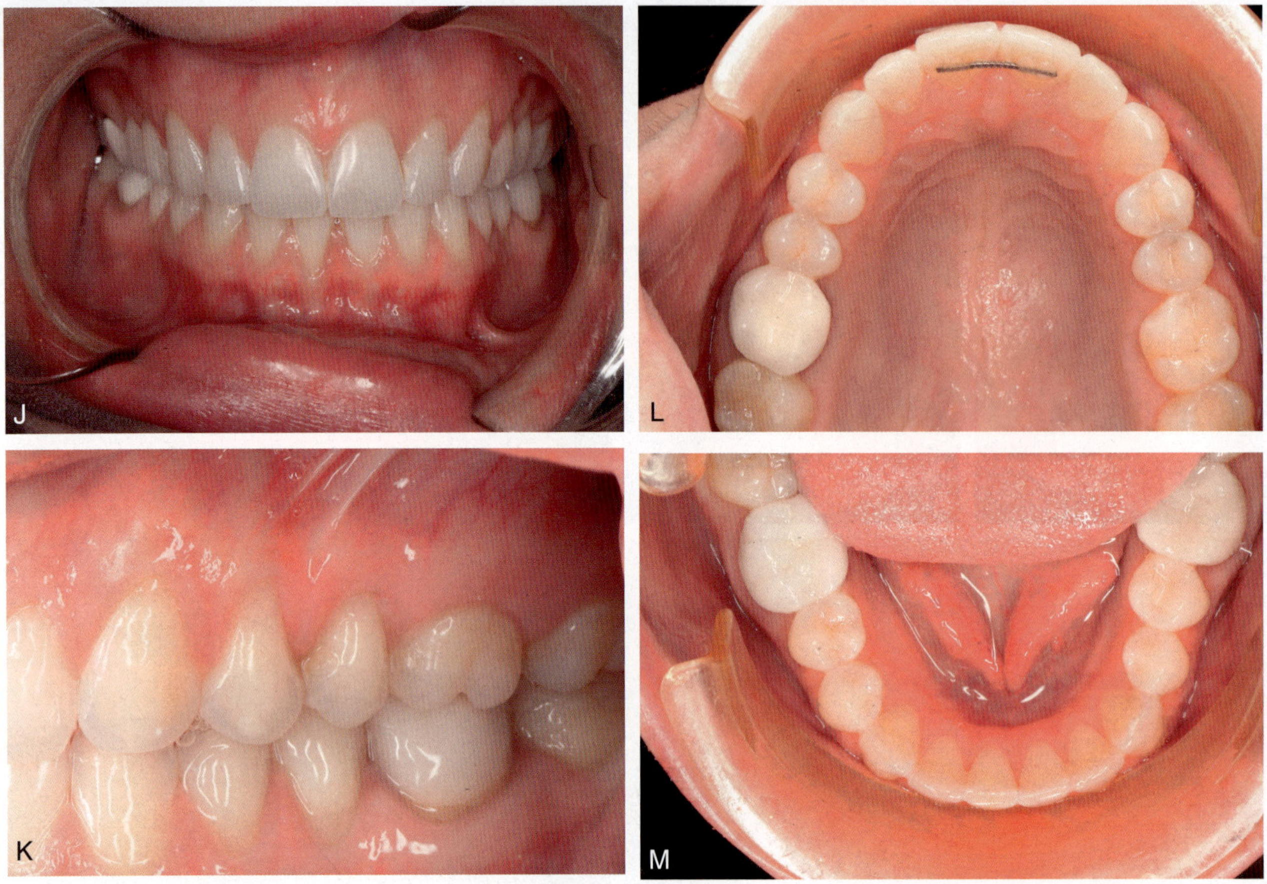

• **Fig. 7.35, cont'd**

a discussion regarding the most frequent things that are likely to occur with patients during treatment: pain and discomfort and how to address it; root resorption; the possible damage to the teeth from inadequate hygiene with resulting white spot lesions; gingival inflammation, infection and deterioration also due to inadequate oral hygiene; and the need to have posttreatment retention appliances. These issues are often poorly understood by patients.[30] Additionally, patients need to be alerted to the need for trauma prevention in the form of mouth guards, especially during treatment.

Pain occurs during efforts to move teeth in three-quarters or move of patients. The pain usually begins in roughly 12 hours or less and peaks at approximately 24 hours, with a gradual decline over 3 to 5 days. Some report pain after 1 week. When the blood vessels are occluded in the periodonital ligament by the force, the inflammatory reaction recruits leukocytes that release inflammatory mediators and cytokines that recruit monocytes and macrophages to remodel bone. As mediators bond to nerve sites pain is encountered. Pain occurs at the beginning of treatment when teeth are separated for band fitting and placement. Then the forces of fixed and removable intraoral appliances, extraoral applinces (facmasks and headgear) and auxiliary components like elastics cause additional pain. Because the pain with all but the fixed appliances can be avoided by noncooperation, this can hinder treatment progress and has caused a movement by many practitioners to various fixed correctors (MARA and Herbst appliances for example). The pain is predictable when adjustments are made to the appliances. Because pain has emotional and cognitive properties as well, it can be combatted in several ways. Pharmacologically, nonsteroidal antiinflammatories seem to help, but there are some data to suggest they may slow tooth movement, so acetaminophen is an alternative choice. Some suggest chewing on bite wafers, which has only limited data for support. The effectiveness of low level laser therapy to the affected arch is somewhat cloudy due to differences in the methods of use. Finally, behavioral approaches that distract or reassure patients can be effective, such as structured telephone calls.[32]

Root resorption to some extent occurs in most patients, with incisors and molars affected most often. Severe resorption affecting say 5 mm or incisor root length is not often observed, but has not been demonstrated routinely to cause early tooth loss. Long treatment durations and heavy forces seem to cause resoptive problems. It seems advisable to obtain a panoramic image at about 9 months into treatment to check for significant active resorption. A 2 to 3 month rest period may be helpful in limiting the resorption, before proceeding. Other options to timely treatment completion can be restoration placement to close spaces and interproximal enamel reduction to obtain space.[33]

Inadequate oral hygiene will impact the teeth and supporting soft and hard tissue. Patients should have oral hygiene under control prior to beginning treatment. White spot lesions on the teeth can proceed rapidly in the presence of poor hygiene and appliances. White spot lesions in orthodontic patients have an incidence of nearly 46% and a prevalence in orthodontic patients of 68%. The lesions are the result a demineralized surface and a subsurface lesion, which, if untreated will lead to caries. The white and opaque lesions appear at the margins of the appliances and the gingival margins during treatment (see Fig 6.6), especially the maxillary anterior teeth. Most agree the lesions are more prevalent and severe in males, more frequent in adolescents than adults and accompany longer treatment. If patients are compliant, fluoride toothpaste and mouth rinses can reduce the incidence of lesions. There is some evidence that a spontaneous reduction in the severity of the lesions occurs during the year following appliance removal due to either abrasion of the effected enamel and/or remineralization.[34] Treatments that appear to be the most highly rate include self-assembling (SAP) P_{11}-4 in combination with fluoride varnish (FV) and resin infiltration (RI).[35] The SAP +FV is applied to isolated and clean dry enamel. The RI method involves isolated, cleaned, etched enamel, which is air and chemically dried. The lesion is then infiltrated with a low viscosity resin and light cured.

Periodontal disease signs such as bleeding upon probing, excess pocket depth, recession and tooth mobility are also usually related to poor oral hygiene (see Fig 6.7). If these are under control prior to treatment, and arise later, a periodontal consult in addition to introducing and reinforcing adjuncts to tooth cleaning, is indicated as is the possibly of suspending treatment or removing some appliances until the condition improves. Termination of treatment is always a possibility.

Certainly the end of orthodontic treatment is a welcome milestone, but it is really just the beginning of another phase of orthodontics. Retention is the stage of maintaining the correction achieve by the dental and skeletal changes. Compliance with instruction is critical and that mostly involves appliance wear and care. Returning irregularity or crowding can and will occur in nearly all patients following tooth movement. This is important for patients and parent to understand and expect. This topic is addressed in Chapter 19.

All patients should understand that trauma during orthodontics can have impact on their teeth and soft tissues immediately and in the long run. Immediately, orthodontic appliances can support adjacent traumatized teeth, as they spread the impact force to more teeth. The appliances can cause injury to the lips, tongue and cheeks as they become embedded in the tissue at impact. Teeth that have been injured can experience root resorption, require endodontic treatment or become ankylosed (stuck to the bone) and either not continue to erupt while the patient is growing or be unable to be moved. To minimize this possibility, it is essential that patients involved in vigorous activity that can cause impact to the face and teeth wear an appropriate mouth guard during these activities and later to preserve their dentition.

The correct mouth guard for an orthodontic patient to wear includes one with coverage of each arch that has appliances in place. The guard should be comfortable and have smooth channels to surround the teeth without indentations to inhibit tooth movement. These are usually sold as orthodontic mouth guards (Fig. 7.36). Again, they should not be for fit to the teeth. Although there are many designs on the market, the most important thing is that the patient will wear it. Following treatment conventional mouth guards adapted to the teeth are appropriate.

Next it is necessary to have discussions about other issues unique to *this* patient—for instance, missing teeth, impacted teeth, or the need for temporary anchorage devices (TADs). For many patients an issue is arch expansion versus extraction to solve crowding problems (discussed earlier). A second frequent problem requiring input from the patient is whether to begin treatment for a skeletal problem before adolescence or wait until the adolescent growth spurt. In this situation, two aspects must be discussed: the efficacy of beginning treatment early versus waiting for adolescence, and if early treatment is chosen, the mode of treatment.

The patient's desire for treatment and potential cooperation also must be taken into account when treatment timing is considered. For patients with Class II problems, there is little reason to proceed with headgear or functional appliance treatment for a child who has no intention of wearing the device. Treatment results with the two methods are not precisely the same but are more similar than different, and if the patient would wear one but not the other, it would be wise to select the one he or she would

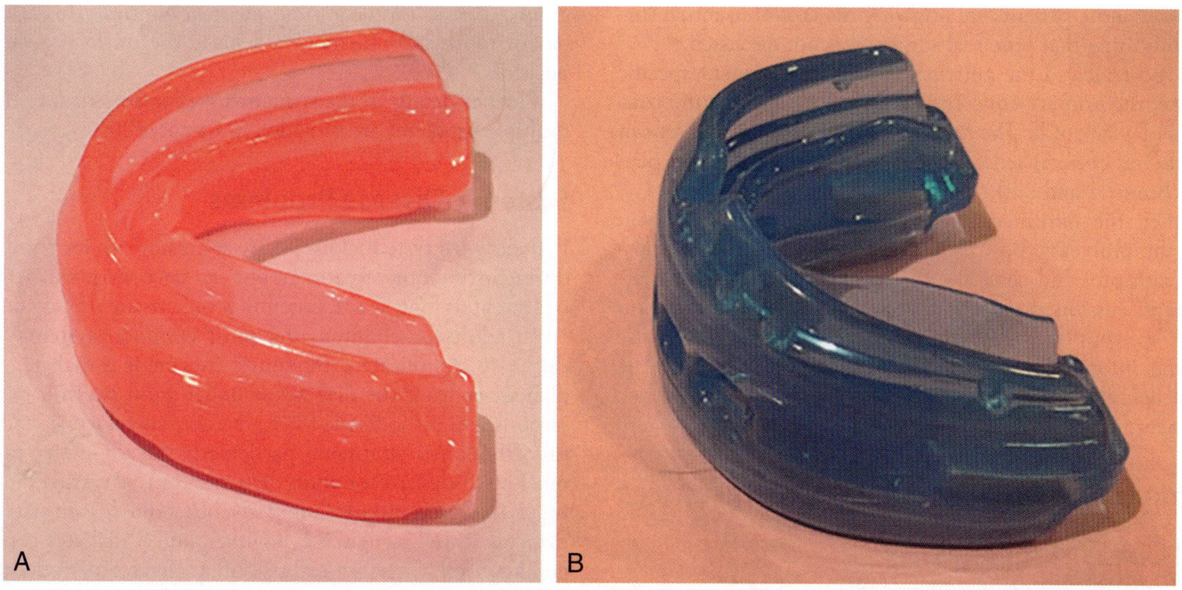

• **Fig. 7.36** Here are two mouth guards appropriate for orthodontics. (A) covers the maxillary arch only and has the flat occlusal surfaces and no indentations for teeth on any surface, so they can easily move. (B) This mouth guard covers both arches and has a set of breathing holes in the anterior portion. It has the same features in the tooth channels and good facial surface coverage.

prefer. For our example patient, her level of sexual maturation indicates that she is approaching the ideal time for treatment, and headgear was the preferred approach, but the patient and parent need to understand why these are the recommendations and what alternatives exist. There are a variety of choices for Class II correction. That also is true for other types of jaw discrepancies.

When a severe skeletal problem exists, a third frequent issue for discussion with the patient and parents is whether orthodontic treatment alone would produce an acceptable result, or whether orthognathic surgery should be selected. Sometimes this difficult decision revolves around jaw function and stability. In most instances, however, it is primarily an esthetic decision or which treatment will address multiple problems. The facial appearance is likely to be better if the jaw relationship is corrected. Is that improvement worth the additional risk, cost, and morbidity of surgery? In the final analysis, only the patient and parents can—or should—make that decision. In decisions such as surgery versus orthodontic camouflage and whether to expand the dental arches or extract, a picture is worth a thousand words (see Fig. 7.28).

Sometimes, involving patients in treatment planning discussions is interpreted as allowing the patient and parent to make all the decisions. Clearly, this is not the case. It is the doctor's responsibility to explain the options to the patient and parents and to negotiate with them the final treatment plan. It is not the doctor's responsibility to do anything the patient wants. Just as any patient has the right to refuse to accept treatment, the doctor has the right to refuse to carry out treatment that he or she considers not in the patient's best interest or not consistent with the standard of care. Establishing the concept of the final treatment plan is and must be an interactive process between the doctor and the patient.

In our example case, the patient and her parents understood the importance of correcting the Class II malocclusion and deep bite if a better facial appearance was to be achieved, accepted the suggestion that headgear during the adolescent growth spurt would be the best approach, and acknowledged that a change in the treatment plan to include extraction or even orthognathic surgery might be needed if the patient did not respond well to the more conservative initial treatment plan. This is currently a key issue because more patients are litigating the cost of eventual surgery by indicating that potential surgery was not discussed.[36]

They also reviewed the anticipated risks of treatment specific to her case, the primary concern being cooperation and the consequences of a lack of it. The result was both informed consent in the broad (and correct) sense and approval of the treatment plan concept (Boxs 7.7 and 7.8).

So, when the informed consent discussion occurs and you reiterate the problems, positive attributes, goals, treatment possibilities with pros and cons, no treatment and the risks of treatment, the discussion should be familiar to the patient and you can refer to your previous comments. New issues that arise during the informed consent discussion should be rare. The approach described should provide true understanding and risk management.

• BOX 7.8 Patient F.P.: Final Treatment Plan

Treatment Concept

- Align maxillary incisors and correct their inclination without increasing overjet.
- During adolescent growth, headgear to correct skeletal Class II, reduce overjet.
- Correct anterior deep bite by controlling lower incisor eruption as vertical growth occurs.
- Correct midlines

Treatment Details

- Delay start of treatment until level of maturation indicates onset of adolescent growth.
- Stress need for excellent oral hygiene.
- High-pull headgear.
- Level mandibular arch with reverse curve archwires.
- Alignment of maxillary anterior teeth preserving the smile arc
- Lingual root torque to maxillary incisors.
- Class II elastics as needed.
- Retainer wear.

Treatment Planning in Special Circumstances

Dental Disease Problems

Until the late 20th century, there was concern that endodontically treated teeth could not be moved. It is now clear that if the periodontal ligament remains normal, endodontically treated teeth respond to orthodontic force in the same way as teeth with vital pulps. Although some investigators have suggested that root-filled teeth are more subject to root resorption, the current consensus is that this is not a major concern.[37] Occasionally, hemisection of a posterior tooth, with removal of one root and endodontic treatment of the remaining root, is desirable. It is perfectly feasible to orthodontically reposition the remaining root of a posterior tooth, should this be necessary, after the endodontics is completed.

Essentially all periodontal treatment procedures may be used in bringing a pre-orthodontic patient to the point of satisfactory maintenance, with the exception of osseous surgery. Scaling, curettage, flap procedures, and gingival grafts should be employed as appropriate, so that progression of periodontal problems during orthodontic treatment can be avoided. Children or adults with a lack of adequate attached gingiva in the mandibular anterior region should have free gingival grafts to create attached gingiva before the beginning of orthodontics. This is especially true if tooth movement would place the teeth in a more facial position.

Further details in the sequencing of treatment for adults with multiple problems are provided in Chapter 20.

Systemic Disease Problems

Patients with systemic disease are at greater risk for complications during orthodontic treatment but can have successful orthodontic treatment as long as the systemic problems are under control.

In adults or children, the most common systemic problem that may complicate orthodontic treatment is diabetes or a prediabetic state. If the diabetes is under good control, periodontal responses to orthodontic force are essentially normal, and successful orthodontic treatment, particularly the adjunctive procedures most often desired for adult diabetics, can be carried out successfully. The rapid progression of alveolar bone loss in patients with diabetes is well recognized, however, and if diabetes is not under good control, there is a real risk of accelerated periodontal breakdown (Fig. 7.37). For this reason, careful monitoring of a diabetic patient's compliance with medical therapy is essential during any phase of orthodontic treatment. Prolonged comprehensive orthodontic treatment should be avoided in these patients.

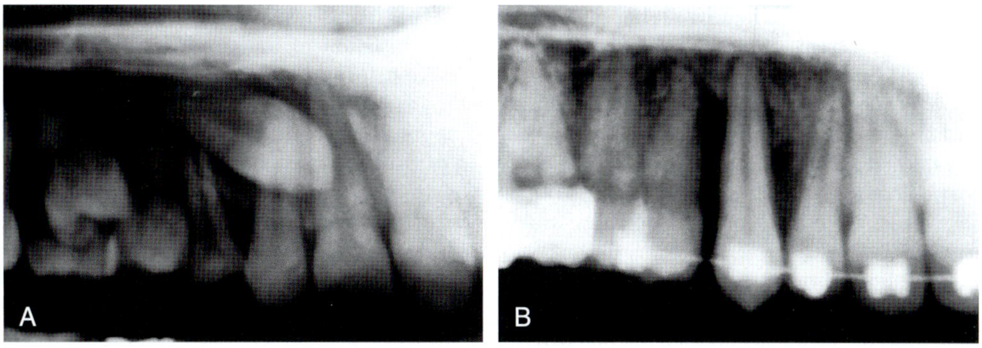

• **Fig. 7.37** Patients with uncontrolled diabetes may experience rapid bone loss during orthodontic tooth movement. (A) Impacted canine in a 13-year-old girl. (B) One year later. Note the extent of bone loss around the tooth as it was being moved. During the year of active treatment, the patient had great difficulty in controlling her diabetes and was hospitalized for related problems on two occasions. (Courtesy Dr. G. Jacobs.)

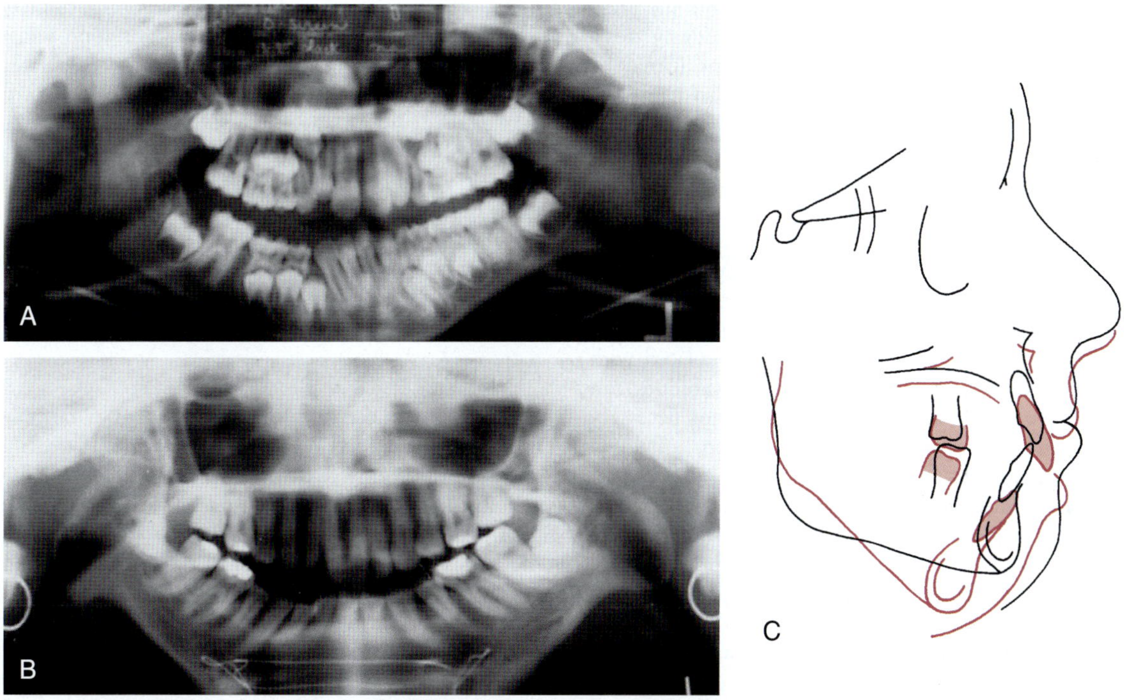

• **Fig. 7.38** Rheumatoid arthritis can affect the condylar process and in the worst case can lead to loss of the entire condylar process. (A) Panoramic radiograph of a child with rheumatoid arthritis. Note the early degenerative changes in the condyle on the left side (compare the left with the as yet unaffected right side). (B) Panoramic radiograph of a young adult with complete destruction of the condylar processes. (C) Cephalometric superimpositions for a patient with severe degeneration of the condylar process of the mandible because of rheumatoid arthritis. Age 18, after uneventful orthodontic treatment *(black);* age 29 *(red)*, by which time the condylar processes had been destroyed. Note the downward-backward rotation of the mandible. (B, Courtesy Dr. M. Goonewardene; C, Courtesy Dr. J. R. Greer.)

Arthritic degeneration may also be a factor in orthodontic planning. Juvenile idiopathic arthritis (JIA) can produce severe skeletal mandibular deficiency, and adult-onset rheumatoid arthritis can destroy the condylar process and create a deformity (Fig. 7.38). Reduced mandibular growth has been reported after steroid injections into the temporomandibular joint in JIA treatment,[38] and long-term administration of steroids as part of the medical treatment may increase the possibility of periodontal problems during orthodontics. Keep in mind that children on steroids may also be taking bisphosphonates, which make orthodontic tooth movement almost impossible. Prolonged orthodontic treatment should be avoided in patients with either type of rheumatoid arthritis because the potential for harm is at least as great as the potential benefit.

Comprehensive orthodontic treatment for children with other systemic diseases also is possible if the disease is controlled but requires careful judgment about whether the benefit to the patient warrants the orthodontic treatment. It is not uncommon for the parents of a child with a severe systemic problem (for instance, cystic fibrosis) to seek orthodontic consultation in their bid to do everything possible for their child. With the increasing long-term survival after childhood malignancies and other major problems, parents now are increasingly likely to view children with complex medical backgrounds (such as radiation therapy, long-term steroid use, and drugs to prevent loss of bone mass) as potential orthodontic patients. If treatment is feasible, a limited scope may be the best acceptable compromise. For patients with a poor long-term prognosis it is usually good judgment to limit the scope of treatment plans, accepting some compromises, while adjusting the treatment time and intensity.

Finally, although orthodontic treatment can be carried out during pregnancy, there are risks involved. Gingival hyperplasia is likely to be a problem, and the hormonal variations in pregnancy sometimes can lead to surprising results from otherwise predictable treatment procedures. Because of bone turnover issues during pregnancy and lactation, an orthodontist theoretically should be vigilant about loss of alveolar bone and root resorption during pregnancy, but radiographs to check on the status of bone and tooth roots are not permissible then. Treatment for a potential patient who is already pregnant should be deferred until the pregnancy is completed. If a patient becomes pregnant during treatment, the possible problems should be discussed, and it may be wise to place her in a holding pattern during the last trimester, limiting the amount of active tooth movement.

Dental and Jaw Injuries

In general, prior endodontic treatment does not contraindicate orthodontic tooth movement, but teeth with a history of severe trauma may be at greater risk of root resorption, whether they have received endodontic treatment or not. Some posttraumatic injury teeth ankylose, require decoronation or are replaced with transplanted teeth (see Chapter 12). All these possibilities can require an altered approach to treatment, but do not necessary preclude orthodontic treatment to the affected (except ankylosed teeth) or adjacent teeth.

Fortunately, severe injuries to the maxilla in children are rare, because their consequences are difficult to manage. If the maxilla is displaced by trauma, it should be repositioned immediately if this is possible. When immediate attention to a displaced maxilla is impossible because of other injuries, protraction force from a facemask before fractures have completely healed can successfully reposition it.

The causes of asymmetric mandibular deficiency are discussed in Chapter 14, and the information on hemifacial microsomia versus condylar injury should be reviewed at this point. In planning treatment, it is important to evaluate whether the affected condyle can translate normally. If it can, as one would expect in a mild-to-moderate form of hemifacial microsomia or after a condylar fracture, a functional appliance could be helpful and should be tried first. If translation of the condyle is severely restricted by posttraumatic scarring, a functional appliance will be ineffective and should not be attempted until the restriction on growth has been removed.

Mandibular asymmetry with deficient growth but some translation on that side is a particular indication for custom-designed "hybrid" functional appliances (see Fig. 10.9) because requirements for the deficient side will be different from those for the normal or more normal side. Often, it is desirable to incorporate a bite block between the teeth on the normal side while providing space for eruption on the deficient side so that the vertical component of the asymmetry can be addressed. In the construction bite, the mandible would be advanced more on the deficient side than on the normal side.

The severe restriction of growth that accompanies little or no translation of the condyle can lead to a progressively more severe deformity as growth of other parts of the face continues. Progressive deformity of this type is an indication for early surgical intervention. There is nothing to be gained by waiting for such a deformity to become worse. The goal of surgery is to create an environment in which growth is possible, and orthodontic treatment with a hybrid functional appliance usually is needed after surgery to release ankylosis to guide the subsequent growth.

Sleep Apnea

Sleep apnea carries that name because affected individuals stop breathing while asleep, typically missing several cycles of respiration before waking up abruptly, gasping for breath. The problem is a blockage or collapse of the airway, which can occur at any point between the nostrils and lungs. Sleep apnea has been recognized recently as a more frequent problem than had been appreciated previously (see Chapters 5 and 6). It is important to remember that dentists and dental specialists do not appropriately diagnose obstructive sleep apnea (OSA) or other sleep related problems. The dentist screens for these problems and refers for diagnosis and management by primary care, otolaryngology or sleep medicine providers.

Here we will explore surgical and orthodontically related treatment possibilities for OSA with some more detail in Chapters 13, 20, and 22.

Treatment of OSA in Children

Adenotonsillectomy

Hypertrophy of the tonsils and adenoids is by far the greatest risk factor for OSA in children. The first line of treatment remains adenotonsillectomy. Results of robust clinical trials support the effectiveness of surgery for significant improvements in behavior, quality of life, and objective sleep breathing parameters, including the apnea-hypopnea index (AHI).[39] However, it has been shown that roughly 80% of children will not see resolution of their OSA symptoms following surgery, and patients with severe disease or obesity experiencing much lower levels of treatment success.

In situations where the lymphoid tissue is not hypertrophic and adenotonsillectomy is not indicated, or if significant symptoms persist postsurgery, the alternative options such as continuous positive airway pressure (CPAP) secondary airway surgeries such as lingual tonsillectomy, or weight management may be considered.

Maxillary Expansion

As the maxilla comprises both the roof of the mouth and floor of the nose, it is reasonable to expect that maxillary expansion may increase the nasal cavity volume and therefore improve respiration during sleep. Early evidence seemed to suggest that RME may be an effective and important treatment in the management of OSA in children.[40] However more recent studies have tempered this optimism somewhat.[41] The overall level of evidence showing benefit of expansion is not high and mainly stems from case reports or uncontrolled studies. The lack of control groups for comparison in OSA treatment in children is particularly important as high quality data from RCTs of surgical interventions in both preschool and school-aged children demonstrate that roughly 50% of children will see spontaneous normalization of their AHI after a period of 7 to 12 months. As such with the lack of untreated controls groups for comparison, it is unclear how much of the reported improvement is from the expansion rather than spontaneous resolution.

Representative of this disconnect between maxillary width, airway size and function, a significant proportion of children will not see an improvement and some have a worsening of their OSA following maxillary expansion. In a retrospective case review of 45 children treated with what was called a bimaxillary expansion protocol, where the mandibular arch was also expanded to allow for even greater amounts of maxillary expansion, one-third of the patients reported objectively worse levels of OSA when comparing pre and post orthodontic treatment sleep studies.[42] At this point the evidence is lacking for maxillary expansion performed for the sole purpose of attempting to improve sleep disordered breathing, especially in the absence of posterior crossbite or maxillary deficiency.

Mandibular Advancement Appliances

As mandibular advancing appliances have been proven effective in a large proportion of adults with OSA, it would be reasonable to expect that similar appliances—such as functional appliances used to treat Class II malocclusions, would be useful in the management of pediatric OSA. If worn during sleep in a retrognathic child, would such an appliance be effective at reducing the collapsibility of the upper airway? Unfortunately the evidence to support this is rather limited, with the latest Cochrane Review on the subject concluding that there is insufficient evidence to support or refute the effectiveness of such appliances for the treatment of OSA in children.[43]

A more recent systematic review, which included both controlled and uncontrolled studies of children with OSA treated with mandibular advancing appliances, was more supportive of this form of treatment.[44] However, the meta-analysis calculated mean difference in AHI attributed to treatment from the two high quality studies was an unimpressive −1.75 events/h. The small sample sizes, unclear inclusion criteria of the degree of retrognathia or overjet, variable treatment protocols and observation periods were criteria that future studies should address.

Myofunctional Therapy

Due to the clear contribution of neuromuscular impairment of the upper airway in the etiology of the disease, myofunctional therapy would seem like a reasonable approach to OSA treatment. To date, good long-term evidence to support the effectiveness of myofunctional therapy or related appliances in treating OSA, especially in children, is lacking. While a good idea in theory, there are significant challenges that prevent the widespread applicability of myofunctional therapy in OSA management. First, there is a significant training effect with exercises to enhance the stamina or strength of the orofacial muscles. Similar to any other form of conditioning (like running, for example), once the training stops there can be a quick regression to baseline.[45] This would imply then that any myofunctional therapy would require long-term, perhaps of many months or years, adherence by the patient for lasting effectiveness. Any such requirement, especially in children can be impractical and perhaps the source of the lack of high quality data supporting this form of treatment for OSA. This absence of adherence was highlighted in a non-controlled trial which enrolled 54 children with OSA into a myofuctional therapy program. After 6 months only 10 children had good compliance, and at the 1 year follow-up almost all participants had stopped the program.[46]

Treatment of OSA in Adults

Effectiveness of Oral Sleep Appliance Treatment

As the name suggests, while worn during sleep these oral appliances work to protrude the mandible and associated soft tissues which increases the caliber of the airway, especially in the transverse dimension, thus reducing airway collapsibility. It is important to note, however, that despite the significant change in mandibular position and apparent increase in airway volume, only 29% to 71% of patients will have their OSA resolve completely with appliance use,[47] and roughly one-third of patients will see no therapeutic effect at all. It is now standard protocol that after the appliance is fitted and optimally titrated, a follow-up assessment is made by the referring physician, with polysomnography used to verify treatment efficacy.

Due to the significant number of OSA patients ineffectively treated with mandibular advancing appliances, they have been considered an inferior treatment option to CPAP for managing OSA. However, while CPAP is more effective than mandibular advancing appliances at lowering the number of apneas during sleep, this may be offset by improved patient tolerance and adherence with oral appliance therapy. This concept of mean disease alleviation, where oral appliances are generally less effective, but used more, whereas CPAP is very effective but used much less often, is thought to be why more recent data have pointed to equivalent outcomes for cardiovascular and quality of life measures of disease even in cases of severe OSA.

Dental Side Effects of OSA Treatment

It should come as no surprise that mandibular advancing appliances used to manage obstructive sleep apnea, much like functional appliances to treat Class II malocclusions, can cause significant tooth movement. The short term and temporary side effects of these appliances can include tooth or muscle soreness, dry mouth or alternatively excess salivation, and intraoral soft tissue irritation. Over the long term—and it is important to remember that for many patients prescribed mandibular advancing oral appliances, this can mean for the rest of their lives, the weight of holding the mandible and associated soft tissues forward is transmitted by the appliance to the dentition resulting in tooth movement. Studies examining occlusal changes after a period of 10 or more years have reported reductions in overjet and overbite of 2 to 3 mm with a wide amount of individual variation. The formation of anterior crossbites is common, and the reductions in overjet appear to be progressive with each year of appliance use.[48] Interestingly, there is little skeletal movement or change in mandibular position observed over similar time periods, though significant proclination of the mandibular incisors and uprighting of the maxillary incisors can be expected.[49]

Perhaps less well recognized are the dental changes resulting from prolonged CPAP use. Most commonly seen in patients who use a nasal mask type interface for their CPAP therapy, dental spacing due to proclination of the anterior teeth has been reported.[50] It is thought that as air is forced through the nose and down the pharynx, the tongue is pushed forward against the teeth leading to their movement over time. As such it would be reasonable for patients who are prescribed this type of CPAP to be also provide orthodontic retainers to prevent this unwanted side effect. Managing appliance therapy for sleep apnea is discussed in Chapter 20.

Maxillomandibular Surgery

Orthognathic surgery, normally has been used to treat significant skeletal discrepancies to improve facial esthetics and dental occlusion. It has also been employed specifically to increase the dimensions of the upper airway as a treatment for obstructive sleep apnea. The goal is to maximize the lumen and minimize the collapsibility of the upper airway, irrespective of the presence of any underlying malocclusion.

Maxillomandibular advancement surgery (MMA) involves the advancement of both upper and lower jaws upwards of 10 mm, depending on the initial occlusion. In the absence of an underlying deformity, esthetics can be compromised and in at least one study 31% of patients self-reported a negative esthetic outcome following MMA.[51] However, advances in surgical techniques, which employ a counterclockwise rotation of the occlusal plane with the advancement have improved esthetic outcomes, especially in patients with convex pretreatment profiles due to bimaxillary protrusion and increased mandibular plane angles.[52]

In a systematic review that included data from 518 adult patients who underwent MMA, 85% of patients experienced a more than 50% reduction of their AHI, however a complete resolution or OSA cure occurred less than 40% of the time.[53] Highlighting the significant non-anatomical etiologies to the disease, it should be noted that 73% of the patients in this systematic review also had some form of upper airway soft tissue surgery, which was deemed unsuccessful in treating their OSA, prior to undergoing the MMA procedure. Meaning for some patients, despite multiple and relatively large changes to airway morphology, the disease persists. MMA for OSA is most effective for patients with severe levels (AHI >60) of the disease, ideally with an underlying skeletal discrepancy. In this way, as complete resolution of symptoms is not certain, they will at a minimum appreciate significant improvements to their occlusion and facial profile.

In recognition of the effects of orthognathic surgery on the upper airway, isolated mandibular setback for management of prognathism and a Class III malocclusion have been reconsidered. Is there at greater risk of developing OSA from such procedures? A prospective study of 50 skeletal Class III patients undergoing mandibular set back surgery with or without Lefort 1 osteotomy (maxillary advancement) had full sleep studies (PSG) performed at baseline and 3 months postoperatively.[54] Roughly half of the sample had mandibular setbacks greater than 10 mm, including some patients with 15 mm or more, which resulted in significant reductions in oropharyngeal, hypopharyngeal, and total airway volumes measured from cone beam computed tomography (CBCT) imaging. However despite the substantial magnitude of movement, on average no changes were observed in subjective symptoms of sleep quality, and no significant changes in AHI were reported from the postsurgical sleep studies. It should be noted that three patients were found to have considerable increases in their AHI of greater than 10 events per hour following surgery, and so the potential for deterioration of sleep quality should be discussed with patients planned for such procedures, especially with setbacks greater than 10 mm.

Soft Tissue Surgery

Any anatomical variation of the upper airway from the nasal valves to the larynx may impede normal function of respiration during sleep, and as such several soft tissue surgeries have been employed as treatments for OSA. Among these, nasal turbinate reduction and soft palate procedures such as uvulopalatopharyngoplasty (UPPP) are most common. In isolation these procedures have had variable success rates, and case selection is important to maximize surgical outcomes. A recent RCT investigating the effects of combined UPPP and tongue volume reduction surgery in 102 adults with moderate to severe sleep apnea, reported that on average patients experienced a significant reduction in daytime sleepiness and their apea-hypopnea index when compared to the control group.[55] Though it is important to note that despite the invasiveness and significant alteration to upper airway anatomy, most patients did not see a complete resolution to their OSA symptoms, with the treatment group still experience moderate levels of OSA (AHI >15) at the end of the trial.

Hypoglossal Nerve Stimulation

A relatively new treatment for OSA is the electrical stimulation of the tongue causing it to contract and protrude during inspiration, thereby opening up the airway. The surgery involves dissecting the specific efferent of the hypoglossal nerve that leads to the genioglossus muscle causing protrusion, on to which a small electrode is attached. This is led to a pacemaker-like device that is implanted subcutaneously on the chest which senses inspiration and matches the timing of tongue protrusion to inhalation. Prior to sleeping the patient activates the device via remote control on a timed delay, allowing it to activate after they have fallen to sleep.

Case selection is critical to the success of this technique, which often involves nasoendoscopy during drug-induced sleep (DISE) to visualize the pattern of collapse of the upper airway during sleep. Hypoglossal nerve stimulation is contraindicated in patients who experience concentric collapse of the palatal tissues, and who are severely obese (BMI > 35).[56] Though not recommended as a first line of treatment due to invasiveness and cost of the procedure, patients fitting these specific criteria can be expected, on average, to see significant reduction in daytime sleepiness and improvements in AHI and other respiration parameters during sleep[57].

Common Dentofacial and Craniofacial Anomalies

Hemimandibular Hypertrophy

Mandibular and facial asymmetry can also be caused by excessive growth of a mandibular condyle or lengthening of the condylar neck. Growth problems of this type are never symmetric, and in most patients one condyle is normal or nearly so. The excessive growth is not a tumor in which the growing cells are abnormal—it is simply excessive growth on one side of normal condylar tissue, with no histologic difference from normal condyles.[58] The mechanism by which that could happen is not understood. The condition typically appears in the late teens, most frequently in girls, but may begin at an earlier age. Because the body of the mandible is distorted by the excessive growth (usually by bowing downward on the affected side), the condition is appropriately described as hemimandibular hypertrophy; however, because excessive growth at the condyle appears to be the primary cause, the old name for this condition, condylar hyperplasia, was not totally wrong.

There are two possible modes of treatment, both surgical: (1) a ramus osteotomy to correct the asymmetry resulting from unilateral overgrowth, after the excessive growth has ceased; and (2) condylectomy to remove the excessively growing condyle and reconstruct the joint. The reconstruction usually is done with a section of rib incorporating the costochondral junction area but occasionally can be accomplished just by recontouring the condylar head ("condylar shave"). Because surgical involvement of the temporomandibular joint should be avoided if possible, the asymmetric ramus osteotomy is preferable. This implies, however, that the abnormal growth has stopped or, in a younger patient, will stop within reasonable limits. As a practical matter, removal of the condyle is likely to be necessary in the more severe and more rapidly growing cases, whereas a ramus osteotomy is preferred for the less severe problems.

The bone-seeking isotope technetium 99 m (^{99m}Tc) can be used to distinguish an active rapidly growing condyle from an enlarged condyle that has ceased growing. This short-lived gamma-emitting isotope is concentrated in areas of active bone deposition. ^{99m}Tc imaging of the oral structures typically shows high activity in areas around the alveolar ridge, particularly in areas where teeth are erupting. The condyles are not normally areas of intense imaging, and a "hot" condyle is evidence of active growth at that site (Fig. 7.39).

Unfortunately, although false-positive images are rare, false-negative images are not, so a negative bone scan of the condyles cannot be taken as evidence that hyperplastic growth of one condyle is not occurring. A positive unilateral condylar response on a bone scan indicates that condylectomy will probably be required, whereas a negative response means that further observation for continuing growth is indicated before the surgical procedure is selected. Given the progressive nature of this condition, orthodontic treatment should typically be deferred until a surgical plan is finalized.

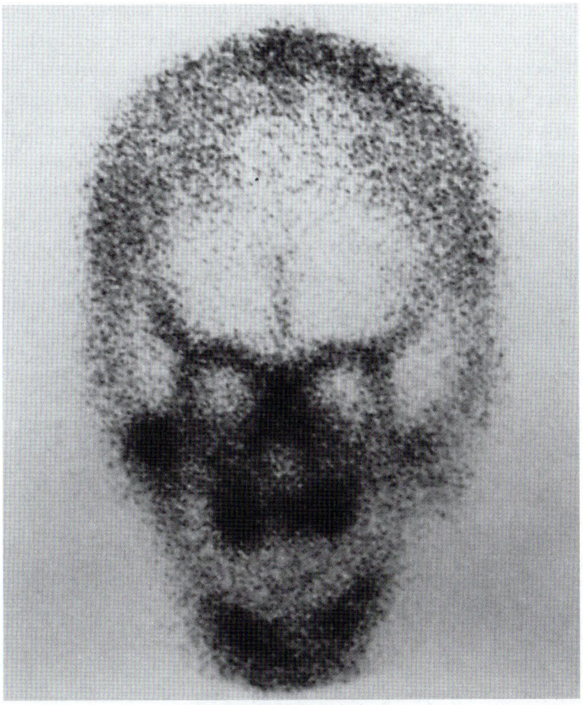

• **Fig. 7.39** Bone scan with technetium 99 m (^{99m}Tc; Towne's view with the mouth open) in a 10-year-old boy with suspected hyperplasia of the mandibular right condyle. Note the "hot spot" in the area of the right condyle and the difference in uptake of the isotope between the right and left sides. Eruption of teeth and apposition of bone at the alveolar processes normally create heavy isotope presence along the dental arches.

Cleft Lip and Palate

Patients with cleft lip and palate routinely require extensive and prolonged orthodontic treatment.[59] Orthodontic treatment may be involved at any or all of four separate stages: (1) in infancy before the initial surgical repair of the lip, (2) during the late primary and early mixed dentition, (3) during the late mixed and early permanent dentition, and (4) in the late teens after the completion of facial growth, with or without orthognathic surgery. Stage 2 revolves around the planning for alveolar bone graft surgery, while definitive orthodontics in Stage 4 often involves orthognathic surgery. The typical sequence of treatment is outlined in Table 7.2, and the treatment procedures are discussed in more detail in the following sections.

In the next section we will focus on the relationship between presurgical infant orthopedics and orthodontics in the patient with nonsyndromic cleft lip and palate.

Infant Orthopedics

An infant with a cleft lip and palate will have an asymmetric maxillary arch at birth in nearly every instance. In patients with a bilateral cleft, the premaxillary segment is often displaced anteriorly while the posterior maxillary segments are lingually collapsed behind it (Fig. 7.40). In the case of a unilateral alveolar cleft, the lesser segment will be collapsed, but to a lesser degree than a bilateral cleft (Fig. 7.41). If the size of the cleft is wide, or the premaxilla is displaced and rotated severely, surgical closure of the lip can be difficult. Orthodontic intervention to reposition the lateral segments of the maxilla and to bring the protruding premaxillary segment back into the arch may be needed to obtain a good surgical repair of the lip.[60] This presurgical infant orthopedics (PSIO) is one of the few instances in which orthodontic treatment for a newborn infant, before eruption of any teeth, may be indicated. The lateral movement of the maxillary segment is accomplished by a nasoalveolar molding plate (NAM plate) and the posterior movement of the premaxilla is achieved by a combination of taping the lip and the NAM plate (Fig.7.42 A–E).

Lip taping either by itself (Fig. 7.43A,B) or in conjunction with NAM utilizes tape placed across the cleft lip segments to approximate them. This creates tension along the labial gap and the alveolar segments. NAM involves a custom orthopedic appliance to aid in the correction of the nose and lip before lip repair;

TABLE 7.2 Sequence of Treatment for Cleft Palate Patients

Age	Treatment
1 week to 3 months	Presurgical Infant Orthopedics (PSIO), if needed
3–4 months	Cleft Lip Repair
9 months to 1 year	Cleft Palate Repair
5–7 years	Orthodontics around alveolar bone graft surgery (before eruption of lateral incisor or canine to provide surgical access to the alveolar cleft)
Adolescence	Comprehensive orthodontics post alveolar bone graft surgery Lip/nose revision, if needed
Late adolescence/ Post pubertal	Presurgical comprehensive orthodontics and orthognathic surgery, if needed

with the added benefit of approximation of the alveolar segments. Several studies have concluded that the biggest benefit to NAM is improved outcomes in nasal esthetics.[61] The additional benefit of NAM is to reduce the number of surgeries required for lip repair. However, there is an increased burden on families with frequent visits for adjustments and evaluation of progress while undergoing NAM treatment.[62]

Soon after this treatment, the infants who had presurgical orthopedics look much better than those who did not. With each passing year, however, it becomes more difficult to tell which patients had segments repositioned in infancy and which did not.[63] The short-term benefit is more impressive than the long-term benefit. For some infants with extremely malpositioned segments, presurgical infant orthopedics remains useful. Many craniofacial surgeons may also plan lip repair in two stages, first with a lip adhesion to provide an elastic force from the lip itself (Fig. 7.43C), followed at a somewhat later stage by definitive lip repair (Fig. 7.43D).

At some centers, primary bone grafts to stabilize the position of the segments were placed across the cleft alveolus soon after infant orthopedics and lip and palate repair. Although few clinicians still advocate this procedure, there is evidence that early primary grafting of the alveolar process is contraindicated because it tends to restrict later growth of the maxilla. Alveolar bone grafts are better deferred until the early mixed dentition timed with the eruption of the permanent lateral incisor or the permanent canine.[64]

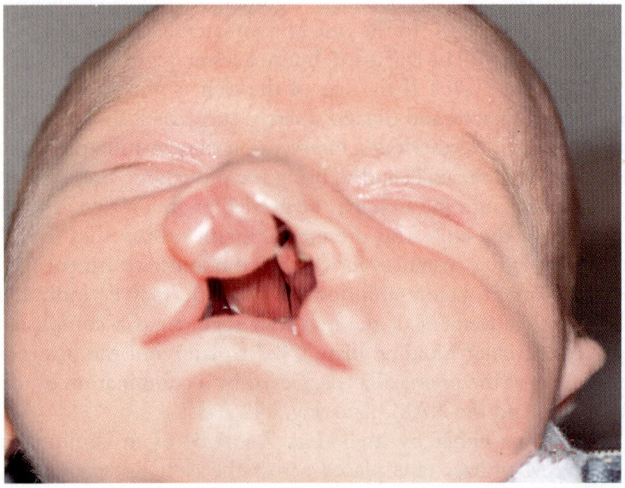

• **Fig. 7.40** This infant with a bilateral cleft of the lip and palate shows forward displacement of the premaxillary segment and medial collapse of the lateral maxillary segments. This displacement of the segments nearly always is seen in infants with a bilateral cleft lip and palate.

Late Primary and Early Mixed Dentition Treatment

Many of the orthodontic problems of children with cleft lip and palate in the late and early mixed dentition result not from the cleft itself, but from the effects of surgical repair. Although the techniques for repair of cleft lip and palate have improved tremendously in recent years, closure of the lip inevitably creates some constriction across the anterior part of the maxillary arch, and closure of a cleft palate causes some degree of lateral and anterior/posterior constriction. As a result, surgically treated cleft lip and palate patients have a tendency toward both anterior and posterior crossbites, which is not seen in patients with untreated clefts. This result is not an argument against surgical repair of the lip and palate, which is necessary for functional (speech) reasons and restoring normal anatomy. It simply means that orthodontic treatment must be considered a necessary part of the overall treatment of the malocclusions that arise because of surgical intervention.

Orthodontic intervention is often unnecessary until the permanent incisor teeth begin to erupt but is usually imperative at that point if the goal is to bone graft for the canine eruption. As the permanent teeth come in, there is a strong tendency for the maxillary incisors to erupt rotated and often in crossbite. The major goal of orthodontic treatment at this time is to prepare the cleft site for alveolar bone graft surgery through expansion or limited bracketing. Incisor alignment is *not a goal* prior to alveolar bone graft surgery and can be detrimental if teeth are inadvertently moved into the cleft without bony support. If limited bracketing is used, it is to move teeth away from the cleft to allow for adequate surgical access for appropriate grafting. Teeth may continue to be rotated or crowded until after a successful bone graft that provides continuity to the maxilla. For patients with clefting, an expander with more anteriorly than posteriorly expansion has been shown to be effective (Fig. 7.44).[65] W arch and hyrax expanders can also be used depending on the anatomy of the cleft.

The objective of timing alveolar bone graft surgery appropriately, is to have a permanent tooth erupt through the grafted material to stimulate the graft and create a continuous alveolus

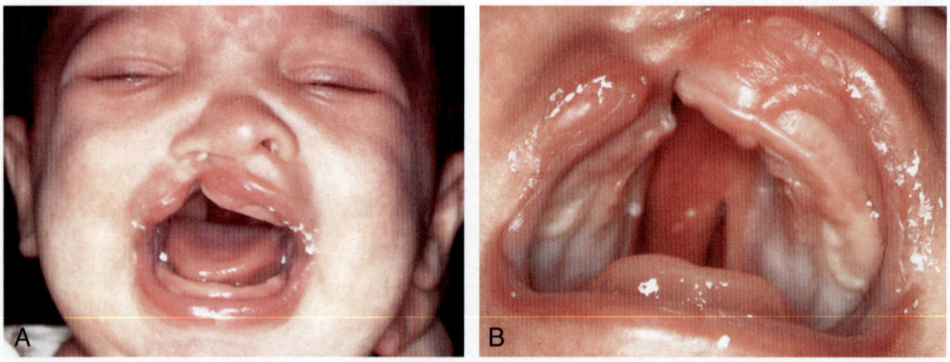

• **Fig. 7.41** This infant, with incomplete unilateral cleft lip and cleft palate, has notching of the alveolar segments. Additionally, notice the displacement of the greater and lesser alveolar segments into a tapered asymmetric V-shape. (A) The frontal extraoral image shows the depression of the ala of the nose on the cleft side. (B) In the intraoral image, the wide cleft of the palate allows direct visualization of the vomer of the nose indicative of the oral/nasal communication prior to palate repair.

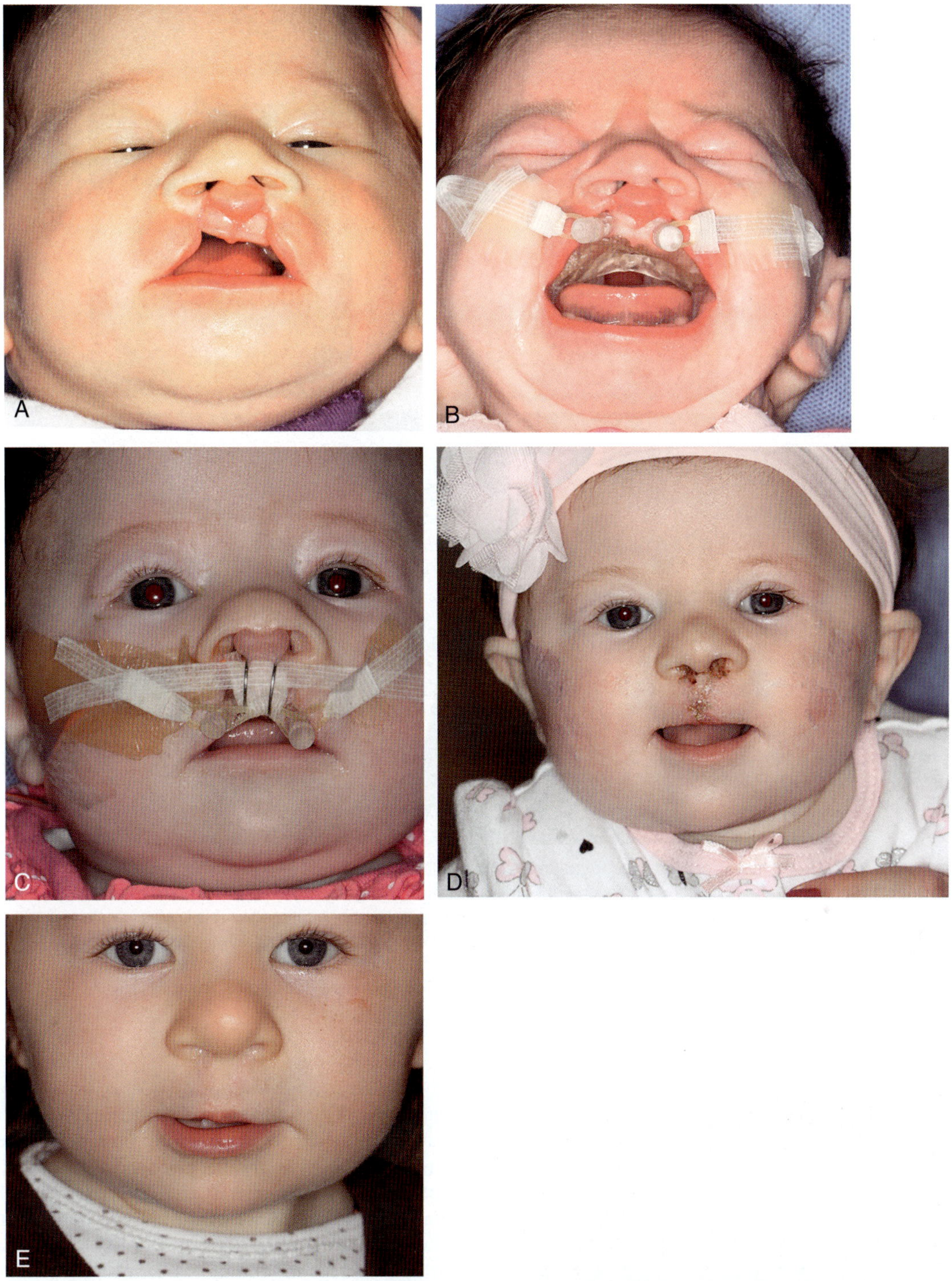

• **Fig. 7.42** Nasoalveolar molding or NAM is one option for presurgical infant orthopedics. (A) An infant with a bilateral cleft lip and palate. Notice displacement of the premaxilla. (B) This demonstrates the application of the introral plate of NAM. Through application of this plate the premaxilla is centered and partially retracted. (C) Here, the intraoral portion of the NAM appliance is seen with the nasal stents added. The nasal stent is used to elongate the columella and project the nasal tip to aid in surgical repair. (D) The patient 1 month following surgical repair of the lip. (E) The patient 1 year postsurgery. The tissue is well healed, and the scar is barely visible.

(Fig. 7.45A). An erupting tooth brings bone with it, augmenting and stimulating the previously grafted material. Appropriate diagnostic imaging should be taken to determine the timing for bone grafting based on development of the permanent canine or the permanent lateral incisor. [66,67] If the permanent lateral incisors are present and unerupted, grafting can be planned before they erupt or when root form is ½ to ⅔ complete. If the laterals are missing, the graft can be delayed but should be completed before

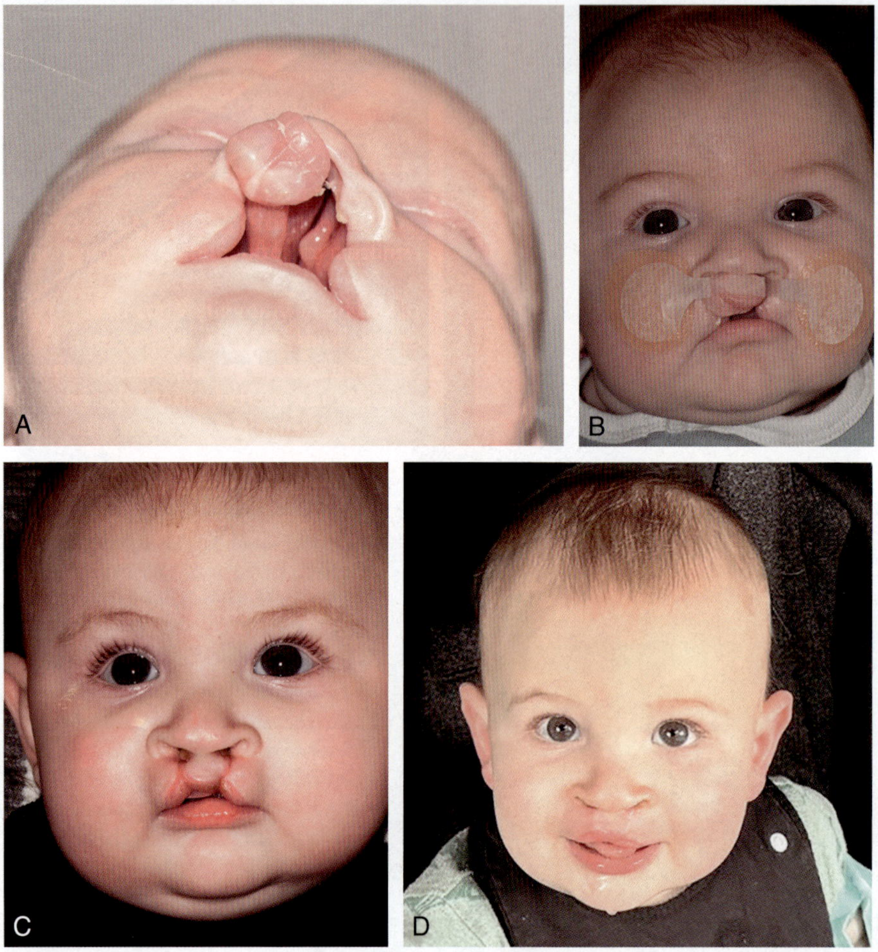

• **Fig. 7.43** Lip taping can be used in the treatment of infants with a cleft. (A) This infant has a bilateral cleft lip and palate. Notice the displacement of the premaxilla. (B) Lip taping is applied to help rotate and retract the premaxilla to aid in surgical repair. There is no intraoral component to this. This is an example of lip taping using a skin protectant under the Dynacleft lip tape. (C) Lip adhesion is often used prior to final lip repair surgery. This infant has had lip taping and lip adhesion surgery. The goal of adhesion is to narrow the cleft and place the nose in a more normal position. (D) Four months following final lip repair.

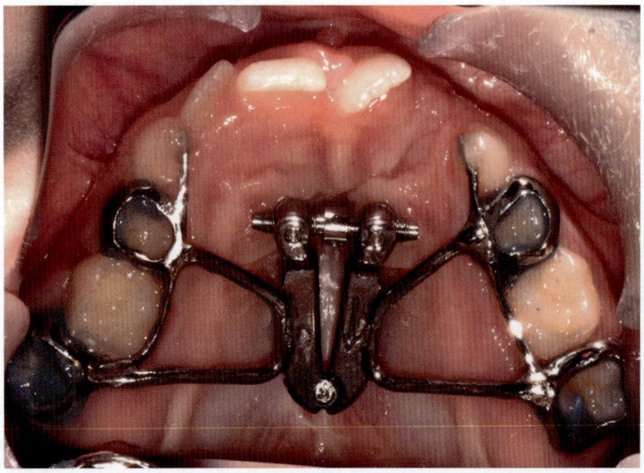

• **Fig. 7.44** A fan expander is commonly used in preparation for alveolar bone grafting. This expander opens more anteriorly than posteriorly, creating greater surgical access to the graft site. In this example, the patient has a left cleft lip and palate treated with a custom 3D printed 4 bonded expander.

the permanent canines erupt with ½ to 2/3 root formation completed as well. Any necessary alignment of incisors to move them away from the cleft or expansion of posterior segments should be completed before the alveolar grafting. Additionally, any necessary extractions of supernumerary teeth or teeth within the cleft should be completed in advance of the alveolar bone graft procedure, if possible. Alveolar bone graft surgery is a routine part of contemporary treatment and timing of treatment is critically important to the long-term success of surgical and orthodontic outcomes. The success of alveolar bone graft surgery is determined by postsurgical imaging 3 to 6 months after surgery. A panoramic x-ray with an occlusal film can be taken, but more commonly a CBCT is used to determine bone graft success (Fig. 7.45B).

Early Permanent Dentition Treatment

As the canine and premolar teeth erupt, a posterior crossbite is likely to develop, particularly on the cleft side in a unilateral cleft patient, and the teeth are likely to be malaligned (Fig. 7.46). The more successful the surgery, the fewer the problems, but in essentially every instance, fixed appliance orthodontic treatment is necessary in the late mixed or early permanent dentition. New bone

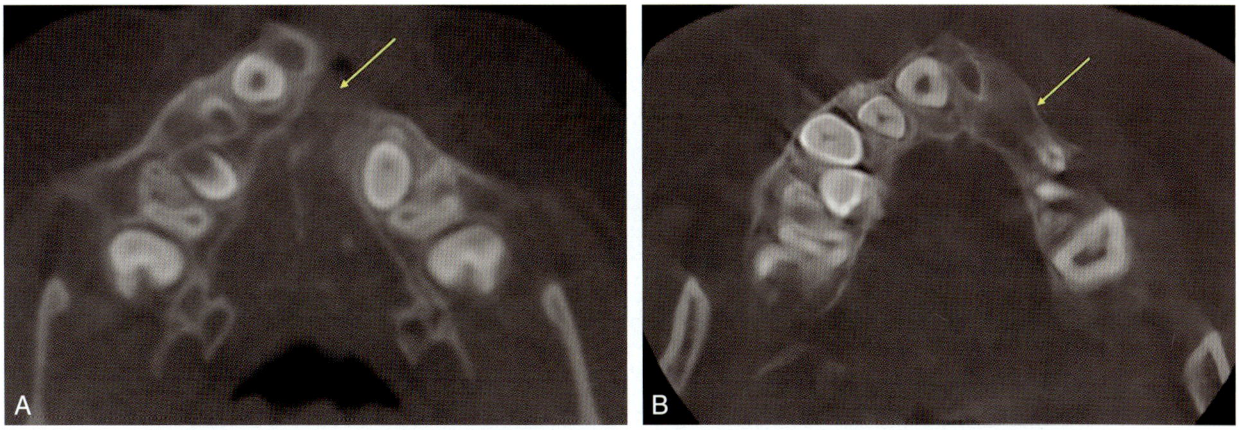

• **Fig. 7.45** Imaging is required to determine success of alveolar bone graft surgery. This small field CBCT was taken to determine graft success. An occlusal film also can be used. (A) Axial slice of the anterior maxilla showing the area of deficient bone in the cleft prior to alveolar bone graft surgery (*yellow arrow*). (B) Axial slice of same area following alveolar bone surgery with a continuous maxilla and successful bone graft.

fills in the grafted cleft as the canine erupts, which makes it possible to close spaces due to missing teeth, and this now is a major objective of this phase of treatment.

If space closure is not possible, orthodontic tooth movement may be needed to position teeth as abutments for eventual fixed prosthodontics. In that circumstance, a resin-bonded bridge that provides a semipermanent replacement for missing teeth can be extremely helpful. Orthodontic treatment is often completed at age 14, but a permanent bridge in many instances cannot be placed until age 17 or 18. The semipermanent fixed bridge is preferable to prolonged use of a removable retainer with a replacement tooth. Alternatively, as patient's age, space can be maintained for future implant placement. In those cases, patients will often need additional bone augmentation prior to implant placement.

Orthognathic Surgery for Patients With Cleft Lip and Palate

In some patients with cleft lip and palate, more often in males than females, continued mandibular growth after the completion of active orthodontic treatment leads to the return of anterior and lateral crossbites. This result is not so much from excessive mandibular growth as from deficient maxillary growth, both anteroposterior and vertically, and it is seen less frequently now because of the improvements in cleft lip and palate surgery in recent years. Orthognathic surgery to bring the deficient maxilla downward and forward may be a necessary last stage in treatment of a patient with cleft lip or palate, typically at about age 18 if required. Occasionally, surgical mandibular setback also may be needed. After this, the definitive restorative work to replace any missing teeth can be carried out. A pharyngeal flap to control leakage of air through the nose often is needed after maxillary advancement in cleft patients.

There has been a striking decrease in recent years in the number of teenage cleft patients needing either prosthodontic replacement of missing teeth or orthognathic surgery to correct maxillary deficiency. Contemporary palatal surgery minimizes interferences with growth and closure of the space where teeth are missing and is made possible by alveolar grafts in the early mixed dentition. Improvements in the United States have been promoted by and documented in the Americleft program, an organized way to gather data from multiple sites of cleft care so that superior procedures can be selected.[68,69] This program is an excellent example of the way in which good data from treatment outcomes can be used to improve the quality of treatment.

Cleft Palate Only

Of note, cleft palate only can occur in isolation or in the context of a syndrome. The most common syndromes associated with cleft palate only are Pierre Robin Sequence, Stickler Syndrome and 22Q11.2 deletion syndrome. Orthodontic management of children with cleft palate only depends on the severity of the cleft meaning involvement of the soft palate only or the soft and hard palate named Veau 1 and Veau 2 cleft, respectively. Patients with cleft palate only can often have a skeletal class III malocclusion presentation due to maxillary growth restriction secondary to palate repair. These patients should be evaluated for orthodontic care around 7 years of age as a child without a cleft would be evaluated. Management of crowding and class III skeletal appearance can be treated with similar modalities of facemask, class III bone anchored maxillary protraction, camouflage orthodontics or possible orthognathic surgery if a severe skeletal discrepancy persists.

Hemifacial Microsomia

Hemifacial microsomia (HFM) or craniofacial microsomia is characterized by unilateral underdevelopment of the facial structures arising from the first and second brachial arches. Typically, the mandible, maxilla, ear, orbit, soft tissue, or facial nerve can be impacted. Underdevelopment of these structures can disrupt hearing, feeding, and the upper airway. HFM occurs in 1:3000 to 1:5000 live births.[70]

The etiology of the HFM is unknown, but is believed to be caused by ischemia, injury or genetic causes contributing to disruption in structures innervated by cranial nerves V and VII.[71]

From an orthodontic standpoint, the role is intricately tied to the severity of the underdevelopment of the mandible and midface. Changes in occlusion from HFM can be managed with orthodontics alone while more severe cases involve orthognathic surgery in conjunction with orthodontics. If severity of mandibular underdevelopment impacts the airway in infancy, distraction osteogenesis is indicated early in life otherwise infants may require a tracheostomy. The distraction screws and

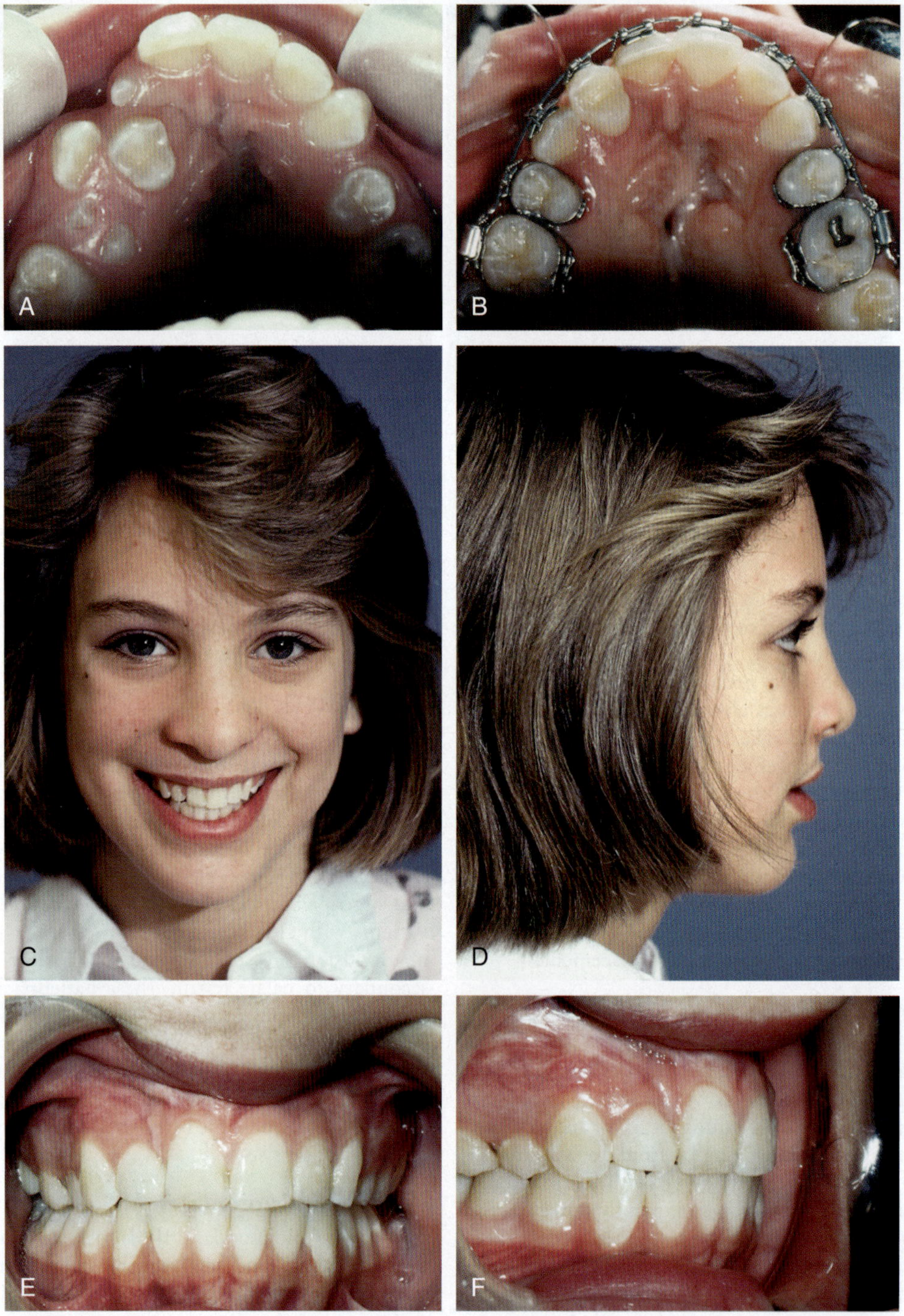

• **Fig. 7.46** Long term observation of a patient with cleft lip and palate. A) Age 11, transposed first premolar erupting in the grafted area. (B) First premolar in lateral incisor position toward the end of active orthodontics, age 12. A tooth that erupts in a grafted area or that is moved orthodontically into the area stimulates formation of new bone that eliminates the cleft and forms a continuous maxilla. (C and D) Facial and (E and F) intraoral photos, age 12. (G and H) Facial and (I and J) intraoral photographs, age 21. At this point the occlusion is stable and both the facial and alveolar cleft can hardly be discerned. Although the palate repair is obvious on intraoral examination, it does not affect appearance or function.

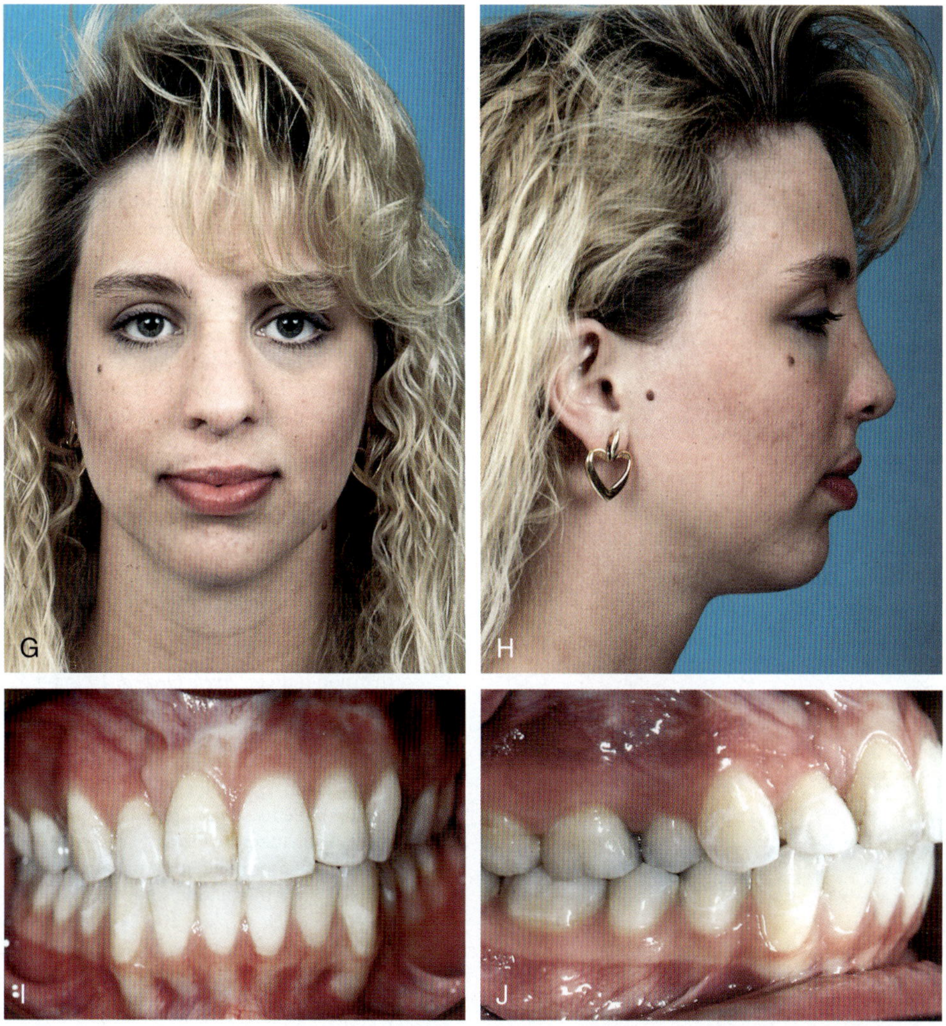

• **Fig. 7.46, cont'd**

plates may impact permanent first molar development. The molars may present with hypoplastic enamel requiring crowns or may not erupt leading to extractions with potential second molar substitution.

Craniosynostosis

Craniosynostosis is characterized by premature fusion of one or more of the cranial sutures leading to abnormal head shape. Craniosynostosis occurs in 1 in 2000 to 2500 live births.[72] Normal cranial sutures fuse between 20 and 30 years of age, except the metopic which fuses during the first year of life. Craniosynostosis has a significant impact on the growing brain as the sutures normally allow for adequate bony protection of the brain and increased head size to accommodate the growing brain.

The majority of craniosynostosis cases fall under the nonsyndromic category. Typically the most common suture affected in nonsyndromic craniosynostosis is the sagittal suture. Roughly, 25% of cases are syndromic, many of which are associated with a mutation in the Fibroblast Growth Factor Receptor. Advances in genetics have identified new mutations associated with craniosynostosis, but the majority have an unknown genetic cause. There are some known environmental causes such as prenatal exposure to teratogens, oligohydramnios, fetal intrauterine constraint and family history.

Craniosynostosis is typically diagnosed within the first year of life. Children with craniosynostosis are often managed by multiple team members including craniofacial surgeons, ophthalmologists, and otolaryngologists.

The role of the orthodontist in treatment of patients with craniosynostosis is key in monitoring dentofacial growth and development, as well as management of crowding. Often, orthodontics is required in conjunction with orthognathic surgery due to maxillary hypoplasia for patients with syndromic craniosynostosis. These patients may require Lefort III distraction to help with eye support and midface retrusion. At skeletal maturity these patients may also require a finishing Lefort I osteotomy to idealize occlusion as the Lefort III procedure is for airway and eyes, and not the occlusion. There can be orthodontic challenges in all three planes of space: anteroposterior, transverse and vertical. For example, some patients, depending on the type of craniosynostosis, can exhibit maxillary retrusion, a steep mandibular plane and an anterior openbite (Fig. 7.47). Appropriate diagnosis and treatment with orthodontics alone or with additional surgical management may be necessary for ideal outcomes depending on severity.

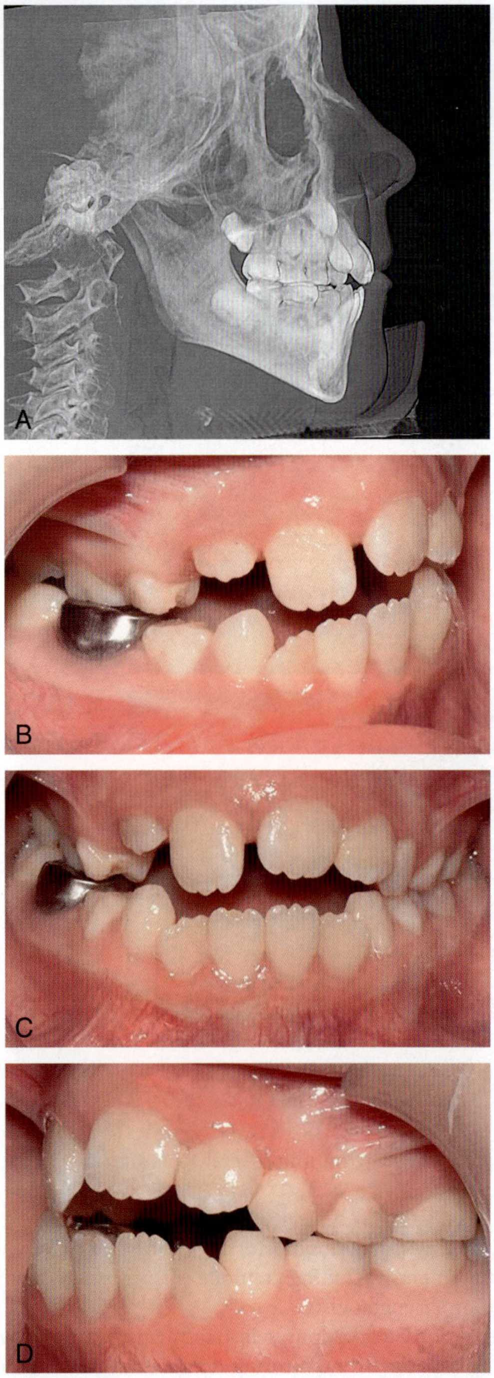

• Fig 7.47 Records from an 8-year-old child with multisuture craniosynostosis. (A) Lateral cephalogram reveals a hyperdivergent, class II skeletal profile with and increased anterior lower face height. (B-D) show the anterior openbite and maxillary constriction, as well as signs of crowding.

References

1. Bowman SJ, Johnston LE. *Angle Orthod*. 2000;70(1):3–10.
2. Hagler BL, Lupini J, Johnston LE. Long-term comparison of extraction and nonextraction alternatives in matched samples of African American patient. *Am J Orthod Dentofac Orthop*. 1998;114:393–403.
3. Paquette DE, Beattie JR, Johnston LE. A long-term comparison of non-extraction and premolar extraction edgewise therapy in "borderline" Class II patients. *Am J Orthod Dentofac Orthop*. 1992;102(1):1–14. https://doi.org/10.1016/0889-5406(92)70009-Y.
4. Meyer AH, Woods MG, Manton DJ. Maxillary arch width and buccal corridor changes with orthodontic treatment. Part 2: attractiveness of the frontal facial smile in extraction and nonextraction outcomes. *Am J Orthod Dentofac Orthop*. 2014;145:296–304.
5. Iared W, Koga da Silva EM, Iared WG, Macedo CM. Esthetic perception of changes in facial profile resulting from orthodontic treatment with extraction of premolars: a systematic review. *J Am Dent Assoc*. 2017;148:9–16.
6. Anthony A, Gianelly AA. Leeway space and the resolution of crowding in the mixed dentition. *SemOrthod*. 1995;1(3):188–194.
7. Little RM. Stability and relapse: early treatment of arch length deficiency. *Am J Orthod Dentofac Orthop*. 2002;121(6):578–581.
8. Dugoni SA, Lee JS, Varela J, Dugoni AA. Early mixed dentition treatment: postretention evaluation of stability and relapse. *Angle Orthod*. 1995;65(5):311–320.
9. BeGole EA, Fox DL, Sadowsky C. Analysis of change in arch form with premolar expansion. *Am J Orthod Dentofac Orthop*. 1998;113(3):307–315. https://doi.org/10.1016/s0889-5406(98)70302-6.
10. Betts NJ, Vanarsdall RJ, Barber HD, et al. Diagnosis and treatment of transverse maxillary deficiency. *Int J Adult Orthodon Orthognath Surg*. 1995;10:75–96.
11. Nimkarn Y, Miles PG, O'Reilly MT, et al. The validity of maxillary expansion indices. *Angle Orthod*. 1995;65:321–326.
12. Phillips C, Hill BJ, Cannac C. The influence of video imaging on patients' perceptions and expectations. *Angle Orthod*. 1995;65:263–270.
13. Chamberland S, Proffit WR, Chamberland PE. Genioplasty in growing patients. *Angle Orthod*. 2015;85:360–373.
14. Troy BA, Shanker S, Fields HW, Vig KWL, Johnston W. A comparison of incisor inclination in patients with Class III malocclusion treated with orthognathic surgery or orthodontic camouflage. *Am J Orthod Dentofac Orthop*. 2009;135:146. e1-146.e9.
15. Potts B, Shanker S, Fields HW, Vig KWL, Beck FM. Description of dental and skeletal changes associated with Class II surgical-orthodontic treatment. *Am J Orthod Dentofac Orthop*. 2009;135(5):566. e1-7; discussion 566-7.
16. Springer NC, Chang C, Fields HW, et al. Smile esthetics from the patients' perspective. *Am J Orthod Dentofac Orthop*. 2011;139:e91–e101.
17. Dickens S, Sarver DM, Proffit WR. The dynamics of the maxillary incisor and the upper lip: a cross-sectional study of resting and smile hard tissue characteristics. *World J Orthod*. 2002;3:313–320.
18. Parekh S, Fields HW, Beck FM, Rosenstiel S. Acceptability of Variations in the Smile Arc and Buccal Corridor Space. *Orthod Craniofac Res*. 2007;10:15–21.
19. Benedetto AV. Asymmetrical smiles corrected by botulinum toxin serotype A. *Dermatol Surg*. 2007;33(1 Spec No.):S32–S36. https://doi.org/10.1111/j.1524-4725.2006.32329.x.
20. Kokich VO, Kinzer GA. Managing congenitally missing lateral incisors. Part I. Canine substitution. *J Esthet Restor Dent*. 2005;17:5–10.
21. Alexander R. Readability of published dental educational materials. *J Am Dent Assoc*. 2000;131:937–942.
22. Scott, Brian. "Readability Calculator." ReadabilityFormulas.com, 17 Aug. 2024, https://readabilityformulas.com/free-readability-calculators/.
23. Miller G. The magical number seven plus or minus two: some limits on our capacity for processing information. *Psychol Rev*. 1956;63(2):81–97.
24. Pawlak CE, Fields HW Jr, Beck FM, Firestone AR. Orthodontic informed consent considering information load and serial position effect. *Am J Orthod Dentofac Orthop*. 2015;147(3):363–372.
25. Hadden KB, Prince LY, Moore TD, James LP, Holland JR, Trudeau CR. Improving readability of informed consents for research at an academic medical institution. *J Clin Transl Sci*. 2017;1(6):361–365. https://doi.org/10.1017/cts.2017.312. PMID: 29707258; PMCID: PMC5915809.

26. National Center for Education Statistics. National Assessments of Adult Literacy (NAAL). https://nces.ed.gov/naal/index.asp
27. Agency for Healthcare Research and Quality, Health Literacy Universal Precautions Toolkit, 3rd edition. *Use the Teach-Back Method: Tool #5*. Content last reviewed September 2020. https://www.ahrq.gov/health-literacy/improve/precautions/tool5.html.
28. Kutner M, Greenberg E, Jin Y, et al. *The Health Literacy of America's Adults: Results From the 2003 National Assessment of Adult Literacy*. US Department of Education, National Center for Education Statistics. NCES; 2006:483.
29. Carr KM, Fields Jr HW, Beck FM, et al. Impact of verbal explanation and modified consent materials on orthodontic informed consent. *Am J Orthod Dentofac Orthop*. 2012;141:174–186.
30. Desman AR, Fields HW, Ni Ai, Robinson FG, Skulski B, Firestone AR, Heinlein D. Rehearsal's effect on long-term recall and comprehension of orthodontic informed consent. *Am J Orthod Dentofac Orthop*. 2021:e1–e13. https://doi.org/10.1016/j.ajodo.2021.06.013.
31. Bandura A, Barbaranelli C, Capara GV, et al. Self-efficacy beliefs as shapers of children's aspirations and career trajectories. *Child Dev*. 2001;72:187–206.
32. Long H, Wang Y, Jian F, Liao LN, Yang X, Lai WL. Current advances in orthodontic pain. *Int J Oral Sci*. 2016;8(2):67–75. https://doi.org/10.1038/ijos.2016.24. PMID: 27341389; PMCID: PMC4932774.
33. Weltman B, Vig, et al.Fields HW, et al. Root resorption associated with orthodontic tooth movement: A systematic review. *Am J Orthod Dentofac Orthop*. 2010;137:462–476.
34. Sundararaj D, Venkatachalapathy S, Tandon A, Pereira A. Critical evaluation of incidence and prevalence of white spot lesions during fixed orthodontic appliance treatment: A meta-analysis. *J Int Soc Prev Community Dent*. 2015;5(6):433–439. https://doi.org/10.4103/2231-0762.167719. PMID: 26759794; PMCID: PMC 4697225.
35. Xie Z, Yu L, Li S, et al. Comparison of therapies of white spot lesions: a systematic review and network meta-analysis. *BMC Oral Health*. 2023;23:346. https://doi.org/10.1186/s12903-023-03076-x.
36. AAOIC eNews. Manage malpractice exposure in orthognathic surgery cases. *eNews Fall* 2019. https://aaoic.com/aaoic-enews-fall-2019.
37. Llamas-Carreras JM, Amarilla A, Solano E, et al. Study of external root resorption during orthodontic treatment in root filled teeth compared with their contralateral teeth with vital pulps. *Int Endod J*. 2010;43:654–662.
38. Stostrup P, Kristensen KD, Kuseler A, et al. Reduced mandibular growth in experimental arthritis in the TM joint treated with intra-articular corticosteroids. *Eur J Orthod*. 2008;30:111–119.
39. Marcus CL, Moore RH, Rosen CL, et al. A randomized trial of adenotonsillectomy for childhood sleep apnea. *N Engl J Med*. 2013;368(25):2366–2376.
40. Camacho M, Chang ET, Song SA, Abdullatif J, Zaghi S, Pirelli P, et al. Rapid maxillary expansion for pediatric obstructive sleep apnea: A systematic review and meta-analysis. *Laryngoscope*. 2017;127(7):1712–1719. https://doi.org/10.1002/lary.26352.
41. Fernández-Barriales M, Lafuente-Ibáñez de Mendoza I, Alonso-Fernández Pacheco JJ, Aguirre-Urizar JM. Rapid maxillary expansion versus watchful waiting in pediatric OSA: A systematic review. *Sleep Med Rev*. 2022 Apr;62:101609. https://doi.org/10.1016/j.smrv.2022.101609. Epub 2022 Feb 11. PMID: 35286895.
42. Quo SD, Hyunh N, Guilleminault C. Bimaxillary expansion therapy for pediatric sleep-disordered breathing. *Sleep Med*. 2017;30:45–51. https://doi.org/10.1016/j.sleep.2016.03.011.
43. Carvalho FR, Lentini-Oliveira DA, Prado LBF, Prado GF, Carvalho LBC. Oral appliances and functional orthopaedic appliances for obstructive sleep apnoea in children. *Cochrane Database Syst Rev*. 2016(Issue 10): https://doi.org/10.1002/14651858.CD005520.pub3. Art. No.: CD005520.
44. Yanyan M, Min Xuemei G. Mandibular advancement appliances for the treatment of obstructive sleep apnea in children: a systematic review and meta-analysis. *Sleep Med*. 2019;60:145–151. https://doi.org/10.1016/j.sleep.2018.12.022.
45. Kaede K, Kato T, Yamaguchi M, Nakamura N, Yamada K, Masuda Y. Effects of lip-closing training on maximum voluntary lip-closing force during lip pursing in healthy young adults. *J Oral Rehabil*. 2016;43:169–175. https://doi.org/10.1111/joor.12358.
46. Huang Y-S, Chuang L-C, Hervy-Auboiron M, Paiva T, Lin C-H, Guilleminault C. Neutral supporting mandibular advancement device with tongue bead for passive myofunctional therapy: a long term follow-up study. *Sleep Med*. 2019;60:69–74. https://doi.org/10.1016/j.sleep.2018.09.013.
47. Bamagoos AA, Sutherland K, Cistulli PA. Mandibular advancement splints. *Sleep Med Clin*. 2016;11(3):343–352. https://doi.org/10.1016/j.jsmc.2016.04.002.
48. Pliska BT, Nam H, Chen H, Lowe AA, Almeida FR. Obstructive sleep apnea and mandibular advancement splints: occlusal effects and progression of changes associated with a decade of treatment. *J Clin Sleep Med*. 2014;10(12):1285–1291. https://doi.org/10.5664/jcsm.4278.
49. Hamoda MM, Almeida FR, Pliska BT. Long-term side effects of sleep apnea treatment with oral appliances: nature, magnitude and predictors of long-term changes. *Sleep Med*. 2019;56:184–191. https://doi.org/10.1016/j.sleep.2018.12.012.
50. Pliska BT, Almeida FR. Tooth movement associated with CPAP Therapy. *J Clin Sleep Med*. 2018;14(4):701–702. https://doi.org/10.5664/jcsm.7080.
51. Islam S, Aleem F, Ormiston IW. Subjective assessment of facial aesthetics after maxillofacial orthognathic surgery for obstructive sleep apnea. *Br J Oral Maxillofac Surg*. 2015;53(3):235–238. https://doi.org/10.1016/j.bjoms.2014.11.018.
52. Wei S, Zhang Y, Guo X, Yu W, Wang M, Yao K, et al. Counterclockwise maxillomandibular advancement: a choice for Chinese patients with severe obstructive sleep apnea. *Sleep Breath*. 2017;21(4):853–860. https://doi.org/10.1007/s11325-017-1484-7.
53. Zaghi S, Holty J-EC, Certal V, Abdullatif J, Guilleminault C, Powell NB, et al. Maxillomandibular advancement for treatment of obstructive sleep apnea a meta-analysis. *JAMA Otolaryngol - Head Neck Surg*. 2016;142:58–66. https://doi.org/10.1001/jamaoto.2015.2678.
54. On SW, Kim HJ, Cho DH, Moon YR, Song IS. Silent changes in sleep quality following mandibular setback surgery in patients with skeletal class III malocclusion: a prospective study. *Nat Publ Group*. 2019;9(1):9737. https://doi.org/10.1038/s41598-019-46166-z.
55. MacKay S, Carney AS, Catcheside PG, Chai-Coetzer CL, Chia M, Cistulli PA, et al. Effect of multilevel upper airway surgery vs medical management on the apnea-hypopnea index and patient-reported daytime sleepiness among patients with moderate or severe obstructive sleep apnea: the SAMS randomized clinical trial. *J Am Med Assoc*. 2020;324(12):1168–1179. https://doi.org/10.1001/jama.2020.14265.
56. Olson MD, Junna MR. Hypoglossal nerve stimulation therapy for the treatment of obstructive sleep apnea. *Neurotherapeutics*. 2021;18(1):91–99. https://doi.org/10.1007/s13311-021-01012-x. Epub 2021 Feb 8. PMID: 33559036; PMCID: PMC8116425.
57. Costantino A, Rinaldi V, Moffa A, et al. Hypoglossal nerve stimulation long-term clinical outcomes: a systematic review and meta-analysis. *Sleep Breath*. 2020;24:399–411. https://doi.org/10.1007/s11325-019-01923-2.
58. Eslami B, Behnia H, Javadi H, et al. Histopathologic comparison of normal and hyperplastic condyles. *Oral Surg Oral Med Oral Pathol Oral Radiol Endod*. 2003;96:711–717.
59. Bennun RD, Harfin JF, Sándor GKB, Genecov D. *Cleft Lip and Palate Management: A Comprehensive Atlas*. John Wiley & Sons; 2015.
60. Bongaarts CAM, Prahl-Andersen B, Bronkhorst EW, et al. Infant orthopedics and facial growth in complete unilateral cleft lip and palate until six years of age (Dutchcleft). *Cleft Palate Craniofac J*. 2009;46:654–663.

61. Peanchitlertkajorn S, Mercado A, Daskalogiannakis J, et al. An inter-center comparison of nasolabial appearance including a center using nasoalveolar molding. *Cleft Palate Craniofac J*. 2018;55(5):655–663.
62. Singer E, Daskalogiannakis J, Russell KA, et al. Burden of care of various infant orthopedic protocols for improvement of naso-labial esthetics in patients with cuclp. *Cleft Palate Craniofac J*. 2018;55(9):1236–1243.
63. Vig KWL, Mercado AM. Overview of orthodontic care for children with cleft lip and palate, 1915-2015. *Am J Orthod Dentofac Orthop*. 2015;148:543–556.
64. Weissler EH, Paine KM, Ahmed MK, Taub PJ. Alveolar bone grafting and cleft lip and palate: a review. *Plast Reconstr Surg*. 2016;138:1287–1295.
65. Garib D, Lauris RC, Calil LR, et al. Dentoskeletal outcomes of a rapid maxillary expander with differential opening in patients with bilateral cleft lip and palate: a prospective clinical trial. *Am J Orthod Dentofac Orthop*. 2016;150:564–574.
66. Boyne PJ, Sands NR. Secondary bone grafting of residual alveolar and palatal clefts. *J Oral Surg*. 1972;30(2):87–92.
67. Precious DS. A new reliable method for alveolar bone grafting at about 6 years of age. *J Oral Maxillofac Surg*. 2009;67(10):2045–2053.
68. Long Jr RE, Hathaway R, Daskalogiannakis J, et al. The Americleft study: an inter-center study of treatment outcomes with unilateral cleft and palate, part 5. General discussion and conclusions. *Cleft Palate Craniofac J*. 2011;48:265–270.
69. Ruppel K, Long Jr RE, Oliver DR, et al. The Americleft project: a comparison of short- and longer-term secondary bone graft out-comes in two centers using the standardized way to assess grafts scale. *Cleft Palate Craniofac J*. 2016;53:508–515.
70. Rooijers W, Tio PAE, van der Schroeff MP, Padwa BL, Dunaway DJ, Forrest CR, Koudstaal MJ, Caron CJJM. Hearing impairment and ear anomalies in craniofacial microsomia: a systematic review. *Int J Oral Maxillofac Surg*. 2022;51(10):1296–1304.
71. Birgfeld CB, Heike C. Craniofacial microsomia. *Semin Plast Surg*. 2012;26(2):91–104.
72. Greenwood J, Flodman P, Osann K, Boyadjiev SA, Kimonis V. Familial incidence and associated symptoms in a population of individuals with nonsyndromic craniosynostosis. *Genet Med*. 2014;16(4):302–310.

SECTION 3

Biomechanics, Mechanics, and Contemporary Orthodontic Appliances

Orthodontic therapy depends on the reaction of the teeth, and more generally the facial structures, to gentle but persistent force. In an orthodontic context, *biomechanics* is commonly used in discussions of the reaction of the dental and facial structures to orthodontic force, whereas *mechanics* is reserved for the properties of the strictly mechanical components of the appliance system. In this section, the biologic responses to orthodontic force that underlie biomechanics are discussed in Chapter 8, and the potential for various drugs to either inhibit or accelerate the rate of tooth movement is reviewed. Other proposed methods to accelerate tooth movement by impacting the biology are also evaluated. Chapter 9, which is concerned with the design and application of orthodontic appliances, is largely devoted to mechanics but also includes some biomechanical considerations and introduces the application of temporary skeletal anchorage. The ways that foundation biomechanical principles can be applied to both fixed and removable appliances are emphasized, including the use of clear aligners.

Contemporary orthodontic treatment involves the use of both fixed and removable appliances. The first part of Chapter 10 describes all types of removable appliances that are used in clinical care and outlines the considerations that are important in clear aligner therapy. The section on growth modification includes a discussion on the components approach to designing functional appliances for individual patients.

In the early decades of the 21st century there have been major changes in fixed appliances, and these are reviewed in the second part of Chapter 10. The principle of the edgewise appliance, control of tooth movement via rectangular archwires in a rectangular slot, remains the basis of contemporary fixed appliance therapy, but changes in brackets and archwire fabrication are occurring as computer-aided design/computer-aided manufacturing (CAD/CAM) design and production become more and more important. The major problems that limited the use of fixed lingual appliances have largely been overcome. Skeletal anchorage, based on both multiscrew miniplates and alveolar bone screws, has quickly become an important part of contemporary treatment. A major goal of Chapter 10 and the subsequent chapters on comprehensive treatment is to evaluate these changes in appliances in the context of data for clinical outcomes with their use.

8

The Biologic Basis of Orthodontic Therapy

BRENT E. LARSON, MATTHEW E. LARSON, AND WILLIAM R. PROFFIT

CHAPTER OUTLINE

Periodontal and Bone Response to Normal Function

Orthodontic movement of teeth is based on the observation that if prolonged light pressure is applied to a tooth, tooth movement will occur as the bone around the tooth remodels. Bone is selectively removed in some areas and added in others. In essence, the tooth moves through the bone carrying its attachment apparatus with it, as the socket of the tooth migrates. Because the bony response is mediated by the periodontal ligament (PDL), tooth movement is primarily a PDL phenomenon.

Forces applied to the teeth can also affect the pattern of bone apposition and resorption at sites distant from the teeth, particularly the sutures of the maxilla and bony surfaces on both sides of the temporomandibular joint. In addition, it is possible now to apply force to implants in the maxilla or mandible to influence growth at maxillary sutures and at the mandibular condyle, affecting skeletal growth with minimal or no tooth movement. Thus the biologic response to orthodontic therapy includes not only the response of the PDL but also the response of growing areas distant from the dentition. It is not possible to move bones in the same way teeth are moved, because pressure against sutures, synchondroses, or joints does not stimulate similar remodeling of adjacent bone, but it is possible to generate formation of new bone by distraction osteogenesis, and the pattern of skeletal growth can be modified.

In this chapter, the focus is on the response of periodontal structures to orthodontic force, with consideration of potential deleterious effects including enamel decalcification. Growth modification of skeletal areas distant from the dentition as a component of orthodontic treatment is discussed in detail in Chapters 13 and 14, drawing on the background of normal growth provided in Chapters 2 to 4 and etiologic considerations in Chapter 5. Applications of distraction osteogenesis to generate new bone are described in the clinical chapters for children, adolescents, and adults.

Periodontal Ligament Structure and Function

Each tooth is attached to and separated from the adjacent alveolar bone by a heavy collagenous supporting structure, the PDL. Under normal circumstances, the PDL occupies a space approximately 0.2 to 0.4 mm in width around all parts of the root. By far the major component of the ligament is a network of parallel collagenous fibers, inserting into cementum of the root surface on one side and into a relatively dense bony plate, the lamina dura, on the other side. These supporting fibers run at an angle, attaching farther apically on the tooth than on the adjacent alveolar bone. This arrangement, of course, resists the displacement of the tooth expected during normal function (Fig. 8.1).

Although most of the PDL space is taken up with the collagenous fiber bundles that constitute the ligamentous attachment, two other major components of the ligament must be considered. These are (1) the cellular elements, including mesenchymal cells of

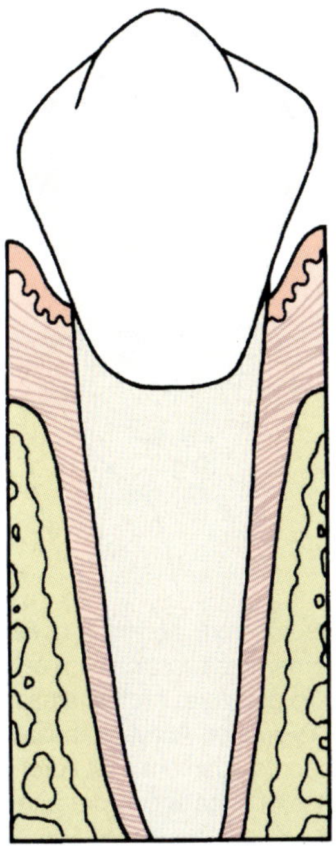

• **Fig. 8.1** Diagrammatic representation of periodontal structures *(pale red)*. Note the angulation of the periodontal ligament fibers.

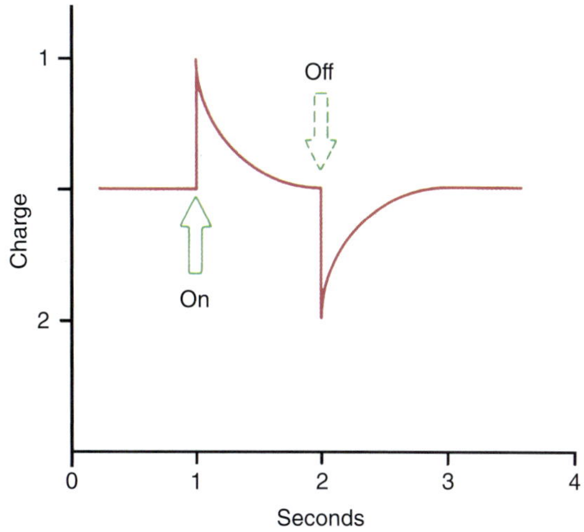

• **Fig. 8.2** Piezoelectricity: When a force is applied to a crystalline structure such as bone or collagen, a flow of current is produced that quickly dies away. When the force is released, an opposite current flow is observed. This piezoelectric effect results from migration of electrons within the crystal lattice as it is distorted by applied force and then returns to its original form when the force is removed.

various types along with vascular and neural elements, and (2) the tissue fluids. Both play an important role in normal function and in making orthodontic tooth movement possible.

The principal cellular elements in the PDL are undifferentiated mesenchymal cells and their progeny in the form of fibroblasts and osteoblasts. The collagen of the ligament is constantly being remodeled and renewed during normal function. The same cells can serve both as fibroblasts, producing new collagenous matrix materials, and fibroclasts, destroying previously produced collagen.[1] Remodeling and recontouring of the bony socket and the cementum of the root is also constantly being carried out, although on a smaller scale, as a response to normal function.

Fibroblasts in the PDL have properties similar to those of osteoblasts, and new alveolar bone probably is formed by osteoblasts that differentiated from the local cellular population. Recent research indicates that differentiation of PDL fibroblasts is dependent on the amount of mechanical strain, and that calcitonin induces this differentiation.[2] Bone and cementum are removed by specialized osteoclasts and cementoclasts, respectively. These multinucleated giant cells are quite different from the osteoblasts and cementoblasts that produce bone and cementum. Despite years of investigation, their origin remains controversial. Most are of hematogenous origin, differentiating within the PDL space from circulating precursor cells; some may be derived from stem cells found in the local area.[3]

Although the PDL is not highly vascular, it does contain blood vessels and cells from the vascular system. Nerve endings are also found within the ligament, both the unmyelinated free endings associated with perception of pain and the more complex receptors associated with pressure and positional information (proprioception).

Finally, it is important to recognize that the PDL space is filled with fluid. This fluid is the same as that found in all other tissues, ultimately derived from the vascular system. A fluid-filled chamber with retentive but porous walls is a description of a shock absorber, and in normal function the fluid allows the PDL space to play just this role.

Response to Normal Function

During masticatory function, the teeth and periodontal structures are subjected to intermittent heavy forces. Tooth contacts last for 1 second or less; forces are quite heavy, ranging from 1 or 2 kg while soft substances are being chewed to as much as 50 kg against a more resistant object. When a tooth is subjected to heavy loads of this type, quick displacement of the tooth within the PDL space is prevented by the incompressible tissue fluid. Instead, the force is transmitted to the alveolar bone, which bends in response.

The extent of bone bending during normal function of the jaws (and other skeletal elements of the body) is often not appreciated. The body of the mandible bends as the mouth is opened and closed, even without heavy masticatory loads. On wide opening, the distance between the mandibular molars decreases by 2 to 3 mm. In heavy function, individual teeth are slightly displaced as the bone of the alveolar process bends to allow this to occur, and bending stresses are transmitted over considerable distances. Bone bending in response to normal function generates piezoelectric currents (Fig. 8.2) that appear to be an important stimulus to skeletal regeneration and repair (see further discussion later in this chapter). This is the mechanism by which bony architecture is adapted to functional demands.

Very little of the fluid within the PDL space is squeezed out during the first second of pressure application. If pressure against a tooth is maintained, however, the fluid is rapidly expressed, and the tooth displaces within the PDL space, compressing the ligament itself against adjacent bone. Not surprisingly, this hurts. Pain is normally felt after 3 to 5 seconds of heavy force application, indicating that the fluids are expressed and crushing pressure is applied against the PDL in this amount of time (Table 8.1). The resistance provided by tissue fluids allows normal mastication, with its force applications of 1 second or less, to occur without pain.

TABLE 8.1 Physiologic Response to Heavy Pressure Against a Tooth

Time (seconds)	Event
<1	PDL fluid incompressible, alveolar bone bends, piezoelectric signal generated
1–2	PDL fluid expressed, tooth moves within PDL space
3–5	PDL fluid squeezed out, tissues compressed; immediate pain if pressure is heavy

PDL, Periodontal ligament.

Although the PDL is beautifully adapted to resist forces of short duration, it rapidly loses its adaptive capability as the tissue fluids are squeezed out of its confined area. Prolonged force, even of low magnitude, produces a different physiologic response—remodeling of the adjacent bone. Orthodontic tooth movement is made possible by the application of prolonged forces. In addition, light prolonged forces in the natural environment—forces from the lips, cheeks, or tongue resting against the teeth—have the same potential as orthodontic forces to cause the teeth to move to a different location (see the discussion of equilibrium factors in Chapter 5).

Role of the Periodontal Ligament in Eruption and Stabilization of the Teeth

The phenomenon of tooth eruption makes it plain that forces generated within the PDL itself can produce tooth movement. After a tooth emerges into the mouth, further eruption depends on metabolic events within the PDL, including but perhaps not limited to formation, cross-linkage, and maturational shortening of collagen fibers (see Chapter 3). This process continues, although at a reduced rate, into adult life. A tooth whose antagonist has been extracted will often begin to erupt again after many years of apparent quiescence.

The continuing presence of this mechanism indicates that it may produce not only eruption of the teeth under appropriate circumstances but also active stabilization of the teeth against prolonged forces of light magnitude. It is commonly observed that light prolonged pressures against the teeth are not in perfect balance, as would seem to be required if tooth movement were not to occur (Fig. 8.3). The ability of the PDL to generate a force and thereby contribute to the set of forces that determine the equilibrium situation probably explains this.

Active stabilization also implies a threshold for orthodontic force, because forces below the stabilization level would be expected to be ineffective. The threshold, of course, would vary depending on the extent to which existing soft tissue pressures were already being resisted by the stabilization mechanism. In some experiments, the threshold for orthodontic force, if one was found at all, appeared to be extremely low. In other circumstances, a somewhat higher threshold, but still one of only a few grams, seems to exist. The current concept is that active stabilization can overcome prolonged forces of a few grams at most, perhaps up to the 5 to 10 g often observed as the magnitude of unbalanced soft tissue resting pressures.

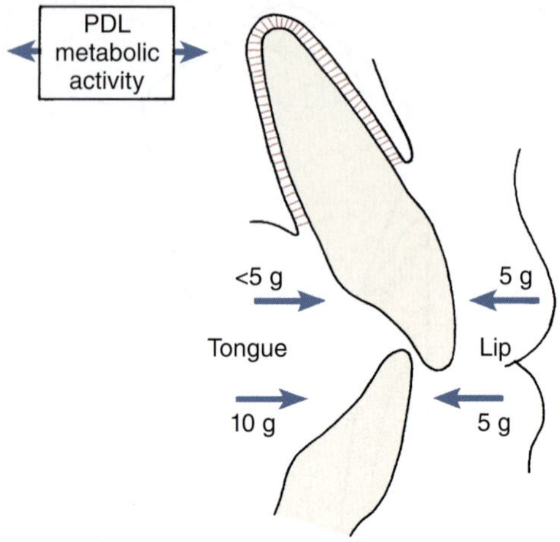

• **Fig. 8.3** Resting pressures from the lips or cheeks and tongue are usually not balanced. In some areas, as in the mandibular anterior, tongue pressure is greater than lip pressure. In other areas, as in the maxillary incisor region, lip pressure is greater. Active stabilization produced by metabolic effects in the periodontal ligament *(PDL)* probably explains why teeth are stable in the presence of imbalanced pressures that would otherwise cause tooth movement.

Periodontal Ligament and Bone Response to Sustained Force

The response to sustained force against the teeth is a function of force magnitude: heavy forces lead to rapidly developing pain, necrosis of cellular elements within the PDL, and the phenomenon (discussed in more detail later) of "undermining resorption" of alveolar bone near the affected tooth. Lighter forces are compatible with survival of cells within the PDL and a remodeling of the tooth socket by a relatively painless "frontal resorption" of the tooth socket. In orthodontic practice, the objective is to produce tooth movement as much as possible by frontal resorption, recognizing that some areas of PDL necrosis and undermining resorption will probably occur despite efforts to prevent this.

Biologic Control of Tooth Movement

Before discussing in detail the response to orthodontic force, it is necessary to consider the biologic control mechanisms that lead from the stimulus of sustained light force to the response of alveolar bone remodeling that allows tooth movement. Two possible control elements, biologic electricity and pressure—tension in the PDL that affects blood flow, are contrasted in the two major theories of orthodontic tooth movement. The bioelectric theory relates tooth movement at least in part to changes in bone metabolism controlled by biologic electricity that are produced by light pressure against the teeth. The pressure-tension theory relates tooth movement to cellular changes produced by chemical messengers, traditionally thought to be generated by alterations in blood flow through the PDL and/or release of chemical messengers from damaged cells in the PDL. Pressure and tension within the PDL, by reducing (pressure) or increasing (tension) the diameter of blood vessels in the ligament space, could certainly alter blood flow, and disruption of cells occurs when soft tissues are stressed. The electricity and chemical messenger theories are neither incompatible nor mutually exclusive, and it appears that both mechanisms may play a part in the biologic control of tooth movement, but chemical messengers play a dominant role.

Biologic Electricity

Electric signals that might initiate tooth movement initially were thought to be piezoelectric. Piezoelectricity is a phenomenon observed in many crystalline materials in which a deformation of the crystal structure created by external force produces a flow of electric current as electrons are displaced from one part of the crystal lattice to another. The piezoelectricity of many inorganic crystals, including those in bone, has been recognized for many years. Organic crystals also can be piezoelectric, and collagen crystals in the PDL have this property.

Piezoelectric signals have two unusual characteristics: (1) a quick decay rate (i.e., when a force is applied, a piezoelectric signal is created in response that quickly dies away to zero even though the force is maintained) and (2) the production of an equivalent signal, opposite in direction, when the force is released (see Fig. 8.2).

Both of these characteristics are explained by the migration of electrons within the crystal lattice as it is distorted by pressure. When the crystal structure is deformed, electrons migrate from one location to another and an electric current flow is observed. As long as the force is maintained, the crystal structure is stable and no further electric events are observed. When the force is released, however, the crystal returns to its original shape, and a reverse flow of electrons is seen. With this arrangement, rhythmic activity would produce a constant interplay of current flows in one direction and then the other that would be measured as amperes, whereas occasional application and release of force would produce only occasional signal of this type.

Ions in the fluids that bathe living bone interact with the complex electric field generated when the bone bends, causing electric signals in the form of volts as well as temperature changes. As a result, both convection and conduction currents can be detected in the extracellular fluids, and the currents are affected by the nature of the fluids. The small voltages that are observed are called the "streaming potential." These voltages, although different from piezoelectric current flows, have in common their rapid onset and alteration as changing stresses are placed on the bone.

There is also a reverse piezoelectric effect. Not only will the application of force cause distortion of crystalline structure and with it an electric signal, but also application of an electric field can cause a crystal to deform and produce force in doing so. Reverse piezoelectricity has no place in natural control systems, at least as far as is presently known, but there are intriguing possibilities for use of external electric fields to promote bone healing and regeneration after injury.[4]

There is no longer any doubt that piezoelectricity is important in the general maintenance of the skeleton. Without such signals, bone mineral is lost and general skeletal atrophy ensues—a situation that has proved troublesome for astronauts, whose bones no longer flex in a weightless environment as they would under normal gravity. Signals generated by the bending of alveolar bone during normal chewing almost surely are important for maintenance of the bone around the teeth.

On the other hand, sustained force of the type used to induce orthodontic tooth movement does not produce piezoelectric or other types of stress-generated signals. As long as the force is sustained, nothing happens. If stress-generated signals were important in producing the bone remodeling associated with orthodontic tooth movement, a vibrating application of pressure would be advantageous. Although earlier experiments indicated little or no advantage in using vibration to generate piezoelectric signals over sustained force for the movement of teeth,[5] this idea was revived in the early 21st century and has been heavily promoted in recent years. It is discussed later in the section of this chapter on possibilities for accelerating tooth movement, where the conclusion still is that vibratory signals have little if anything to do with the response to orthodontic force and the rate of tooth movement.

Electromagnetic fields also can affect cell membrane potentials and permeability and thereby trigger changes in cellular activity. In animal experiments, a pulsed electromagnetic field increased the rate of tooth movement, apparently by shortening the initial "lag phase" before tooth movement begins,[6] but this has not been demonstrated in human subjects. It was hoped 25 years ago that the fields generated by small magnets attached to the teeth could change the basic biology of the response to force. It is clear now that is not the case. The idea that moving teeth with magnetic force reduces pain and mobility is not supported by evidence and is no longer taken seriously.

Pressure-Tension Effects in the Periodontal Ligament Space

Chemical messengers are known to be important in the cascade of events that lead to remodeling of alveolar bone and tooth movement, and both mechanical compression of tissues and changes in blood flow can cause their release. Because the sequence of chemical changes after orthodontic force is applied does explain the course of events in tooth movement reasonably well, it remains the basis of the following discussion.

There is no doubt that sustained pressure against a tooth causes the tooth to shift position within the PDL space, compressing the ligament in some areas while stretching it in others. The mechanical effects on cells within the ligament cause the release of cytokines, prostaglandins, and other chemical messengers. In addition, blood flow is decreased where the PDL is compressed (Fig. 8.4), while it is maintained or increased where the PDL is under tension (Fig. 8.5). These alterations in blood flow also quickly create changes in the chemical environment. For instance, oxygen levels decrease on the compressed area and carbon dioxide (CO_2) levels increase, while the reverse occurs on the tension side. These chemical changes, acting either directly or by stimulating the release of other biologically active agents, then would stimulate cellular differentiation and activity. In essence, this view of tooth movement shows three stages: (1) initial compression of tissues and alterations in blood flow associated with pressure within the PDL, (2) the formation and/or release of chemical messengers, and (3) activation of osteoblasts and osteoclasts, leading to remodeling of alveolar bone.

Effects on the Response to Orthodontic Force

Sequence of Events

The heavier the sustained pressure, the greater should be the reduction in blood flow through compressed areas of the PDL, up to the point that the vessels are totally collapsed and no further blood flows (Fig. 8.6). That this theoretical sequence actually occurs has been demonstrated in animal experiments, in which increasing the force against a tooth causes decreasing perfusion of the PDL on the compression side (see Figs. 8.4 and 8.5).[7] Let us consider the time course of events after application of orthodontic force, contrasting what happens with heavy versus light force (Table 8.2).

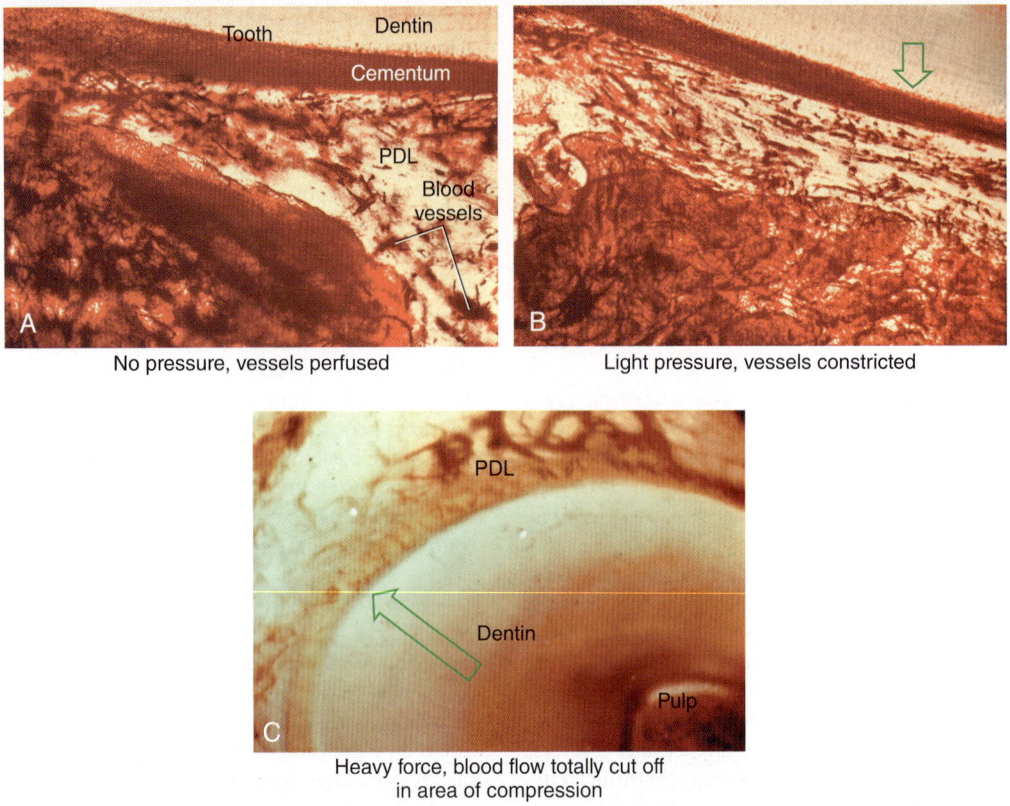

• **Fig. 8.4** In experimental animals, changes in blood flow in the periodontal ligament *(PDL)* can be observed by perfusing India ink into the vascular system while the animal is killed. The vessels are filled with India ink, so their size can be seen easily. (A) Normal perfusion of the PDL. Note the dark areas indicating blood flow. (B) A 50-g force is compressing the PDL. Note the decreased amount of perfusion, but there still is blood flow through the compressed area. (C) Heavy force with almost complete obliteration of blood flow in the compressed area. This specimen is seen in horizontal section, with the tooth root on the left and the pulp chamber just visible in the upper left. The PDL is below and to the right. Cells disappear in the compressed areas, and the area is sometimes said to be hyalinized because of its resemblance to hyaline cartilage. (Courtesy Dr. F.E. Khouw.)

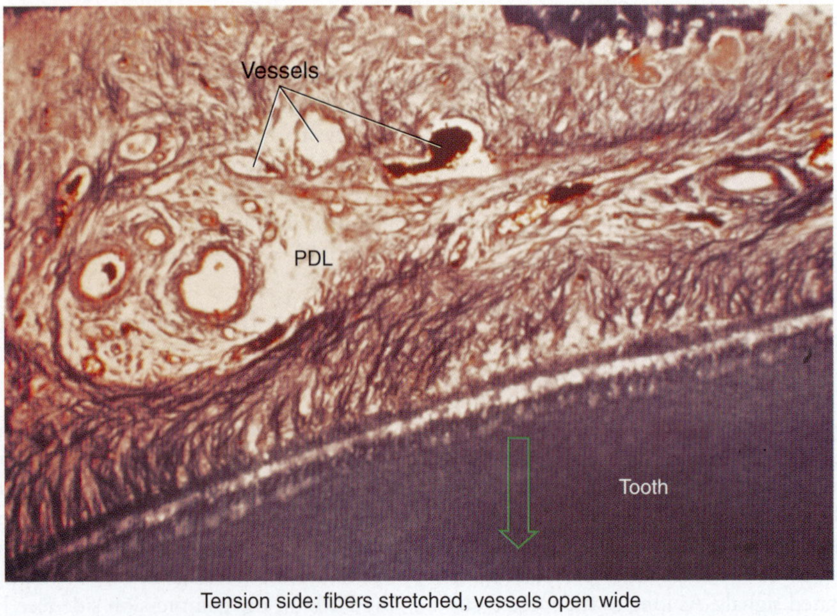

• **Fig. 8.5** On the side away from the direction of tooth movement, the periodontal ligament *(PDL)* space is enlarged and blood vessels dilate. Expanded vessels that are only partially filled can be seen on the tension side of the PDL. (Courtesy Dr. F.E. Khouw.)

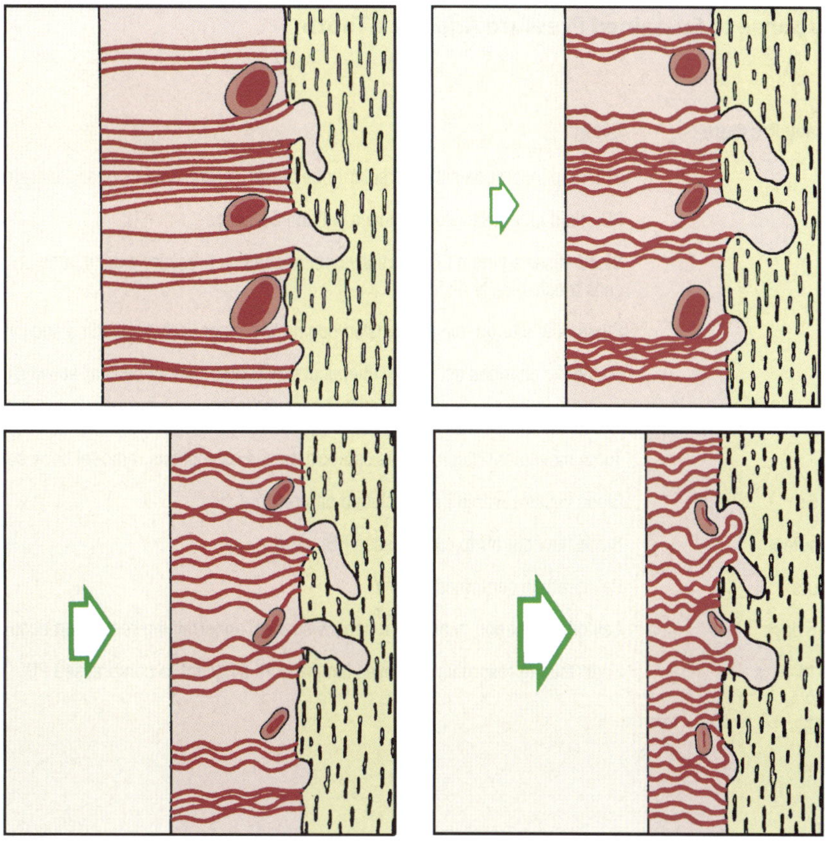

• **Fig. 8.6** Diagrammatic representation of the increasing compression of blood vessels as pressure increases in the periodontal ligament. At a certain magnitude of continuous pressure, blood vessels are totally occluded and a sterile necrosis of periodontal ligament tissue ensues.

When light but prolonged force is applied to a tooth, blood flow through the partially compressed PDL decreases as soon as fluids are expressed from the PDL space and the tooth moves in its socket (i.e., in a few seconds). Within a few hours at most, the resulting change in the chemical environment produces a different pattern of cellular activity. Animal experiments have shown that increased levels of cyclic adenosine monophosphate (cAMP), the "second messenger" for many important cellular functions and cell differentiation, appear after about 4 hours of sustained pressure. This amount of time to produce a response correlates rather well with the human response to removable appliances. If a removable appliance is worn less than 4 to 6 hours per day, it will produce no orthodontic effects. Above this duration threshold, tooth movement does occur.

What happens in the first hours after sustained force is placed against a tooth, between the onset of pressure and tension in the PDL and the appearance of second messengers a few hours later? Experiments have shown that prostaglandin and interleukin-1 beta levels increase within the PDL within a short time after the application of pressure, and it is clear now that both are important mediators of the cellular response. Because prostaglandins are released when cells are mechanically deformed, it appears that prostaglandin release is a primary rather than a secondary response to pressure. At the molecular level, we are beginning to understand how these effects are created. Focal adhesion kinase (FAK) appears to be the mechanoreceptor in PDL cells, and its compression is at least part of the reason that prostaglandin E_2 (PgE_2) is released.[8] Experiments have shown that concentrations of the receptor activator of nuclear factor kappa-B ligand (RANKL) and osteoprotegerin (OPG) in gingival crevicular fluid increase during orthodontic tooth movement, which suggests that PDL cells under stress may induce the formation of osteoclasts through upregulation of RANKL.[9] Other chemical messengers, particularly members of the cytokine family but also nitric oxide (NO) and other regulators of cellular activity, also are involved. Because drugs of various types can affect both prostaglandin levels and other potential chemical messengers, pharmacologic modification of the response to orthodontic force is more than just a theoretical possibility (see further discussion later).

For a tooth to move, osteoclasts must be formed so that they can remove bone from the area adjacent to the compressed part of the PDL. Osteoblasts also are needed to form new bone on the tension side and remodel resorbed areas on the pressure side. Prostaglandins have the interesting property of stimulating both osteoclastic and osteoblastic activity, making them particularly suitable as a mediator of tooth movement. If parathyroid hormone is injected, osteoclasts can be induced in only a few hours, but the response is much slower when mechanical deformation of the PDL is the stimulus, and it can be up to 48 hours before the first osteoclasts appear within and adjacent to the compressed PDL. Studies of cellular kinetics indicate that they arrive in two waves, implying that some (the first wave) may be derived from a local cell population, whereas others (the larger second wave) are brought in from distant areas via blood flow.[10] These cells attack the lamina dura, the layer of dense bone on the outer wall of the tooth socket, removing bone in the process of "frontal resorption,"

TABLE 8.2 Physiologic Response to Sustained Pressure Against a Tooth

TIME		
Light Pressure	**Heavy Pressure**	**Event**
<1 s		PDL fluid incompressible, alveolar bone bends, piezoelectric signal generated
1–2 s		PDL fluid expressed, tooth moves within PDL space
3–5 s		Blood vessels within PDL partially compressed on pressure side, dilated on tension side; PDL fibers and cells mechanically distorted
Minutes		Blood flow altered, oxygen tension begins to change; prostaglandins and cytokines released
Hours		Metabolic changes occurring: chemical messengers affect cellular activity, enzyme levels change
~4 h		Increased cAMP levels detectable, cellular differentiation begins within PDL
~2 days		Tooth movement beginning as osteoclasts and osteoblasts remodel bony socket
	3–5 s	Blood vessels within PDL occluded on pressure side
	Minutes	Blood flow cut off to compressed PDL area
	Hours	Cell death in compressed area
	3–5 days	Cell differentiation in adjacent narrow spaces, undermining resorption begins
	7–14 days	Undermining resorption removes lamina dura adjacent to compressed PDL, tooth movement occurs

cAMP, Cyclic adenosine monophosphate; *PDL*, periodontal ligament.

and tooth movement begins soon thereafter. At the same time, but lagging somewhat behind so that the PDL space becomes enlarged, osteoblasts (recruited locally from progenitor cells in the PDL) form bone on the tension side and begin remodeling activity on the pressure side.[11]

The course of events is different if the sustained force against the tooth is great enough to totally occlude blood vessels and cut off the blood supply to an area within the PDL. When this happens, rather than cells within the compressed area of the PDL being stimulated, a sterile necrosis ensues within the compressed area. In clinical orthodontics it is difficult to avoid pressure that produces at least some avascular areas in the PDL, and it has been suggested that releasing pressure against a tooth at intervals, while maintaining the pressure for enough hours to produce the biologic response, could help in maintaining tissue vitality. This seems to be the mechanism by which chewing on a plastic wafer or chewing gum after orthodontic force is applied reduces pain—chewing force briefly displaces the tooth and allows a spurt of blood into compressed areas, thereby reducing the size of necrotic areas in the PDL.

Because of its histologic appearance as the cells disappear, an avascular area in the PDL traditionally has been referred to as *hyalinized* (see Fig. 8.4). Despite the name, the process has nothing to do with the formation of hyaline connective tissue. It represents the inevitable loss of all cells when the blood supply is totally cut off. When this happens, remodeling of bone bordering the necrotic area of the PDL must be accomplished by cells derived from adjacent undamaged areas.

After a delay of several days, cellular elements begin to invade the necrotic (hyalinized) area. More importantly, osteoclasts appear within the adjacent bone marrow spaces and begin an attack on the underside of the bone immediately adjacent to the necrotic PDL area (Fig. 8.7). This process is appropriately described as *undermining resorption*, because the attack is from the underside of the lamina dura. When hyalinization and undermining resorption occur, an inevitable delay in tooth movement results. This is caused first by a delay in stimulating differentiation of cells within the marrow spaces, and second because a considerable thickness of bone must be removed from the underside before any tooth movement can take place. The different time course of tooth movement when frontal resorption is compared with undermining resorption is shown graphically in Fig. 8.8.

Not only is tooth movement more efficient when areas of PDL necrosis are avoided, but pain is also lessened. However, even with light forces, small avascular areas are likely to develop in the PDL, and tooth movement will be delayed until these can be removed by undermining resorption. The smooth progression of tooth movement with light force shown in Fig. 8.8 may be an unattainable ideal when continuous force is used. In clinical practice, tooth movement usually proceeds in a more stepwise fashion because of the inevitable areas of undermining resorption.

Effects of Force Distribution

From the previous discussion, it is apparent that the optimum force levels for orthodontic tooth movement should be just high enough to stimulate cellular activity without completely occluding blood vessels in the PDL. Both the amount of force delivered to a tooth and the area of the PDL over which that force is distributed are important in determining the biologic effect. The PDL response is determined not by force alone, but by force per unit area, or pressure. Because the distribution of force within the PDL, and therefore the pressure, differs with different types of tooth movement, it is necessary to specify the type of tooth movement as well as the amount of force in discussing optimum force levels for orthodontic purposes.

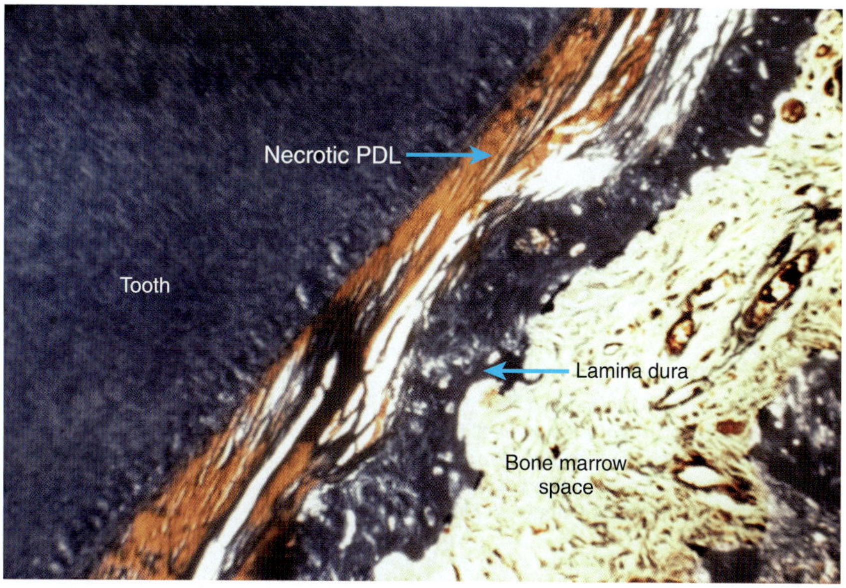

• **Fig. 8.7** Histologic specimen of compressed periodontal ligament *(PDL)* area after several days. When the PDL is compressed to the point that blood flow is totally cut off, differentiation of osteoclasts within the PDL space is not possible. After a delay of several days, osteoclasts within adjacent marrow spaces attack the underside of the lamina dura in the process called *undermining resorption*. The scalloped underside seen in this image indicates active osteoclast activity against that area. (Courtesy Dr. F.E. Khouw.)

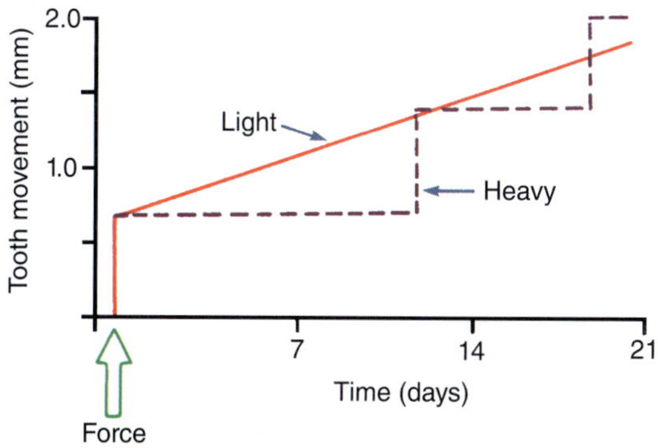

• **Fig. 8.8** Diagrammatic representation of the time course of tooth movement with frontal resorption versus undermining resorption. With frontal resorption, a steady attack on the outer surface of the lamina dura results in smooth continuous tooth movement. With undermining resorption, there is a delay until the bone adjacent to the tooth can be removed. At that point, the tooth "jumps" to a new position, and if heavy force is maintained, there will again be a delay until a second round of undermining resorption can occur.

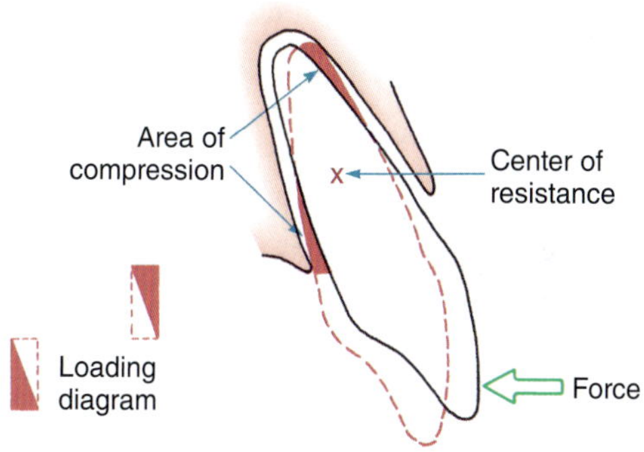

• **Fig. 8.9** Application of a single force to the crown of a tooth creates rotation around a point approximately halfway down the root. Heavy pressure is felt at the root apex and at the crest of the alveolar bone, but pressure decreases to zero at the center of resistance. The loading diagram therefore consists of two triangles as shown.

The simplest form of orthodontic movement is tipping. Tipping movements are produced when a single force (e.g., a spring extending from a removable appliance) is applied against the crown of a tooth. When this is done, a tipping moment is created, and the tooth rotates around its *center of resistance*, a point located about halfway down the root. (A further discussion of the center of resistance and its control follows in Chapter 9.) When the tooth rotates in this fashion, the PDL is compressed near the root apex on the same side as the spring and at the crest of the alveolar bone on the opposite side from the spring (Fig. 8.9). Maximum pressure in the PDL is created at the alveolar crest and at the root apex. Progressively less pressure is created as the center of resistance is approached, and there is minimum pressure at that point.

In tipping, only one-half of the PDL area that could be loaded actually is. As shown in Fig. 8.9, the "loading diagram" consists of two triangles, covering half of the total PDL area. On the other hand, pressure in the two areas where it is concentrated is high in relation to the force applied to the crown. For this reason, forces used to tip teeth must be kept quite low. Both experiments with animals and clinical experience with humans suggest that tipping forces for a single-rooted tooth should not exceed approximately 50 g, and lighter forces are better for smaller teeth (which have a smaller PDL).

If two forces are applied simultaneously to the crown of a tooth so that there is no net tipping moment, the tooth can be moved bodily (translated)—that is, the root apex and crown move in the

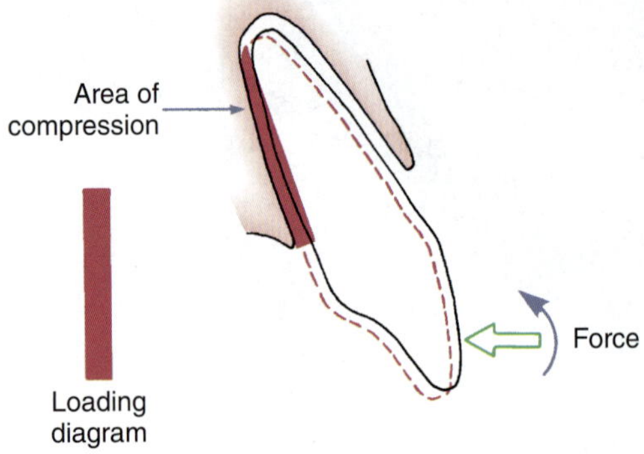

• **Fig. 8.10** Translation or bodily movement of a tooth requires that the periodontal ligament space be loaded uniformly from alveolar crest to apex, creating a rectangular loading diagram. Twice as much force applied to the crown of the tooth would be required to produce the same pressure within the periodontal ligament for bodily movement as compared with tipping.

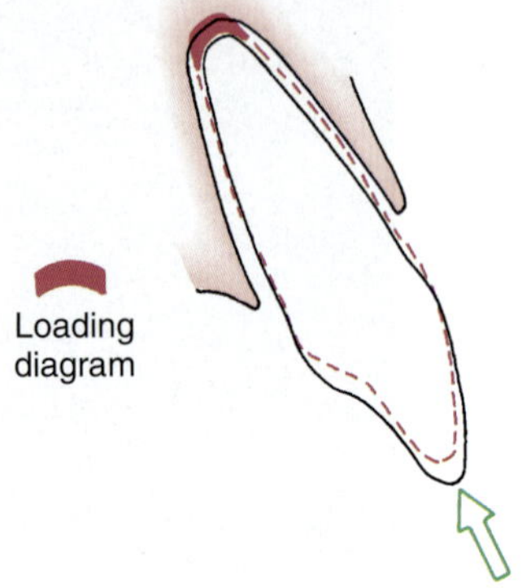

• **Fig. 8.11** When a tooth is intruded, the force is concentrated over a small area at the apex. For this reason, extremely light forces are needed to produce appropriate pressure within the periodontal ligament during intrusion.

TABLE 8.3 Optimum Forces for Orthodontic Tooth Movement

Type of Movement	Force[a] (g)
Tipping	35–60
Bodily movement (translation)	70–120
Root uprighting	50–100
Rotation	35–60
Extrusion	35–60
Intrusion	10–20

[a]Values depend in part on the size of the tooth: smaller values are appropriate for incisors, higher values for multirooted posterior teeth.

same direction the same amount. In this case, the total PDL area is loaded uniformly (Fig. 8.10). It is apparent that to produce the same pressure in the PDL and therefore the same biologic response, twice as much force would be required for bodily movement as for tipping. To move a tooth so that it is partially tipped and partially translated would require forces intermediate between those needed for pure tipping and bodily movement (Table 8.3).

In theory, forces to produce rotation of a tooth around its long axis could be much larger than those to produce other tooth movements, because the force could be distributed over the entire PDL rather than over a narrow vertical strip. In fact, however, it is essentially impossible to apply a rotational force so that the tooth does not also tip in its socket, and when this happens, an area of compression is created just as in any other tipping movement. For this reason, appropriate forces for rotation are similar to those for tipping.

Extrusion and intrusion are also special cases. Extrusive movements ideally would produce no areas of compression within the PDL, only tension. Like rotation, this is more a theoretical than a practical possibility, because if the tooth tipped at all while being extruded, areas of compression would be created. Even if compressed areas could be avoided, heavy forces in pure tension would be undesirable unless the goal was to extract the tooth rather than to bring alveolar bone along with the tooth. Extrusive forces, like rotation, should be about the same magnitude as those for tipping.

For many years, it was considered essentially impossible to produce orthodontic intrusion of teeth. Now it is clear that clinically successful intrusion can be accomplished, but only if very light forces are applied to the teeth. Light force is required for intrusion because the force will be concentrated in a small area at the tooth apex (Fig. 8.11). As with extrusion, the tooth probably will tip somewhat as it is intruded, but the force still will be concentrated at the apex. Only if the force is kept very light can intrusion be expected.

Effects of Force Duration and Force Decay

The key to producing orthodontic tooth movement is the application of sustained force, which does not mean that the force must be absolutely continuous. It does mean that the force must be present for a considerable percentage of the time, certainly hours rather than minutes per day. As we have noted previously, animal experiments suggest that only after force is maintained for approximately 4 hours do cyclic nucleotide levels in the PDL increase, indicating that this duration of pressure is required to produce the "second messengers" needed to stimulate cellular differentiation.

Clinical experience suggests that there is a threshold for force duration in humans in the 4- to 8-hour range and that increasingly effective tooth movement is produced if force is maintained for longer durations. Although no firm experimental data are available, a plot of efficiency of tooth movement as a function of force duration would probably look like Fig. 8.12. Continuous forces, produced by fixed appliances that are not affected by what the patient does, produce more tooth movement than removable appliances unless the removable appliance is present almost all the time. Removable appliances worn for decreasing fractions of time produce decreasing amounts of tooth movement.

Duration of force has another aspect, related to how force magnitude changes as the tooth responds by moving. Only in theory is it possible to make a perfect spring, one that would deliver the same force day after day, no matter how much or how little the tooth moved in response to that force. In reality, some decline in force magnitude (i.e., force decay) is noted with even the springiest device after the tooth has moved a short distance (although with the superelastic nickel–titanium materials discussed in Chapter 9,

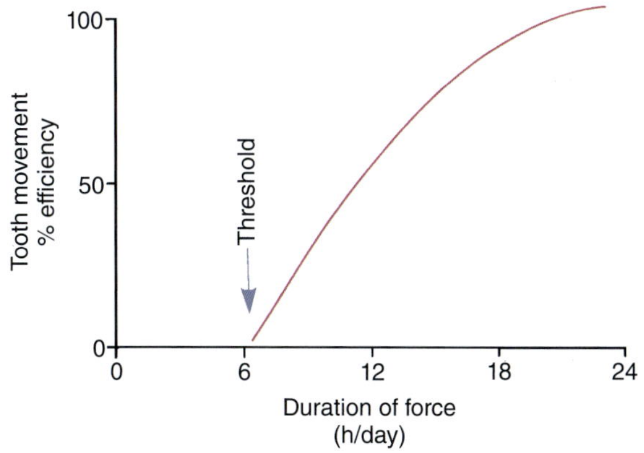

• **Fig. 8.12** Theoretical plot of tooth movement efficiency versus duration of force in hours per day. Continuous force, 24 h/day, produces the most efficient tooth movement, but successful tooth movement can be produced by shorter durations, with a threshold at about 6 hours.

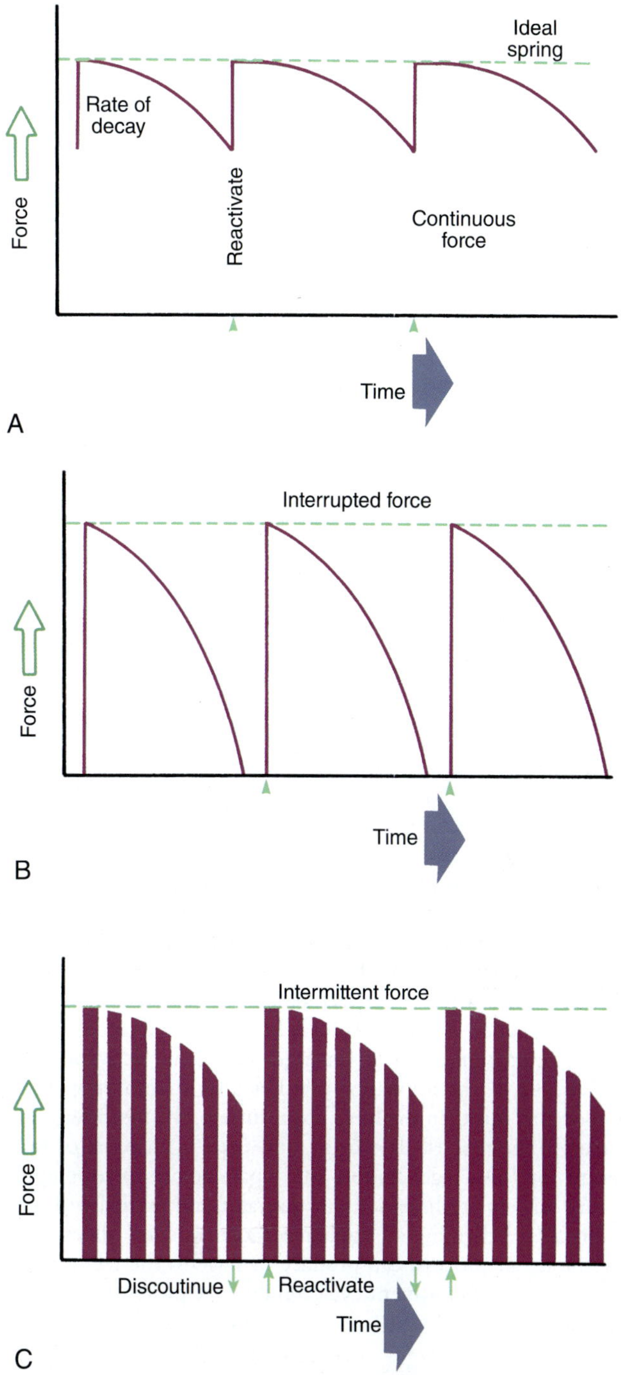

• **Fig. 8.13** Diagrammatic representation of force decay. (A) An ideal spring would maintain the same amount of force regardless of distance a tooth had moved, but with real springs the force decays at least somewhat as tooth movement occurs. Forces that are maintained between activations of an orthodontic appliance, even though the force declines, are defined as continuous. (B) In contrast, interrupted forces drop to zero between activations. (C) Intermittent forces fall to zero when a removable appliance is taken out, only to resume when the appliance is reinserted into the mouth. These forces also decay as tooth movement occurs.

the decrease is amazingly small). With many orthodontic devices, the force may drop all the way to zero. From this perspective, orthodontic force duration is classified (Fig. 8.13) by the rate of decay as:

- Continuous—force maintained at some appreciable fraction of the original from one patient visit to the next
- Interrupted—force levels decline to zero between activations

Both continuous and interrupted forces can be produced by fixed appliances that are constantly present.

- Intermittent—force levels decline abruptly to zero intermittently, when a removable orthodontic appliance or elastic traction to a fixed appliance is removed by the patient, and then return to the original level some time later when the appliance is reinserted or the elastics are replaced. When tooth movement occurs, force levels with a removable appliance will decrease as they would with a fixed appliance (i.e., force decay occurs, often all the way to zero before the removable appliance is reactivated). It is quite possible, therefore that intermittent force can also be interrupted.

Intermittent forces are produced by all removable appliances such as clear aligners, functional appliances, headgear, and elastics. Forces generated during normal function (e.g., chewing, swallowing, speaking) can be viewed as a special case of intermittently applied forces, most of which are not maintained for enough hours per day to have significant effects on the position of the teeth.

There is an important interaction between force magnitude and how rapidly the force declines as the tooth responds. Consider first the effect of a nearly continuous force. If this force is quite light, a relatively smooth progression of tooth movement will result from frontal resorption. If the continuous force is heavy, however, tooth movement will be delayed until undermining resorption can remove the bone necessary to allow the tooth movement. At that time, the tooth will change its position rapidly, and the constant force will again compress the tissues, preventing repair of the PDL and creating the need for further undermining resorption and so on. Such a heavy continuous force can be quite destructive to both the periodontal structures and the tooth itself.

Consider now the effect of forces that decay fairly rapidly, so that the force declines to zero after the tooth moves only a short distance. If the initial force level is relatively light, the tooth will move a small amount by frontal resorption and then will remain in that position until the appliance is activated again. If the force level is heavy enough to produce undermining resorption, the tooth will move when the undermining resorption is complete. Then, because the force has dropped to zero at that point, it will remain in that position until the next activation. Although the original force is heavy, after the tooth moves there is a period for regeneration and repair of the PDL before force is applied again.

Theoretically, there is no doubt that light continuous forces produce the most efficient tooth movement. Despite the clinician's best efforts to keep forces light enough to produce only frontal resorption, some areas of undermining resorption are probably produced in every clinical patient. The heavier forces that produce this response are physiologically acceptable only if the force level quickly drops to zero so that there is a period of repair and regeneration before the next activation or if the force decreases at least to the point that no second and third rounds of undermining resorption occur.

The bottom line: heavy continuous forces are to be avoided; heavy intermittent forces, although less efficient, can be clinically acceptable. To say it another way: the more perfect the spring in the sense of its ability to provide continuous force, the more careful the clinician must be that only light force is applied. Some of the cruder springs used in orthodontic treatment have the paradoxical virtue of producing forces that rapidly decline to zero and are thus incapable of inflicting the biologic damage that can occur from heavy continuous forces. Several clinical studies have indicated that heavy force applications may produce more tooth movement than lighter force, which can be understood only from consideration of force decay characteristics.

Experience has shown that orthodontic appliances should not be reactivated more frequently than at 3-week intervals. A 4- to 6- or 8-week appointment cycle is the usual minimum in clinical practice, and now a 6- or 8-week cycle is more typical. Undermining resorption requires 7 to 14 days (longer on the initial application of force, shorter thereafter). When this is the mode of tooth movement and when force levels decline rapidly, tooth movement is essentially complete in this length of time. The wisdom of the interval between adjustments now becomes clear. If the appliance is springy and light forces produce continuous frontal resorption, there is no need for further activation for 6 to 8 weeks. If the appliance is stiffer and undermining resorption occurs, but then the force drops to zero, the tooth movement occurs in the first 10 days or so, and there is an equal or longer period for PDL regeneration and repair before force is applied again. This repair phase is highly desirable and needed with many appliances. Activating an appliance too frequently, short-circuiting the repair process, can produce damage to the teeth or bone that a longer appointment cycle would have prevented or at least minimized.

Drug Effects on the Response to Orthodontic Force

At present, drugs that stimulate tooth movement are unlikely to be encountered, although efforts to produce them continue. A major problem is how they would be applied to the local area where an effect on tooth movement is desired. Direct injection of prostaglandin into the PDL has been shown to increase the rate of tooth movement, but this is quite painful (a bee sting is essentially an injection of prostaglandin) and not very practical. Relaxin, a "pregnancy hormone" discovered in the 1980s, facilitates birth by causing a softening and lengthening of the cervix and pubic symphysis. It works by simultaneously reducing collagen synthesis and increasing collagen breakdown. Preliminary data in rats showed faster tooth movement with relaxin treatment, but a well-done, double-blinded clinical trial at the University of Florida, in which relaxin or just physiologic saline was injected adjacent to a tooth to be moved, did not show a consistent positive effect,[12] and further clinical trials were abandoned.

In the future, it is possible that drugs to facilitate tooth movement will become clinically useful—but there is no way to know how long it will take to develop them. Drugs aimed at increasing brain levels of acetylcholine (ACH), the key neurotransmitter in the brain, now are widely used to maintain neural function in patients with cognitive decline. Such drugs (e.g., donepezil [Aricept]) have widespread effects on other bodily functions, and perhaps might accelerate tooth movement by affecting circulating hormone levels. There is no solid information as to the effect of these powerful drugs on PDL activity, but given their effect on brain activity, using them to affect tooth movement would be hard to justify. The problem, of course, is to find something that primarily works locally.

Drugs that inhibit tooth movement as a side effect of their use for other problems, however, already are encountered frequently, although not yet prescribed for their tooth-stabilizing effect. Two types of drugs are known to depress the response to orthodontic force and may influence current treatment: prostaglandin inhibitors for pain control (especially the more potent members of this group that are used in treatment of arthritis, such as indomethacin), and the bisphosphonates used in treatment of osteoporosis (e.g., alendronate [Fosamax], ibandronate [Boniva], risedronate [Actonel]).

Nonsteroidal Antiinflammatory Drugs and Other Prostaglandin Inhibitors

If PgE plays an important role in the cascade of signals that leads to tooth movement, one would expect inhibitors of its activity to affect tooth movement. Drugs that affect prostaglandin activity fall into two categories: (1) corticosteroids and nonsteroidal antiinflammatory drugs (NSAIDs) that interfere with prostaglandin synthesis and (2) other agents that have mixed agonistic and antagonistic effects on various prostaglandins.

In the body, prostaglandins are formed from arachidonic acid, which in turn is derived from phospholipids. Corticosteroids reduce prostaglandin synthesis by inhibiting the formation of arachidonic acid; NSAIDs inhibit the conversion of arachidonic acid to prostaglandins. Most over-the-counter analgesics are NSAIDs and therefore are prostaglandin inhibitors (aspirin, ibuprofen, naproxen [Aleve], and many others). The major exception is acetaminophen (Tylenol), which acts centrally rather than peripherally. This raises the interesting possibility that the medication used by many patients to control pain after orthodontic appointments could interfere with tooth movement. Fortunately, with the low doses and short durations of analgesic therapy in orthodontic patients, this does not occur, but it can become a problem in adults or children being treated chronically for arthritis pain. Control of pain related to orthodontic treatment is discussed later in more detail.

Several other classes of drugs can decrease prostaglandin levels and therefore could slow the response to orthodontic force. Tricyclic antidepressants (doxepin, amitriptyline, imipramine), antiarrhythmic agents (procaine), antimalarial drugs (quinine, quinidine, chloroquine), and methylxanthines fall into this category. In addition, the anticonvulsant drug phenytoin has been reported to decrease tooth movement in rats, and some tetracyclines (e.g., doxycycline) inhibit osteoclast recruitment, an effect similar to that of bisphosphonates.[13] It is possible that an unusual lack of response to orthodontic force could be encountered in patients taking any of these medications, and as mentioned earlier, there could also be an increased response with some drugs that affect neurotransmitters.

Bisphosphonates

Osteoporosis is a problem particularly in postmenopausal women but is associated with aging in both sexes and now also is being observed in children who require long-term steroids after cancer therapy or other medical treatment. Estrogen therapy, which was used frequently in the past to prevent loss of bone in older women, now has been shown to carry significant risks and is not widely used. Estrogens have little or no effect on orthodontic treatment, but pharmacologic agents that inhibit bone resorption are a potential problem. At present, bisphosphonates, synthetic analogues of pyrophosphate that bind to hydroxyapatite in bone, are the major class of drugs for control of osteoporosis. They act as specific inhibitors of osteoclast-mediated bone resorption, so it is not surprising that the bone remodeling necessary for tooth movement is slower in patients who are taking this medication.

Bisphosphonates are a special concern for two reasons:

1. Their use has been associated with an unusual necrosis of mandibular bone. This typically occurs after extraction of a tooth or other injury to the bone, which fails to heal and becomes the center of an expanding necrotic area. Fortunately, this is rare and occurs most often in patients with metastatic bone cancer who receive high doses of potent bisphosphonates, but elective extractions for orthodontic purposes should be avoided for a patient who has been taking any of these drugs.
2. They are incorporated into the structure of bone, then slowly eliminated over a period of years—so stopping the drug does not eliminate all of its effects. It appears that there are two elimination rates: a fast elimination from the surface of the bones within some weeks, and slower elimination from bone structure. Fortunately, most of the drug is only on the surface, which makes orthodontic treatment possible after about 3 months with no further bisphosphonate therapy.[14] Obviously, treatment would be possible only if the physician were willing for the patient to have a drug holiday or if the patient could be switched to raloxifene (Evista; the estrogen analogue with the greatest effect on bone), at least temporarily.

Could distraction osteogenesis (discussed in detail later) be used to move teeth in a patient who had been taking bisphosphonates for a long time? The situation then would be similar to ankylosis of all the teeth, and presumably could be approached by moving alveolar bone segments as shown in Fig. 8.14 in a patient with ankylosis of a central incisor after trauma. But bone healing in patients taking bisphosphonates is problematic, and distraction osteogenesis would be a risky procedure, probably unacceptably so. Distraction also could be considered in a patient with primary failure of eruption (PFE; see Chapter 3), but this is feasible only if PFE developed after a tooth had erupted at least partially and is difficult to impossible when several posterior teeth in a quadrant are involved. In short, distraction osteogenesis to reposition an isolated ankylosed tooth or teeth is acceptable; when all or many of the teeth are affected by bisphosphonates or a syndrome, it rarely would be useful.

Other Medications

Several other medications that orthodontic patients may be taking have been investigated for their impact on tooth movement.[15] Most of these reports are from animal studies and as such may not be directly generalizable to humans. ACE inhibitors, like Losartan, were found to reduce the rate of orthodontic tooth movement by potentially reducing osteoclastic activity. Some antihistamines have also demonstrated a negative impact on osteoclastic activity and a subsequent slowing of tooth movement. The administration of beta-blockers in low doses have slowed tooth movement by interfering with the RANKL mediated differentiation of osteoclasts. In light of the broad range of medications that may impact tooth movement, it is important to have a thorough understanding of all medications an orthodontic patient is taking.

Local Injury to Accelerate Tooth Movement

Because remodeling of alveolar bone is the key component of orthodontic tooth movement and bone remodeling is accelerated during wound healing (via the regional acceleratory phenomenon described by Frost),[16] the idea that teeth could be moved faster after local injury to the alveolar process first appeared early in the history of orthodontics. The pioneer American oral surgeon Hullihan is said to have experimented with moving teeth after making cuts in alveolar bone in the late 19th century, and sporadic experiments with this continued into the early 20th century. The approach was not widely adopted, however, for several reasons that included concerns about infections and bone loss in this pre-antibiotic era.

Corticotomy

In the mid-20th century, the German surgeon Köle revived the idea that cuts between teeth could produce faster tooth movement and introduced the term *corticotomy* to describe the technique.[17] After flap surgery to reflect the gingiva all the way around the arch, vertical cuts were made facially and lingually between the teeth. A banded orthodontic appliance (placed before the surgery) was activated as soon as possible, using relatively stiff archwires and wire ties to generate enough force to create greenstick fractures of the bone around the root apex and bring the teeth into alignment almost instantly. The root apex did not move, so the teeth were tipped into position, not moved bodily. The time for alignment was minutes and hours, not days and weeks. It was not used widely because many surgeons and most orthodontists thought it was too invasive, and it did not allow precise positioning of the teeth.

More recently, corticotomy was revived and reconsidered as a stimulus to a regional acceleration of bone remodeling that allows faster tooth movement, rather than movement of blocks of bone that contain a tooth. The surgical technique, with a large flap to fully expose the alveolar bone and cuts between the teeth, still is similar to Köle's, but now lighter force to move teeth more physiologically is recommended, and the surgical approach has been broadened into "periodontal accelerated osteogenic orthodontics" (PAOO) by adding decortication of the facial surfaces of alveolar bone. The exposed bone is then covered with demineralized freeze-dried bone or a mixture of this with bovine bone or allograft bone; Fig. 8.15.[18] One of the risks of expansion of the dental arches, of course, is fenestration of the alveolar bone, and the PAOO approach is said to generate new bone that allows facial movement of teeth without this risk. In order to evaluate the outcomes of corticotomy-assisted orthodontics, as with any other type of treatment, an analysis of benefit versus cost and risk is needed. The primary benefit claimed for corticotomy is a reduction in treatment time, with facilitation of arch expansion via PAOO as a secondary benefit.

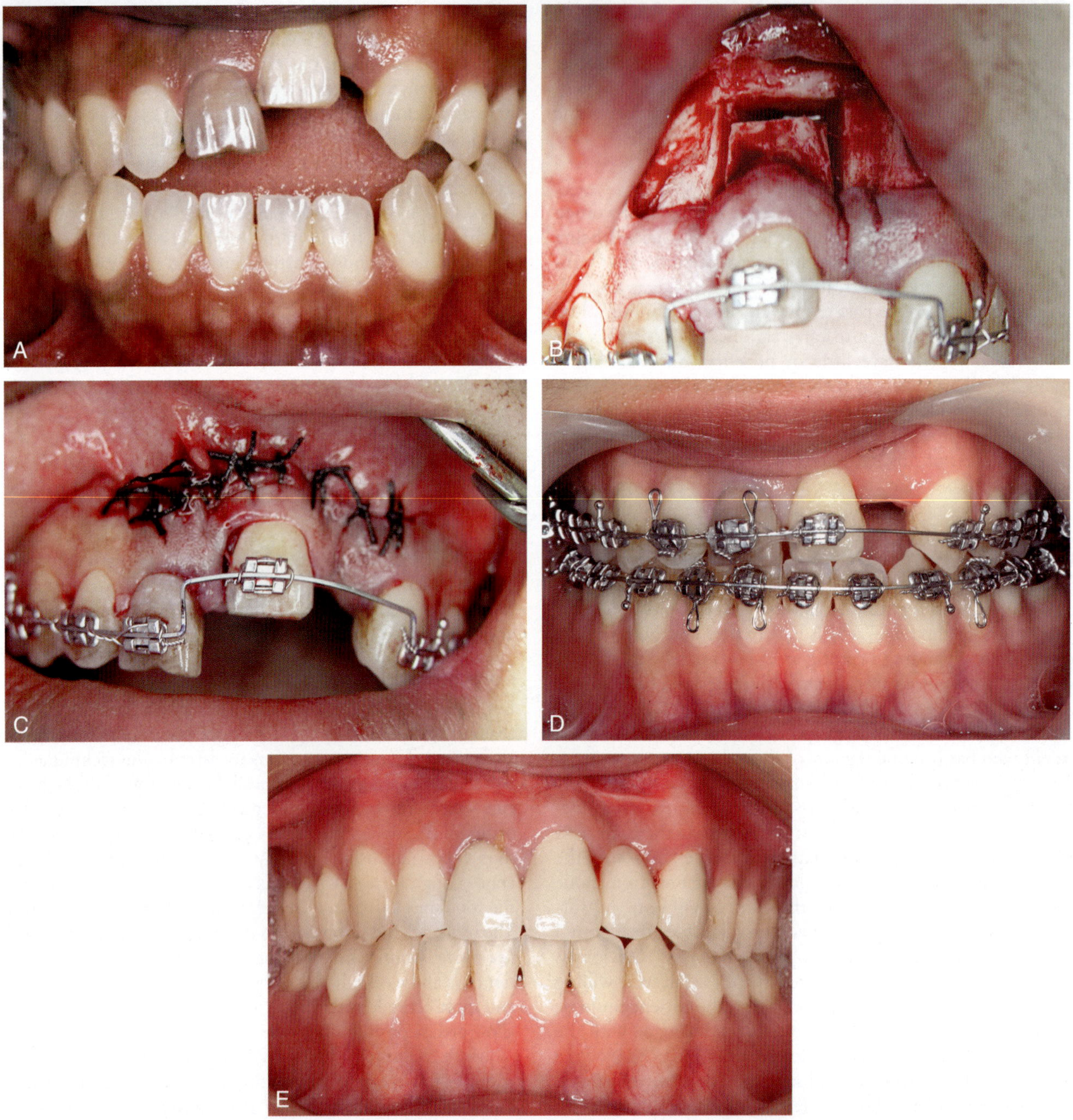

• **Fig. 8.14** An ankylosed tooth can be moved only by moving the bone to which it is attached. Distraction osteogenesis allows that to be done. (A) Age 21, maxillary central incisor that ankylosed after an accident at age 8 (the lateral incisor was lost at that time). (B) Creation of the bony segment to be moved. (C) Closure of the wound. A period of initial healing, usually 5–7 days, is allowed before the archwire is activated to begin movement of the segment. (D) The tooth nearly in final position, 3 weeks later. (E) Treatment completed, with prosthetic replacement of the missing lateral incisor. (Courtesy Dr. H. Chen; Reprinted from *Am J Orthod Dentofacial Orthop*. 2019;138:829–838.)

A recent meta-analysis found that PAOO does result in more canine retraction during the 1 to 3 months after the surgical procedure compared to conventional orthodontic treatment. This analysis also found that the bone grafting procedure added an additional 0.4 mm of buccal bone thickness.[19] The overall treatment time was found to be reduced when bone grafting was included, but not when corticotomy alone was done.

When considering the significant surgical intervention required for PAOO and the modest gains in treatment time and buccal bone, this procedure has not gained widespread acceptance. It may be considered for the individual patient for whom these potential benefits are critical but its use must include a robust informed consent discussion to review the risks and benefits.

In short, the benefit of PAOO and corticotomy is primarily in reduction of the time to align crowded teeth or to close extraction spaces. As with any procedure, the benefits must be evaluated relative to the cost and risk of the treatment. Cost, of course, includes all aspects of the "burden of treatment." In addition

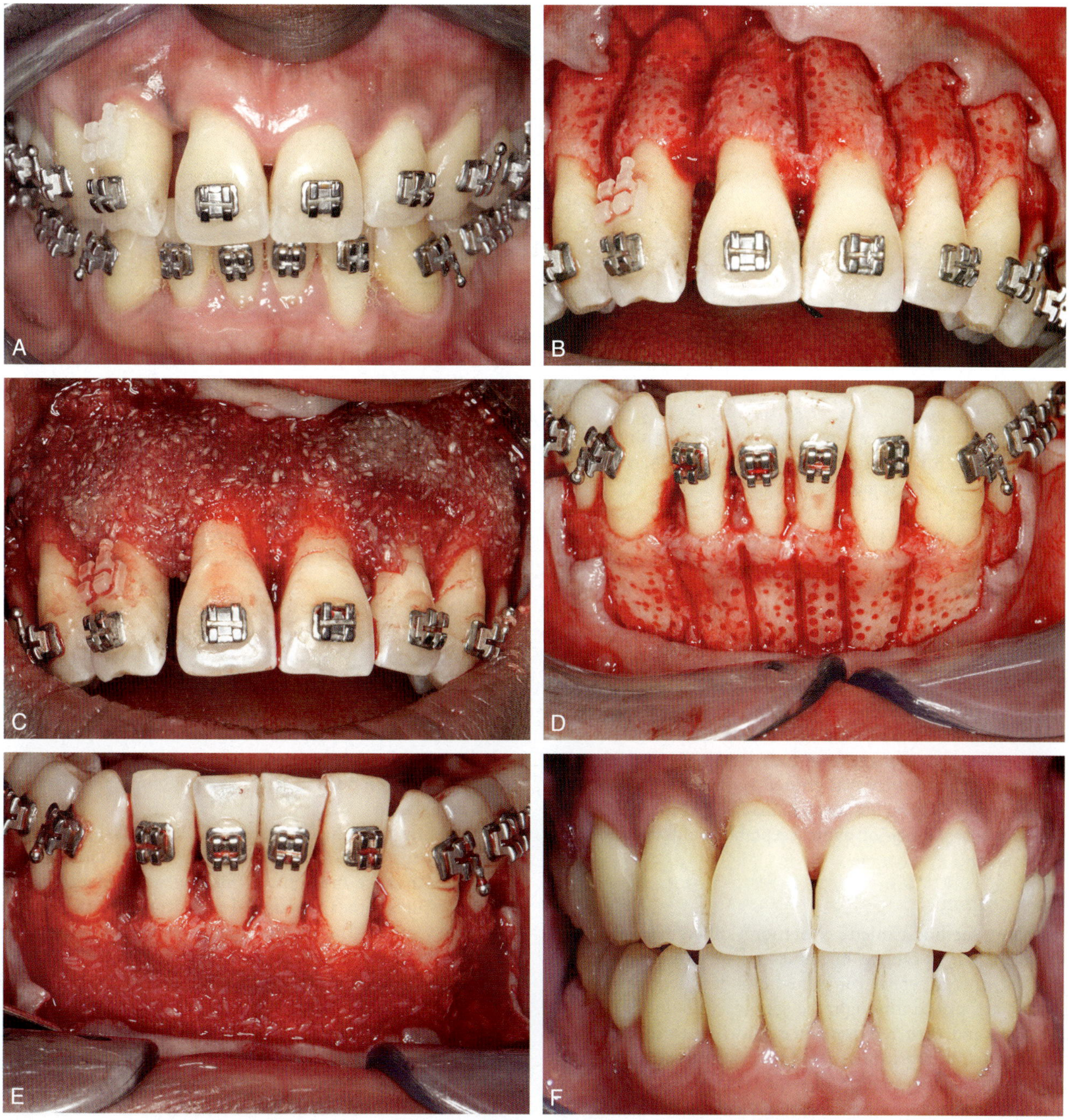

• **Fig. 8.15** (A) For this adult with an upper incisor that was brought down into position and crowding in the lower incisor region, corticotomy and bone grafting on the facial surface (accelerated osteogenic orthodontics [AOO]) was planned. (B) After reflection of a flap, corticotomy cuts between the teeth were made and small circular depressions were placed in the facial surface of the bone over the maxillary anterior teeth. (C) Bone graft material in the form of a slurry of demineralized freeze-dried bone was placed over the facial surface. (D) Corticotomy and preparation of the bone over the lower incisor was done at the same time, and (E) bone graft material was placed to reduce the chance of bone loss as the lower incisors were advanced. (F) Eleven months later, after completion of treatment that required 6 months, with good healing of the alveolar bone. (Courtesy Dr. S. Dibart.)

to the economic cost of the surgery (which can require several hours), morbidity and inconvenience of all types must be considered. Risk includes the possibility of loss of alveolar bone height, which occurs when corticotomy is done without bone grafting[20]; unsightly facial bruising; unfavorable changes in the appearance of the gingiva after the extensive flaps; and the possibility of gingival stripping (Fig. 8.16).

Modified Corticotomy: Piezocision

Given the extensive surgery and flap reflection needed for corticotomy, a reasonable question is whether less invasive surgery could be equally effective in producing faster tooth movement. In 2009 Dibart, a periodontist at Boston University, introduced a technique he called *piezocision*. In this technique, gingival incisions between crowded incisors are used only on the facial side and

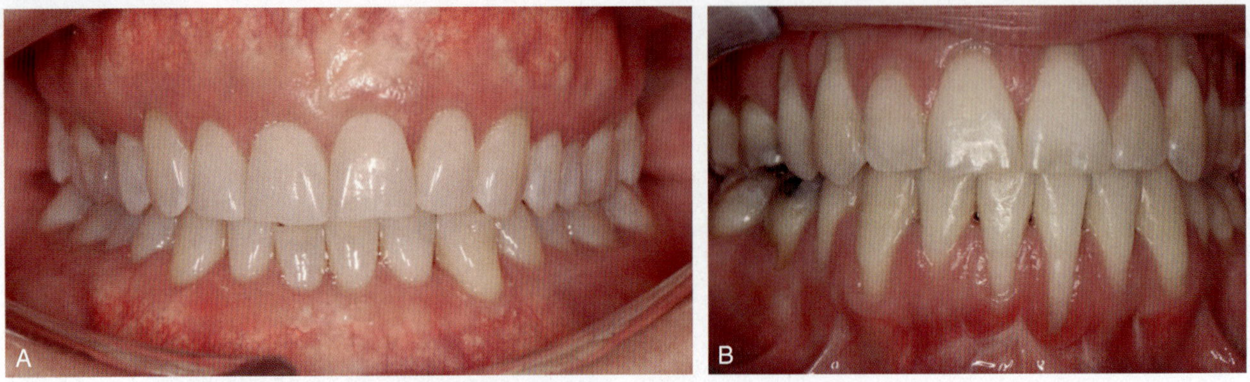

• **Fig. 8.16** Corticotomy complications include (A) whitening of the gingiva after reflection of the large flap and (B) fenestration of incisor roots after labial movement of these teeth, which can happen even after placing particulate bone grafts. (Courtesy Dr. S. Dibart.)

injury to the bone in that area is performed with a vibrating piezoelectric knife (Fig. 8.17).[21] Tunneling beneath the gingiva allows placement of a slurry bone graft.

In a randomized clinical trial (RCT) with a small sample of patients treated with the sequence of archwires in the standard Damon technique (see Chapter 10), Charavet et al. documented a statistically significant shortening of treatment time[22] and concluded that replacing corticotomy with this approach can be recommended for adults. It also is true that there is remarkably little information about possible complications with piezocision. A 2017 report from Australian investigators noted that in 5 of 14 patients in a split-mouth study in whom premolars were extracted for examination with microcomputed tomography after 4 weeks of buccal tipping, root damage from contact with the piezoelectric knife was evident, and there was greater tooth remodeling in the piezocision group.[23] Being less invasive than corticotomy does not necessarily qualify piezocision as an acceptable tool for accelerated tooth movement.

Microperforation

A third injury method, "microperforation", differs from the previous two in that it can be implemented by orthodontists. In this method, special screws (or miniscrews designed for skeletal anchorage) are placed through the gingiva into interproximal alveolar bone and then removed. It is said that three such perforations in each interproximal area between teeth are enough to generate a regional acceleration of bone remodeling and thereby produce faster tooth movement. Although this method was highly promoted for the past several years, a recent scoping review concluded that the evidence for microperforations increasing the rate of tooth movement was inconclusive.[24]

For the injury methods, perhaps a fair summary is that for some but certainly not all patients, the cost–benefit and risk–benefit ratios are favorable, and controlled injury would be a valuable adjunct to orthodontic treatment. The extent of injury with modified corticotomy is less, and it seems to be as effective as and more efficient than the original method, but caution in recommending it still seems prudent. Microperforation, if it is effective, would appear to be limited to specific areas rather than a whole arch or even all the anterior teeth because of the increased effort needed to place so many screw holes.

Other Physical Effects to Accelerate Tooth Movement

Three other methods intended to accelerate tooth movement have been marketed since the onset of the 21st century: vibration of the teeth, application of light to the alveolar process, and application of therapeutic ultrasound to the teeth and adjacent bone. Vibration may or may not really be another way to injure alveolar bone; penetrating light and therapeutic ultrasound are not injurious (at least as far as we know at present), but the mechanism by which they may work is not understood.

Vibrational Forces

The vibrational systems that have been designed for at home use by orthodontic patients, unlike the efforts 40 years ago to induce piezoelectric currents with vibration that we have already discussed, are based on delivery of high-frequency vibration to the teeth for approximately 20 minutes per day. The proposed rationale is that this stimulates cell differentiation and maturation so that the bone remodeling necessary for tooth movement occurs more quickly.

A recently published Cochrane Collaboration review specifically evaluated the evidence for acceleration of tooth movement using non-invasive methods.[25] This review concluded that there was no evidence that vibrational adjuncts increased the rate of tooth movement. The studies they considered looked at overall treatment time, time for alignment, speed of canine retraction and the time in treatment with aligners. Although the level of evidence for most of these studies is relatively low, we can conclude that at the present time there is no advantage to using vibrational forces when moving teeth.

Tissue-Penetrating Light

The same Cochrane review mentioned above also looked at the evidence for the application of light to the teeth and alveolus to increase the speed of movement. They assessed the evidence for the use of low level laser therapy (LLLT) and light-emitting diode (LED) use. With both the light applying techniques, small differences in the rate of tooth movement were seen during canine retraction and space closure. These differences were unlikely to have significant clinical benefits, but they indicate that a small benefit of light application may occur during certain stages of treatment. The level of evidence was again low for this part of the review so further development of these techniques and better evidence for their impact would be needed before using light therapy as a regular adjunct for orthodontic treatment.

Therapeutic Ultrasound

Low-intensity therapeutic ultrasound has also been proposed as a method to increase the speed of tooth movement. SmileSonica

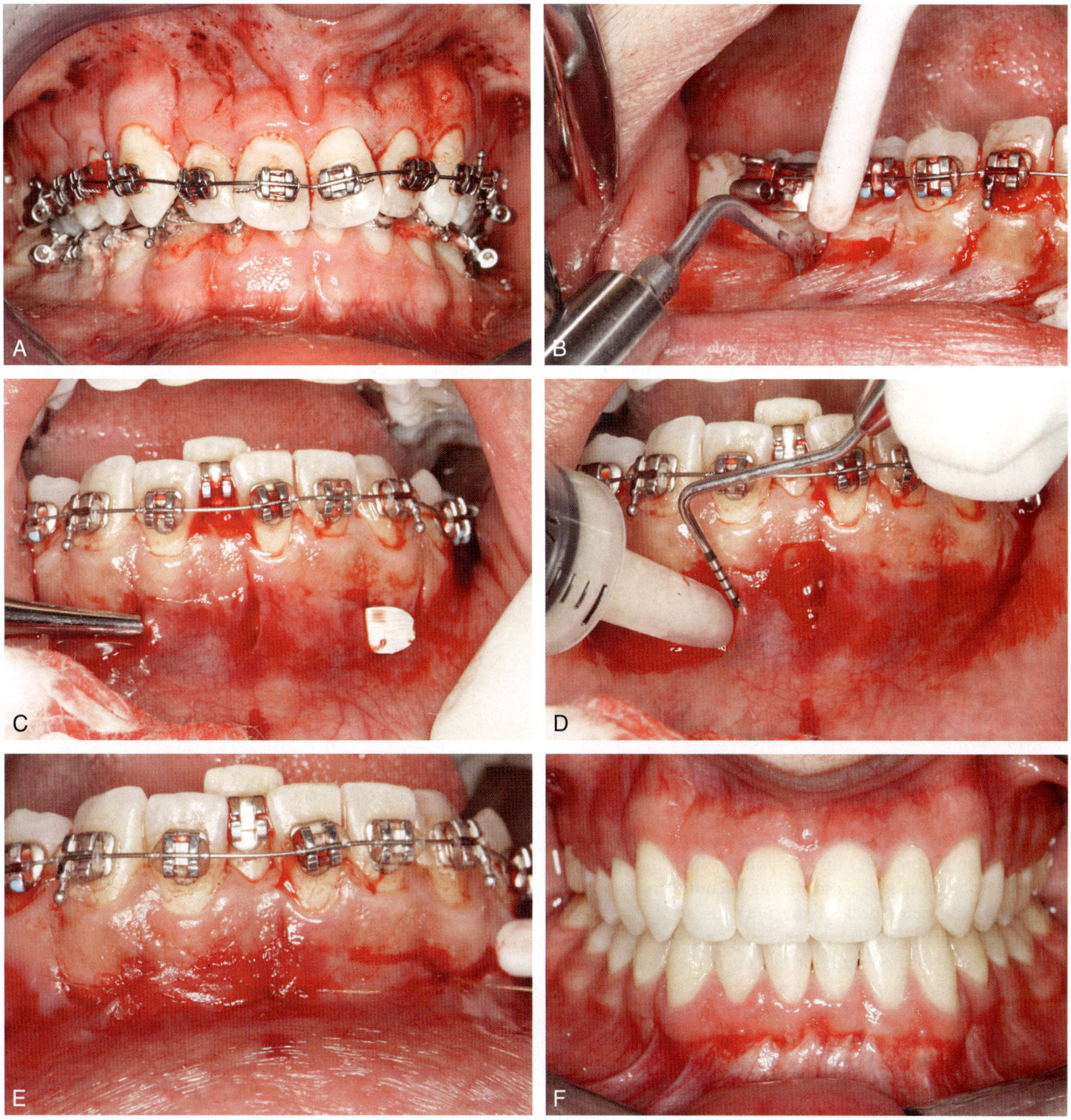

• **Fig. 8.17** (A) Modified corticotomy avoids reflecting a flap, using thin micro-incisions through the facial tissue. (B) A piezoelectric knife is used to penetrate the cortical bone and extend into the medullary bone between the teeth. (C) If a bone graft is desired, a tunnel under the soft tissue is established, and (D) the graft slurry is placed into the area with a syringe. (E) Appearance at the end of the procedure, with the graft material in place. (F) Ten months later. (Courtesy Dr. S. Dibart.)

of Canada markets theAevo device in Canada and Europe for this purpose., It is known that therapeutic ultrasound (which is different from diagnostic ultrasound) increases blood flow in treated areas; indeed, it is used routinely in physical therapy to increase blood flow in muscles. The theory is that increased blood flow in the PDL would increase the rate of bone remodeling and tooth movement and also could decrease root resorption. This is plausible, especially because an important aspect of injury to bone is an increase in blood flow to the healing area. Perhaps ultrasound could provide the major effect of injury to alveolar bone without surgical intervention. At this time, however, there is no convincing demonstration of effectiveness or efficiency in accelerating tooth movement.

Anchorage and Its Control

Anchorage: Resistance to Unwanted Tooth Movement

The term *anchorage*, in its orthodontic application, is defined in an unusual way: the definition as "resistance to unwanted tooth movement" includes a statement of what the dentist desires. The usage, although unusual, is clearest when presented this way. The dentist or orthodontist always constructs an appliance to produce certain desired tooth movements. For every (desired) action, there is an equal and opposite reaction. Inevitably, reaction forces can move other teeth as well if the appliance contacts them. Anchorage, then, is the resistance to reaction forces that is provided usually by other teeth, occasionally by the palate, sometimes by the head or neck (via extraoral force), and more and more often by anchors screwed into bones.

At this point, let us focus first on controlling unwanted tooth movement when some teeth are to serve as anchors. In planning orthodontic therapy, it is simply not possible to consider only the teeth whose movement is desired. Reciprocal effects throughout the dental arches must be carefully analyzed, evaluated, and controlled. An important aspect of treatment is maximizing the tooth movement that is desired, while minimizing undesirable side effects.

An obvious strategy for anchorage control would be to concentrate the force needed to produce tooth movement where it is desired, and then to dissipate the reaction force over as many other teeth as possible, keeping the pressure in the PDL of anchor teeth as low as possible. A threshold, below which pressure would produce no reaction, could provide perfect anchorage control, because it would only be necessary to be certain that the threshold for tooth movement was not reached for teeth in the anchorage unit. A differential response to pressure, so that heavier pressure produced more tooth movement than lighter pressure, would make it possible to move some teeth more than others, even though some undesired tooth movement occurred.

In fact, the threshold for tooth movement appears to be quite low, but there is a differential response to pressure, so this strategy of "divide and conquer" is reasonably effective. As Fig. 8.18 indicates, teeth behave as if orthodontic movement is proportional to the magnitude of the pressure, up to a point. When that point is reached, the amount of tooth movement becomes more or less independent of the magnitude of the pressure, so that a broad plateau of orthodontically effective pressure is created.[26] The optimum force level for orthodontic movement is the lightest force and resulting pressure that produces a near-maximum response (i.e., it is found at the edge of the plateau). Forces greater than that, although equally effective in producing tooth movement, would be unnecessarily traumatic and, as we will see, unnecessarily stressful to anchorage.

Control of Anchorage

Anchorage Situations

From this background, we can now define several anchorage situations.

Reciprocal Tooth Movement

In a reciprocal situation, the forces applied to teeth and to arch segments are equal, and so is the force distribution in the PDL. A simple example is what would occur if two maxillary central incisors separated by a diastema were connected by an active spring (Fig. 8.19). The essentially identical teeth would feel the same force distributed in the same way through the PDL and would move toward each other by the same amount.

A somewhat similar situation would arise if a spring were placed across a first premolar extraction site, pitting the central incisor, lateral incisor, and canine in the anterior arch segment against the second premolar and first molar posteriorly. Whether this would really produce reciprocal tooth movement requires some thought. The same force would be felt by the three anterior teeth and the

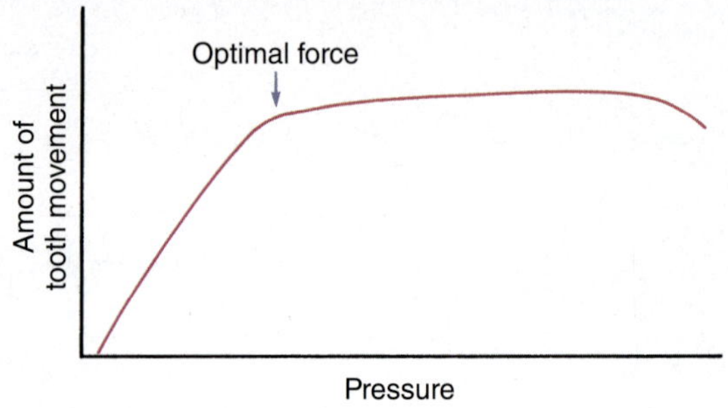

• **Fig. 8.18** Theoretical representation of the relationship of pressure within the periodontal ligament (PDL) to the amount of tooth movement. Pressure in the PDL is determined by the force applied to a tooth divided by the area of the PDL over which that force is distributed. The threshold for tooth movement is very small. Tooth movement increases as pressure increases up to a point, remains at about the same level over a broad range, and then may actually decline with extremely heavy pressure. The best definition of the optimum force for orthodontic purposes is the lightest force that produces a maximum or near-maximum response (i.e., that brings pressure in the PDL to the edge of the nearly constant portion of the response curve). The magnitude of the optimum force will vary, depending on the way it is distributed in the PDL (i.e., it is different for different types of tooth movement [tipping, bodily movement, intrusion, and so on]).

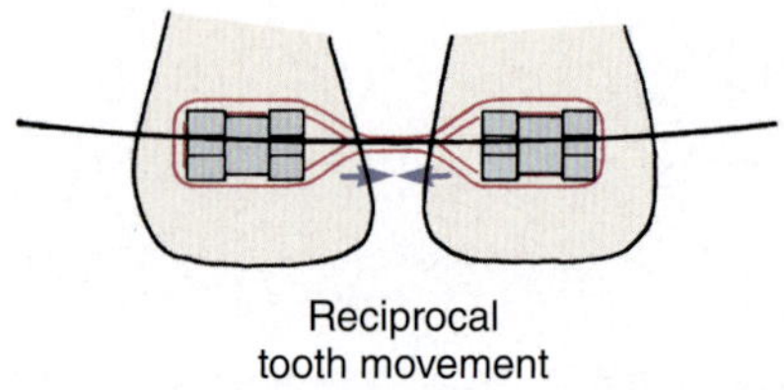

• **Fig. 8.19** Reciprocal tooth movement is produced when two teeth or resistance units of equal size pull against each other, as in this example of the reciprocal closure of a maxillary midline diastema.

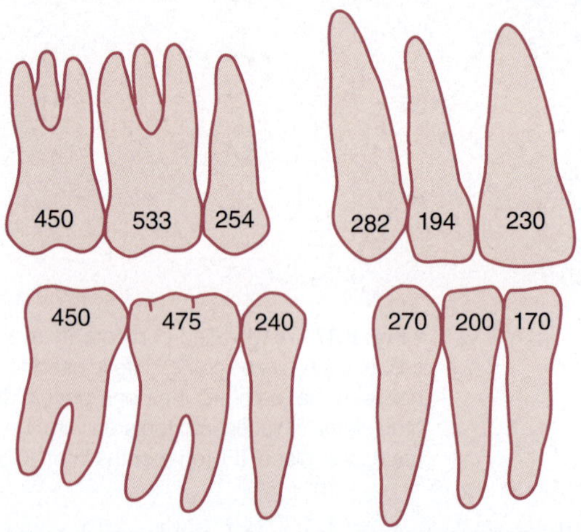

• **Fig. 8.20** The "anchorage value" of any tooth is roughly equivalent to its root surface area. As this diagram shows, the first molar and second premolar in each arch are approximately equal in surface area to the canine and two incisors. (Modified from Freeman DC. [Master's thesis.] University of Tennessee Department of Orthodontics; 1965.)

two posterior teeth, because the action of the spring on one segment has an equal and opposite reaction on the other. Reciprocal movement would require the same total PDL area over which the force was distributed.

Conceptually, the "anchorage value" of a tooth, that is, its resistance to movement, can be thought of as a function of its root surface area, which is the same as its PDL area. The larger the root, the greater the area over which a force can be distributed, and vice versa. As Fig. 8.20 shows, the PDL area for the two posterior teeth in this example is slightly larger than the total anterior PDL area. Therefore, with a simple spring connecting the segments, the anterior teeth would move slightly more than the posterior teeth. The movement would not be truly reciprocal but would be close to it.

Reinforced Anchorage

Continuing with the extraction site example, if it is desired to differentially retract the anterior teeth, the anchorage of the posterior teeth could be reinforced by adding the second molar to the posterior unit (see Fig. 8.20). This would change the ratio of the root surface areas so that there would be relatively more pressure in the PDL of the anterior teeth and therefore relatively more retraction of the anterior segment than forward movement of the posterior segment.

Note that reinforcing anchorage by adding more resistance units is effective because with more teeth (or extraoral structures) in the anchorage, the reaction force is distributed over a larger area. This reduces the pressure on the anchor teeth, moving them down the slope of the pressure-response curve. Now the shape of the pressure-response curve becomes important. Keeping the force light has two virtues. Not only does this minimize trauma and pain, but it also makes it possible to create anchorage by taking advantage of different PDL areas in the anchor segments. As Fig. 8.21 illustrates, too much force destroys the effectiveness of reinforced anchorage by pulling the anchor teeth up onto the flatter portion of the pressure-response curve. Then the clinician is said to have slipped, burned, or blown the anchorage by moving the anchor teeth too much.

Stationary Anchorage

The term *stationary anchorage*, traditionally used although inherently less descriptive than the term *reinforced anchorage*, refers to the advantage that can be obtained by pitting bodily movement of one group of teeth against tipping of another (Fig. 8.22). Using our same example of a premolar extraction site, if the appliance were arranged so that the anterior teeth could tip lingually while the posterior teeth could only move bodily, the optimum pressure for the anterior segment would be produced by about half as much force as if the anterior teeth were to be retracted bodily. This would mean that the reaction force distributed over the posterior teeth would be reduced by half, and these teeth would move half as much.

If PDL areas were equal, tipping the anterior segment while holding the posterior segment for bodily movement would have the effect of doubling the amount of anterior retraction compared with posterior forward movement. It is important to note again, however, that successful implementation of this strategy requires light force. If the force were large enough to bring the posterior teeth into their optimum movement range, it would no longer matter whether the anterior segment tipped or was moved bodily. Using too much force would disastrously undermine this method of anchorage control.

If tooth movement were actually impeded by very high levels of pressure, it might be possible to structure an anchorage situation so that there was more movement of the arch segment with the larger PDL area. This result could happen, of course, if such high force were used that the smaller segment was placed beyond the greatest tooth movement range, while the larger segment was still in it (see Fig. 8.21). Because the effect would be highly traumatic, it would be an undesirable way to deliberately manage anchorage.

In fact, it is not certain that the amount of tooth movement in response to applied force really decreases with very high force levels in any circumstance, and so this type of differential movement may not really exist. By using too much force, however, it is certainly possible to produce more movement of the anchor segment than was expected, even if the mechanism is merely a differential movement of the anchor segment up the slope of the pressure-response curve rather than a decline in the response of the movement segment. Differential force is understood best in

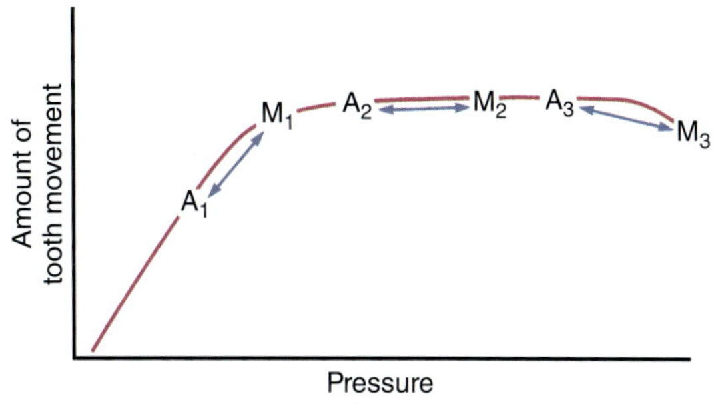

• **Fig. 8.21** Consider the response of anchor teeth (A on the chart) and teeth to be moved (M) in three circumstances. In each case, the pressure in the periodontal ligament (PDL) of the anchor teeth is less than the pressure in the PDL of the teeth to be moved because there are more teeth in the anchor unit. In the first case (A_1–M_1), the pressure for the teeth to be moved is optimal, whereas the pressure in the anchor unit is suboptimal, and the anchor teeth move less (anchorage is preserved). In the second case (A_2–M_2), although the pressure for the anchor teeth is less than for the teeth to be moved, both are on the plateau of the pressure-response curve, and the anchor teeth can be expected to move as much as the teeth that are desired to move (anchorage is lost). With extremely high force (A_3–M_3), the anchor teeth might move more than the teeth it was desired to move. Although the third possibility is theoretical and may not be encountered clinically, both the first and second situations are seen in clinical orthodontics. This principle explains the efficacy of light forces in controlling anchorage, and why heavy force destroys anchorage.

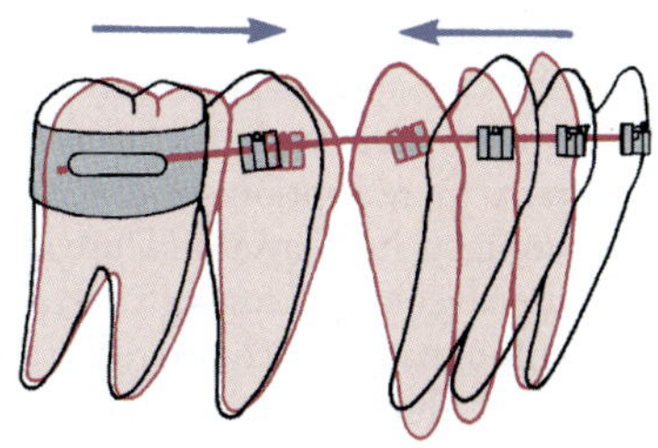

• **Fig. 8.22** Displacement of anchor teeth can be minimized by arranging the force system so that the anchor teeth must move bodily if they move at all, while movement teeth are allowed to tip, as in this example of retracting incisors by tipping them posteriorly. The crowns of the incisors moved back much more than the posterior teeth moved forward because the lighter force for tipping the incisors decreased the periodontal ligament pressure for the anchor teeth. The approach is called stationary anchorage. In this example, treatment is not complete because the roots of the lingually tipped incisors will have to be uprighted at a later stage, but two-stage treatment with tipping followed by uprighting can be used as a means of controlling anchorage.

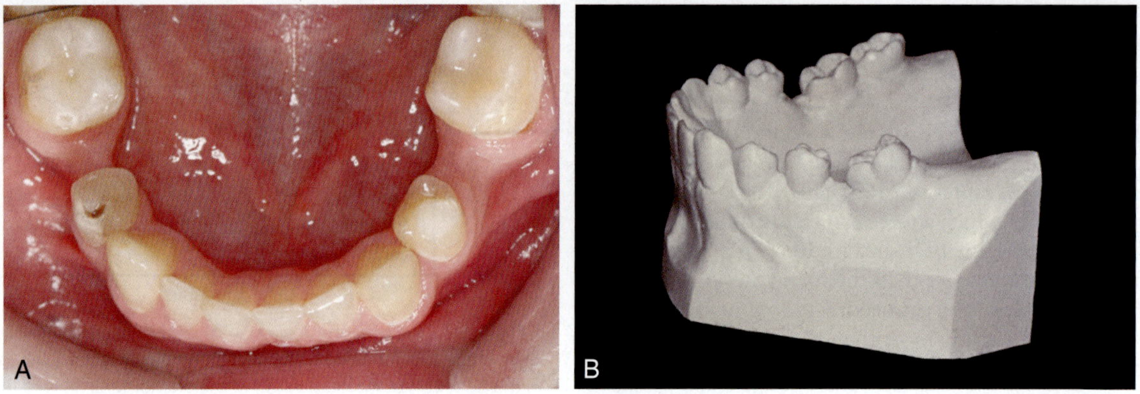

• **Fig. 8.23** Loss of alveolar bone at an old extraction site can create an area of cortical bone between adjacent teeth, as the alveolar process resorbs and narrows. (A) This child lost second primary molars early and was congenitally missing the second premolars. The greater ridge resorption on the right than the left side indicates that the right second primary molar was lost first. This is one situation in which "cortical anchorage" definitely can be a factor. Closing such an extraction site is extremely difficult because of the resistance of cortical bone to remodeling, and the result often is as much retraction of the anterior teeth as forward movement of the posterior teeth. (B) In adults who had a permanent first molar extracted during childhood or adolescence, the second molar tips mesially, but resorption of alveolar bone at the extraction site narrows the ridge. Closing these spaces also is difficult and slow because remodeling of cortical bone is required.

terms of the plateau portion of the curve in Figs. 8.18 and 8.21, not the questionable decline at the far right.

Cortical and Skeletal Anchorage

Another consideration in anchorage control is the different response of cortical compared with medullary bone. Cortical bone is more resistant to resorption, and tooth movement is slowed when a root contacts it. A layer of dense cortical bone that has formed within the alveolar process can certainly affect tooth movement. This situation may be encountered at an old extraction site—for example, in an adult in whom a molar or premolar was lost many years previously (Fig. 8.23). Another frequent example is an area in which a permanent tooth never erupted, as when a mandibular second premolar was congenitally missing. It can be very difficult to close such a space in the dental arch because tooth movement is slowed to a minimum as the roots encounter cortical bone along the resorbed alveolar ridge.

As a general rule, torquing movements are limited by the facial and lingual cortical plates. If a root is persistently forced against either of these cortical plates, tooth movement is greatly slowed and root resorption is likely. A common example is the difficulty in obtaining an ideal inclination of maxillary incisors when there is little space between their roots and cortical bone of the palate. At one time, deliberately creating root contact of lower molars against the buccal cortical plate was suggested as a way to increase their resistance to forward movement when Class II elastics were employed. Like excessive torquing of maxillary incisors, this is now recognized more as a prescription for root resorption than as a good way to reinforce anchorage.

It has long been realized that if structures other than the teeth could be made to serve as anchorage, it would be possible to produce tooth movement or growth modification without unwanted side effects. Until the turn of the 21st century, extraoral force (headgear) and to a lesser extent the anterior palate were the only ways to obtain anchorage that was not from the teeth. Although headgear can be used to augment anchorage, there are two problems: (1) it is impossible for a patient to wear headgear all the time, and most wear it half the time at best, and (2) when headgear is worn, the force against the teeth is greater than optimal. The result is a force system that is far from ideal. Heavy intermittent force from headgear is simply not a good way to counterbalance the effect of light continuous force from the orthodontic appliance. It is not surprising that headgear to the anchor segment of a dental arch usually does not control its movement very well. In theory, additional anchorage can be obtained from the rugae area of the palate; in fact, this is not very effective (see Chapter 16).

With the development of successful bone implant techniques to replace missing teeth, it was quickly realized that implants also could be used for orthodontic anchorage. A successful implant is like an ankylosed tooth: it does not move unless pathologic degeneration of the bone around it develops. It has become apparent that the osseointegration needed for long-term implant success is not necessary, and perhaps not desirable, for temporary attachments to bone to provide orthodontic anchorage. A number of options for skeletal anchorage exist at present, the principal ones being titanium screws that penetrate through the gingiva into alveolar bone (Fig. 8.24A) and bone plates held by multiple screws that are placed beneath the soft tissue, usually in the zygomatic buttress area of the maxilla (Fig. 8.24B).

At this point, application of bone screws or plates for skeletal anchorage has become a routine aspect of clinical orthodontics, and in many ways has superseded extraoral devices for control of anchorage. These devices are discussed further in Chapters 9 and 10, and their current applications are illustrated in most of the clinical chapters that follow.

Skeletal Effects of Orthodontic Force: Growth Modification

Orthodontic force directly affects the teeth and alveolar bone, but it also can have indirect effects on the jaws more generally. Force against maxillary teeth is greatly attenuated before it reaches the sutures above and behind the maxilla that are sites of maxillary growth, but sustained light force can inhibit or enhance the maxilla's normal downward and forward growth. Force against

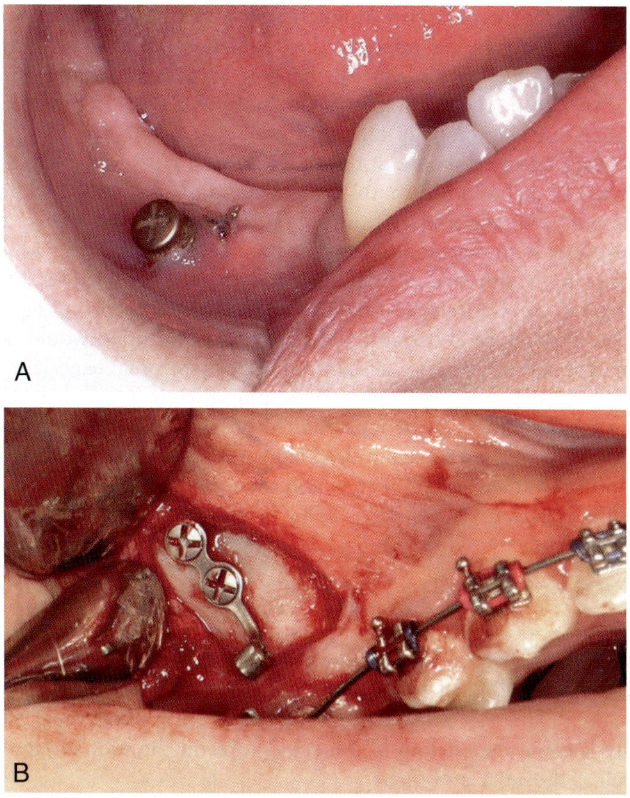

• **Fig. 8.24** Skeletal (absolute) anchorage can be provided in two major ways: (A) screws placed through the gingiva into the alveolar bone, as in this patient in whom the screw will be used for anchorage so that the lower incisors can be aligned before prosthodontic replacement of the missing teeth; or (B) bone anchors placed beneath the soft tissue, usually at the base of the zygomatic arch, so that the posterior teeth can be intruded or the anterior teeth retracted. After soft tissues are sutured back over the plate and screws, only the tube for attachment of springs will extend into the oral cavity.

mandibular teeth similarly can affect the direction, and perhaps the amount, of growth at the mandibular condyles (see Chapter 4). It is possible now to place force directly against the maxilla or mandible by using implants in the bone, and as one might have predicted, heavy force is not needed to affect growth.

Growth modification is the subject of Chapters 13 and 14, and the skeletal effects of force against the jaws is discussed there in detail.

Deleterious Effects of Orthodontic Force

Mobility and Pain Related to Orthodontic Treatment

Orthodontic tooth movement requires not only a remodeling of bone adjacent to the teeth but also a reorganization of the PDL itself. Collagen fibers become detached from the bone and cementum, then reattach at a later time. Radiographically, it can be observed that the PDL space widens during orthodontic tooth movement. The combination of a wider ligament space and a somewhat disorganized ligament means that some increase in mobility will be observed in every patient.

A moderate increase in mobility is an expected response to orthodontic treatment. The heavier the force, however, the greater the amount of undermining resorption expected, and the greater the mobility that will develop. Excessive mobility is an indication that excessive forces are being encountered. This may occur because the patient is clenching or grinding against a tooth that has moved into a position of traumatic occlusion. If a tooth becomes extremely mobile during orthodontic treatment, it should be taken out of occlusion and all force should be discontinued until the mobility decreases to moderate levels. Unlike root resorption, excessive mobility will usually correct itself without permanent damage.

If heavy pressure is applied to a tooth, pain develops almost immediately as the PDL is literally crushed. There is no excuse for using force levels for orthodontic tooth movement that produce immediate pain of this type. If appropriate orthodontic force is applied, the patient feels little or nothing immediately. Several hours later, however, pain usually appears. The patient feels a mild aching sensation, and the teeth are quite sensitive to pressure, so that biting a hard object hurts. The pain typically lasts for 2 to 4 days, then disappears until the orthodontic appliance is reactivated. At that point, a similar cycle may recur, but for almost all patients, the pain associated with the initial activation of the appliance is the most severe. It is commonly noted that there is a great deal of individual variation in any pain experience, and this is certainly true of orthodontic pain. Some patients report little or no pain even with relatively heavy forces, whereas others experience considerable discomfort with quite light forces.

The pain associated with orthodontic treatment is related to the development of ischemic (hyalinized) areas in the PDL that will undergo sterile necrosis. The increased tenderness to pressure suggests inflammation at the apex, and the mild pulpitis that usually appears soon after orthodontic force is applied probably also contributes to the pain. There does seem to be a relationship between the amount of force used and the amount of pain: all other factors being equal, the greater the force, the greater the pain. This is consistent with the concept that ischemic areas in the PDL are the major pain source, because greater force would produce larger areas of ischemia.

If the source of pain is the development of ischemic areas, strategies to temporarily relieve pressure and allow blood flow through compressed areas should help. In fact, if light forces are used, the amount of pain experienced by patients can be decreased by having them engage in repetitive chewing (of sugarless gum, a plastic wafer placed between the teeth, and so on) during the first 8 hours after the orthodontic appliance has been activated. Presumably this works by temporarily displacing the teeth enough to allow some blood flow through compressed areas, thereby preventing buildup of metabolic products that stimulate pain receptors. Light forces, however, are the key to minimizing pain as a concomitant feature of orthodontic treatment.

As we have noted previously, many drugs used to control pain have the potential to affect tooth movement because of their effects on prostaglandins. It has been suggested that acetaminophen (Tylenol) should be a better analgesic for orthodontic patients than aspirin, ibuprofen, naproxen, and similar prostaglandin inhibitors because it acts centrally rather than as a prostaglandin inhibitor. There are two counterarguments against acetaminophen. First, inflammation in the PDL contributes to the pain. Acetaminophen does not reduce inflammation, but the peripherally acting agents such as ibuprofen do, so they may offer more effective pain control (i.e., lower doses would suffice). Second, prolonged use of acetaminophen now has been shown to have the potential to cause serious damage to renal function. Based on clinical studies, it now is widely accepted that acetaminophen and the over-the-counter NSAIDs are equally acceptable for controlling pain over the 3 to 4 days after an orthodontic appliance has been activated. Given the recently discovered potential for liver damage from acetaminophen, the choice for orthodontic pain now has swung toward the prostaglandin inhibitors, although neither type of drug would be used for orthodontic pain in large enough quantities or long enough to create problems.

It also is of interest that there is a strong placebo effect: reassuring patients and calling them at home the evening after appliances were placed was as effective in reducing pain as either type of drug in a recent and well-done study.[27] Physicians now often make an end-of-the-day phone call after surgery, and many orthodontic practice management consultants now recommend a personal phone call after appliance placement.

Metal or Latex Allergy

It is rare but not impossible for orthodontic patients to develop pain and inflammation of soft tissues, not because of the orthodontic force, but because of an allergic reaction. There are two major culprits when this occurs: a reaction to the latex in gloves or elastics and a reaction to the nickel in stainless steel bands, brackets, and wires. Latex allergies can become so severe as to be life-threatening. Extreme care should be taken to avoid using latex products in patients reporting a latex allergy.

Nickel is allergenic, and nearly 20% of the U.S. population show some skin reaction to nickel-containing materials (such as cheap jewelry and earrings). Fortunately, most children with a skin allergy to nickel have no mucosal response to stainless steel orthodontic appliances (which are about 8% nickel) and tolerate treatment perfectly well, but some do not. The typical symptoms of nickel allergy in an orthodontic patient are widespread erythema and swelling of oral tissues, developing 1 to 2 days after a stainless steel appliance is placed. For such patients (see further discussion in Chapter 10), titanium brackets and tubes can be substituted for stainless steel, and beta-titanium archwires can be used instead of nickel–titanium (NiTi) or steel wires.[28]

If there is doubt about how a patient with a known nickel allergy will react to an orthodontic appliance, it is wise to bond one or two steel brackets and wait for a week or two to see if there will be an allergic response before placing a complete appliance. A true mucosal allergy is rare enough that in most such patients, there will be no response and a completely titanium appliance would not be necessary.

Effects on the Dental Pulp

Although pulpal reactions to orthodontic treatment are minimal, there is probably a modest and transient inflammatory response within the pulp, at least at the beginning of treatment. As we have noted previously, this may contribute to the discomfort that patients often experience for a few days after appliances are placed, but the mild pulpitis has no long-term significance.

There are occasional reports of loss of tooth vitality during orthodontic treatment. Usually there is a history of previous trauma to the tooth, but poor control of orthodontic force also can be the culprit. If a tooth is subjected to heavy continuous force, a sequence of abrupt movements occurs, as undermining resorption allows increasingly large increments of change. A large enough abrupt movement of the root apex could sever the blood vessels as they enter. Loss of vitality has also been observed when incisor teeth were tipped distally to such an extent that the root apex, moving in the opposite direction, was moved outside the alveolar process. This also can happen with excess torque (Fig. 8.25). Again, such movements probably would sever the blood vessels entering the pulp canal.

Because the response of the PDL, not the pulp, is the key element in orthodontic tooth movement, moving endodontically treated teeth is perfectly feasible. Endodontic treatment may be necessary before orthodontics after trauma at any age or in adults receiving adjunctive orthodontic treatment (see Chapter 20). There is no contraindication to going ahead with orthodontics soon after the pulp therapy, and severe root resorption would not be expected. One special circumstance is a tooth that experienced severe intrusive trauma and required pulp therapy for that reason. If such a tooth must be repositioned orthodontically, resorption seems less likely if a calcium hydroxide fill is maintained until the tooth movement is completed, and then the definitive root canal filling is placed.[29]

Root Resorption

Orthodontic treatment requires remodeling of bone adjacent to the tooth roots. For many years, it was thought that the roots were not remodeled in the same way as bone. More recent research has made it plain that when orthodontic forces are applied, there usually is some remodeling of the cementum on the root surface as well as the adjacent bone.

Brudvik and Rygh have shown that cementum adjacent to hyalinized (necrotic) areas of the PDL is "marked" by this contact and that clast cells attack this marked cementum when the PDL area is repaired.[30] This observation helps explain why heavy continuous orthodontic force can lead to severe root resorption. Even with the most careful control of orthodontic force, however, it is difficult to avoid creating some hyalinized areas in the PDL. It is not surprising, therefore, that careful examination of the root surfaces of teeth that have been moved reveals repaired areas of resorption of both cementum and dentin of the root (Fig. 8.26). It appears that cementum (and dentin, if resorption penetrates through the cementum) is removed from the root surface, then cementum is restored in the same way that alveolar bone is removed and then replaced. Root remodeling, in other words, is a constant feature of orthodontic tooth movement, but permanent loss of root structure would occur only if repair did not replace the initially resorbed cementum.

Repair of the damaged root restores its original contours, unless the attack on the root surface produces large defects at the apex that eventually become separated from the root surface (Fig. 8.27). Once an island of cementum or dentin has been cut totally free from the root surface, it will be resorbed and will not be replaced. On the other hand, even deep defects in the form of craters into the root surface will be filled in again with cementum once orthodontic movement stops, so permanent loss of root structure related to orthodontic treatment occurs primarily at the apex.

Apical root resorption (loss of root length) during orthodontic treatment occurs in three distinct forms that must be distinguished when its etiology is considered.

Moderate Generalized Resorption

Despite the potential for repair, careful radiographic examination of individuals who have undergone comprehensive orthodontic treatment shows that most of the teeth have some loss of root

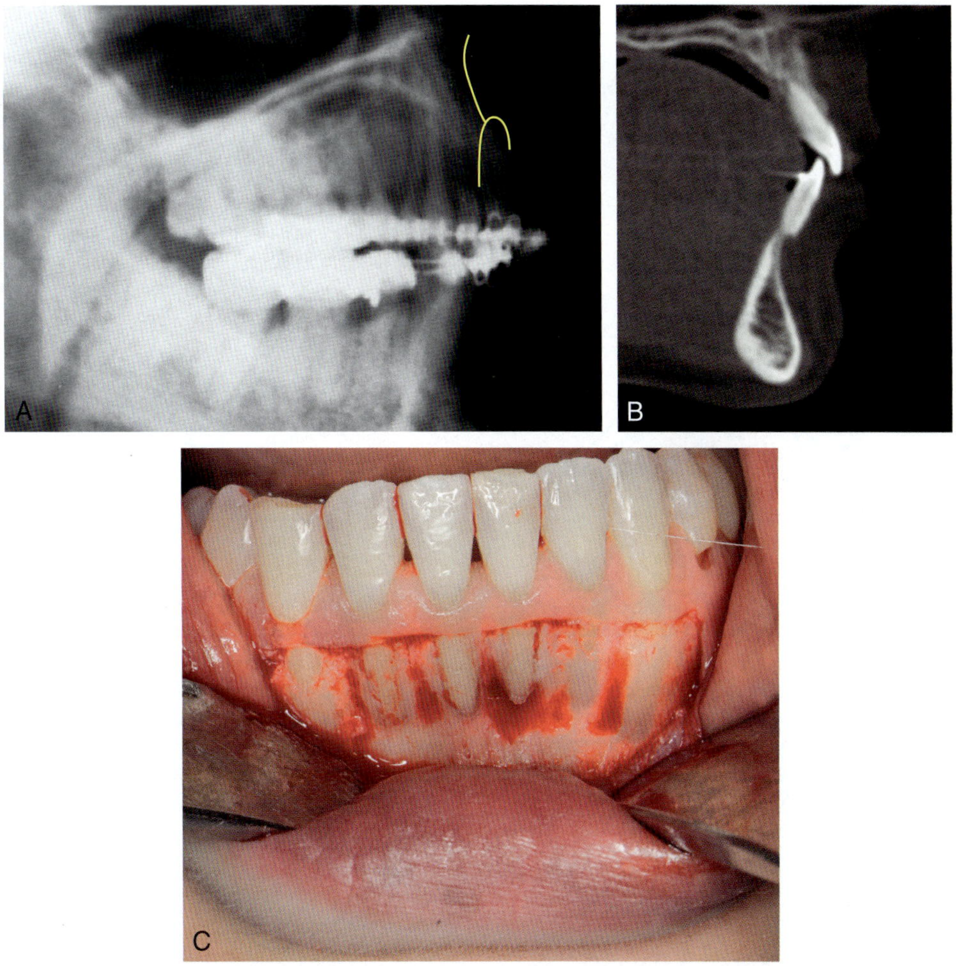

• **Fig. 8.25** (A) Extreme tipping of maxillary incisor teeth from excessive and poorly controlled orthodontic forces. In this patient, the apices of all four maxillary incisors were carried through the labial cortical plate, and pulp vitality was lost. Mandibular incisor root shown out of bone in cone beam computed tomography image (B) and clinical photograph (C).

length, and this is greater in patients whose treatment duration was longer (Table 8.4). The average shortening of root length of maxillary incisors is somewhat greater than for other teeth, but all teeth included in the typical fixed orthodontic appliance show slight average shortening. In the Seattle study from which the data of Table 8.4 were derived, all teeth except upper second molars were banded. Note that these were the only unaffected teeth. Although 90% of maxillary incisors and over half of all teeth show some loss of root length during treatment, for the great majority of the patients, this modest shortening is almost imperceptible and is clinically insignificant (Fig. 8.28A and B).

Occasionally, however, loss of one-third or one-half or more of the root structure is observed in patients who received what seemed to be only routine orthodontic therapy. To understand this, it is important to distinguish between two forms of severe resorption.

Severe Generalized Resorption

Severe root resorption of all the teeth, fortunately, is rare. Some individuals are prone to root resorption, even without orthodontic treatment—severe generalized resorption has been observed many times in individuals who never were orthodontic patients. If there is evidence of root resorption before orthodontic treatment, the patient is at considerable risk of further resorption during orthodontic treatment, much more so than a patient with no pretreatment resorption. Although hormonal imbalances and other metabolic derangements have been suspected in these susceptible patients, little evidence supports these theories.

Various reports have suggested that above-average resorption can be anticipated if the teeth have conical roots with pointed apices, distorted tooth form (dilaceration), or a history of trauma (with or without endodontic treatment). These characteristics, however, are best considered indicators of possible moderate resorption than as risk factors for severe resorption.

At this point the etiology of severe generalized resorption must be considered entirely unknown—but at least we know that it is not a complication of orthodontic treatment.

Severe Localized Resorption

In contrast to severe generalized resorption, severe localized resorption (i.e., severe resorption of a few teeth) (see Fig. 8.28C) usually is caused by orthodontic treatment. It has been known for many years that excessive force during orthodontic treatment increases the risk of root resorption, particularly if heavy continuous forces are used. Prolonged duration of orthodontic treatment also increases the amount of resorption.

It is increasingly apparent that some individuals are more susceptible to root resorption. It seems reasonable to presume that

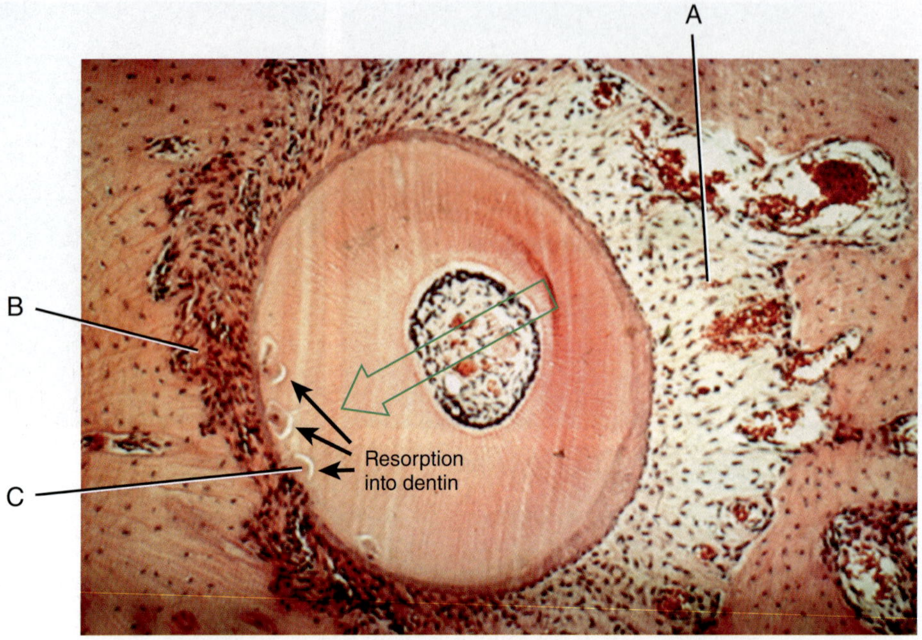

• **Fig. 8.26** Coronal section of alveolar bone through the root of a premolar being moved to the left *(arrow)*. Note the zone of periodontal ligament (PDL) compression to the left and tension to the right. Dilation of blood vessels and osteoblastic activity (A) can be seen on the right. Osteoclasts removing bone are present on the left (B). Areas of beginning root resorption that will be repaired by later deposition of cementum also can be seen on the left (C). If resorption penetrates through the cementum and into the dentin, the result will be cementum repair that fills in craters in the dentin. (Courtesy Professor B. Melsen.)

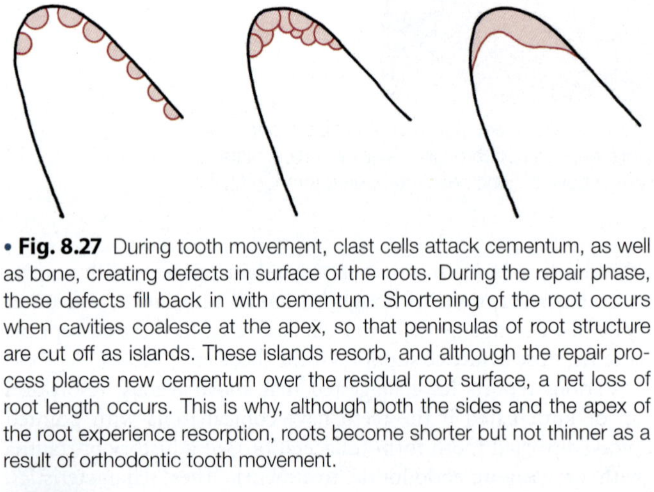

• **Fig. 8.27** During tooth movement, clast cells attack cementum, as well as bone, creating defects in surface of the roots. During the repair phase, these defects fill back in with cementum. Shortening of the root occurs when cavities coalesce at the apex, so that peninsulas of root structure are cut off as islands. These islands resorb, and although the repair process places new cementum over the residual root surface, a net loss of root length occurs. This is why, although both the sides and the apex of the root experience resorption, roots become shorter but not thinner as a result of orthodontic tooth movement.

the large individual differences relate to genetic factors, although there is not yet any way to use genetic testing to evaluate resorption risk. Perhaps the best way to detect those who are likely to experience unusually large amounts of resorption is to take a panoramic radiograph 6 to 9 months into treatment and evaluate the amount of resorption during this time. Patients who show significant resorption in the initial stage of treatment are likely to have greater resorption at the end of treatment.[31]

The risk of severe localized resorption is much greater for maxillary incisors (3% affected versus <1% for all other teeth; Table 8.5). Kaley and Phillips reported a 20-fold increase in the risk of severe resorption for maxillary incisors if the roots were forced against the lingual cortical plate during treatment (Table 8.6).[32] This is likely to occur during camouflage treatment for skeletal problems, when the maxillary incisors are torqued (as in Class

TABLE 8.4 Average Root Length Change

	MAXILLARY		MANDIBULAR	
	Serial Ext Plus	Late Ext	Serial Ext Plus	Late Ext
Central incisor	−1.5	−2.0	−1.0	−1.5
Lateral incisor	−2.0	−2.5	−1.0	−1.0
Canine	−1.0	−1.5	−0.5	−1.0
Second premolar	−0.5	−1.5	−0.5	−1.5
First molar (mesial)	−0.5	−1.0	−0.5	−1.5

Data from Kennedy DB, Joondeph DR, Osterburg SK, et al. The effect of extraction and orthodontic treatment on dentoalveolar support. *Am J Orthod.* 1983;84:183.
ext, Extraction.

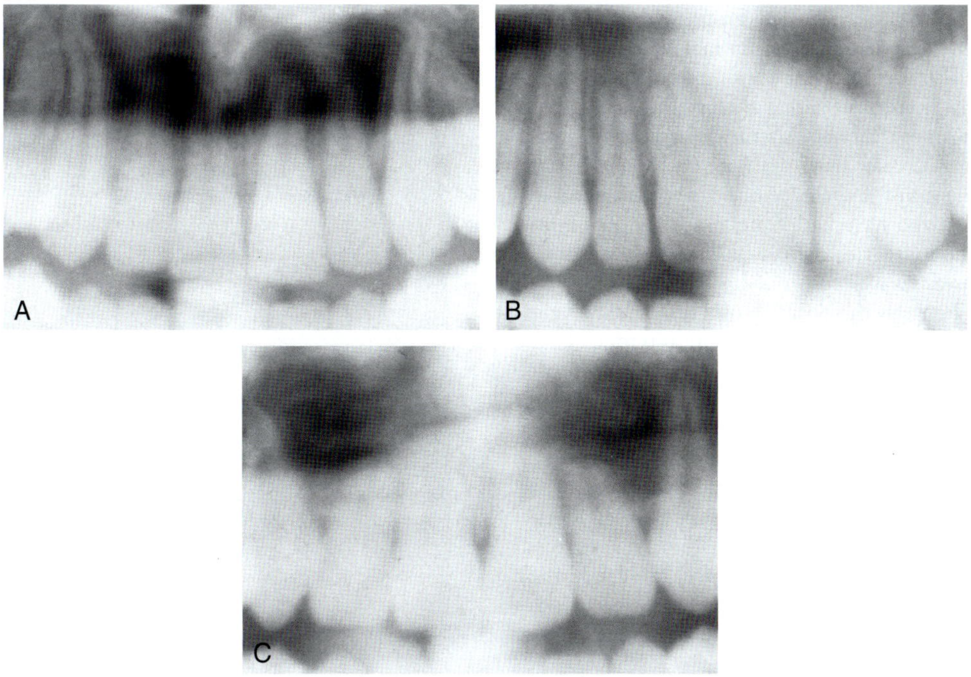

• **Fig. 8.28** Root resorption accompanying orthodontic treatment can be placed into three categories as illustrated here for maxillary central and lateral incisors: (A) category 1, slight blunting; (B) category 2, moderate resorption, up to ¼ of root length; (C) category 3, severe resorption, greater than ¼ of root length. See Table 8.5 for data for prevalence of these levels of resorption. (From Kaley JD, Phillips C. Factors related to root resorption in edgewise practice. *Angle Orthod*. 1991;61:125–131.)

TABLE 8.5 Percentage of Patients With Root Resorption by Degree of Resorption (200 Consecutive Full-Treatment Patients)

	RESORPTION CATEGORY[a]			
Tooth	0	1	2	3
Maxillary				
Central incisor	8	45	44	3
Lateral incisor	14	47	37	3
Second premolar	51	45	4	0.5
Mandibular				
Central incisor	16	63	20	0.5
Second premolar	55	38	6	0.5

Data from Kaley JD, Phillips C. Factors related to root resorption in edgewise practice. *Angle Orthod.* 1991;61:125–131.

[a]Values are for the right tooth in each instance (no significant right–left differences): 0 = no apical root resorption; 1 = slight blunting of the root apex; 2 = moderate resorption, up to of root length; 3 = severe resorption, greater than of root length (see Fig. 8.28).

II patients) or tipped (as in Class III treatment) so that the root apices are thrust against the lingual cortical plate. Contact with the cortical plates also can explain other patterns of localized root resorption, such as resorption of lower molar roots when buccal root torque is used in an effort to augment anchorage.

TABLE 8.6 Risk Factors for Severe Root Resorption, Maxillary Incisors

Factor	Probability	Odds Ratio
Lingual plate approximation	.001	20
Maxillary surgery	.002	8
Torque	.01	4.5
Extraction	.01	.5
Mandibular surgery	.05	3.6

Data from Kaley JD, Phillips C. Factors related to root resorption in edgewise practice. *Angle Orthod.* 1991;61:125–131.

Lingual plate approximation largely explains the other risk factors.

Effects of Treatment on Alveolar Bone Height

Pressure in the PDL space is at its peak, except when tipping of the tooth is perfectly controlled, at the root apex and the alveolar bone crest. For that reason alone, it would seem logical to suspect that another side effect of orthodontic treatment might be loss of alveolar bone height. In addition, there are two other potential risk factors: the blood supply at the bone crest is diminished relative to the thicker bone beneath it, and the presence of orthodontic appliances increases the amount of gingival inflammation, even with good hygiene.

Fortunately, excessive loss of crestal bone height is almost never seen as a complication of orthodontic treatment. Loss of alveolar crest height in one large series of patients averaged less than 0.5 mm and almost never exceeded 1 mm, with the greatest changes occurring at extraction sites.[33] Minimal effects on crestal alveolar bone levels also are observed on long-term follow-up of orthodontic patients. The reason is that the position of the teeth determines the position of the alveolar bone. When teeth erupt or are moved, they bring alveolar bone with them. The only exception is tooth movement in the presence of active periodontal disease, and even adults who have had bone loss from periodontal disease can have orthodontic treatment with good bone responses if the periodontal disease is well controlled.

The relationship between the position of a tooth and alveolar bone height can be seen clearly when teeth erupt too much or too little. In the absence of pathologic factors, a tooth that erupts too much simply carries alveolar bone with it, often for considerable distances. It does not erupt out of the bone. But unless a tooth erupts into an area of the dental arch, alveolar bone will not form there. If a tooth is congenitally absent or extracted at an early age, a permanent defect in the alveolar bone will occur unless another tooth is moved into the area relatively rapidly. This is an argument against very early extraction, as in, for instance, the enucleation of an unerupted premolar. Early removal of teeth poses a risk of creating an alveolar bone defect that cannot be overcome by later orthodontic treatment.

Because an erupting tooth brings alveolar bone with it, orthodontic tooth movement can be used to create the alveolar bone needed to support an implant to replace a congenitally missing tooth. For instance, if a maxillary lateral incisor is missing and a prosthetic replacement is planned, it is advantageous to have the permanent canine erupt mesially, into the area of the missing lateral incisor, and then to move it back into its proper position toward the end of the growth period. This stimulates the formation of alveolar bone in the lateral incisor region that otherwise would have not formed.

The same effects on alveolar bone height are seen with orthodontic extrusion as with eruption: as long as the orthodontic treatment is carried out with reasonable force levels and reasonable speed of tooth movement, a tooth brought into the dental arch by extrusive orthodontic forces will bring alveolar bone with it. The height of the bone attachment along the root will be about the same at the conclusion of movement as at the beginning. In some circumstances, it is possible to induce bone formation where an implant will be required, by extruding the root of an otherwise hopelessly damaged tooth, so that new hard and soft tissue forms in the area. If a tooth is intruded, bone height tends to be lost at the alveolar crest, so that about the same percentage of the root remains embedded in bone as before, even if the intrusion was over a considerable distance.

In most circumstances, this tendency for alveolar bone height to stay at the same level is a therapeutic plus. Occasionally, it would be desirable to change the amount of tooth embedded in bone, either to expose more of the crown to facilitate restoration after an injury, or to create better bone support after bone loss due to periodontal disease. In theory, very rapid orthodontic extrusion to expose more of the crown would not be followed by alveolar bone. The effect, however, is greater trauma for an already compromised tooth, and it is better to extrude more slowly and then recontour the alveolar bone.

For a patient who had lost alveolar bone height because of periodontal disease, if it were possible to intrude teeth without compensatory changes in alveolar height, pocket depths would decrease and bony support for the teeth would be improved as the roots moved deeper into the bone. Otherwise, intrusion would just create additional loss of bone height, which is what usually happens. There are reports of therapeutic benefit from intruding periodontally involved teeth,[34] and that can be an important part of comprehensive treatment for a patient with severe periodontal problems (see Chapter 20). But when reduced pocketing occurs in those patients, it relates to the formation of a long junctional epithelium, not to reattachment of the PDL or more extensive bony support.

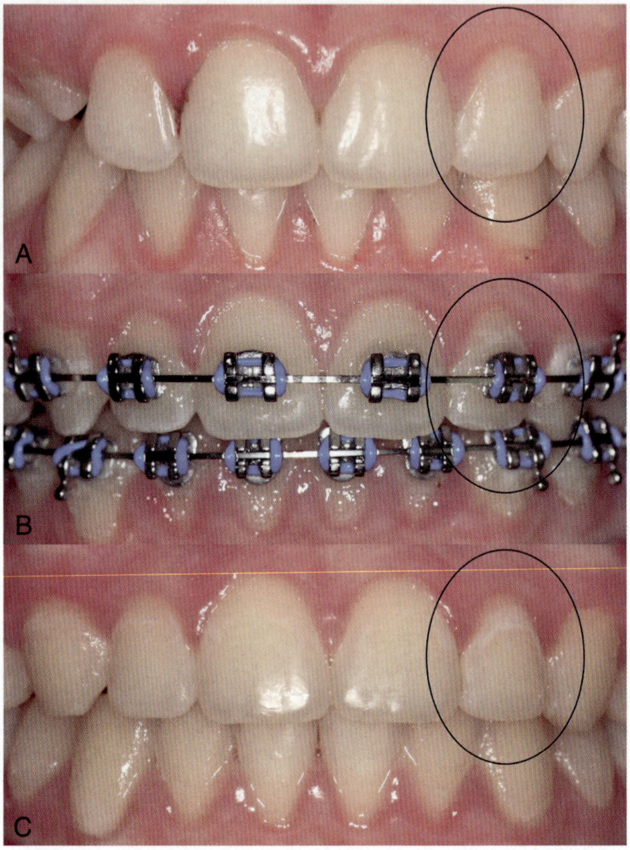

• **Fig. 8.29** Enamel demineralization, or white spot lesions, are most frequently seen in the maxillary anterior teeth around bonded orthodontic brackets. Note the maxillary left lateral incisor (*circled in black*) in this adolescent before orthodontic treatment (A), during orthodontic treatment with a bonded bracket in place (B), and after treatment showing a typical mild white spot lesion gingival to where the bracket was positioned (C).

Enamel Demineralization

Enamel demineralization around the gingival edge of bands was a well-known problem when most teeth were banded, but banding only molar teeth and using glass ionomer rather than zinc phosphate cement largely solved this problem. Unfortunately, bonding brackets has made it worse. Although bonded brackets do not directly damage the teeth, the contours of a bracket make it a trap for food debris and more difficult to clean—which increases the risk of unsightly white spot lesions around the areas where brackets were (Fig. 8.29A–C).

Maxillary incisors, particularly lateral incisors, have the greatest likelihood of obvious demineralization. In a group of 338 patients treated in a university orthodontic clinic, clinical examinations revealed that 36% had at least one clearly visible lesion on a maxillary incisor tooth at the end of treatment despite preventive efforts. Risk factors were young age at the beginning of treatment,

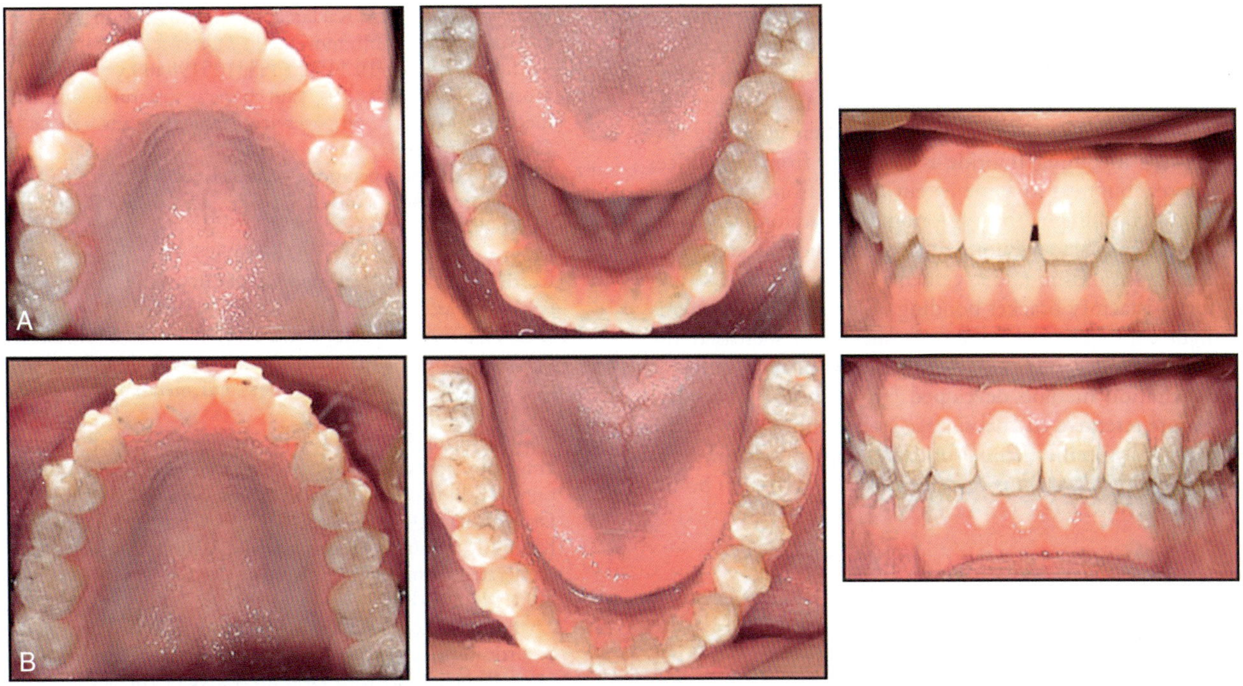

• **Fig. 8.30** Enamel demineralization is possible when clear aligners are used for orthodontic treatment as well. (A) Top row of photos shows patient prior to aligner treatment. (B) Bottom row shows the same patient in treatment with demineralized enamel visible on nearly all tooth surfaces not covered by attachments. (From Moshiri, et al. *J Clin Orthod*. 2013;47(8):494–498.)

poor hygiene before the start of treatment, and citations for poor hygiene during treatment.[35] Light-induced fluorescence reveals less completely decalcified areas, and with this method Boersma et al. found that that all but 2 of 62 patients (97%) examined immediately after comprehensive orthodontic treatment had evidence of demineralization around or adjacent to bracket sites.[36] A less obvious but also quite prevalent problem: demineralization beneath the occlusal-coverage portion of a bonded maxillary expander, in which the cusp tips of nearly all the teeth may be affected.[37]

The adoption of clear aligners for orthodontic treatment brought the promise of less demineralization because, unlike traditional brackets and wires, the aligners could be removed for routine cleaning. A cohort study comparing demineralization of traditional patients and aligners patients did find significantly fewer white spot lesions in aligner patients – only about 2%.[38] Although demineralization is less with aligners, it is not zero, and drinking acidic soda products with the aligners in place can result in very widespread demineralization due to the acid being trapped against the enamel surface, preventing the natural buffering effect of the saliva (Fig. 8.30).

The lesions can be carious or noncarious. Carious lesions are rough and porous, noncarious ones are smooth and shiny white spots. Some natural remineralization occurs, and the carious lesions have a better prognosis for this because the surface is porous. Nevertheless, the lesions are not likely to completely correct themselves. One 14-year follow-up study showed that most of the white spot lesions noted at the end of treatment were still there.[39]

Fluoridated water and a fluoride-containing toothpaste are effective as caries-controlling measures in the general population and should be considered an essential part of a program to prevent white spot lesions. There is some evidence that a daily 0.05% neutral sodium fluoride rinse is effective in preventing white spots. The major problem with the toothpaste and rinse, of course, is sporadic or no compliance. Optimal prevention requires a constant fluoride application to the area around the bracket. For caries-prone patients in general, a fluoride varnish application at 6-month intervals is recommended; for noncompliant orthodontic patients who are developing lesions, more frequent fluoride varnish applications may be helpful, although the evidence to support this is weak. A short-term daily chlorhexidine rinse program (usually 14 days) could be a last resort approach to a noncompliant patient with persistent plaque accumulation, despite the staining of teeth that occurs.

A number of fluoride-releasing bonding materials (usually composite resins impregnated with sodium fluoride) have been offered commercially in the hope that they would control demineralization around brackets, but a 2013 review of the published data, updated in 2019, concluded that there was no good evidence that any were effective against white spot formation around brackets.[40] The problem is that the fluoride release is large initially, then dwindles to little or nothing long before a typical 18- to 24-month orthodontic treatment is completed.

One way to control obvious white spot lesions is to put brackets on the lingual, not the labial, surface of the teeth. Although demineralization does occur on the lingual surface, there is good evidence that it is significantly less than on the labial surface, probably because of greater saliva flow on the lingual side of the teeth.[41] A German study found that in lingual orthodontics for children and adolescents, the addition of a layer of hydrophilic resin decreased the number of white spot lesions by 70% and the remaining lesions were minor,[42] so this change can be recommended.

Fluoride release from the glass-ionomer cements that now are the standard material for band cementation (see Chapter 10) is more sustained over time than release from fluoride-impregnated bonding resins, because the glass-ionomer cement "recharges" by absorbing fluoride when it is available, and then gradually discharges it. This incoming fluoride is primarily from dentifrices and oral rinses, but also to some extent comes from fluoridated drinking water. Bonding with glass ionomers, therefore, would be a way to obtain satisfactory fluoride release around brackets.

Unfortunately, glass-ionomer cements are simply not strong enough for satisfactory bracket bonding. Glass-ionomer cements with a small component of adhesive resin added increased the bond strength, but it was still unsatisfactory until a different surface preparation method developed by Justus and coworkers allowed a more retentive enamel surface after etching.[43]

This potentially useful method for decreasing or even eliminating enamel demineralization is presented in the section on bonding in Chapter 10.

References

1. Jacobs C, Grimm S, Ziebart T, et al. Osteogenic differentiation of periodontal fibroblasts is dependent on the strength of mechanical strain. *Arch Oral Biol.* 2013;58:896–904.
2. Wei Y, Ye Q, Tang Z, et al. Calcitonin induces collagen synthesis and osteoblastic differentiation in human periodontal ligament fibroblasts. *Arch Oral Biol.* 2017;74:114–122.
3. Thilander B. Tissue reactions in orthodontics. In: Graber LW, Vanarsdall R, Vig KWL, Huang GJ, eds. *Orthodontics: Current Principles and Techniques.* 6th ed. Elsevier; 2017.
4. Pilla AA. Low-intensity electromagnetic and mechanical modulation of bone growth and repair: are they equivalent? *J Orthop Sci.* 2002;7:420–428.
5. Shapiro E. Orthodontic movement using pulsating force-induced piezoelectricity. *Am J Orthod.* 1979;73:59–66.
6. Darendeliler MA, Zea A, Shen G, et al. Effects of pulsed electromagnetic field vibration on tooth movement induced by magnetic and mechanical forces: a preliminary study. *Aust Dent J.* 2007;52:282–287.
7. Khouw FE, Goldhaber P. Changes in vasculature of the periodontium associated with tooth movement in the rhesus monkey and dog. *Arch Oral Biol.* 1970;15:1125–1132.
8. Kang YG, Nam JH, Kim KH, et al. FAK pathway regulates PGE_2 production in compressed periodontal ligament cells. *J Dent Res.* 2010;89:1444–1449.
9. Yamaguchi M. RANK/RANKL/OPG during orthodontic tooth movement. *Orthod Craniofac Res.* 2009;12:113–119.
10. Chen YW, Wang HC, Gao LH, et al. Osteoclastogenesis in local alveolar bone in early decortication-facilitated orthodontic tooth movement. *PLoS ONE.* 2016;11(4):e0153937.
11. Roberts WE. Bone physiology, metabolism, and biomechanics in orthodontic practice. In: Graber LW, Vanarsdall RL, Vig KWL, Huang GH, eds. *Orthodontics: Current Principles and Techniques.* 6th ed. Elsevier; 2017.
12. McGorray SP, Dolce C, Kramer S, et al. A randomized, placebo-controlled clinical trial on the effects of recombinant human relaxin on tooth movement and retention. *Am J Orthod Dentofac Orthop.* 2012;141:196–203.
13. Bartzela T, Turp JC, Motschall E, et al. Medication effects on the rate of orthodontic tooth movement: a systematic literature review. *Am J Orthod Dentofac Orthop.* 2009;135:16–26.
14. Zahrowski JJ. Optimizing orthodontic treatment in patients taking bisphosphonates for osteoporosis. *Am J Orthod Dentofac Orthop.* 2009;135:361–374.
15. Makrygiannakis MA, Kaklamanos EG, Athanasiou AE. Medication and orthodontic tooth movement. *J Orthod.* 2019;46(1_suppl):39–44. https://doi.org/10.1177/1465312519840037.
16. Frost HM. Wolff's Law and bone's structural adaptations to mechanical usage: an overview for clinicians. *Angle Orthod.* 1994;64:175–188.
17. Köle H. Surgical operations of the alveolar ridge to correct occlusal abnormalities. *Oral Surg Oral Med Oral Pathol.* 1959;12:515–529.
18. Patterson BM, Dalci O, Darendeliler MA, Papadopoulou AK. Corticotomies and orthodontic tooth movement: a systematic review. *J Oral Maxillofac Surg.* 2016;74:453–473.
19. Gao J, Nguyen T, Oberoi S, Oh H, Kapila S, Kao RT, Lin GH. The significance of utilizing a corticotomy on periodontal and orthodontic outcomes: a systematic review and meta-analysis. *Biol (Basel).* 2021;10(8):803.
20. Yang C, Wang B, Deng F, et al. Biomechanical effects of corticotomy approaches on dentoalveolar structures during canine retraction: a 3-dimensional finite element analysis. *Am J Orthod Dentofac Orthop.* 2015;148:457–465.
21. Keser EI, Dibart S. Sequential piezocision: a novel approach to accelerated orthodontic treatment. *Am J Orthod Dentofac Orthop.* 2013;144:879–889.
22. Charavet C, Lecloux G, Bruwier A, et al. Localized piezoelectric decortication for orthodontic treatment in adults: a randomized controlled clinical trial. *J Dent Res.* 2016;95:1003–1009.
23. Patterson BM, Dalci O, Papadopoulou AK, et al. Effect of piezocision on root resorption associated with orthodontic force: a microcomputer tomography study. *Am J Orthod Dentofac Orthop.* 2017;151:53–62.
24. Maspero C, Cappella A, Dolci C, Cagetti MG, Inchingolo F, Sforza C. Is orthodontic treatment with microperforations worth it? A scoping review. *Child (Basel).* 2022;9(2):208.
25. El-Angbawi A, McIntyre G, Fleming PS, Bearn D. Non-surgical adjunctive interventions for accelerating tooth movement in patients undergoing orthodontic treatment. *Cochrane Database Syst Rev.* 2023;6(6):CD010887.
26. Quinn RS, Yoshikawa DK. A reassessment of force magnitude in orthodontics. *Am J Orthod.* 1985;88:252–260.
27. Murdock S, Phillips C, Khondker Z, et al. Treatment of pain after initial arch wire placement: a noninferiority randomized clinical trial comparing over-the-counter analgesics and bite-wafer use. *Am J Orthod Dentofac Orthop.* 2010;137:316–323.
28. Pazzini CA, Pereira LJ, Marques LS, Ramos-Jorge J, Aparecida da Silva T, Paiva SM. Nickel-free vs conventional braces for patients allergic to nickel: gingival and blood parameters during and after treatment. *Am J Orthod Dentofac Orthop.* 2016;150:1014–1019.
29. Llamas-Carreras JM, Amarilla A, Solano E, et al. Study of external root resorption during orthodontic treatment in root filled teeth compared with their contralateral teeth with vital pulps. *Int Endod J.* 2010;43:654–662.
30. Brudvik P, Rygh P. Transition and determinants of orthodontic root resorption-repair sequence. *Eur J Orthod.* 1995;17:177–188.
31. Artun J, Van t'Hullenaar R, Doppel D, et al. Identification of orthodontic patients at risk of severe apical root resorption. *Am J Orthod Dentofac Orthop.* 2009;135:448–455.
32. Kaley JD, Phillips C. Factors related to root resorption in edgewise practice. *Angle Orthod.* 1991;61:125–131.
33. Kennedy DB, Joondeph DR, Osterburg SK, et al. The effect of extraction and orthodontic treatment on dentoalveolar support. *Am J Orthod.* 1983;84:183–190.
34. Melsen B, Agerbaek N, Markenstam G. Intrusion of incisors in adult patients with marginal bone loss. *Am J Orthod Dentofac Orthop.* 1989;96:232–241.
35. Chapman JA, Roberts WE, Eckert GJ, et al. Risk factors and severity of white spot lesions during treatment with fixed orthodontic appliances. *Am J Orthod Dentofac Orthop.* 2010;138:188–194.

36. Boersma JG, van der Veen MH, Lagerweij MD, et al. Caries prevalence measured with quantitative light-induced fluorescence after treatment with fixed orthodontic appliances: influencing factors. *Caries Res*. 2005;39:41–47.
37. Yagci A, Korkmaz YN, Buyuk SK, et al. White spot lesion formation after treatment with full-coverage maxillary expanders. *Am J Orthod Dentofac Orthop*. 2016;149:331–338.
38. Buschang PH, Chastain D, Keylor CL, Crosby D, Julien KC. Incidence of white spot lesions among patients treated with clear aligners and traditional braces. *Angle Orthod*. 2019; 89(3):359–364.
39. Shungin D, Olsson DI, Persson M. Orthodontic treatment-related white spot lesions: a 14-year prospective quantitative follow-up, including bonding material assessment. *Am J Orthod Dentofacial Orthop*. 2010;138:136e1–136e8. discussion 136–137.
40. Benson PE, Parkin N, Dyer F, Millett DT, Germain P. Fluorides for preventing early tooth decay (demineralised lesions) during fixed brace treatment. *Cochrane Database Syst Rev*. 2019.
41. Wiechmann D, Klang E, Helms HJ, Knosel M. Lingual appliances reduce the incidence of white spot lesions during orthodontic multi-bracket treatment. *Am J Orthod Dentofac Orthop*. 2015;148:414–422.
42. Beyling F, Schwestka-Polly R, Wiechmann D. Lingual orthodontics for children and adolescents: improvement of the indirect bonding protocol. *Head Face Med*. 2013;927.
43. Justus R, Cubero T, Ondarza R, et al. A new technique with sodium hypochlorite to increase bracket shear bond strength of fluoride-releasing resin-modified glass ionomer cements: comparing shear bond strength of two adhesive systems with enamel surface deproteinization before etching. *Semin Orthod*. 2010;16:66–75.

9

Mechanical Principles in Orthodontic Force Control

BRENT E. LARSON, MATTHEW E. LARSON, AND WILLIAM R. PROFFIT

CHAPTER OUTLINE

Optimum orthodontic tooth movement is produced by light, continuous force. The challenge in designing and using an orthodontic appliance is to produce a force system with these characteristics, creating forces that are neither too great nor too variable over time. It is particularly important that light forces do not decrease rapidly, decaying away either because the material itself loses its elasticity or because a small amount of tooth movement causes a larger change in the amount of force delivered. Both the behavior of elastic materials and mechanical factors in the response of the teeth must be considered in the design of an orthodontic appliance system through which mechanotherapy is delivered.

Elastic Materials and the Production of Orthodontic Force

The Basic Properties of Elastic Materials

Elastic materials are materials able to resist external distorting force and to return to their original position after applied load is removed. This allows a consistent amount of applied force based on the amount of deflection, whether an aligner flexing over teeth or an archwire activated into a bracket slot. This response depends on the material composition, the material processing, and the geometry in which it is loaded.

For analysis, orthodontic archwires and springs can be considered as beams, supported either only on one end (e.g., a spring projecting from a removable appliance) or on both ends (the segment of an archwire spanning between attachments on adjacent teeth) (Fig. 9.1). If a force is applied to such a beam, its response can be measured as the deflection (bending or twisting) produced by the force (Fig. 9.2). Force and deflection are external measurements and are significantly affected by the geometry of the material. *Stress* and *strain* refer to the internal state of the material being studied: stress is the internal distribution of the load, defined as force per unit area, whereas strain is the internal distortion produced by the load, defined as deflection per unit length. Internal stress and strain can be calculated from force and deflection by considering the cross-sectional area and length of the beam. This can be used to generate a stress-strain curve (Fig. 9.3), which show internal characteristics of the material independent of geometry.

For orthodontic purposes, three major properties of beam materials are critical in defining their clinical usefulness: strength, stiffness, and range. Each can be defined by appropriate reference to a force-deflection or stress-strain diagram (Figs. 9.2 and 9.3).

Three different points on a stress-strain diagram can be taken as representative of the strength of a material (see Fig. 9.3). Each represents, in a somewhat different way, the maximum load that the material can resist. The first two points attempt to describe the elastic limit of the material, the point at which any permanent deformation is first observed. The most conservative measure is the *proportional limit*, the highest point where stress and strain still have a linear relationship (this linear relationship is known as *Hooke's law*). Precisely determining this point can be difficult, so a

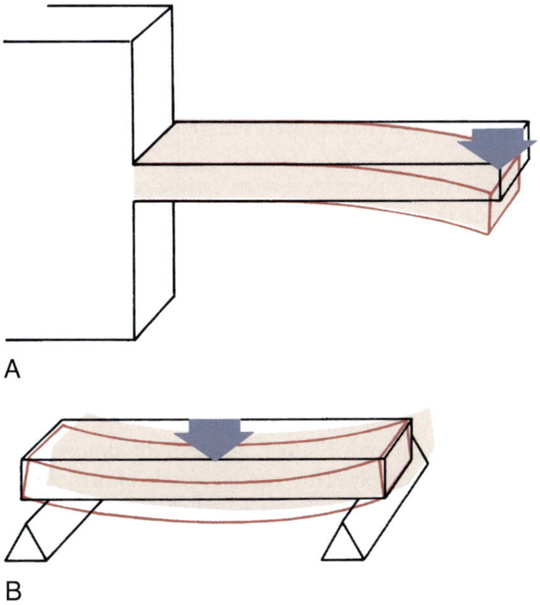

• **Fig. 9.1** Cantilever (A) and supported beams (B).

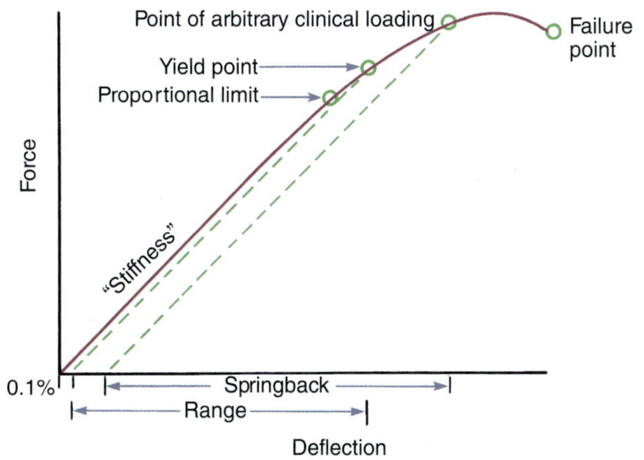

• **Fig. 9.2** A typical force-deflection curve for an elastic material like an orthodontic archwire. The stiffness of the material is given by the slope of the linear portion of the curve. The range is the distance along the x-axis to the point at which permanent deformation occurs (usually taken as the yield point, at which 0.1% permanent deformation has occurred). Clinically useful springback occurs if the wire is deflected beyond the yield point (as to the point indicated here as "arbitrary clinical loading"), but it no longer returns to its original shape. At the failure point, the wire breaks.

more practical indicator is the *yield strength*—the intersection of the stress-strain curve with a parallel line offset at 0.1% strain. Typically, the true *elastic limit* lies between these two points, but both serve as good clinical estimates of how much force or deflection a wire can withstand before permanent deformation occurs. The maximum load the wire can sustain—the *ultimate tensile strength*—is reached after some permanent deformation and is greater than the yield strength. This ultimate strength determines the maximum force the wire can deliver if used as a spring, so it also is important clinically, especially because yield strength and ultimate strength differ much more for the newer titanium alloys than for steel wires.

Strength is measured in units of stress—the SI (International System of Units) unit is the pascal (Pa), but English units such as g/cm^2 may still be encountered. Data in megapascals (MPa) now appear in orthodontic journals, and MPa will be used in the rest of this text. Other units of stress such as g/cm^2 and psi can easily be converted to MPa (1 MPa = 10,197 g/cm^2 = 145 psi).

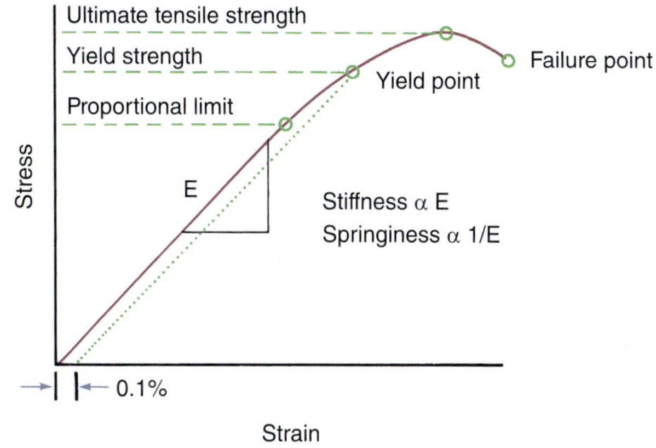

• **Fig. 9.3** Stress and strain are internal characteristics that can be calculated from measurements of force and deflection, so the general shapes of force-deflection and stress-strain curves are similar. Three different points, as noted here on a stress-strain diagram, can be taken as representing the strength. The slope of the stress-strain curve *(E)* is the modulus of elasticity, to which stiffness and springiness are proportional.

Stiffness is proportional to the slope of the elastic portion of the force-deflection curve (see Fig. 9.2). The more vertical the slope, the stiffer the wire, the more horizontal the slope, the more flexible the wire.

Range is defined as the distance that the wire will bend elastically before permanent deformation occurs. For orthodontics, this distance is measured in millimeters (see Fig. 9.2). If the wire is deflected beyond this point, it will not return to its original shape, but clinically useful springback will still occur unless the failure point is reached. This springback is measured along the horizontal axis as shown in Fig. 9.2. Orthodontic wires often are deformed beyond their elastic limit, so springback properties are important in determining clinical performance.

These three major properties have an important relationship:

$$\text{Strength} = \text{Stiffness} \times \text{Range}$$

Two other characteristics of some clinical importance also can be illustrated with a stress-strain diagram: resilience and formability (Fig. 9.4). *Resilience* is the area under the stress-strain curve out to the proportional limit. It represents the energy storage capacity of the wire, which is a combination of strength and springiness. *Formability* is the amount of permanent deformation that a wire can withstand before failing. It represents the amount of permanent bending the wire will tolerate (while being formed into a clinically useful spring, for instance) before it breaks.

The properties of an ideal wire material for orthodontic purposes can be described largely in terms of these criteria: it should possess (1) high strength, (2) low stiffness (in most applications), (3) high range, and (4) high formability. In addition, the material should be weldable or solderable, so that hooks or stops can be attached to the wire. It should also be reasonable in cost. In contemporary practice, no one archwire material meets all these requirements, and the best results are obtained by using specific archwire materials for specific purposes (Table 9.1).

In the United States, orthodontic appliance dimensions, including wire sizes, are specified in thousandths of an inch. For simplicity in this text, they are given in mils (i.e., 0.016 inch =

16 mil). In Europe and many other areas of the world, appliance dimensions are specified in millimeters. For the range of orthodontic sizes, a close approximation of sizes in millimeters can be obtained by dividing the dimensions in mils by 40 (i.e., 16 mil = 0.4 mm; 40 mil = 1.0 mm).

Orthodontic Archwire Materials

Precious Metal Alloys

In the first half of the 20th century, precious metal alloys were used routinely for orthodontic purposes, primarily because nothing else would tolerate intraoral conditions. Gold itself is too soft for nearly all dental purposes, but alloys (which often included platinum and palladium along with gold and copper) could be useful orthodontically. The introduction of stainless steel made precious metal alloys obsolete for orthodontic purposes even before precious metals became prohibitively expensive. Currently, the only considerable advantage to gold is the ease of fabricating cast appliances, such as custom-fit bonding pads used with fixed lingual appliances (see Chapter 10).

Stainless Steel and Cobalt-Chromium Alloys

Stainless steel, or a cobalt-chromium alloy (Elgiloy; Rocky Mountain Co.) with similar properties, replaced precious metal in orthodontics because of considerably better strength and springiness with equivalent corrosion resistance. Stainless steel's rust resistance results from a relatively high chromium content. A typical formulation for orthodontic use has 18% chromium and 8% nickel (thus the material is often referred to as an 18-8 stainless steel).

The properties of these steel wires can be controlled over a reasonably wide range by varying the amount of cold working and annealing during manufacture. Steel is softened by annealing and hardened by cold working. Fully annealed stainless steel wires are soft and highly formable. The steel ligatures used to tie orthodontic archwires into brackets on the teeth are made from such "dead soft" wire. Steel archwire materials are offered in a range of partially annealed states, in which yield strength is progressively enhanced at the cost of formability. The steel wires with the most impressive yield strength ("super" grades) are almost brittle and will break if bent sharply. The "regular" grade of orthodontic steel wire can be bent to almost any desired shape without breaking. If sharp bends are not needed, the super wires can be useful, but it is difficult to show improved clinical performance that justifies either their higher cost or limited formability.

Elgiloy, the cobalt-chromium alloy, has the advantage that it can be supplied in a softer and therefore more formable state, and the wires can be hardened by heat treatment after being shaped. The heat treatment decreases the formability but increases the range significantly. After heat treatment, the softest Elgiloy becomes equivalent to regular stainless steel, while harder initial grades are equivalent to the "super" steels. This material, however, had almost disappeared by the end of the 20th century because of its additional cost relative to stainless steel and the extra step of heat treatment to obtain optimal properties, and it is used only rarely at present.

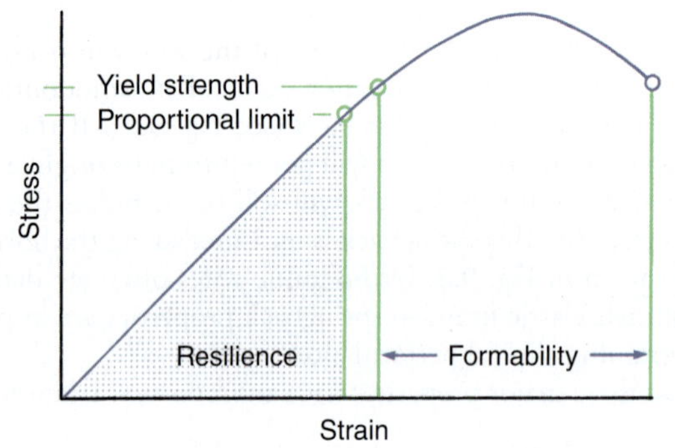

• **Fig. 9.4** Resilience and formability are defined as an area under the stress-strain curve and a distance along the x-axis, respectively, as shown here. Because the plastic deformation that makes a material formable also may be thought of as cold work, formability alternatively can be interpreted as the area under that part of the stress-strain curve.

Nickel-Titanium Alloys

Properties of Nickel-Titanium Alloys

Nickel-titanium alloys have an exceptional ability to deliver light force over a large range of activation, making these archwires the material of choice during initial alignment in modern orthodontics. The first nickel-titanium alloy was developed for the space program and named *Nitinol* (Ni, nickel; Ti, titanium; NOL, Naval Ordnance Laboratory). In this book, the term *NiTi* is used subsequently to refer to the family of nickel-titanium wire materials (*nitinol*, with the word not capitalized, is used in the same way

TABLE 9.1 Comparative Properties of Orthodontic Wires

	Strength	Stiffness	Range	Formability	Clinical Use
Desired Ideal	Good	High	High	Good	
Material					
Gold (historic)	Intermediate	Intermediate	Low	Good	Not used - Expensive
Stainless Steel	Good	High	Low	Good	Finishing wires
Co-Cr (Elgiloy)	Good	High	Low	Good	Finishing wires
Beta-Titanium (B-Ti)	Intermediate	Intermediate	Intermediate	Good	Large finishing wires or intermediate wires
Nickel-Titanium (NiTi)	Intermediate	Low	High	Poor	Initial alignment

in some other publications). Reference to a specific material is by its trademark (capitalized) name.

The properties of NiTi alloys cannot be discussed without first understanding that these alloys can exist in more than one crystal structure at intraoral temperature. At higher temperatures and lower stress, the alloy exists in a simple cubic structure called *austenite*. At lower temperatures and higher stress, the alloy is more stable in a monoclinic phase called *martensite*. Although many metal alloys exist in different crystal structures, the uniqueness of NiTi is that the transition between the two structures is fully reversible and may occur at or near intraoral temperature. This phase transition allows certain NiTi alloys to exhibit two remarkable properties found in no other archwire materials—heat-activation and superelasticity.

Heat-activation refers to the ability of the material to go from a martensitic state to an austenitic state when its temperature is increased. This temperature-induced change in crystal structure (called *thermoelasticity*) was important to the original Nitinol used in the space program but proved difficult to exploit in orthodontic applications. Many companies still heavily promote heat-activation properties of their wires, but keep in mind that clinicians do not add slow, controlled temperature change during this initial alignment stage to incrementally move the material to its austenitic phase. These wires typically express other desirable properties and are still highly useful, but the most clinically applicable property is not the thermoelastic phase transformation.

One unique property of some alloys that go through a heat-activated phase transformation is shape memory. *Shape memory* refers to the ability of the material to "remember" its original shape after being plastically deformed while in the martensitic form. In a typical application, a certain shape is set while the alloy is maintained at an elevated temperature, above the martensite-austenite transition temperature. When the alloy is cooled below the transition temperature, it can be easily deformed in the martensitic state, but the original shape is restored when it is heated enough to regain an austenitic structure.

Superelasticity refers to the very large reversible strains that certain NiTi wires can withstand due to the martensite-austenite phase transition. This reversible deformation can be over 10 times greater than similar dimension archwires in other materials. In engineering applications, it also is frequently described as pseudoelasticity, owing to the nonlinear stress-strain curve (Fig. 9.5), which does not display classic elastic behavior obeying the linear stress-strain relationship of Hooke's Law. Materials displaying superelasticity are austenitic alloys that undergo a transition to martensite in response to stress—a stress-induced analog to the thermally induced shape memory effect. This is possible because the transition temperature is very close to room temperature. Most archwire materials can be reversibly deformed only by stretching interatomic bonds (which creates the linear region of the stress-strain curve), while superelastic materials can undergo a reversible change in internal structure after a certain amount of deformation. This stress-induced martensitic transformation manifests in the almost flat section of the load-deflection curve. This means that an initial archwire can exert about the same force whether it was deflected a relatively small or large distance, which is a unique and extremely desirable characteristic (Fig. 9.6). For a change, superelasticity is not just another advertising term.

Although shape memory is a thermal reaction and superelasticity is a mechanical one, they are inherently linked. Superelastic materials must exhibit a reversible phase change at a close transition temperature, which must be lower than intraoral temperature

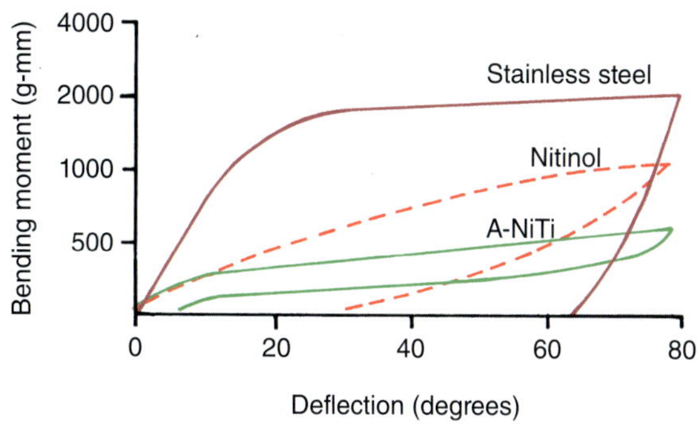

• **Fig. 9.5** Bending moment versus deflection plotted for 16-mil orthodontic wires (*solid red*, stainless steel; *dashed red*, stabilized martensitic nickel-titanium [M-NiTi]; *green*, austenitic NiTi [A-NiTi]). Note that after an initial force level is reached, A-NiTi has a considerably flatter load-deflection curve and greater springback than M-NiTi, which in turn has much more springback than steel. (Redrawn from Burstone CJ, Qin B, Morton JY. Chinese NiTi wire-a new orthodontic alloy. *Am J Orthod*. 1985;87:445–452.)

for the austenite phase to exist clinically once placed in the mouth. Shape memory alloys only have exceptional range clinically if stress-induced transformation also occurs. Otherwise, in order to keep the force light, the temperature would have to be slowly increased as the teeth come closer to alignment—which, again, does not occur clinically. Because of the close interaction of these properties, wires displaying martensite-austenite transitions are subsequently referred to as *austenitic nickel-titanium* (*A-NiTi*). All other NiTi wires are stabilized in the martensitic form without undergoing intraoral phase transformations and are subsequently referred to as *martensitic nickel-titanium* (*M-NiTi*).

Nickel-Titanium Wires in Clinical Orthodontics

The original Nitinol wires marketed under that name in the late 1970s by Unitek were M-NiTi wires, with no application of phase transition effects. As supplied for orthodontic use, Nitinol is exceptionally springy and quite strong but has poor formability (Table 9.2). In the late 1980s, new nickel-titanium wires with an austenitic grain structure (A-NiTi) appeared. These wires (Sentinol, GAC; Copper NiTi, Ormco/Sybron; and several other trade names from other suppliers) exhibit superelasticity and/or shape memory in various degrees. Without laboratory data, however, it is dangerous to assume that wires advertised as superelastic really are,[1] so care in purchasing is advised. Data for performance under controlled conditions, not testimonials from prominent clinicians, should be the basis for choosing a specific wire.

Part of the unusual nature of a superelastic material such as A-NiTi is that its unloading curve differs from its loading curve (i.e., the reversibility has an energy loss associated with it [hysteresis]) (Fig. 9.7). This means the force that it delivers is not the same as the force applied to activate it. The different loading and unloading curves produce the even more remarkable effect that the force delivered by an A-NiTi wire can be changed during clinical use merely by releasing and retying it after movement (Fig. 9.8).

For the orthodontist, wire bending in the classic sense is all but impossible with A-NiTi wires because they do not undergo plastic deformation until remarkably deformed (see Fig. 9.5). The wires can be shaped and their properties can be altered, however, by heat treatment. This can be done in the orthodontic office by passing an electric current between electrodes attached to the wire or a segment of it. Miura et al. were the first to show that it is possible

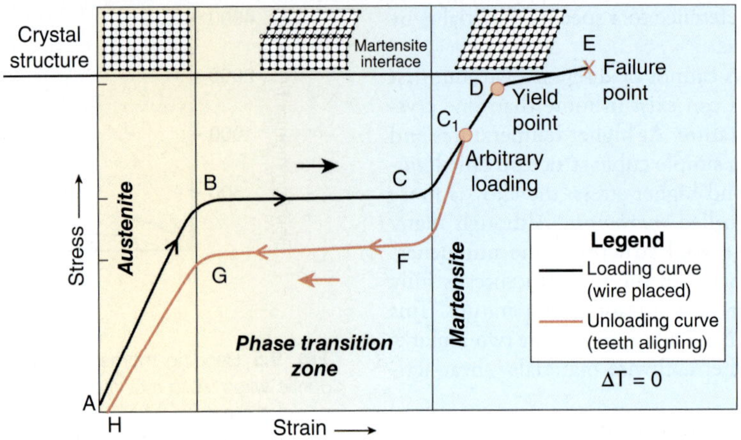

• **Fig. 9.6** A stress-strain curve illustrating superelasticity due to the stress-induced transformation from the austenitic to the martensitic phase, as in an austenitic nickel-titanium (A-NiTi) archwire. Section A–B represents purely elastic deformation of the austenitic phase (note in Fig. 9.5 that in this phase A-NiTi is stiffer than martensitic nickel-titanium [M-NiTi]). The stress corresponding to point B is the minimum stress at which transformation to the martensitic phase starts to occur. At point C, the transformation is completed. The difference between the slopes of A–B and B–C indicates the ease with which transformation occurs. After the transformation is completed, the martensitic structure deforms elastically, represented by section C–D (but orthodontic archwires are almost never stressed into this region, and this part of the graph usually is not seen in illustrations of the response of orthodontic archwires). At point D, the yield stress of the martensitic phase is reached, and the material deforms plastically until failure occurs at E. If the stress is released before reaching point D (as at point C^1 in the diagram), elastic unloading of the martensitic structure occurs along the line C^1–F. Point F indicates the maximum stress on which the stress-induced martensitic structure on unloading can exist, and at that point the reverse transformation to austenite begins, continuing to point G, where the austenitic structure is completely restored. G–H represents the elastic unloading of the austenite phase. A small portion of the total strain may not be recovered because of irreversible changes during loading or unloading.

TABLE 9.2 Comparative Properties of Orthodontic Wires

	Modules of Elasticity (GPa)	Material Stiffness Relative to Steel
Gold (heat-treated)	83	0.41
Stainless steel	200	1.00
Cobalt-chromium	193	0.97
Beta-titanium	72	0.36
A-NiTi	83[a]	0.41
M-NiTi	33	0.17

A-NiTi, Austenitic nickel-titanium; M-NiTi, martensitic nickel-titanium.
[a]From initial elastic part of force-deflection curve.

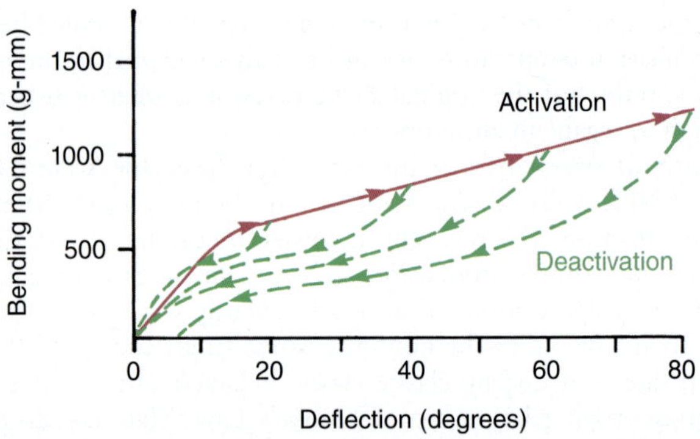

• **Fig. 9.7** Activation *(solid)* and deactivation *(dashed)* curves for austenitic nickel-titanium (A-NiTi) wire. Note that the unloading curves change at different activations (i.e., the unloading stiffness is affected by the degree of activation). In contrast, the unloading stiffness for steel, beta-titanium (beta-Ti), and martensitic nickel-titanium (M-NiTi) wires is the same for all activations. (Redrawn from Burstone CJ, Qin B, Morton JY. Chinese NiTi wire-a new orthodontic alloy. *Am J Orthod*. 1985;87:445–452.)

to reposition the teeth on a dental cast to the desired posttreatment occlusion, bond brackets to the set-up, force an A-NiTi wire into the brackets, and then heat-treat the wire so that it "memorizes" its shape with the teeth in the desired position.[2] The wire then incorporates all of what would otherwise be the "finishing bends" usually required in the last stages of treatment.

In theory at least, this allows certain types of treatment to be accomplished with a single wire, progressively bringing the teeth toward their predetermined position. The concept is exactly the same as Edward Angle's original approach to arch expansion, which implies that the same limitations would be encountered. At present, however, this approach is used primarily in computer-assisted fabrication of the initial archwires for lingual orthodontics (see later section in this chapter), and there is no attempt to do everything with one archwire.

The properties of A-NiTi have quickly made it the preferred material for orthodontic applications in which a long range of activation with relatively constant force is needed (i.e., for initial tooth alignment and coil springs). M-NiTi remains useful, primarily in the later stages of treatment when flexible but larger and somewhat stiffer wires are needed. At this point, small round nickel-titanium wires usually should be A-NiTi to take advantage of its large range. Rectangular A-NiTi wires, however, do not have enough torsional stiffness to be efficient torquing arches, so larger rectangular wires used for more detailed positioning of teeth perform better if made from a stiffer archwire material.

Beta-Titanium

In the early 1980s, after Nitinol but before A-NiTi, a quite different titanium alloy, beta-titanium (beta-Ti), was introduced into orthodontics. This beta-Ti material (TMA, Ormco/Sybron [the name is an acronym for *titanium-molybdenum alloy—the addition of molybdenum stabilizes the stiffer body centered cubic beta phase of titanium desirable for archwires*]), was developed primarily for orthodontic use. It offers a highly desirable combination of strength and springiness (i.e., excellent resilience), as well as reasonably good formability. This makes it an excellent choice for auxiliary springs and for intermediate and finishing archwires, especially rectangular wires for the late stages of edgewise treatment.

Composite Plastics

The new orthodontic materials of recent years have been adapted from those used in aerospace technology. The high-performance aircraft of the 1980s and 1990s were titanium-based, but their replacements are being built (with some difficulty) of composite plastics (e.g., Boeing's 787 or the US military's Lockheed Martin F-35). Orthodontic technology tends to trail aerospace technology by 15 to 20 years, and orthodontic "wires" of composite materials were shown in the laboratory more than 10 years ago to have desirable properties[3] but have not yet come into clinical use because of problems with stability and performance under intraoral conditions.[4,5] It was more than a decade before the first NiTi wires went from clinical curiosity to regular use, but it appears now that composite wires may never be a useful replacement for metal wires for routine clinical care.

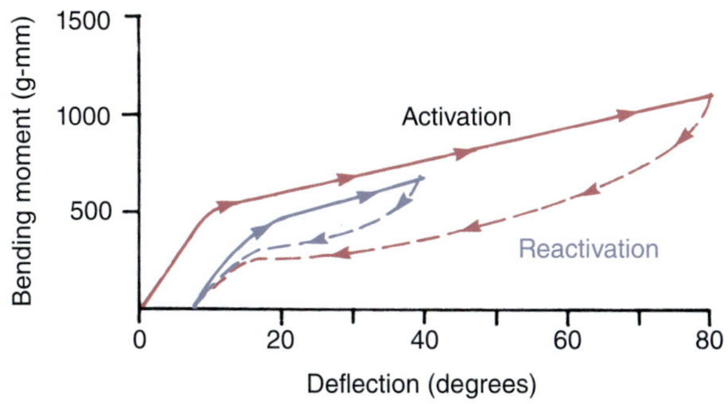

• **Fig. 9.8** Red lines, activation to 80 degrees (*solid line*) and deactivation (*dashed line*) for superelastic nickel-titanium (NiTi) wire; blue lines, reactivation of the wire to 40 degrees. In each case, the deactivation (unloading) curve indicates the force that would be delivered to a tooth. Note that the amount of force exerted by a piece of austenitic nickel-titanium (A-NiTi) wire that had previously been activated to 80 degrees (shown by the upper deactivation curve) could be considerably increased by untying it from a bracket and then retying it—again, a unique property of this alloy. (Redrawn from Burstone CJ, Qin B, Morton JY. Chinese NiTi wire-a new orthodontic alloy. *Am J Orthod*. 1985;87:445–452.)

Comparison of Contemporary Archwires

Strength, stiffness, and range for stainless steel, beta-Ti, and M-NiTi wires are compared in Fig. 9.9 (also see Table 9.2 for other comparative data). Note that in many ways the properties of beta-Ti are intermediate between stainless steel and M-NiTi, and all three archwire materials are important in contemporary orthodontic practice. Their comparative properties explain why specific wires are preferred for specific clinical applications (which are discussed further in Chapters 15 to 19). Hooke's law (which defines the linear elastic behavior of materials illustrated in Figs. 9.2–9.4) applies to all orthodontic wires except superelastic A-NiTi. For everything else, a useful method for comparing two archwires of various materials, sizes, and dimensions is the use of ratios of the major properties (strength, stiffness, and range):

$$\text{Strength A/Strength B} = \text{Strength ratio}$$

$$\text{Stiffness A/Stiffness B} = \text{Stiffness ratio}$$

$$\text{Range A/Range B} = \text{Range ratio}$$

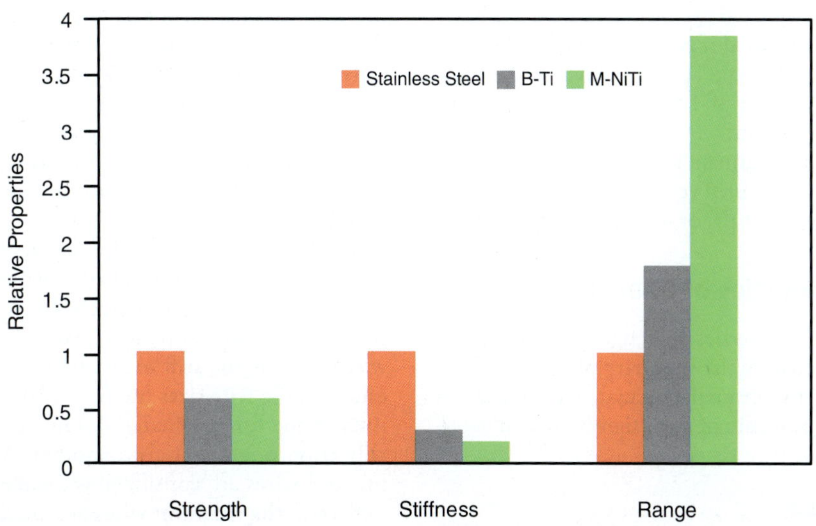

• **Fig. 9.9** The relative strength, stiffness, and range for stainless steel, B-Ti, and martensitic nickel-titanium (M-NiTi) wires (which would be the same for any wire size). Note that both B-Ti and M-NiTi have half the strength of steel; M-NiTi has slightly less stiffness but much more range than B-Ti.

These ratios were calculated for many different wires by the late Robert Kusy,[6] and the data presented here are taken from his work. When the comparative properties of wires are considered, it is important to keep two things in mind:

1. Bending describes round wires reasonably completely in orthodontic applications, but both bending and torsional stresses are encountered when rectangular wires are placed into rectangular attachments on teeth. The fundamental relationships for torsion are analogous to those in bending but are not the same. Appropriate use of the equations for torsion, however, allows torsion ratios to be computed in the same way as bending ratios.
2. The ratios apply to the linear portion of the load-deflection curve and thus do not accurately describe the behavior of wires that are stressed beyond their elastic limit but still have useful springback. This is an increasingly significant limitation as consideration passes from steel or chromium-cobalt to beta-Ti to M-NiTi. The nonlinear response of A-NiTi makes calculation of ratios for it all but impossible. Nevertheless, the ratios offer an initial understanding of the properties of traditional steel wires as compared with the newer titanium alloys, and they can be quite helpful in appreciating the effects of changing wire size and geometry in a typical archwire sequence.

An efficient method for comparing different wire materials and sizes (within the limitations described earlier) is the use of bar charts such as Fig. 9.10 that show the strength, stiffness, and range of stainless steel, M-NiTi, and beta-Ti relative to a common reference, in this case 12-mil stainless steel. Note that because all wire types and sizes are compared with the same reference, wires of different materials, as well as different sizes, can be compared. Fig. 9.11 gives comparative information for torsion in a similar way.

These bar charts are particularly helpful in allowing one to assess at a glance a set of relationships that would require pages of tables. For example, let's use Fig. 9.11 to compare 21 × 25 M-NiTi with 21 × 25 beta-Ti in torsion (the appropriate comparison if the wires would be used to produce a torquing movement of the root of a tooth).

- The 21 × 25 beta-Ti has a torsional stiffness value of 6, whereas 21 × 25 M-NiTi has a value of 3, so the beta-Ti wire would deliver twice the force at a given deflection.
- The strength value for 21 × 25 beta-Ti wire is 4, whereas the value for this size M-NiTi wire is 6, so the NiTi wire is less likely to become permanently distorted if twisted into a bracket.
- The range value for 21 × 25 beta-Ti is 0.7, whereas the same size M-NiTi has a range value of 1.9, so the NiTi could be twisted nearly three times as far.

The bar charts contain the information to allow a similar comparison of any one of the wire sizes listed versus any other wire shown on the chart, in bending (see Fig. 9.10) or torsion (see Fig. 9.11).

Effects on Elastic Properties of Beams

Each of the major elastic properties—strength, stiffness, and range—is substantially affected by the geometry of a beam. Both the cross-section (whether the beam is circular, rectangular, or square) and the length of a beam are of great significance in determining its properties.

Geometry: Size and Shape

Relative changes in elastic properties related to size and shape are independent of the material. In other words, decreasing the diameter of a steel beam by 50% would reduce its strength to a specific percentage of what it had been previously (the exact reduction would depend on how the beam was supported, as we discuss later). Decreasing the diameter of a similarly supported TMA beam by 50% would reduce its strength by exactly the same percentage as the steel beam. But keep in mind that the performance of a beam, whether beneath a highway bridge or between two teeth in an orthodontic appliance, is determined by the combination of material properties and geometric factors.

Cantilever Beams

Let us begin by considering a cantilever beam supported on only one end. In orthodontic applications, this is the type of spring often used in removable appliances, in which a wire extends from the plastic body of the removable appliance as a fingerspring. When a round wire is used as a fingerspring, doubling the diameter of the wire increases its strength eight times (i.e., the larger wire can resist eight times as much force before permanently deforming or can deliver eight times as much force). Doubling the diameter, however, increases stiffness by a factor of 16 and decreases range by a factor of 2.

More generally, for a round cantilever beam, the strength of the beam changes as the third power of the ratio of the larger to the smaller beam; stiffness changes as the fourth power of the ratio of the larger to the smaller; and range changes directly as the ratio of the smaller to the larger (Fig. 9.12).

Supported Beams

The situation is somewhat more complex for a beam supported on both ends, as is the case for a segment of archwire between two teeth. Supporting both ends makes the beam stronger and less flexible, particularly if the ends are tightly anchored as opposed to being free to slide. If a rectangular beam is evaluated, its dimension in the direction of bending is the primary determinant of its properties. The principle with any supported beam, however, is the same as with a cantilever beam: as the beam size increases, strength increases as a cubic function, whereas stiffness increases as a fourth power function and range decreases proportionately, not exponentially.

Although round beams can be placed in torsion in engineering applications, torsion is of practical importance in orthodontics only for rectangular wires that can be twisted into rectangular slots. In torsion, the analytic approach is basically similar to that in bending, but shear stress rather than bending stress is encountered, and the appropriate equations are all different. The overall effect is the same, however: Decreasing the size of a wire decreases its strength and stiffness in torsion while increasing its range, just as in bending.

As the diameter of a wire decreases, its strength decreases so rapidly that a point is reached at which the strength is no longer adequate for orthodontic purposes. As the diameter increases, its stiffness increases so rapidly that a point is reached at which the wire is simply too stiff to be useful. These upper and lower limits establish the wire sizes useful in orthodontics. The phenomenon is the same for any material, but the useful sizes vary considerably from one material to another. As Table 9.3 indicates, useful steel wires are considerably smaller than the gold wires they replaced. The titanium wires are much springier than steel wires of equal sizes but not as strong. Their useful sizes therefore are larger than steel and quite close to the sizes for gold.

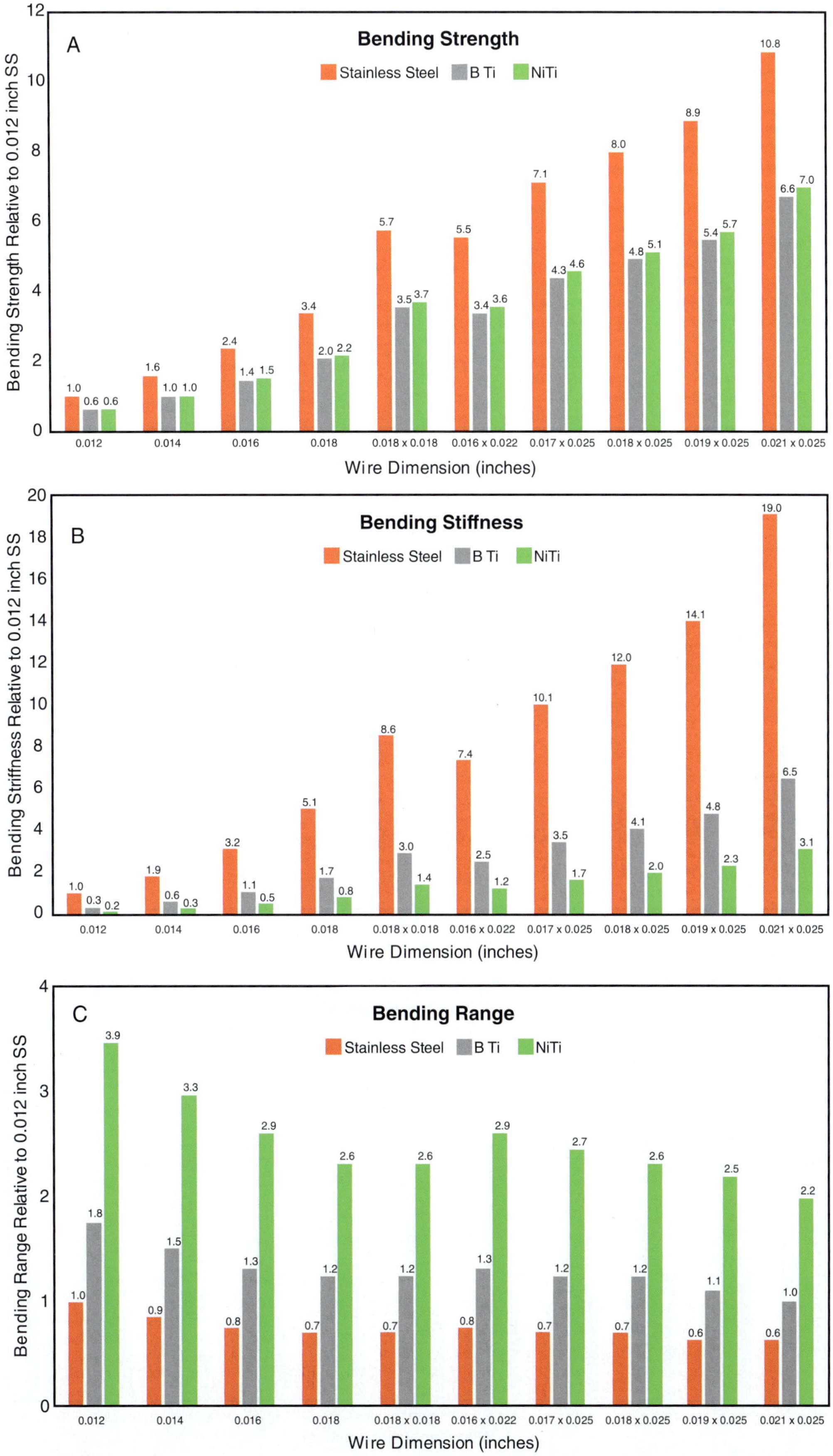

• **Fig. 9.10** Strength (A), stiffness (B), and range (C) comparisons in bending for stainless steel, martensitic nickel-titanium (M-NiTi; Nitinol), and beta-titanium (TMA; B Ti) wires. The index for all three comparisons, with an assigned value of 1, is 12 mil steel, so all values are comparable.

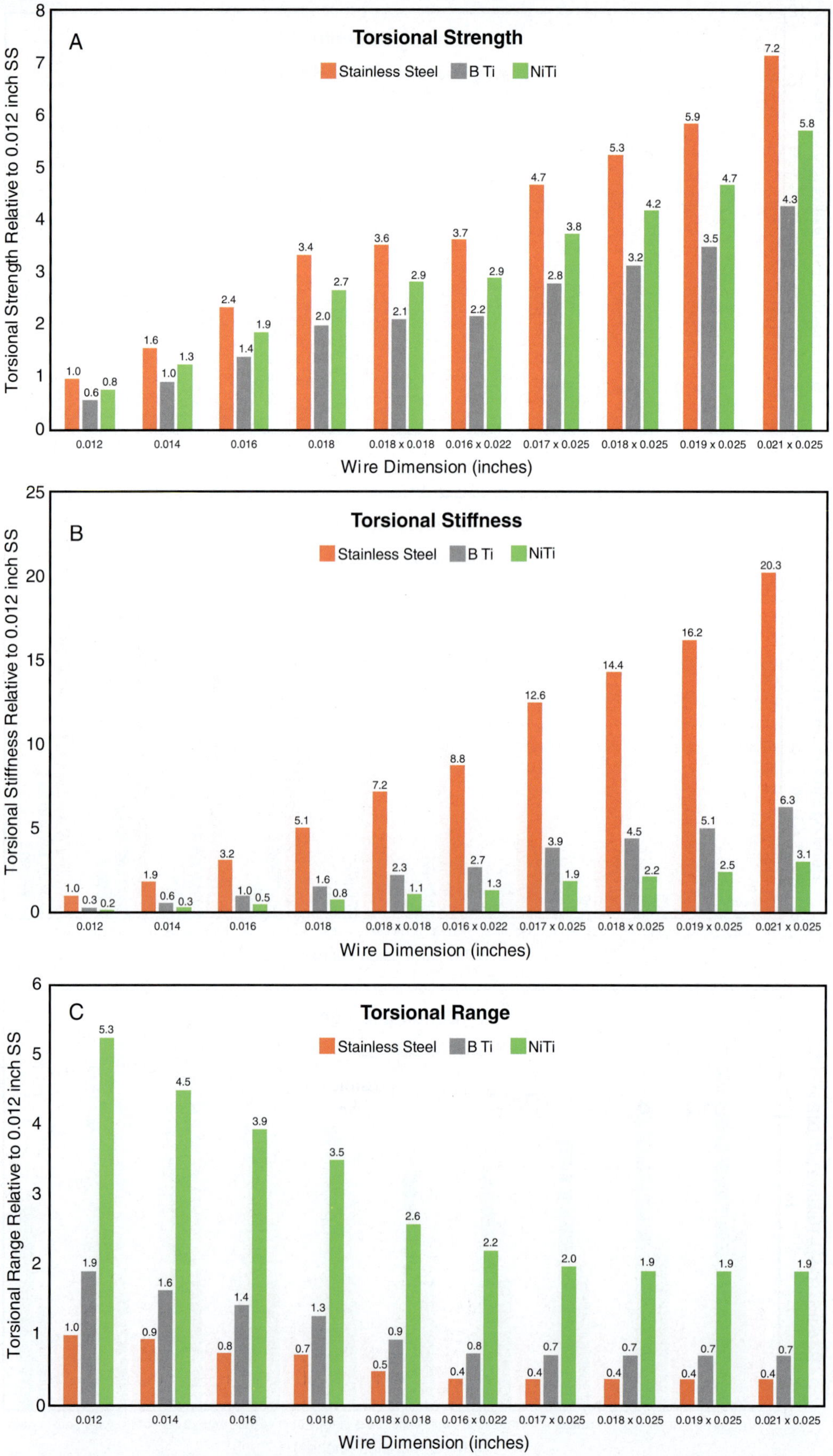

• **Fig. 9.11** Strength (A), stiffness (B), and range (C) comparisons in torsion for stainless steel, martensitic nickel-titanium (M-NiTi; Nitinol), and beta-titanium (TMA; B Ti) wires. For all three comparisons, the index wire is the same, making all values comparable.

TABLE 9.3 Useful Wire Sizes in Various Materials (Dimensions in Mil)

	Gold	Steel	Cobalt-Chromium	Beta-Ti	M-NiTi	A-NiTi
Stranded archwire		6–9				
Archwire						
Round	20–22	12–20	12–20	16–20	16–20	14–20
Rectangular	22 × 28	16 × 16 to 19 × 25	16 × 16 to 19 × 25	16 × 22 to 21 × 25	16 × 22 to 21 × 25	16 × 22 to 21 × 25
Removable appliance	30–40	22–30	22–30			
Lingual arch	40	30, 36, 32 × 32	30, 36	32 × 32		
Headgear		45, 51				
Auxiliary expansion arch		36, 40				

A-NiTi, Austenitic nickel-titanium; *beta-Ti*, beta-titanium; M-NiTi, martensitic nickel-titanium.

Geometry: Length and Attachment

Changing the length of a beam, whatever its size or the material from which it is made, also dramatically affects its properties (Fig. 9.13). If the length of a cantilever beam is doubled, its bending strength is cut in half, its stiffness decreases eight times, and its range increases four times. More generally, when the length of a cantilever beam increases, its strength decreases proportionately, its stiffness decreases as the cubic function of the ratio of the length, and its range increases as the square of the ratio of the length. Length changes affect torsion quite differently from bending: stiffness decreases and range increases proportionally with length, whereas torsional strength is not affected by length.

Changing from a cantilever to a supported beam, although it complicates the mathematics, does not affect the big picture: as beam length increases, there are proportional decreases in strength, exponential decreases in stiffness, and exponential increases in range.

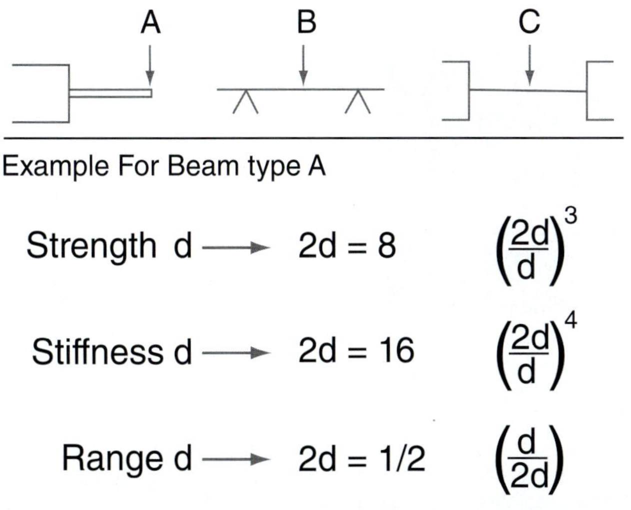

• **Fig. 9.12** Changing the diameter (*d*) of a beam, no matter how it is supported, greatly affects its properties. As the figures below the drawing indicate, doubling the diameter of a cantilever beam makes it 8 times as strong and 16 times as stiff and reduces the range by half. More generally, when beams of any type made from two sizes of wire are compared, strength changes as a cubic function of the ratio of the two cross-sections; springiness changes as the fourth power of the ratios; range changes as a direct proportion (but the precise ratios are different from those for cantilever beams).

The way in which a beam is attached also affects its properties. An archwire can be tied tightly or loosely, and the point of loading can be any point along the span. As Fig. 9.13 shows, a supported beam such as an archwire is four times less stiff if it can slide over the abutments (in clinical use, through a bracket into which it is loosely tied) rather than if the beam is firmly attached (tied tightly). With multiple attachments, as with an archwire tied to several teeth, the gain in springiness from loose ties of an initial archwire is less dramatic but still significant.[7]

Controlling Orthodontic Force by Varying Materials and Size and Shape of Archwires

Obtaining enough orthodontic force is rarely a problem. The difficulty is in obtaining light but sustained force. A spring or archwire strong enough to resist permanent deformation may be too stiff, which creates two problems: the force is likely to be too heavy initially and then will decay rapidly when the tooth begins to move. A very flexible wire with excellent range may nevertheless fail to provide a sustained force if it distorts from inadequate strength the first time the patient has lunch. The best balance of strength, stiffness, and range must be sought among the almost innumerable possible combinations of beam materials, diameters, and lengths.

The first consideration in spring design is adequate strength: the wire that is selected must not deform permanently in use. As a general rule, fingersprings for removable appliances are best constructed using steel wire. Great advantage can be taken of the fact that fingersprings behave like cantilever beams: springiness increases as a cubic function of the increase in length of the beam, whereas strength decreases only in direct proportion. Thus a relatively large wire, selected for its strength, can be given the desired spring qualities by increasing its length.

In practice, this lengthening often means doubling the wire back on itself or winding a helix into it to gain length while keeping the spring within a confined intraoral area (Fig. 9.14). The same technique can be used with archwires, of course; the effective length of a beam is measured along the wire from one support to the other, and this does not have to be in a straight line (Fig. 9.15). Bending loops in archwires can be a time-consuming chairside procedure, which is the major disadvantage.

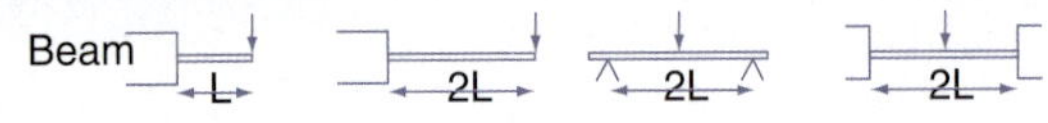

Strength	1/2	1/4	1	2
Stiffness	1	1/8	1	4
Range	1	4	1	1/2

• **Fig. 9.13** Changing either the length of a beam or the way in which it is attached dramatically affects its properties. Doubling the length of a cantilever beam cuts its strength in half, reduces its stiffness by 8 times, and gives it 4 times the range. More generally, strength varies inversely with length, whereas stiffness varies as a cubic function of the length ratios and range as a second power function. Supporting a beam on both ends makes it much stronger but also much stiffer than supporting it on only one end. Note that if a beam is rigidly attached on both ends, it is twice as strong and 4 times as stiff as a beam of the same material and length that can slide over the abutments. For this reason, the elastic properties of an orthodontic archwire are affected by whether it is tied tightly or held loosely in a bracket.

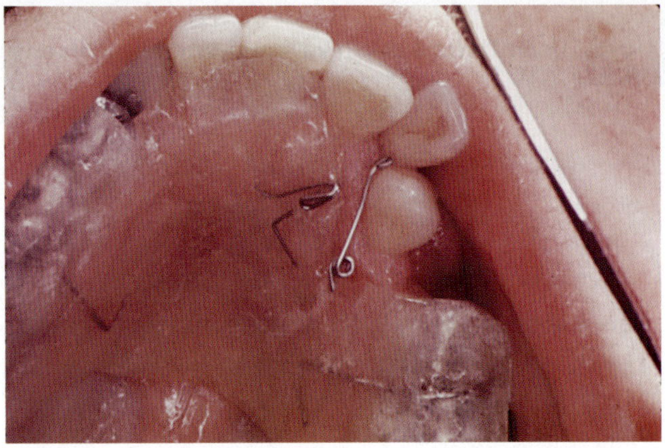

• **Fig. 9.14** A removable appliance incorporating a cantilever spring for initial tipping of a maxillary canine toward a premolar extraction site. Note that a helix has been bent into the base of the cantilever spring, effectively increasing its length to obtain more desirable mechanical properties.

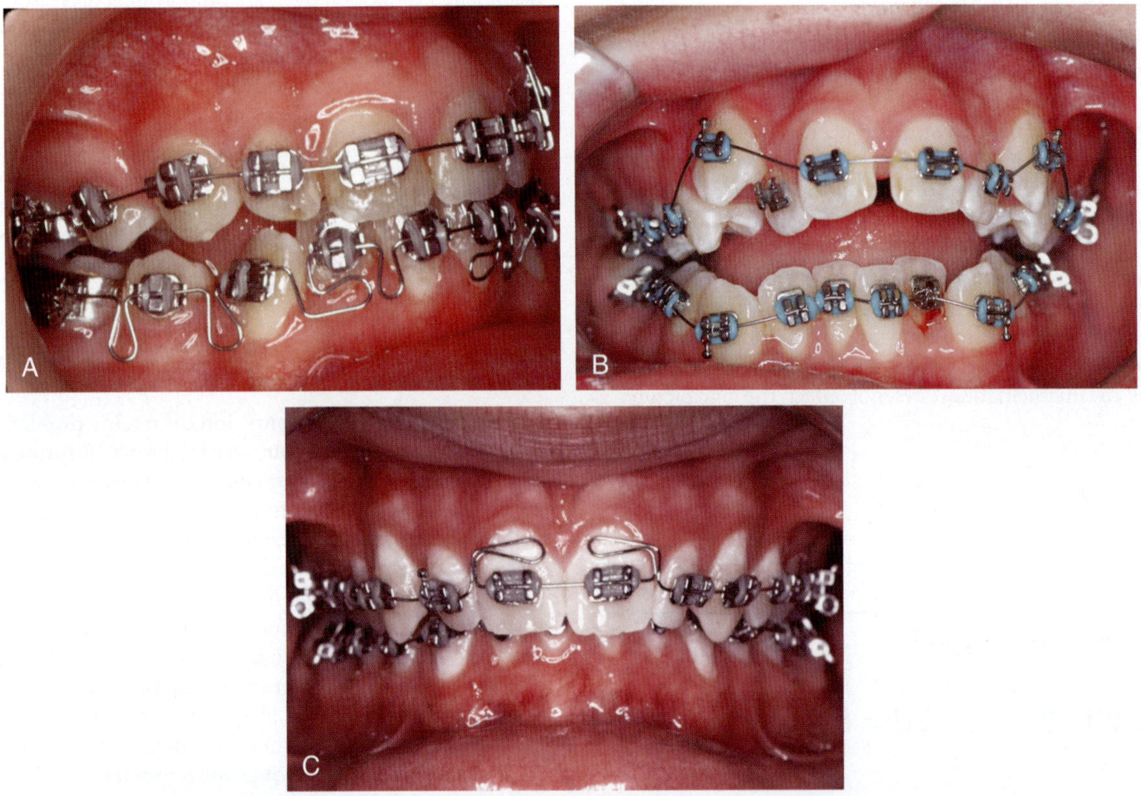

• **Fig. 9.15** (A) Improved springiness and range with steel archwires can be obtained by either of two strategies: bending loops into the archwire, as shown in the lower arch here, to increase the length of the beam segments between adjacent teeth; or using multistranded or small-diameter steel wires, as shown in the upper arch. (B) The exceptional range and flat force-deflection curve of modern superelastic austenitic nickel-titanium (A-NiTi) wire make it possible to use a single strand of 14- or 16-mil wire for initial alignment. Using these wires is more efficient than using multistrand steel wires because of the greater range of A-NiTi and takes less clinical time than bending loops, so A-NiTi has almost totally replaced both the steel alternatives. (C) A round steel wire can be used advantageously to change the axial inclination of incisors if this is needed at the initial stage of treatment (as it may be in patients with Class II division 2 malocclusion), by bending loops that contact the gingival area of the teeth when the wire is tied in place. If the end of the wire is free to slide forward, the result is facial tipping of the incisors; if the end of the wire is bent over behind the molar tube, the incisor crowns cannot tip facially and the result is lingual root torque.

Another way to obtain a better combination of stiffness and strength is to combine two or more strands of a small and therefore more flexible wire. Two 10-mil steel wires in tandem, for instance, could withstand twice the load as a single strand before permanently deforming, but if each strand could bend without being restrained by the other, the reduced stiffness is maintained. The genesis of the "twin wire" appliance system (see Chapter 10) was just this observation: that a pair of 10-mil steel wires offered proper stiffness and range for aligning teeth and that two wires gave adequate strength, although a single wire did not. Later, three or more strands of smaller steel wires, twisted into a cable, came into common use. The properties of the multistrand wire depend both on the characteristics of the individual wire strands and on how tightly they have been woven together. Multistrand steel wires offer an impressive combination of strength and spring qualities but now have been displaced for most applications by NiTi wires.

The exceptional flexibility of A-NiTi makes it a particularly attractive alternative to steel wires in the initial phases of treatment when the teeth are severely malaligned. A continuous NiTi archwire of either type will have better properties than multistrand steel wires and properties similar to a steel archwire with loops. TMA, as an intermediate between NiTi and steel, is less useful than either in the first stage of full-appliance treatment. Its excellent overall properties, however, make it quite useful in the later stages of treatment. It is possible and frequently desirable to carry out orthodontic treatment with a series of wires of approximately the same size, using a sequence from NiTi to TMA to steel. Archwire selection in varying circumstances is discussed in more detail later in this chapter and in Chapters 15–17.

Other Sources of Elastic Force

Plastic Materials: Clear Aligners

The increased use of clear aligners for orthodontic treatment has made it important to understand the elastic properties of the materials that are delivering the orthodontic force. A variety of thermoplastic polymers including polyethylene, polypropylene, and polyurethane have been used to fabricate clear aligners designed to move teeth. These materials generally are 0.75 to 1.0 mm in thickness before being thermoformed over a modified plaster cast or three-dimensional (3D) printed model. The process of thermoforming stretches the material over the cast or model and thins it to a variable degree that may affect the force delivery characteristics of the aligner.

Just as for the archwire materials discussed earlier, it is possible to develop a stress-strain curve for these clear aligner materials, and this has been done for some of the available materials as shown in Fig. 9.16. From this, it is possible to determine an elastic modulus from the slope of the curve. The modulus values, however, are not directly comparable to archwire properties because aligners are not delivered in a standardized geometric configuration such as a wire. But it is clear that these materials can store enough elastic energy to create tooth movement.

A large difference exists between the elastic range of the aligner materials and NiTi wires. A NiTi wire has an effective force-delivering range of several millimeters, whereas the range of a plastic aligner is generally limited to about 0.2 mm. What this means practically is that an incisor displaced 3 mm from its ideal position in the arch would require a minimum of five aligner trays for each millimeter it needs to travel, in this case 15 trays (3 mm × 5 trays/mm), plus any additional trays needed to create space for the moving tooth or to help with root movement. This explains why a single NiTi wire can be used with brackets to align irregular incisors, whereas doing this with aligners could take up to 20 individual trays.

Plastics for aligners also are subject to stress relaxation and water absorption that may affect their ability to deliver tooth-moving forces over time. Several suppliers of aligners and aligner materials have developed polymers that demonstrate less stress relaxation and relatively constant force delivery over a 14-day period (Fig. 9.17). Shaping aligners so that they deliver the desired force for the next movement in the sequence of aligners remains a not-yet-achieved goal.

Rubber and Elastomeric Materials

From the beginning, rubber bands were used in orthodontics to transmit force from the upper arch to the lower. Rubber has the particularly valuable quality of a great elastic range, so the extreme

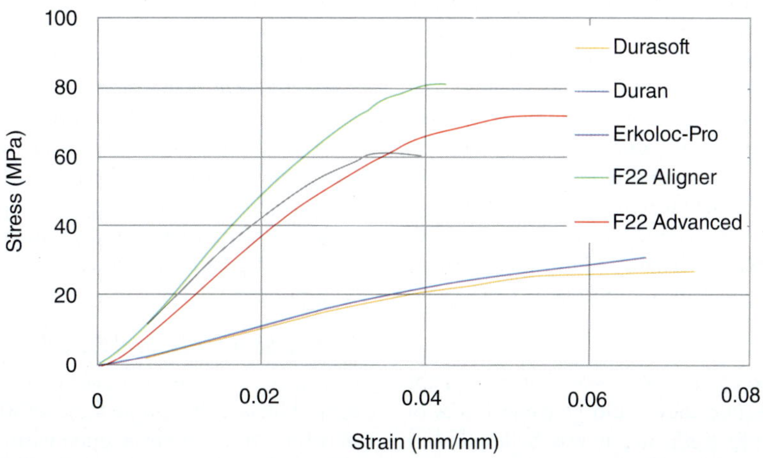

• **Fig. 9.16** Representative loading-unloading curves for several thermoplastic materials made from various polymers. Both F22 materials are polyurethane (TPU), Duran is polyethylene terephthalate glycol-modified (PET-G), Erkoloc-Pro is a dual layer PET-G/TPU and Durasoft is a dual layer TPU/polycarbonate(PC) (From Albertini P, Mazzanti V, Mollica F, Pellitteri F, Palone M, Lombardo L. Stress relaxation properties of five orthodontic aligner materials: a 14-day in-vitro study. *Bioengineering (Basel)*. 2022;9(8):349.)

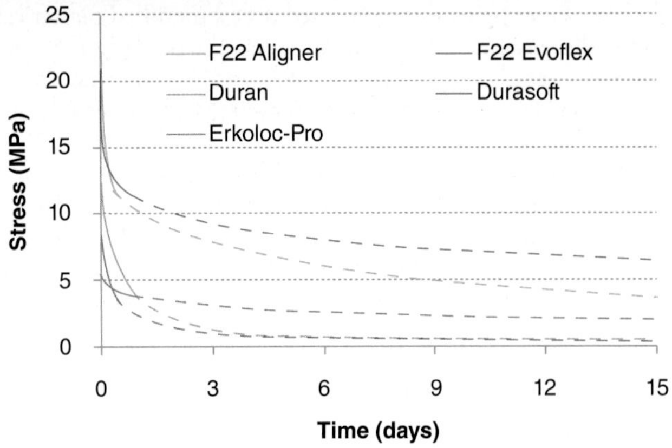

• **Fig. 9.17** Diagram showing the stress relaxation properties of the same 5 thermoplastic materials shown in Fig. 9.16. The stress decay was greatest in the first 3 days with more gradual loss up until day 15. The total stress decay was between 60% and 95% for the materials over the 15 days. (From Albertini P, Mazzanti V, Mollica F, Pellitteri F, Palone M, Lombardo L. Stress relaxation properties of five orthodontic aligner materials: a 14-day in-vitro study. *Bioengineering (Basel)*. 2022;9(8):349.)

stretching produced when a patient opens the mouth while wearing rubber bands can be tolerated without destroying the appliance. Rubber bands are also easier for a patient to remove and replace than, for instance, a heavy coil spring.

The greatest problem with orthodontic use of all types of rubber is that they absorb water and deteriorate under intraoral conditions. Gum rubber, which is used to make the rubber bands commonly used in households and offices, begins to deteriorate in the mouth within a couple of hours, and much of its elasticity is lost in 12 to 24 hours. Although orthodontic elastics once were made from this material, they have been superseded by latex elastics, which have a useful performance life four to six times as long. In contemporary orthodontics, only latex rubber elastics or a suitable nonlatex substitute should be used.

Elastomeric plastics for orthodontic purposes are marketed under a variety of trade names, A-lastic being the best known. Small elastomeric modules replace wire ligature ties to hold archwires in the brackets in many applications (see Fig. 9.15B), and also can be used to apply a force to close spaces within the arches. Like rubber, however, these elastomers tend to deteriorate in elastic performance after a relatively short time in the mouth. This does not prevent them from performing quite well in holding archwires in place, nor does it contraindicate their use to close small spaces. It simply must be kept in mind that when elastomers are used to move teeth, the forces decay rapidly and so can be characterized better as interrupted rather than continuous (see Fig. 8.13).[8] Although larger spaces within the dental arch can be closed by sliding teeth with rubber bands or elastomeric chains, the same tooth movement can be done much more efficiently with A-NiTi springs, which provide a more constant force over quite a large range.

Magnets

Rare earth magnets developed in the 1980s were promoted for orthodontic force delivery because they could generate forces of the magnitude needed to move teeth and it was believed they would have a biologic effect that would speed tooth movement and reduce pain. These biologic effects have proven not to be true,[9] so the dramatic changes in force as the distance between magnets in attraction or repulsion change have all but eliminated them from contemporary treatment.[10]

Basic Biomechanics: Foundation Concepts

Two-Point Contact for Control of Root Position

Definition of Terms

Before beginning to discuss control of root position, it is necessary to understand some basic physical terms that must be used in the discussion:

Force—a load applied to an object that will tend to move it to a different position in space. Force, though rigidly defined in units of newtons (mass × the acceleration of gravity), is usually measured clinically in weight units of grams or ounces. In this context, for all practical purposes, 1.0 N ≅ 100 g

Center of resistance—a point at which resistance to movement can be concentrated for mathematical analysis. For an object in free space, the center of resistance is the same as the center of mass. If the object is partially restrained, as is the case for a fence post extending into the earth or a tooth root embedded in bone, the center of resistance will be determined by the nature of the external constraints. The center of resistance for a tooth is at the approximate midpoint of the embedded portion of the root (i.e., about halfway between the root apex and the crest of the alveolar bone; Fig. 9.18).

Moment—a measure of the tendency to rotate an object around some point. A moment is generated by a force acting at a distance. Quantitatively, it is the product of the force times the perpendicular distance from the point of force application to the center of resistance and thus is measured in units of gram-millimeters (or equivalent). If the line of action of an applied force does not pass through the center of resistance, a moment is necessarily created. Not only will the force tend to translate the object, moving it to a different position, it also will tend to rotate the object around the center of resistance. This, of course, is precisely the situation when a force is applied to the crown of a tooth (see Fig. 9.18). Not only is the tooth displaced in the direction of the force, it also rotates around the center of resistance—thus the tooth tips as it moves.

Couple—two forces equal in magnitude and opposite in direction but not on the same line. The result of applying two forces in this way is a pure moment, because the translatory effect of the forces cancels out. A couple will produce pure rotation, spinning the object around its center of resistance; the combination of a force and a couple can change the way an object rotates while it is being moved (Fig. 9.19).

Center of rotation—the point around which rotation actually occurs when an object is being moved. When two forces are applied simultaneously to an object, the center of rotation can be controlled and made to have any desired location. The application of a force and a couple to the crown of a tooth, in fact, is the mechanism by which bodily movement of a tooth, or even greater movement of the root than the crown, can be produced.

Forces, Moments, and Couples in Tooth Movement

Consider the clinical problem posed by a protruding maxillary central incisor. If a single force of 50 g is applied against the crown of this tooth, as might happen with a spring on a maxillary removable appliance, a force system will be created that includes a 750 g-mm moment (see Fig. 9.18). The result will be that the crown will be retracted more than the root apex, which might actually move slightly in the opposite direction. (Remember that a force will tend to displace the entire object, despite the fact that

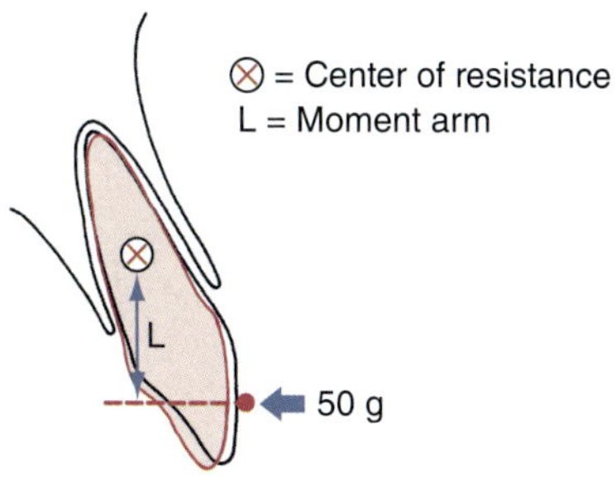

• **Fig. 9.18** The center of resistance (C_R) for any tooth is at the approximate midpoint of the embedded portion of the root. If a single force is applied to the crown of a tooth, the tooth will not only translate but also rotate around C_R because a moment is created by applying a force at a distance from C_R. The perpendicular distance from the point of force application to the center of resistance is the moment arm *(L)*. Pressure in the periodontal ligament will be greatest at the alveolar crest and opposite the root apex (see Fig. 8.9).

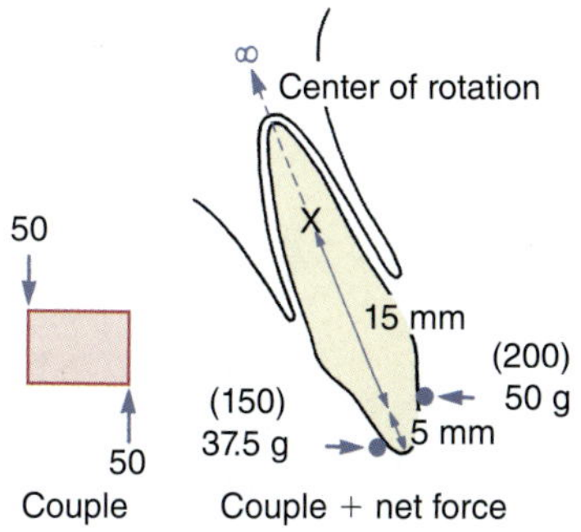

• **Fig. 9.19** A couple, as shown on the left, is defined as two forces equal in magnitude and opposite in direction. The application of a couple produces pure rotation. In clinical application, two unequal forces applied to the crown of a tooth to control root position can be resolved into a couple and a net force to move the tooth. If a 50-g force were applied to a point on the labial surface of an incisor tooth 15 mm from the center of resistance, a 750 g-mm moment (the moment of the force, or M_F) would be produced, tipping the tooth. To obtain bodily movement, it is necessary to apply a couple to create a moment (the moment of the couple, or M_C) equal in magnitude and opposite in direction to the original moment. One way to do this would be to apply a force of 37.5 g pushing the incisal edge labially at a point 20 mm from the center of resistance. This creates a 750 g-mm moment in the opposite direction, so the force system is equivalent to a couple with a 12.5-g net force to move the tooth lingually. With this force system, the tooth would not tip, but with so light a net force, there would be only a small amount of movement. To achieve a net 50 g for effective movement, it would be necessary to use 200 g against the labial surface and 150 g in the opposite direction against the incisal edge. Controlling forces of this magnitude with a removable appliance is very difficult, almost impossible—effective root movement is much more feasible with a fixed appliance.

its orientation will change via simultaneous rotation around the center of resistance.) If it is desired to maintain the inclination of the tooth while retracting it, it will be necessary to overcome the moment created when the force was applied to the crown.

One way to decrease the magnitude of the moment is to apply the force closer to the center of resistance. In orthodontics, it is impractical to apply the force directly to the root, but a similar effect could be achieved by constructing a rigid attachment

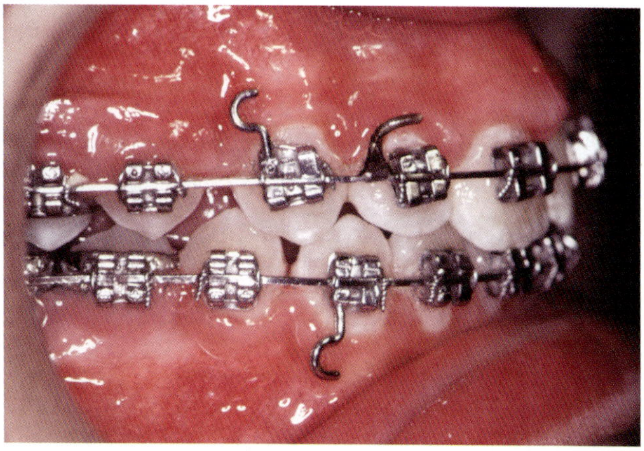

• **Fig. 9.20** Attachments extending toward the center of resistance, seen here as hooks integrated into the canine brackets, can be used to shorten the moment arm and thereby decrease the amount of tipping when elastics or springs are used to slide teeth mesiodistally along an archwire. This idea from the 1920s was reintroduced as part of the early straight-wire appliance. Unfortunately, the longer the hook, the more effective it is mechanically but the greater the chance of oral hygiene problems leading to gingival irritation and/or decalcification. Other methods for controlling tipping are more practical.

that projected upward from the crown. Then the force could be applied to the attachment such that its line of action passed near or through the center of resistance. If the attachment were perfectly rigid, the effect would be to reduce or eliminate the moment arm and thereby the tipping (Fig. 9.20). Because it is difficult to make the arms long enough to totally eliminate tipping, this procedure is only a partial solution at best, and it creates problems with oral hygiene.

Another way to control or eliminate tipping is to create a second moment opposite in direction to the first one. If a second counterbalancing moment could be created equal in magnitude to the moment produced by the first force application, the tooth would remain upright and move bodily. A moment can be created only by application of a force at a distance, however, so this would require that a second force be applied to the crown of the tooth.

In our example of the protruding central incisor, the tendency for the incisor to tip when it was being retracted could be controlled by applying a second force to the lingual surface of this tooth, perhaps with a spring in a removable appliance pushing outward from the lingual near the incisal edge (see Fig. 9.19). As a practical matter, it can be difficult to maintain removable appliances in place against the displacing effects of a pair of springs with heavy activation. The usual orthodontic solution is a fixed attachment on the tooth, constructed so that forces can be applied at two points. With round wires in bracket slots, an auxiliary spring is needed to produce a torquing couple (Fig. 9.21). A rectangular archwire fitting into a rectangular bracket slot on the tooth is most widely used because the entire force system can be produced with a single wire (Fig. 9.22).

It should be noted that with this approach, the two points of contact are the opposite edges of the rectangular wire. The moment arms of the couple therefore are quite small, which means that the forces at the bracket necessary to create a countervailing moment are quite large. If a rectangular archwire is to be used to retract a central incisor bodily, the net retraction force should be small, but the twisting forces on the bracket must be large in order to generate the moment.

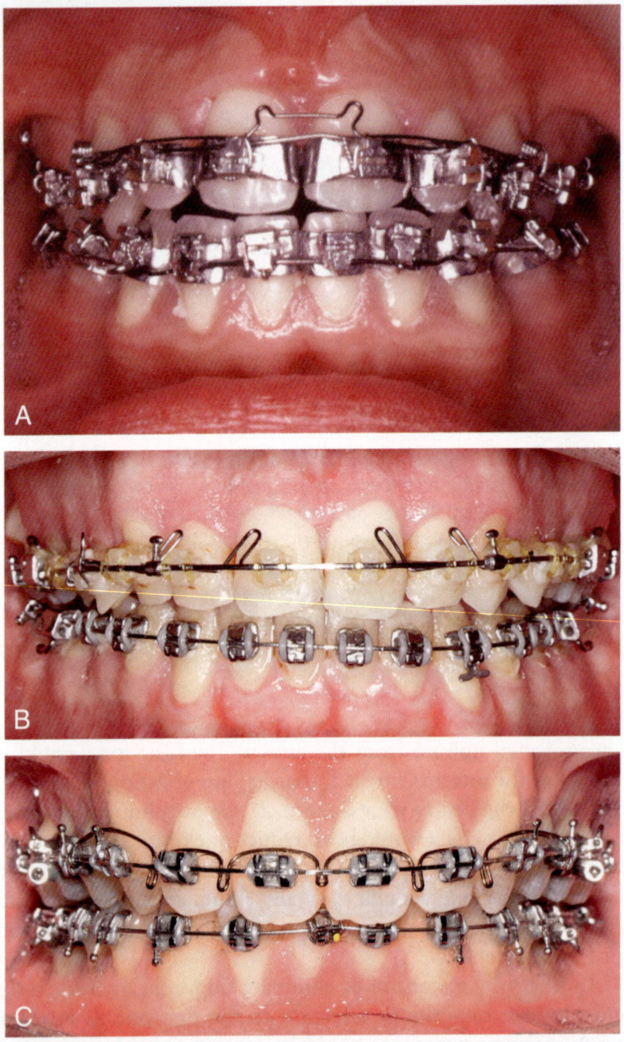

• **Fig. 9.21** (A) Auxiliary root positioning springs and auxiliary torquing springs were used routinely with the Begg appliance, and both can be seen in the maxillary arch of this patient being treated with an early (1980s) Begg-edgewise combination appliance. The torquing spring contacts the facial surface of the central incisors; uprighting springs are present bilaterally on the canines. Note that the base wires are pinned in the Begg slot, and the edgewise slot is not used at this point in treatment. (B) An auxiliary torquing spring in use with the Tip-Edge appliance, the current version of a combination Begg-edgewise appliance. (C) An ART Auxiliary root torqueing spring placed for lingual root torque of all four maxillary incisors (American Orthodontics, Sheboygan, WI). (A, Courtesy Dr. W.J. Thompson; B, Courtesy Dr. D. Grauer.)

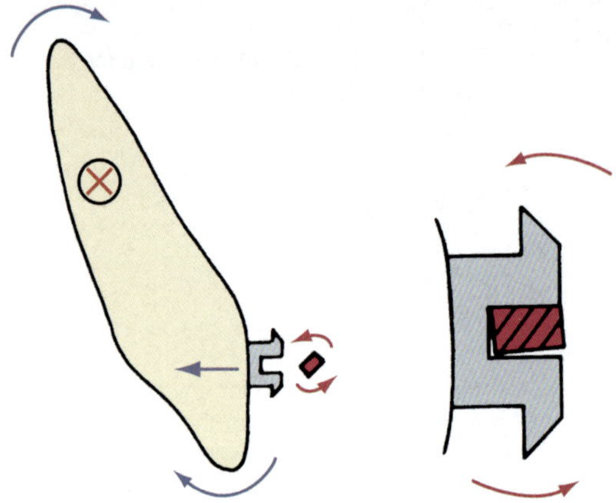

• **Fig. 9.22** A rectangular archwire fitting into a rectangular slot can generate the moment of a couple (M_C) necessary to control root position. The wire is twisted (placed into torsion) as it is put into the bracket slot. The two points of contact are at the edge of the wire, where it contacts the bracket. The moment arm therefore is quite small, and forces must be large to generate the necessary M_C. Using the same tooth dimensions indicated in Fig. 9.19, a 50-g net lingual force would generate a 750 g-mm moment. To balance it by creating an opposite 750 g-mm moment within a bracket with a 0.5 mm slot depth, a torsional force of 1500 g is required.

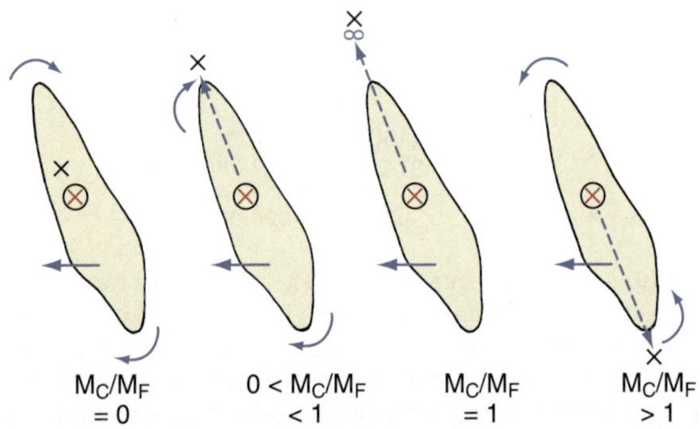

• **Fig. 9.23** The ratio between the moment produced by the force applied to move a tooth (M_F) and the counterbalancing moment produced by the couple used to control root position (M_C) determines the type of tooth movement. With no M_C ($M_C/M_F = 0$), the tooth rotates around the center of resistance (pure tipping). As the moment-to-force ratio increases ($0 < M_C/M_F < 1$), the center of rotation is displaced further and further away from the center of resistance, producing what is called *controlled tipping*. When $M_C/M_F = 1$, the center of rotation is displaced to infinity and bodily movement (translation) occurs. If $M_C/M_F > 1$, the center of rotation is displaced incisally and the root apex will move more than the crown, producing root torque.

M_C/M_F Ratios and Control of Root Position

The previous analysis demonstrates that control of root position during movement requires both a force to move the tooth in the desired direction and a couple to produce the necessary counterbalancing moment for control of root position. The heavier the force, the larger the counterbalancing movement must be to prevent tipping, and vice versa.

Perhaps the simplest way to determine how a tooth will move is to consider the ratio between the moment created when a force is applied to the crown of a tooth (the moment of the force [M_F]), and the counterbalancing moment generated by a couple within the bracket (the moment of the couple [M_C]). Then it can be seen (Fig. 9.23) that the following possibilities exist:

$M_C/M_F = 0$	Pure tipping (tooth rotates around center of resistance)
$0 < M_C/M_F < 1$	Controlled tipping (inclination of tooth changes but the center of rotation is displaced away from the center of resistance, and the root and crown move in the same direction)
$M_C/M_F = 1$	Bodily movement (equal movement of crown and root)
$M_C/M_F > 1$	Torque (root apex moves further than crown)

The moment of the force is determined by the magnitude of the force and the distance from the point of force application to the center of resistance. For most teeth, this distance is 8 to 10 mm, so M_F will be 8 to 10 times the force. In other words, if a 100-g net force were used to move such a tooth, a balancing moment of 800 to 1000 g-mm would be needed to obtain bodily movement. In the orthodontic literature, the relationship between the force and the counterbalancing couple often has been expressed in this way, as the "moment-to-force" ratio. In those terms, moment-to-force ratios of 1 to 7 would produce controlled tipping, ratios of 8 to 10 (depending on the length of the root) would produce bodily movement, and ratios greater than that would produce torque. Because the distance from the point of force application to the center of resistance can and does vary, moment-to-force ratios must be adjusted if root length, amount of alveolar bone support, or point of force application differs from the usual condition. M_C/M_F ratios more precisely describe how a tooth will respond.

Remember that when a force is applied to a bracket to slide it along an archwire, as often is the case in clinical orthodontics, the force felt by the tooth will be less than the force applied to the bracket because of resistance to sliding within the bracket (see later discussion). The *net* force (after resistance to sliding is subtracted) and the moment associated with the net force are what is important. In contrast, when a couple is created within a bracket, friction rarely is a factor.

It is easy to underestimate the magnitude of the forces needed to create the balancing couple. In the example presented previously, if a 50-g net force was used to retract a central incisor, a 500 g-mm moment would be needed to keep it from tipping as the crown moved lingually. To produce a moment of this magnitude within the confines of an 18-mil (0.45-mm) bracket would require opposite forces of 1100 g, derived from twisting the archwire. These forces within the bracket produce only a pure moment, so the periodontal ligament (PDL) does not feel heavy force, but the necessary magnitude can come as a considerable surprise. The wire must literally snap into the bracket.

Root Control With Clear Aligners

The increased use of clear aligner treatment in orthodontics has led to innovations to increase their application to a greater range of malocclusions. The designers of these innovations have recognized that teeth don't just follow plastic, but that the plastic must exert tooth-moving forces just as fixed appliances do. In an attempt to control root position, has aligner systems have been developed that creates two-point contact for mesiodistal and buccolingual root movement, which is mechanically the same as what we previously saw with the use of two springs in contact with the crown of a tooth (see Fig. 9.19). For example, to provide a moment for lingual root movement of an upper incisor, a plastic ridge may provide a lingual force on the facial surface near the gingival margin while a facial force is applied on the lingual surface near the incisal edge. For distal root movement of a premolar, two attachments can be placed on the facial surface of the tooth, which exert a distal force near the gingival margin and a mesial force closer to the cusp tip (see chapter 18). Although these two-point force systems can theoretically provide better root control with aligners, the extent to which they are clinically effective in doing so is still not clear.

Narrow Versus Wide Brackets in Fixed Appliance Systems

Control of root position with an orthodontic appliance is especially needed in two circumstances: when the root of a tooth needs to be torqued facially or lingually (as in the previous example) and when mesiodistal root movement is needed for proper paralleling of teeth when spaces are closed (as at extraction sites). In the former instance, the necessary moment is generated within the bracket, and the key dimensions are those of the archwire; in the latter circumstance, the moment is generated across the bracket, and bracket width determines the length of the moment arm.

The wider the bracket, all other things being equal, the easier it will be to generate the moments needed to bring roots together at extraction sites or to control mesiodistal position of roots in general. Consider retracting the root of a canine tooth into a first premolar extraction site (Fig. 9.24). With a retraction force of 100 g and a 10-mm distance from the bracket to the center of resistance, a 1000 g-mm counterbalancing moment will be needed. If the bracket on this tooth is 1 mm wide, 1000 g of force will be needed at each corner of the bracket, but if the bracket is 4 mm wide, only 250 g of force at each corner will be necessary.

This assumes even greater practical significance when the extraction site is to be closed by sliding teeth along an archwire, and binding between the wire and bracket is encountered. Binding of the wire against the corners of the bracket is affected by the force with which the bracket contacts the archwire and the contact angle between the wire and the bracket (see Fig. 9.24). The wider bracket reduces both the force needed to generate the moment and the contact angle and is thus advantageous for space closure by sliding.

Despite their advantage when spaces are to be closed by sliding teeth on an archwire, wide brackets have a partially offsetting disadvantage. The wider the bracket on a tooth, the smaller the interbracket span between adjacent teeth, and therefore the shorter the effective length of the archwire segments between supports. Reducing the span of the wire segments in this way (reducing the length of the beam, in the terminology of our previous discussion) greatly increases the stiffness of the archwire and decreases its range of action. For this reason, the use of extremely wide brackets is contraindicated. The maximum practical width of a wide bracket is about half the width of a tooth, and narrower brackets have an advantage when teeth are malaligned because the greater interbracket span reduces stiffness of any type of wire.

Effect of Bracket Slot Size in the Edgewise System

The use of rectangular archwires in rectangular bracket slots was introduced by Edward Angle in the late 1920s with his edgewise arch mechanism (see Chapter 10). The original appliance was designed for use with gold archwires, and the 22 × 28 mil bracket slot size was designed to accommodate rectangular archwires of

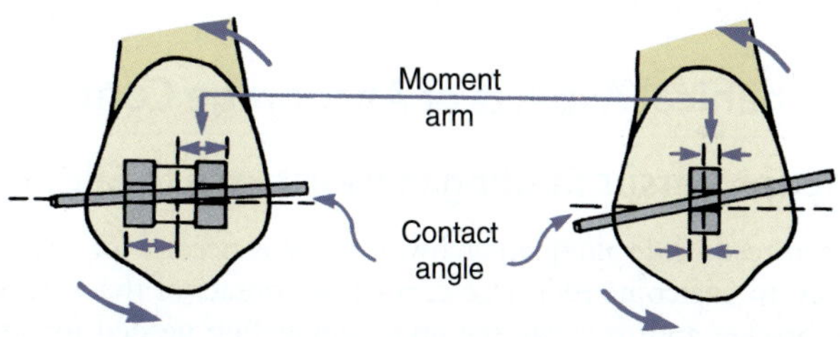

• **Fig. 9.24** The width of the bracket determines the length of the moment arm (half the width of the bracket) for control of mesiodistal root position. Bracket width also influences the contact angle at which the corner of the bracket meets the archwire. The wider the bracket, the smaller the contact angle.

approximately the same dimension. In Angle's concept of treatment, sliding teeth along archwires to close extraction sites was unnecessary because extractions for orthodontic purposes simply were not done. Torquing movements, on the other hand, were important, and a major goal of the appliance design was efficient torque. The appliance was engineered to produce appropriate force and a reasonable range of action in torsion when gold archwires of 22 × 28 dimension were used with narrow brackets.

When steel archwires replaced gold, Angle's original engineering calculations were no longer valid because steel wire of the same size was so much stiffer. An alternative was to redesign the edgewise appliance, optimizing the bracket slot size for steel. A reduction in slot size from 22 to 18 mil was advocated for this purpose. Even with this smaller slot size, full-dimension steel wires still produce slightly greater forces than the original edgewise system did, but the properties of the appliance system are close to the original. Good torque is possible with steel wires and 18-mil edgewise brackets.

On the other hand, using undersized archwires in edgewise brackets is a way to reduce the frictional component of resistance to sliding teeth along an archwire, which was an important consideration by the time steel wire replaced gold. As a practical matter, sliding teeth along an archwire requires at least 2 mil of clearance to minimize friction, and even more clearance may be desirable. The greater strength of an 18-mil archwire compared with a 16-mil wire can be an advantage in sliding teeth. The 18-mil wire would, of course, offer excellent clearance in a 22-slot bracket but fit tightly in an 18-slot bracket. The original 22-slot bracket therefore would have some advantage during space closure but would be a definite disadvantage when torque was needed later.

With steel archwires of 21 mil as the smaller dimension (close enough to the original 22-mil bracket slot size to give a good fit), springiness and range in torsion are so limited that effective torque with the archwire is essentially impossible. Using wide brackets to help with space closure would make the torque problem worse. Exaggerated inclinations of smaller rectangular wires (e.g., 19 × 25) are one alternative, but torquing auxiliaries (see Fig. 9.21) are often necessary with undersized steel wires in 22-slot edgewise brackets.

In this situation, a role for the titanium archwires becomes clearer. If only steel wires are to be used, the 18-mil slot system has considerable advantage over the larger bracket slot size. With their excellent springback and resistance to permanent deformation, A-NiTi wires overcome some of the alignment limitations of steel wires in wide 22-mil slot brackets; rectangular NiTi and beta-Ti wires offer advantages over steel for the finishing phases of treatment and torque control. In short, titanium archwires greatly help overcome the major problems associated with continued use of the original edgewise slot size.

Mechanical Aspects of Anchorage Control

Friction Versus Binding in Resistance to Sliding

When teeth slide along an archwire, force is needed for two purposes: to overcome resistance created by contact of the wire with the bracket and to create the bone remodeling needed for tooth movement. As we pointed out in Chapter 8, controlling the position of anchor teeth is accomplished best by minimizing the reaction force that reaches them. It is tempting for the clinician to use heavier force when moving a tooth along an archwire to overcome the friction and binding of the wire in the bracket. The prudent decision when anchorage control is critical is to err on the side of lighter force so that differential anchorage is possible (see Fig. 8.22) or to use an approach, such as closing loops, that does not require sliding a bracket along the wire.

Because of the increasing use of passive self-ligating brackets and other techniques designed to reduce friction (which are discussed in detail in Chapter 10), it has become important to clearly distinguish between the contributions of friction and binding to resistance to sliding.

Friction in Fixed Appliance Treatment

When one object moves relative to another, friction at their interface produces resistance to the direction of movement. Friction ultimately is derived from electromagnetic forces between atoms—it is not a fundamental force that can be defined independently of local conditions. It is proportional to the force with which the contacting surfaces are pressed together and is affected by the nature of the surface at the interface (e.g., rough or smooth, chemically reactive or passive, modified by lubricants). It is interesting to note that friction is independent of the apparent area of contact. This is because all surfaces, no matter how smooth, have irregularities that are large on a molecular scale, and real contact occurs only at a limited number of small spots at the peaks of the surface irregularities (Fig. 9.25). These spots, called *asperities*, carry all the load between the two surfaces. Even under light loads, local pressure at the asperities may cause appreciable plastic deformation of those small areas. Because of this, the true contact area is to a considerable extent determined by the applied load and is directly proportional to it.[11]

When a tangential force is applied to cause one material to slide past the other, the junctions begin to shear. The coefficient of friction then is proportional to the shear strength of the junctions and is inversely proportional to the yield strength of the materials (because this determines the extent of plastic deformation at the asperities). At low sliding speeds, a "stick-slip" phenomenon may occur as enough force builds up to shear the junctions and a jump occurs, then the surfaces stick again until enough force again builds to break them.

Two other factors affect friction: the interlocking of surface irregularities, which obviously becomes more important when the asperities are large or pointed, and the extent to which asperities on a harder material plow into the surface of a softer one. Thus the total frictional resistance will be the sum of three components: (1) the force necessary to shear all junctions, (2) the resistance caused

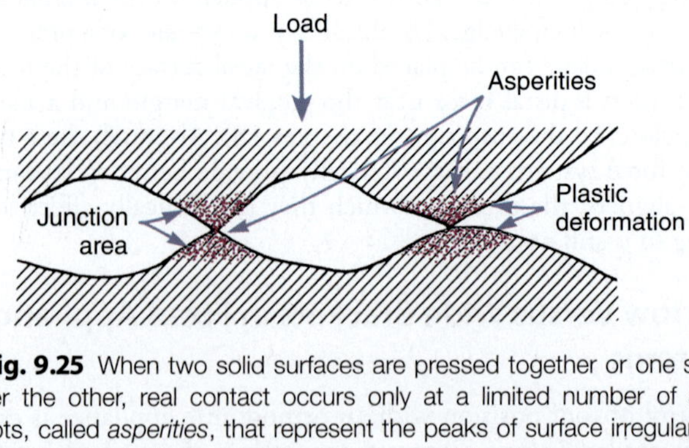

• **Fig. 9.25** When two solid surfaces are pressed together or one slides over the other, real contact occurs only at a limited number of small spots, called *asperities*, that represent the peaks of surface irregularities. These junctions shear as sliding occurs, and the force to produce this plastic deformation of the surface irregularities is the frictional resistance. (Redrawn from Jastrzebski ZD. *The Nature and Properties of Engineering Materials*. 3rd ed. Wiley; 1987.)

by the interlocking of roughness, and (3) the plowing component of the total friction force.[12] In practice, if the two materials are relatively smooth and not greatly dissimilar in hardness, friction is largely determined by the shearing component.

The concept that surface qualities are an important variable in determining friction has been emphasized by experience in recent years with both titanium wires and ceramic or plastic brackets. Stainless steel brackets slide reasonably well on steel wires, but the situation is not so fortunate with some other possible combinations.

Friction Related to Surface Qualities of Wires

When NiTi wires were first introduced, manufacturers claimed that they had an inherently slick surface compared with stainless steel, so that all other factors being equal, there would be less interlocking of asperities and thereby less frictional resistance to sliding a tooth along a NiTi wire than a stainless steel one. This is erroneous—the surface of NiTi is rougher (because of surface defects, not the quality of polishing) than that of beta-Ti, which in turn is rougher than steel. More important, however, is that there is little or no correlation for orthodontic wires between the coefficients of friction and surface roughness[13] (i.e., interlocking and plowing are not significant components of the total frictional resistance). Although NiTi has greater surface roughness, beta-Ti has greater frictional resistance. It turns out that as the titanium content of an alloy increases, its surface reactivity increases, and the surface chemistry is a major influence. Thus beta-Ti, at 80% titanium, has a higher coefficient of friction than NiTi at 50% titanium, and there is greater frictional resistance to sliding with either than with steel. With beta-Ti, there is enough titanium reactivity for the wire to "cold-weld" itself to a steel bracket under some circumstances, making sliding all but impossible.

A possible solution to this problem is alteration of the surface of the titanium wires by implantation of ions into the surface. Ion implantation (with nitrogen, carbon, and other materials) has been done successfully with beta-Ti and has been shown to improve the characteristics of beta-Ti hip implants. In clinical orthodontics, however, implanted NiTi and beta-Ti wires failed to show improved performance in initial alignment or sliding space closure respectively, and are no longer marketed.

Friction Related to Surface Qualities of Brackets

Bracket surfaces also are important in friction. Most modern orthodontic brackets are either cast or milled from stainless steel and, if properly polished, have relatively smooth surfaces comparable with steel wires. Titanium brackets are now promoted as particularly needed for patients who have a nickel allergy, but are rarely needed for that reason (see Chapter 8). At best, the surface properties of titanium brackets are like those of titanium wires, and polishing the interior of bracket slots is difficult enough that these critical areas may be rougher than wires. Sliding with titanium brackets therefore may be problematic, particularly if titanium archwires also are used.

Ceramic brackets became quite popular in the 1990s because of their improved esthetics, but their surface properties are far from ideal. The ones made from polycrystalline ceramics have considerably rougher surfaces than steel brackets. The rough but hard ceramic material is likely to penetrate the surface of even a steel wire during sliding, creating considerable resistance, and of course, this is worse with titanium wires. Although single crystal brackets are quite smooth, these brackets also can damage wires during sliding, and so they also have increased resistance to sliding.[14] As a result, ceramic brackets with metal slots and with rounded corners in the slot have been introduced, a rather explicit recognition of the problems created by friction against ceramic surfaces (see further discussion of esthetic appliances in Chapter 10).

It is possible that composite plastic brackets will begin to be used in orthodontics within the next few years. They have the advantages of being tooth colored and nonallergenic, and at least in theory should have surface properties that would not be as troublesome as ceramics. As with composite plastic wires, however, their fabrication is difficult and their development has been slow.

Elastic and Inelastic Binding in Resistance to Sliding

The amount of force between the wire and the bracket strongly influences the amount of resistance to sliding. This resistance is determined primarily by two things: friction as the wire contacts the walls or bottom of the bracket and elastic or inelastic binding as the wire contacts the corners of the bracket. As we will see, binding, not friction, is the major component of resistance to sliding.

In theory, a wire could move through a bracket or tube with no friction whatever, if it were small relative to the bracket and did not contact any part of the bracket (Fig. 9.26A). Even in the laboratory, this is very difficult—unless everything is aligned perfectly, the wire will contact the bottom of the bracket or some other area, but friction will be small if nothing forces the wire against the bracket.

This, however, has no resemblance to what happens in the mouth. In fact, contact of the wire against the bracket is necessary to control rotation and root position by generating couples to offset the moments created by the forces to move the teeth. When a wire shaped to arch form fits through multiple brackets, contact with the base of the bracket and/or bracket walls is inevitable (Fig. 9.26B). If a tooth is pulled along an archwire, the resistance to sliding will be only friction until the tooth tips enough to bring the corners of the bracket into contact with the wire. The tooth tips, of course, because the force is applied to a bracket on its crown, and the center of resistance is halfway down the root. As soon as the corners of the bracket engage the wire, which happens after a very small movement of the tooth, a moment is generated that opposes further tipping (Fig. 9.27). This generates elastic binding between the bracket and the wire, which is different from friction.

The greater the angle at which the wire contacts the corners of the bracket, the greater the force between the wire and bracket—so, as we noted previously, there is greater resistance to sliding with narrow than wide brackets. As can be seen from Fig. 9.28, resistance to sliding includes elastic binding almost immediately when tooth movement begins and goes up rapidly as the angle between the bracket and the wire increases.[15]

A series of experiments in Kusy's laboratory help to put into perspective the importance of binding versus friction as components of resistance to sliding.[16] In the experiments, 21 × 25 M-NiTi and steel wires were tied into a 22-slot steel twin bracket with 200-g ligature force, so there was a lot of friction. Then the resistance to sliding was evaluated as a function of the angle of contact between the wire and the bracket. As Fig. 9.29 shows, with a 3-degree contact angle, most of the resistance to sliding was binding with a steel wire, and nearly half was binding with an M-NiTi wire. At a 7-degree or greater angle, almost all the resistance was due to binding with both wires.

The conclusion: For very early alignment of teeth, resistance to sliding is due to a combination of friction and binding, but almost

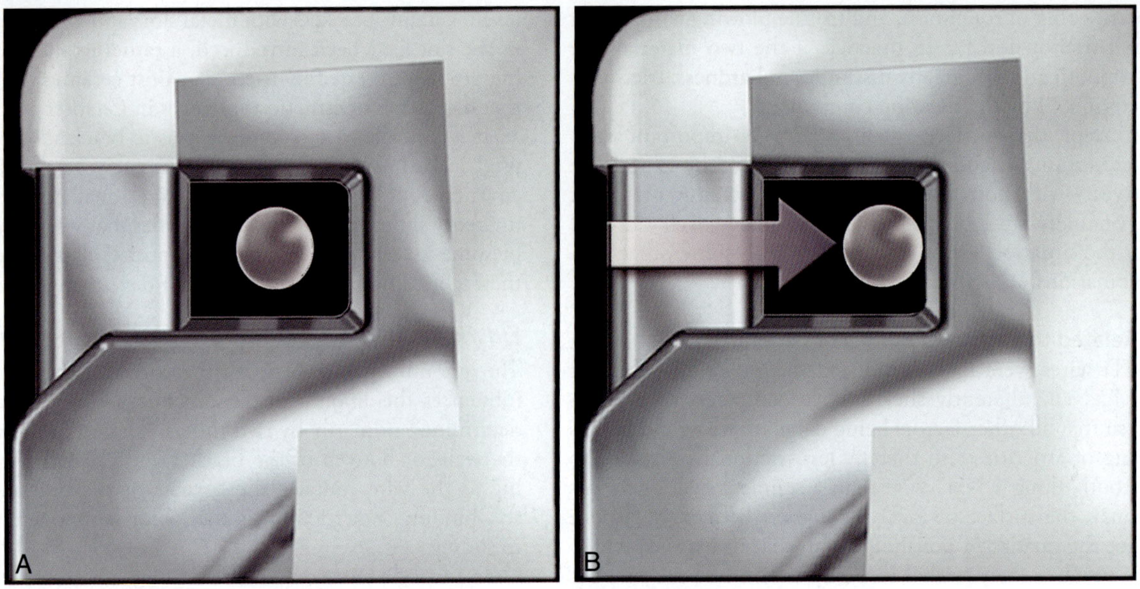

• **Fig. 9.26** (A) It is possible in the laboratory to orient a small wire within a bracket (or tube) so that it does not touch any of the walls, and therefore there would be no frictional resistance to moving the wire relative to the bracket. (B) In the mouth, a curved archwire passing through a series of brackets will inevitably contact the bottom of the bracket, so there will be some friction.

immediately, unless the tooth is allowed to tip to keep the contact angle low, the frictional component becomes so low that it is negligible, and resistance to sliding is due almost totally to elastic binding.

During orthodontic tooth movement, inelastic binding also is likely to be encountered. This occurs when notching of the edge of the wire occurs (Fig. 9.30). When a notch encounters the edge of the bracket, tooth movement stops until displacement of the tooth during function releases the notch (remember, teeth move during function as alveolar bone bends under the heavy loads and return to their original position as the bone springs back when the heavy loading is released). Given the presence of both types of binding, it is not surprising that observations of tooth movement show that it happens almost entirely in a series of steps, not in a smooth flow.

Magnitude of Resistance to Sliding

Perhaps the most important information to be gained from a consideration of resistance to sliding is an appreciation of its magnitude, even under the best of circumstances. If a canine tooth is to slide along an archwire as part of the closure of an extraction space, and a 100-g net force is needed for tooth movement, approximately another 100 g will be needed to overcome the effects of binding and friction. The total force needed to slide the tooth therefore is twice as great as might have been expected. Because this resistance is due mostly to binding, replacing a conventional edgewise bracket and elastomeric ligature tie with a self-ligating bracket so that the wire is not forced against the bottom of the bracket does not lead to faster space closure.[17]

In terms of the effect on orthodontic anchorage, the problem created by resistance to sliding is not so much its presence as the difficulty of knowing its magnitude. To slide a tooth or teeth along an archwire, the clinician must apply enough force to overcome the resistance and produce the biologic response. As mentioned earlier, it is difficult to avoid the temptation to estimate the resistance to sliding generously and add additional force to be certain that tooth movement will occur. The effect of any force beyond what was really needed to overcome resistance to sliding is to bring the anchor teeth up onto the plateau of the tooth movement curve (see Fig. 8.21). Then either unnecessary movement of the anchor teeth occurs or additional steps to maintain anchorage are necessary (such as headgear or bone screws).

If a springy loop is bent into the archwire, activated to produce tooth movement, and then tied tightly, archwire segments move, taking the teeth with them instead of the teeth moving relative to the wire. Springs of this type are called *retraction springs* if they attach to only one tooth or *closing loops* if they connect two archwire segments (Fig. 9.31). Incorporating springs into the archwire makes the appliance more complex to fabricate and use clinically but eliminates the difficulty in predicting resistance to sliding.

Methods to Control Anchorage

From the previous discussion of the biologic aspects of anchorage in Chapter 8 and the earlier review in this chapter of the effects of friction and binding, it is apparent that several potential strategies could be used to control anchorage. Nearly all the possible approaches are actually used in clinical orthodontics, and all are affected by whether resistance to sliding will be encountered and, if so, how much. Let us consider these strategies in more detail.

Anchorage Types

Reinforcement

The extent to which anchorage should be reinforced (by adding teeth to the anchorage unit) depends on the tooth movement that is desired. In practice, this means that anchorage requirements must be established individually in each clinical situation. Once it has been determined that reinforcement is desirable, however, this typically involves including as many teeth as possible in the anchorage. For significant differential tooth movement, the ratio of PDL area in the anchorage unit to PDL area in the tooth movement unit should be at least 2 to 1 without sliding and 4 to 1 with it. Anything less produces something close to reciprocal movement, especially if force levels are not well controlled.

Satisfactory reinforcement of anchorage may require the addition of teeth from the opposite dental arch to the anchor unit. For

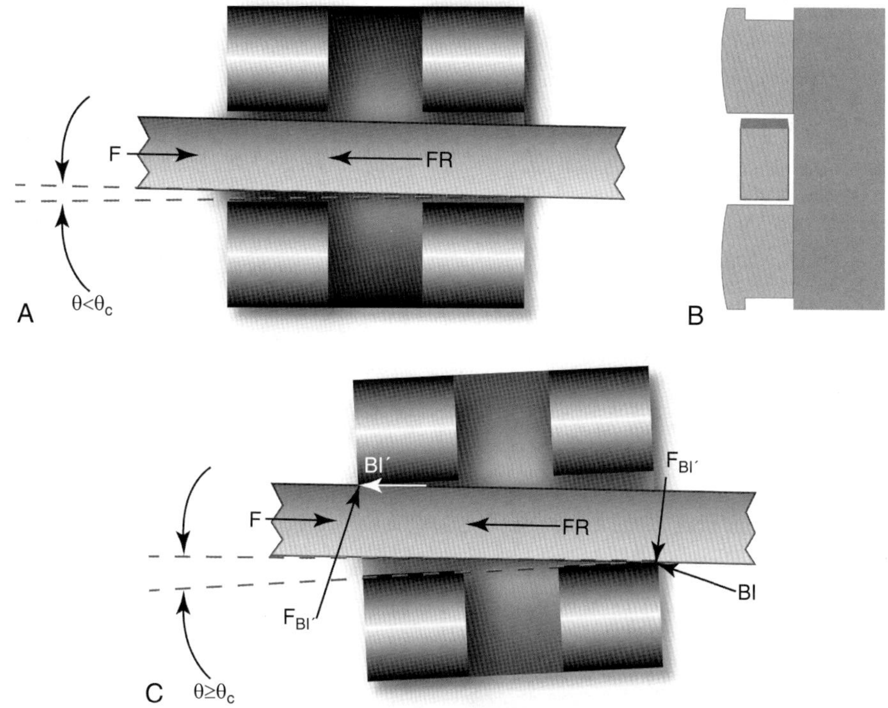

• **Fig. 9.27** (A) and (B) The force *(F)* to move a bracket along an archwire initially will be resisted only by friction *(FR)* because of contact of the wire with the bottom or sides of the bracket slot. (C) Because the root of a tooth resists movement, the tooth tips until the corners of the bracket contact the wire, and at that point, elastic binding *(BI)* of the wire against the corner of the bracket adds to the resistance to sliding.

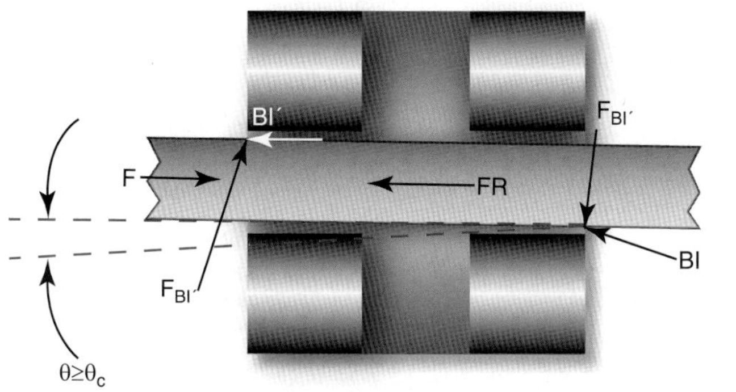

Very early alignment: RS = FR + BI
Almost immediately: RS = BI

• **Fig. 9.28** Because binding creates most of the resistance to sliding *(RS)* as the angle of contact between the wire and the corner of the bracket increases, resistance to sliding in very early alignment is the sum of elastic binding *(BI)* and friction *(FR)*, but almost immediately the proportion of resistance from binding exceeds friction by so much that the frictional component can be disregarded—for all practical purposes, the resistance to sliding is due just to binding (see Fig. 9.29).

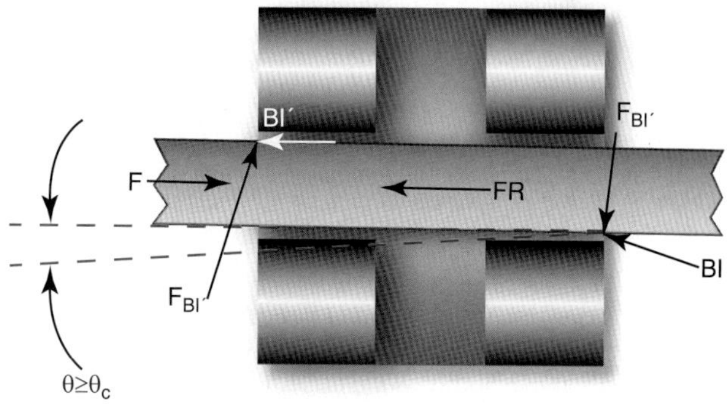

Steel Wire	NiTi Wire
3° RS = 73% BI	3° RS = 45% BI
7° RS = 94% BI	7° RS = 93% BI
11° RS = 97% BI	11° RS = 95% BI

• **Fig. 9.29** Laboratory studies in which the bracket was allowed to tip relative to the wire along which it was being moved have shown that with a 21 × 25 steel wire that was tied into a steel bracket with a 200-g force (so there was a lot of friction), 73% of the resistance to sliding *(RS)* was due to binding *(BI)* at a contact angle of 3 degrees, and over 90% was due to binding at 7 degrees or higher angles. With a martensitic nickel-titanium (M-NiTi) wire of the same size, there was less binding at 3 degrees but similar binding at higher angles. The component of resistance attributed to friction can be seen to be negligible at contact angles that are reached quickly in sliding a tooth along a wire. (From Articolo LC, Kusy RP. Influence of angulation on the resistance to sliding in fixed appliances. *Am J Orthod Dentofacial Orthop*. 1999;115:39–51.)

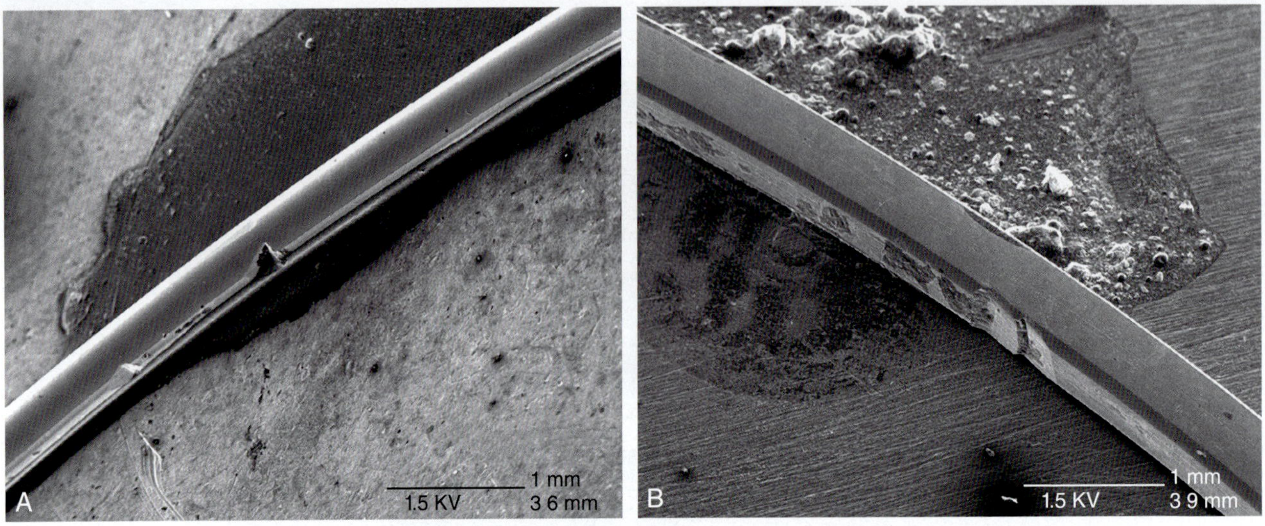

• **Fig. 9.30** Scanning electron microscope images show that sliding a bracket along a wire (or a wire through a bracket) causes surprising amounts of distortion of the wire surface. (A) A 16-mil steel wire after sliding through a bracket. Note the significant tear in the wire. (B) A 21 × 25 steel wire after sliding. Note the series of indentations. When the corner of the bracket catches on damaged areas such as these, tooth movement stops until the notching is released by masticatory function. (Courtesy Dr. Robert Kusy.)

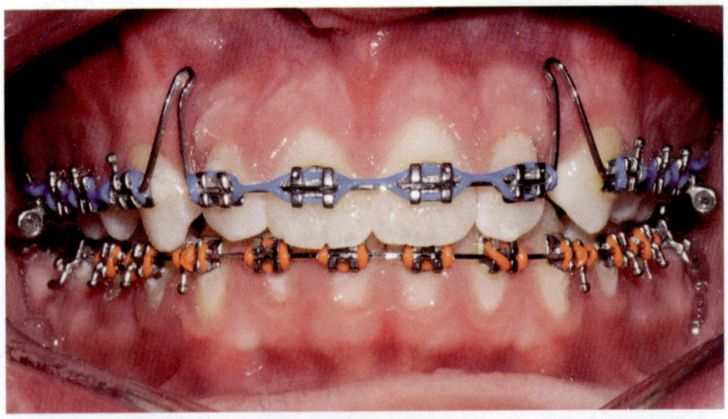

• **Fig. 9.31** Closing loops are being use bilaterally to close the remaining spaces between the upper lateral incisors and canines. Note that the anterior segment of four incisors can move to close the space without having to slide along the wire—the loops will close and the segment will retract to meet the canines without friction.

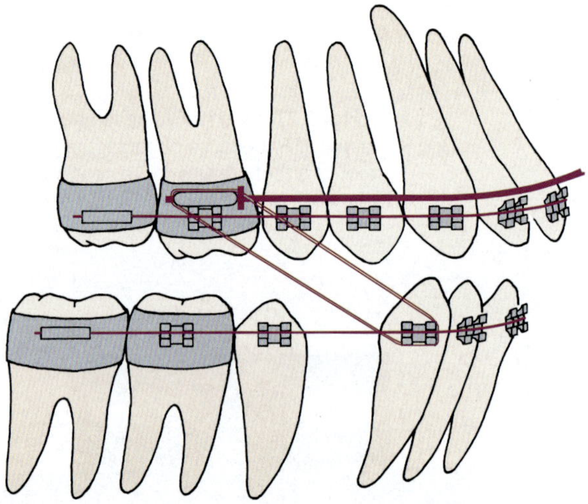

• **Fig. 9.32** Reinforcement of anchorage can be obtained by adding additional teeth within the same arch to the anchor unit, or by using elastics from the opposite arch to help produce desired tooth movement, as with the interarch elastic shown here. Additional reinforcement can be obtained with extraoral force, as with addition of a facebow to the upper molar to resist the forward pull of the elastic.

example, to close a mandibular premolar extraction site, it would be possible to stabilize all the teeth in the maxillary arch so that they could only move bodily as a group and then to run an elastic from the upper posterior to the lower anterior, thus pitting forward movement of the entire upper arch against distal movement of the lower anterior segment (Fig. 9.32). This addition of the entire upper arch would greatly alter the balance between retraction of the lower anterior teeth and forward slippage of the lower posterior teeth.

This anchorage could be reinforced even further by having the patient wear an extraoral appliance (headgear) placing backward force against the upper arch. The reaction force from the headgear is dissipated against the bones of the cranial vault, thus adding the resistance of these structures to the anchorage unit. The only problem with reinforcement outside the dental arch is that springs within an arch provide constant forces, whereas elastics from one arch to the other tend to be intermittent, and extraoral force is likely to be even more intermittent. Although this time factor can significantly decrease the value of cross-arch and extraoral reinforcement, both can be quite useful clinically.

Subdivision of Desired Movement

A common way to improve anchorage control is to pit the resistance of a group of teeth against the movement of a single tooth, rather than dividing the arch into more or less equal segments. In our same extraction site example, it would be perfectly possible to reduce the strain on posterior anchorage by retracting the canine individually, pitting its distal movement against mesial movement of all other teeth within the arch (Fig. 9.33). After the canine tooth had been retracted, one could then add it to the posterior anchorage unit and retract the incisors. This approach has the advantage of dissipating the reaction force over a large PDL area in the anchor unit—but only if the retraction force is kept light, as

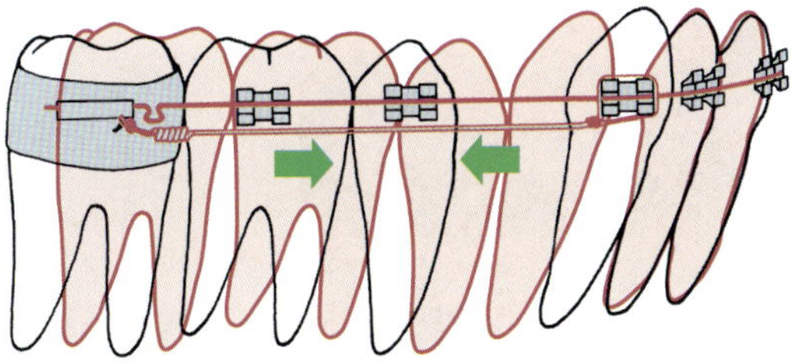

• **Fig. 9.33** Retraction of the canine by itself, as the first step in a two-stage space closure, often is used to conserve anchorage, particularly when sliding teeth along an archwire.

discussed in Chapter 8. Its disadvantage is that closing the space in two steps rather than one takes nearly twice as long.

Subdivision of tooth movement improves the anchorage situation regardless of whether sliding is involved and where a space in the arch is located. If it is desired to slip all the posterior teeth forward (in which case the anterior teeth are the anchor unit), bringing them forward one at a time is the most conservative way to proceed. Again, keeping the force levels light is the key to producing the differential tooth movement.

Tipping and Uprighting

Another possible strategy for anchorage control is to tip the teeth and then upright them, rather than moving them bodily. In our familiar extraction site example, this would again require two steps in treatment. First, the anterior teeth would be tipped distally by being pitted against mesial bodily movement of the posterior segment (see Fig. 8.22). Using a bracket that allows the teeth to tip as they slide along an archwire reduces binding and therefore keeps resistance to sliding small. As a second step, the tipped teeth would be uprighted, moving the canine roots distally and torquing the incisor roots lingually, again with stationary anchorage in the posterior segments. It would be extremely important to keep forces as light as possible during both steps, so that the teeth in the posterior segment were always below the optimum force range, while the anterior teeth received optimum force.

Anchorage Control in Space Closure

At this point, let's begin by considering a relatively typical extraction situation, in which it is desirable to close the extraction space 60% by retraction of the anterior teeth and 40% by forward movement of the posterior segments (Fig. 9.34). This outcome would be expected from any of three possible approaches: (1) one-step space closure with no sliding (via closing loops so that segments of wire are moved with the teeth attached, rather than sliding); (2) a two-step closure sliding the canine bodily along the archwire, then retracting the incisors (as in the original Tweed technique); or (3) two-step space closure, tipping the anterior segment with some friction, then uprighting the tipped teeth (as in the Begg technique). (See Chapter 16 for a detailed discussion of these techniques.)

This example makes the cost of binding and friction in a clinical setting more apparent: the greater strain on anchorage when brackets slide along an archwire must be compensated for by a more conservative approach to anchorage control. The price therefore is paid in increased treatment time. The closing loop approach, although more difficult to fabricate and manipulate, will result in the same space closure significantly more quickly.

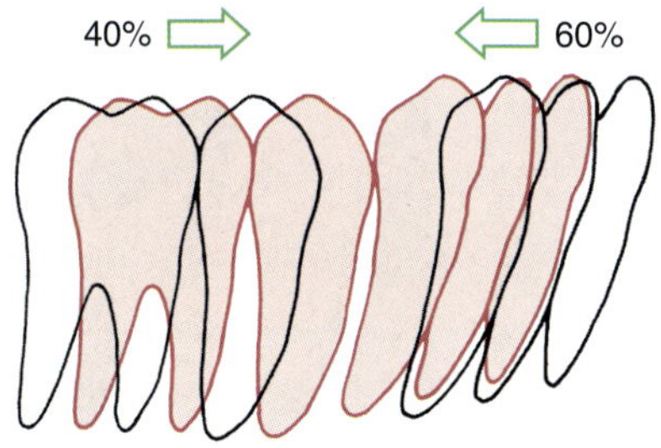

• **Fig. 9.34** Closure of a premolar extraction site often is desired in a ratio of 60% retraction of incisors, 40% forward movement of molar and second premolar. This result can be obtained straightforwardly in three ways: (1) one-step space closure with no sliding (closing loop); (2) two-step space closure with sliding mechanics, retracting the canine individually, and then retracting the four incisors in a second step (the classic Tweed approach); or (3) two-step sliding with distal tipping of the canine and incisors initially, followed by uprighting of these teeth (the classic Begg approach). Good clinical results can be obtained with all three methods. The cost of resistance to sliding in space closure, with well-managed orthodontic appliances, is paid more in increased treatment time than in decreased quality of result.

Note that strategies for anchorage control are associated with particular orthodontic appliances; indeed, they are literally built into the appliance in many instances. The approach to anchorage control that is implicit in the appliance design is sometimes called the *appliance philosophy*, not quite so strange a term when viewed in this way.

Skeletal Anchorage

Skeletal anchorage is derived from bone screws, which differ from implants to support replacement teeth in that osseointegration with the screw is not desired, simply because it is to be removed when it is no longer needed as an orthodontic anchor. They can be used either as single screws or, when greater anchorage is needed for more complex tooth movement, as miniplates attached with screws to basal bone of the maxilla or mandible (Fig. 9.35). Collectively, these devices are referred to as *temporary anchorage devices* (TADs). They make tooth movement possible now that simply could not be accomplished without them. With properly designed skeletal anchorage, there is no concern about moving teeth that were not intended to be moved, but the amount of force to teeth that are to be moved still must be determined with resistance to sliding in mind, and the desired treatment outcome must be determined with some precision before bone anchors are placed so that they can be positioned to provide the proper force directions.

From a broad perspective, the indication for skeletal anchorage is inadequate intraoral and extraoral anchorage to obtain the desired tooth movement. At that point, the key consideration is whether individual bone screws that the orthodontist can place would be satisfactory, or whether miniplates that require raising a flap for placement (more surgery than many orthodontists would wish to perform) would be required. The relative advantages and disadvantages of screws alone versus miniplates have been the subject of some controversy,[18,19] but it seems clear that the more anchorage that would be needed, the greater the indication for miniplates and their multiple screws.

For missing teeth that eliminate the usual dental anchorage possibility, impacted teeth, and other problems that require movement of only a few teeth, alveolar bone screws are adequate

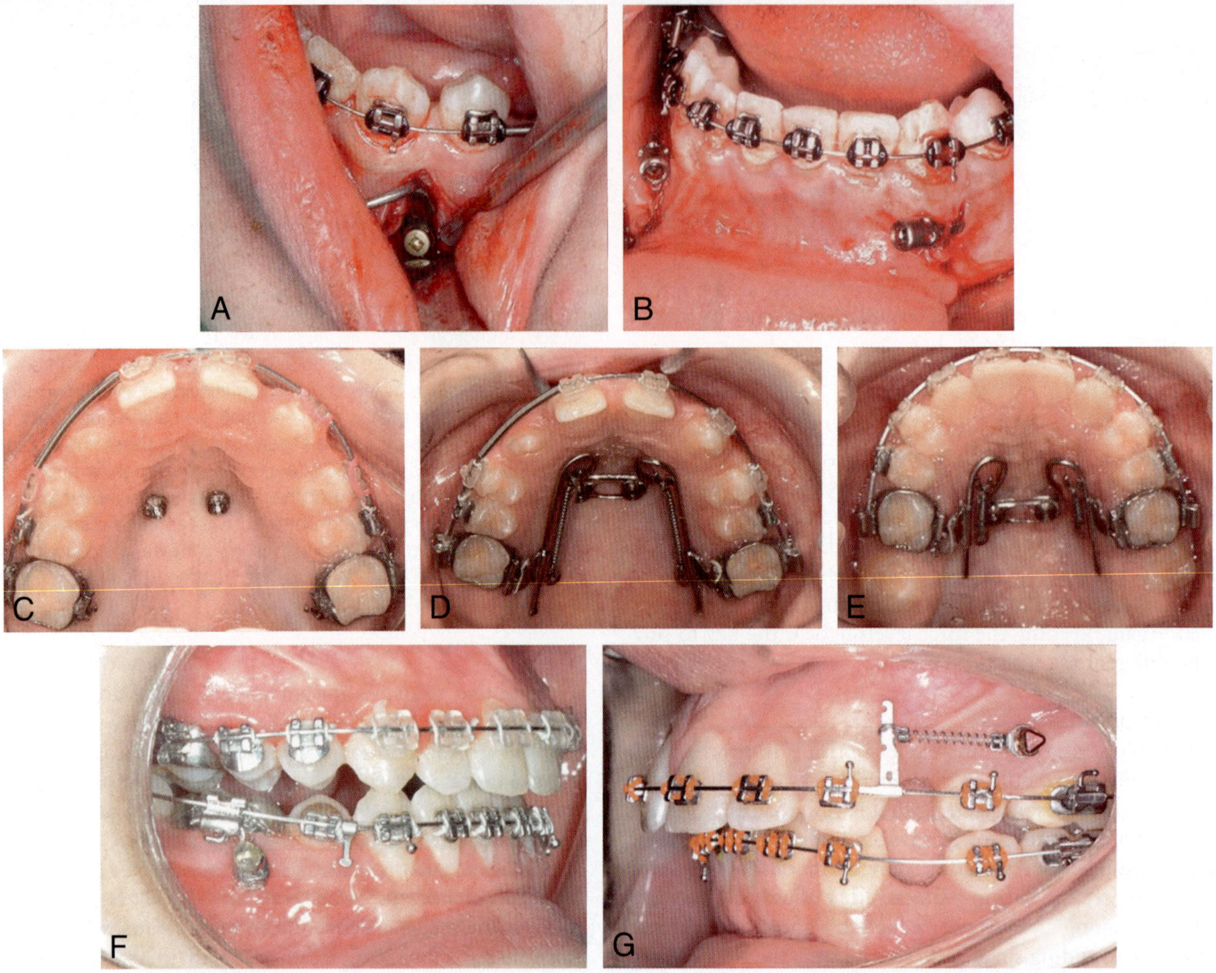

• **Fig. 9.35** Bone anchors retained by screws, or screws with a head that extends into the mouth can be placed in both the mandibular and maxillary arches to provide skeletal anchorage for tooth movement. This makes it possible to produce tooth movement that otherwise would be impossible. (A) Placement of screws to hold a bone anchor in the mandible. (B) Bone anchors in place bilaterally. (C) Two palatal screws placed to provide anchorage for space closure in the maxillary arch. (D) Same patient with appliance attached to palatal screws designed to close spaces by protracting posterior teeth (E) Patient with spaces now successfully closed using skeletal anchorage to avoid unwanted retraction of the incisors. (F) An example of indirect skeletal anchorage showing a screw mesial to the lower first molar and attached to the molar to prevent mesial movement of the molar (G) An example of direct skeletal anchorage with a screw placed mesial to the upper first molar used to anchor a spring for retraction of incisors. (C–F, Courtesy Drs. P. Medland and W. Medland.)

and indicated. It is interesting that single bone screws also can be satisfactory for intrusion of multiple teeth, as when maxillary posterior teeth are to be intruded to close an anterior open bite, because a requirement for intrusion is light force. For more complex tooth movement—for example, moving the entire maxillary arch distally for Class II camouflage—or when the desired force direction cannot be obtained with alveolar screws, miniplates that are attached with two or three screws and can be placed above or below tooth apices are needed.

Skeletal anchorage is used in two ways: direct or indirect. Direct anchorage is when the tooth or teeth to be moved are attached directly to the bone anchor; indirect anchorage is when another tooth or teeth are attached to the bone anchor to hold them in position while they serve as anchorage. With indirect anchorage there is nothing different from what has been discussed previously. With direct anchorage the location of the bone anchor must be carefully considered, because the line of force from it almost always is above or below the line of force from anchorage teeth. Miniplates are better for direct anchorage, even though they are likely to be even further from the teeth than isolated bone screws, because attachments to miniplates usually allow placing a wire through the attachment so that the line of force can be varied.

In many areas around the dentition, the bone where skeletal anchors might be placed is not nearly as thick or dense as one might think. Such areas are not good sites for single screws, although they might be satisfactory if a miniplate in that area were placed with multiple screws. The bone above the maxillary posterior teeth, where miniplates are preferred, is the best example, but this also applies more generally if heavy force would be used—the heavier the force, the greater the need for bone density if a single screw is to be satisfactory. The bone of the palate is more dense than alveolar bone, which makes it a favored site for screws rather than plates.

Age also is a factor in the use of skeletal anchorage: adequate bone density for most orthodontic procedures is not attained until early adolescence, so bone anchors cannot be used for most mixed dentition treatment.

The skeletal anchorage devices themselves are discussed and illustrated in Chapter 10, and their use to accomplish tooth movement that was very difficult or impossible previously is described in detail in Chapters 15–17 and 20.

Advanced Biomechanics: Clinical Applications

Determinate Versus Indeterminate Force Systems

The laws of equilibrium require not only that for every force there is an equal and opposite reactive force, but also that the sum of the moments around any arbitrary point is equal to zero. In other words, the moments, as well as the forces, generated by an orthodontic appliance system must be balanced, in all three planes of space. It can be very difficult to visualize the total force system when multiple teeth are involved, but unexpected and unwanted tooth movement easily can result when an important component of the system is overlooked.

Force systems can be defined as statically *determinate*, meaning that the moments and forces can readily be discerned, measured, and evaluated, or as *indeterminate*. Statically indeterminate systems are too complex for precisely calculating all forces and moments involved in the equilibrium. Typically, only the direction of net moments and approximate net force levels can be determined.

This is more of a problem in orthodontics than in most engineering applications because the eventual action of an orthodontic appliance is affected by the biologic response. For instance, the amount of tooth movement will be determined largely by the magnitude of the forces felt by anchor teeth and teeth whose movement is intended, not just by the differential between those forces. If the force applied to the anchor teeth is high enough to pull them up onto the plateau of the pressure-response curve, reciprocal tooth movement will occur despite a difference in PDL pressures (see Fig. 8.21). Similarly, whether intrusion of incisor teeth or extrusion of posterior teeth occurs is almost totally a function of the magnitude of intrusive versus extrusive forces, not their direction or the difference between them. Determinate force systems therefore are particularly advantageous in orthodontics when control of force magnitudes is necessary to produce the desired biologic response.

For all practical purposes, determinate systems in orthodontics are those in which a couple is created at one end of an attachment, with only a force (no couple) at the other (i.e., a one-couple system). This means that a wire that will serve as a spring can be inserted into a tube or bracket at one end but must be tied so that there is only one point of contact on the other (Fig. 9.36). When the wire is tied into a bracket on both ends, a statically indeterminate two-couple system has been created.

One-Couple Systems

In orthodontic applications, one-couple systems are found when two conditions are met: (1) a cantilever spring or auxiliary archwire is placed into a bracket or tube(s) and typically attaches to a tooth or teeth that are part of a stabilized segment (i.e., reinforced anchorage is being used), and (2) the other end of the cantilever spring or auxiliary archwire is tied to a tooth or group of teeth that are to be moved, with a single point of force application.[20]

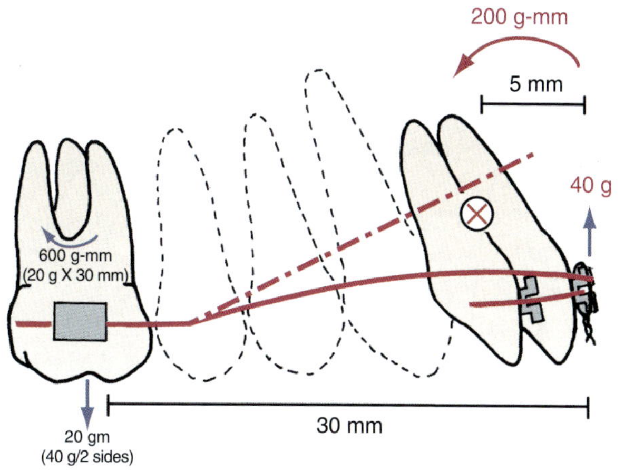

• **Fig. 9.36** An intrusion arch made from rectangular wire, which fits into a rectangular tube on the molars and is tied to one point of contact on the incisor segment, is an example of a determinate one-couple system. If the archwire is activated by pulling it down and tying it to the incisor segment so that it delivers 40 g of intrusion force (10 g per incisor, 20 g per side), and if the distance from the molar tube to the point of attachment is 30 mm, each molar will feel a 20-g extrusive force in reaction and a 600 g-mm moment to tip the crown distally. At the incisor segment, the force will create a 200-g-mm moment to rotate the incisor crowns facially. At each molar, the extrusive force also would create a moment to roll the crown lingually. If the buccal tube were 4 mm buccal to the center of resistance, the magnitude of this moment would be 80 g-mm.

For analysis, the teeth in the anchor unit are considered as if stabilization had created a single large multirooted tooth, with a single center of resistance. It is important to tie teeth in an anchor unit tightly together with as rigid a stabilizing wire segment as possible. Often the posterior teeth on both sides are tied together with a rigid lingual/palatal arch, so that a single posterior stabilizing segment is created. If the goal is to move more than one tooth, the tooth movement segment similarly must be tied so the teeth become a single unit.

Cantilever Spring Applications

Cantilever springs are used most frequently to bring severely displaced (impacted) teeth into the arch (Fig. 9.37). These springs have the advantage of a long range of action, with a minimal decrease in force as tooth movement proceeds and excellent control of force magnitude. There are two disadvantages: (1) as with most devices with a long range of action, cantilever springs do not fail safely—if they are distorted by the patient, significant tooth movement in the wrong direction is quite possible—and (2) the moment of the force on an unerupted tooth rotates the crown lingually as the tooth is brought toward the occlusal plane, which is undesirable if the tooth is already lingual to its proper position (as most unerupted teeth are). Although an additional force can be added to overcome this, the system rapidly becomes extremely complex, making it hard to know what forces and couples exist. If the cantilever spring is tied into a bracket on the unerupted tooth so that a couple can be created for better control, the force system becomes statically indeterminate and force magnitudes are no longer known with certainty.

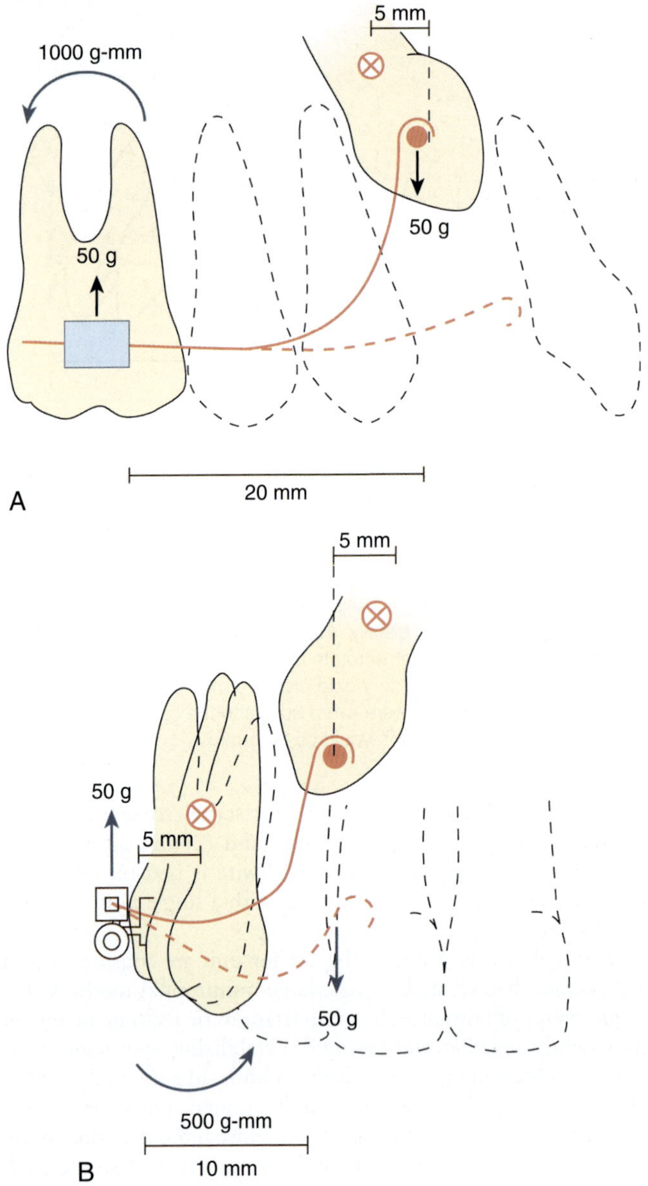

• **Fig. 9.37** A cantilever spring, made from a rectangular wire that fits into a rectangular tube (or bracket) on one end and is tied to one point of contact on the other, produces a determinate one-couple system in which the forces and moments can be known precisely. (A) Lateral view of the force system created by a cantilever spring to extrude an impacted maxillary canine. If the distance between the molar tube and a button on the canine to which the spring is tied is 20 mm, placing a 50-g extrusive force on the canine creates a 50-g intrusive force on the molar and also a 1000 g-mm moment to rotate the molar crown forward around its center of resistance. (B) Frontal view of the same force system. Consider the buccolingual (torque) moments created by the force on the molar and canine. Since the 50 g vertical forces at the canine and molar do not pass through the center of resistance of those teeth, associated moments are also produced. If the force on the canine in the frontal view is applied 5 mm buccal to the center of resistance as shown, a 250 g-mm moment will tend to rotate the crown lingually (typically not desired). At the molar, the intrusive 50 g force will produce a 250 g-mm moment rotating the crown facially - this will partially offset the 500 g-mm moment of a couple produced by the wire to a net 250 g-mm moment rotating the crown lingually.

Auxiliary Intrusion or Extrusion Arches

The major use of one-couple systems is for intrusion, typically of incisors that have erupted too much. For this purpose, light force against the teeth to be intruded is critical. An intrusion arch typically employs posterior (molar) anchorage against two or four incisors (Fig. 9.38). Because the intrusive force must be light, the reaction force against the anchor teeth also is light, well below the force levels needed for extrusion and tipping that would be the reactive movements of the anchor teeth. Tying the molar teeth together with a rigid lingual/palatal arch prevents buccal tipping of the molars. In adults, usually the premolar teeth are also added to the anchor unit.

It would be easy enough to activate an auxiliary archwire to produce extrusion of incisors rather than intrusion. This is rarely done clinically, however. The force needed for extrusion is four to five times higher than for intrusion, so the reactive force against the anchor teeth also would be higher and the anchor teeth would not be as stable. Perhaps more important, the precise control of force magnitude that is the major advantage of a one-couple system is less critical when extrusion is desired. The additional complexity of stabilizing segments and an auxiliary archwire may not be cost-effective if extrusion is the goal.

Two-Couple Systems

Utility Arches for Intrusion

An easy way to see the effect of changing from a determinate one-couple to an indeterminate two-couple system is to observe the effect of tying an intrusion arch into brackets on incisor teeth, rather than tying it with one-point contact.[21] The utility arch, popularized by Ricketts and recommended for incisor intrusion, makes just this change. It is formed from rectangular wire so that it will not roll in the molar tubes, bypasses the canine and premolar teeth, and (unlike a one-couple intrusion arch) is tied into the incisor brackets (i.e., it is a 2 × 4 archwire attached to two molars and four incisors). The resulting long span provides excellent load-deflection properties, so the light force necessary for intrusion can be created. One-couple intrusion arches can look quite similar. The difference comes when the utility arch is tied into the incisor brackets, creating a two-couple system.

When the utility arch is activated for intrusion, the moment of the intrusive force tips the crowns facially (Fig. 9.39). One way to prevent the facial tipping is to apply a force to retract the incisors, which would create a moment in the opposite direction. This could be done by cinching or tying back the intrusion utility arch. Although the retraction force could be light, any force to bring the anchor teeth mesially is likely to be undesirable.

Another strategy to control the facial tipping is immediately apparent: place a twist in the anterior segment of the utility arch, to torque the incisors lingually, and accentuate the torque by cinching the end of the wire at the molar tube. Let us examine the effect of doing this (see Fig. 9.39B and C). An effect of the couple within the bracket is to increase the intrusive force on the incisors and also the reactive extrusive force on the molars. Although one can be sure that the magnitude of the intrusive force would increase, it is impossible to know how much. An increase in the magnitude of the intrusive force often is not anticipated from such an apparently unrelated change in the archwire. In addition, now the magnitude of the reactive forces is not known with certainty, which makes it impossible to accurately adjust the archwire even if

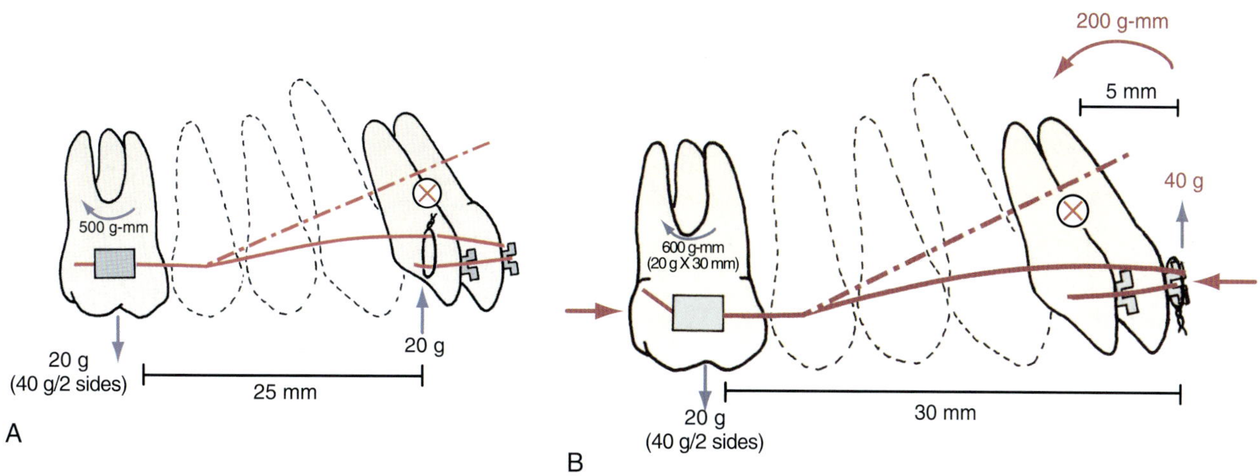

• **Fig. 9.38** Two factors in the action of an intrusion arch are the relationship of the point of force application relative to the center of resistance of the incisor segment and whether the incisor teeth are free to tip facially as they intrude or whether the arch is cinched back to produce lingual root torque. (A) An intrusion arch can be tied at any point along the incisor segment. If it is tied behind the lateral incisor bracket, the force is applied in line with the center of resistance, and there is no moment to rotate the incisors faciolingually. The effect on the anchor molar would be slightly less than if the intrusion arch were tied in the midline (see Fig. 9.36). (B) If the intrusion arch were tied in the midline and cinched back so it could not slide forward in the molar tube, the effect would be lingual root torque on the incisors as they intruded. Equilibrium requires that both moments and forces be balanced, so any lingual force exerted by the wire to restrain the incisors would be balanced by a mesial force on the molar *(red arrows)*.

you do anticipate the increase. Both effects help explain why utility arches often produce disappointing amounts of incisor intrusion relative to molar extrusion.

Symmetric and Asymmetric Bends

When a wire is placed into two brackets, the forces of the equilibrium always act at both brackets. For analysis, two groups of teeth that have been tied together to create the equivalent of a single multirooted tooth can be treated as if there were just one bracket for each group. There are three possibilities for placing a bend in the wire to activate it:

- *Symmetric V-bend,* which creates equal and opposite couples at the brackets (Fig. 9.40). The associated equilibrium forces at each bracket are also equal and opposite, and therefore cancel each other out. A symmetric V-bend is not necessarily halfway between two teeth or two groups of teeth; the important quality is that it generates equivalent couples at both ends. These couples are affected by both bracket width and bracket alignment, so care must be taken if placing symmetric V-bends before the teeth are well aligned. In addition, if a symmetric V-bend is to be placed between posterior and anterior teeth, studies have shown that the bend must be placed closer to the posterior segment owing to the curve of the archwire. Finally, equal and opposite couples have the benefit of no net reaction forces, but these equal couples will not generate equivalent tooth movement if the anchorage of one section is much greater.
- *Asymmetric V-bend,* which creates unequal and opposite couples, and net equilibrium forces that would intrude one unit and extrude the other (Fig. 9.41). Although the absolute magnitude of the forces involved cannot be known with certainty (this is, after all, an indeterminate system), the relative magnitude of the moments and the direction of the associated equilibrium forces can be determined. The bracket with the larger moment will have a greater tendency to rotate than the bracket with the smaller moment, and this will indicate the direction of the equilibrium forces. Placing the short segment of the wire in the bracket is a good way to visualize the direction of the equilibrium forces. As the bend moves closer to one of two equal units, the moment increases on the closer unit and decreases on the distant one, while equilibrium forces increase.
- In most studies of asymmetric V-bends, a location is found where no moment is felt at the distant bracket, only a single force. When the bend moves closer than this to one bracket, moments at both brackets are in the same direction, and equilibrium forces increase further. The location of this point, however, varies in different studies, ranging from one-third of the distance along the wire to not being found even when the bend is placed right by one anchor unit. The difficulty of locating this point and therefore of confidently predicting the effect of placement of the bend is another illustration of why it is important to watch clinically for undesired side effects.
- *Step bend,* which creates two couples in the same direction regardless of its location between the brackets (Fig. 9.42). The location of a V-bend is a critical variable in determining its effect, but the location of a step bend has little or no effect on either the magnitude of the moments or the equilibrium forces.

The general relationship between bend location and the forces and moments that are produced is shown in Table 9.3. Note that for V-bends, the force increases steadily as the beam moves off-center. For step bends, because both couples are in the same direction, the force is increased over what an asymmetric V-bend would produce.

Forces and Couples Created by Interbracket Bends

Under laboratory conditions, the forces and couples created in a two-couple system by interbracket bends can be evaluated experimentally.[22] With a 16-mil steel wire and an interbracket distance of 7 mm (about what would be found between central incisors with twin brackets or between narrow canine and premolar brackets), a

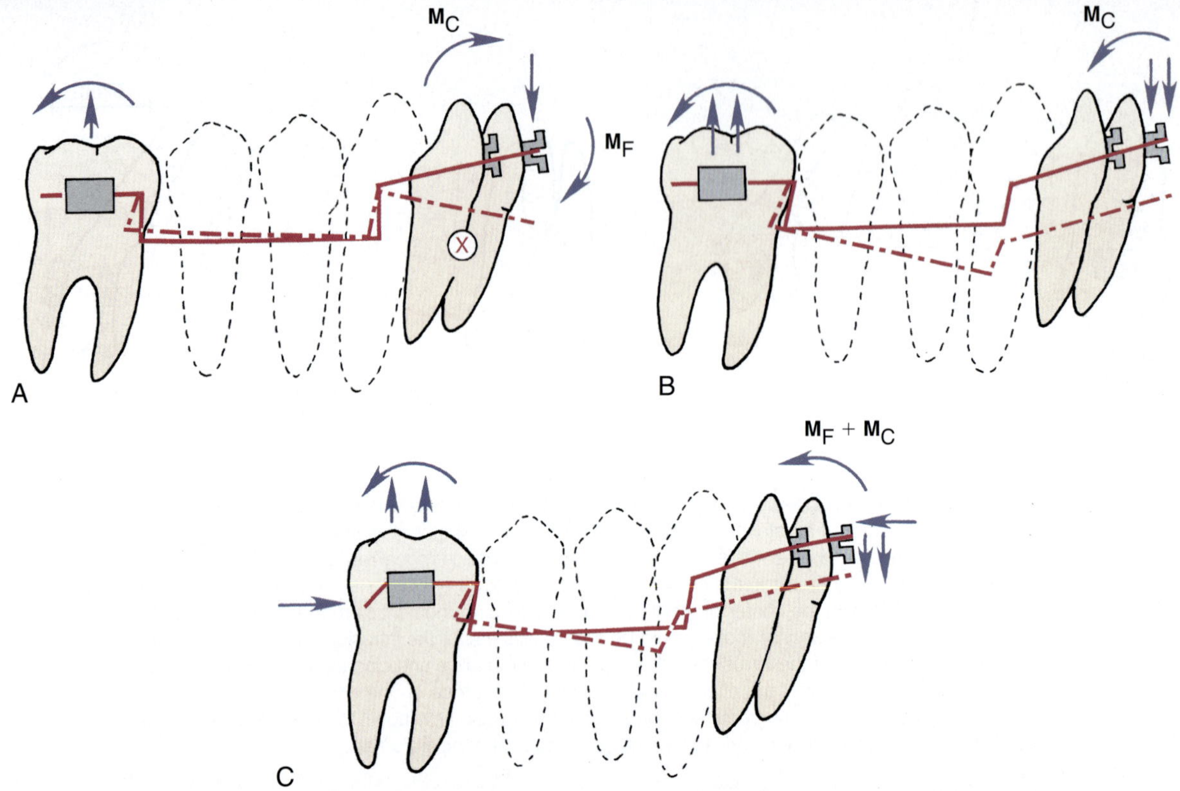

• **Fig. 9.39** A utility arch often is an intrusion arch in a two-couple configuration, created by tying the rectangular intrusion arch into the brackets on the incisors. When this is done, the precise magnitude of forces and couples cannot be known, but the initial activation of the arch should be to provide about 40 g to the incisor segment for intrusion. (A) Activating the utility arch by placing it in the brackets creates the intrusion force, with a reactive force of the same magnitude on the anchor molar and a couple to tip its crown distally. At the incisors, a moment to tip the crowns facially (M_F) is created by distance of the brackets forward from the center of resistance, and an additional moment in the same direction is created by the couple within the bracket (M_C) as the inclination of the wire is changed when it is brought to the brackets. The moment of this couple cannot be known, but it is clinically important because it affects the magnitude of the intrusion force. (B) Placing a torque bend in the utility arch creates a moment to bring the crown lingually, controlling the tendency for the teeth to tip facially as they intrude, but it also increases the magnitude of the intrusive force on the incisor segment and the extrusive force and couple on the molar. (C) Cinching back the utility arch creates a force to bring the incisors lingually, and a moment of this force opposes the moment of the intrusion force. At the molar, a force to bring the molar mesially is created, along with a moment to tip the molar mesially. Especially if a torque bend still is present, it is difficult to be certain which of the moments will prevail or whether the intrusion force is appropriate. With this two-couple system, the vertical forces easily can be heavier than desired, changing the balance between intrusion of the incisors and extrusion of the molars. (Redrawn from Davidovitch M, Rebellato J. Utility arches: a two-couple intrusion system. *Semin Orthod*. 1995;1:25–30.)

step bend of only 0.35 mm would produce intrusive and extrusive forces of 347 g and 1210 g-mm couples in the same direction (see Table 9.4). Permanent distortion of the wire would occur with a step bend of 0.8 mm. Because this force magnitude is far too great for intrusion, it is clear that extrusion would prevail.

The heavy vertical forces produced by what orthodontists would consider modest bends in a light archwire such as 16-mil steel explain why extrusion is the response to step bends in continuous archwires. An asymmetric V-bend that places the apex of the bend 0.35 mm above the plane of the brackets produces 803 g-mm couples with no net intrusive or extrusive forces at the one-third position. At the one-sixth position, intrusive and extrusive forces over 900 g occur, with very large moments (see Table 9.4), so the result here also would be extrusion in addition to root movement.

The moments and forces are greatly reduced as interbracket distances increase. For instance, the same 0.35-mm step bend that produced 347 g with a 7-mm interbracket span produces only 43 g with a 14-mm span (which is still too high for intrusion). Even with flexible archwires, an interbracket span equivalent to the distance from the first molar to the lateral incisor usually is needed to obtain the light force necessary for intrusion (which is why intrusion arches are designed to bypass the premolars and canines).

Longer spans also make the location of V-bends less critical. With a 7-mm interbracket span, moving a V-bend only 1.2 mm from a centered position would put it at the one-third position that totally eliminates the moment on the distant bracket. With a 21-mm span, the same error would be almost negligible. It is much easier therefore to control two-couple systems when the distances between attachments are relatively large, as they are when

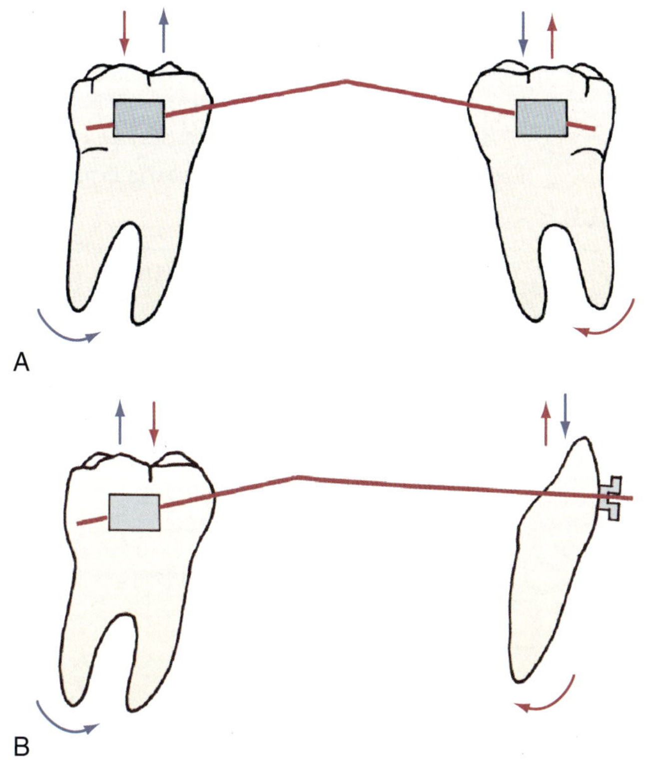

• **Fig. 9.40** (A) When a symmetric V-bend is placed halfway between two units with equal resistance to movement, it creates equal and opposite moments *(red and blue curved arrows)*, and the intrusive-extrusive forces indicated by the red and blue vertical arrows cancel each other. (B) To create equal and opposite couples between two units with unequal resistance to movement, a V-bend must be displaced toward the unit with greater resistance, so a symmetric V-bend between an incisor and molar would be offset toward the molar. One must know the approximate anchorage value of teeth or units of the dental arch to calculate the appropriate location of symmetric or asymmetric V-bends.

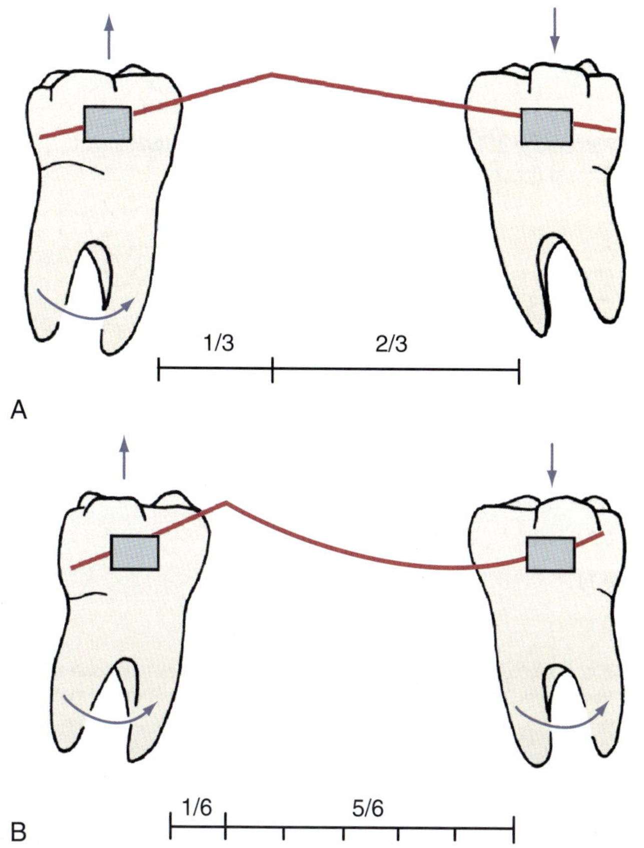

• **Fig. 9.41** (A) An asymmetric V-bend creates a greater moment on one tooth or unit than the other. As the bend moves toward one tooth, the moment on it increases and the moment on the distant tooth decreases. When the bend is one-third of the way along the interbracket span, the distant tooth (on the right in this drawing) receives only a vertical force, with no moment. (B) If the V-bend moves closer than the one-third point to one of the teeth, a moment in the same direction is created on both teeth, instead of opposite moments. A V-bend placed to parallel the roots of the adjacent teeth would not do so if the bend were too close to one of the teeth.

wires connect only to molars and incisors in a 2 × 4 arrangement, or to anterior and posterior segments.

Still another level of complexity exists for a 2 × 4 two-couple wire, because 3D effects are produced when the wire goes around the arch from the molars to the incisors. This makes the analysis of torque bends particularly difficult. Using finite analysis modeling, Isaacson et al have shown that the general principles of two-dimensional (2D) analysis remain valid when 3D analysis is done.[23] In a long-span wire such as a utility arch, however, a V-bend at the molar produces significantly less moment and associated equilibrium forces than the same V-bend located at the same distance from the incisor segment. In addition, the reversal of moments so that the moment is in the same direction on the molar and the incisor does not occur in the 3D analysis when the V-bend moves closer than one-third of the distance to the molar or incisors. This makes the effect of utility arches with complex bends even less predictable.

Two-Couple Archwires to Change Incisor Inclination

A two-couple system to change the inclination of incisors can be arranged to produce either tipping or torque.[24] The change in inclination is the same for tipping or torque; the difference is crown movement or root movement. If a wire spanning from the molars to the incisors is activated to rotate incisors around their center of resistance, the crowns will move facially when the wire is free to slide

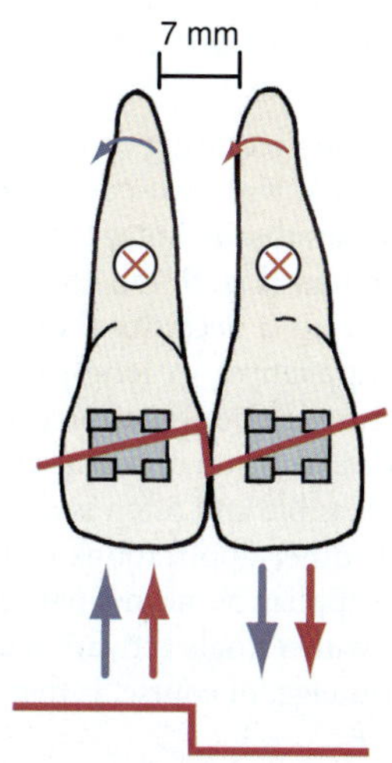

• **Fig. 9.42** A step bend between two teeth produces intrusive force on one tooth and extrusive force on the other and creates couples in the same direction. In contrast to V-bends, there is little effect on either the force or the couples when the step bend is moved off-center.

TABLE 9.4 Force Systems From Step and V-Bends

Percentage of Total Span to Closest Bracket	Moment Far Tooth/Moment Near Tooth	Force General Condition	DATA FROM EXPERIMENT 16 STEEL, 7-MM SPAN, 0.35-MM BEND	
			Force (g)	Moment (g-mm)
Step Bend				
Any	1.0	XX	347	1210/1210
V-Bend				
0.5	−1.0	None	0	803/803
0.4	−0.3	X		
0.33	0	XX		
0.29			353	2210/262
0.2	0.3	XXX		
0.14			937	4840/1720
0.1	0.4	XXXX		

X, XX, XXX, XXXX indicate relative force levels generated at the various V-bend locations.
From Burstone CJ, Koenig HA. Creative wire bending—the force system from step and V bends. *Am J Orthod Dentofacial Orthop*. 1988;93:59–67.

through the molar tube (Fig. 9.43A). Occasionally, this provides a convenient way to tip maxillary incisors facially to correct anterior crossbite in the mixed dentition (see Chapters 15–17 and 19).

If the wire is cinched back (Fig. 9.43B), the effect will be to torque the incisor roots lingually, and a reaction force to bring the molar mesially is created. The incisors also will extrude, while the molars will intrude and roll facially. For incisor root torque, the long range of action provided by a 2 × 4 two-couple system is not necessarily an advantage, particularly when there is nothing to control the vertical side effects on the incisors. In patients with severely upright maxillary central incisors (as in Class II division 2 malocclusion), a one-couple torquing arch with all the other teeth as anchorage can be used to advantage (Fig. 9.44).

Posterior Crossbite Correction: Transverse Movement of Posterior Teeth

Dental posterior crossbite, requiring expansion or constriction of molars, can be approached with two-couple archwires.[25] Then the anterior segment becomes the anchorage and movement of one or both first molars is desired (Fig. 9.45). Incorporating the canines into the anchor segment is a necessity (i.e., this requires a 2 × 6 rather than a 2 × 4 appliance). A long-span bypassing the premolars still is needed for appropriate force levels and control of moments. Asymmetric expansion or constriction to correct unilateral crossbite is quite feasible and often is the indication for using this method. As with other applications of two-couple systems, the large range of the appliance means that teeth can be moved a considerable distance with a single activation of the appliance. The corresponding disadvantage, of course, is that the system has poor fail-safe properties.

Lingual Arches as Two-Couple Systems

Still another example of a two-couple appliance system is a transpalatal lingual arch (or a mandibular lingual arch that does

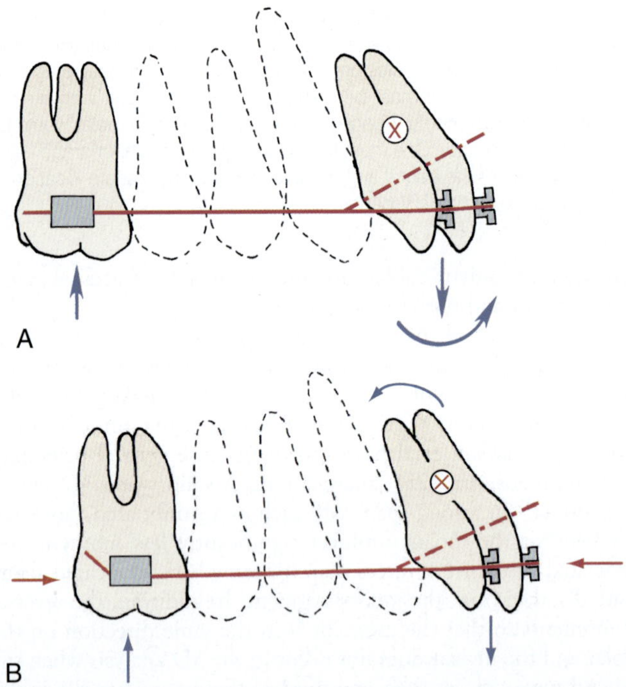

• **Fig. 9.43** An asymmetric V-bend in a rectangular wire spanning from the first molars to the incisor segment produces a moment to rotate the incisors faciolingually, with an intrusive force but no moment on the molars and an extrusive force on the incisors. (A) If the archwire is free to slide forward through the molar tube, the result is anterior tipping and extrusion of the incisors. Occasionally, this is desirable in the correction of anterior crossbite in the mixed dentition. (B) If the archwire is cinched behind the molar so that it cannot slide, the effect is lingual root torque and extrusion for the incisors. As noted in Fig. 9.38B, any lingual force exerted by the wire to restrain the incisors would be balanced by a mesial force on the molar *(red arrows)*.

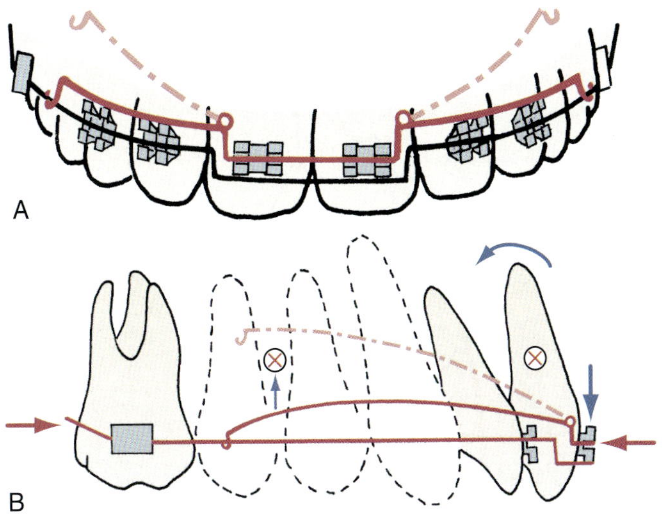

• **Fig. 9.44** For torque of very upright maxillary central incisors (as in Class II division 2 malocclusion), a one-couple torquing arch designed by Burstone can be very effective. (A) A heavy stabilizing arch is placed in all the teeth but the central incisors, contoured so that it steps below the brackets on the central incisors and contacts the facial surface of these teeth, and tied back against the molars. A wire tied into the central incisor brackets and activated by bending it down and hooking it between the first molar and second premolar then produces the desired moment. (B) Because the stabilizing archwire resists facial tipping and extrusion of the central incisors, the result is lingual root torque with optimum force over a long range. The reaction force to intrude the remaining teeth and bring them anteriorly is distributed over all the other teeth, minimizing the reaction.

not contact the anterior teeth).[26] Lingual arches often are employed to prevent tooth movement rather than create it. The need for a lingual arch to stabilize posterior segments in many situations has been noted previously. When a lingual arch is used to move teeth, spring properties are required, which means that either a different wire size or different material is needed for an active rather than a stabilizing lingual arch. Whatever a lingual arch is made of and however it is attached, its two-couple design predicts the effect of symmetric V, asymmetric V, and step bends. Often, it is desirable to rotate maxillary first molars so that the mesiobuccal cusp moves facially. This can be accomplished bilaterally with symmetric bends or unilaterally with an asymmetric bend (Fig. 9.46). An asymmetric activation tends to rotate the molar on the side closest to the bend and move it mesially, while the molar on the other side is displaced distally.

It is tempting to think that net distal movement of an upper molar can be accomplished routinely with this type of activation of a transpalatal lingual arch, and it has been suggested that a clinician can distalize one molar while rotating the other, then reverse the process, moving both of them back. However, the evidence indicates that significant distal movement beyond rotation of the buccal cusps is unlikely—mesial movement of the anchor molar is entirely possible and indeed quite likely.[27]

A lingual arch also can be activated to torque roots facially or lingually (Fig. 9.47). Symmetric torque when molars are expanded provides bodily movement rather than tipping. An interesting approach to unilateral crossbite is the use of a lingual arch with buccal root torque (lingual crown torque) on one side pitted against buccal tipping on the other side. As Ingervall and coworkers have shown quite convincingly, significant expansion on the tipping side can be produced, perhaps more effectively if the appliance is converted to a one-couple device by placing a round rather than rectangular wire in the bracket on the tipping side.[28]

A somewhat unusual application of a lingual arch would be to tip one molar distally, uprighting it. The reciprocal, of course, would be mesial tipping of the opposite molar. This activation would require a twist in the lingual wire. The location of this twist bend is not critical. The relative moments on the molar teeth will be equal and opposite, wherever the twist bend is placed.

Segmented Arch Mechanics

What is often called *segmented arch mechanics* is best considered an organized approach to using one-couple and two-couple systems for most tooth movements, so that an engineering analysis can provide an approximation of both forces and moments. This would allow use of more favorable force levels and potentially provide better control. The essence of the segmented arch system is the establishment of units of teeth, so that anchorage and movement segments are clearly defined. The desired tooth movement is accomplished with cantilever springs where possible, so that the precision of the one-couple approach is available, or with the use of two-couple systems through which at least net moments and the direction of equilibrium forces can be known (as they cannot be with the multicouple force system created by a continuous rectangular archwire tied into brackets on all teeth in a dental arch).

In segmented arch treatment, lingual arches are used for stabilization in a majority of the patients, and stabilizing wire segments in the brackets of teeth in anchor units also are used routinely. The requirements for stabilization, of course, are just the opposite of those for tooth movement: the heaviest and most rigid available wires are desired. For this reason, the 22-slot edgewise appliance is favored for segmented arch treatment. The wires used for stabilizing segments usually are 21 × 25 steel, which is far too stiff for tooth movement. The stabilizing lingual arches usually are 36 steel, soldered to the molar bands or with doubled-over ends that fit into rectangular sheaths.

Typical segmented arch treatment would call for initial alignment within anterior and posterior segments, the creation of appropriate anchorage and tooth movement segments, vertical leveling using intrusion or extrusion as needed, space closure with differential movement of anterior and posterior segments, and perhaps the use of auxiliary torquing arches. Sliding archwires through brackets almost always is avoided in this technique because resistance to sliding hampers efforts to control anchorage and introduces uncertainties into the calculation of appropriate force levels. Continuous archwires, particularly rectangular wires, would be reserved for the final stages of treatment when quite small but precise movements are required.

The advantages of the segmented arch approach are the control that is available and the possibility of tooth movements that would be impossible with continuous archwires. The disadvantages are the greater complexity of the orthodontic appliance and the greater amount of the doctor's time needed to install, adjust, and maintain it. It is an interesting paradox that simplifying the engineering analysis of the appliance, by dealing insofar as possible with identifiable one- and two-couple systems, complicates the appliance rather than making it simpler.

An excellent example of the segmented arch approach is the design of an appliance to simultaneously retract and intrude protruding maxillary central incisors. This is difficult to accomplish because lingual tipping of the incisors tends to move the crown

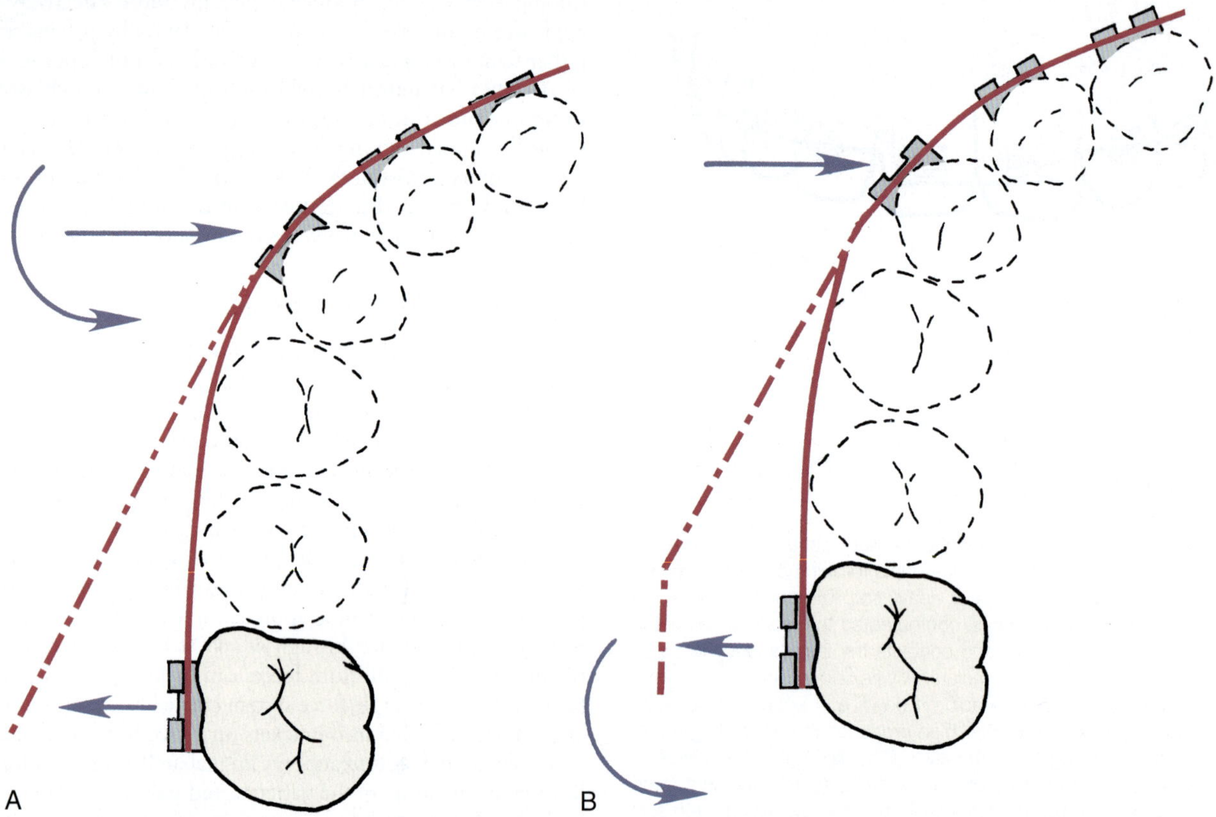

• **Fig. 9.45** A 2 × 6 appliance can be used to produce transverse movement of first permanent molars. In this circumstance, the anterior segment becomes the anchorage and it is important to add the canines to the anchor unit, but the premolars cannot be tied to the archwire without destroying its effectiveness. The long span between the canine and molar is needed to produce the desired forces and moments in this two-couple system. (A) An outward bend a few millimeters behind the canine bracket results primarily in expansion of the molar, with little or no rotation (with the unequal segments, this approximates the one-third position between the units of the two-couple system). (B) An outward bend behind the canine combined with a toe-in bend at the molar results in expansion and mesial-out rotation of the molar. (Redrawn from Rebellato J. Two-couple orthodontic appliance systems: activations in the transverse dimension. *Semin Orthod*. 1995;1:37–43.)

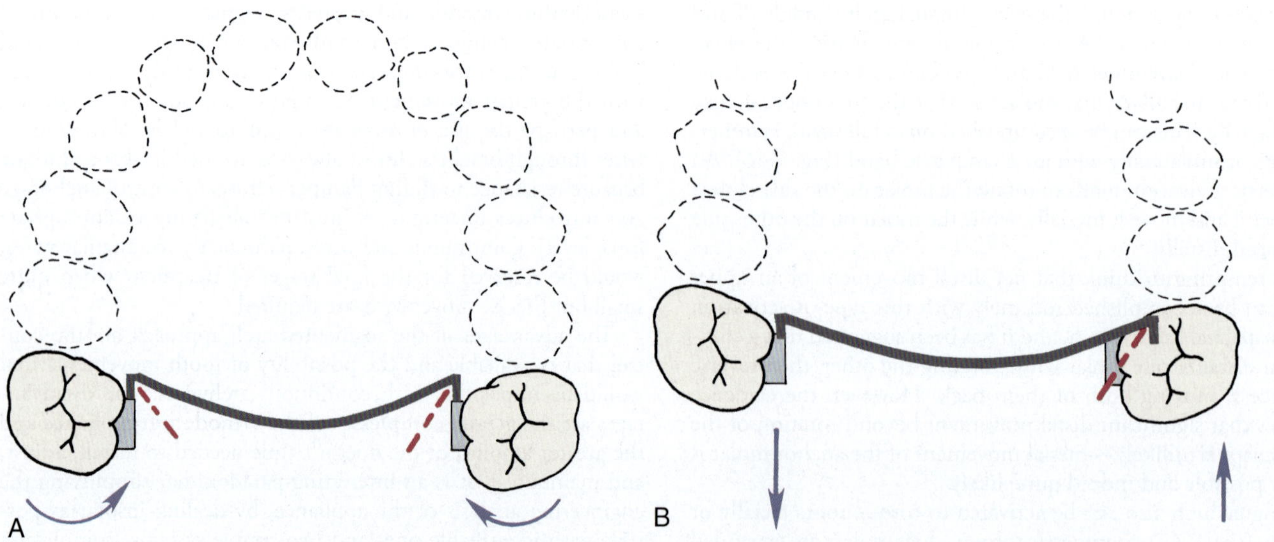

• **Fig. 9.46** (A) Bilateral toe-in bends at the first molars create equal and opposite couples, so the mesiodistal forces cancel and the teeth are rotated to bring the mesiobuccal cusp facially. When space has been lost in the maxillary arch or when a Class II molar relationship exists, this type of rotation often is desired, but a flexible rather than a rigid lingual arch is needed to obtain it. (B) A unilateral toe-in bend rotates the molar on the side of the bend, and creates a force to move the other molar distally. Although mesial movement of the molar on the side of the bend is limited by contact with the other teeth, mesial movement may occur. Although net distalization of both molars has been claimed by bends of this type on first one side, then the other, significant distal movement of both teeth is unlikely.

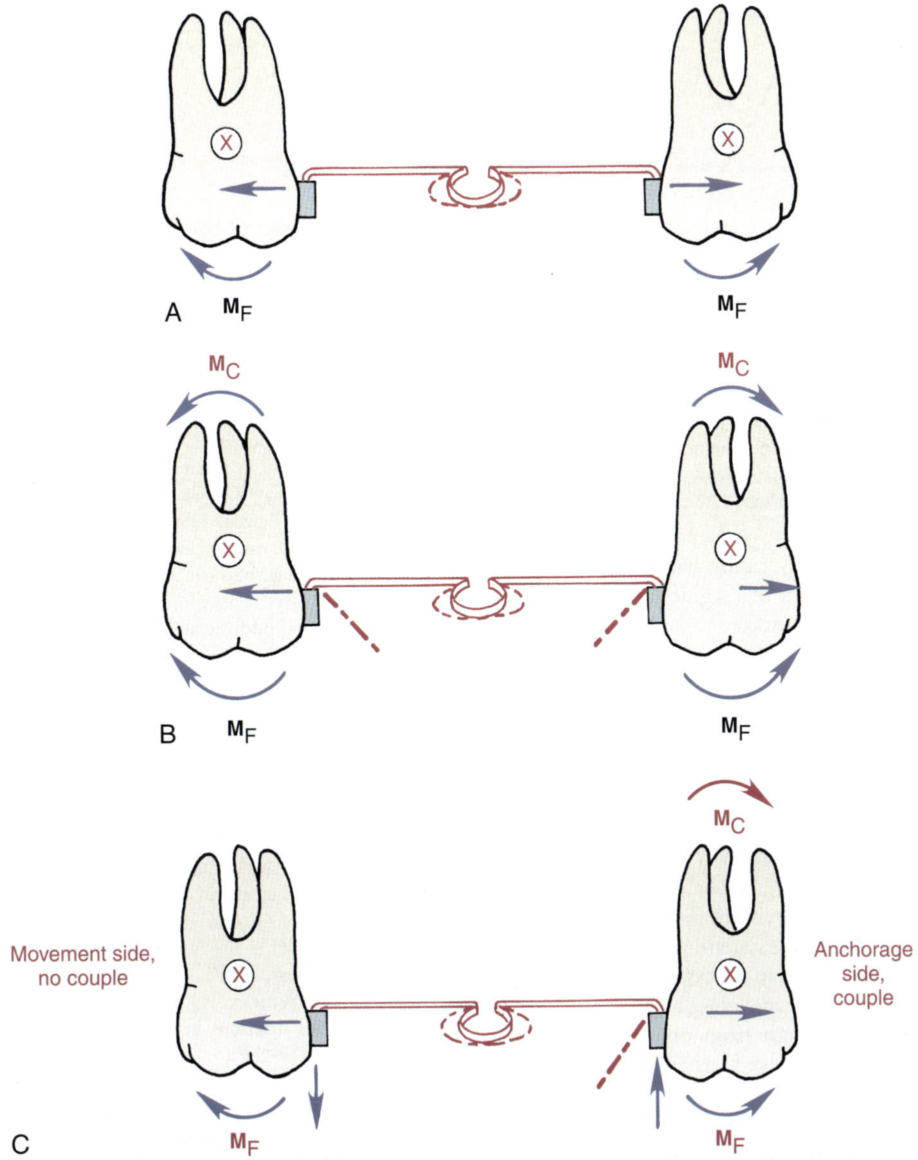

• **Fig. 9.47** (A) Bilateral expansion of molars can be created by expansion of a transpalatal arch, which typically is achieved by opening a loop in the middle. The moment of the expansion force tips the crowns facially. (B) Placing a twist in the wire creates a moment to torque the roots facially. The moment of the couple must be greater than the moment of the force for this to occur. Unless a flexible wire is used for the lingual arch, it can be difficult to insert the activated lingual arch with enough twist to produce the desired torque. (C) A twist in the wire on one side can be used to create stationary anchorage to tip the opposite molar facially. This is particularly effective if the wire is rounded on the movement side, so that a one-couple rather than two-couple system exists in the faciolingual plane of space. (A and B, Redrawn from Rebellato J. Two-couple orthodontic appliance systems: transpalatal arches. *Semin Orthod*. 1995;1:44–54; C, Modified from Ingervall B, Gollner P, Gebauer U, et al. A clinical investigation of the correction of unilateral molar crossbite with a transpalatal arch. *Am J Orthod Dentofacial Orthop*. 1995;107:418–425.)

downward as the tooth rotates around its center of resistance. Intrusion of the root apex is necessary to keep the crown at the same vertical level relative to the lip and other teeth. This problem can be solved by creating anterior and posterior segments, using a rigid bar to move the point of force application distal to the center of resistance of the incisor segment, and applying separate intrusion and retraction forces (Fig. 9.48).[29] This could be done much more easily now, however, by using TADs as illustrated in Chapter 15. Skeletal anchorage has the potential to replace many of the more complex applications of segmented arch treatment.

Complex segmented arch treatment carries with it two other potential disadvantages that must be kept in mind. First, even with the most careful engineering analysis, it can turn out that something was overlooked in the determination of the likely outcome. The application of engineering theory to orthodontics is imperfect enough that a unique force system for an individual patient may not produce the expected outcome. Second, most segmented arch mechanisms contain little or nothing to control the distance that teeth can be displaced if something goes wrong. If precisely calibrated springs with a long range of action encounter something

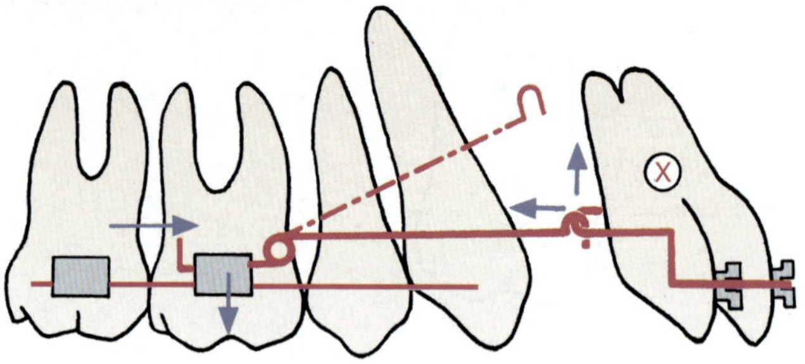

• **Fig. 9.48** A segmented arch approach allows simultaneous retraction and intrusion of an anterior segment. A rigid bar in the anterior segment can be extended posteriorly so that the point of application of an intrusive force is at or distal to the center of resistance of the incisor segment. If a cantilever spring is used to apply an intrusive force at that point, the tendency of a retraction force to elongate the anterior segment can be overcome. (Redrawn from Shroff B, et al. Simultaneous intrusion and retraction using a three-piece base arch. *Angle Orthod*. 1997;67:455–462.)

that distorts them (such as a sticky candy bar), major problems can occur. The mechanical efficiency of a segmented appliance can be both an advantage and a disadvantage.

Continuous Arch Mechanics

Engineering analysis of the effects of a continuous archwire, one that is tied into the brackets on all the teeth, is essentially impossible. All that can be said is that an extremely complex multicouple force system is established when the wire is tied into place. The initial result is a small movement of one tooth. As soon as that occurs, the force system is changed, and the new system causes a small movement of another tooth (or a different movement of the first tooth). Either way, the result is still another complex force system, which causes another movement, leading to another change in the system, and so on.

Sometimes, orthodontic tooth movement is conceived as a slow, smooth transition of the teeth from one arrangement to another, but the force systems involved, particularly those with continuous arch mechanics, make it plain that this is far from the case. If it were possible to take time-lapse photographs of teeth being moved into position, we undoubtedly would see "the dance of the teeth," as the complex force systems formed and changed, producing varied effects in sequence, and Hayashi et al. have shown just this sort of movement.[30] It is a saving grace that a continuous archwire usually does not allow the teeth to move very far from the desired endpoint.

The advantages and disadvantages of the continuous arch approach are just the reverse of those with the segmented arch approach. Continuous arch treatment is not as well defined in terms of the forces and moments that will be generated at any one time and certainly is less elegant from an engineering perspective. But continuous archwires often take less chair time because they are simpler to make and install, and they have excellent fail-safe properties in most applications. In modern orthodontics, often the clinician must evaluate the trade-off between segmented and continuous arch approaches to specific problems. For those who use primarily the segmented approach, some use of continuous archwires simplifies life. For those who use primarily continuous archwires, some use of the segmented approach is necessary to meet specific objectives. Quite literally, you consider the benefits versus the cost (time) and risks, and make your choice.

The development of contemporary fixed appliances and their characteristics are discussed in the next chapter (Chapter 10). Clinical applications of the mechanical principles reviewed in this chapter and further information about the use of specific treatment methods are provided in some detail in Chapters 13 to 18 and 20–22.

References

1. Gurgel J, Kerr S, Powers JM, et al. Force-deflection properties of superelastic nickel-titanium archwires. *Am J Orthod Dentofacial Orthop*. 2001;120:378–382.
2. Miura F, Mogi M, Okamoto Y. New application of superelastic NiTi rectangular wire. *J Clin Orthod*. 1990;24:544–548.
3. Cacciafesta V, Sfondrini MF, Scribante LA, et al. Force levels of fiber-reinforced composites and orthodontic stainless steel wires: a 3-point bending test. *Am J Orthod Dentofacial Orthop*. 2008;133:410–413.
4. Spendlove J, Berzins DW, Pruszynski JE, Ballard RW. Investigation of force decay in aesthetic, fibre-reinforced composite orthodontic archwires. *Eur J Orthod*. 2015;37:43–48.
5. Chang JH, Berzins DW, Pruszynski JE, Ballard RW. The effect of water storage on the bending properties of esthetic, fiber-reinforced composite orthodontic archwires. *Angle Orthod*. 2014;84:417–423.
6. Kusy RP. On the use of nomograms to determine the elastic property ratios of orthodontic archwires. *Am J Orthod*. 1983;83:374–381.
7. Adams DM, Powers JM, Asgar K. Effects of brackets and ties on stiffness of an arch wire. *Am J Orthod Dentofacial Orthop*. 1987;91:131–136.
8. Masoud AI, Tsay TP, BeGole E, Bedran-Russo AK. Force decay evaluation of thermoplastic and thermoset elastomeric chains: a mechanical design comparison. *Angle Orthod*. 2014;84:1026–1033.
9. Linder-Aronson A, Lindskog S, Rygh P. Orthodontic magnets: effects on gingival epithelium and alveolar bone in monkeys. *Eur J Orthod*. 1992;14:255–263.
10. Darendeliler MA, Darendeliler A, Mandurino M. Clinical application of magnets in orthodontics and biological implications: a review. *Eur J Orthod*. 1997;19:431–442.
11. Jastrzebski ZD. *The Nature and Properties of Engineering Materials*. 3rd ed. Wiley; 1987.
12. Kusy RP, Whitley JQ. Effects of surface roughness on the coefficients of friction in model orthodontic systems. *J Biomech*. 1990;23:913–925.
13. Kusy RP, Whitley JQ, Gurgel J. Comparisons of surface roughnesses and sliding resistances of 6 titanium-based or TMA-type archwires. *Am J Orthod Dentofacial Orthop*. 2004;126:589–603.
14. Saunders CR, Kusy RP. Surface topography and frictional characteristics of ceramic brackets. *Am J Orthod Dentofacial Orthop*. 1994;106:76–87.
15. Kusy RP, Whitley JQ. Assessment of second-order clearances between orthodontic archwires and bracket slots via the critical contact angle for binding. *Angle Orthod*. 1999;69:71–80.
16. Articolo LC, Kusy RP. Influence of angulation on the resistance to sliding in fixed appliances. *Am J Orthod Dentofacial Orthop*. 1999;115:39–51.
17. Burrow SJ. Canine retraction rate with self-ligating brackets vs conventional edgewise brackets. *Angle Orthod*. 2010;80:438–445.
18. Baumgaertel S. Temporary skeletal anchorage devices: the case for miniscrews. *Am J Orthod Dentofacial Orthop*. 2014;145:558–564.
19. Sugawara J. Temporary skeletal anchorage devices: the case for miniplates. *Am J Orthod Dentofacial Orthop*. 2014;145:559–565.
20. Lindauer SJ, Isaacson RJ. One-couple systems. *Semin Orthod*. 1995;1:12–24.
21. Davidovitch M, Rebellato J. Utility arches: a two-couple intrusion system. *Semin Orthod*. 1995;1:25–30.
22. Burstone CJ, Koenig HA. Creative wire bending—the force system from step and V bends. *Am J Orthod Dentofacial Orthop*. 1988;93:59–67.
23. Isaacson RJ, Lindauer SJ, Conley P. Responses of 3-dimensional archwires to vertical V-bends: comparisons with existing 2-dimensional data in the lateral view. *Semin Orthod*. 1995;1:57–63.

24. Isaacson RJ, Rebellato J. Two-couple orthodontic appliance systems: torquing arches. *Semin Orthod.* 1995;1:31–36.
25. Rebellato J. Two-couple orthodontic appliance systems: activations in the transverse dimension. *Semin Orthod.* 1995;1:37–43.
26. Rebellato J. Two-couple orthodontic appliance systems: transpalatal arches. *Semin Orthod.* 1995;1:44–54.
27. Dahlquist A, Gebauer U, Ingervall B. The effect of a transpalatal arch for correction of first molar rotation. *Eur J Orthod.* 1996;18:257–267.
28. Ingervall B, Gollner P, Gebauer U, et al. A clinical investigation of the correction of unilateral molar crossbite with a transpalatal arch. *Am J Orthod Dentofacial Orthop.* 1995;107:418–425.
29. Davoody AR, Posada L, Utreja A, et al. A prospective comparative study between differential moments and miniscrews in anchorage control. *Eur J Orthod.* 2013;35:568–576.
30. Hayashi K, DeLong R, Mizoguchi I. Comparison of the finite helical axis and the rectangular coordinate system in representing orthodontic tooth movement. *J Biomech.* 2006;39:2925–2933.

10

Contemporary Orthodontic Appliances

BRENT E. LARSON, MATTHEW E. LARSON, WILLIAM R. PROFFIT, AND TORO DEGUCHI

CHAPTER OUTLINE

Orthodontic appliances have evolved steadily since the development of the specialty, but the pace of change has accelerated significantly in recent years. Technologic advances have brought both changes and some improvements in existing appliance systems (for instance, new brackets and wires for the edgewise appliance) and new ways of correcting malocclusion (such as clear aligners formed on 3D-printed models and temporary skeletal anchorage). Improved technology has greatly increased the productivity of orthodontists. Charles Tweed suggested in the 1950s that an orthodontist should not start treatment for more than 50 patients per year because there would not be enough time to manage more than that and to achieve high-quality results. This number has greatly increased since then, but so has average treatment quality—and comprehensive orthodontic treatment that cost about the same as a new car at that time now costs far less.

Although at this point an orthodontist could use one fixed appliance system to treat all of their patients, it is better to select among appliance systems to fit the needs of individual patients. Modern removable appliances can do some things better than fixed appliances, and variants within fixed appliance systems do some things better than others. The purpose of this chapter is to provide an overview of modern appliances and put them in perspective in a way that helps in choosing the best appliance for specific situations—a goal that extends into the clinical chapters that follow.

Removable Appliances

Removable orthodontic appliances have two immediately apparent advantages: (1) They are fabricated in the laboratory and adjusted extraorally rather than directly in the patient's mouth, reducing the dentist's chair time, and (2) they can be removed on socially sensitive occasions if wires on the facial part of the teeth would be visible, or can be made almost invisible if fabricated from clear plastic materials. This makes them (at least initially) more acceptable to adult patients. In addition, removable appliances allow some types of growth guidance treatment to be carried out more readily than is possible with fixed appliances. These advantages for both the patient and the dentist have ensured a continuing interest in removable appliances for both children and adults.

There are also two significant disadvantages: (1) The response to treatment is heavily dependent on patient compliance, because the appliance can only be effective when the patient chooses to wear it, and (2) it is difficult to obtain the two-point contacts on teeth necessary to produce complex tooth movements, which means that the appliance itself may limit the possibilities for treatment. Because of these limitations, fixed appliances dominate modern treatment.

Modern removable appliance therapy consists largely of the use of:

1. Active appliances with springs for tooth movement, used primarily in preadolescents (they have been largely replaced by clear aligners in adolescent and adult treatment).
2. Various types of functional appliances for growth guidance in adolescents and, less frequently, in children.
3. Clear plastic aligners for tooth movement in children, adolescents, and adults.

The focus of this part of the chapter is, accordingly, on the characteristics of the appliances used for these purposes.

Development of Active Appliances for Alignment

In the United States, the original removable appliances were rather clumsy combinations of vulcanite bases and precious metal or nickel-silver wires. In the early 1900s, George Crozat developed a removable appliance fabricated entirely of precious metal that consisted of an effective clasp for first molar teeth, heavy gold wires as a framework, and lighter gold fingersprings to produce the desired tooth movement (Fig. 10.1). The Crozat appliance attracted a small but devoted following and was still being used in the late 20th century for comprehensive treatment by a few practitioners. Its limitation was that, like almost all removable appliances, it produced mostly tipping of teeth. It had little impact on the mainstream of US orthodontic thought and practice, however, which from the beginning was focused on fixed appliances.

Development of removable appliances for tooth movement continued in Europe despite their neglect in the United States. There were three interesting reasons for this trend: (1) Angle's dogmatic approach to occlusion, with its emphasis on precise positioning of each tooth, had less impact in Europe than in the United States; (2) social welfare systems developed much more rapidly in Europe, which tended to place the emphasis on limited orthodontic treatment for large numbers of people, often delivered by general practitioners rather than orthodontic specialists; and (3) precious metal for fixed appliances was less available in Europe, both as a consequence of the social systems and because the use of precious metal in dentistry was banned in Germany in the early 1930s. This forced German orthodontists to focus on removable appliances that could be made with available materials, primarily acrylic plastics for baseplates and brass (later, stainless steel) wires for springs.

The result was that in the 1925 to 1965 era, US orthodontics was based almost exclusively on the use of fixed appliances (partial or complete banding), whereas fixed appliances were essentially unknown in Europe and all treatment was done with removables. Two European orthodontists deserve special mention for their contributions to removable appliance techniques for moving teeth. Martin Schwarz in Vienna developed and publicized a variety of "split plate" appliances, which were effective for expanding the dental arches (Fig. 10.2). Philip Adams in Belfast modified the arrowhead clasp favored by Schwarz into the Adams crib (Fig. 10.3), which is still an effective clasp to keep a removable appliance in position when springs are used to move teeth.

Tooth movement with removable appliances in children falls almost always into one of two major categories: (1) arch expansion, in which groups of teeth are moved to expand the arch perimeter, and (2) repositioning of individual teeth within the arch.

Active Plates for Arch Expansion

The framework of an active plate is a baseplate that serves as a foundation in which screws or springs are embedded and to which clasps are attached. The active element is sometimes a jackscrew placed so that it holds the parts of the plate together (see Fig. 10.2). Opening the screw then separates the sections of the plate. The screw offers the advantage that the amount of movement can be controlled, and the baseplate remains rigid despite being cut into two parts. The disadvantage is that the force system is very different from the ideal one for moving teeth. Rather than providing a light and continuous force, activation of the screw produces a heavy force that rapidly decays. This is acceptable for arch expansion if activation is slow, but not for moving individual teeth. Activating the screw too rapidly results in the appliance being progressively displaced away from the teeth rather than the arch being expanded as desired.

Removable Acrylic Appliances With Springs for Tooth Movement

In contrast to the heavy, rapidly decaying forces produced by a screw, near optimum light continuous forces can be produced by springs in a removable appliance. Like the edges of an active plate, however, these springs contact the tooth surface at only one point, and it is difficult to use them for anything but tipping tooth movements. The guideline for tooth movement with a spring from a

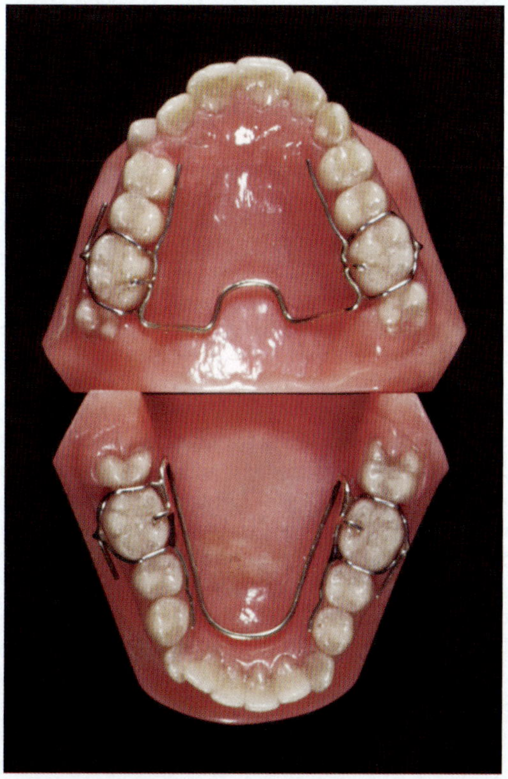

• Fig. 10.1 Crozat appliances for the upper and lower arch, showing the transverse connectors that allow lateral expansion. The Crozat clasps on the molars use fingers that extend into the mesiobuccal and distobuccal undercuts.

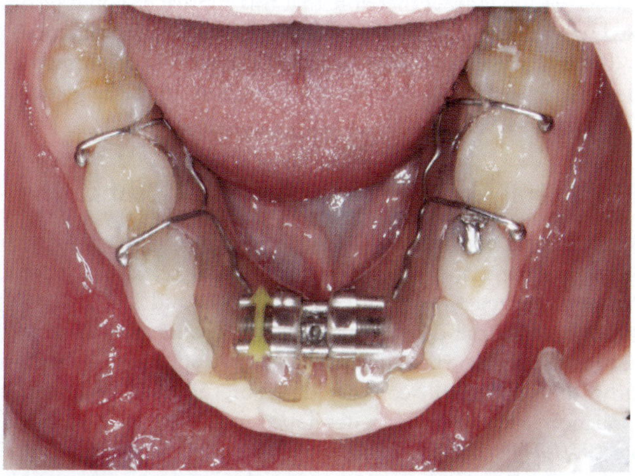

• Fig. 10.2 A removable appliance of the "Schwarz plate" type used a jackscrew to separate the parts of the acrylic plate and expand the dental arch. They were used in the maxillary or mandibular dental arch—this one was designed to expand across the lower incisors to provide more space for the crowded teeth. The force system created by turning a screw is far from ideal, and plates of this type are now obsolete, but they can create small amounts of tooth movement.

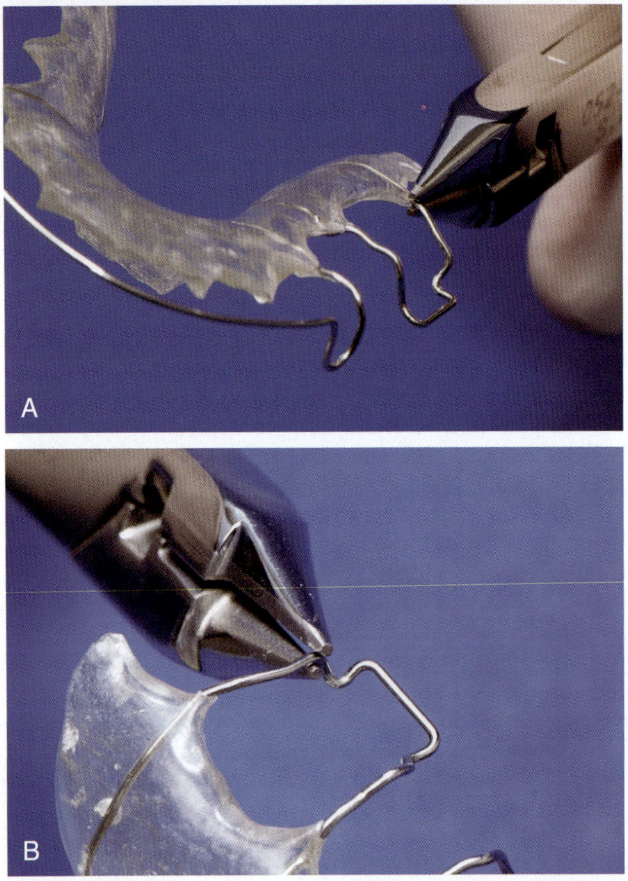

• **Fig. 10.3** Clinical adjustments of an Adams clasp. (A) Tightening the clasp by bending it gingivally at the point where the wire emerges from the baseplate. This is the usual adjustment for a clasp that has become loose after repeated insertions and removals of an appliance. (B) Adjustment of the clasp by bending the retentive points inward. This alternative method of tightening a clasp is particularly useful during the initial fitting of an appliance. This bend can also be made with the plier positioned slightly closer to the appliance body.

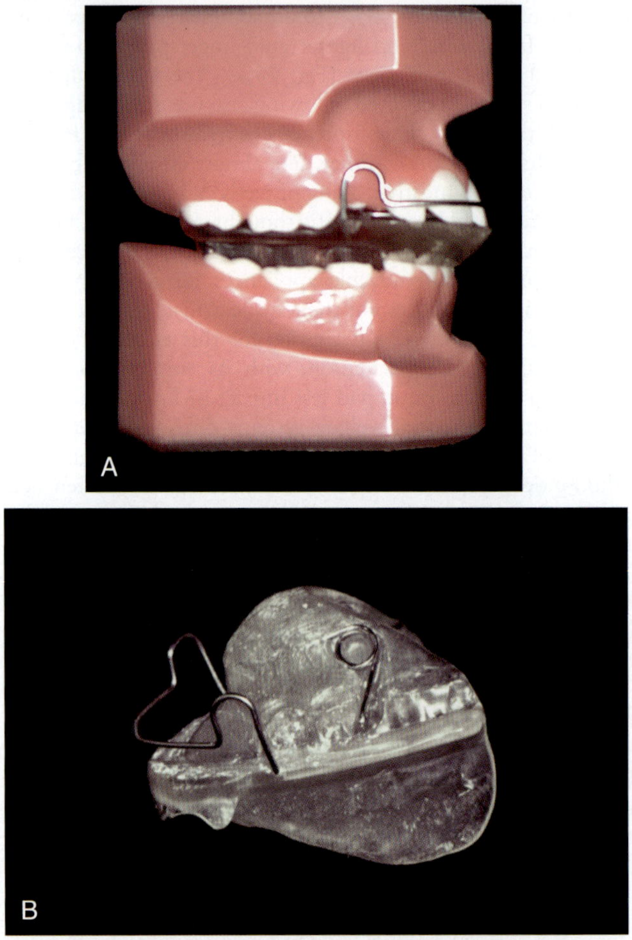

• **Fig. 10.4** (A) The activator, a tooth-borne passive appliance, was the first functional appliance to be widely used. It opens the bite, and the mandible is advanced for Class II correction as the patient is forced to move it forward to avoid contact of the lingual flanges with the lingual soft tissues. (B) The design of the original Andresen activator reflects the concept that stimulating activity of the jaw muscles was the key to altering mandibular growth; the large spring in the palate is to keep the appliance from staying in place except when the patient is biting against it. Whenever the patient relaxes, the appliance drops down and the patient has to bite against it, so the muscles are activated repeatedly while it is being worn. As that concept disappeared, so did the displacement springs (which were often replaced with clasps to help hold the activator in position), but complete coverage of the palate continued.

removable appliance is therefore that this approach should be only used when a few millimeters of tipping movement are acceptable.

Because these appliances are used primarily for minor tooth movement in children, they are discussed in more detail in Chapters 11 and 12.

Functional Appliances for Growth Modification

By definition, a functional appliance is one that changes the posture of the mandible, holding it open or open and forward. Pressures created by stretch of the muscles and soft tissues are transmitted to the dental and skeletal structures, moving teeth and modifying growth. The monobloc developed by Robin in the early 1900s is generally considered the forerunner of all functional appliances, but the activator developed in Norway by Andresen in the 1920s (Fig. 10.4) was the first to be widely accepted.

Andresen's activator became the basis of the "Norwegian system" of treatment. Both the appliance system and its theoretical underpinnings were improved and extended elsewhere in Europe, particularly by the German school led by Haupl, who believed that the only stable tooth movement was produced by natural forces and that alterations in function produced by these appliances would give stable corrections of malocclusion. This philosophic approach was diametrically opposite to that espoused by Angle and his followers in the United States, who emphasized fixed appliances to precisely position the teeth and presumed that if they were in ideal occlusion, that would keep them there. These opposing beliefs contributed to the great differences between European and US orthodontics at the mid-20th century.

Functional appliances were introduced into US orthodontics in the 1960s through the influence of orthodontic faculty members with a background in Europe (of whom Egil Harvold was prominent) and later from personal contact by US orthodontists with their European counterparts. (Fixed appliances spread to Europe at the same time through similar personal contacts.) A major boost to functional appliance treatment in the United States came from the results of animal experiments in the 1970s showing that skeletal changes really could be produced by posturing the mandible to a new position and holding out the possibility

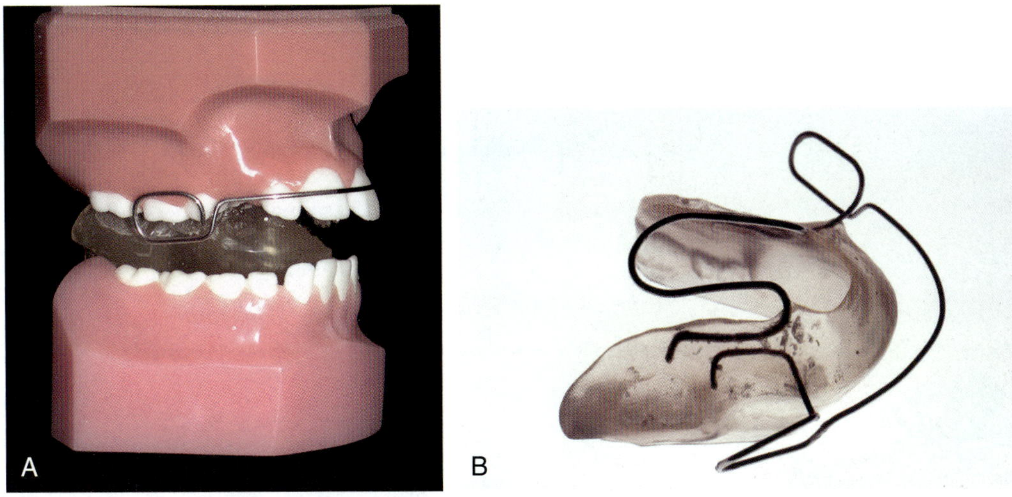

• **Fig. 10.5** (A) The Bionator design, which removes much of the bulk of the activator and is more comfortable for the patient to wear, also uses lingual flanges to force the patient to hold the mandible forward. (B) It can include posterior facets or acrylic occlusal stops to control the amount or direction of tooth eruption and is still used occasionally, although it has largely been displaced by the twin block appliance or other more modern removable functional appliances.

that true stimulation of mandibular growth could be achieved (see Chapter 14).

Some of the enthusiasm for functional appliance treatment resulting from the favorable animal experiments has faded in the light of less impressive results from human clinical trials and retrospective clinical studies, but functional appliances have achieved a major place in contemporary growth modification treatment. In modern use, primarily because the patient has no choice but to wear them full-time, fixed functional appliances are now more widely used than the removable alternatives. These include the Herbst appliance, which became quite popular after Pancherz documented in the 1970s that it could be quite effective,[1] and variants introduced more recently. They are grouped here with the removable functionals because they are quite different from traditional fixed appliances but have much in common with removable appliances. Both fixed and removable functionals are fabricated from identical construction bites. This advances the mandible in patients with Class II malocclusion and rotates it downward in those with Class III malocclusion. In addition, vertical stops or bite blocks are used to control the vertical dimension in both.

Functional appliances are best understood when viewed as falling into one of four broad categories:

- *Passive tooth-borne.* These appliances have no intrinsic force-generating capacity from springs or screws and depend only on soft tissue stretch and muscular activity to produce treatment effects. In current use, the Bionator (Fig. 10.5), twin block (Fig. 10.6), and Herbst appliance (Fig. 10.7A) are examples of passive tooth-borne appliances. The Bionator is always removable, the twin block usually is removable but can be fixed, and the Herbst appliance is usually fixed but can be constructed to be removable.
- *Active tooth-borne.* In removable form, these are largely modifications of activator and Bionator designs that include expansion screws or springs to move teeth. Some current fixed functionals have evolved in this same direction in that, like their removable predecessors, they produce tooth movement that often replaces jaw growth modification with camouflage tooth movement. For that reason, although removables of this type were once the mainstay of European orthodontics, they are now rarely used. It seems likely that fixed functionals with active springs will have the same fate.
- *Tissue-borne.* The Frankel appliance (which Frankel called the *function regulator*) is the only tissue-borne functional appliance (Fig. 10.8). Insofar as possible, contact of the appliance with the teeth is avoided, reflecting the goal of inducing tooth movement from soft tissue pressures rather than pressures directly moving the teeth. Much of the appliance is located in the vestibule, holding the lips and cheeks away from the dentition. This makes it an arch expansion appliance in addition

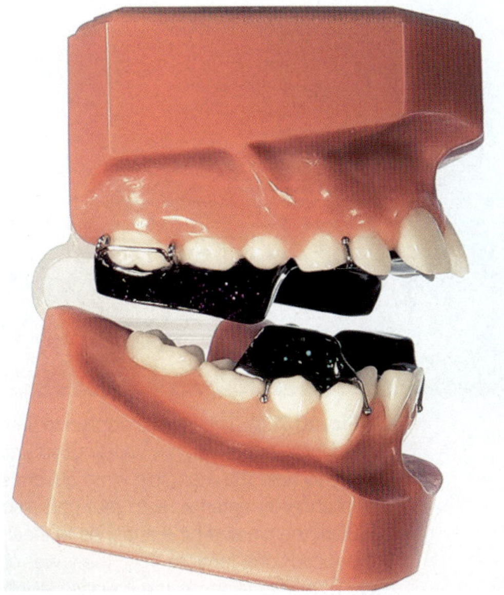

• **Fig. 10.6** The twin-block appliance consists of individual maxillary and mandibular plates with ramps that guide the mandible forward when the patient closes down. The maxillary plate incorporates tubes for attachment of a headgear and often includes an expansion screw to increase posterior arch width. (Courtesy AOA Laboratories, Sturtevant, WI.)

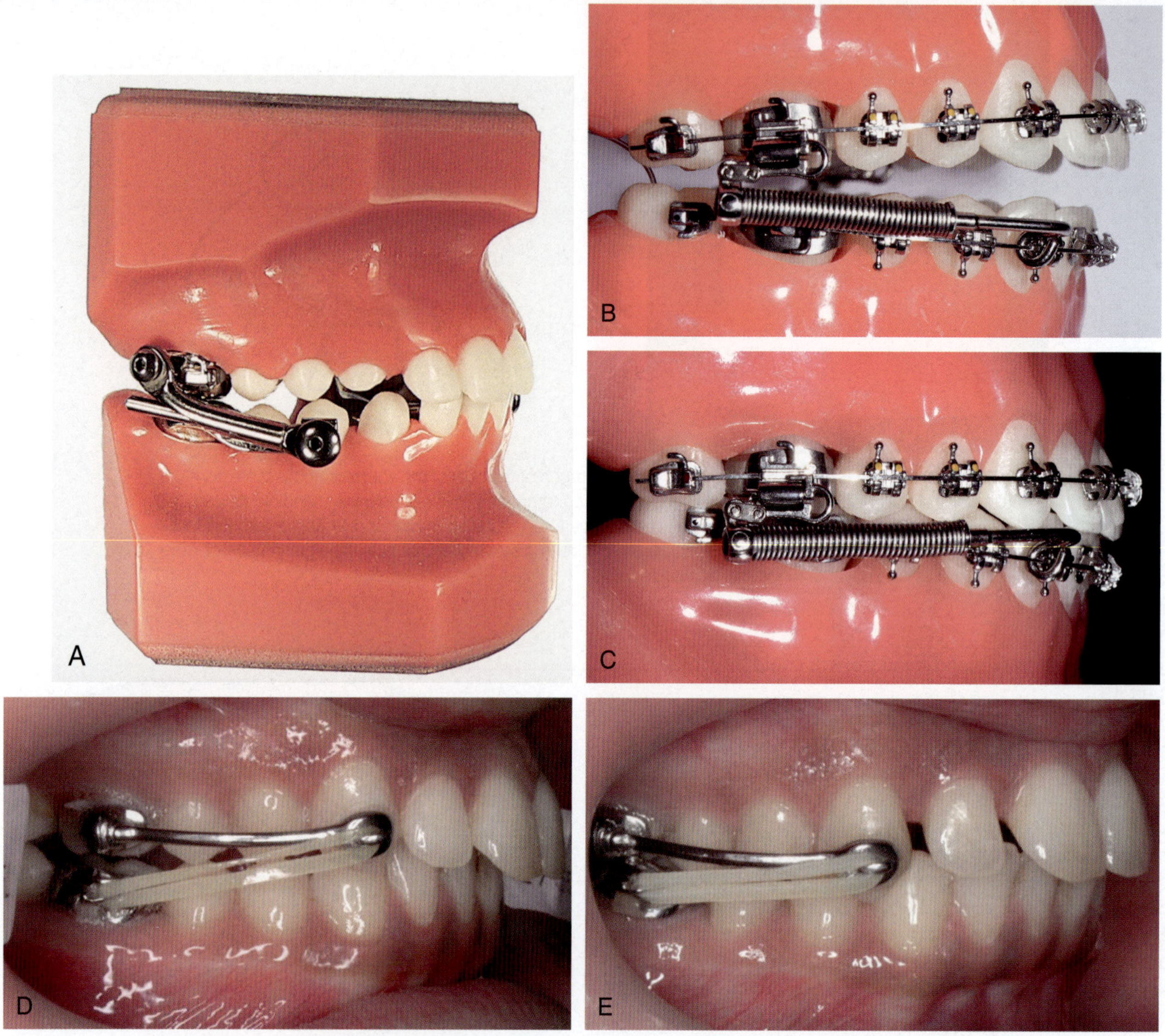

• **Fig. 10.7** (A) The Herbst appliance, introduced by Herbst in the 1920s, was the original fixed functional appliance, but it was not widely used until it was reintroduced in the 1970s. It uses a pin and tube apparatus to hold the mandible in an advanced position and is quite compatible with the presence of a fixed appliance on anterior teeth (but can also be used with bonded or removable splints). Note that for this patient the pin and tube attaches to steel crowns on the molars, which are sturdier than molar bands, and the extensions forward from the lower crowns are bonded to the lower premolars. In current use, there are many variations in the precise design of the appliance. (B and C) The Forsus appliance, offered as a modern alternative to the Herbst appliance, uses springs to maintain the mandible (and mandibular teeth) forward; the reaction is a distal force on the maxilla. In theory, the effect would be similar to that of the Herbst appliance; in fact, studies have shown that it has a greater skeletal effect on maxillary growth than the Herbst and produces more forward movement of the mandibular dentition but less skeletal mandibular advancement. (D) The Carriere motion appliance similarly creates a distal force against the maxilla while pushing the mandible forward so that (E) the molar relationship is corrected. Then the maxillary incisors are retracted. It has the advantage of minimal restriction of lateral excursions of the mandible. In theory, it is also creating forces similar to the Herbst appliance that would create similar effects; in that case, no data beyond selected case reports are available to show what it really does skeletally and dentally. The same can be said of a number of other currently advertised appliances to correct Class II malocclusion. (D and E, Courtesy Henry Schein Co., Carlsbad, CA.)

to its effects on jaw growth because the arches tend to expand when lip and cheek pressure is removed making tongue pressure dominant.

- *Hybrid.* Hybrid functionals are composed of components that are common to functional appliances but are combined to meet a specific need, and are used primarily in the treatment of jaw asymmetry (Fig. 10.9).

The components of functional appliances are shown in Table 10.1. They can be combined as needed for individual patients. Functional appliances are used primarily in late preadolescent

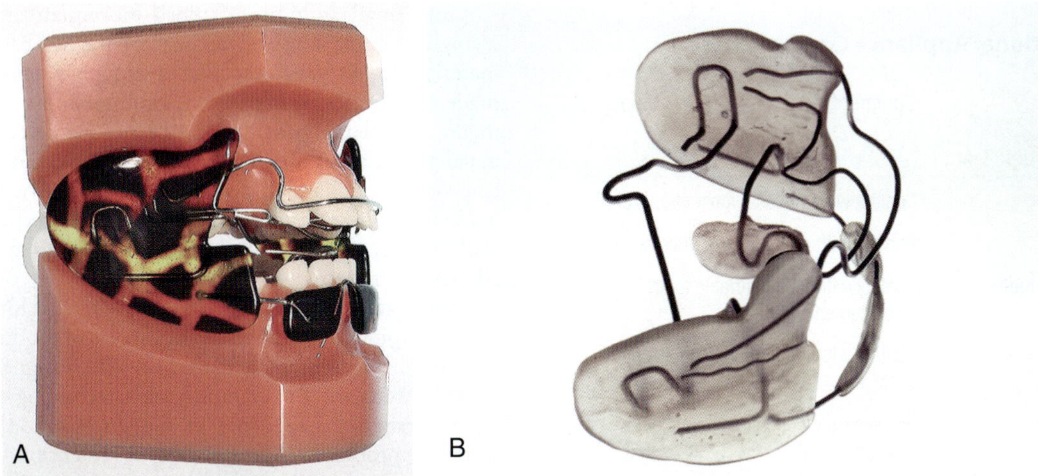

• **Fig. 10.8** (A) The Frankel appliance on dental casts and (B) as it would look before being placed in the mouth. It is the only functional appliance that is primarily tissue-borne rather than tooth-borne, and is the expression of the German theory that the only stable tooth movement was produced by changing the soft tissue environment of the jaws. It was offered in Class II, Class III, and open bite versions, but its primary use was Class II treatment with the Frankel-II design shown here. Its active components are the large buccal shields and lip pads that reduce cheek and lip pressure on the dentition and provide the expansion of the maxillary arch that is usually needed as part of Class II correction; the small lower lingual pad behind the lower incisors that holds the mandible forward, and the facial pad in front of the lower incisors that holds the lower lip forward. The appliance looks bulky, but for the most part, it is restricted to the buccal vestibule, and therefore it interferes less with speech and is more compatible with 24-h wear than other removable functional designs. (Courtesy AOA Laboratories, Sturtevant, WI.)

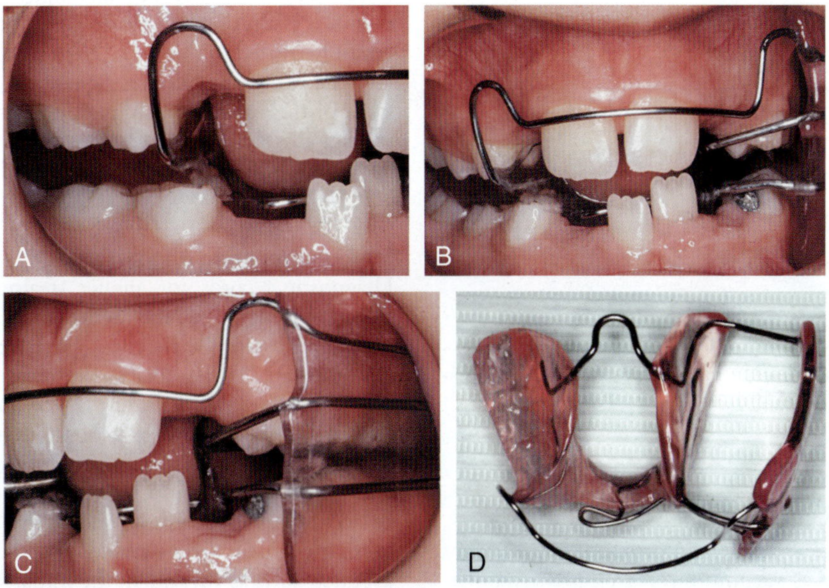

• **Fig. 10.9** A hybrid functional appliance consists of the components of one type of functional on one side and components of another type on the other. For a child with a facial asymmetry, an appliance of the type shown here can be effective in improving both the vertical and anteroposterior aspects of the problem. Note that in (A) a bite block impedes eruption of teeth on the left side, while (B and C) the teeth are free to erupt on the left side, where (D) a lingual, as well as a buccal, side is required to keep the patient's tongue out of the space where eruption is required. The bite is taken to bring the jaw to the midline, advancing the deficient side (here, the left) more than the other. (From Proffit WR, White RP, Sarver DM. *Contemporary Treatment of Dentofacial Deformity*. Mosby; 2003.)

TABLE 10.1 Functional Appliance Components

Component	Comment
Functional Components	
Lingual flanges	Contact with mucosa; most effective
Lingual pad	Contact with mucosa; less effective
Sliding pin and tube	Contact with teeth; variable tooth displacement
Tooth-supported ramps	Contact with teeth; tooth displacement likely
Lip pads	Secondary effect only on mandibular position
Tooth-controlling Components	
Arch Expansion	
Buccal shields	Passive, effective
Buccinator bow, other wire shield	Passive, less effective
Expansion screws and/or springs	Must activate slowly; questionable stability
Vertical Control	
Occlusal or incisal stops	Prevent eruption in discrete area
Bite blocks	Prevent eruption of all posterior teeth
Lingual shield	Facilitate eruption
Stabilizing Components	
Clasps	No effect on growth modification
Labial bow	Keep away from incisors, lingual tipping undesirable
Anterior torquing springs	Needed to control lingual tipping, especially with headgear-activator combination

children and during the adolescent growth spurt. They are discussed in more detail in Chapter 14.

Clear Aligner Therapy

Development of Clear Aligners

The use of a sequence of clear aligners in orthodontic treatment for adults became possible as vacuum-formed clear thermoplastic sheets were introduced into orthodontics in the 1980s. These "suck-down" materials were used initially as retainers and still are important for this purpose (see Chapter 19). It became apparent rather quickly, however, that if teeth were reset slightly and the vacuum-formed sheet was made to fit the reset teeth, a tooth moving device rather than a retainer would be the result.[2] The device could now be, and quickly was, called a "clear aligner" because the typical use was to bring mildly displaced teeth back into alignment, as, for instance, when mild irregularity of maxillary or mandibular incisors occurred in an orthodontic patient after retainers were discontinued.

Only small amounts of tooth movement are possible with a single aligner, however, because of the stiffness of the plastic material. It became clear that a sequence of several aligners, made on a series of casts with some teeth reset in small increments (less than 1 mm), would be needed to correct even mild malalignment. Although a sequence of modified dental casts can be produced by hand and a short sequence of two to five aligners made from these casts works for minor tooth movement, this is prohibitively time-consuming and difficult if more than a few aligners are required.

In the late 1990s, a new company, Align Technology, obtained venture capital to computerize the process of producing a sequence of casts with incremental changes on which aligners could be fabricated. With careful planning, this technology supported the digital design of a sequence of aligners that could correct more complex problems. Because aligner retention improves with greater exposed tooth surface and growth changes are difficult to predict, the method was targeted primarily for treatment of adults or late adolescents. Thankfully, these are the patients most interested in an invisible or minimally visible orthodontic appliance.

The early days of Invisalign treatment were fraught with problems because the unique biomechanics of aligner treatment, including staging of treatment, optimal rates of tooth movement in each plane of space, and indications for use of attachments on the teeth were all being developed. Due the significant early limitations, initial professional acceptance of the method was spotty. The technique has matured, however, as clinical evaluation has clarified the best sequence of steps in treatment and the amount of tooth movement in each stage that should be attempted, and as the use of tooth-colored attachments bonded to the teeth has improved retention and predictability of more challenging movements. It is clear now that even complex malocclusions can be successfully treated in this way.[3] Now that patents are expiring, other companies are also offering sequenced aligners based on modifications of the current techniques, and orthodontists are beginning to digitally design aligners and utilize three-dimensional (3D) printing in their own labs to produce clear aligners.[4]

Aligner Production Process

Steps in Preparing Aligners

Diagnostic records for aligner treatment are the same photographs, radiographs, and dental casts as for any other type of orthodontic treatment. For aligners, either an intraoral optical scan (see Fig. 10.10, which also records the initial occlusion) is obtained or polyvinylsiloxane (PVS) impressions and a bite registration are made and digitized. The resulting digital model needs to have any obvious artifacts removed and then be segmented so each tooth can be moved independently (see Fig. 10.11) Once an accurate, segmented 3D model in occlusion has been created, tooth movement can be added. When using a commercial aligner product, such as Invisalign, the initial staging of the tooth movement is created by a digital technician using the doctor's prescription and applying any saved doctor preferences. When using an in-house software, this movement can be staged by an assistant or the doctor themselves using the software tools provided. With either method, final doctor approval of the planned movements is needed to verify that the desired movements are staged within biological limits. This need for the treating doctor to assess the biologic reality of the treatment plan is the reason that full diagnostic records are needed, even though the required submission materials for any particular aligner system may not include radiographs or clinical photographs.

After approval of the virtual treatment plan, digital models of each stage are exported and 3D printed. This process is shown for in-house fabrication with an on-site printer in Fig. 10.12. The 3D printer cures the resin layer by layer to produce a 3D model for each stage in the aligner process. Those models are then rinsed in isopropyl alcohol and cured in a light box as a postprocessing operation to ensure all excess uncured resin is removed. Once printed and post-processed, these models can be used to fabricate aligners using a thermoformed plastic, as shown in Fig. 10.13. This manufacturing process can be done more efficiently for complex cases requiring more aligners at commercial production facilities with larger printers and more automated processes, so most orthodontists still have comprehensive cases produced in this way.

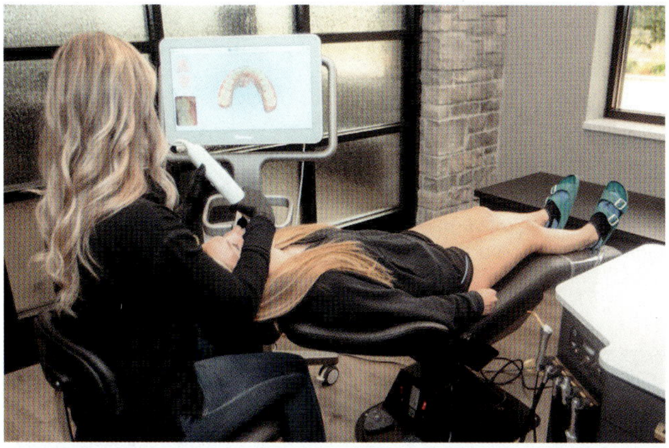

• **Fig. 10.10** A photo of an intraoral scan being done on a patient to obtain a direct 3D digital representation of the teeth. On the scanner screen, the digital dental model is built in real time as the doctor or assistant proceeds with the scan, and any missing areas can be filled in before the digital models are saved. Once both the upper and lower arches are captured, the teeth are scanned on the sides while the patient is biting together to capture the interocclusal record.

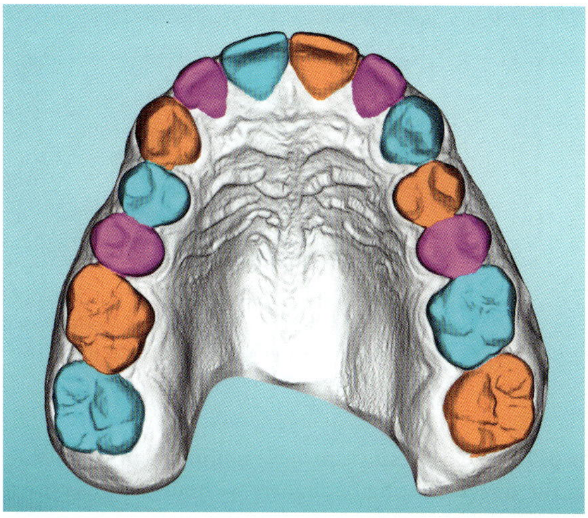

• **Fig. 10.11** Once the digital model is provided by the scanner, it must be segmented into individual teeth in order to proceed with any tooth movement simulation. This screen capture shows a maxillary arch with the teeth now segmented from the gingival tissue and from each other so that they are ready to be digitally moved to represent the desired tooth movement (uLab systems). Most systems now provide for this segmentation process to be largely automated, but some manual touch-up may be required to provide the most accurate simulation.

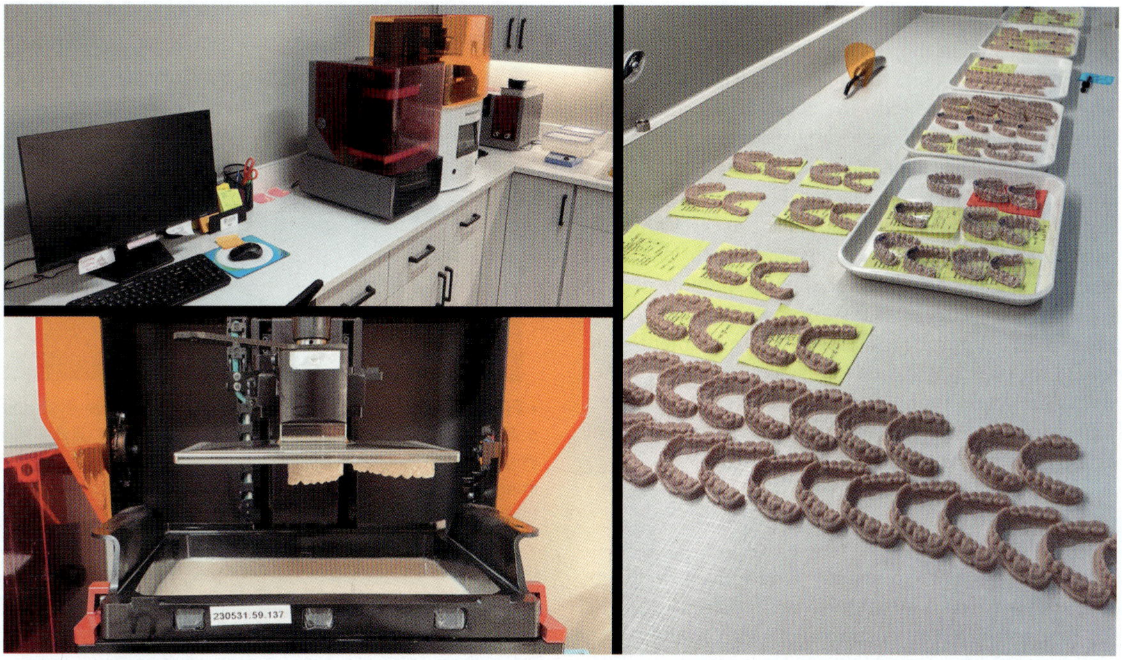

• **Fig. 10.12** An example of a setup for in-office production of aligners. The top left image shows the computer for treatment design, two different 3D printers for model fabrication, and in the corner the postprocessing wash units to remove uncured resin. The bottom left image is a close-up of just completed models hanging below the print platform of the 3D printer before moving to the postprocessing stage. The right image show completed models ready for making aligners or retainers by thermoforming. Note that in a busy office, there are many models that must be properly identified and organized for efficient management of these processes.

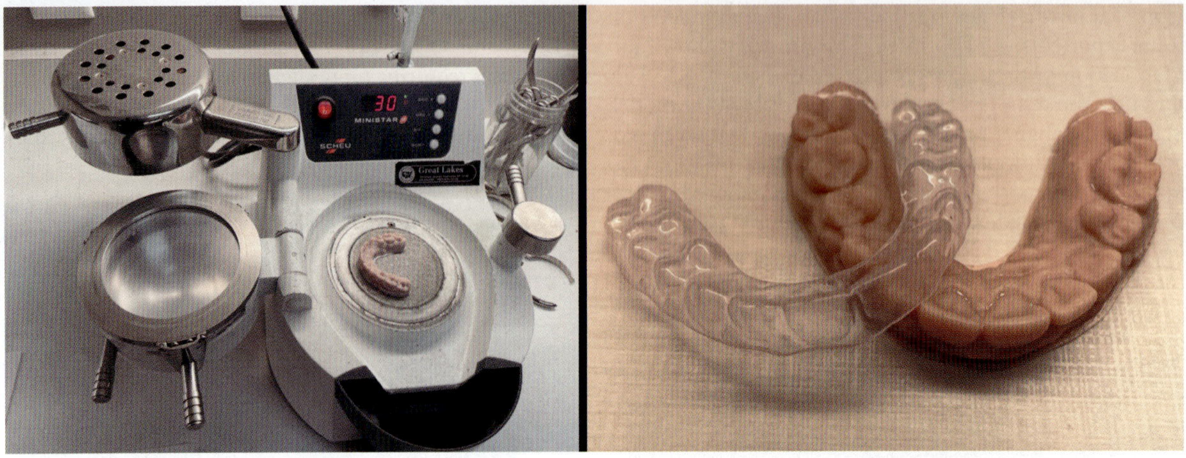

• **Fig. 10.13** The final step in creating aligners or retainers from 3D-printed models is thermoforming. The left side image shows a typical thermoforming machine produced for in office use (Ministar, Great Lakes Dental Technologies, Tonowanda, NY). The right side shows a completed aligner and the printed model on which it was made.

Some 3D printing resins are now commercially available that allows the direct printing of aligners without the need for model fabrication and thermoforming, but the material properties and clinical efficiencies are still being investigated.

Clinician's Role in Digital Setups, Staging, and Sequencing

There are several important aspects for a clinician to verify when modifying and approving a digital plan. First, the final planned position of the teeth needs to be set. Software controls in representative software systems are shown in Fig. 10.14. This creates a final aligner in that shape, but it is critical to remember that shape alone may not produce a sufficient force system to arrive at that final position. Therefore, overcorrection of certain movements is recommended, which is discussed in more depth in Chapters 18 and 21. Once the final positioning is set, the staging and sequencing of movements should also be reviewed. The actual tooth movement that occurs depends on how well each progressive step along the way provides the required force for movement—the teeth do not care how perfect the final digital plan was setup! A great deal of this staging is set by computer algorithms to move teeth at certain velocities through the stages, but changes are often made by the clinician. This also includes planning any interproximal reduction needed during treatment. Finally, attachments—tooth-colored composite material bonded to the surface of teeth to help movement—are frequently needed for predictable tooth movement. Again, further discussion of clinical applications during clear aligner treatment is described in Chapters 18 and 21, but examples of two different treatment-planning programs are shown in Fig. 10.15.

Fixed Appliances

Contemporary fixed appliances are mostly variations of the edgewise appliance system, using rectangular archwires for precise positioning of the teeth after initial treatment with round wires. The Begg appliance, which used only round wires and auxiliary springs, morphed into the Tip-Edge appliance in the early 21st century so that rectangular wires could easily be used in finishing. Although Tip-Edge treatment stages are shown in Chapters 16 and 17, the focus in this and the succeeding chapters is almost entirely on the contemporary edgewise appliance, which continues to evolve as digitally assisted design and manufacturing develops.

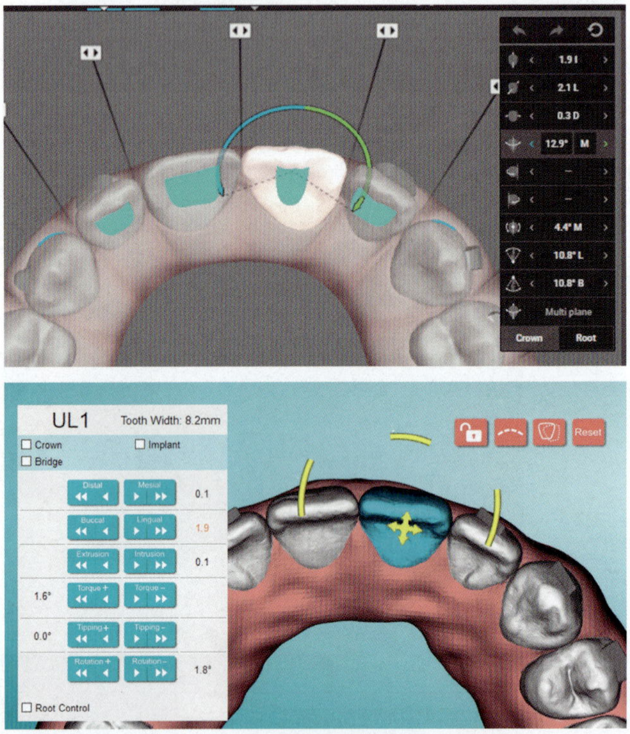

• **Fig. 10.14** Screenshots from two representative systems showing the software controls available to doctors for doing digital setups. The top image is the ClinCheck Pro software provided by Invisalign and the bottom image is uDesign provided by uLab Systems. Both images show movement being made to the upper left central incisor. Each provides a virtual handle to drag and drop the tooth to its desired position, an objective readout of the movement completed in all three translational and all three rotational dimensions and tools to create and monitor any interproximal reduction being planned.

The Development of Contemporary Fixed Appliances

Angle's Progression to the Edgewise Appliance

Edward Angle's position as the "father of modern orthodontics" is based not only on his contributions to classification and diagnosis

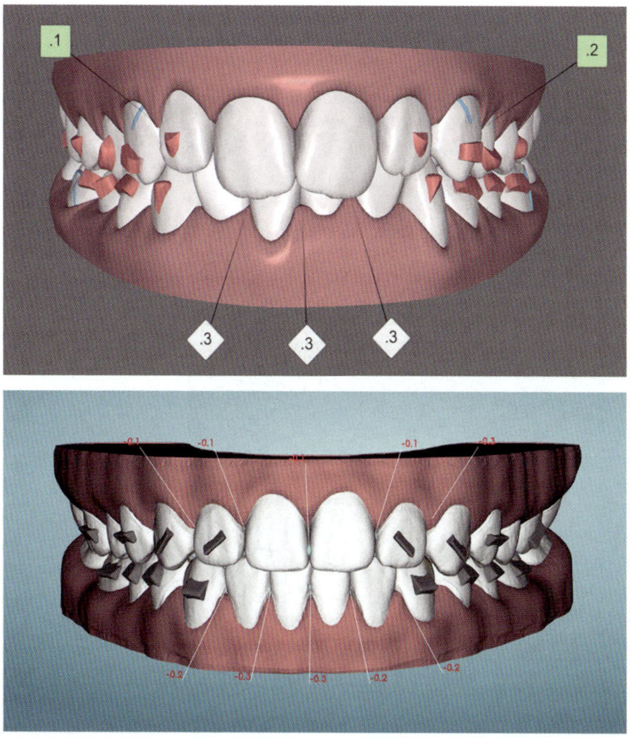

• **Fig. 10.15** The same two virtual planning software systems shown in Fig. 10.14, but this time showing a frontal view of both arches. The top image is a ClinCheck image of the start of treatment showing the amount of interproximal reduction, a visual representation of the attachments planned and planned cuts for elastic hooks. The bottom image is the uDesign software showing the expected finish of treatment with the planned IPR and the planned attachments. Most aligner systems provide similar visualization and tools.

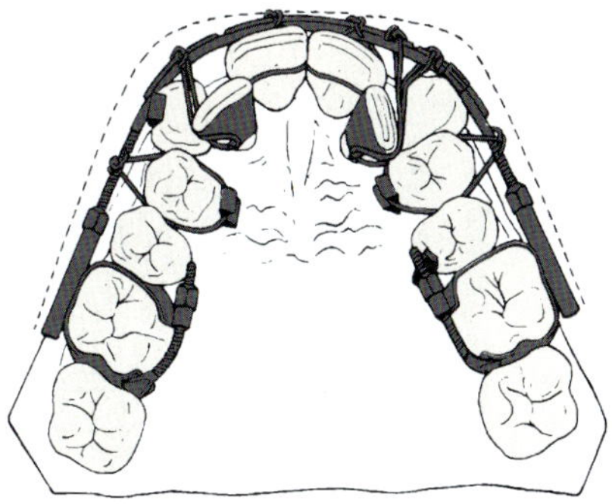

• **Fig. 10.16** Edward Angle's E-arch from the early 1900s. Ligatures from a heavy labial arch were used to bring malposed teeth to the line of occlusion.

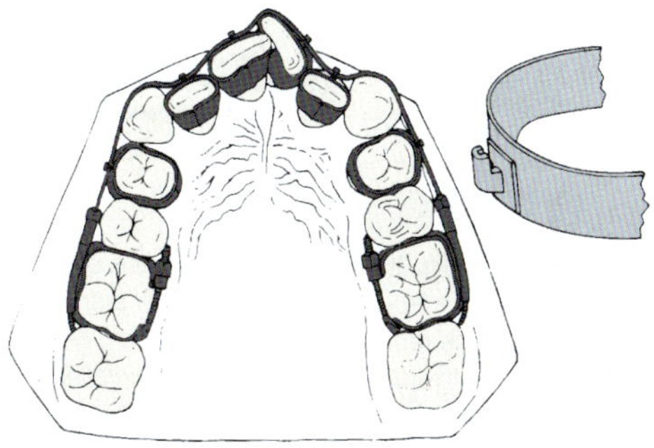

• **Fig. 10.17** Angle's ribbon arch appliance, introduced about 1910, was well adapted to bring teeth into alignment but was too flexible to allow precise positioning of roots.

but also on his creativity in developing new orthodontic appliances. With few exceptions, the fixed appliances used in contemporary orthodontics are based on Angle's designs from the early 20th century. Angle developed four major appliance systems:

- *E-arch.* In the late 1800s, a typical orthodontic appliance depended on some sort of rigid framework to which the teeth were tied so that they could be expanded to the arch form dictated by the appliance. Angle's first appliance, the E-arch, was an improvement on this basic design (Fig. 10.16). Bands were placed on molar teeth, and a heavy labial archwire extended around the arch. The end of the wire was threaded, and a small nut placed on the threaded portion of the arch allowed the archwire to be advanced so that the arch perimeter increased. Individual teeth were simply ligated to this expansion arch. This appliance could still be found in the catalogs of some mail-order orthodontic laboratories as late as the 1980s, perhaps because of its simplicity, and despite the fact that it can deliver only heavy interrupted force.
- *Pin and tube.* The E-arch was capable only of tipping teeth to a new position. It was not able to precisely position any individual tooth. To overcome this difficulty, Angle began placing bands on other teeth and used a vertical tube on each tooth into which a soldered pin from a smaller archwire was placed. With this appliance, tooth movement was accomplished by repositioning the individual pins at each appointment. An incredible degree of craftsmanship was involved in constructing and adjusting this pin and tube appliance, and although it was theoretically capable of great precision in tooth movement, it proved impractical in clinical use. It is said that only Angle himself and one of his students ever mastered the appliance. The relatively heavy base arch meant that spring qualities were poor, and the problem therefore was compounded because many small adjustments were needed.
- *Ribbon arch.* Angle's next appliance modified the tube on each tooth to provide a vertically positioned rectangular slot behind the tube. A ribbon archwire of 10 × 20 gold wire was placed into the vertical slot and held with pins (Fig. 10.17). The ribbon arch was an immediate success, primarily because the archwire, unlike any of its predecessors, was small enough to have good spring qualities and therefore was quite efficient in aligning malpositioned teeth. Although the ribbon arch could be twisted as it was inserted into its slot, the major weakness of the appliance was that it provided relatively poor control of root position. The resiliency of the ribbon archwire simply did not allow generation of the moments necessary to torque roots to a new position.
- *Edgewise.* To overcome the deficiencies of the ribbon arch, Angle reoriented the slot from vertical to horizontal and inserted a rectangular wire rotated 90 degrees to the orientation it had with the ribbon arch, thus the name "edgewise" (Fig. 10.18). The dimensions of the slot were altered to 22 × 28 mil, and a 22 × 28 precious metal wire was used. These dimensions, arrived at after extensive experimentation, did allow excellent control of crown and root position in all three planes of space. After its introduction in 1928, this appliance became the mainstay of multibanded fixed appliance therapy, although the ribbon arch continued in common use for another decade.

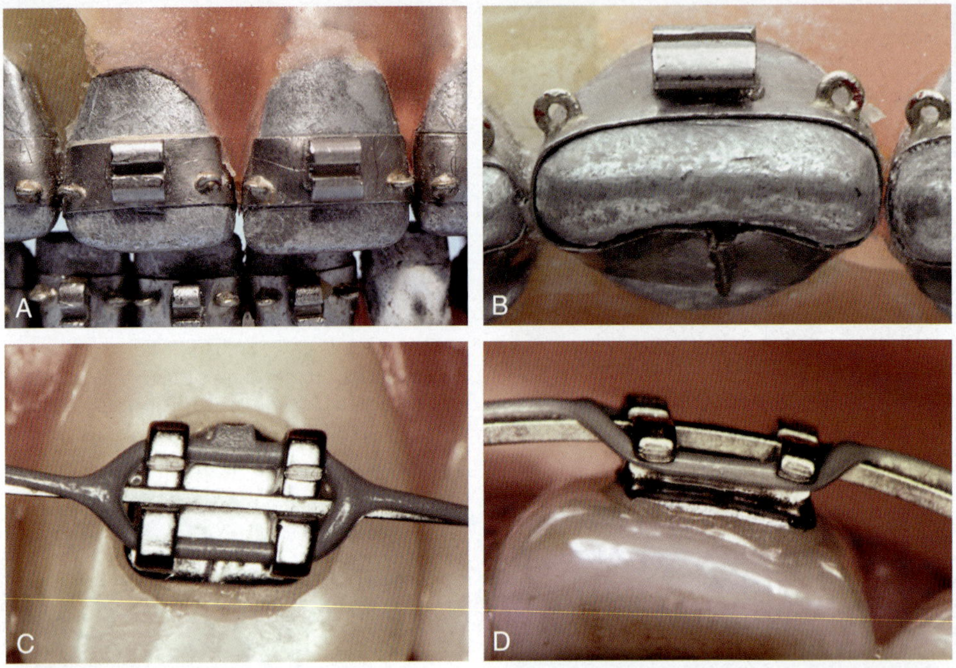

• **Fig. 10.18** (A and B) Angle's edgewise appliance received its name because the archwire was inserted at a 90-degree angle to the plane of insertion of the ribbon arch, which made it wider than it was tall. The rectangular wire could be twisted to create torque (see Fig. 10.29). It was tied into a rectangular slot with wire ligatures, making excellent control of root position possible. The original appliance is seen here on a typodont. Note the narrow brackets (double width on the maxillary centrals, which are wider teeth), which were soldered to gold bands. Also note the eyelets soldered on the corners of the bands. These were used for ligature ties to the archwire as needed for rotational control. (C and D) Close-up views of a modern edgewise twin bracket with a rectangular archwire in place. The wire is held in the bracket by an elastomeric ligature, here part of a chain of ligatures that also keep spaces closed between the teeth.

Other Early Fixed Appliance Systems

Labiolingual, Twin Wire

Before Angle, placing attachments on individual teeth simply had not been done, and Angle's concern about precisely positioning each tooth was not widely shared during his lifetime. In addition to a variety of removable appliances using fingersprings for repositioning teeth, there were two major competing appliance systems in the first half of the 20th century. The labiolingual appliance used bands on first molars and a combination of heavy lingual and labial archwires to which fingersprings were soldered to move individual teeth. The twin-wire appliance used bands on incisors as well as molars and featured twin 10-mil steel archwires for alignment of the incisor teeth. These delicate wires were protected by long tubes that extended forward from the molars to the vicinity of the canines. Neither of these appliances, however, was capable of more than tipping movements except with special and unusual modifications. They have disappeared from contemporary use.

Begg Appliance

Given Angle's insistence on expansion of the arches rather than extraction to deal with crowding problems, it is ironic that his appliances finally provided the control of root position necessary for successful extraction treatment. The edgewise appliance was being used for this purpose within a few years of its introduction. Charles Tweed, one of Angle's last students, was the leader in the United States in adapting the edgewise appliance for extraction treatment. In fact, little adaptation of the appliance was needed. Tweed moved the teeth bodily and used the subdivision approach for anchorage control, first sliding the canines distally along the archwire, then retracting the incisors (see Fig. 9.33).

Raymond Begg had been taught use of the ribbon arch appliance at the Angle school before his return to Australia in the 1920s. Working independently in Adelaide, Begg also concluded that extraction of teeth was often necessary, and set out to adapt the ribbon arch appliance so that it could be used for better control of root position.

Begg's adaptation took three forms: (1) He replaced the precious metal ribbon arch with high-strength 16-mil round stainless steel wire when this became available from an Australian company in the late 1930s; (2) he retained the original ribbon arch bracket, but turned it upside down so that the bracket slot pointed gingivally rather than occlusally; and (3) he added auxiliary springs to the appliance for control of root position. In the resulting Begg appliance (Fig. 10.19),[5] friction was minimized because the area of contact between the narrow ribbon arch bracket and the archwire was very small and the force of the wire against the bracket was also small. Binding was minimized because Begg's strategy for anchorage control was tipping and uprighting (see Fig. 8.22), and tipping minimizes the angle of contact between the wire and corner of the bracket.

Although the progress records with his approach looked vastly different, it is not surprising that Begg's overall result in anchorage control was similar to Tweed's, because both used two steps to compensate for resistance to sliding. The Begg appliance is now rarely seen in contemporary use, although as we noted earlier, it still appears now in the hybrid Tip-Edge appliance, with brackets that allow the use of rectangular wires in finishing (Fig. 10.20).[6] Unlike labiolingual, twin-wire, and other partially banded fixed

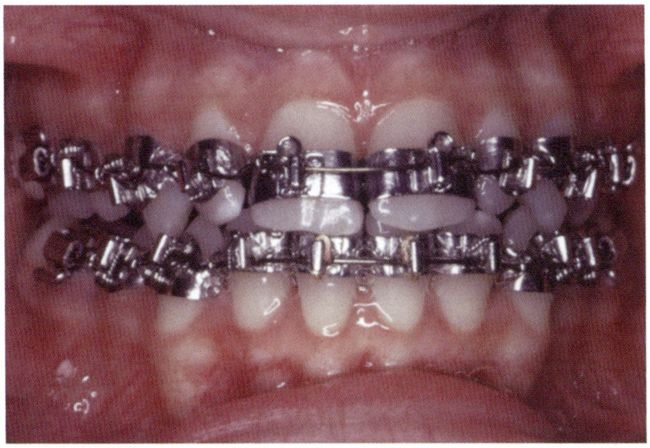

• **Fig. 10.19** The Begg appliance uses a modification of the ribbon arch attachment, into which round archwires are pinned. A variety of auxiliary archwires are used in this system to obtain control of root position. For this patient late in treatment, the mandibular archwire is held in place in the central incisors with brass pins, and auxiliary springs (placed in the vertical slot and also serving as pins to retain the archwire) are being used to position the roots of several teeth (they are seen clearly in the maxillary central incisors, activated to move the roots distally).

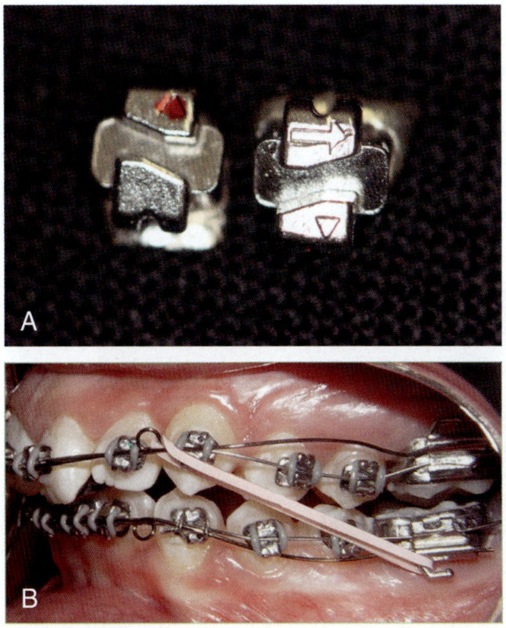

• **Fig. 10.20** The Begg appliance now is rarely used in the form in which Dr. Begg developed it, but his ideas survive in the Tip-Edge bracket (A), which has a rectangular slot cut away on one side to allow crown tipping in that direction with no incisal deflection of the archwire. This allows a tooth to be tipped during space closure and uprighted afterward with auxiliary springs, but a rectangular wire can be used for torque in finishing. (B) Tip-Edge brackets in the initial stage of treatment, with small-diameter steel archwires. (Courtesy Dr. D. Grauer.)

appliances, the Begg appliance was a complete treatment system in the sense that it allowed good control of crown and root position in all three planes of space.

Contemporary Edgewise

The Begg appliance became widely popular in the 1960s because it was more efficient than the edgewise appliance of that era, in the sense that equivalent results could be produced with less investment of the clinician's time. Developments have since then reversed the balance. The contemporary edgewise appliance has evolved far beyond the original design while retaining the basic principle of a rectangular wire in a rectangular slot, and now is more efficient than the Begg appliance, which is the reason for its almost universal use now.

Major steps in the evolution of the edgewise appliance include:

- *Automatic rotational control.* In the original appliance, Angle soldered eyelets to the corners of the bands, so a separate ligature tie could be used as needed to correct or control rotations as a tooth was moved (see Fig. 10.18). Now rotation control is achieved without the necessity for an additional ligature, by using either twin brackets or single brackets with extension wings that contact the underside of the archwire (Lewis or Lang brackets). Both types of brackets to make it easier to obtain the necessary moment in the rotational plane of space.
- *Alteration in bracket slot dimensions.* The significance of reducing Angle's original slot size from 22 to 18 mil and the implications of using the larger slot with undersize steel wires have been discussed in Chapter 9. There are now two modern edgewise appliances, because the 18- and 22-slot appliances are used rather differently. The introduction of a 20-slot appliance with greater precision than the existing ones has been discussed for many years but only recently has been implemented by some of the digitally assisted systems discussed later in this chapter. Chapters 15 to 17 discuss the differences in using the 18- and 22-slot appliances in detail.
- *Straight-wire bracket prescriptions.* Angle used the same bracket on all teeth, as did the other appliance systems. In the 1980s, bonding made it much easier to have different brackets for each tooth, and Andrews developed bracket modifications for specific teeth to eliminate the many repetitive bends in archwires that were necessary to compensate for differences in tooth anatomy. The result was the "straight-wire" appliance.[7] This was the key step in improving the efficiency of the edgewise appliance.

In the original edgewise appliance, faciolingual bends in the archwires (*first-order*, or *in-out, bends*) were necessary to compensate for variations in the contour of labial surfaces of individual teeth. In the contemporary appliance, this compensation is built into the base of the bracket itself, by varying the thickness of the base depending on which tooth it will be attached to. This reduces the need for compensating bends but does not eliminate them because of individual variations in tooth thickness.

Angulation of brackets relative to the long axis of the tooth is necessary to achieve proper positioning of the roots of most teeth. Originally, this mesiodistal root positioning required angled bends in the archwire, called *second-order*, or *tip*, bends. Angulating the bracket or bracket slot decreases or removes the necessity for these bends.

Because the facial surface of individual teeth varies markedly in inclination to the true vertical, in the original edgewise appliance it was necessary to place a varying twist (referred to as *third-order*, or *torque*, bends) in segments of each rectangular archwire, to make the wire fit passively. Torque bends were required for every patient in every rectangular archwire, not just when roots needed to be moved facially or lingually, to avoid inadvertent movements of properly positioned teeth. The bracket slots in the contemporary edgewise appliance are inclined to compensate for the inclination of the facial surface, so that third-order bends are less necessary.

The angulation and torque values built into the bracket are often referred to as the *appliance prescription*. Obviously, any prescription based on a group average would precisely position only the average tooth and would not be correct for outliers in a normal population.

The edgewise appliance continues to evolve. Current commercially available edgewise appliances are reviewed in some detail at the end of this chapter, along with the possibilities of custom prescriptions for each tooth using digital techniques for individualized appliance fabrication. Before getting to this, let us examine banding versus bonding as the means for positioning the appliance on the teeth.

Bands for Attachments

Indications for Banding

Until the 1980s, the only practical way to place a fixed attachment was to put it on a band that could be cemented to a tooth. The pioneer orthodontists of the early 1900s used clamp bands, which were tightened around molar teeth by screw attachments. Only with the advent of custom-fitted gold bands that were fabricated with special pliers was it practical to place fixed attachments on more than a few teeth. Preformed steel bands came into widespread use during the 1960s but are used now primarily for molar teeth.

There are many advantages to bonding brackets, so it is no longer appropriate to routinely place bands on all teeth. However, indications still exist for use of a band rather than a bonded attachment, including:

- *Heavy intermittent forces against the attachments.* This is the primary indication for banding. An excellent example is an upper first molar against which extraoral force will be placed via a headgear. The twisting and shearing forces often encountered when the facebow is placed or removed are better resisted by a steel band than by a bonded attachment.
- *Teeth that will need both labial and lingual attachments,* such as a molar with both headgear and lingual arch tubes. Isolated bonded lingual attachments that are not tied to some other part of the appliance can be swallowed or aspirated if something comes loose.
- *Teeth with short clinical crowns,* so that bonded brackets are difficult to place correctly. If attached to a band, a tube or bracket can slightly displace the gingiva as it is carried into proper position. It is much more difficult to do this with bonded attachments. The decision to band rather than bond second premolars in adolescents is often based on the length of the clinical crown.

Although there are exceptions, the rule in contemporary orthodontics is that bonded attachments are almost always preferred for anterior teeth and premolars. Bands are usually preferred for first molars, especially if both buccal and lingual attachments are needed. Second molars are bonded if exposure of the crown allows it, and banded if not.

Steps in Banding

Separation

Tight interproximal contacts make it impossible to properly fit a band, which means that some device to separate the teeth must usually be used before banding. Although there are many types of separators, the principle is the same for all of them: A device to force or wedge the teeth apart is left in place long enough for initial tooth movement to occur, so that the teeth are slightly separated when bands are to be fitted.

Two main methods of separation are used for posterior teeth: (1) separating springs (Fig. 10.21), which exert a scissors action above and below the contact, typically opening enough space for banding in approximately 1 week; and (2) elastomeric separators

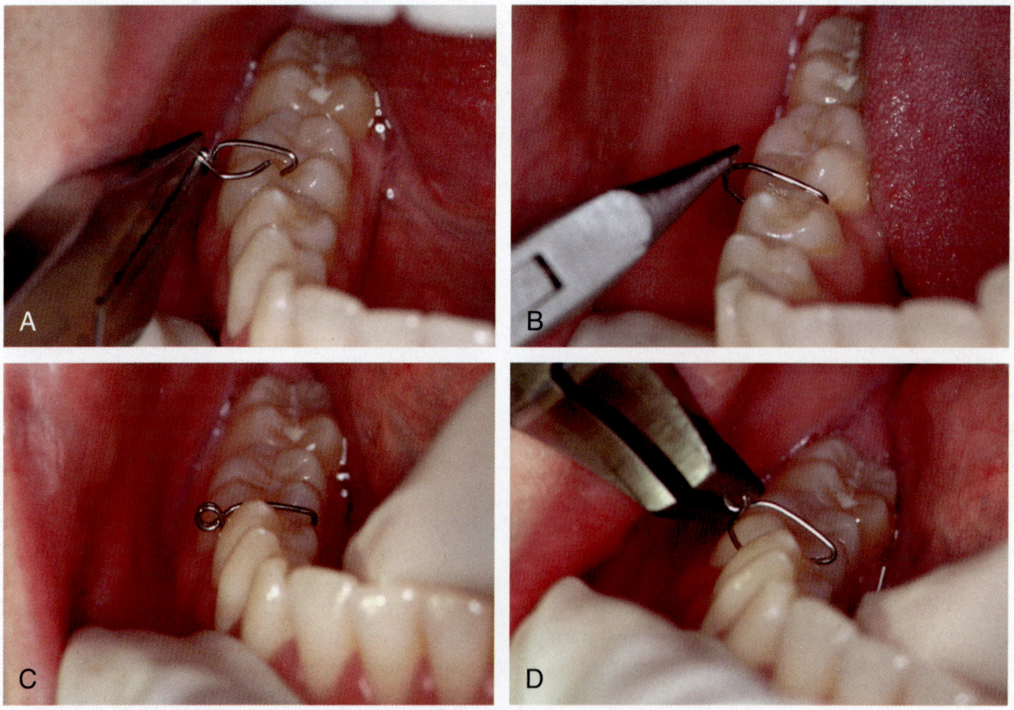

• **Fig. 10.21** Separation with steel separating springs. (A) The spring is grasped at the base. (B) The bent-over end of the longer leg is placed in the lingual embrasure, and the spring is pulled open so the shorter leg can slip beneath the contact. (C) The spring in place, with the helix to the buccal. (D) The spring can be removed most easily by squeezing the helix, forcing the legs apart.

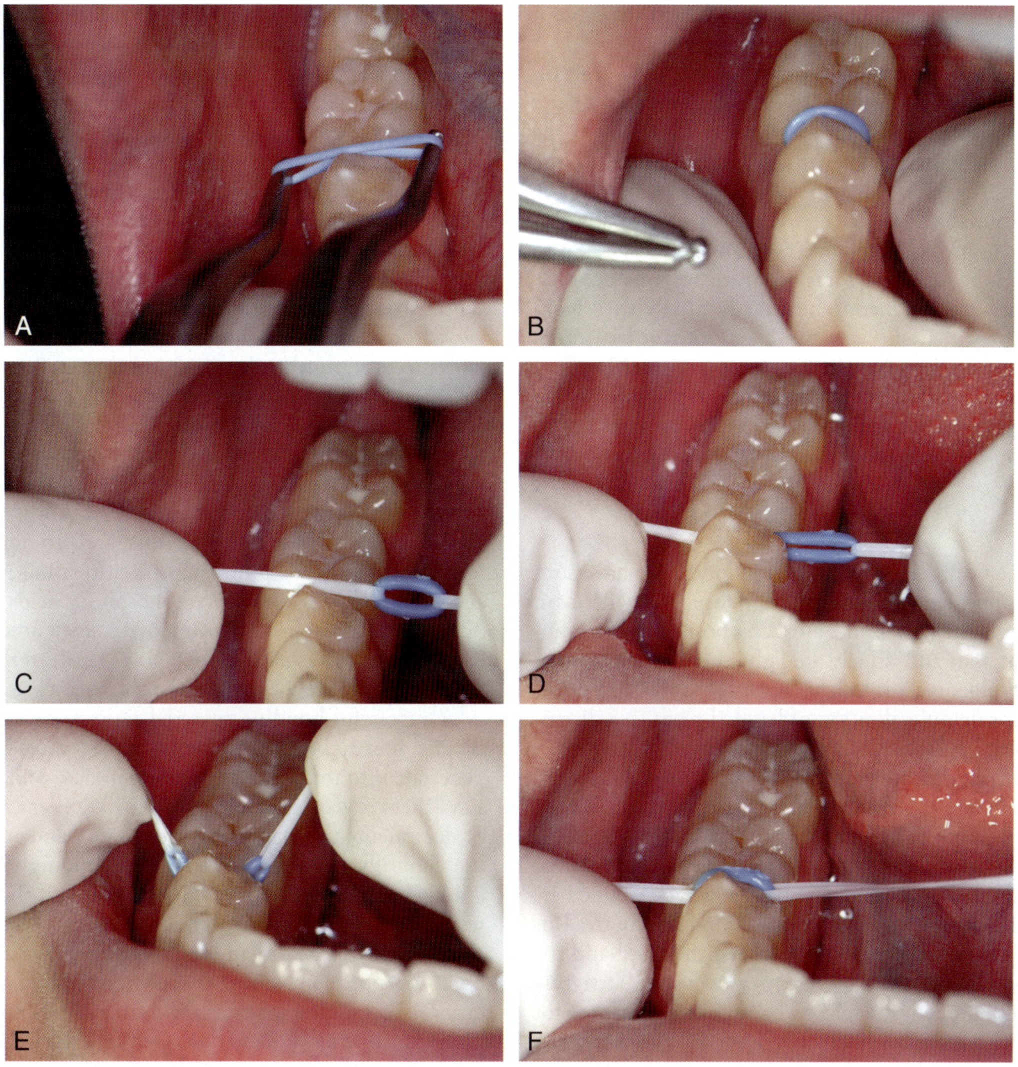

• **Fig. 10.22** Separation with an elastomeric ring or "doughnut." (A) The elastomeric ring is placed over the beaks of a special pliers and stretched, then (B) one side is snapped through the contact and the pliers slipped out so that the doughnut now surrounds the contact; (C) an alternative to the special pliers is two loops of dental floss, placed so they can be used to stretch the ring. (D) The dental floss is snapped through the contact and the doughnut is pulled underneath the contact; (E) the doughnut is pulled upward, and (F) the doughnut is snapped into position. At that point, the dental floss is removed.

("doughnuts"), applied as shown in Fig. 10.22, which surround the contact point and squeeze the teeth apart over a period of several days.

From the patient's perspective, separation of teeth before banding may be the worst part of orthodontics—it hurts, especially if multiple teeth are to be banded. Steel spring separators may be easier to place when interproximal contacts are tight or when poorly contoured restorations result in very broad interproximal contact areas. These separators tend to come loose and may fall out as they accomplish their purpose, which is their main disadvantage and the reason for leaving them in place only a few days, and not for more than a week.

Elastomeric separators may be more difficult to insert but are usually retained well once placed around the interproximal contact and so may be left in position for somewhat longer periods. They exert heavy force initially that decays quickly, but pain medication may be required for the first 24 to 36 hours. Because elastomeric separators are radiolucent, a serious problem can arise if one is lost into the interproximal space or gingival crevice. It is wise to use a brightly colored elastomeric material to make a subgingivally displaced separator more visible, and elastomeric separators should generally not be left in place for more than 2 weeks.

Fitting Bands

With the wide availability of preformed bands now, forming bands clinically is too inefficient. Almost all bands are supplied with prewelded attachments. This saves clinical time and allows the use of templates to ensure accurate placement of the attachment.

Fitting a preformed band involves stretching the stainless steel material over the tooth surface. This simultaneously contours and work-hardens the initially rather soft band material. It follows that heavy force is needed to seat a preformed band. This force should be supplied by the masticatory muscles of the patient, not by the arm strength of the dentist or dental assistant. Patients can bite harder and with much greater control, a fact best appreciated on the rare occasions when a patient is unable to bite bands to place and the orthodontist has to do it with hand pressure.

Preformed bands are designed to be fitted in a certain sequence, and it is important to follow the manufacturer's instructions. A typical maxillary molar band is designed to be placed initially by hand pressure on an instrument placed on the mesial and distal surfaces. This brings the band down close to the height of the marginal ridges. Then it is driven to place by biting pressure on the mesiobuccal and distolingual surfaces. The final seating is with heavy biting force on the distolingual corner. Lower molar bands are designed to be seated initially with hand pressure on the proximal surfaces and then with heavy biting force along the buccal but not the lingual margins. Maxillary premolar bands are usually seated with alternate pressure on the buccal and lingual surfaces; mandibular premolar bands, like mandibular molars, are designed for heavy pressure on the buccal surface only.

Cementation

New cements specifically designed for orthodontic use have supplanted the zinc phosphate and early glass ionomer cements used in the 20th century. The newer ones are a composite of glass ionomer and resin materials and usually are light-cured. Their use has greatly reduced problems with leakage beneath bands that previously was a risk for demineralization of banded teeth (see discussion in Chapter 8).

All interior surfaces of an orthodontic band must be coated with cement before it is placed, so that there is no bare metal. As the band is carried to place, the occlusal surface should be covered so that cement is expressed from the gingival as well as the occlusal margins of the band (Fig. 10.23). Bands are largely retained by the elasticity of the band material as it fits around the tooth. This is augmented by the cement that seals between the band and the tooth, but a band retained only by cement was not fitted tightly enough. It is good judgment to replace a band that comes loose for the second time with a smaller sized one.

Bonded Attachments

The Basis of Bonding

Bonding of attachments, eliminating the need for bands, was a dream for many years before rather abruptly becoming a routine clinical procedure in the 1980s. Bonding is based on the mechanical locking of an adhesive to irregularities in the enamel surface of the tooth and to mechanical locks formed in the base of the orthodontic attachment. Successful bonding therefore requires careful attention to three components of the system: the attachment base, the tooth surface and its preparation, and the bonding material itself.

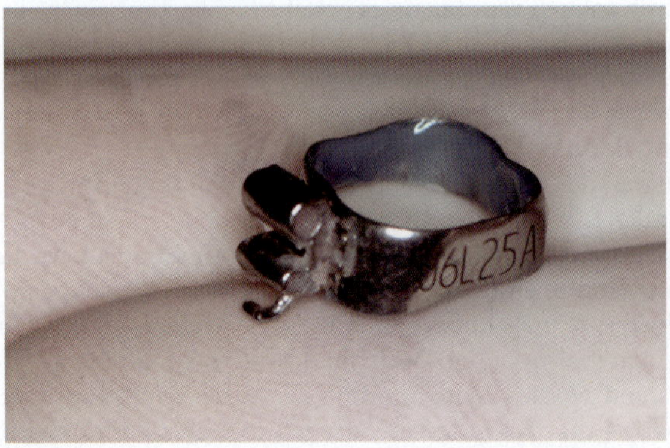

• **Fig. 10.23** Molar band ready to cement. The cement must cover all the interior surface of the band. We recommend placing a gloved finger over the top of the band when it is carried to place, to help in keeping cement on the gingival aspect of the band.

The base of a metal bonded bracket or tube is manufactured so that a mechanical interlock between the bonding material and the attachment surface is achieved. The objective is to obtain a stronger attachment of the bonding material to the bracket than to the tooth surface, so that on debonding the bonding material breaks away from the tooth rather than the bracket. This is not necessary with most ceramic brackets because an unpolished ceramic surface has enough irregularity.

Before bonding of an orthodontic attachment, it is desirable to remove the enamel pellicle (the thin layer of protein material that coats the teeth) and then create irregularities in the enamel surface. In the standard technique that still is widely used, this is accomplished by gently cleaning and drying the enamel surface (avoiding heavy pumicing), then treating it with an etching agent, usually 37% unbuffered phosphoric acid (H_3PO_4) for 20 to 30 seconds.[8] The effect is to remove a small amount of the softer interprismatic enamel and open pores between the enamel prisms, so the adhesive can penetrate into the enamel surface (Fig. 10.24).

A successful bonding material must meet a set of formidable criteria: it must be dimensionally stable; it must be fluid enough to penetrate into the prepared enamel surface, while tacky enough to stay where it was placed; it must have excellent inherent strength, as documented by laboratory testing[9,10]; and it must be easy to use clinically. The most widely used bonding material at present is a light-activated composite resin, although chemically activated resins still are widely available.

Especially in treatment of adults, it occasionally is necessary to bond to a porcelain veneer or crown, or to gold or amalgam restorations. Techniques for bonding to these restorative materials have been developed,[11] and are described in Chapter 20.

Direct Bonding

During direct bonding, bracket position is determined intraorally by the clinician during the bonding procedure. This technique can be used quite successfully as a routine clinical procedure. Even when most attachments are bonded indirectly (as described later), direct bonding may be more efficient whenever a single bracket must be repositioned. The major difficulty with direct bonding is that the dentist must be able to judge the proper position for the attachment and must carry it to place rapidly and accurately. There is less opportunity for precise measurements of bracket position or detailed adjustments than there would be at the laboratory bench. For this reason, it is generally conceded that direct bonding does not provide as accurate a placement of brackets as indirect bonding. On the other hand, direct bonding is easier, faster (especially if only a few teeth are to be bonded), and less expensive (because the laboratory fabrication steps are eliminated).

Steps in the direct bonding technique when using a light-activated resin for each bracket are illustrated in Fig. 10.25. Light-cured resins now are used more frequently than chemically activated resins because the newer light-cured materials have more flexibility in working time and usually have higher bond strengths.

As we have noted in Chapter 8, demineralization around brackets is a significant problem in fixed appliance treatment at present, and glass ionomer materials offer the possibility of enough sustained fluoride release to protect the enamel around the

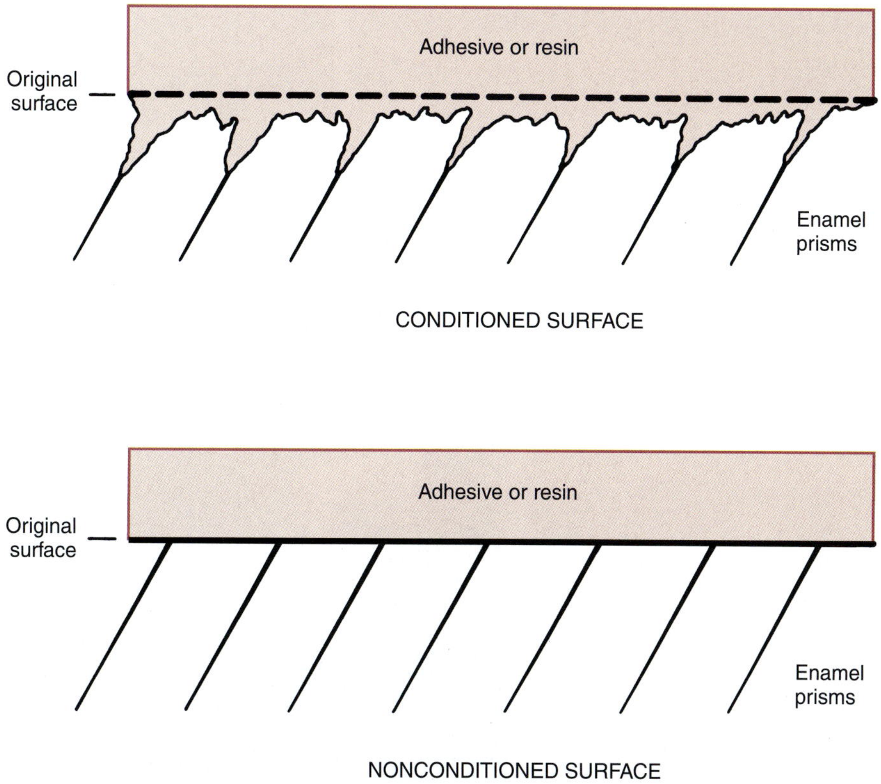

• **Fig. 10.24** Diagrammatic representation of the effect of preparation of the enamel surface before bonding. Pretreatment with phosphoric acid creates minute irregularities in the enamel surface, allowing the bonding material to form penetrating "tags" that mechanically interlock with the enamel surface.

edges of brackets. Trials with modified glass ionomers for bonding showed that even when some composite resin was included in the bonding material, the bond strength still was not adequate. Justus and coworkers have advocated a way to improve the bond strength of a modified glass ionomer to the point that it should be adequate for bonding.[12]

The Justus method involves deproteinization of the enamel surface with 5% NaOCl (sodium hypochlorite, widely sold as Clorox), and then a 15- to 20-second etch time with phosphoric acid. With this approach, the debonding rate is said to be about 5%, roughly comparable to rates with composite resin bonding materials.

Does this use of resin-modified glass ionomer cement really reduce the incidence of demineralization and white spots? The ideal evidence would be outcomes from a randomized clinical trial, which has not been done, but the clinical data presented by Justus are impressive. It appears that the improved fluoride release from the resin-modified glass ionomer can provide useful protection against demineralization, and the glass ionomer component allows the ability to "recharge" the fluoride content of the resin by in-office fluoride treatment.

Indirect Bonding

Indirect bonding is done by accurately placing the brackets on dental casts in a laboratory or in virtual space, then using a template or tray to transfer this bracket position to the patient. The result is more precise location of brackets because the limitations of cheeks that partially obstruct the view of the teeth are removed, salivary contamination of prepared surfaces is easier to control, and direct transfer to a tooth location determined from virtual bonding in a computer system is straightforward.[13]

Indirect setups can be completed by the clinician in the office laboratory by creating a stone cast from an impression or by printing a 3D model from an intraoral scan. Indirect bracket setups can also be done by a service laboratory by using a stable impression material suitable for digital scanning at a distant site or, more likely in today's digital world, by sending a direct intraoral scan from the office scanner to the lab. Laboratory and clinical steps in indirect bonding are illustrated in Fig. 10.26.

Producing indirect bonding bracket setups and transfer trays in the office remains a rapid and cost-effective method. After producing an accurate stone cast, a layer of separator is placed on the cast. The brackets are then placed on the cast by using a light-activated composite resin in the desired location and are checked by the orthodontist for positioning accuracy. Once the brackets are in position, any excess flash is removed and they are secured in this location by exposing them to an appropriate curing light in a light box (such as the Triad unit [Dentsply Sirona, York, PA]). Less efficiently, this also can be done with a hand-held curing light. This process creates a custom composite base for each bracket that fits each tooth surface precisely. A transfer tray is then made using a PVS putty that covers the brackets and provides occlusal/incisal stops. The tray is trimmed to remove excess tray material and sectioned into quadrants. This makes it easier to insert and to see clearly that the trays are fully seated during the clinical bonding procedure. A frequently used but more time-consuming alternative (because of the greater effort to trim these trays) is to vacuum-form the transfer trays from an aligner-type material.

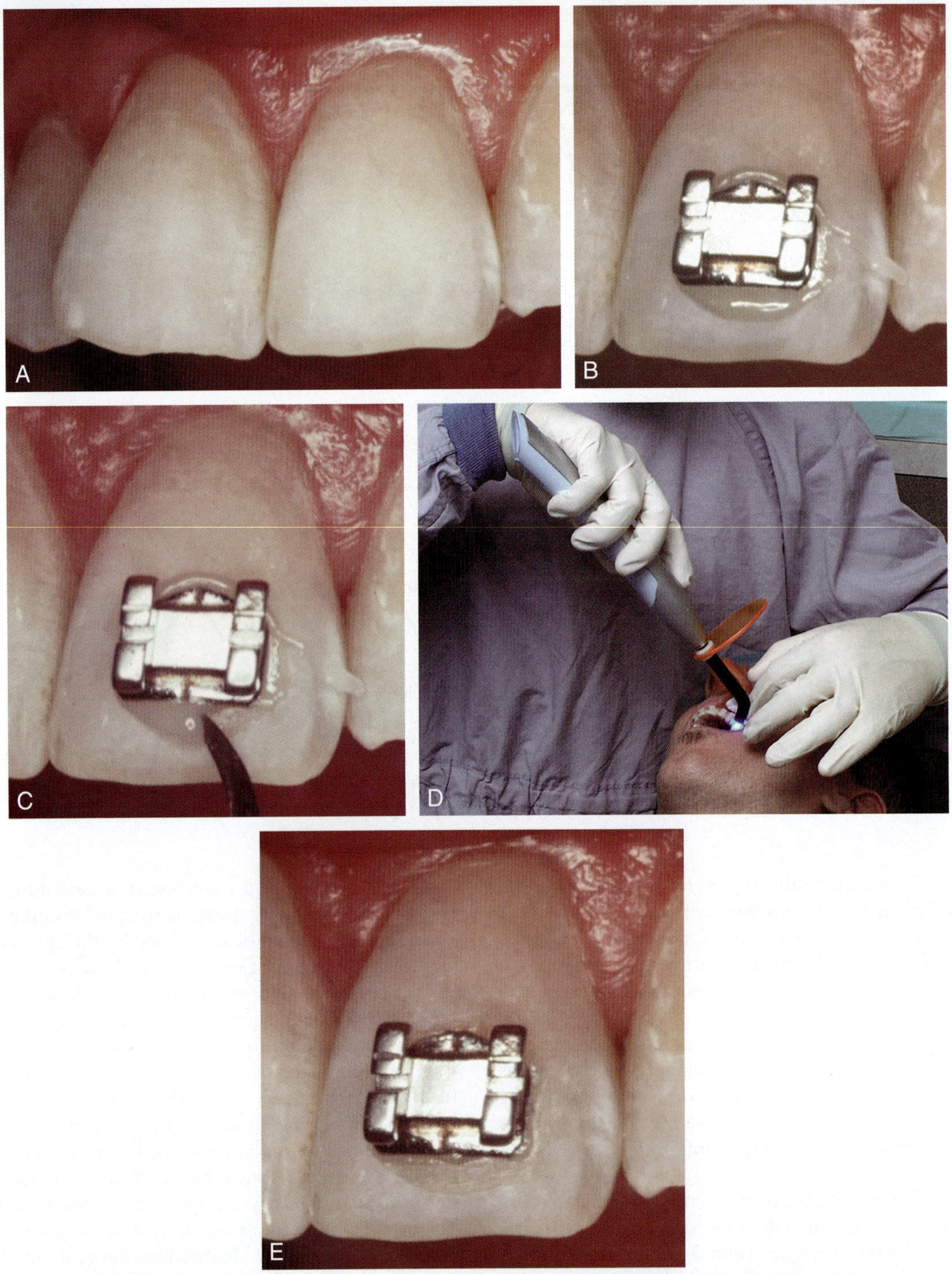

• **Fig. 10.25** Steps in direct bonding. (A) After etching, the tooth surface has a somewhat chalky or frosted appearance if dried (drying is no longer necessary with modern tooth preparation materials, but the tooth surface must be etched). (B) A small amount of the bonding agent is squeezed into the mesh on the back of the bracket, and it is pressed to place on the tooth surface. (C) Excess bonding material is removed from around the bracket. (D) For light-cured materials, a cordless light now is the most convenient way to activate the adhesive bonding process. (E) The bracket bonded in place.

The trays are clinically used by placing a lightly filled sealant on the patient's teeth and on the bracket backs and then seating the trays in the patient's mouth. The lightly filled sealant used for bonding can be a chemical-cured resin, a "no-mix" resin, or a light-activated resin. A chemical cure resin that is mixed before application to the brackets and teeth is efficient because all brackets cure simultaneously, but care must be taken to minimize excess resin to avoid flash after tray removal. A "no-mix" resin has an advantage in minimizing flash; a composite resin is placed on the tooth surface in unpolymerized form, and the polymerization catalyst is placed on the back of the brackets. When the tray carrying the brackets is placed against the tooth surface, the resin immediately

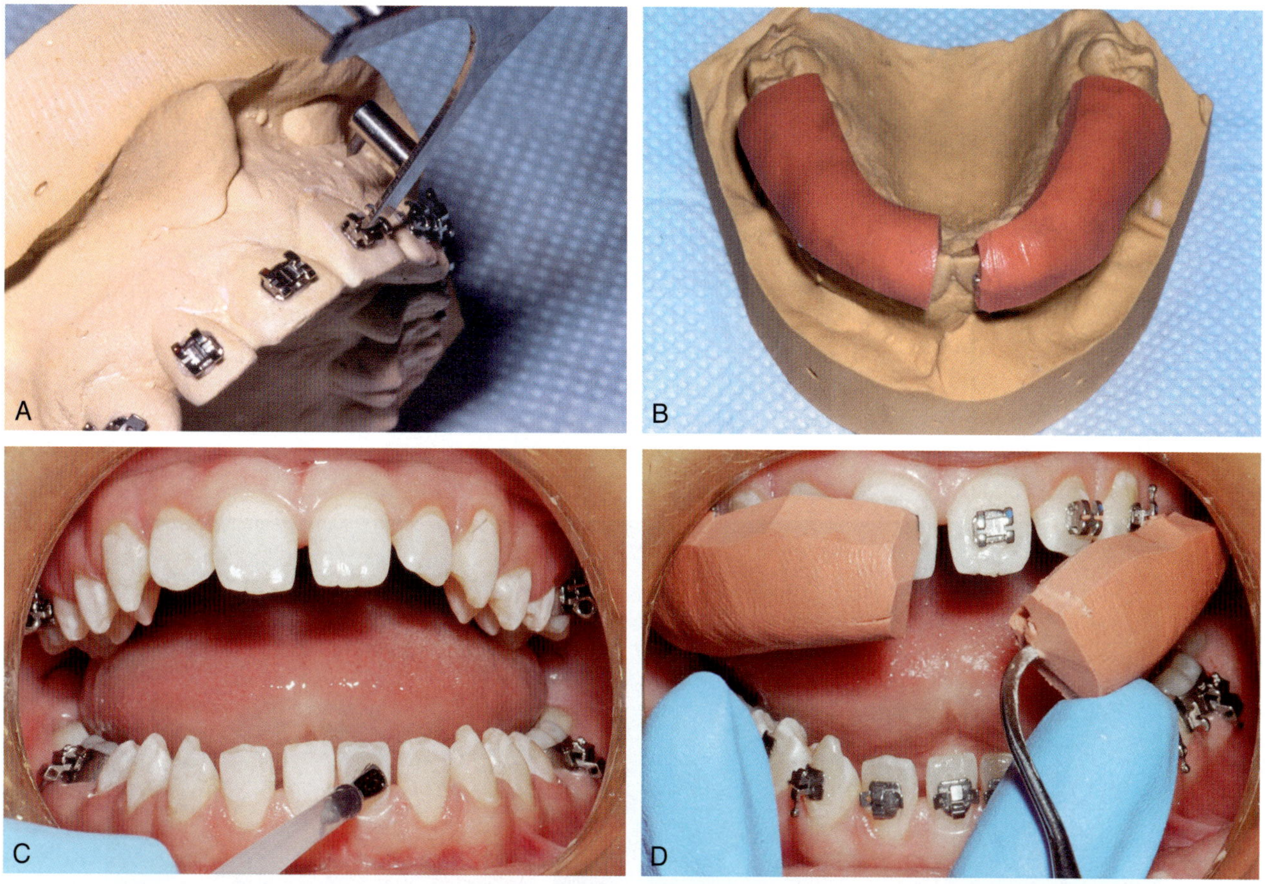

• **Fig. 10.26** Steps in indirect bonding. (A) Brackets are placed precisely as desired on a cast of the teeth and held in place with a filled resin. (B) After the brackets are cured in the ideal position, a transfer tray is formed from a vinyl polysiloxane putty. The trays are removed from the working cast after soaking in warm water and trimmed. (C) The teeth are isolated and etched, and a chemically cured two-paste resin is painted on the etched enamel and the brackets; alternatively, a light-cured resin can be used, but only with translucent trays. Then the transfer trays are inserted. (D) After the resin has completely set, the trays are carefully removed, leaving the brackets bonded to the teeth.

beneath the bracket is activated and polymerizes, but excess resin around the margins of the brackets does not polymerize and can be easily cleared away when the bracket tray is removed. Some studies, however, have found increased bond failures with this technique because it relies on diffusion for proper polymerization. Finally, a flowable light-cured material can be used with a translucent tray, but polymerizing the resin at each bracket through or around the tray takes more time than using a chemical cure. With any of these techniques, proper isolation to prevent saliva contamination is critical for obtaining adequate bond strength.

There are now several digitally assisted methods to produce indirect bonding trays for the clinician. Some of these simply duplicate the in-office process described earlier. Others provide a value-added service by producing transfer trays based on bracket position determined from a digital treatment simulation (Fig. 10.27). This is meant to ensure that the bracket position will provide optimal alignment. In this case the digital models are segmented into movable teeth and virtually aligned following the arch form prescribed by the orthodontist. Virtual brackets are then placed on the teeth in such a position that a straight wire of the proper arch form will engage all the bracket slots. This "ideal" bracket position is then digitally transferred back to the original cast and a tray is fabricated to produce this bracket position in the patient. Some of these trays are directly 3D printed so the brackets can be snapped into place. To gain the benefits of indirect bonding, the transfer process itself must be accurate, and we now have some evidence that this is the case.[14]

At present, indirect bonding is the preferred technique for placement of a complete fixed appliance. Custom brackets that were manufactured for an individual patient require precise placement that can be achieved only by indirect bonding. More generally, the poorer the visibility, the more difficult direct bonding becomes and the greater the indication for an indirect approach. For this reason, indirect bonding is a necessity for lingual attachments. Bonding an isolated lingual hook or button is not difficult, but precisely positioning the brackets for a lingual appliance is, and even the placement of a fixed lingual retainer is easier with indirect technique and a transfer tray.

Characteristics of Contemporary Fixed Appliances

Appliance Materials

Stainless Steel Brackets

The brackets and tubes for an edgewise appliance must be precisely manufactured so that the internal slot dimensions are accurate to at least ±1 mil. Until the recent introduction of ceramic and

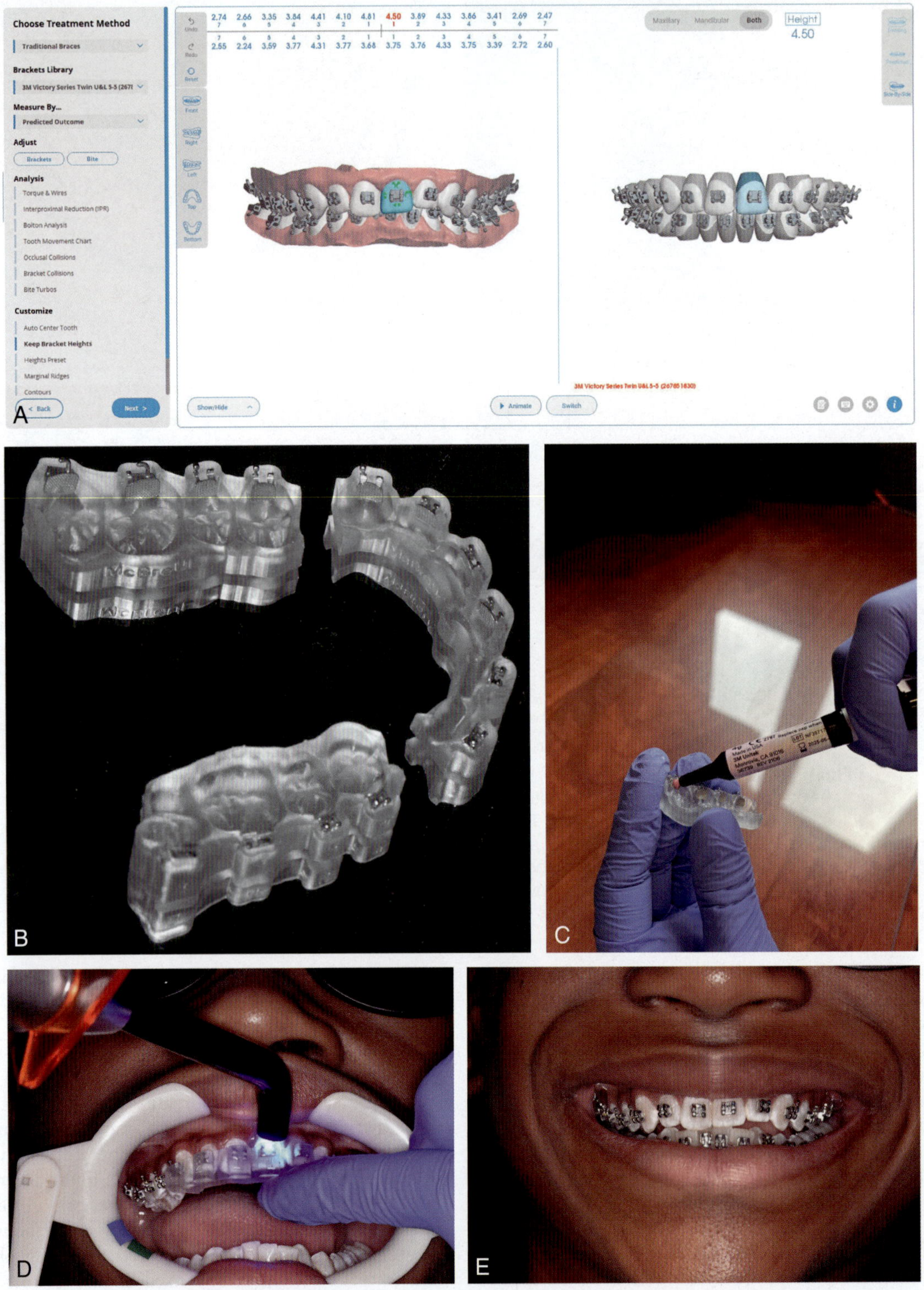

• **Fig. 10.27** Indirect bonding using a digitally assisted bracket placement system (DIBS AI, OrthoSelect). (A) The software interface used to plan the bracket placement. (B) The 3D-printed transfer trays with the brackets inserted. (C) Light-cure resin placed on the bracket pads prior to insertion. (D) The anterior tray section placed in the patient's mouth and a curing light used to harden the adhesive to attach the bracket to the tooth. The light is used to cure each bracket individually. (E) The patient immediately after removal of the final transfer tray showing the brackets now in place in the digitally planned position.

titanium brackets, fixed appliances had been fabricated entirely from stainless steel for many years, and stainless steel remains the standard material for appliance components.

There are now three contemporary ways to produce edgewise brackets and tubes: by metal-injection molding (MIM), casting, or 3D printing (which is possible with metals and ceramics, as well as plastics). Most of the brackets and tubes for contemporary appliances still are produced by MIM, but an increasing percentage are cast. Better precision of bracket slot size is achieved by milling the slot of a cast bracket, which corrects errors introduced by shrinkage of the casting as it cools. The use of 3D printing offers the possibility of significantly better bracket slot precision, and 3D brackets are now available for some of the newest digitally assisted appliance systems (see later). It is likely that 3D printing, using a variety of resins, metals or ceramics, will gradually replace the older technology for bracket production.

Titanium as an Alternative to Stainless Steel

Titanium edgewise brackets have been commercially available for some years now and can be used for comprehensive treatment. A major indication for titanium brackets and wires is to eliminate the possibility of an allergic response to the 8% nickel content in stainless steel (see Chapter 8). In addition to their greater safety in an increasingly allergic population, titanium brackets have an important advantage over steel brackets—and also a potentially important disadvantage.

The major advantage is better bond reliability—that is, a lower chance that a bonded bracket will be lost during active treatment. The greater reliability of titanium brackets is primarily because titanium has the same strength as stainless steel, but is half as stiff.

Titanium also has an inherently rougher surface than stainless steel, and all other things being equal, that means potentially greater resistance to sliding a tooth along an archwire if the wire or the bracket is titanium. The area of contact of an archwire against a bracket slot is quite small under most circumstances, and a titanium bracket is not a problem when small round wires are used. Titanium also has a chemically active surface, and this can contribute to difficulty in sliding, especially with a TMA wire in a titanium bracket. Clinically, that means that when titanium brackets are used, small spaces should be closed by sliding along undersized steel wires, and extraction sites preferably would be closed with closing loops in steel or TMA wires.

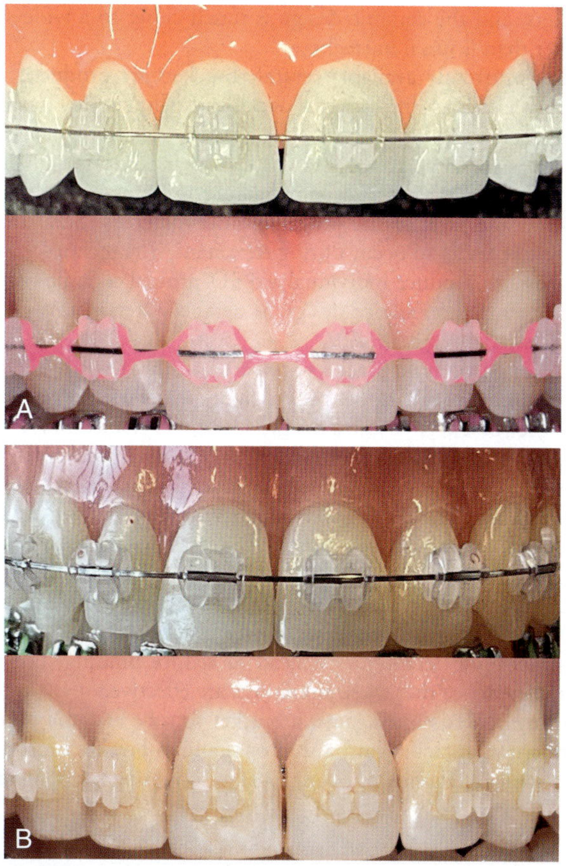

• **Fig. 10.28** Representative ceramic brackets that are used to provide a more esthetic fixed appliance. (A) Symetri Clear by Ormco. The top image shows the ceramic brackets on a demonstration model using clear elastic ligatures to keep a small-diameter archwire securely in place. The bottom panel show the same brackets on a patient with a rectangular archwire held in place by a colored elastic chain. (B) 3M Clarity Advanced Ceramic Brackets. The top image again shows the brackets on a demonstration model with clear elastic ligatures to keep a rectangular archwire in place. The bottom image shows a patient with Clarity brackets with the archwire out and discolored adhesive around the brackets from poor bonding technique and flash removal. This demonstrates that it is not just the bracket selection that makes an appliance more esthetic, but the care that's taken during bonding and the patient's hygiene habits throughout treatment.

Nonmetallic Appliance Materials: Plastics, Ceramics, and Composite Plastics

Recurring efforts have been made to make fixed appliances more esthetic by eliminating their metallic appearance. A major impetus to the development of bonding for orthodontic attachments was elimination of the unsightly metal band. Tooth-colored or clear brackets for anterior teeth (Fig. 10.28) became practical when successful systems for direct bonding were developed. Although plastic brackets were introduced with considerable enthusiasm in the 1980s and have retained a small market share ever since, they have four largely unresolved problems:

- Staining and discoloration, particularly in patients who smoke or drink coffee
- Poor strength, so that brackets are likely to break when large archwires are used
- Poor dimensional stability, so that it is not possible to provide precise bracket slots or build in all the straight-wire features
- Friction and binding between the plastic bracket and metal archwires that makes it very difficult to slide teeth to a new position

Using a metal slot in the plastic bracket helps with the last three problems, but even with this modification, plastic brackets are useful only when complex tooth movements are not required.

Ceramic brackets, which became available in the late 1980s, largely overcome the esthetic limitations of plastic brackets in that they are quite durable and resist staining (see Fig. 10.28). In addition, they can be custom-molded to fit individual teeth and are dimensionally stable, so the precise bracket angulations and slots of the straight-wire appliance can be incorporated.

Ceramic brackets were received enthusiastically and immediately achieved widespread use, but problems with fractures, friction within bracket slots, wear on teeth contacting a bracket, and enamel damage from bracket removal soon became apparent. Fractures of ceramic brackets occur in two ways: (1) loss of part of the brackets (e.g., tie wings) during archwire changes or eating and (2) cracking of the bracket when torque forces are applied. Ceramics are a form of glass, and like glass, ceramic brackets tend to be brittle. Because the fracture toughness of steel is much greater, ceramic brackets must be bulkier than stainless steel brackets, and the ceramic design is much closer to a wide single bracket than is usual in steel.

Most currently available ceramic brackets are produced from alumina, either as single-crystal or polycrystalline units. In theory, single-crystal brackets should offer greater strength, which is true until the bracket surface is scratched. At that point, the small surface crack tends to spread, and fracture resistance is reduced to or below the level of the polycrystalline materials. Scratches, of course, are likely to occur during treatment. The technology now also exists to produce individualized 3D-printed ceramic brackets for customized appliance design as detailed later in this chapter (see Figs. 10.36 and 10.37).

Although ceramic brackets are better in this regard than plastics, resistance to sliding has proved to be greater with ceramic than with steel brackets. Because of the multiple crystals, polycrystalline alumina brackets have relatively rough surfaces in the bracket slots. Even though monocrystalline alumina is as smooth as steel, these brackets also do not allow good sliding, perhaps because of a chemical interaction between the wire and bracket material. For this reason, many second-generation ceramic brackets were supplied with an integrated metal slot. Most current brackets now have eliminated the metal slot, using corner-rounding and surface-smoothing techniques instead to reduce binding, but with limited evidence that these alterations are effective.

Many patients bite against a bracket or tube at some point in treatment. Contact against a steel or titanium bracket causes little or no wear of enamel, but contact of an opposing tooth against a ceramic bracket can abrade enamel quite rapidly. This risk is largely avoided if ceramic brackets are placed only on the upper anterior teeth, where improved esthetics is most important. Most patients who want the esthetic effect will accept steel or titanium brackets elsewhere if ceramic brackets are used on the most visible teeth.

Debonding ceramic brackets also can be a challenge when it comes time for bracket removal. Most manufacturers now offer debonding pliers designed to fracture the bracket along a feature engineered into the bracket. An alternative is to use a diode laser or thermal instrument to weaken the adhesive by heating it. This is quite effective in reducing the chance of enamel damage.[15] Unfortunately, it introduces the chance of damaging the tooth pulp if the heat application is not controlled quite precisely, and for that reason has not been widely adopted. Debonding techniques are discussed in greater detail in Chapter 17.

Straight-Wire Concept in Bracket and Tube Design

Modern edgewise appliances use brackets or tubes that are custom-made for each tooth, with the goal of minimizing the number of bends in archwires needed to produce an ideal arrangement of the teeth, hence the "straight-wire" name. In Angle's terminology for his appliance, first-order bends were used to compensate for differences in tooth thickness, second-order bends to position roots correctly in a mesiodistal direction, and third-order (torque) bends to position roots in a faciolingual direction (Fig. 10.29). Let's view these bracket and tube compensations for bends in archwires in more detail.

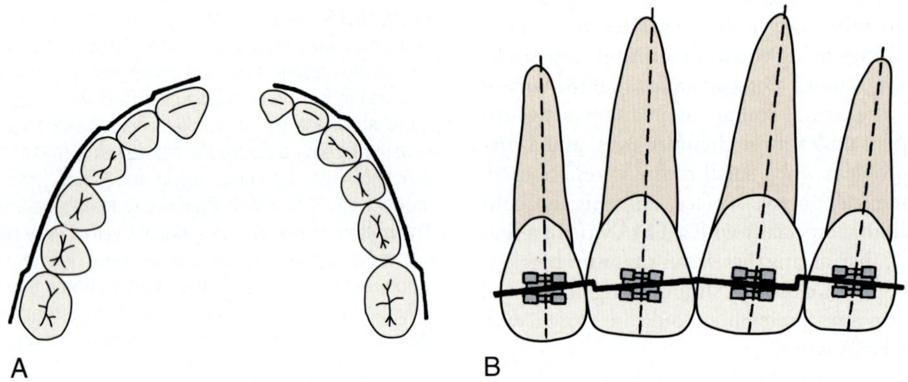

• **Fig. 10.29** First-, second-, and third-order bends in edgewise wires. (A) First-order bends in a maxillary *(left)* and mandibular *(right)* archwire. Note the lateral inset required in the maxillary archwire and the canine and molar offset bends that are required in both. (B) Second-order bends in the maxillary incisor segment to compensate for the inclination of the incisal edge of these teeth relative to the long axis of the tooth. (C) Third-order bends for the maxillary central incisors and maxillary first molars showing the twist in the archwire to provide a passive fit in a bracket or tube on these teeth. Twist in an archwire provides torque in a bracket; the torque is positive for the incisor, negative for the molar.

Compensations for First-Order Bends

For anterior teeth and premolars, varying the bracket thickness eliminates in-out bends in the anterior portions of each archwire, but an offset position of molar tubes is necessary to provide correct molar rotation (Fig. 10.30). For good occlusion, the buccal surface must sit at an angle to the line of occlusion, with the mesiobuccal cusp more prominent than the distobuccal cusp. For this reason, the tube or bracket specified for the upper molar should have at least a 10-degree offset, as should the tube for the upper second molar. The offset for the lower first molar should be 5 to 7 degrees, about half as much as for the upper molar. The offset for the lower second molar should be at least as large as for the first molar.

Compensations for Second-Order Bends

In the original edgewise appliance, second-order bends, sometimes called *artistic positioning bends*, were an important part of the finishing phase of treatment. These bends were necessary because the long axis of each tooth is inclined relative to the plane of a continuous archwire (Fig. 10.31). Contemporary edgewise brackets have a built-in tip for maxillary incisor teeth, which varies among the appliances that are now available. A distal tip of the upper first molar is also needed to obtain good interdigitation of the posterior teeth. If the upper molars are too vertically upright, even though a proper Class I relationship apparently exists, good interdigitation cannot be achieved. Tipping upper molars distally brings their distal cusps into

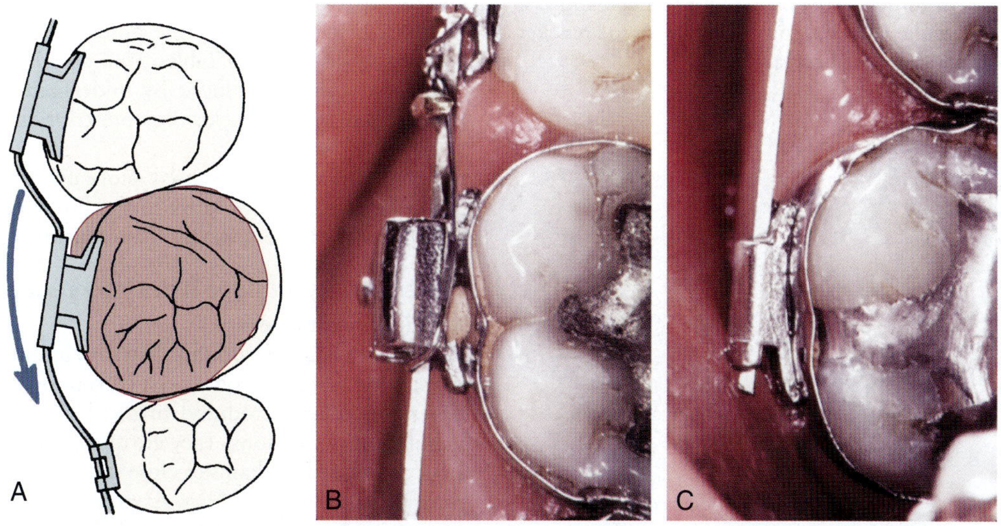

• **Fig. 10.30** (A) The rhomboidal surface of the upper, and to a lesser extent the lower, molars means that placing a springy archwire through attachments that were flat against the facial surface would produce a mesiolingual rotation of these teeth, causing them to take up too much space in the arch. Compensation requires a bend in the archwire, or placing the tube at an angle offset to the facial surface. (B) Rectangular and headgear tubes for the upper first molar and (C) rectangular tube for the lower second molar in a contemporary appliance. Note the offset position of the tubes so that a first-order bend in the wire is unnecessary.

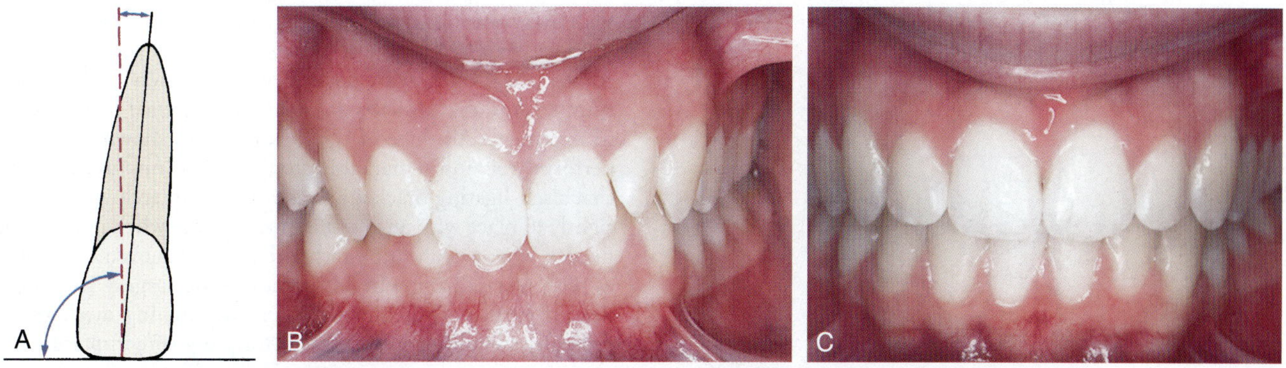

• **Fig. 10.31** (A) A second-order bend, or an inclination of the bracket slot to produce the same effect, is necessary for the maxillary incisors because the long axes of these teeth are inclined relative to the incisal edge. The angle between the dotted red line and the long axis of the tooth is the bracket angulation. The term "bracket tip" refers to the same angle. (B) and (C) Malaligned maxillary incisors before and after treatment using straight-wire brackets to facilitate both mesiodistal (tip) and faciolingual (torque) root positioning. (A, Redrawn from Andrews LF. The straight-wire appliance. Explained and compared. *J Clin Orthod*. 1976;10(3):174–195.)

occlusion and creates the space needed for proper relationships of the premolars (Fig. 10.32).

Compensations for Third-Order Bends

If the bracket for a rectangular archwire is placed flat against the labial or buccal surface of any tooth, the plane of the bracket slot will twist away from the horizontal, often to a considerable extent. With the original edgewise appliance, it was necessary to place a twist in each rectangular archwire to compensate for this. Failure to place third-order bends meant that in the anterior region, the teeth would become too upright, while posteriorly the lingual cusps of molars would be elevated relative to the occlusal plane (Fig. 10.33). Compensation for this can be done by cutting the bracket slot into the bracket at an angle or forming the base so that the face of the bracket is at an angle. This is called placing torque in the bracket or torque in the base, respectively. It allows a horizontally flat rectangular archwire to be placed into the bracket slots without incorporating twist bends.

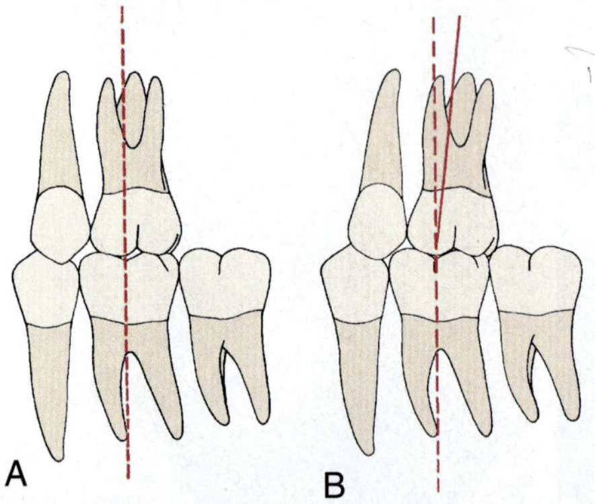

• **Fig. 10.32** A distal inclination or tip of the maxillary first molar is important for proper posterior occlusal interdigitation. If the mesiobuccal cusp occludes in the mesial groove of the mandibular first molar, creating an apparently ideal Class I relationship, proper interdigitation of the premolars still cannot be obtained if the molar is positioned too upright (A). Tipping the molar distally (B) allows the premolars to interdigitate properly. (Redrawn from Andrews LF. The straight-wire appliance. Explained and compared. *J Clin Orthod*. 1976;10(3):174–195.)

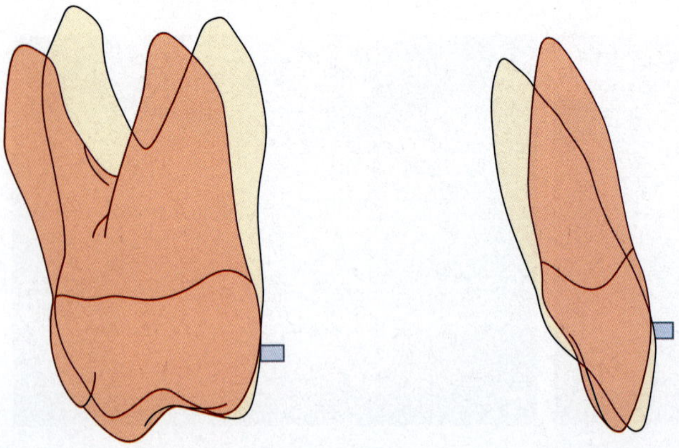

• **Fig. 10.33** The plane of a flat rectangular archwire relative to a maxillary incisor and molar is shown in red. To produce the proper faciolingual position of both anterior and posterior teeth, either a rectangular archwire must be twisted (torqued), or the bracket slot must be cut at an angle to produce the same torque effect. Otherwise, the improper inclination shown in red will be produced. Proper torque is necessary not to move teeth but to prevent undesired movement.

The amount of torque recommended in the various appliance prescriptions varies more than any other feature of contemporary edgewise appliances. Although a number of factors are important in establishing the appropriate torque, four are particularly germane to how much torque is used for any particular bracket:

- The value that the developer of the appliance chose as the average normal inclination of the tooth surface. (This varies considerably among individuals and therefore can be different in "normal" samples.)
- Where on the labial surface (i.e., how far from the incisal edge) the bracket is intended to be placed. The inclination of the tooth surface varies depending on where the measurement is made, so an appliance meant to be placed more gingivally would require different torque values than would one placed more incisally.
- The expected "play" between the wire and the bracket slot, which is determined by the difference between the wire size and the slot size. As Tables 10.2 and 10.3 demonstrate, the effective torque produced by undersized rectangular wires is far less than the bracket slot prescription might lead one to expect.[16]
- The resistance to unwanted movements, such as a negative torque prescribed for lower incisors to resist the expected proclination from nonextraction alignment.

Contemporary Straight-Wire Brackets and Tubes

Self-Ligating Brackets

Placing wire ligatures around tie wings on brackets to hold archwires in the bracket slot is a time-consuming procedure. The elastomeric modules introduced in the 1970s largely replaced wire ligatures for two reasons: They are quicker and easier to place, and they can be used in chains to close small spaces within the arch or prevent spaces from opening. At present, brackets with a built-in ligating mechanism are widely used. They are called "self-ligating" but most really aren't, because manually opening or closing the mechanism is still required (Fig. 10.34).

A variety of claims have been made as advantages of self-ligating brackets, but it is clear now that almost all have been proved incorrect when clinical outcomes are reviewed. A definitive review of claims versus evidence concluded that self-ligating brackets save a little time in ligation but do not produce a saving of treatment time or better results.[17]

That should not be taken to mean that there is anything wrong with these brackets. The problem has been the advertising, not the product. As a group, the self-ligating brackets perform as well as conventional ones, with no evidence that their latching mechanism makes any positive or negative difference in the outcome of treatment. All three of the ligation types shown in Fig. 10.34 perform well and remarkably similarly. It is important, however, that a self-ligating bracket is made so that an archwire can be tied tightly in place with an external steel ligature when needed. This is needed when stabilization rather than tooth movement is needed, as with a stabilizing wire for orthognathic surgery patients. It is needed even more frequently when the latching mechanism has difficulty in holding a rectangular torquing wire in place.

Individually Customized Brackets

Because of individual variations in the contours of the teeth, no appliance prescription can be optimal for all patients, and compensatory bends in finishing archwires often are necessary. Custom brackets for the facial surface of teeth offer the prospect of eliminating almost all archwire bending (i.e., they could

TABLE 10.2 Bracket/Tube Prescription: Incisors Through Premolars, Bracket Prescription

	CENTRAL		LATERAL		CANINE		FIRST PREMOLAR		SECOND PREMOLAR	
	Torque	Tip	Torque	Tip	Torque	Tip	Torque	Tip	Torque	Tip
Maxillary										
Alexander	15	5	9	9	–3	10	–6	0	–8	4
Andrews	7	5	3	9	–7	11	–7	2	–7	2
Damon (standard torque)	15	5	6	9	7	5	–11	2	–11	2
MBT	17	4	10	8	–7	8	–7	0	–7	0
Ricketts	22	0	14	8	7	5	0	0	0	0
Roth	12	5	8	9	–2	9	–7	0	–7	0
Mandibular										
Alexander	–5	2	–5	6	–7	6	–7	0	–9	0
Andrews	–1	2	–1	2	–11	5	–17	2	–22	2
Damon (standard torque)	–3	2	–3	4	7	5	–12	4	–17	4
MBT	–6	0	–6	0	–6	3	–12	2	–17	2
Ricketts	0	0	0	0	7	5	0	0	0	0
Roth	0	0	0	0	–11	7	–17	0	–22	0

TABLE 10.3 Molar Tube/Bracket Prescriptions

	FIRST MOLAR			SECOND MOLAR		
	Torque	Tip	Rotation	Torque	Tip	Rotation
Maxillary						
Alexander	–10	0	13	–10	0	10
Andrews	–9	5	10	–9	0	10
Damon (standard torque)	–18	0	12	–27	0	6
MBT	–14	0	10	–14	0	10
Ricketts	0	0	0	0	0	0
Roth	–14	0	14	–14	0	14
Mandibular						
Alexander	–10	0	0	0	0	5
Andrews	–25	2	0	–30	0	0
Damon (standard torque)	–28	2	2	–10	0	5
MBT	–20	0	0	–10	0	0
Ricketts	0	0	0	0	0	0
Roth	–30	1	4	–30	0	4

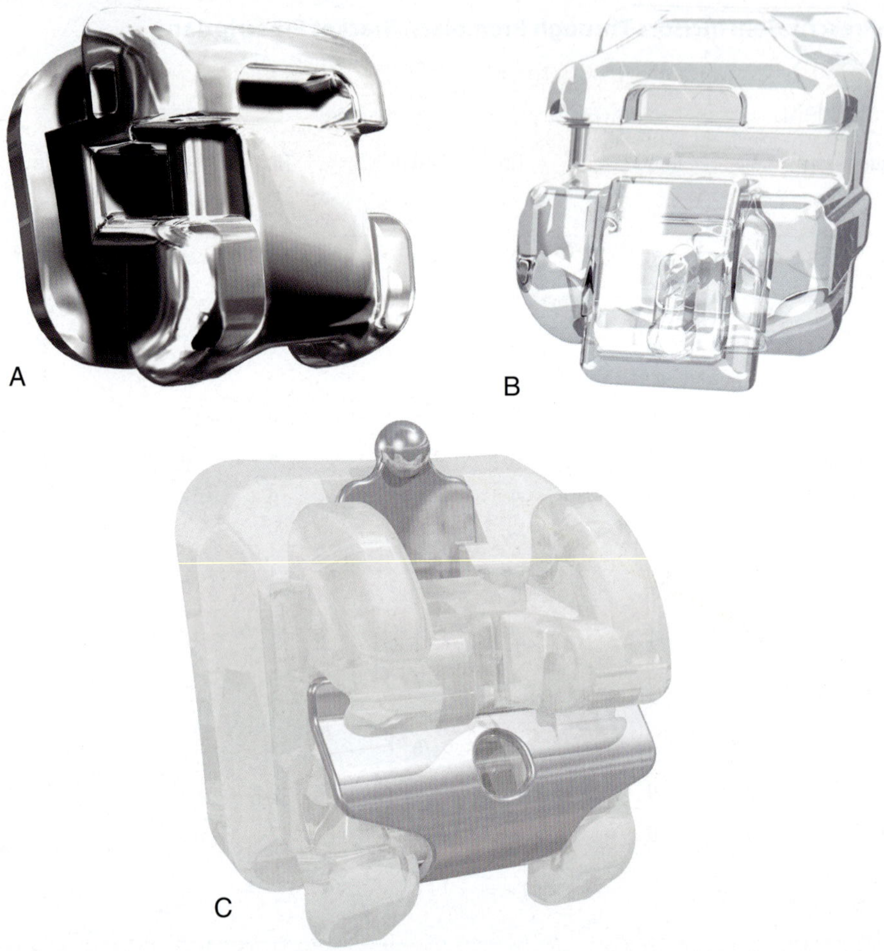

• **Fig. 10.34** Self-ligating brackets have either a rigid clip, or spring clip to hold an archwire in the bracket slot. Demonstration of a bracket with a rigid clip that is closed ([A] Damon-Q) to passively hold the archwire in place. The clip contacts the wire when required to control rotation and facial-lingual tooth position. (B) The In-Ovation-X bracket, which has a spring clip that does not put pressure on small round wires but does tightly hold rectangular wires in place. Esthetic nonmetal brackets are available now in most self-ligating bracket designs. (C) The Empower Clear bracket is an example of a ceramic bracket combined with a spring clip for a more esthetic option. (A, Courtesy Ormco Corporation, Monrovia, CA; B, Courtesy Dentsply Sirona, Cupertino, CA; C, Courtesy American Orthodontics, Sheboygan, WI.

provide the perfect straight-wire appliance). Two approaches have recently been taken to provide a customized bracket set for each patient. The first approach could be called a semi-custom solution and consists of a patient-specific selection of brackets from finite number of stock options combined with precise positioning with advanced indirect bonding. The second approach is a fully-custom solution that designs and manufactures a unique bracket for each tooth on each patient.

A good example of the semi-custom approach are the brackets and bonding system provided by KL Owen (Fig. 10.35). By using a finite number of brackets placed in an infinite number of positions, the first-, second-, and third-order control can be uniquely designed for each patient while avoiding the high costs of individually manufactured brackets. As with all custom systems, the process starts with a digital intraoral scan representing the tooth surfaces and the interocclusal relationship. The teeth are then segmented and a digital setup, or simulation, of the final desired tooth positions is completed. The best brackets are selected from the options available and virtually placed on the teeth using the ability to vary base thickness to provide the exact torque and in-out compensations required. Once these precise bracket positions are determined, indirect bonding trays are 3D printed to allow the practitioner to transfer these precise positions to the patient. These indirect bonding trays may be commercially printed and delivered to the provider, or the dentist or orthodontist may choose to print the trays in the office and load the prescribed brackets from their stock.

The KL Owen system also minimizes the "slop" between the bracket and wire by use of a 19 × 25 mil wire in a very precise 19.5 mil slot. This tight tolerance allows for more full expression of the 3rd order correction prescribed in the brackets.

A fully customized bracket solution designed and manufactured for each tooth is represented by the LightForce system (Figs. 10.36 and 10.37). This system consists of an integrated software and hardware solution that represents cutting-edge technology for manufacturing. The software is much like other technology assisted solutions that uses an intraoral scan to create a digital model for treatment simulation, or setup. Once again the teeth are segmented to allow individual movement and the patient's final alignment and occlusion are simulated.

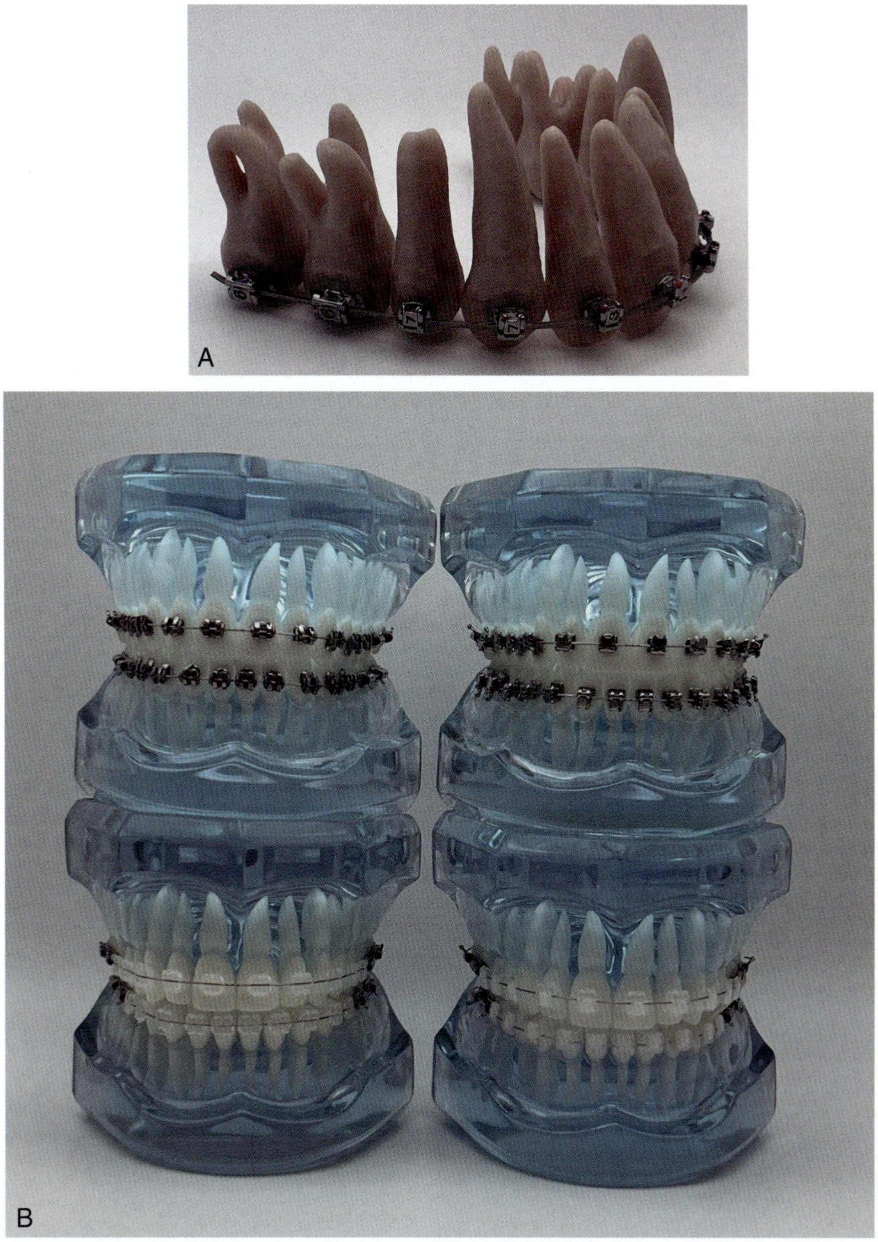

• **Fig. 10.35** The KL Owen bracket system provides individual customization for each patient by combing a finite series of brackets with precise indirect bonding. The system uses a digital setup to identify the proper brackets for each tooth and uses variable base thickness to provide minor adjustments to the rotation and torque, a digital solution that is sometimes called semi-custom. The promised result is precise root control as shown in (A). The full expression of the wire/bracket slot combination to provide this root control is a result of only 2 degrees of "slop" with the full-sized archwire. (B) This system provides a full selection of metal and ceramic brackets with both available in a self-ligating design if the doctor desires. (A and B, Courtesy Dr. Brandon Owen, founder KL Owen.)

Once the final desired position of the teeth is known, a custom bracket is designed for each tooth to allow a straight wire to connect all the bracket slots. Each bracket is designed with a base that fits the exact tooth morphology where it is being place—not depending on variable adhesive thickness for customization. These custom brackets are 3D printed in ceramic and provided with an indirect bonding tray to positon them precisely where planned. This may be the most elegant custom appliance available, but the fully-custom manufacturing process translates into increased laboratory costs compared to a semi-custom system.

There are other custom systems that are available, and certainly more that will become available in the future. What they share in common is personalized design in a digital world using an intraoral scan, they require a digital technician (or in-office staff) to do a virtual treatment setup, and they all rely on indirect bonding to precisely position the brackets on the patient. Some systems also allow a CBCT scan to be added so that the root position in the bone can be visualized while doing the setup, and there is some evidence from a study done at the University of Minnesota that this visualization may change treatment-planning decisions.[18]

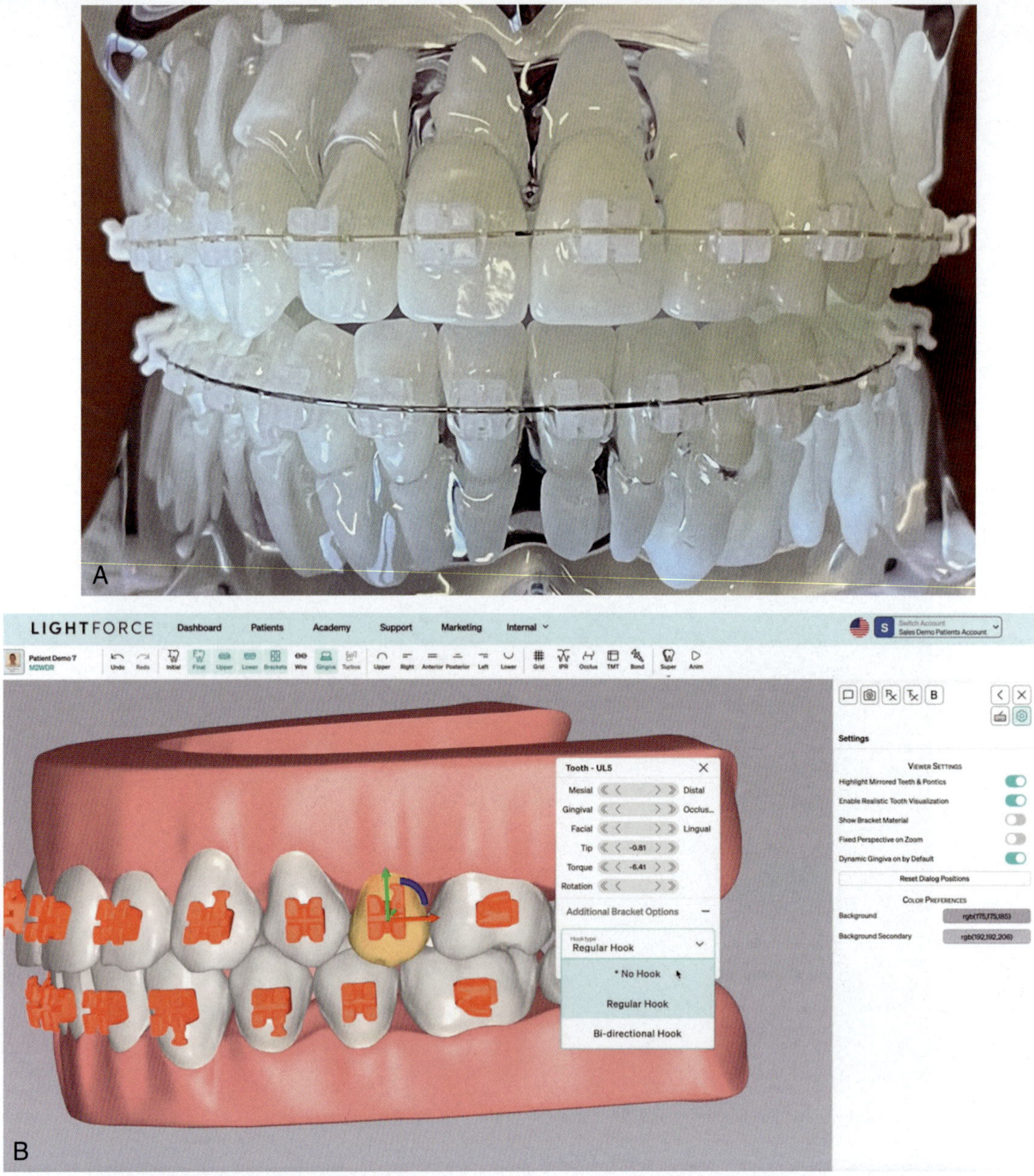

• **Fig. 10.36** A fully customized fixed appliance produced by LightForce shown on a demonstration model (A). This is a 3D-printed ceramic bracket system where each bracket is individually designed for the patient based on a digital setup done on their propriety cloud-based software called LightPlan (B). Because each bracket is manufactured for the individual patient, any desired slot prescription can be produced along with a bracket base customized for that patient's particular tooth shape.

In a study at the University of North Carolina (UNC), the use of a custom bracket system (Insignia SL; Ormco) did result in a significant decrease in both treatment time and the number of archwire changes compared with directly or indirectly bonded conventional brackets, but more of the decrease was attributed to indirect bonding than the custom brackets.[19] That leads to the interesting thought that careful indirect bonding has an excellent cost-benefit ratio, and that custom brackets add to the efficiency of treatment, but perhaps with a less favorable cost-benefit ratio.

It is important to remember that even with the evolution of custom bracket systems, the custom brackets and archwires do not make the dental arches fit together. That relies on interarch relationships, which usually are provided by interarch elastics and are mostly under the control of the patient.

Lingual Appliances

A major objection to fixed orthodontic appliances always has been their visible placement on the facial surface of the teeth. This is one reason for using removable appliances and is the major reason for the current popularity of clear aligners. The introduction of bonding in the 1970s made it possible to place fixed attachments on the lingual surface of teeth to provide an invisible fixed appliance, and brackets designed for the lingual surface were first offered soon after bonding was introduced. However, there were multiple challenges encountered with lingual braces, including difficulty producing a low-profile bracket that minimized tongue irritation, challenging access for bonding and adjustments, and difficulty placing finishing bends with the reduced interbracket spans. In

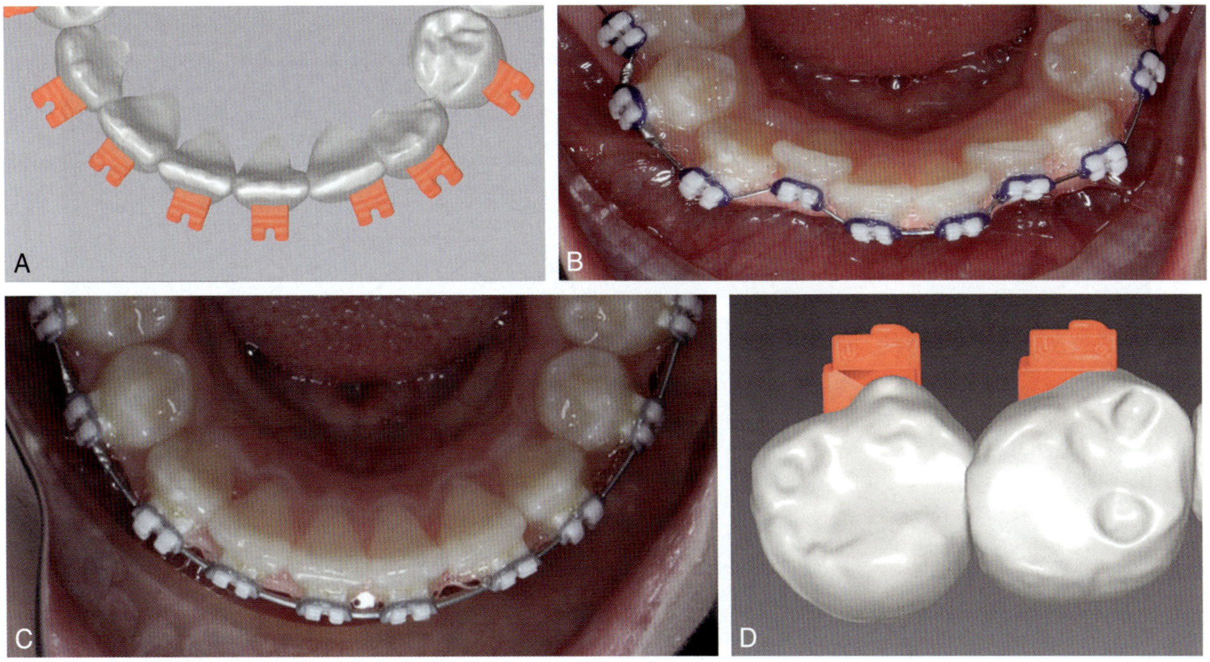

• **Fig. 10.37** More details of the LightForce system shown in Fig. 10.36. (A) An example of the custom digital design of lower incisors brackets—note the distal position designed for the placement of the lower left lateral incisor bracket. (B) The initial bonding and activation of the brackets planned in (A). Note the rotated left lateral incisor which is the reason the bracket was designed to be placed on the available distal facial surface of the tooth. A conventional bracket placed in this location would not allow full derotation of the incisor, but the customized bracket does without placing compensating bends in the archwire (C). The fully customized bracket base allows for easy bracket placement on teeth that can normally be a significant clinical challenge such as the facial surface of an upper second molar that has an extra cusp (D).

the United States, most clinicians in the 1980s abandoned lingual appliances until new versions utilizing more advanced technology were introduced.

One successful German appliance design, Incognito, was purchased by 3M-Unitek in 2012 and widely marketed. It uses a custom precious metal pad for each tooth that covers a large area on the lingual surface. Low-profile brackets designed so the archwire can be inserted easily from the top are attached to the pad. Wire bending is eliminated by using wire-bending robots to form the archwires. This custom lingual system revitalized interest in lingual braces, but the precious metal pads and design process made the system fairly expensive.

A German successor to Incognito (Fig. 10.38) called the WIN appliance uses a different bracket design, 3D printing for production of brackets with precise slots (its first commercial use in orthodontics), and computer-formed archwires. It has been shown to significantly decrease treatment time compared with Incognito,[20] and to compare favorably with Incognito in producing the planned outcomes.[21]

In the United States, the InBrace system reimagined lingual bracket and archwire design to enable tooth movement via programmed non-sliding mechanics rather than traditional sliding mechanics. Its unique patient-specific archwire (shown in Fig. 10.39) allows programmed crown and root movement in all directions, while also allowing engagement into the brackets without additional ligation. This custom archwire and bracket design is digitally setup by the doctor as shown in Fig. 10.40, promising excellent control and efficient clinical outcomes.

A major test for any of the computer-assisted appliance systems is the accuracy with which the planned outcome (established during manufacture of the customized appliance) actually is achieved. A 2011 study, using a new method for analyzing the difference between the computer template and the actual result, showed that Incognito outcomes were quite accurate representations of

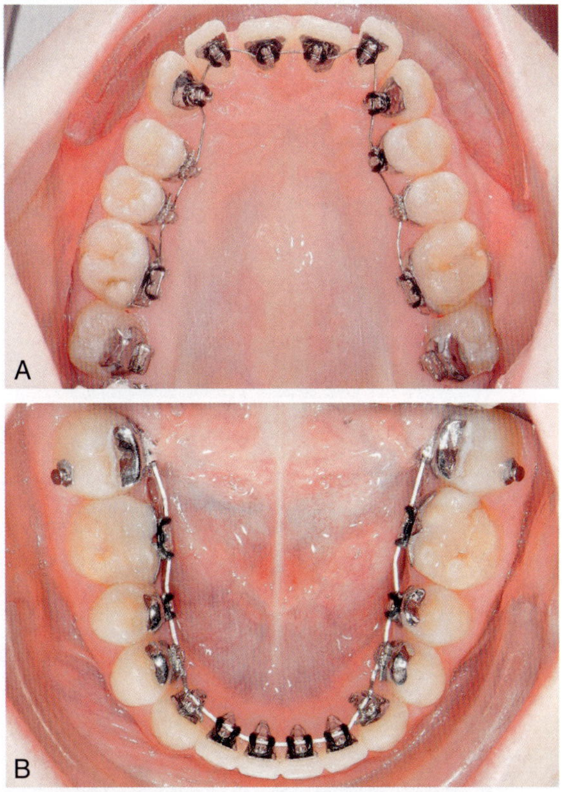

• **Fig. 10.38** The WIN appliance, a successor to an earlier lingual design, uses low-profile metal brackets produced by 3D printing with a proprietary alloy. The greater precision of this technique allows smaller tolerances in bracket slot size. (A) Maxillary arch with a computer-formed nickel-titanium (NiTi) archwire for initial alignment. (B) Mandibular arch with a computer-formed steel toward the end of treatment. Note the bonded attachments on the second molars for Class II attachments and the partial occlusal coverage for better bonding of the molar tube. (Courtesy Dr. D. Wiechmann.)

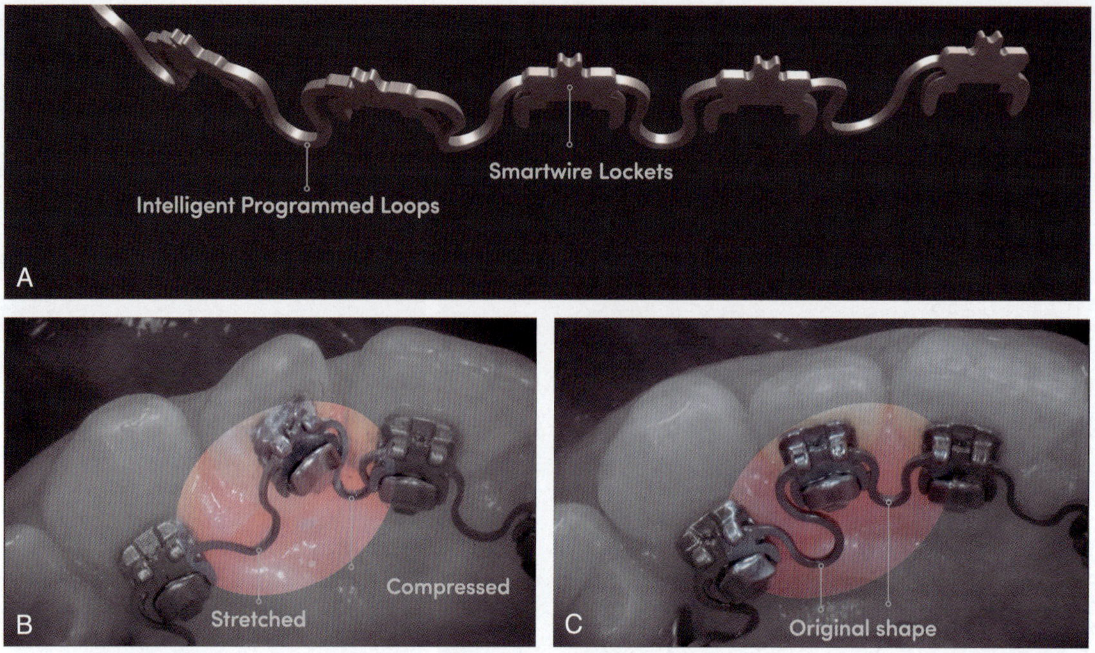

• **Fig. 10.39** A novel lingual fixed appliance system from inbrace. This system uses a customized looped wire that snaps tightly into modified lingual brackets (A). The loops in the wire compensate for the reduced interbracket span that is found on the lingual side of teeth, and the lockets snap into the brackets and eliminate the need for ligation. The precise registration of the lockets into the brackets theoretically allow full expression of the programmed tooth movements by eliminating the typical "slop" between archwire and bracket (B and C).

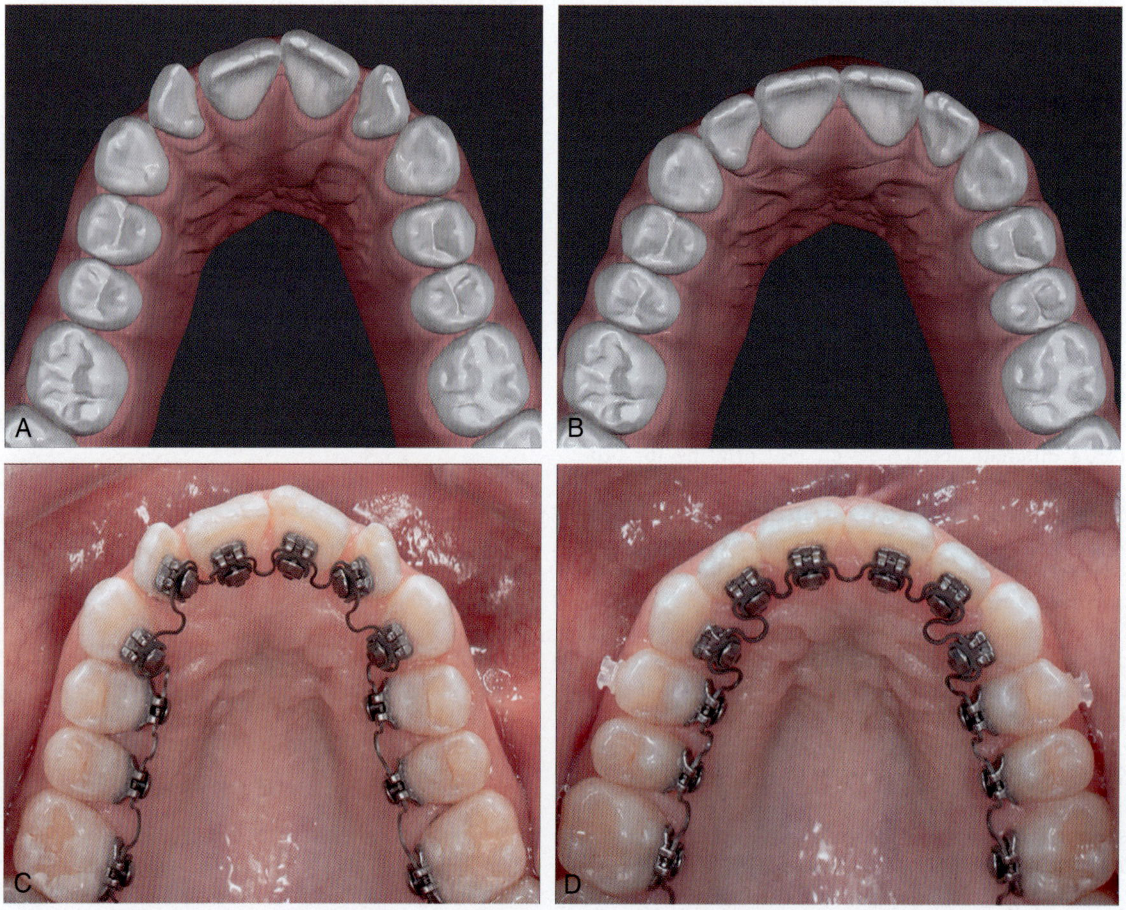

• **Fig. 10.40** The inbrace lingual system mentioned in Fig. 10.39 demonstrated for alignment of a complete maxillary arch. (A) The digital representation of crooked maxillary teeth. (B) The same maxillary arch shown after virtual planning with alignment and space closure. (C) The inbrace appliance inserted into the arch at the start of treatment. (D) The clinical expression of the archwire that was programmed to provide the position shown in (B). Note the ceramic brackets placed on the facial surface of the premolars for use with interarch elastics to correct the occlusion.

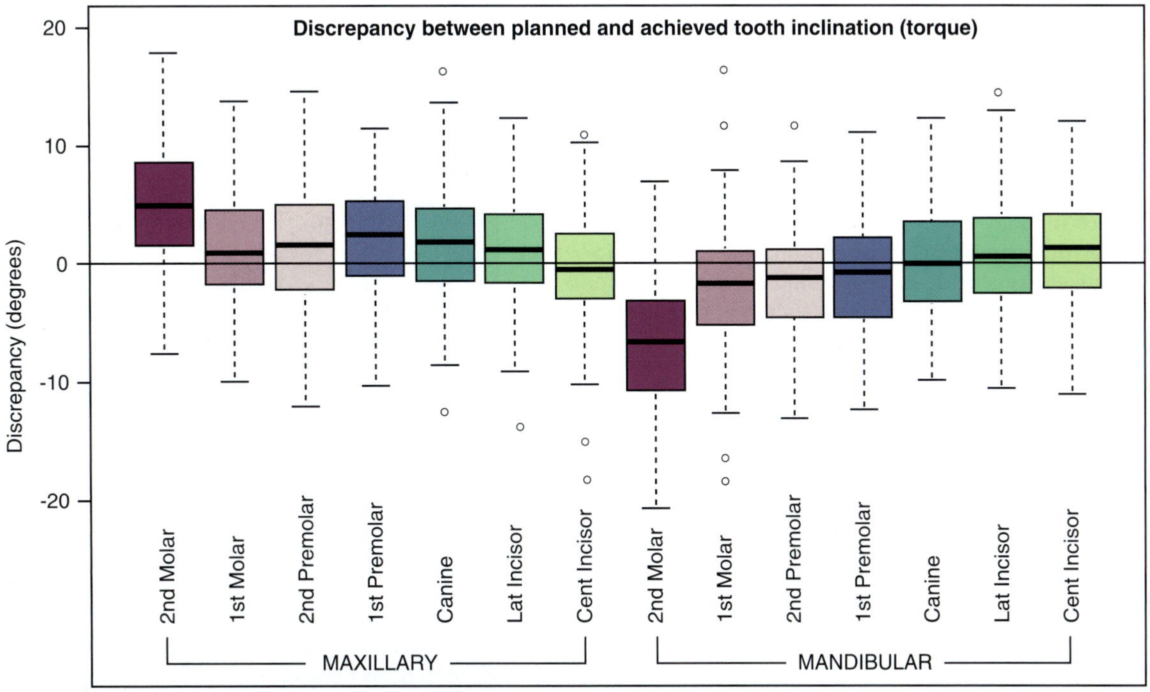

• **Fig. 10.41** Box plots depicting the difference between the planned and achieved inclination (torque) by tooth type in a sample of 94 patients treated using the Incognito lingual appliance (from TopService GMBH, Bad Essen, Germany). Each box shows the median difference from the plan *(dark line)* and the amount of deviation for the median 50% of the patients. Range and extreme outliers are shown by the whiskers and small circles, respectively. Note that for most of the sample and for all teeth except second molars, mean inclination differences were very small and differences of greater than 6 degrees of inclination were rare. (Courtesy Dr. D. Grauer.)

the template, except that second molars were not positioned as precisely as the other teeth (Fig. 10.41).[22] That led to algorithm changes to improve second molar positions. Feedback of that type is needed for all the computer-assisted appliances, both to improve the accuracy of the system and to allow better evaluation of the method.

Making Appliance Choices Based on Patient Preference

There are considerable differences in what patients feel is the most attractive appliance, the one they would prefer to have.[23] Most notably, this is related to patient age, but there are some minor gender differences. For 9- to 11-year-olds, the preference is either shaped brackets such as WildSmiles (WildSmiles Braces, Omaha, NE) with or without colored elastomeric ties, or mini-twin brackets with colored elastomeric ties. Inconspicuous esthetic brackets are not a high priority for this group. In the 12- to 14-year age group, clear aligners and esthetic brackets are more highly prized, but mini-twin brackets with colored ties and the shaped brackets all are rated similarly. Clear aligners rarely are compatible with partially erupted teeth and continuing growth.

For 15- to 17-year-olds, clear aligners or esthetic brackets with a clear wire (see discussion later) are considered most attractive. For this group, clear aligners can make sense because the permanent teeth are fully erupted and rapid growth is completed. Adults prefer lingual appliances, clear aligners, or esthetic brackets, especially when combined with a clear wire. The spectrum changes from unique and colorful for children to esthetic appliances with older adolescents and adults. With this combination of acceptable alternatives, it is possible to meet esthetic demands and accomplish the biomechanics for almost every patient.

Arch Form and Archwire Fabrication

Selection of Arch Form for Individual Patients

Preformed Arch Wires. As another contributor to increased efficiency, preformed archwires are an important part of the modern edgewise appliance, whether individualized custom brackets are used or not. When NiTi and beta-titanium (beta-Ti, sold commercially as TMA) wires are needed, there is no choice but to use preformed archwires because these wires are almost impossible to shape to arch form without special tools. What arch form should be employed?

The concept that dental arch form varies among individuals is driven home to most dentists in full-denture prosthodontics, where it is taught that the dimensions and shape of the dental arches are correlated with the dimensions and shape of the face. The same variations in arch form and dimensions of course exist in the natural dentition, and it is not the goal of orthodontic treatment to produce dental arches of a single ideal size and shape for everyone.

The basic principle of arch form in orthodontic treatment is that within reason, the patient's original arch form should be preserved. Most thoughtful orthodontists have assumed that this would place the teeth in a position of maximum stability, and long-term retention studies support the view that posttreatment changes are greater when arch form is altered than when it is maintained (see Chapter 19).

As a more general guideline, if the maxillary and mandibular arch forms are incompatible at the beginning of treatment, the mandibular arch form should be used as a basic guide. In many patients with Class II malocclusion, the maxillary arch is narrow across the canines and premolars and should be expanded to match the lower arch as overjet is reduced. Obviously, this guideline would not apply when mandibular arch form is distorted. That can happen in many ways, the most common being lingual displacement of the mandibular incisors by habits or heavy lip pressures. Although some judgment is required, the arch form desired at the end of orthodontic treatment should be determined at the beginning, and the patient's occlusal relationships should be established in the context of this arch form.

An excellent mathematical description of the natural dental arch form is provided by a catenary curve, which is the shape that a loop of chain would take if it were suspended from two hooks. The length of the chain and the width between the supports determine the precise shape of the curve. When the width across the first molars is used to establish the posterior attachments, a catenary curve fits the dental arch form of the premolar-canine-incisor segment of the arch very nicely for most individuals. For all patients, the fit is not as good if the catenary curve is extended posteriorly from the first molars, because the dental arch normally curves slightly lingually in the second and third molar region (Fig. 10.42A). When they were first offered, most preformed archwires were based on a catenary curve, with average intermolar dimensions. With this arch form, modifications by the orthodontist to accommodate for a generally more tapering or squarer morphology are appropriate, and the second molars must be "tucked in" slightly.

Another mathematical model of dental arch form, originally advocated by Brader and often called the *Brader arch form*, is based on a trifocal ellipse. Its anterior segment closely approximates the anterior segment of a catenary curve, but the trifocal ellipse gradually constricts posteriorly in a way that the catenary curve does not (Fig. 10.42B). The Brader arch form therefore will more closely approximate the normal position of the second and third molars. It also differs from a catenary curve in producing somewhat greater width across the premolars.

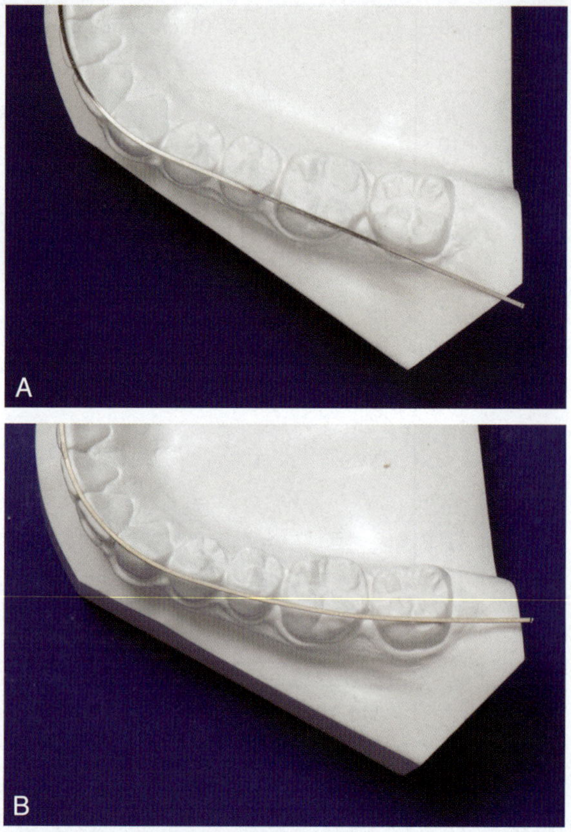

• **Fig. 10.42** (A) Preformed archwire with catenary arch form on a lower dental cast from an untreated patient. Note the good correspondence between the arch form and the line of occlusion, except for the second molars. (B) The Brader arch form for preformed archwires is based on a trifocal ellipse, which slightly rounds the arch in the premolar region compared with a catenary curve and constricts it posteriorly. An archwire formed to the Brader curve fits much better in the second molar region for this untreated patient than a catenary curve.

Recently, several manufacturers have offered preformed archwires that appear to be variations of the Brader arch, with advertisements that suggest these wires are more compatible with arch expansion therapy. Expansion across the premolars often is thought to have esthetic advantages; whether the modified arch form to produce this has any effect on stability is unknown. More refined mathematical descriptions of typical human arch forms have been proposed,[24] and it is likely that better mathematical models will improve the arch forms for preformed archwires in the future.

It is important to keep in mind that neither the ligation method nor the prescription adjustments placed in straight-wire brackets have anything to do with arch form, which is still established by the shape of the archwires. Arch form is particularly important during the finishing stage of treatment, when heavy rectangular archwires are employed. Preformed archwires are best considered as "arch blanks" and are sometimes listed in the catalogs in that way. The name is appropriate, because this properly implies that a degree of individualization of their shape will be required to accommodate the needs of patients.

Wire-Bending Robots. Another approach to the goal of reducing the amount of clinical time spent bending archwires is to use a computer-controlled machine to shape the archwire as desired. If the effort to fabricate a complex archwire were eliminated, inexpensive "plain vanilla" brackets could be used instead of going to the trouble of producing custom brackets with a specific prescription for every tooth. A less complex bracket also could be smaller and have a lower profile.

For labial or lingual orthodontics, SureSmile (OraMetrix, Richardson, TX) uses data acquired via a direct intraoral scan or CBCT to shape finishing archwires to the desired arch form and adjust it at each bracket to provide correct in-out, angulation, and torque bends (Fig. 10.43).

A study done at the University of Minnesota used digital superimposition techniques to carefully compare the actual final tooth position obtained by using the robotically formed archwires versus the predicted and desired position. In general, the final tooth position was remarkably close to what had been prescribed, but there tended to be a lack of full expression of arch form and torque on second molars. As we have noted previously, rectangular superelastic archwires provide lower moments within brackets than are ideal for both tip and torque, and they have less stiffness for arch form control, so it is not surprising that full expression of arch form and terminal torque may not be realized.[25]

Clear Polymer Archwires. Orthodontic archwires formed from clear polymers offer two potential advantages over stainless

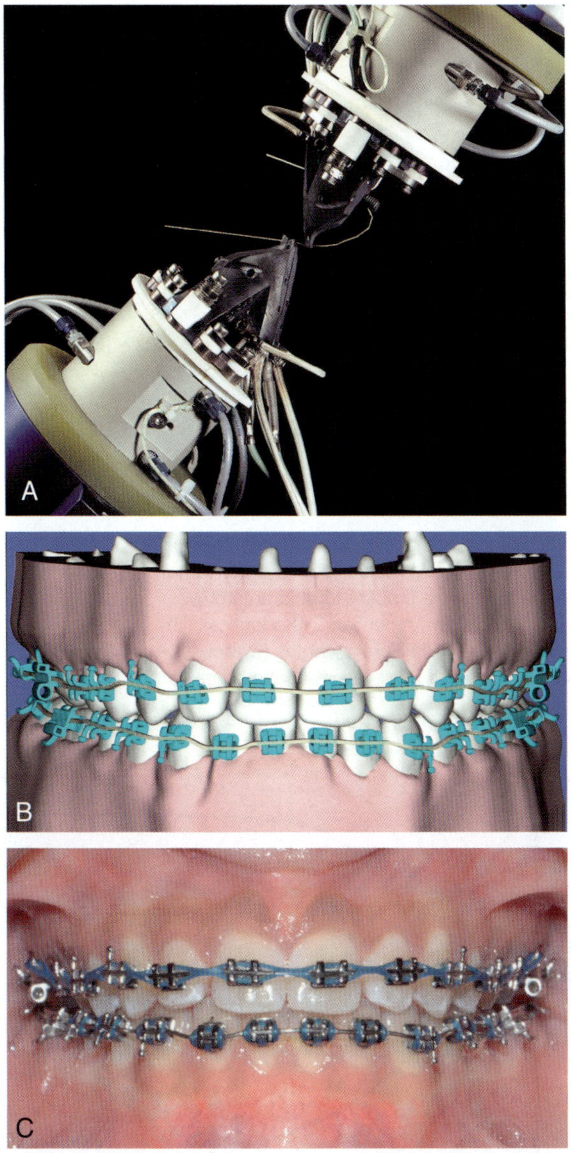

• **Fig. 10.43** Various stages of the SureSmile system, which uses digital technologies for treatment simulation and treatment assistance by robotically bent archwires. (A) A wire-bending robot capable of making the precise bends in a custom wire designed as shown in the following images. (B)The final SureSmile plan in which the teeth are virtually moved into the desired finished position to obtain ideal alignment, root position, and occlusion and the custom wire designed to achieve the final tooth position in the plan. (C) The wire designed in (B) and fabricated by the robot, after placement in the patient's mouth.

steel or titanium: better esthetics because the wire can be clear or the same color as the teeth, so the wire becomes almost invisible when used with ceramic brackets, and physical properties that may equal or exceed those of metal archwires. From 2010 to 2012 they were marketed enthusiastically—and then problems with wire stability and discoloration diminished the enthusiasm to the point that further progress will be needed to make them an acceptable choice in clinical treatment.[26,27]

Coated Archwires. Another option for esthetics is archwires coated with white or more tooth-colored materials. White wires are rated as highly as clear wires by adults. Initially, these coatings were easily lost. More recently the coatings have become better, but their esthetic value still is at risk over time.

At this point, it seems likely that most fixed orthodontic appliances of the not-too-distant future will be individualized with scans of the tooth surfaces and computer technology. It is still too soon to tell which of the competing technologies will prevail. Will it be custom brackets that allow the use of preformed archwires with little or no manual wire bending, custom archwires formed by a wire-bending robot, or a sequence of nonadjustable custom wires produced for that patient? Or something we haven't even thought of yet?

Temporary Anchorage Devices

With the rapid development and commercialization of bone screws and miniplates for orthodontic anchorage devices, there is now a remarkable diversity in these items. The key characteristics of any orthodontic temporary anchorage device (TAD) are (1) its short- and long-term stability, the major indicator of success or failure, and (2) its ease of use, which includes both its placement and the features of the attachment that extends into the oral cavity. The goal here is to discuss what has been learned about desirable and undesirable features of this increasingly important part of the orthodontist's armamentarium.

Bone Screws

A wide variety of bone screws for use as intraoral TADs now are available. It is interesting that use of bone screws now has somewhat declined as clinicians have become more aware of the situations in which they perform well and no longer try to solve almost all problems with them.

A variety of typical screws for use as TADs are shown in Fig. 10.44, and desirable characteristics are summarized in Box 10.1. Although stainless steel screws were marketed initially, most screws are now formed from titanium (purity grades I to IV) to take advantage of its greater biocompatibility. From the perspective of both stability and ease of use, it is now clear that screws for alveolar bone should have different characteristics than screws for the denser bone of the palate or mandible.

Stability

Short-term or primary stability is determined by mechanical retention of the screw in bone, which depends on bone properties, the engineering design of the screw, and placement technique. *Long-term or secondary stability* is defined by the biologic union of the screw to the surrounding bone. It is determined by the implant surface, bone characteristics, and bone turnover (especially in the context of cortical versus medullary bone) and is affected by the implant surface and the mechanical system used. To obtain good secondary stability it is important to limit micromovements that could lead to bone resorption and formation of a fibrous capsule. Over time, primary stability decreases while secondary stability increases; clinical stability is the sum of primary and secondary stability and is the major factor in clinical success (Fig. 10.45).

Factors in stability-related success that have been shown to be important are:

- *The pitch of the screw threads* (i.e., how close the threads are to one another). A tight pitch means the threads are close, a loose pitch means they are farther apart. The denser the bone, the closer the threads should be. It has become apparent that most of a screw's resistance to being dislodged comes from contact

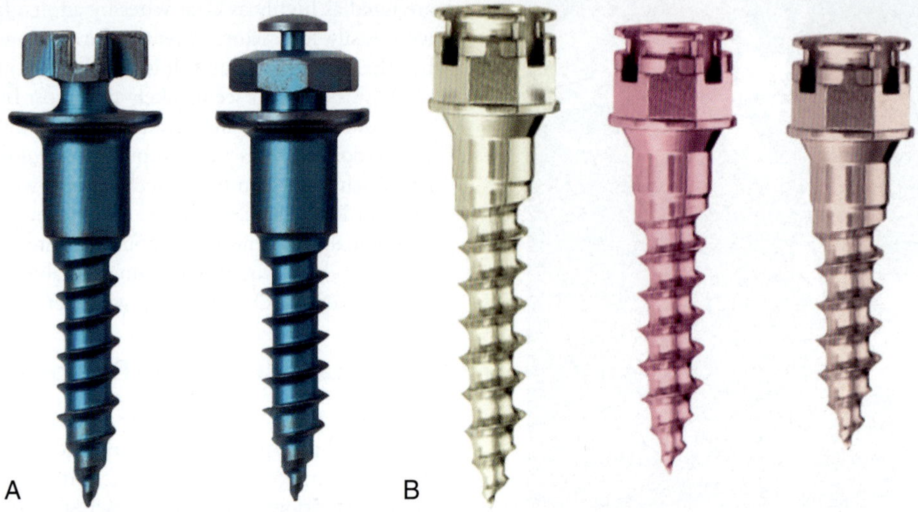

• **Fig. 10.44** Examples of bone screws used as orthodontic temporary anchorage devices (TADs). Different head shapes, different diameters, and different length screws are available. (A) Shows the same diameter and length screw with two different head types—one that is like a bracket to hold an archwire and the second that is a button to attach a spring or elastic (Aarhus system, American Orthodontics). (B) Demonstrates screws with the same head design and diameter, but in three different lengths (Orthoeasy, Forestadent). Optimal length is often determined by the thickness of the soft tissue overlying the bone, so a longer screw may be needed on the palate compared to the alveolus.

• BOX 10.1 Design Factors for Bone Screws

Related to Stability and Success

- Pitch of screw threads: tight, not loose
- Length of screw
  - Alveolar bone, approximately 6 mm
  - Palatal or mandibular bone, approximately 4 mm
  - Base of zygomatic bone, 6 to 8 mm
- Diameter of screw
  - Minimum 1.3 mm
  - Maximum 2.0 mm
- Shape of screw: conical preferred
- Form of tip: thread-cutting preferred
- Bicortical versus monocortical: monocortical preferred
  - Minimal stability advantage for bicortical
  - Decreased ease of use

Related to Ease of Use

- Pilot hole: better if not necessary
- Soft tissue punch: better if not necessary
- Insertion torque: better if low
- Insertion device: better if simple
- Direct versus indirect anchorage: both acceptable

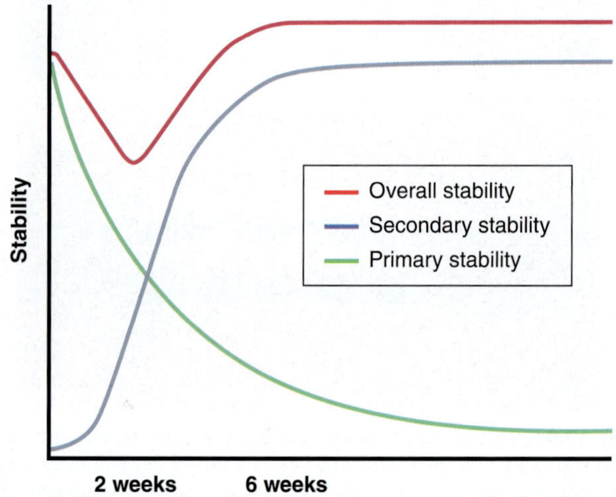

• **Fig. 10.45** Primary stability, which is created by mechanical retention of a bone screw in bone, is maximal immediately after the screw has been placed and declines rapidly as bone remodeling occurs around the screw. Secondary stability, created by a biologic union between the screw and bone, increases over time. Clinical stability is the sum of primary and secondary stability. Note that clinical stability declines to a minimum at about 2 weeks after insertion, then (if all goes well) stabilizes at a somewhat larger value than the initial primary stability at about 6 weeks.

with cortical bone and relatively little from medullary bone. Because the layer of cortical bone is thin in the dental alveolus, a tighter pitch of the threads near the head of the screw gives greater contact with the cortical bone, higher pull-out strength, and better primary stability.[28]

- *The length of the screw.* If the amount of contact with cortical bone is the major factor in stability, and the amount of contact with medullary bone makes little difference, it seems apparent that short screws should perform as well as longer ones. But the amount of soft tissue overlying the bone is an important consideration; screws extending into the base of the zygomatic process need to be longer to reach some cortical bone. A long screw that passes all the way through the alveolus to reach cortical bone on the other side (called a *bicortical screw*) does provide greater stability,[29] but for most applications this is not worth the greater invasiveness.
- *The diameter of the screw.* A screw that is to be placed into the alveolar process must be narrow enough to fit between the teeth. Bone screw TADs currently on the market can be as narrow as 1.3 mm and as wide as 2 mm. The success rate drops when the screw is narrower than 1.3 mm. Within the 1.3- to

2.0-mm diameter range, stability and survival are much more strongly related to the amount of cortical bone contact rather than the screw diameter, but a larger diameter screw does show better primary stability when heavy force is applied.

- *Root proximity.* Root proximity once was thought to have less effect on screw failure. However, recent clinical[30,31] and histological[32] studies have suggested that root proximity is one of the major reasons for screw failure. Studies that evaluated in 2D with dental radiographs[30] and in 3D CBCT[31] have both shown that the distance between the screw and the root was more significantly correlated with screw failure (Fig. 10.46). This tendency was more obvious in the mandible. Histologic studies has indicated that screws contacting adjacent roots resulted in less bone and a greater volume of soft tissue. Therefore, it is important to place screws far from the roots by using screws with smaller diameters and shorter length that have enough resistance to withstand orthodontic forces. Diameters of 1.3 to 1.5 mm and length of 5 to 7 mm are recommended for interradicular areas.[33]
- *The form of the tip.* All orthodontic miniscrews are self-tapping (i.e., they create their own thread as they advance). There are two self-tapping designs: thread-forming and thread-cutting. The difference is the presence of a cutting flute on the tip of the thread-cutting screw. A thread-forming screw compresses the bone around the thread as the screw advances, obtains better bone-to-screw contact, and is better adapted for use with alveolar bone. The flutes on a thread-cutting screw improve penetration into denser bone. It appears that thread-cutting screws perform better in the mandibular ramus, mandibular buccal shelf, zygomatic buttress, and palate.[34]

For a more detailed review of the factors that influence clinical stability and success rates in major tooth movement, see Lee et al.[35]

Ease of Use

For bone screws, ease of use has two components: how easy or difficult it is to place the screw (Fig. 10.47) and how easy it is to use the exposed screw head as an attachment for springs or wires.

Factors in ease of screw placement include:

- *Whether a pilot hole is needed.* Self-drilling screws do not need a pilot hole beyond the cortical plate and can penetrate the cortical plate if it is thin.[36] Screws of this type now have largely replaced screws that require a pilot hole because they can be used either way, with the decision being made at the time of insertion. If the cortical plate is difficult to penetrate, a pilot hole can decrease insertion torque and potential for screw fracture.
- *Whether a tissue punch is needed.* A tissue punch through the gingiva is rarely needed unless a pilot hole is to be drilled but frequently is needed in unattached tissue to keep gingival tissue from wrapping around the screw thread.
- *The ease or difficulty of turning the screw as it is inserted, while keeping pressure on it.* Once the screw threads engage, pressure on it is no longer needed, but strong resistance to turning the screw at that point reflects high insertion torque. This increases primary stability, but it can lead to fracture of the screw, increased microdamage to the bone, and decreased secondary stability. Moderate insertion torque provides enough primary stability without causing excessive bone compression and subsequent remodeling. A driver made to fit around the head of the specific screw type is needed for insertion, and some systems offer a torque-controlled instrument for placement of their bone screws.
- *The design of the area of the head to which a wire, spring, or elastomeric will be attached.* It is desirable to have an attachment that locks this force delivery device in place. A slot in the head that would allow insertion of a heavy wire would make it possible

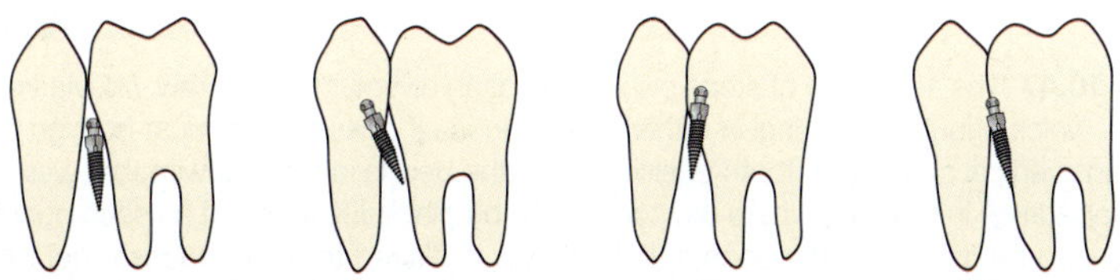

Screw root proximity and successful rate		A Success rate	A n	B Success rate	B n	C Success rate	C n	D Success rate	D n
CT	Maxilla	95.0%	85	80.0%	5	100.0%	1	50.0%*	2
	Mandible	92.0%	25	33.3%*	3	0%*	1	0%*	5
	Total	94.5%	110	62.5%*	8	50.0%*	2	14.3%*	7
Dental	Maxilla	100.0%	37	85.0%*	7	88.9%*	27	91.0%	22
	Mandible	85.7%	14	40.0%	5	88.9%	9	33.3%*†	6
	Total	96.1%	51	66.7%*	12	88.9%	36	78.0%*	28

*p<0.05 vs A, †p<0.05 vs C

• **Fig. 10.46** Success rate of bone screws related to root proximity. Classification of the radiographs from A to D according to the proximity of the miniscrew and the root. (A) The miniscrew was completely separated from the root surface. (B) Only apex of the miniscrew was in contact with the root surface. (C) The neck at alveolar bone level or middle part of the miniscrew was in contact, and the apex was separated from the root surface. (D) The entire body of the miniscrew was in contact with the root surface.

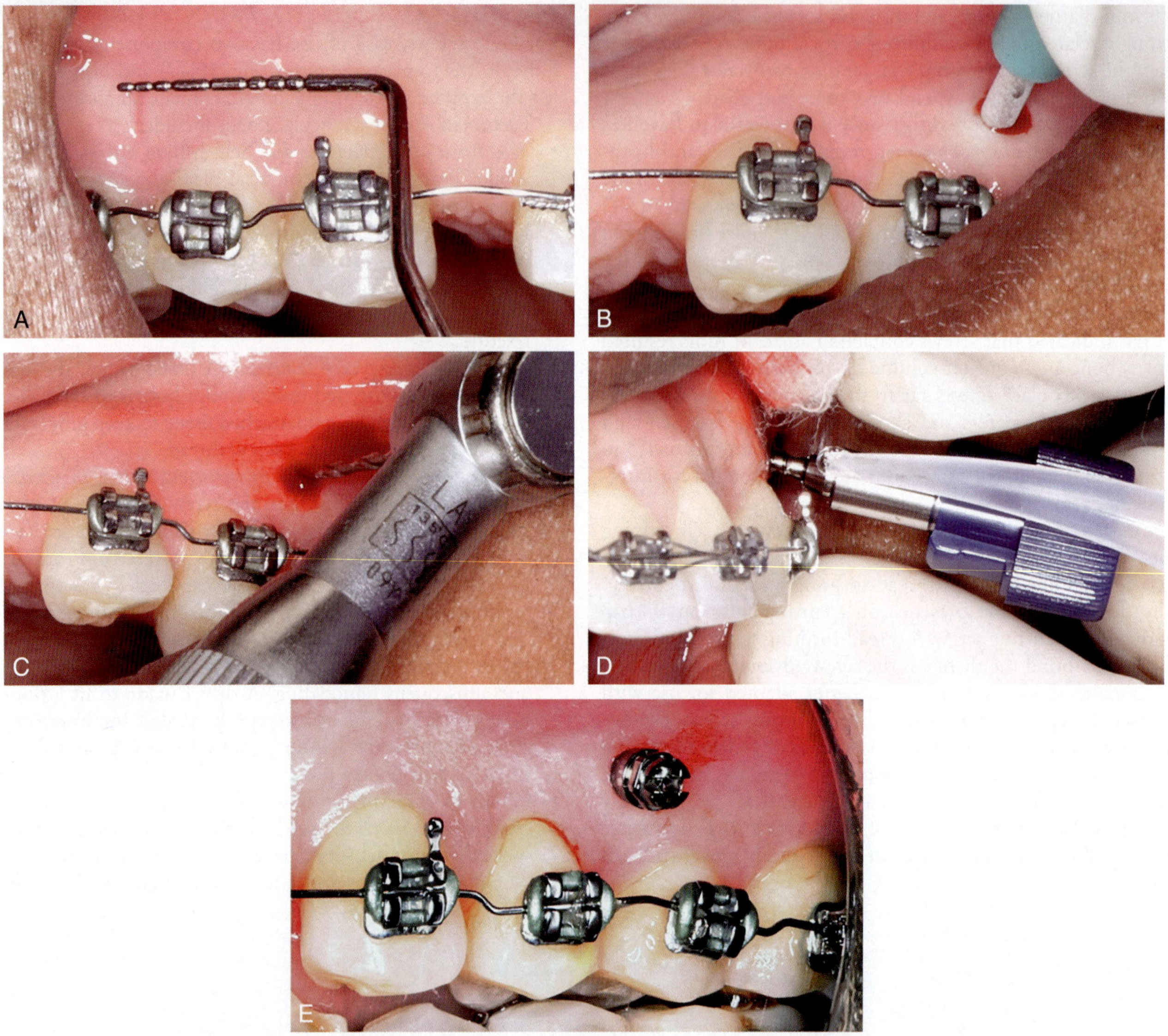

• **Fig. 10.47** The sequence of steps in insertion of an alveolar bone screw. (A) Marking the location for the screw, which should be in gingiva rather than mucosa if possible but must be high enough to accommodate any vertical changes in tooth position. Note the bends in the archwire that were used to create some root separation in the area where the screw is to be placed. (B) Use of a tissue punch, which is needed if a hole is to be drilled into the bone or if the screw is placed through mucosa, but may not be needed for a screw placed through gingiva. (C) Drilling a pilot hole through the cortical plate (which is needed only if the cortical bone is relatively thick). (D) Placing the screw, which will then be screwed into position using a special driver shaped to fit the screw head. (E) The screw in position, ready for use.

to change the direction of force, but the resulting moment is likely to twist or otherwise loosen the screw.

In summary, bone screws can be used readily as either direct or indirect anchorage (Fig. 10.48). The desirable characteristics of a bone screw TAD are listed in Box 10.1. This serves as a guide in selecting the screw for a specific area and use, and suggests that efficient practice requires having more than one type of bone screw available.

Linked Screws in Palatal Anchorage

As we have noted previously, the dense bone of the palate is an excellent place for bone screws, with the greatest bone density found anteriorly and lateral to the midline.[37] Screws in the palate almost always are used in pairs and often are linked together to stabilize a small plate that has attachments to reach the dentition (Fig. 10.49). This linkage of screws offers the same advantage of greater resistance to force as two or more screws holding a miniplate. Linking palatal screws differs from the miniplates discussed hereafter in that the linked attachment usually does not offer the ability to change the direction of force by adding an extension. With palatal anchorage, direct anchorage usually is employed for intrusion of posterior teeth. For repositioning teeth along the line of the arch (as in the maximum retraction space closure shown here), indirect anchorage is the usual choice.

Miniplates

Miniplates have two major components: the plate itself, which is contoured to fit on the surface of the bone where it attached, and

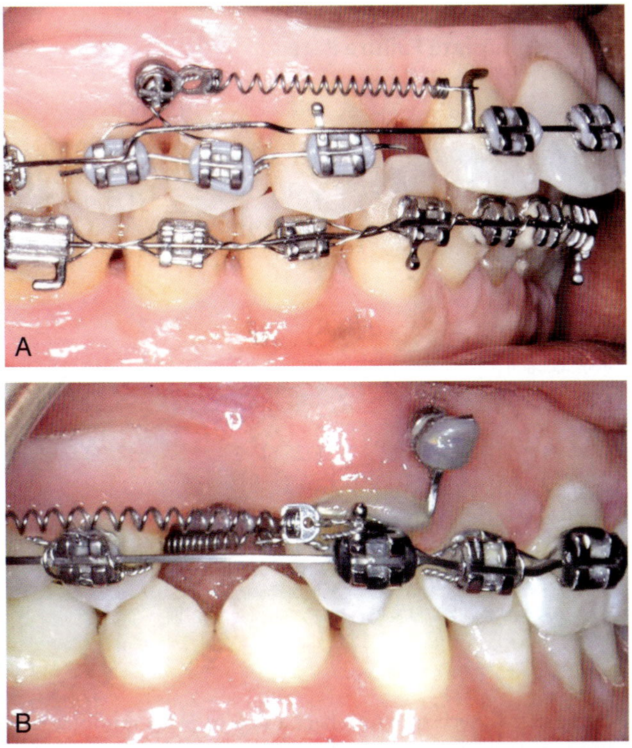

• **Fig. 10.48** (A) An alveolar bone screw used for direct anchorage usually serves as the attachment point for a superelastic nickel-titanium (NiTi) spring, as in this use to retract protruding maxillary incisors. (B) Alveolar bone screws also work well for indirect anchorage, when a rigid attachment from the screw is used to prevent movement of anchor teeth, as in this patient in whom the maxillary posterior teeth are being moved forward via a spring to the stabilized canine.

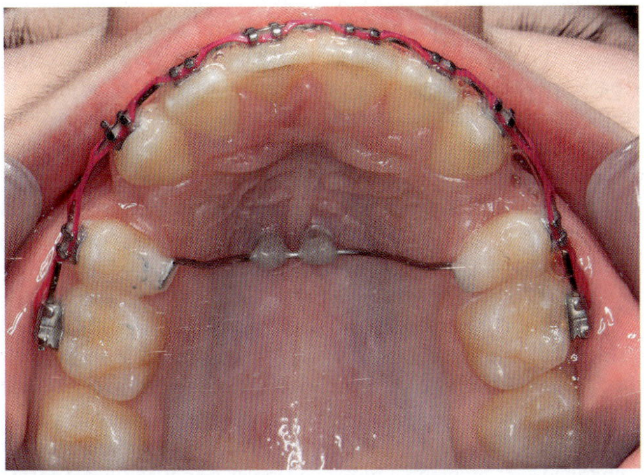

• **Fig. 10.49** Screws in the palate usually are in pairs that are linked by a plate or heavy wire, as shown here. The advantage over using a single screw on each side is that neither screw can rotate when they are tied together, but single screws can rotate, and this greatly increases the chance that the screw will loosen and be lost.

a connector that penetrates into the mouth. Ideally, this is at the junction of the fixed gingival tissue and alveolar mucosa, but the location of the connector is not a critical variable. The connector is designed so that superelastic NiTi springs (or less desirable elastomerics) can be attached to it for direct anchorage, or wires can be attached for indirect anchorage.

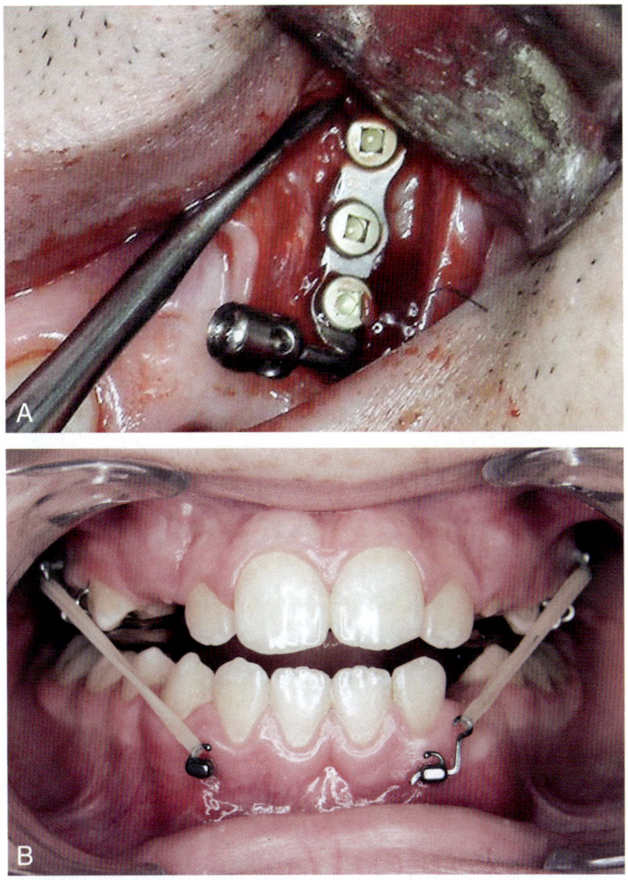

• **Fig. 10.50** (A) A miniplate placed at the base of the zygomatic arch requires creating a flap to expose the bone and must be contoured so it fits closely to the bone surface. In this location it is above the roots of the teeth and is ideally positioned as an anchor for mesiodistal movement of the maxillary teeth. (B) A miniplate on the mandible to serve as an attachment for Class III elastics. Note that a segment of wire has been used on one side to move the attachment point so that the elastic will not impinge on the gingiva. Being able to move the attachment point is a major advantage of using miniplates rather than single screws. (Courtesy Dr. H. DeClerck.)

The most frequent location for miniplates as anchorage for repositioning maxillary teeth vertically or sagittally is at the base of the zygomatic arch (but the linked screws in the palate are used even more often for the same purpose). Anchors in this area combined with anchors on the anterior surface of the mandible below the incisors (Fig. 10.50) also are used for Class III growth modification (as discussed in Chapter 13).

For repositioning multiple mandibular teeth, either bone screws or miniplates are most often placed on the buccal shelf of bone below the lower molars (Fig. 10.51), although the anterior surface of the ramus is an alternate possibility. Miniplates designed for this area are notched so that the vertical component of force direction can be varied.

As with single bone screws, the key characteristics for miniplates are stability and ease of use. The major determinants of stability are:

- The number of screws with which the plate is attached, which really is determined by the bone thickness and density in that area. The success rate for plates of four designs placed by the same clinician at the base of the zygomatic arch is shown in Fig. 10.52. With these designs and with a straight-line plate

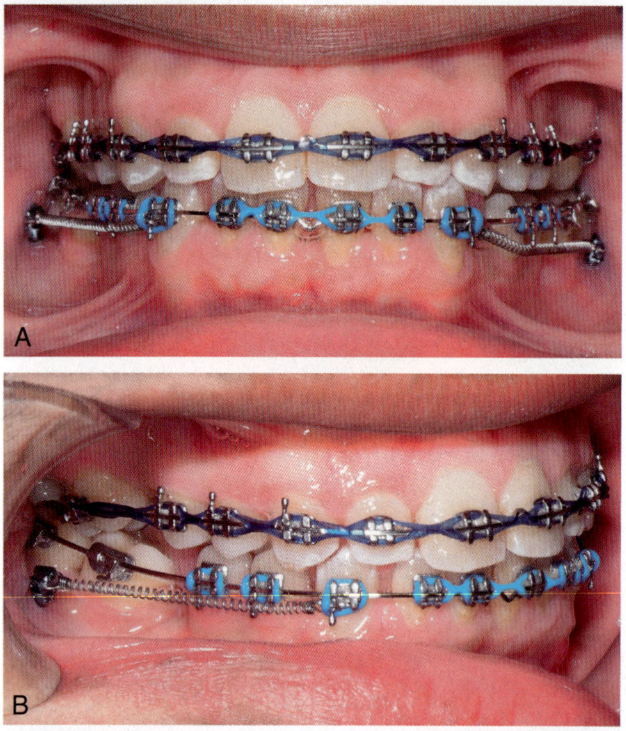

• **Fig. 10.51** A bone screw into the buccal shelf of bone below the mandibular molars provides excellent anchorage for moving or stabilizing mandibular posterior teeth and is easier to use than the anterior surface of the ramus.

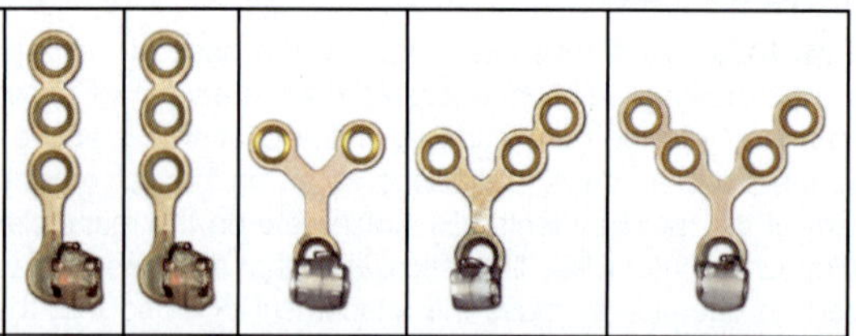

Screw Number	2	3	2	3	4
Success Rate	23/26 88%	11/11 100%	25/26 96%	69/69 100%	20/20 100%

• **Fig. 10.52** Success rates for plates of different designs and number of screws placed at the base of the zygomatic arch by the same clinician. Note that success rates were quite high in all these applications, but failures were more likely with three screws than with two, and no better with four screws than with three—so three screws are preferred. (Courtesy Dr. T. Wu.)

for that area, it appears that three screws provide more stability than two, but nothing additional is gained with four screws. For the palate, two linked screws usually are adequate.

- The age of the patient. As Table 10.4 shows, the number of failures with miniplates at the base of the zygomatic arch or on the anterior mandible in both North Carolina and Belgium was much greater in young patients who had not yet entered puberty. This determines when to use Class III elastics to maxillary and mandibular miniplates (see Chapter 13): bone maturity does not reach the level for good retention of the screws before approximately age 11 (obviously, maturational rather than chronologic age). The denser bone of the mandible and palate is available at somewhat younger ages, but age still is a limitation.

TABLE 10.4 Miniplate Failure Rate

	UNC	UCL
Number of miniplates	59	141
Number of failures	4 (7%)	11 (8%)
Due to mobility	2	5
Soft tissue ulceration	0	4
Anchor breakage	1	2
Poor location	1	0
In growing patients	3 (75%)	8 (73%)
In adults	1 (25%)	3 (27%)
In mandible	NA	6 (56%)

UCL, Université de Catholique de Louvain; *UNC*, University of North Carolina.
Adapted from Cornelis MA, Scheffler NR, Nyssen-Behets C, et al. Patients' and orthodontists' perceptions of miniplates used for temporary skeletal anchorage: a prospective study. *Am J Orthod Dentofac Orthop.* 2008;133(1):18–24.

Because it is necessary to reflect a flap to place miniplates and then suture the soft tissue incision, their surgical placement is significantly more difficult than placement of screws. It is important to contour the miniplates to fit closely against the bone of the base of the zygoma and maintain bone contact at the point of emergence to prevent excessive moments against the proximal screw. As a general rule, orthodontists can place bone screws into alveolar bone quite satisfactorily, but miniplates are better done by those with more extensive surgical training. From the surgeon's perspective, this is a relatively short surgical procedure that can be performed under local anesthesia without significant complications.[38]

Once the plates are in place, however, they are well accepted by patients and providers and are a safe and effective adjunct for complex orthodontic treatment.[39] They are as easy for the orthodontist to use as alveolar TADs. Compared with individual alveolar screws, miniplates have three major advantages:

- The amount of force that the miniplate can tolerate is significantly larger because the plate is held by multiple screws and usually is placed in an area with thicker cortical bone.
- If the miniplate connector has a locking mechanism (as it should), the direction of pull can be changed readily and the source of the force can be moved a considerable distance by extending wire hooks from end of the connector (Fig. 10.53; also see Fig. 10.50). With the vertical posts that are part of the mandibular buccal shelf plate, the angle of force can be changed just by using a higher or lower notch to tie the spring. This also can be done with individual screws that have a slot for a wire extension, but as we noted earlier, putting a force on the extension introduces a moment that can overtighten or loosen the screw, greatly increasing the chance of screw failure. With multiple screws holding the miniplate, this is not a problem.
- The miniplates can be placed well above the roots of the maxillary teeth, so an interdental screw does not become a barrier to moving all the teeth mesially or distally.

In comparing alveolar bone screws with miniplates (Table 10.5), a reasonable conclusion is that individual screws are less invasive and are indicated wherever they can provide adequate anchorage. This is the case when a few teeth need to be repositioned. A long

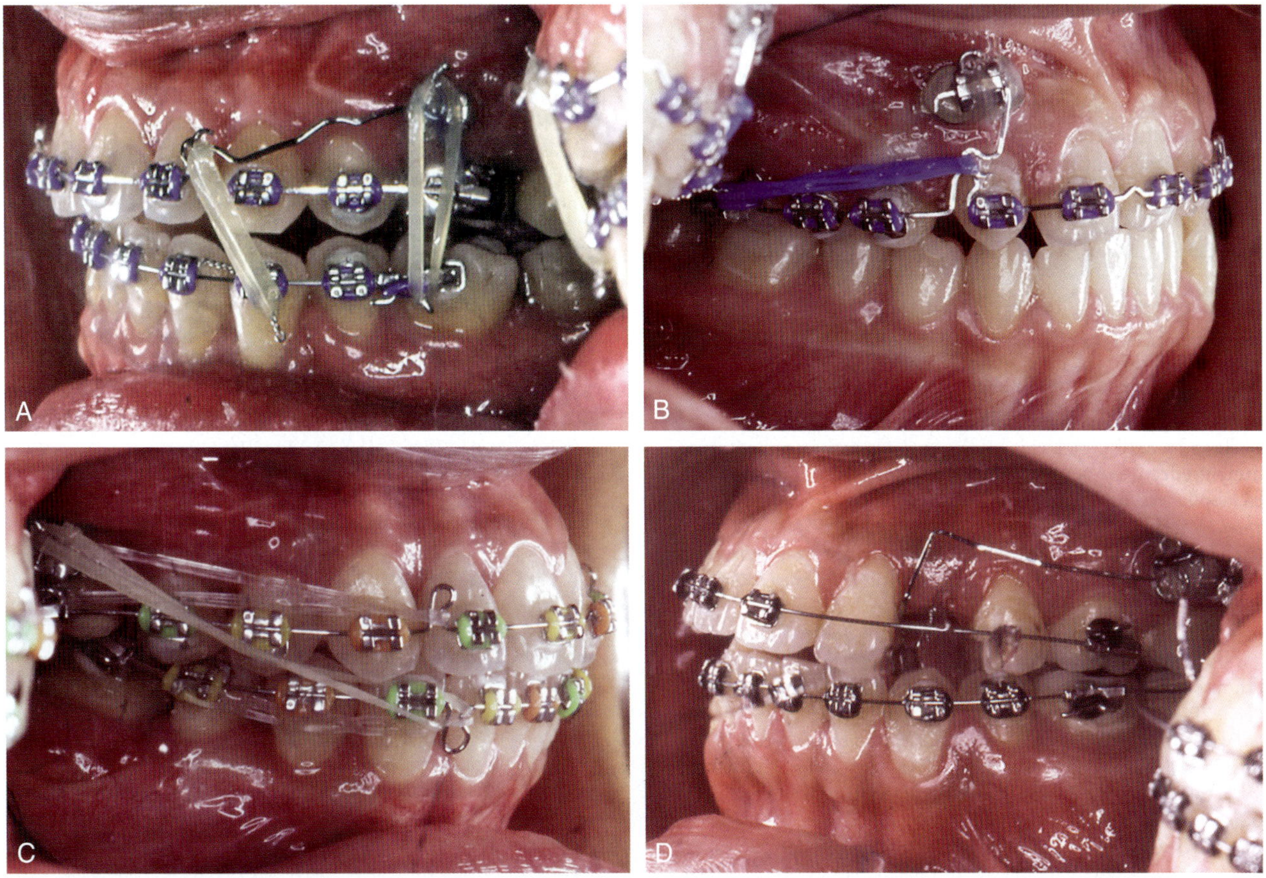

• **Fig. 10.53** (A) to (D) A variety of attachment points can be created with wire extensions from miniplate connectors, as illustrated in this series of variations in force directions using miniplates in the same location at the base of the zygoma. (Courtesy Dr. T. Wu.)

TABLE 10.5 Bone Screws Versus Miniplates

Single Alveolar Screws	Palatal Screws Linked by Plate	Maxillary or Mandibular Miniplates
Advantages		
Less invasive, lower cost	Excellent stability and resistance	Excellent stability and resistance
Orthodontist can place and remove	Orthodontist can place and remove	Can be placed above and below roots to allow en masse movement
Multiple sites for placement	Useful for vertical and anteroposterior movements	Useful for vertical and anteroposterior movements
		Easy to activate unilaterally
		well tolerated during therapy
Disadvantages		
Limited anchorage amount, move one or two teeth but not more	Framework in palate can be difficult for patient to tolerate	Experienced surgeon needed, not for typical orthodontist
No way to alter force direction without risk of losing screw	Bilateral screws needed	Surgery to place and remove
Vertical movement limited	Moderately difficult placement	Cost of surgery and device
Major Indications for Use		
Repositioning or rotating single teeth	Indirect anchorage primarily, for retracting protrusive incisors	Direct anchorage primarily, for retraction and/or intrusion of incisors
Bringing impacted canine(s) into the arch while preserving arch form	Indirect anchorage for intrusion of posterior teeth	Direct anchorage for intrusion of posterior teeth
	Indirect anchorage to bring posterior teeth forward	Direct anchorage for skeletal Class III growth modification

screw at the base of the alveolar arch can be used if intrusion of maxillary posterior teeth (which requires light force) is desired (see Chapter 20), and shorter screws in the palate also can be used for maxillary posterior intrusion. For more complex and extensive movement of multiple teeth, with distalization of an entire dental arch being the best example, miniplates offer better control and are less likely to loosen or need to be replaced.

References

1. Pancherz H. Treatment of Class II malocclusions by jumping the bite with the Herbst appliance: a cephalometric investigation. *Am J Orthod.* 1979;76:423–442.
2. Sheridan JJ, Armbruster P, Nguyen P, et al. Tooth movement with Essix molding. *J Clin Orthod.* 2004;38:435–441.
3. Gu J, Tang JS, Skulski B, Fields Jr HW, et al. Evaluation of Invisalign treatment effectiveness and efficiency compared with conventional fixed appliances using the Peer Assessment Rating Index. *Am J Orthod Dentofacial Orthop.* 2017;151:259–266.
4. Chen YJ, Chan LY, Chung-Chen JY. Clear aligner treatment with "in-office" virtual model set-up and 3D printing. *J Dent Oral Care.* 2017;3:1–5.
5. Begg PR, Kesling PC. *Begg Orthodontic Theory and Technique.* 3rd ed. WB Saunders; 1977.
6. Parkhouse RC. Current products and practice: Tip-Edge Plus. *Int J Orthod.* 2008;19:17–24.
7. Andrews LF. *Straight Wire: The Concept and Appliance.* LA Wells; 1989.
8. Hobson RS, Rugg-Gunn AJ, Booth TA. Acid etch patterns on the buccal surface of human permanent teeth. *Arch Oral Biol.* 2002;47:407–412.
9. Finnema KJ, Ozcan M, Post WJ, et al. In vitro orthodontic bond strength testing: a systematic review and meta-analysis. *Am J Orthod Dentofacial Orthop.* 2010;137:615–622.
10. Al-Saleh M, El-Mowafy O. Bond strength of orthodontic brackets with new self-adhesive resin cements. *Am J Orthod Dentofacial Orthop.* 2010;137:528–533.
11. Maryanchik I, Brendlinger EJ, Fallis DW, Vandewalle KS. Shear bond strength of orthodontic brackets bonded to various esthetic pontic materials. *Am J Orthod Dentofacial Orthop.* 2010;137:684–689.
12. Justus R, Cubero T, Ondarza R, et al. A new technique with sodium hypochlorite to increase bracket shear bond strength of fluoride-releasing resin-modified glass ionomer cements: comparing shear bond strength of two adhesive systems with enamel surface deproteinization before etching. *Semin Orthod.* 2010;16:66–75.
13. Nichols DA, Gardner G, Carballeyra AD. Reproducibility of bracket positioning in the indirect bonding technique. *Am J Orthod Dentofacial Orthop.* 2013;144:770–776.
14. Grunheid T, Lee M, Larson BE. Transfer accuracy of vinyl polysiloxane trays for indirect bonding. *Angle Orthod.* 2016;86:468–474.
15. Feldon PJ, Murray PE, Burch JG, et al. Diode laser debonding of ceramic brackets. *Am J Orthod Dentofacial Orthop.* 2010;138:458–462.
16. Lombardo L, Arreghini A, Bratti E, et al. Comparative analysis of real and ideal wire-slot play in square and rectangular archwires. *Angle Orthod.* 2015;85:848–858.
17. Marshall SD, Currier GF, Hatch NE, et al. Self-ligating bracket claims. *Am J Orthod Dentofacial Orthop.* 2010;138:128–131.
18. A. Grünheid T, Kirk DC, Larson BE. The effect of root and bone visualization on perceptions of the quality of orthodontic treatment simulations. *Angle Orthod.* 2017;87(3):384–390. https://doi.org/10.2319/082416-634.1. Epub 2016 Nov 22. PMID: 27874283; PMCID: PMC8381983.
19. Brown MW, Koroluk L, Ko C-C, et al. Effectiveness and efficiency of a CAD/CAM orthodontic bracket system. *Am J Orthod Dentofacial Orthop.* 2015;148:1067–1074.
20. Grauer D, Proffit WR. Accuracy in tooth positioning with fully customized lingual orthodontic appliances. *Am J Orthod Dentofacial Orthop.* 2011;140:433–443.
21. Knosel M, Klang E, Helms H-J, Wiechmann D. Lingual orthodontic treatment duration: performance of two different completely customized multi-bracket appliances (Incognito and WIN) in groups with different treatment complexities. *Head Face Med.* 2014;10:46. http://www.head-face-med.com/content/10/1/46.
22. Pauls A, Nienkemper M, Schwestka-Polly R, Wiechmann D. Therapeutic accuracy of the completely customized lingual appliance WIN: a retrospective cohort study. *J Orofac Orthop.* 2017;78:52–61.
23. Walton D, Fields HW, Johnston WM, et al. Orthodontic appliance preferences of children and adolescents. *Am J Orthod Dentofacial Orthop.* 2010;138:698. e1–698.e12.
24. Braun S, Hnat WH, Fender WE, et al. The form of the human dental arch. *Angle Orthod.* 1998;68:29–36.
25. Larson BE, Vaubel CJ, Grunheid T. Effectiveness of computer-assisted orthodontic treatment technology to achieve predicted outcomes. *Angle Orthod.* 2013;83:557–562.
26. Chang J-H, Berzins DW, Pruszynski JE, Ballard RW. The effect of water storage on the bending properties of esthetic, fiber-reinforced composite orthodontic archwires. *Angle Orthod.* 2014;84:417–423.
27. da Silva DL, Mattos CT, de Araujo MCA, et al. Color stability and fluorescence of different orthodontic esthetic archwires. *Angle Orthod.* 2013;83:127–132.
28. Brinley CL, Behrents R, Kim KB, et al. Pitch and longitudinal fluting effects on the primary stability of miniscrew implants. *Angle Orthod.* 2009;79:1156–1161.
29. Chatzigianni A, Keilig L, Reimann S, et al. Effect of mini-implant length and diameter on primary stability under loading with two force levels. *Eur J Orthod.* 2011;33:381–387.
30. Kuroda S, Yamada K, Deguchi T, Hashimoto T, Kyung HM, Takano-Yamamoto T. Root proximity is a major factor for screw failure in orthodontic anchorage. *Am J Orthod Dentofacial Orthop.* 2007;131(4 Suppl):S68–73.
31. Watanabe H, Deguchi T, Hasegawa M, Ito M, Kim S, Takano-Yamamoto T. Orthodontic miniscrew failure rate and root proximity, insertion angle, bone contact length, and bone density. *Orthod Craniofac Res.* 2013 Feb;16(1):44–55.
32. Chen YH, Chang HH, Chen YJ, Lee D, Chiang HH, Yao CC. Root contact during insertion of miniscrews for orthodontic anchorage increases the failure rate: an animal study. *Clin Oral Implants Res.* 2008 Jan;19(1):99–106.
33. Suzuki M, Deguchi T, Watanabe H, Seiryu M, Iikubo M, Sasano T, Fujiyama K, Takano-Yamamoto T. Evaluation of optimal length and insertion torque for miniscrews. *Am J Orthod Dentofacial Orthop.* 2013 Aug;144(2):251–259.
34. Rodriguez JC, Suarez F, Chan H, et al. Implants for orthodontic anchorage: success rates and reasons for failures. *Implant Dent.* 2014;23:155–161.
35. Lee JS, Kim JK, Park YC. Biomechanical considerations with temporary anchorage devices. In: Graber LW, Vanarsdall RL, Vig KWL, Huang GJ, eds. *Orthodontics: Current Principles and Techniques.* 6th ed. Elsevier; 2016:511–568. [Chapter 20].
36. Baumgaertel S. Predrilling of the implant site: is it necessary for orthodontic mini-implants? *Am J Orthod Dentofacial Orthop.* 2010;137:825–829.
37. Holm M, Jost-Brinkmann P-G, Mah J, Bumann A. Bone thickness of the anterior palate for orthodontic miniscrews. *Angle Orthod.* 2016;86:826–831.
38. Cornelis MA, Scheffler NR, Nyssen-Behets C, et al. Patients' and orthodontists' perceptions of miniplates used for temporary skeletal anchorage: a prospective study. *Am J Orthod Dentofacial Orthop.* 2008;133:18–24.
39. Cornelis MA, Scheffler NR, Mahy P, et al. Modified miniplates for temporary skeletal anchorage in orthodontics: placement and removal surgeries. *J Oral Maxillofac Surg.* 2008;66:1439–1445.

SECTION 4

Treatment in Preadolescent Children: What Is Different?

Orthodontic treatment rarely is done in the primary dentition, for three reasons: (1) At some point, movement of primary incisors and canines is likely to lead to accelerated root resorption and premature loss of primary teeth; (2) movement of some of the primary teeth has little effect on where the permanent teeth erupt; and (3) growth modification effects in young children are lost to a resumption of growth in the original pattern. That means there usually is little benefit and some risk from primary dentition treatment, usually called *very early treatment*.

That changes as the permanent incisors erupt and the patient enters the mixed dentition, when a first phase of what usually is called *early treatment* definitely should be done in some situations. This treatment can be beneficial even though a second phase of comprehensive treatment that will be completed during adolescence usually is needed. Among the important points when early treatment is considered are the following.

Focus on "should be done" and obvious treatment. Early treatment will be truly beneficial to the patient when the proposed treatments have proven benefits. For instance, patients who are in the mid- or late-mixed dentition with unerupted incisors have obvious esthetic and dental development problems. This clearly falls into the "should be done" category because good data show that delaying treatment is likely to make things worse. On the other hand, 10 mm of crowding will not resolve itself whether or not a lingual arch is placed in the mixed dentition, and requires more definitive decision-making with long-term consequences. Given a mixed dentition child with dental and facial problems, is it wise to start treatment now for this patient? The child's age and behavior, the family and social situation, and the time commitment and cost must be factored into the decision. This is an age group that has unique psychosocial needs due to teasing and bullying, so esthetics may make crooked front teeth a "should be done" problem. Likewise, trauma risk due to protrusive upper incisor and lip incompetence may be another critical problem not seen in other age groups. The treatment must meet the patient's needs, now.

The goals of early treatment must be clearly outlined and understood. For a child with a complex problem, it is highly likely that a second stage of treatment in the early permanent dentition will be required even if early treatment is carried out effectively and properly (Fig. IV.1). There is a limit to the time and cooperation that patients and parents are willing to devote to orthodontics. Unless appropriate endpoints are set in advance, it is easy for mixed dentition treatment to extend over several years and result in an extremely long period of treatment instead of defined treatment segments that are more advantageous. If mixed dentition treatment takes too long, there are two problems: (1) Patients can be "burned out" by the time they are ready for comprehensive treatment in the early permanent dentition and (2) the chance of damage to the teeth and supporting structures increases as treatment time increases.

This means that diagnosis and treatment planning are just as demanding and important as in comprehensive treatment. Adequate records, a comprehensive examination, a prioritized problems list with positive attributes noted and treatment goals are all required. If the treatment goals are not clear, setting appropriate endpoints will be impossible. In early treatment, all aspects of the occlusion usually are not modified to ideal or near ideal. Final tooth and root positions are not required in most cases unless this is all the treatment the child will ever encounter—a prediction that is hard to make.

In mixed dentition treatment with a partial fixed appliance, there simply are fewer options available. This is mostly due to the transition of the teeth from the primary to permanent dentition—primary molars with resorbing roots are not good candidates for banding or

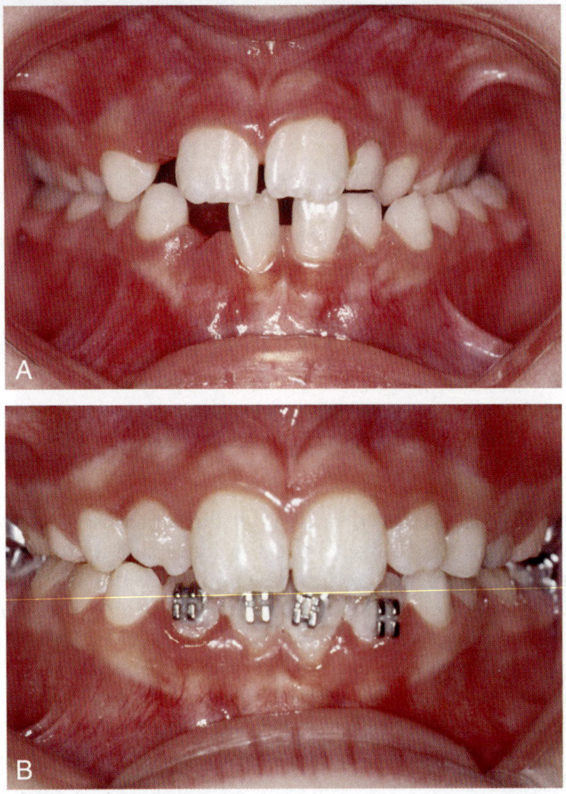

• **Fig. IV.1** Limited treatment in the mixed dentition requires specific objectives but does not require comprehensive objectives. (A) This patient has lower incisor spacing and a posterior crossbite. Both were addressed in the first phase of treatment, but (B) detailed tooth positioning was not attempted (and generally is not required in mixed dentition treatment) because additional teeth will erupt and cause potential problems.

bonding. Immature patients with poor compliance can complicate the problems related to a partial appliance. It is true that numerous fixed correctors are now available that appear to reduce some of the patient compliance variables. So, if a patient will not or does not want to wear a headgear or elastics other appliances can be used, but these types of options are not always available in the mixed dentition. It is still mandatory that certain teeth are available for appliance placement and anchorage. Changing to a different appliance may also change what outcomes can be attained.

In the permanent dentition, full appliances allow more flexibility, and temporary anchorage devices (TADs) can provide more substantial skeletal anchorage. Although some of these options also require cooperation, they often allow immediate adjustment of the treatment approach so it can be completed in an acceptable manner. With a partial appliance and potential compliance problems, the full range of options is just not there.

There are important biomechanical differences between complete and partial appliances. The typical fixed appliance for mixed dentition treatment is a "2 × 4" or "2 × 6" arrangement (2 molar bands, 4 or 6 bonded anterior teeth; Fig. IV.2). When a fixed appliance includes only some of the teeth, archwire spans are longer, large moments are easy to create, and the range of the wires is increased. But, the wires themselves are less stiff and less strong. This can lead to displaced or broken appliances, or to appliances that irritate the soft tissue.

Sometimes only segments of wires are used, like from a maxillary right primary canine to the maxillary left primary canine and including the permanent incisors. When posterior teeth are not

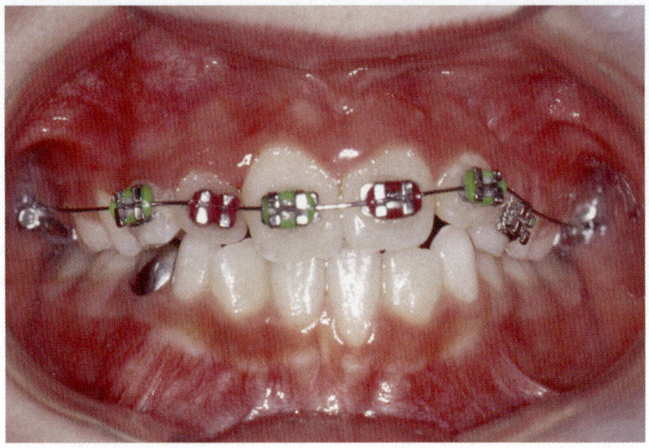

• **Fig. IV.2** This patient has a "2 × 6" appliance in place that includes two molars and six anterior teeth. The "2 × 4" appliance includes two molars and four anterior teeth. This is a typical appliance for the mixed dentition and can include both primary and permanent teeth.

included, it is easy to lose control of arch form and coordination. This is especially true with preformed archwires that are not the appropriate size and configuration.

On the other hand, limited appliances can provide some biomechanical advantages. For example, intrusion of teeth is easier with long spans of wire that keep forces light and allow the appropriate moments to be generated. There is little indication for use of the newer superelastic wires when long unsupported spans exist. Wires with intermediate flexibility and looped configurations or the use of a heavy base wire and a "piggyback" flexible wire are easier to control. Because the available permanent teeth are grouped in anterior (incisor) and posterior (molar) segments, a segmented arch approach to mechanics often is required. The apparently simple fixed appliances used in the mixed dentition can be quite complex to use appropriately. They are better described as deceptively simple.

Anchorage control is both more difficult and more critical. With only the first molars continuously available as anchorage in the posterior segment of the arch, there are limits to the amount of tooth movement that should be attempted in the mixed dentition. Extraoral support from headgear or facemasks can be used, but implant-supported anchorage usually is not practical because of the presence of unerupted teeth and immature bone. The reciprocal effects of an intrusion arch or molar distalizing appliance are accentuated by this reduced anchorage. Stabilizing maxillary and mandibular lingual arches are more likely to be necessary as an adjunct to anchorage.

Beware of unerupted, missing and supernumerary teeth. Although radiographic images of the developing dentition are obtained routinely when early treatment is considered, the effect of tooth movement on unerupted teeth is often overlooked. This is a particular risk when moving lateral incisors that are adjacent to unerupted canines. Care must be taken so that the roots of the lateral incisors are not inadvertently tipped into the path of the erupting canines. Failure to pay attention to this can lead to resorption of considerable portions of the lateral incisor root (Fig. IV.3). It is also wise to make certain that unerupted teeth are present. Discovering their absence at a later time can dramatically alter the course and direction of treatment. Finally, it is important to count the teeth to make certain there are not missing, or extra ones. Five incisors look alot like 4 incisors, but they make a bad occlusion.

Space closure must be managed with particular care. Otherwise, when all teeth are not banded or bonded, the teeth

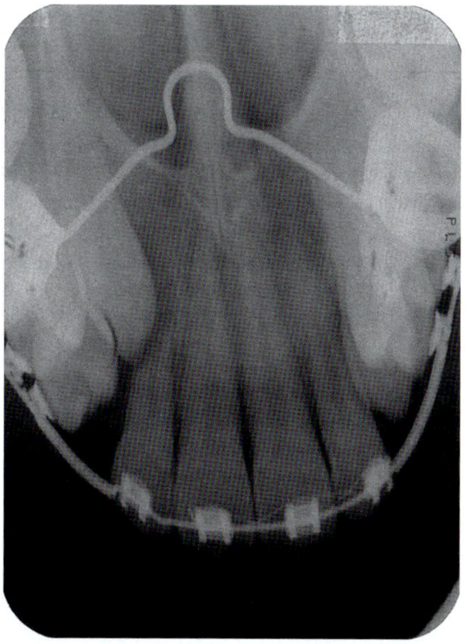

• Fig. IV.3 This patient has resorption of the maxillary right lateral incisor before eruption of the maxillary right canine with appliances in place. This can occur if the canine position is more mesial than normal or, less frequently, the lateral incisor has excessive distal root tip. Early treatment definitely is indicated because the root resorption will get worse if the canine is not repositioned.

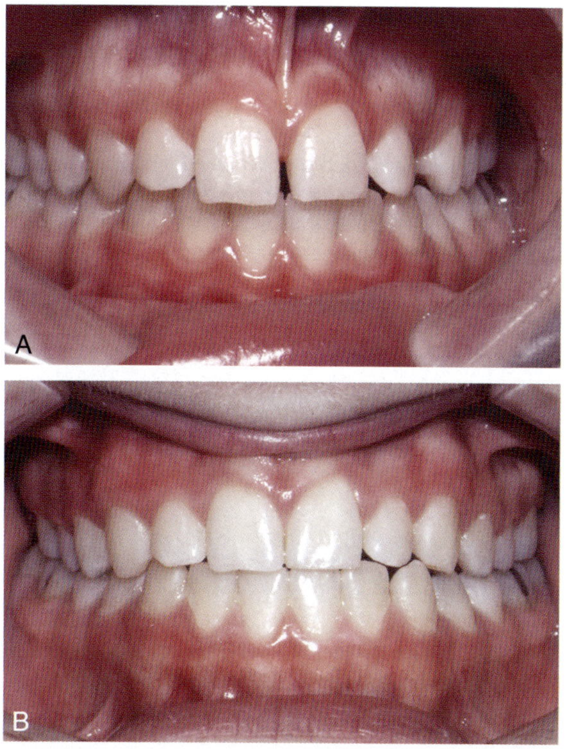

• Fig. IV.4 This shows the limitations of not using interarch mechanics for limited treatment. (A) This patient had limited overbite on the left side where an impacted canine was located, and (B) still has limited overbite after extrusion of the canine because appliances were used only on the maxillary arch, so no interarch vertical elastics could be used.

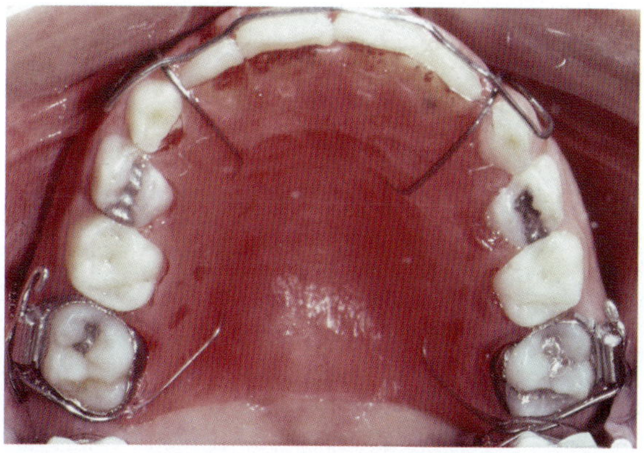

• Fig. IV.5 When retention is used between early (phase 1) and later (phase 2) treatment, creative planning of bow and clasp positions is required to avoid interference with erupting teeth and maintain the effectiveness of clasps. Note that the labial bow crosses the occlusion distal to the lateral incisors rather than in the area where the canines will erupt, and the molar clasps adapt to the bands and headgear tubes.

without attachments will tend to be displaced and squeezed out of the arch. Teeth without attachments may move facially or lingually, or in some instances occlusally. Unanticipated side effects of space closure that would not be encountered with a complete fixed appliance often are a problem in mixed dentition treatment.

Interarch mechanics must be used sparingly, if at all. The side effects of Class II, Class III, or vertical elastics, such as widening or constriction of the dental arches and alteration of the occlusal plane, make them risky with partial fixed appliances and lighter wires like the typical mixed dentition 2 × 4 arrangement. Interarch forces are not recommended under most circumstances unless a complete fixed appliance or heavy stabilizing lingual or buccal wire is present. This also subjects the treatment result to the limitations of not using interarch mechanics (Fig. IV.4). There is one exception: Cross-elastics can be used in the mixed dentition in the treatment of unilateral crossbite, but these teeth can be extruded.

If early treatment is carried out in only one dental arch, the final result is dictated by the untreated teeth and arch. For instance, if the lower arch is not ideally aligned, it will be difficult to ideally align the upper arch and have proper coordination of the teeth without interferences. Likewise, if there is a substantial curve of Spee in the lower arch and only the upper arch is leveled, the overbite and overjet will be excessive. Despite this, early treatment in only one arch, and the interim nonideal tooth positions, can be quite acceptable if the remainder of the total correction is to be accomplished later.

Retention often is needed between mixed dentition treatment and eruption of the permanent teeth. After any significant tooth movement or skeletal change, it is important to maintain the teeth or bone in their new position until a condition of stability is reached. This is as true in the mixed dentition as later. In fact, overcorrection and careful retention may be even more necessary after early treatment. The final stage of transition from the mixed to the permanent dentition is a particularly unstable time. For instance, mesial drift of molars that shortens arch length normally occurs then, but this must be prevented if arch expansion was the goal. Facemask (Cl III) or palatal expansion correction should tend toward overcorrection.

In mixed dentition patients, retention must be planned with two things in mind: the patient's current versus initial condition, and subsequent changes in the dentition and occlusion that will occur as the child matures (Fig. IV.5). With removable retainers, the location of clasps, wires, and labial bows should be chosen carefully, and they should be either modifiable or removable.

Wires through edentulous areas can interfere with eruption of the permanent teeth in that area, and clasps on primary teeth will be of limited use because these teeth will be lost. Preadolescent children, even those who were quite cooperative with active treatment, may not be reliable patients for removable retainers. The greater control provided by fixed retainers must be balanced against their breakage, greater hygiene risk and inability to allow teeth to adapt to adjacent erupting teeth. A prolonged period of retention before comprehensive treatment begins also increases the chance of patient burnout.

In the chapters in this section, our goal is to present the spectrum of early (preadolescent) treatment in the context of this background. Chapter 11 focuses on two things: (1) separating child patients with important but less complex orthodontic problems, who are appropriately treated in a general practice setting, from those with more complex problems who are likely to need treatment by a specialist, and (2) the treatment procedures needed to manage these less complex cases. Chapter 12 is a discussion of more complex treatment in children with nonskeletal problems.

11

Moderate Nonskeletal Problems in Preadolescent Children: Preventive and Interceptive Treatment in General Practice

HENRY W. FIELDS AND WILLIAM R. PROFFIT

CHAPTER OUTLINE

Orthodontic Pretreatment Evaluation: Determining Treatment Complexity and Timing

For a dentist seeing a young patient with a malocclusion, just as with all patients, it is important to begin with the parent or patient's chief concern. Then the initial consultation should seek answers to the key questions: What problems are present? Do they relate to the chief complaint? Are they moderate or complex problems? Is early or limited orthodontic treatment needed? If so, when should it be done? Finally, who should do it? Does this patient need referral to a specialist?

The ability to identify dentofacial problems in children is critical for the general dentist. They are the gatekeepers who determine who gets treated and when. Whether they treat orthodontic problems is not the primary issue, it is recognition of problems and their management (observation, treatment, or referral) that is critical to the patient. Some problems are time sensitive, like ectopic eruption or transpositions, and considerations for transplants or, decoronations. If the generalist is not able to recognize developing problems and has no understanding of the options and timing, opportunities are lost to provide the accepted or highest standard of care.

Sorting out moderate from complex problems is essential because this process determines which patients are appropriately treated within general practice and which are most appropriately referred to a specialist. It is important for the general dentist to be able to distinguish problems that need to be treated soon, as opposed to more routine problems that can wait for later comprehensive care.

As with all components of dental practice, a generalist's decision of whether to include orthodontic treatment as a component of services is an individual one, best based on education, experience, and ability. The principle that moderate problems are handled within the context of general practice and the more complex problems are referred should remain the same, however, regardless of the practitioner's interest in orthodontics. Only the individual practitioner's cutoff points for treating a patient in the general practice or referral should change.

This section presents a logical scheme for orthodontic problem identification and management for children. It is based on the diagnostic approach developed in Chapter 6 and incorporates the principles of determining treatment need that have been discussed. An adequate database and a thorough problem list (including positive attributes), of course, are necessary to carry out the process. Finally, the goals of treatment and a treatment plan are developed in consultation with the patient and parent. A cephalometric radiograph is not required at this point because a facial form analysis is more appropriate in the generalist's office, but appropriate dental radiographs are needed (bitewings supplemented with anterior occlusal radiographs or bitewings and a panoramic radiograph are usually needed depending on the stage of development). Dental casts, photographs, and a space analysis (see later in this chapter) are essential.

Step 1: Syndromes and Developmental Abnormalities

The first step in the problem identification and management process is to separate out patients with facial syndromes or similarly complex dentofacial problems so they can be treated by specialists or teams of specialists. From physical appearance, the medical and dental histories and an evaluation of developmental status, nearly all such patients are easily recognized. Common anomalies and malformations are described and illustrated in Chapter 7. Complex medical treatments, such as radiation, bisphosphonates, and growth hormones, can affect dentofacial development and responses to treatment. Patients who appear to be developing either above the 95th–97th or below the 3rd to 5th percentiles on standard growth charts require special evaluation. Growth disorders may demand that any orthodontic treatment be carried out in conjunction with endocrine, nutritional, or psychologic therapy. For these patients and those with diseases that affect growth, such as juvenile idiopathic arthritis, the proper orthodontic therapy must be combined with identification and control of the disease process.

Patients with significant skeletal asymmetry (not necessarily those whose asymmetry resulting from only a functional shift of the mandible due to dental interferences) always fall into the complex problem category (Fig. 11.1). These patients could have a developmental problem or the growth anomaly that could be the result of an injury. Treatment is likely to involve growth modification and/or surgery, in addition to comprehensive orthodontics. Timing of intervention is affected by whether the cause of the asymmetry is deficient or excessive growth, but early comprehensive evaluation by a specialist is always indicated.

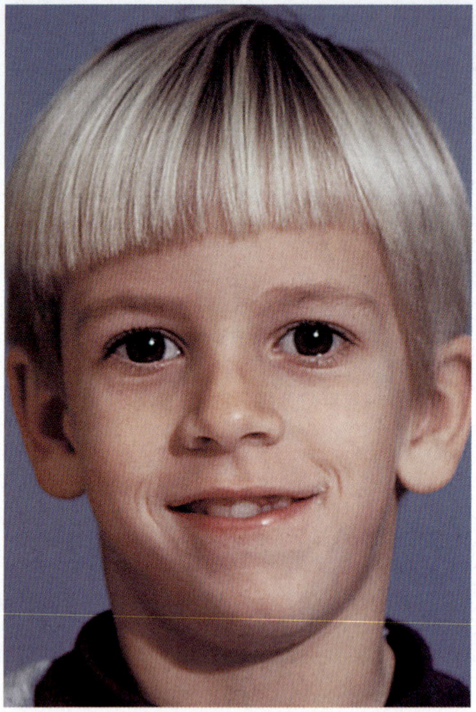

• **Fig. 11.1** At age 8, this boy has a noticeable mandibular asymmetry with the chin several mm off to the left. A problem of this type is likely to become progressively worse and is an indication for referral for comprehensive evaluation by a facial deformities team. (From Proffit WR, White RP, Sarver DM. *Contemporary Treatment of Dentofacial Deformity*. Mosby; 2003.)

Step 2: Facial Form Analysis

Anteroposterior and Vertical Problems

Patients should be evaluated using the Facial Form Analysis method described in Chapter 6 (Fig. 6.15). As mentioned earlier this is an excellent method to screen for maxillary protrusion and retrusion, mandibular protrusion, and retrusion as well as vertical discrepancies. Lip protrusion and competency related to anterior tooth positions should be assessed as well.

Skeletal Class II and Class III problems and their cause (i.e., maxillary protrusion/retrusion or mandibular protrusion/retrusion) and vertical deformities of the long-face and short-face types, regardless of their cause, require thorough cephalometric evaluation to plan appropriate treatment and its timing, and must be considered complex problems (Fig. 11.2). Issues in treatment planning for growth modification are discussed in Chapters 13 and 14.

As a general rule:

- Class II treatment can be deferred until near adolescence because treatment then is equally as effective as earlier treatment.
- Class III treatment for moderate maxillary deficiencies should be addressed earlier. Class III treatment for protrusive mandibles requires either Class III elastics to skeletal anchors during adolescence (the less severe cases) or orthognathic surgery after growth has essentially stopped (see Chapter 22).
    - Treatment of both long- and short-face problems can usually be deferred until adolescence because:
    - Long-face or open bite problems can improve during preadolescent growth but can be aggravated by growth that persists until the late teens and can outstrip early focused intervention.
    - Short-face problems usually can be managed well with comprehensive treatment during adolescence, unless there is maxillary palatal gingival damage due to a deep bite.

As with asymmetry, early evaluation for all of these skeletal problems is indicated even if treatment is deferred, so early referral is appropriate.

Excessive Dental Protrusion or Retrusion

Severe dental protrusion or retrusion, which are also complex treatment problems, should be recognized during the facial form analysis. The urgency for treating these problems usually depends on the esthetic impact or, in the case of protrusion, the potential for traumatic injury. Otherwise, they should be treated as noted earlier.

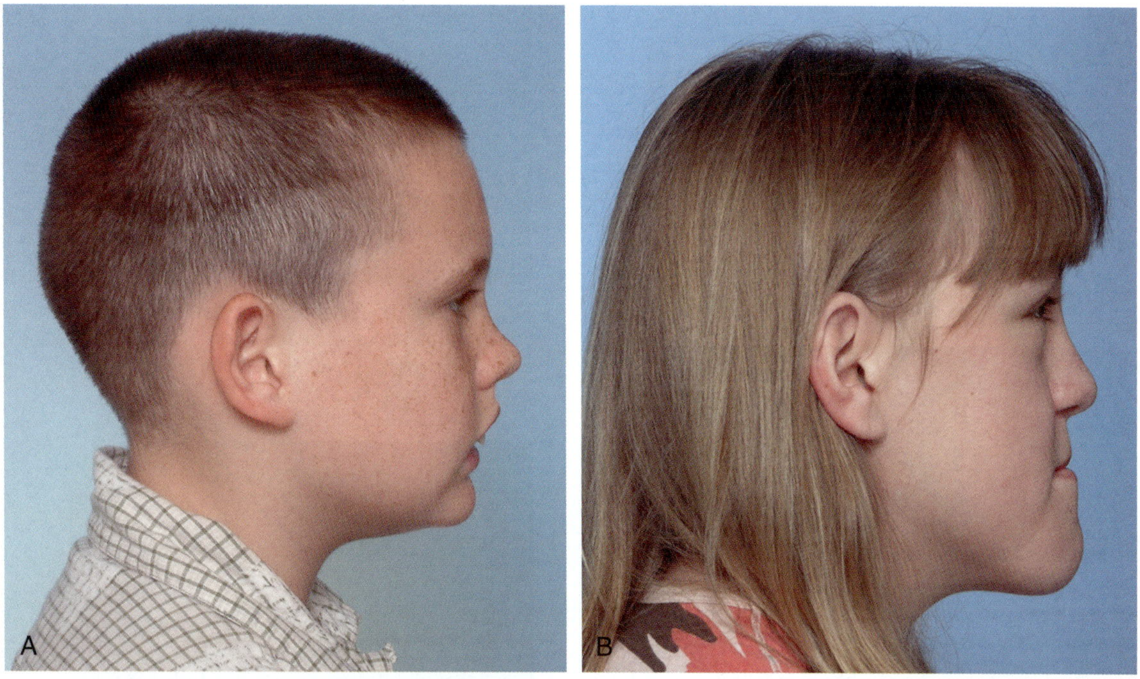

• **Fig. 11.2** A skeletal problem of even moderate severity can easily be picked up from examination of the profile, and a cephalometric radiograph is not necessary. (A) Skeletal Class II malocclusion due to mandibular deficiency. (B) Skeletal Class III malocclusion with a component of both maxillary deficiency and mandibular excess.

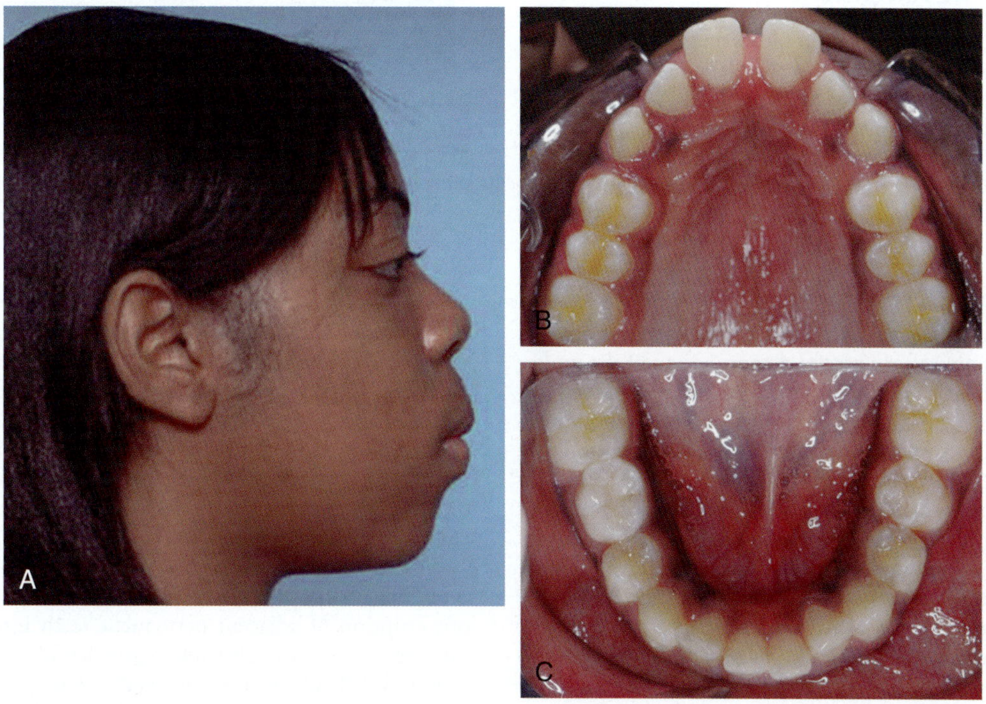

• **Fig. 11.3** (A) Bimaxillary dentoalveolar protrusion. Note the lip strain to bring the lips together over the teeth. The lips were separated at rest by the protruding incisors. (B) and (C) Occlusal views show the spacing in the upper arch and very mild crowding in the lower arch. For this girl, potential crowding of the teeth is expressed almost completely as protrusion.

Some individuals with good skeletal proportions have protrusion of incisor teeth rather than crowding (Fig. 11.3). When this occurs, the space analysis will show a small or nonexistent discrepancy because the incisor protrusion has compensated for the potential crowding. Excessive protrusion of incisors (bimaxillary protrusion, not excessive overjet) is usually an indication for premolar extraction and retraction of the protruding incisors. This is complex and prolonged treatment. Because of the profile changes produced by adolescent growth, it is better for most children to defer extraction to correct protrusion until late in the mixed dentition or early in

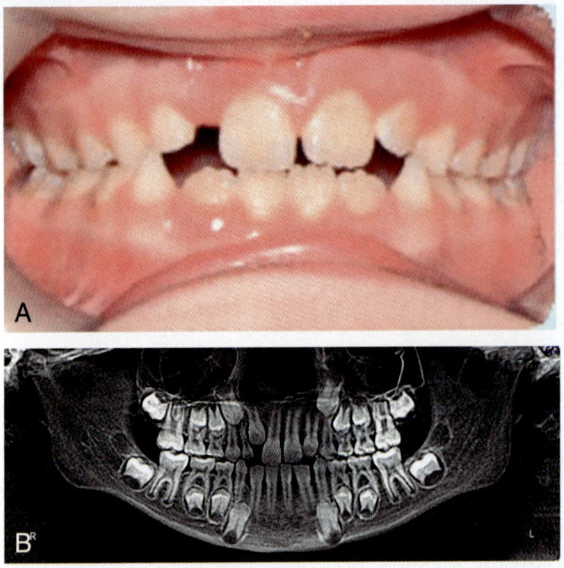

• **Fig. 11.4** (A) At first glance this 8-year-old patient appears quite normal and dental age appropriate. (B) The panoramic radiograph shows the apparent maxillary right lateral is really the primary canine and the permanent lateral incisor is impacted.

the permanent dentition. Techniques for controlling the amount of incisor retraction are described in Chapter 15.

Step 3: Dental Development

Unlike the more complex skeletal problems and problems related to protruding incisors, problems involving dental development (supernumerary teeth, retained or ankylosed teeth, ectopic eruption, or transposition) often need treatment as soon as they are discovered, typically during the early mixed dentition, and can often be handled in general practice. Considerations in making that decision and treatment of the less severe problems of this type are presented in detail in this chapter.

Asymmetric Dental Development

Treatment for an abnormal sequence of dental development should be planned only after a careful determination of the underlying cause. Asymmetric eruption (one side ahead of the other by 6 months or more) is significant (Fig. 11.4). It requires careful monitoring of the situation, and in the absence of outright pathologic conditions, may require early treatment such as selective extraction of primary or permanent teeth. A few patients with asymmetric dental development have a history of childhood radiation therapy to the head and neck or traumatic injury. Surgical and orthodontic treatment for these patients must be planned and timed carefully and may require tooth removal or tooth reorientation. Some of these teeth have severely dilacerated roots and will not be candidates for orthodontic movement. These situations definitely fall into the complex category and usually require early intervention.

Missing or Ankylosed Teeth

Missing primary teeth are extremely rare (0.5%–0.9%). Most likely the missing primary tooth will be a maxillary lateral incisor and subsequently, the permanent maxillary lateral incisor also will be missing. The permanent teeth most likely to be congenitally missing are the maxillary lateral incisors (even when primary lateral incisors are present) and the mandibular second premolars (Fig.11.5). Primary and permanent maxillary central and lateral incisors are the teeth most likely to be lost to trauma.

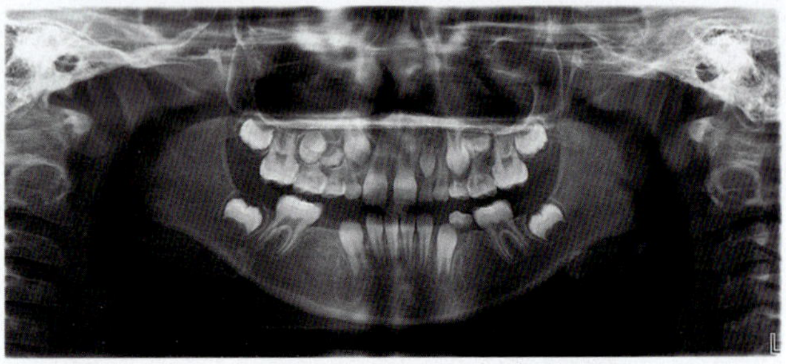

• **Fig. 11.5** A clinical exam will not provide all the information one needs to quantify the status of all the teeth. This patient has a missing 7, peg shaped 10, missing 13, 20, 21, 28 and 29.

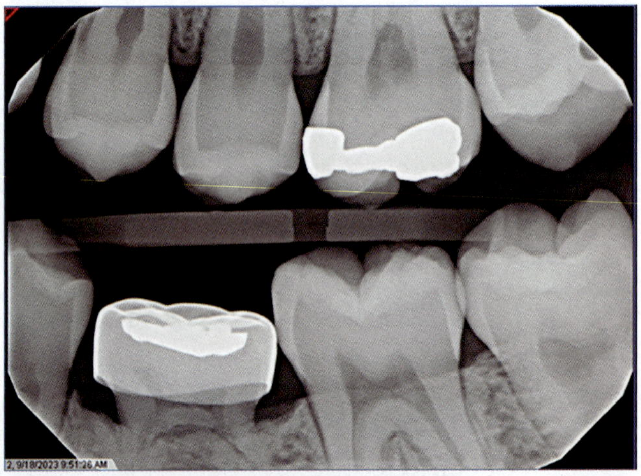

• **Fig. 11.6** This bitewing radiograph shows an ankylosed primary mandibular left second molar. Note the tooth is below the occlusal plane and there are bony defects developing mesially and distally. Given that the other premolars have erupted on the left side, it is probable that the permanent mandibular second premolar is missing.

The treatment possibilities differ slightly for missing permanent anterior and posterior teeth. For missing posterior teeth, it is possible to (1) maintain the primary tooth or teeth, (2) extract the overlying primary teeth and then allow the adjacent permanent teeth to drift, (3) extract the primary teeth followed by immediate orthodontic treatment, (4) decoronate the ankylosed primary tooth with no successor and replace with a later implant, or (5) replace the missing tooth perhaps by transplantation or prosthetically by an implant later.

For missing anterior teeth, maintaining the primary teeth is often less of an option because of the esthetics and the spontaneous eruption of adjacent permanent teeth into the space of the missing tooth with subsequent primary tooth loss. Also, extraction and drift of the adjacent teeth are possible, but less appealing because of the immediate esthetic problems with the missing teeth. Although the anterior edentulous ridges can deteriorate quickly when teeth are missing, subsequent eruption of the drifted permanent teeth will reestablish the bone. As with other growth problems, early evaluation and planning are essential. Treatment of problems related to missing teeth for children in the mixed dentition is discussed in more detail in Chapter 12.

For ankylosed primary teeth with permanent successors, the permanent teeth usually erupt on time but are sometimes malpositioned due to a retained root tip. Ankylosed primary teeth with no successor (Fig. 11.6), as mentioned above, are a complex challenge and offer several treatment options often dependent on timing and are covered in Chapter 12. For all practical purposes, permanent teeth ankylosed at an early age or teeth that fail to erupt for other reasons (such as primary failure of eruption) fall into the same complex category as missing teeth. These severe problems often require a combination of surgery (for extraction or decoronation) and orthodontics, if indeed the condition can be treated satisfactorily at all. After surgical intervention, the ultimate choices are orthodontic space closure, transplantation into the affected area, or prosthetic replacement.

Supernumerary Teeth

Ninety percent of all supernumerary teeth are found in the anterior part of the maxilla (Fig. 11.7). Multiple or inverted supernumeraries and those that are malformed often displace adjacent teeth and cause problems in their eruption. The presence of multiple supernumerary teeth indicates a complex problem and perhaps a syndrome or congenital abnormality such as cleidocranial dysplasia. Early removal of the supernumeraries is indicated, but this must be done carefully to minimize damage to adjacent teeth. If the adjacent permanent teeth have been displaced or severely delayed, surgical exposure, adjunctive periodontal surgery, and possibly orthodontic traction are likely to be required to bring them into the arch after the supernumerary has been removed.

Single supernumeraries that are not malformed often erupt spontaneously, causing crowding problems. If these teeth can be removed before they cause distortions of arch form or eruption problems with adjacent teeth, extraction may be all that is needed.

Other Eruption Problems

Ectopic eruption (eruption of a tooth in the wrong place or along the wrong eruption path) often leads to early loss of a primary tooth (Fig. 11.8), but in severe cases resorption of adjacent permanent teeth can result. Sometimes extraction of adjacent primary teeth can redirect the ectopic tooth. Repositioning of the ectopically erupting tooth may be indicated, either surgically or by exposing the problem tooth, placing an attachment on it, and

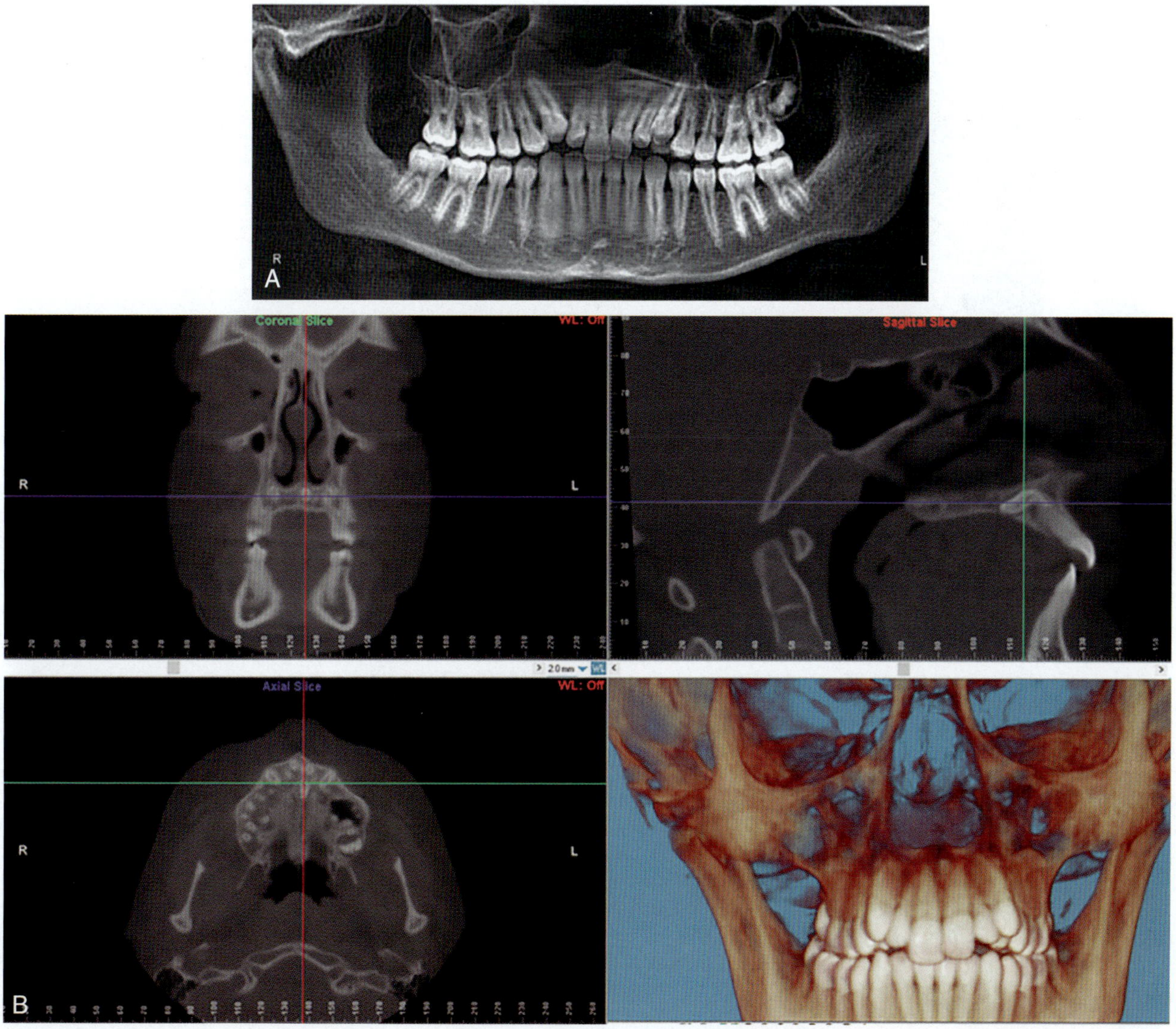

• **Fig. 11.7** When evaluating radiographs for missing and supernumerary teeth, careful attention is required. (A) This panoramic radiograph shows a telltale radiopacity in the maxillary left anterior region. (B) The follow-up CBCT indicates there is a horizontal lingually positioned canine at the crosshairs, that was easily confirmed. A small field CBCT could have provided the same information.

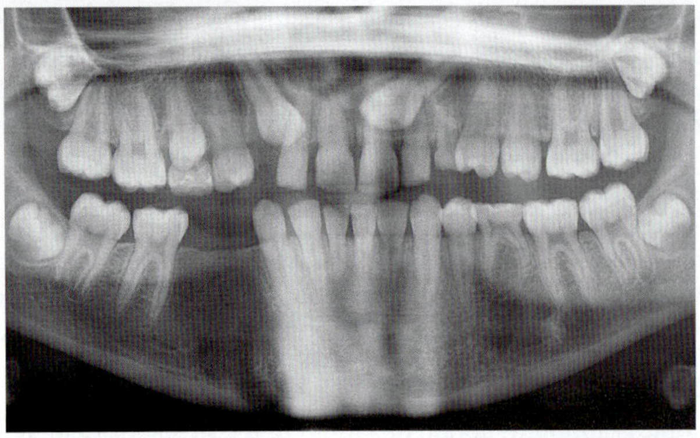

• **Fig. 11.8** This pretreatment panoramic radiograph shows not only several missing teeth (20, 28 and 29), but ectopically erupting maxillary canines and a retained primary maxillary left canine. These findings certainly make the treatment plan more complex than initially imagined.

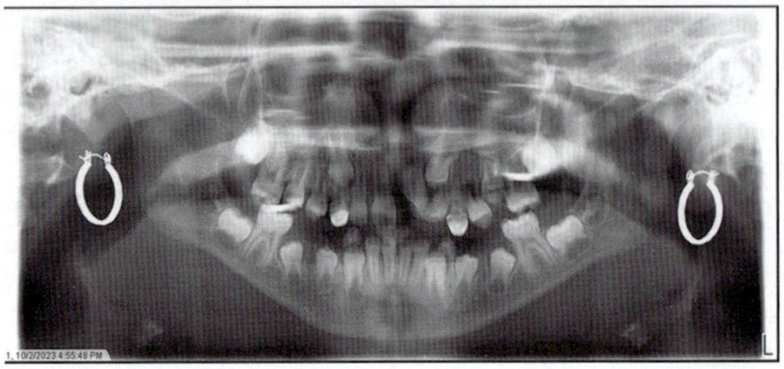

• **Fig. 11.9** This 9-year-old has a transposition already developed between the permanent maxillary left canine and lateral incisor. The transposition has disrupted the permanent maxillary left central and lateral incisor positions (comparison with the normal contralateral side makes this obvious). Given its position, it is probable that there may be some impact on the lateral incisor root development. This can only be defined using a small field CBCT. Then, the possibilities of tooth extraction and/or tooth repositioning can be determined.

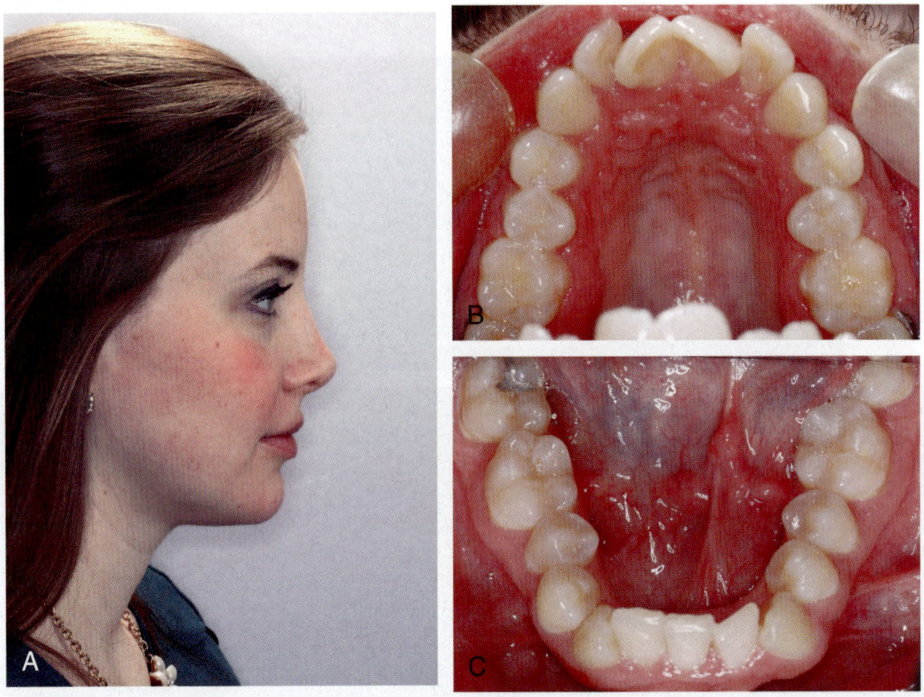

• **Fig. 11.10** In some patients, as in this girl (A) with good lip position, potential crowding is expressed completely as actual crowding (B and C), with no compensation in the form of dental and lip protrusion. In others (see Fig. 11.3), potential crowding is expressed as protrusion. The teeth end up in a position of equilibrium between the tongue and lip forces against them (see Chapter 5).

applying orthodontic traction. A dramatic variation of ectopic eruption is transposition of teeth (Fig. 11.9). Early intervention can reduce the extent to which teeth are malpositioned in some cases. These severe problems often require a combination of surgery and orthodontics and may be genetically linked to other anomalies. They are discussed in Chapter 12.

Step 4: Space Problems

Orthodontic problems in a child with good facial proportions often involve spacing, crowding, irregularity, or malposition of the teeth and become apparent in the mixed dentition. At this stage, the results of space analysis are essential for planning treatment. The presence or absence of adequate space for the teeth must be taken into account when any treatment is planned.

In interpreting the results of space analysis for patients of any age, remember that if space to align the teeth is inadequate, either of two conditions may develop. One possibility is for the incisor teeth to remain upright and well positioned over the basal bone of the maxilla or mandible and then rotate or tip labially or lingually. In this instance, the potential crowding is expressed as actual crowding and is difficult to miss (Fig. 11.10). The other possibility is for the crowded teeth to align themselves completely or partially at the expense of the lips, displacing the lips forward and separating them at rest (see Fig. 11.3). Even if the potential for crowding is extreme, the teeth can align themselves at the expense of the lip, interfering with lip closure. This must be detected during the facial form analysis from the profile examination. If there is already a degree of protrusion in addition to the crowding, it is safe to assume that the natural limits of anterior displacement of incisors have been reached.

Depending on the circumstances, the appropriate response to space deficiencies varies. Remember, a couple of millimeters of crowding during the transition from the primary to permanent dentitions is normal and requires no treatment. For localized space loss of 3 mm or less in a quadrant, lost space can be regained. For total arch space shortage of 4 mm or less or crowding with adequate space, repositioning incisors labially or space management, respectively, during the transition is appropriate. Of these procedures, only treatment to regain space and manage transitional crowding are critical in terms of timing. Treatment planning for these moderate problems is outlined later in this chapter.

Space discrepancies of approximately 5 mm or more, with or without incisor protrusion, constitute complex treatment problems. In these children, if teeth are not extracted, robust mechanics must be employed to align the teeth, and if teeth are extracted, the anchorage considerations are critical to use the extraction space in the most appropriate way, depending upon the dental protrusion or retrusion. Severe crowding of 10 mm or more also requires careful and complex planning and often early intervention so that permanent teeth are not impacted or deflected into eruption paths that affect other permanent teeth or force them into the oral cavity through nonkeratinized tissue.

In general, minor midline diastemas will close and cause little esthetic or developmental problems. Large diastemas, over 2 mm, can be esthetic concerns and inhibit adjacent teeth from erupting properly. They are cause for heightened concern and early treatment.

Step 5: Other Occlusal Discrepancies

Whether crossbite and increased overbite or open bite should be classified as moderate or severe is determined for most children from their facial form. Mixed dentition treatment for all these problems must be discussed in the context of "should be treated" versus "can be treated."

As a general guideline, posterior crossbite in a preadolescent child falls into the moderate category if no other complicating factors (such as severe crowding) are present. It should be treated early if the child shifts laterally from the initial dental contact position (a centric relation-to-centric occlusion [CR-CO] shift). If there is no shift but space in the arch is borderline, early mixed dentition treatment is sometimes recommended to reduce the crowding, but usually it is better to delay until the late mixed dentition so that more teeth can be guided into position. If a skeletal posterior crossbite is treated in adolescence, it will require heavier forces and more complex appliances.

Anterior crossbite involving all or most of the incisors usually reflects a Class III jaw discrepancy, but anterior crossbite of one or two teeth can arise from lingual tipping of the upper incisors or crowding as they erupt. Again, CR-CO shifts, dental abrasion from interferences and developing gingival defects can heighten the concern about the crossbite. Treatment planning for the use of removable versus fixed appliances to correct these simple crossbites early is discussed later.

Excessive overjet, with the upper incisors flared and spaced, often reflects a Class II skeletal problem but can also develop in patients with good jaw proportions. If adequate vertical clearance is present, the upper teeth can be tipped lingually and brought together with a simple removable or limited fixed appliance when the child is almost any age. The timing of treatment often depends on child and parent preference, related to esthetic and psychosocial problems, and the risk of trauma.

Anterior open bite in a young child with good facial proportions usually needs no treatment because there is a good chance of spontaneous correction with additional incisor eruption, especially if the open bite is related to an oral habit such as finger-sucking. A complex open bite (one with skeletal involvement or posterior dental manifestations) or any open bite in an older patient whose permanent teeth have erupted is a severe problem. A deep overbite can develop in several ways (see Chapter 6) but often is caused by or made worse by short anterior face height. This is seldom treated in the mixed dentition unless the lower anterior teeth are damaging the upper palatal tissue (Fig. 11.11).

Traumatically displaced erupted incisors at any age pose a special problem because of the potential resulting occlusal interferences (Fig. 11.12). Mobile teeth displaced into traumatic occlusion should be digitally moved to a better position immediately and then splinted. If they are consolidated in the new

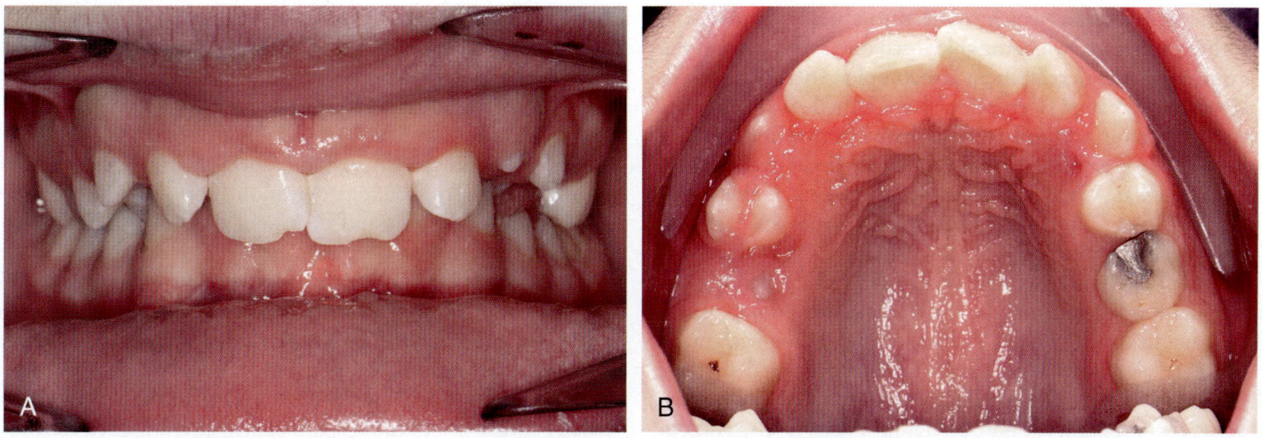

• **Fig. 11.11** This patient has an obvious deep bite, with (A) severe overbite and (B), resulting damage to the palatal tissue adjacent to the maxillary incisors.

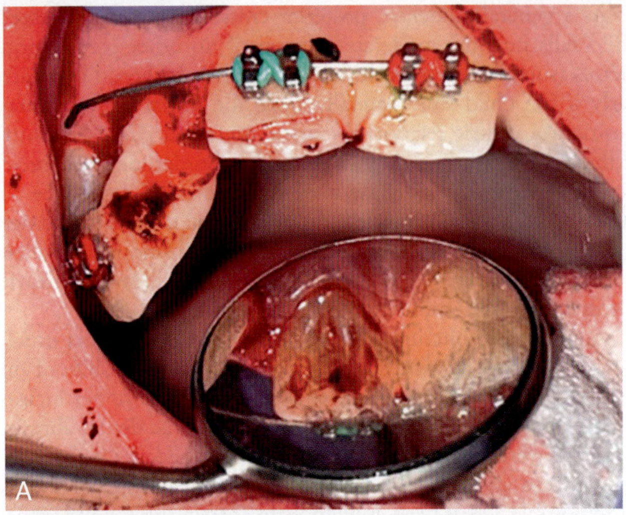

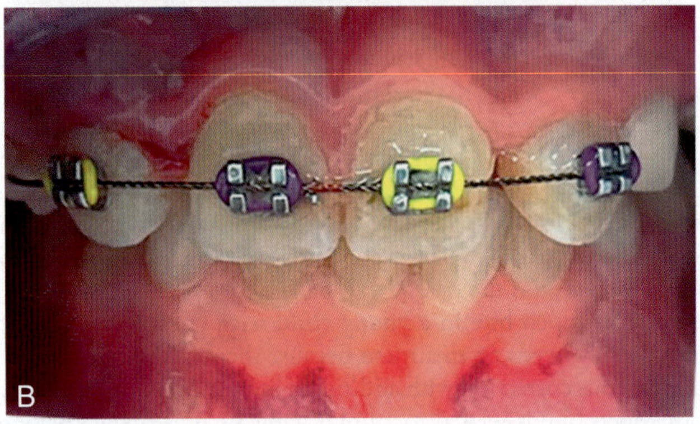

• **Fig. 11.12** (A) This patient was having minor orthodontic tooth movement for alignment in the mixed dentition. (B) The traumatic injury was assess immediately and the partially avulsed maxillary right lateral incisor (retained largely by the orthodontic archwire) was digitally repositioned and stabilized with a light wire. This timely treatment reduced the injury and eliminated the occlusal interference. (Courtesy Dr. B. Schweiger)

position and in traumatic occlusion they should be moved with light forces. If they are consolidated and not in traumatic occlusion, several months of observation followed by orthodontics is recommended.

There is a risk of ankylosis after healing has occurred, especially after traumatic intrusion, which can lead to a serious problem as all the other teeth erupt while the ankylosed one(s) does not. If the apex is open and root development is incomplete in a young child, waiting for spontaneous re-eruption is warranted. If the injuries are in older patients and involve less than 7 mm of intrusion, a short period of observation is also suggested. If the teeth fail to re-erupt, immediate orthodontics is recommended. If the intrusion is greater than 7 mm surgical treatment is needed, and the long-term prognosis must be guarded.

This overall evaluation scheme is oriented toward helping the general practitioner decide which children with orthodontic problems to treat and which to refer. Treatment for children with moderate nonskeletal problems and appropriate for general practice are discussed later in this chapter. Early (preadolescent) treatment of more severe and complex nonskeletal problems is discussed in Chapter 12, and growth modification treatment for skeletal problems is discussed in Chapters 13 and 14.

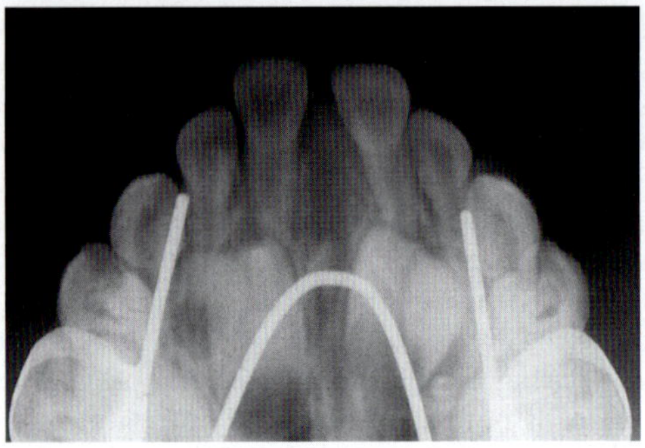

• **Fig. 11.13** In young children, lingual arch maxillary expansion devices (W-arches and quad helices) deliver enough force to open the midpalatal suture, as demonstrated in this maxillary occlusal radiograph.

Management of Occlusal Relationship Problems

Posterior Crossbite

Posterior crossbite in mixed dentition children is reasonably common. In the Third National Health and Nutrition Examination Survey (NHANES III) in 1992, posterior crossbite was noted in 7.1% of US children aged 8 to 11.[1] It usually results from a narrowing of the maxillary arch and is often present in children who have had prolonged sucking habits. The crossbite can be due to a narrow maxilla (i.e., due to skeletal dimensions) or due only to lingual tipping of the maxillary teeth. If the child shifts on closure or if the constriction is severe enough to significantly reduce the space within the arch, early correction is indicated. If not, treatment can be deferred as long as it is corrected before midpalatal suture bridging occurs so lighter forces and simpler, lingual arch–type appliances can be used. Timing is an important consideration for treatment, because the transverse (coronal plane in anatomic and radiographic terms) dimension is the first to complete growth.

It is also important to determine whether any associated mandibular asymmetry is the result of a shift of the lower jaw due to dental interferences or is due to a true maxillary or mandibular asymmetry. Another critical question is whether the posterior crossbite is related to skeletal maxillary retrusion or mandibular protrusion. In these cases, the anteroposterior position of the maxilla or mandible is contributing to the crossbite, and the actual transverse dimension of the palate may be normal.

Correcting posterior crossbites in the mixed dentition increases arch circumference and provides more room for the permanent teeth. On the average, a 1 mm increase in the inter-premolar width increases arch perimeter values by 0.7 mm.[2] Total relapse into crossbite is unlikely in the absence of a skeletal problem, and mixed dentition expansion reduces the incidence of posterior crossbite in the permanent dentition. Early correction also simplifies future diagnosis and treatment by eliminating at least that problem from the list.

Although it is important to determine whether the crossbite is skeletal or dental, in the early mixed dentition years the treatment is usually the same because relatively light forces will move teeth and bones. An expansion lingual arch is the best choice at this age; heavy force from a jackscrew device is needed only when the midpalatal suture has become significantly interdigitated during adolescence (Fig. 11.13; also see further discussion in Chapter 13). Heavy force and rapid expansion are not indicated in the primary

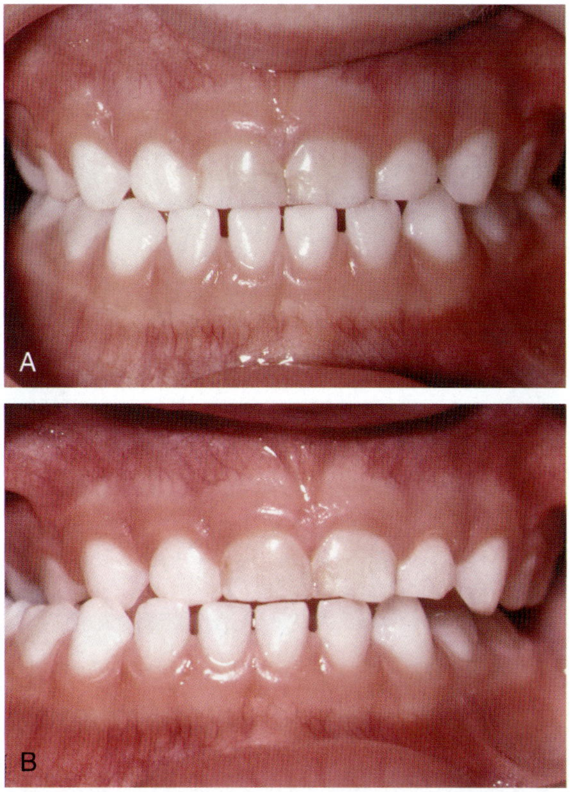

• **Fig. 11.14** Minor canine interferences leading to a mandibular shift. (A) Initial contact; (B) shift into centric occlusion. The slight lingual position of the primary canines can lead to occlusal interferences and an apparent posterior crossbite. This sole cause of posterior crossbite is infrequent and is best treated by occlusal adjustment of the primary canines.

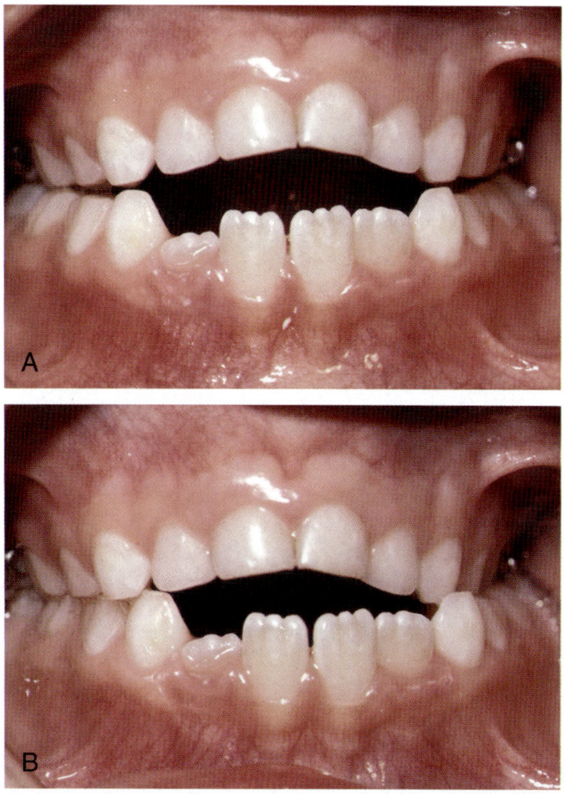

• **Fig. 11.15** Moderate bilateral maxillary constriction. (A) Initial contact; (B) shift into centric occlusion. Moderate bilateral maxillary constriction often leads to posterior interferences on closure and a lateral shift of the mandible into an apparent unilateral posterior crossbite. This problem is also best treated by bilateral maxillary expansion.

or early mixed dentition. There is a significant risk of distortion of the nose if this is done in younger children (see Fig. 13.12).

There are three basic approaches to the treatment of moderate posterior crossbites in children:

1. *Equilibration to eliminate mandibular shift.* In a few cases, mostly observed in the primary or early mixed dentition, a shift into posterior crossbite will be due solely to occlusal interference caused by the primary canines or (less frequently) primary molars. These patients can be diagnosed by carefully positioning the mandible in centric relation; then it can be seen whether the width of the maxilla is adequate and that there would be no crossbite without the shift (Fig. 11.14). In this case, a child requires only limited equilibration of the primary teeth (often, just reduction of the primary canines) to eliminate the interference and the resulting lateral shift into crossbite.[3]
2. *Expansion of a constricted maxillary arch.* More commonly, a lateral shift into crossbite is caused by constriction of the maxillary arch. Even a small constriction creates dental interferences that force the mandible to shift to a new position for maximum intercuspation (Fig. 11.15). Moderate expansion of the maxillary dental arch is needed for correction. The general guideline is to expand to prevent the shift when it is diagnosed, but there is an exception: if the permanent first molars are expected to erupt in less than 6 months, it is better to wait for their eruption so that correction can include these teeth, if necessary. A greater maxillary constriction may allow the maxillary teeth to fit inside the mandibular teeth—if so, there will not be a shift on closure (Fig. 11.16), and there is less reason to provide early correction of the crossbite on this basis. But patients with this amount of constriction generally have a space problem that expansion and correction of the crossbite will improve. Although it is possible to treat posterior crossbite with a split-plate type removable appliance, there are three problems: This treatment relies on patient compliance for success, treatment time is longer, and it is more costly than an expansion lingual arch.[4] The preferred appliance for a preadolescent child is an adjustable lingual arch that requires little patient cooperation. Both the W-arch and the quad helix are reliable and easy to use. The W-arch is a fixed appliance constructed of 36-mil steel wire soldered to molar bands (Fig. 11.17). It is activated simply by opening the apices of the W and is easily adjusted to provide more anterior than posterior expansion, or vice versa, if this is desired. The appliance delivers proper force levels when opened 4 to 6 mm wider than the passive width and should be adjusted to this dimension before being cemented. It is not uncommon for the teeth and maxilla to move more on one side than the other, so precise bilateral expansion is the exception rather than the rule, but acceptable correction and tooth position are almost always achieved. The quad helix (Fig. 11.18) is a more flexible version of the W-arch, although it is made with 38-mil steel wire. The helices in the anterior palate are bulky, which can effectively serve as a reminder to aid in stopping a finger habit if they are positioned correctly. The combination of a posterior crossbite and a finger-sucking habit is the best indication for this appliance. The extra wire incorporated in it gives it a slightly greater range of action than the W-arch, but

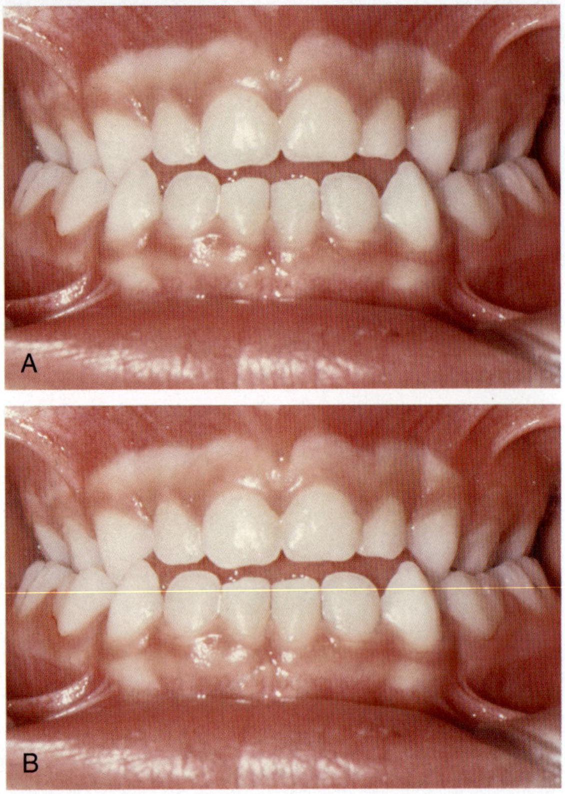

• **Fig. 11.16** Marked bilateral maxillary constriction. (A) Initial contact; (B) centric occlusion (no shift). Severe constriction often produces no interferences on closure, and the patient has a bilateral posterior crossbite in centric relation. This problem is best treated by bilateral maxillary expansion and, unlike with a unilateral crossbite with a mandibular shift, treatment can be delayed until the early permanent dentition.

the forces are equivalent. Soft tissue irritation can become a problem with the quad helix. Both the W-arch and the quad helix leave an imprint on the tongue. Both the parents and the child should be warned about this (Fig. 11.19). The imprint will disappear when the appliance is removed but can take up to a year to totally resolve.

With both types of expansion lingual arches, some opening of the midpalatal suture can be expected for a child in the primary or mixed dentition, so the expansion is not solely dental. Data show an average palatal expansion of 3.9 mm and an average intermolar expansion of 6.5 mm. As with rapid or slow expansion using a jackscrew device, the skeletal change was less than 50% of the total change.[5] Expansion should continue at the rate of 2 mm per month (1 mm on each side) until the crossbite is slightly overcorrected. In other words, the lingual cusps of the maxillary teeth should occlude on the lingual inclines of the buccal cusps of the mandibular molars at the end of active treatment (Fig. 11.20). Intraoral appliance adjustment is possible but may lead to unexpected changes. For this reason, removal and re-cementation are recommended at each active treatment visit. Most posterior crossbites require 2 to 3 months of active treatment (with the patients seen each month for adjustments) and 3 months of retention (during which the lingual arch is left passively in place). This mixed dentition correction appears to be stable in the long term.[6]

3. *Asymmetric repositioning of teeth.* Some children do have a true unilateral crossbite because of unilateral maxillary constriction of the upper arch (Fig. 11.21). In these children the ideal treatment is to move selected teeth on the constricted side. To a limited extent, the goal of asymmetric movement can be achieved by using different length arms on a W-arch or quad helix (Fig. 11.22), but some bilateral expansion must be expected. An alternative is to use a mandibular lingual arch to stabilize the lower teeth and attach cross-elastics to the maxillary teeth that are at fault. This is more complicated and requires cooperation to be successful but is more unilateral in its effect. Both these approaches are preferred to bilateral maxillary expansion and then hoping for unilateral relapse into a normal occlusion.

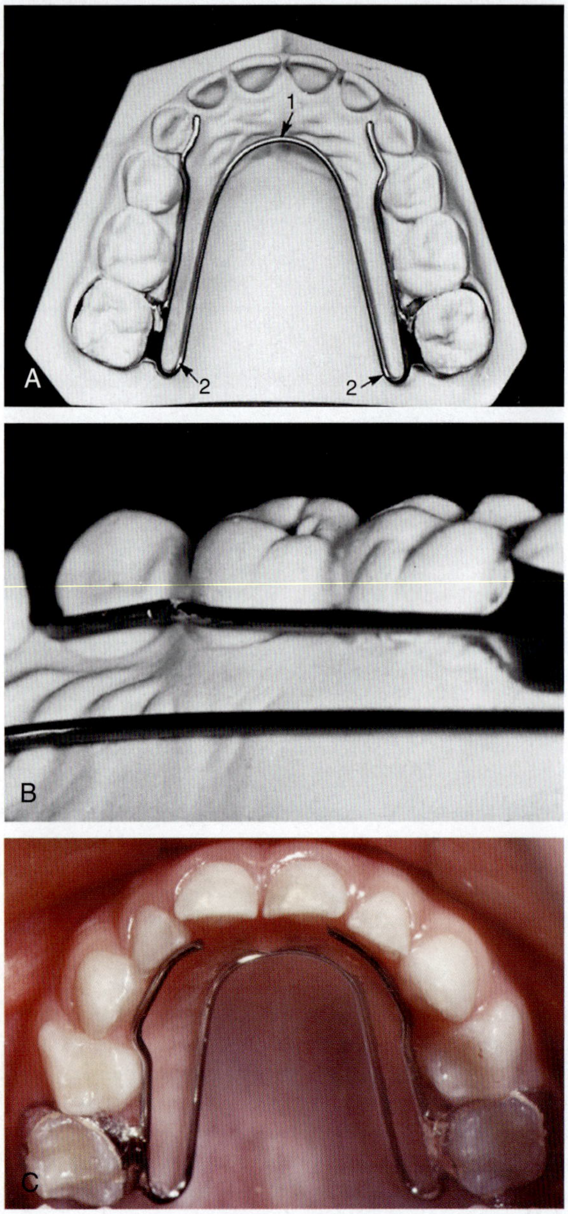

• **Fig. 11.17** The W-arch appliance is ideal for bilateral maxillary expansion. (A) The appliance is fabricated from 36-mil wire and soldered to the bands. The lingual wire should contact the teeth involved in the crossbite and should not extend than 1–2 mm distal to the banded molars to eliminate soft tissue irritation. Activation at point 1 produces posterior expansion and activation at point 2 produces anterior expansion. (B) The lingual wire should remain 1–1.5 mm away from the marginal gingiva and the palatal tissue. (C) This W-arch is being used to correct a bilateral constriction in the primary dentition.

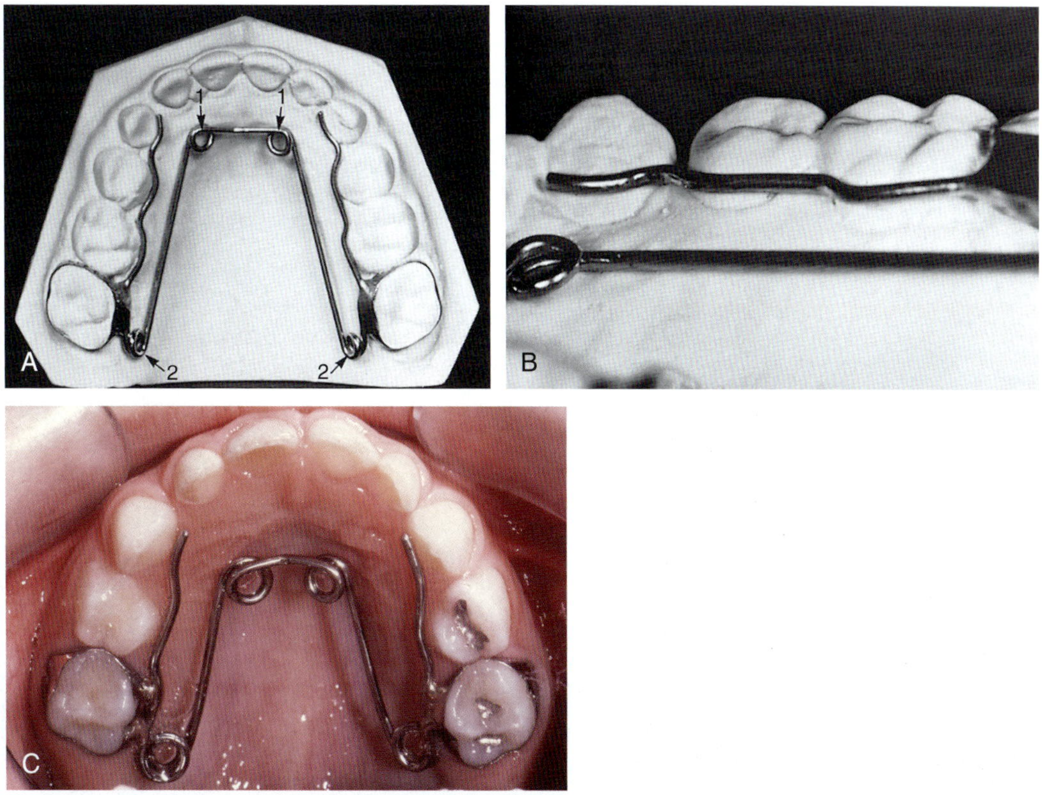

• **Fig. 11.18** A quad helix used to correct bilateral maxillary constriction. (A) The appliance is fabricated from 38-mil wire and soldered to the bands. The lingual wire should contact the teeth involved in the crossbite and extend no more than 1–2 mm distal to the banded molars to eliminate soft tissue irritation. Activation at point 1 produces posterior expansion, whereas activation at point 2 produces anterior expansion. (B) The lingual wire should remain 1–1.5 mm away from the marginal gingiva and palatal tissue. (C) This quad helix is being used to correct a bilateral maxillary constriction in the primary dentition.

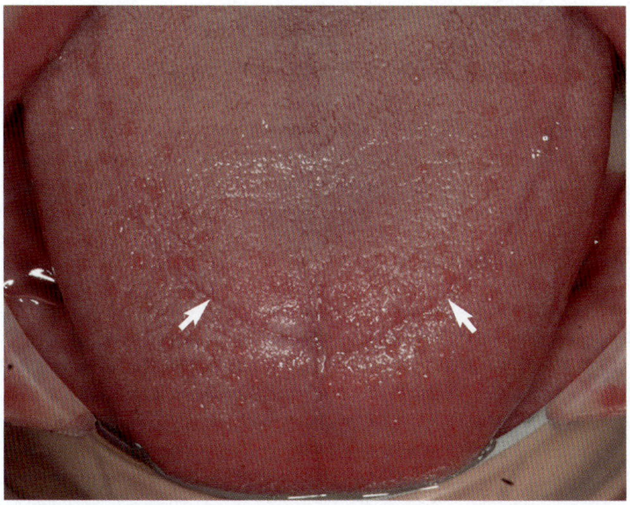

• **Fig. 11.19** W-arches, quad helixes, and habit appliances often leave indentations in the superior surface of the tongue *(arrows)*. These often remain after appliance removal for up to 1 year. No treatment is recommended, but patients and parents should be warned of this possibility.

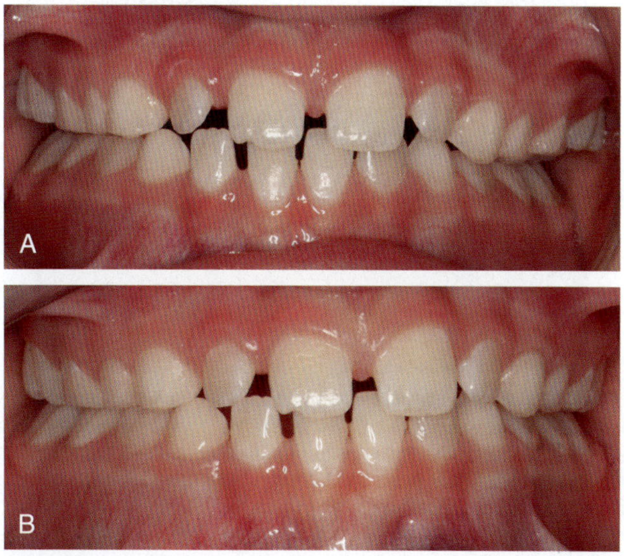

• **Fig. 11.20** (A) Posterior crossbites should be overcorrected until the maxillary posterior lingual cusps occlude with the lingual inclines of the mandibular buccal cusps, as shown here, and then retained for approximately 3 months. (B) After retention, slight lingual movement of the maxillary teeth results in stability.

All the appliances described earlier are aimed at correction of teeth in the maxillary arch, which is usually where the problem is located. If teeth in both arches contribute to the problem, cross-elastics between banded or bonded attachments in both arches (Fig. 11.23) can reposition both upper and lower teeth. The best choice is a latex elastic (unless the patient has a latex allergy, which is an indication for polymer elastics) with a 3/16-inch (5 mm) lumen generating 6 oz (170 g) of force. The force from the elastics

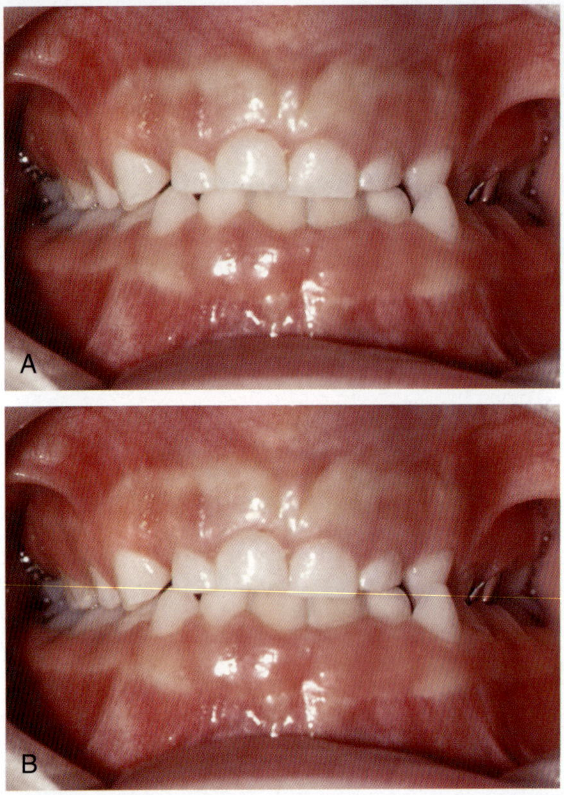

• **Fig. 11.21** True unilateral maxillary posterior constriction. (A) Initial contact. (B) Full occlusion (no shift). True unilateral constriction has a unilateral posterior crossbite in centric relation and in centric occlusion, without a lateral shift. This problem is best treated with asymmetric posterior expansion.

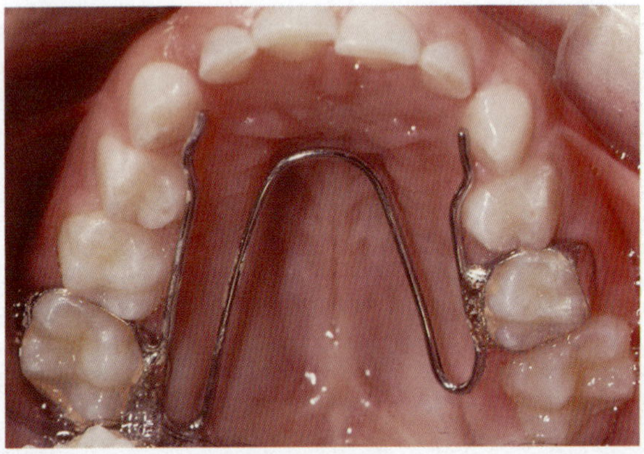

• **Fig. 11.22** An unequal and asymmetric W-arch used to correct a true unilateral maxillary constriction. The side of the arch to be expanded has fewer teeth against the lingual wire than the anchorage unit. Even with this arrangement, both sides can be expected to show some expansion movement, and the extent cannot be predicted.

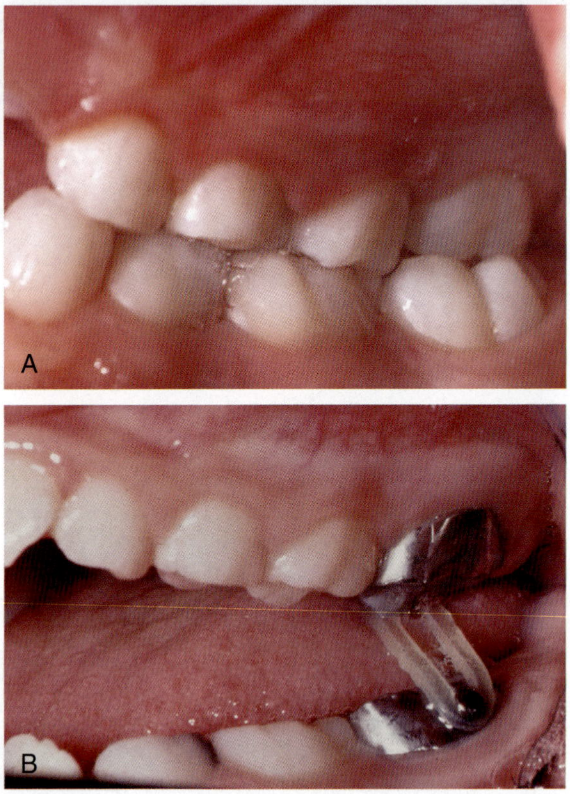

• **Fig. 11.23** (A) This patient's permanent maxillary left first molar is displaced lingually and the permanent mandibular left first molar is displaced facially, which resulted in a posterior crossbite between these teeth. (B) A short and relatively heavy cross-elastic is placed between the buttons welded on the bands. The elastic can be challenging for some children to place, but should be worn full-time, except for eating, and changed frequently.

is directed vertically as well as faciolingually, which will extrude the posterior teeth and reduce the overbite. Therefore cross-elastics should be used with caution in children with increased lower face height or limited overbite.

Crossbites treated with elastics should be overcorrected, and the bands or bonds left in place immediately after active treatment. If there is too much relapse, the elastics can be reinstated without rebanding or rebonding. When the occlusion is stable after several weeks without elastic force, the attachments can be removed. The most frequent problem with this form of crossbite correction is lack of cooperation from the child.

A flowchart is provided to help guide decision-making for posterior crossbites (Fig. 11.24).

Anterior Crossbite

Anterior crossbite of all of the incisors, is rarely found in children who do not have a skeletal Class III jaw relationship. A crossbite relationship of one or two anterior teeth, however, may develop in a child who has good facial proportions. When racial or ethnic groups in the US population are combined, about 3% of children have an anterior crossbite in the mixed dentition (see Chapter 1).

In planning treatment for anterior crossbites, it is critically important to differentiate skeletal problems of deficient maxillary or excessive mandibular growth from crossbites due only to displacement of teeth.[7] If the problem is truly skeletal, simply changing the incisor position is inadequate treatment, especially in more severe cases (see Chapter 13).

Anterior crossbite affecting only one or two teeth almost always is due to lingually displaced maxillary central or lateral incisors. These teeth tend to erupt to the lingual because of the lingual position of the developing tooth buds and may be trapped in that location, especially if there is not enough space

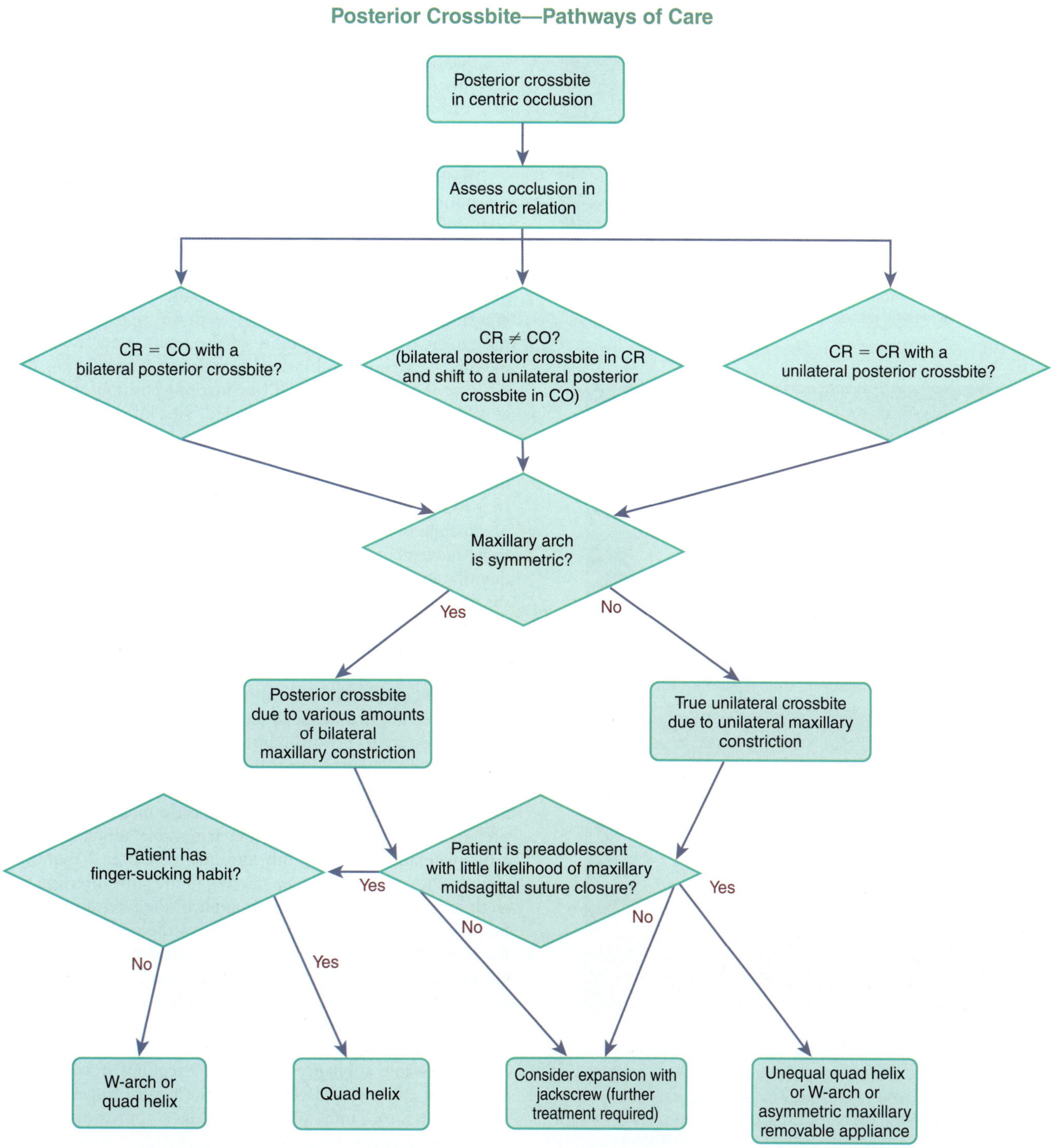

• **Fig. 11.24** This flowchart can be used to aid decision-making regarding possible options for posterior crossbite correction in the primary and mixed dentitions. Answers to the questions posed in the chart should lead to successful treatment pathways. The approaches to skeletal correction of posterior crossbites are described in Chapter 13. *CO*, Centric occlusion; *CR*, centric relation.

(Fig. 11.25). Sometimes, central incisors are involved because they were deflected toward a lingual eruption path by supernumerary anterior teeth or overretained primary incisors. More rarely, trauma to maxillary primary teeth reorients a permanent tooth bud lingually.

The most common etiologic factor for nonskeletal anterior crossbites is lack of space for the permanent incisors, and it is important to focus the treatment plan on management of the total space situation, not just the crossbite. If the developing crossbite is discovered before eruption is complete and overbite has not been established, the adjacent primary teeth can be extracted to provide the necessary space for facial migration of the erupting tooth (Fig. 11.26).

Mandibular anterior crowding can force a lower anterior tooth facially and into crossbite. This position, especially if there is incisal interference in centric relation, will lead to incisal wear, tooth

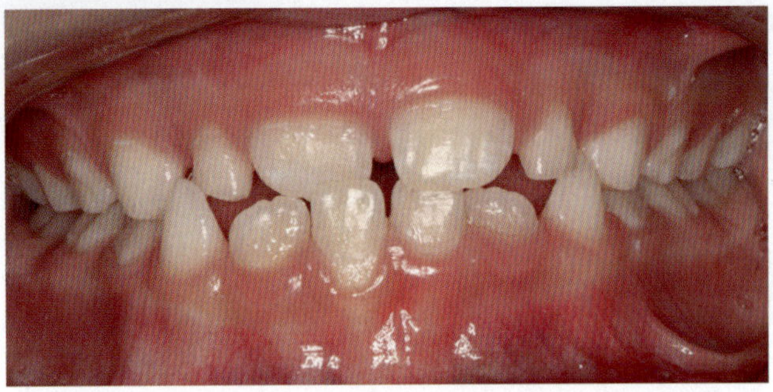

• **Fig. 11.25** Although there was adequate space, this permanent maxillary right central incisor erupted into crossbite. Most likely this was caused by the lingual position of the tooth bud.

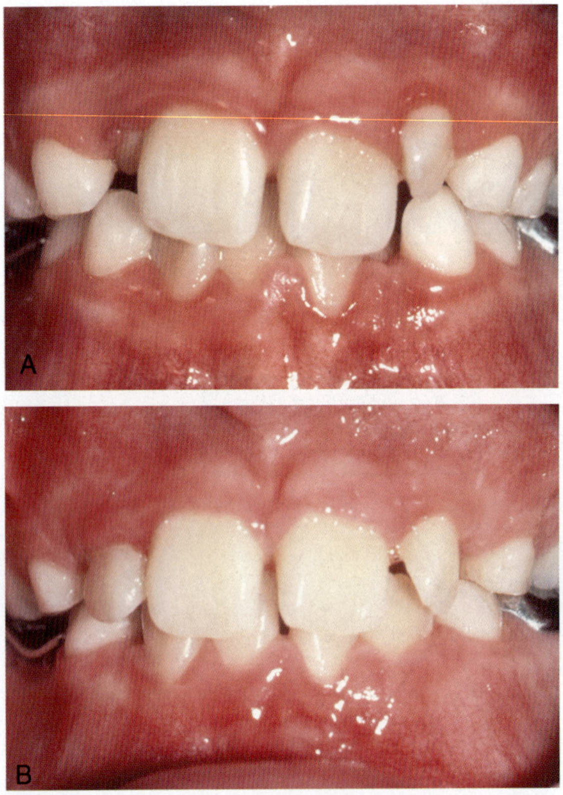

• **Fig. 11.26** An anterior crossbite that is developing as erupting permanent incisors are deflected lingually can be treated by extracting adjacent primary teeth if space is not available for the erupting permanent teeth. (A) The permanent maxillary right lateral incisor is beginning to erupt lingual to the other anterior teeth. (B) Extraction of both primary maxillary canines has allowed spontaneous correction of the crossbite although all the irregularity has not been resolved.

mobility, and possible gingival recession of the affected tooth. Because supernumerary lower incisors can occur, counting these teeth is important. These teeth can cause an increased and more facially positioned arch form and a resultant anterior crossbite.

Treatment of Nonskeletal Anterior Crossbite

In the early mixed dentition, correction of dental anterior crossbites is recommended for two reasons: (1) Lingually positioned maxillary incisors limit lateral jaw movements, and these teeth or their mandibular counterparts sometimes sustain significant incisal abrasion and (2) gingival recession is a risk for anterior teeth in crossbite, especially for the lower incisors, when oral hygiene is less than ideal and gingival inflammation occurs.

Only occasionally, however, is it indicated to correct this type of crossbite in the primary dentition, because crowding severe enough to cause it is rare at that stage and the primary incisors often exfoliate before they can be successfully moved.

The first concern in anterior crossbite treatment is adequate space for tooth movement, which usually requires reducing the width of some adjacent primary teeth, extraction of the adjacent primary teeth, or opening space orthodontically. The diagnostic evaluation should determine whether tipping will provide appropriate correction. Often it will be because the problem arose as eruption paths were deflected. If teeth are tipped when bodily movement is required, stability of the result is questionable. By looking at casts or good intraoral images, it is usually possible to estimate the bodily and axial (inclination) position of the tooth, as well as whether the tooth is rotated. This information is key to selecting a treatment method.

Removable Appliance Therapy

In a young child, one way to tip the maxillary anterior teeth out of crossbite is with a removable appliance, using fingersprings for facial movement of the maxillary incisors (Fig. 11.27). Less frequently, an active labial bow can be used to tip a mandibular incisor lingually. Two maxillary anterior teeth can be moved facially with one 22-mil double-helical cantilever spring. The appliance should have multiple clasps for retention, but a labial bow is contraindicated because it can interfere with facial movement of the incisors and would add little or no retention.

In correction of a dental anterior crossbite in a child, it usually is not necessary to open the bite to prevent incisor interferences that keep the patient in crossbite. Unless the overbite is exceptionally deep, a biteplate would be needed only in a child with a clenching or grinding habit. In the early mixed dentition, the preferred approach is to place the removable appliance without a biteplate and attempt tooth movement. If after 2 months the teeth in the opposing arch are moving in the same direction as the teeth to which the force is being applied, the bite can be opened by adding orthodontic banding resin to the occlusal surfaces of the lower posterior molars. When the crossbite is corrected, the cement can be removed relatively easily, and it does not require alteration of the appliance. Using a biteplate risks the chance that teeth not in contact with the appliance or the opposing arch will erupt excessively.

A removable appliance of this type requires nearly full-time wear to be effective and efficient. If the lingual fingersprings are activated 1.5 to 2 mm, they will produce approximately 1 mm of tooth movement in a month. The offending teeth should be slightly overcorrected and retained until overbite from eruption is adequate to retain the corrected tooth positions. A period of 1 or 2 months of retention with a passive appliance is usually sufficient.

The most common problems associated with these simple removable appliances are lack of patient cooperation, poor appliance design leading to lack of retention, and improper activation. In children asked to wear removable appliances 12 to 15 hours, half of the patients achieved a wear time of 9 hours or more when wearing a monitoring device embedded in the appliance. The wear behaviors showed great variability. Only 15% of the patients wore the appliances every day. Some patients skipped days and then tried to compensate with periods of greater wear time. It is possible that irregular wear can jeopardize treatment success.[8]

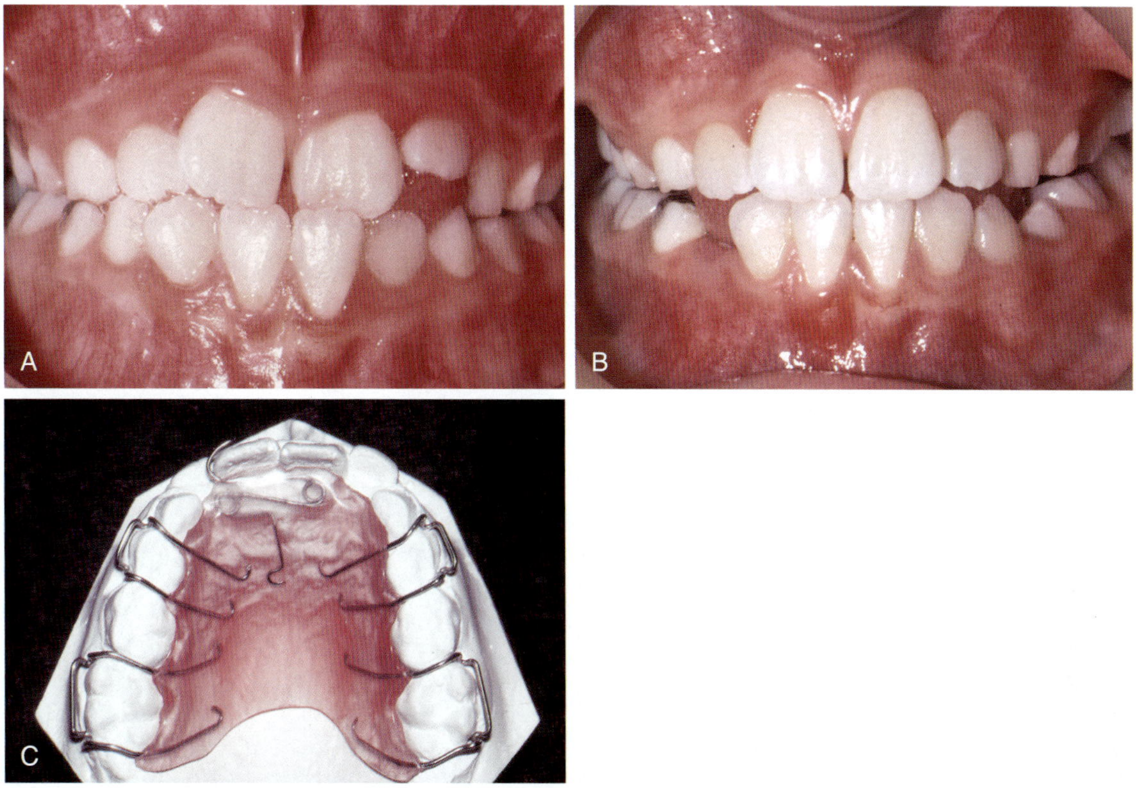

• **Fig. 11.27** Anterior crossbite correction with a removable appliance to tip teeth. (A) The permanent maxillary left central incisor has erupted into crossbite and (B) has been corrected with a removable appliance. (C) This appliance is used to tip both central incisors facially with a 22-mil double-helical fingerspring activated 2 mm per month to produce 1 mm per month of tooth movement. Note that plastic baseplate material extends over the spring to maintain its vertical position (see Chapter 10). The appliance is retained with multiple Adams clasps.

Fixed Appliance Therapy

One of the simplest fixed appliances for correction of maxillary incisors with a moderate anterior crossbite is a maxillary lingual arch with fingersprings (sometimes referred to as whip springs). This appliance (Fig. 11.28) is indicated for a child with whom compliance problems are anticipated. The springs are usually soldered on the opposite side of the arch from the tooth to be corrected, in order to increase their length (and their range). They are most effective if they are approximately 15 mm long. When these springs are activated properly at each monthly visit (advancing the spring about 3 mm), they produce tooth movement at the optimum rate of 1 mm per month. The greatest problems are distortion and breakage from poor patient cooperation and poor oral hygiene, which can lead to decalcification and decay.

It also is possible to tip the maxillary incisors forward with a 2 × 4 or 2 × 6 fixed appliance (2 molar bands with 4 or 6 bonded anterior brackets). In the instance in which there is no skeletal component to the anterior crossbite, this is the best choice for a patient in the mixed dentition with crowding, rotations, the need for bodily movement, or more permanent teeth in crossbite (Fig. 11.29). When the anterior teeth are bonded and moved before permanent canine eruption, it is best to place the lateral incisor brackets with some increased mesial root tip so that the roots of the lateral incisors are not repositioned into the canine path of eruption, with resultant resorption of the lateral incisor roots. If torque or bodily repositioning is needed for these teeth, finishing with a rectangular wire is required even in early mixed dentition treatment. Otherwise, the teeth will tip back into crossbite. This same configuration of a 2 × 4 or 6 appliance can be used in the lower arch to align, derotate or retract lower incisors that are causing the anterior crossbite. When a supernumerary lower incisor is the cause of the crossbite, extracting it and retracting the incisors by closing the space can be accomplished using the same fixed appliance design.

There are several choices to advance the upper incisors using a 2 × 4 or 6 methods after the teeth are aligned with flexible wires. Open coil springs can be used between the molars and incisors or between the incisors and primary canines (Fig. 11.30). The archwires need to be sufficiently strong (TMA or steel) and not larger than 18 mil in a 22 mil bracket slot so the wire can slide. With the archwire cut a little long, but not irritating to the patient, the coil spring moves the anterior teeth facially as the wire slides forward and through the molar tube.

Another approach is to align the incisor and then use a 16 or 18 mil steel wire with loops rolled into it mesial to the permanent maxillary first molars (Fig. 11.31). The loops are stops and the wire between the first molars is a little excessive for the distance so that the archwire must be retracted into the incisor brackets. This will cause the wire to temporarily distort and bow facially between the incisors and molar. Placing a rubber tube over the wire will eliminate some cheek irritation if the activation is not excessive. As the incisors procline, the wire will regain its original arch form. If needed, the loops can be rolled back to increase the arch length, which reactivates the wire and moves the teeth more facially. The appliance can serve as a short-term retainer.

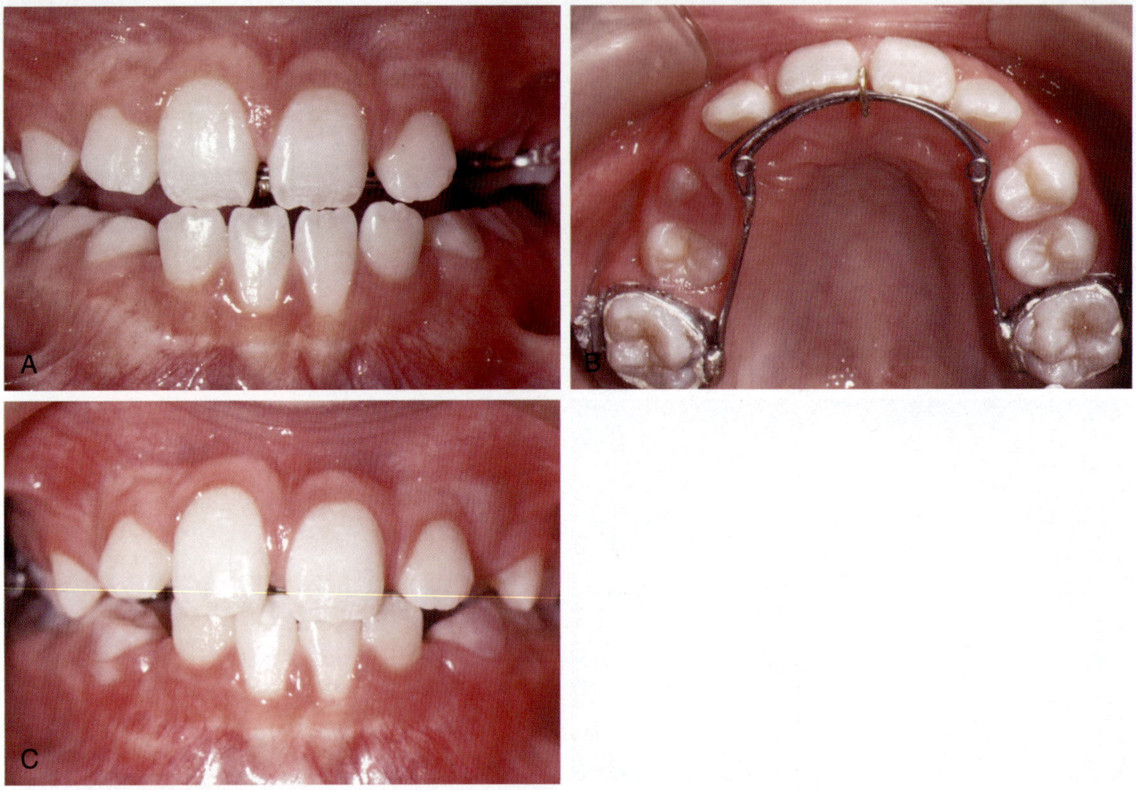

• **Fig. 11.28** (A) An anterior crossbite caused by lingual position of the maxillary incisors can be corrected by using (B) a 36-mil lingual arch with soldered 22-mil fingersprings. A guidewire can be placed between the incisors as shown here to keep the springs from moving incisally. (C) After correction, the appliance can be modified to serve as a retainer by soldering the free ends of the springs to the lingual arch.

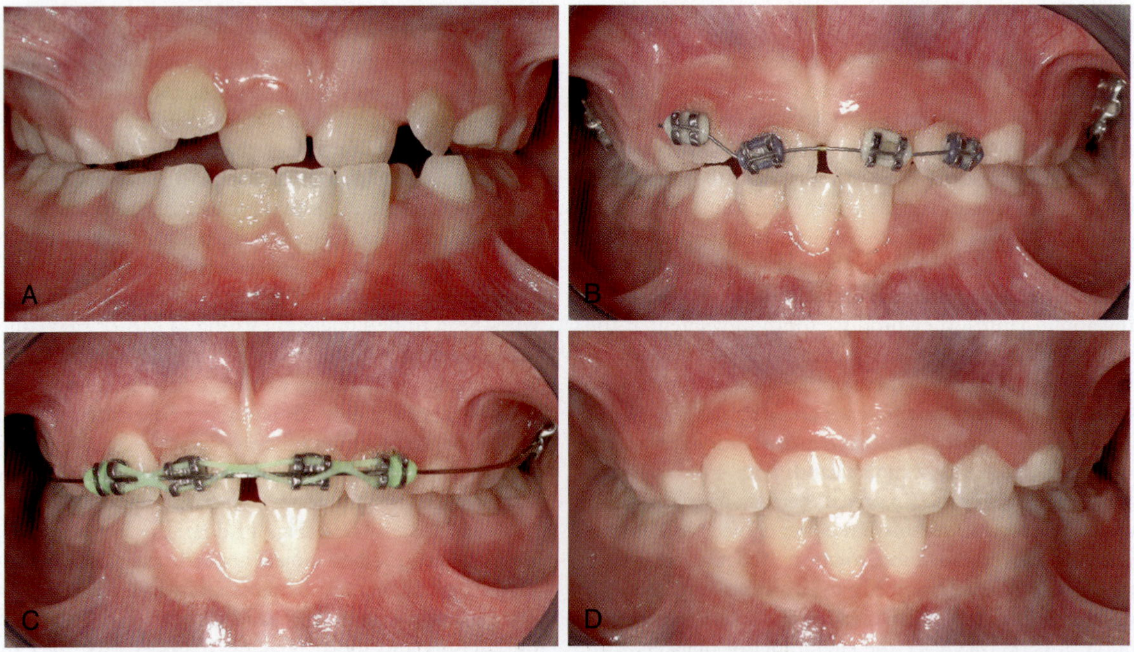

• **Fig. 11.29** (A) This patient has an anterior crossbite and irregular maxillary anterior teeth. (B) A 14 mil segmental nickel-titanium (NiTi) archwire was used from maxillary lateral to lateral incisors to take advantage of the archwire's extreme flexibility for alignment. (C) This was followed by a heavier stainless steel archwire that extended to the molars for more control and stability for diastema space closure with an elastomeric chain as well as (D) final alignment.

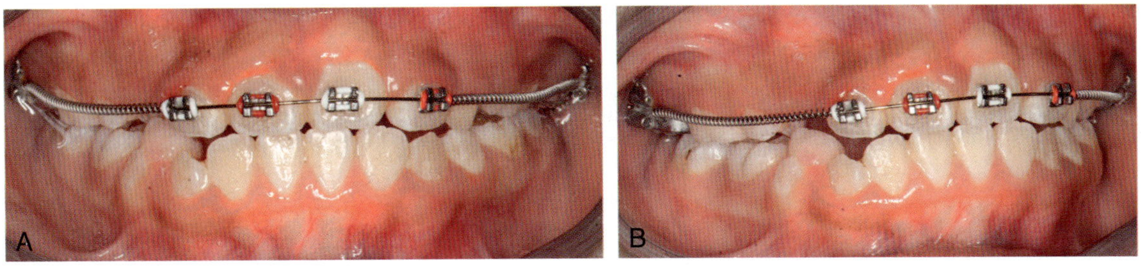

• **Fig. 11.30** Open coil springs can be used to treat an anterior crossbite when multiple anterior teeth are involved. (A) This patient has partial correction of the crossbite using bilateral compressed coil springs between the incisors and molars. As the incisors move facially, the archwire slides through the molar tubes. (B) This view shows the length of the coil spring, which usually should be secured with a steel ligature at its anterior extent. The ligature can be covered by a colored O-tie, if desired.

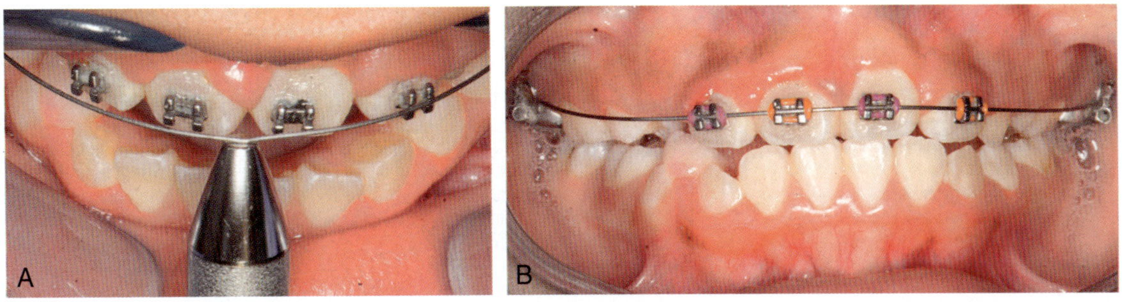

• **Fig. 11.31** An advanced archwire also can move multiple teeth facially to correct an anterior crossbite. (A) When passive the advanced wire will lie facial to the anterior brackets and when engaged place an anterior tipping force on the incisors. (B) The archwire is ligated in place and has rolled loops mesial to the molars to serve as stops with excess wire between the first molars. The excess wire will be displaced buccally between the incisors and molars.

When treatment is complete for fixed appliance anterior crossbite correction, retention can be provided for a couple of months of continued appliance wear to make certain overbite has been established. If rotations or spacing issues were treated in addition to the crossbite, then a Hawley-type appliance with a lateral to lateral incisor labial bow will be needed to hold the tooth position. This appliance has the advantage over a lingual bonded retainer in that the lateral incisors can adjust as the canines erupt.

See Fig. 11.32 for a flowchart to help guide decision-making for anterior crossbites.

Anterior Open Bite

Oral Habits and Open Bites

An open bite in a preadolescent child with normal vertical facial proportions is most likely either a normal transitional open bite from the primary to the permanent dentitions or caused by a habit such as thumb- or finger-sucking, known as nonnutritive sucking. Deviation from the usual transition eruption pattern may have a unique etiologic factor (supernumary, impacted, ectopic, crowded, or missing teeth), but this is less likely. A disproportionately large lower anterior face height with a severe anterior open bite indicates a skeletal problem (excessive vertical growth and rotation of the jaws). All told, these problems affect less than 4% of the mixed dentition population (see Fig. 1.13).

Many of the transitional and habit problems resolve with either time, timely surgical extraction of supernumerary teeth or intervention for ectopic or impacted teeth, or cessation of the sucking habit. Most moderate open bites resolve by adolescence. Open bites that persist into adolescence, except those related to habits, almost always have a significant skeletal component, and careful diagnosis of the contributing factors is required.[9] These are termed *complex open bites*, extend distal to the incisors, and require advanced treatment methods (see Chapter 14).

Effects of Sucking Habits

First, let us consider breastfeeding. Advocates for breastfeeding include a reduced prevalence of malocclusion among its benefits, but in the long-run there appears to be no difference in prevalence of malocclusion between breastfed and nonbreastfed children.[10] It is apparent that longer breastfeeding leads to fewer nonnutritive sucking habits.[11]

During the primary dentition and early mixed dentition years, many children engage in digit- and pacifier-sucking, with these behaviors being more prevalent in girls and nonbreastfed children. Most often children suck digits when they are bored, tired, watching tv, reading, or studying. Some suck exclusively when falling asleep or when sleeping. Although it is possible to deform the alveolus and displace the teeth during the primary dentition years with a prolonged and intense habit, much of the effect is on eruption of the permanent anterior teeth. The extent to which such a habit affects eruption depends on its frequency (hours per day) and duration (months or years) (see Chapter 5). With frequent and prolonged sucking, maxillary incisors are tipped facially, mandibular incisors are tipped lingually, and eruption of some incisors is impeded. As one would expect, overjet increases and

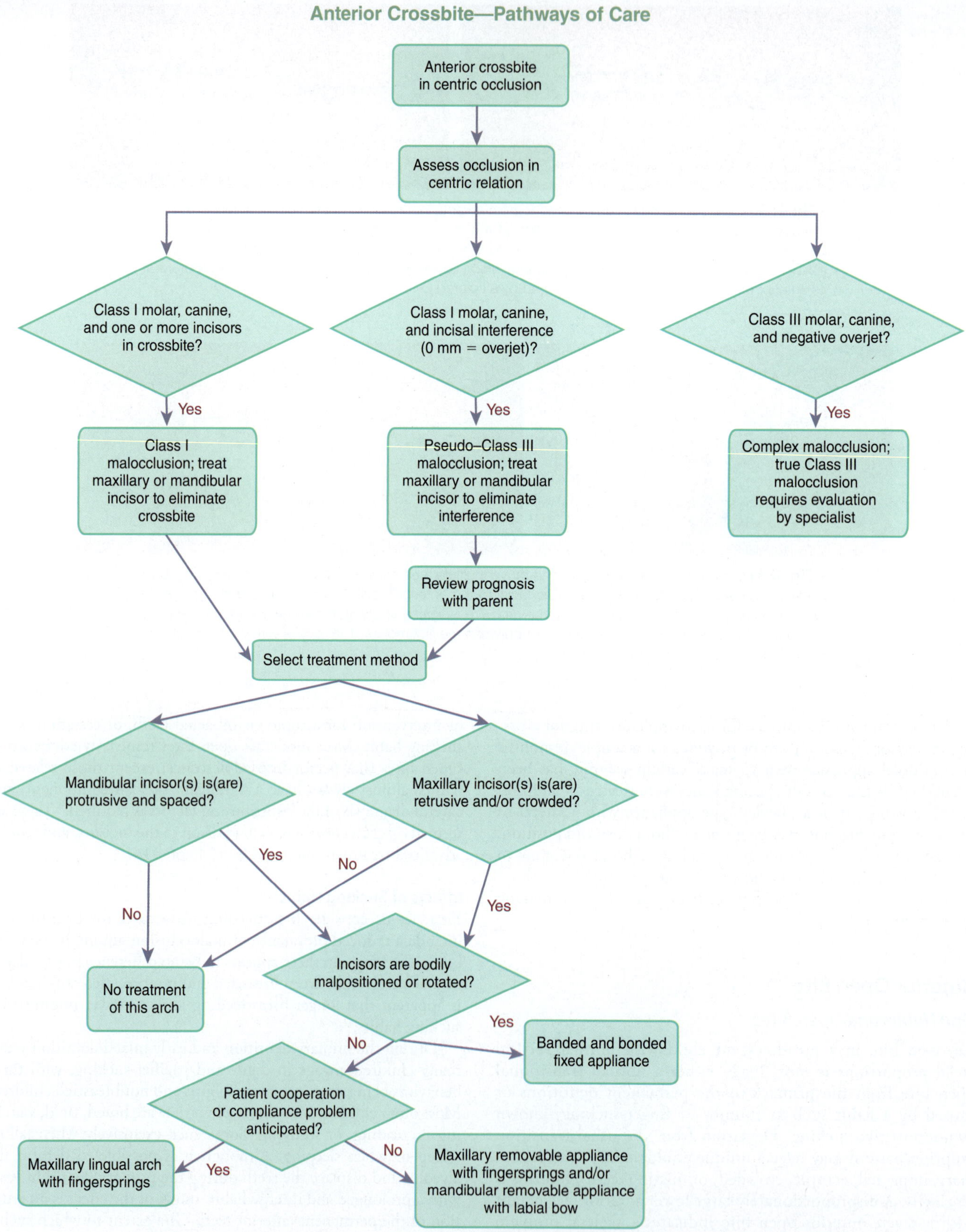

• **Fig. 11.32** This flowchart can be used to aid decision-making regarding possible options for anterior crossbites in the primary and mixed dentitions. Answers to the questions posed in the chart should lead to successful treatment pathways.

overbite decreases. In many children, maxillary intercanine and intermolar width is narrowed, resulting in a posterior crossbite with a V-shaped arch form.

When the effect of digit-sucking is compared with the effect of pacifier use, there is some evidence for increased prevalence of posterior crossbites with pacifiers, and especially with pacifier use for more than 18 months. Pacifier shapes that are designed to produce a more physiologic sucking pattern have not been proven to be beneficial, when compared with other pacifiers or to finger-sucking.[12] Most children have a nonnutritive sucking habit at 24 months, but only 40% have one at 36 months.[13] These habits decrease with age, and pacifier habits are observed less often with older children than digit habits. The social pressures of school are a strong deterrent.

As long as the habit stops before the eruption of the permanent incisors, most of the changes resolve spontaneously with the exception of posterior crossbite (Fig. 11.33).[14] By that time, the majority of children have stopped their sucking habit. Another group still suck but want to stop, and yet another small group who finger suck in mid elementary school or longer do not want to stop and appear to be immune to social pressure. If a child does not want to quit sucking, habit therapy (especially appliance therapy) is not indicated.

Nondental Intervention

As the time of eruption of the permanent incisors approaches, the simplest approach to habit therapy is a straightforward discussion between the child and the dentist that expresses concern and includes an explanation by the dentist of the problems caused by a prolonged finger habit. This "adult" approach (and restraint from intervention by the parents) may be enough to terminate the habit during this first part of the transition to the permanent dentition but is most effective with older children.

Another level of intervention is reminder therapy. This is for the child who wants to quit but needs help. Any one of several reminders that are introduced with an explanation to the child can be useful. One of the simplest approaches is to secure an adhesive bandage with waterproof tape on the finger that is sucked (Fig. 11.34). Alternatively, a tube sock, mitten, or light glove placed

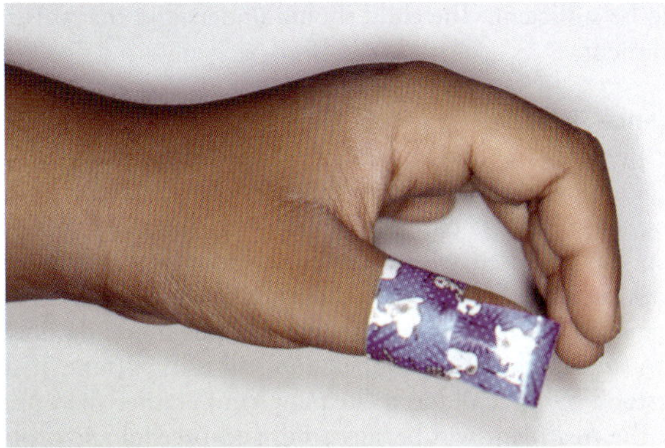

• **Fig. 11.34** An adhesive bandage can be applied over the end of the finger to remind the child not to suck and to reduce the enjoyment. The bandage should be anchored at its base for retention with waterproof tape, so that it will stay in place if sucking is still attempted. (Courtesy Dr. B. Joo.)

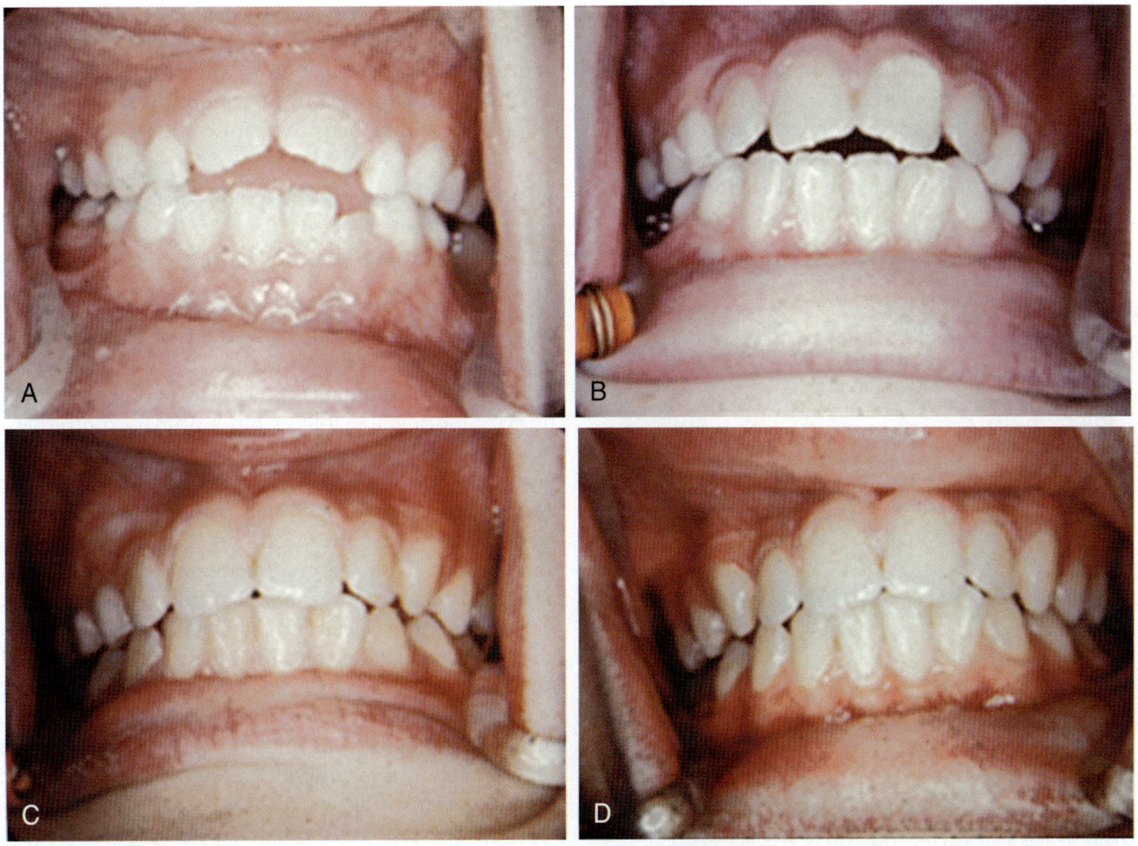

• **Fig. 11.33** (A–D) Photos at 1-year intervals of a child who stopped sucking his thumb at the time of the first photo. Gradual closure of the open bite, without a need for further intervention, usually occurs in patients with normal facial proportions after habits stop.

over the hand and taped around the wrist for security can work. Commercially available fabric or plastic thumb covers as well as bitter tasting nail polishes or liquid preparations can be used successfully.

If the reminder approach fails, a reward system can be implemented that provides a small tangible daily reward for not engaging in the habit. In some cases, a large reward must be negotiated for complete cessation of the habit.

If all these approaches fail and the child really wants to quit, an elastic bandage loosely wrapped around the elbow prevents the arm from flexing and the fingers from being sucked. If this is used, wearing it only at night and 6 to 8 weeks of intervention should be sufficient. The child should understand that this is not punishment.

Appliance Therapy

If the previous methods have not succeeded in eliminating the habit, a removable reminder appliance is contraindicated because lack of compliance is part of the problem. The child who wants to stop can be fitted with a cemented reminder appliance that impedes sucking (Fig. 11.35). These appliances can be deformed and removed by children who are not compliant and do not truly wish to stop the habit, so cooperation still is important. If this is understood by the child as a "helping hand" rather than punishment, the treatment will be successful and psychologic problems will not result.[15] The preferred method is a maxillary lingual arch with an anterior crib device, making it extremely difficult for the child to place the thumb or other object in their mouth. The anterior portion of the quad helix appliance also can be quite useful as a reminder when it is placed in the appropriate position in the palate (see Fig. 11.18).

In about half of the children for whom such a crib is made, thumb-sucking stops immediately and the anterior open bite usually begins to close relatively rapidly. In the remaining children, thumb-sucking persists for a few weeks, but the crib device is eventually effective in extinguishing thumb-sucking in 85% to 90% of patients.[16] It is a good idea to leave the crib in place for 6 months after the habit has apparently been eliminated. Commonly, these cemented reminders, like lingual arch expanders, leave an imprint on the tongue (see Fig. 11.19) that will resolve within 1 year after the appliance is removed. The appliances also trap food and can lead to palatal irritation and mouth odor, so excellent oral hygiene is important.

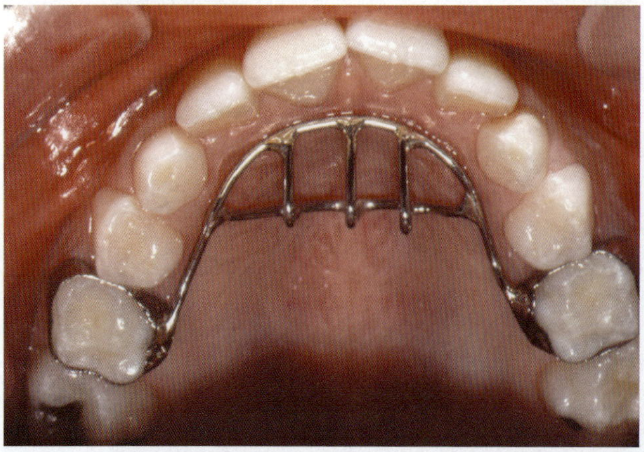

• **Fig. 11.35** A cemented habit crib made of 38- to 40-mil wire can be used as a reminder to interrupt a finger-sucking habit. The appliance can be cemented to either primary or permanent molars and should be extended anteriorly to interfere with the finger position during sucking. The amount of overbite will also help determine the appliance position. A crib is most effective in a child who wants to stop the thumb or finger habit and accepts the crib as a reminder.

The open bites associated with sucking in children with normal jaw relationships often resolve after sucking stops and the remaining permanent teeth erupt (see Fig. 11.33). Other problems that result from sucking habits like a constricted maxilla or flared and spaced incisors will require a maxillary expander or fixed or removable appliance, respectively, to correct. The open bite should require no other treatment in children with good skeletal proportions.

A flowchart is provided to help guide decision-making for open bite problems related to oral habits (Fig. 11.36).

Deep Bite

Before treating an overbite problem, it is necessary to establish its cause. Significant deep bites affect approximately 20% of patients with mixed dentition. The problem may result from reduced lower face height, lack of eruption of posterior teeth, or overeruption of the anterior teeth. The possible treatments are quite different and mutually exclusive.

True reduced lower face height is a skeletal problem and requires more complex treatment (see Chapter 14). Undereruption of posterior teeth or overeruption of anterior teeth also are complex problems that are addressed during comprehensive treatment. They are rarely treated during the mixed dentition years unless there is developing tissue damage (see Fig. 11.11). In those instances as an interim measure, a removable appliance with an anterior bite plane to encourage eruption of the posterior teeth and also provide protection of the affected tissue can be used. Treatment like this is only a temporary solution, and the child will require comprehensive treatment in the permanent dentition.

Management of Eruption Problems

Overretained Primary Teeth

A permanent tooth should replace its primary predecessor when approximately three-fourths of the root of the permanent tooth has formed, whether resorption of the primary roots is or is not to the point of spontaneous exfoliation. Given enough time, the primary tooth will exfoliate, but a primary tooth that is retained beyond this point should be removed because it often leads to gingival inflammation and hyperplasia that cause pain and bleeding and sets the stage for deflected eruption paths of the permanent teeth. These overretained teeth can result in irregularity, crowding, and crossbite. If a portion of the permanent tooth crown is visible and the primary tooth is mobile to the extent that the crown will move 1 mm in the facial and lingual direction, it is probably advisable to encourage the child to "wiggle" the tooth out. If that cannot be accomplished in a few days, extraction is indicated. Most overretained primary maxillary molars have either the buccal roots or the large lingual root intact; most overretained primary mandibular molars have either the mesial or distal root still intact and hindering exfoliation.

Once the primary tooth is out, if space is adequate, moderately abnormal facial or lingual positioning will usually be corrected by the equilibrium forces of the lip, cheeks, and tongue. In general, incisors will erupt lingually and then move facially

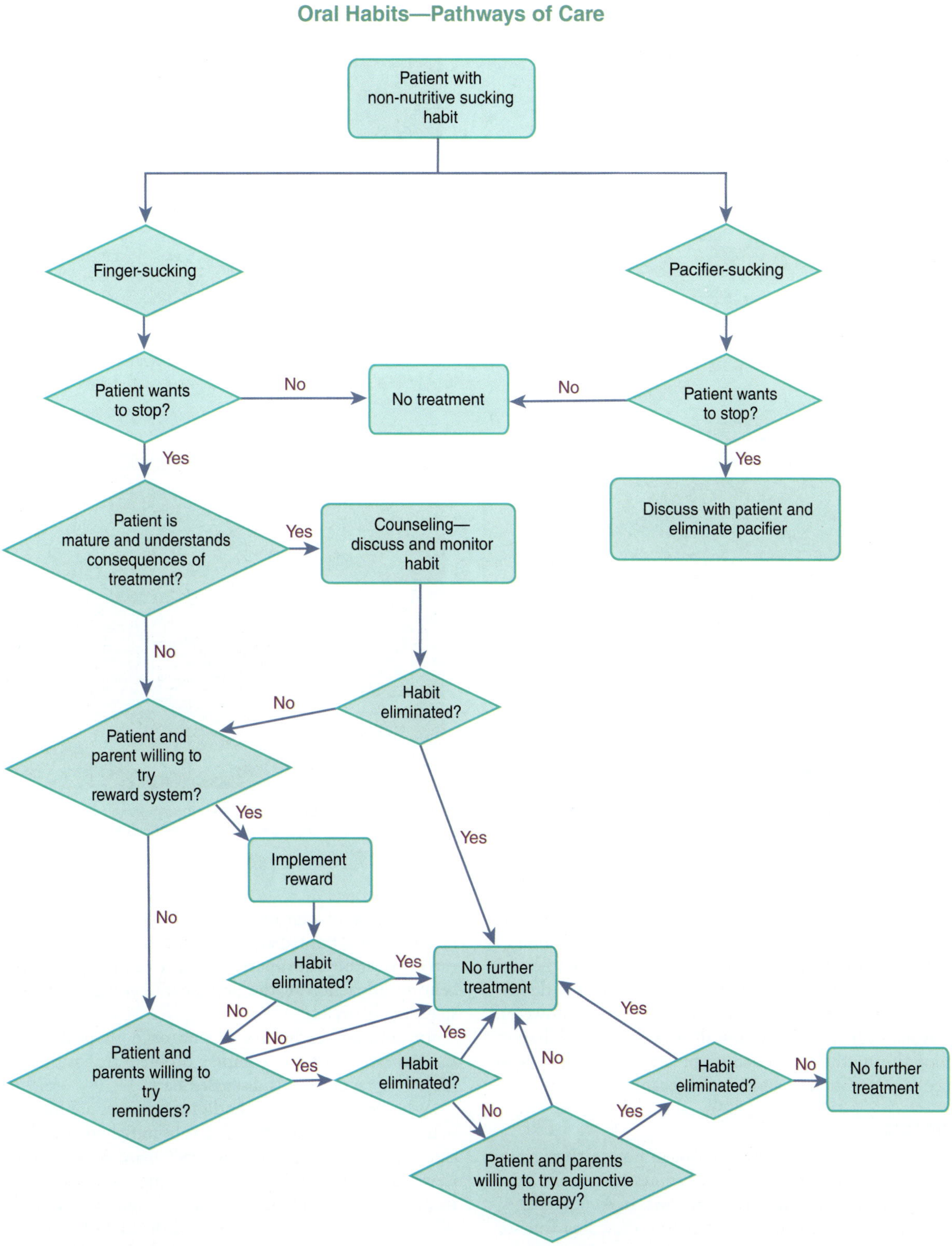

• **Fig. 11.36** This flowchart can be used to aid decision-making regarding possible options for oral habits during the primary and mixed dentitions. Answers to the questions posed in the chart should lead to successful treatment pathways.

when overretained primary incisors exfoliate or are removed (Fig. 11.37). If spontaneous correction has not occurred when overbite is achieved, however, further spontaneous alignment is unlikely in either the anterior or posterior quadrants, and active tooth movement will be required to correct the crossbite.

Ectopic Eruption

The term *ectopic eruption* is used to describe the situation in which a permanent tooth erupts on a deviant eruption path, so it emerges into the mouth at a different point than it should have or becomes totally blocked, and often causes damage to the roots

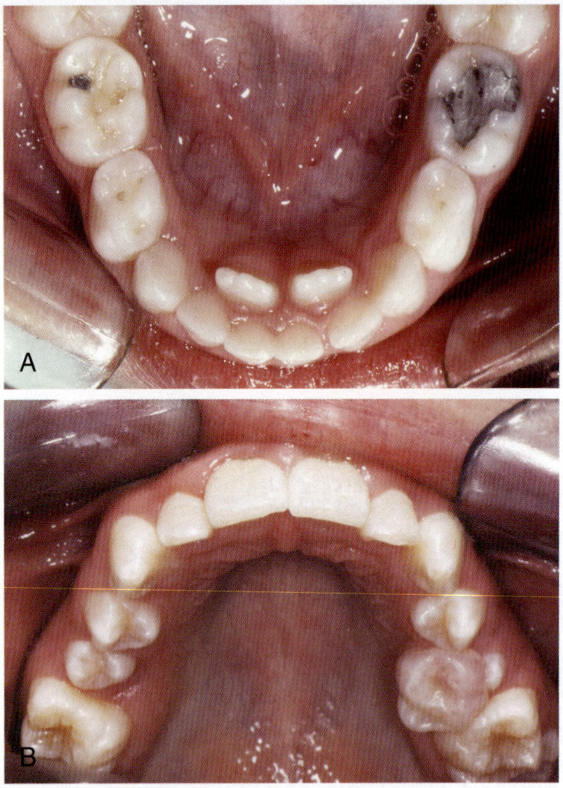

• **Fig. 11.37** Permanent teeth often erupt in abnormal positions as a result of retained primary teeth. (A) These lower central incisors erupted lingually because the permanent incisors have not been lost and their tooth buds are positioned lingual to the primary incisors. This is a common occurrence in this area and is the main reason lingual arches should not be placed until after lower incisors erupt. (B) This maxillary left second premolar has been deflected facially because of the retained primary molar. In both the circumstances shown here, removal of the retained primary tooth or teeth will allow some spontaneous alignment.

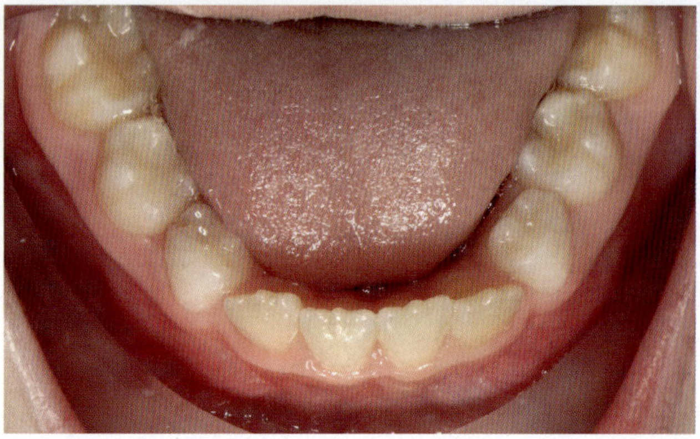

• **Fig. 11.38** This patient lost two primary canines during the eruption of the permanent lower incisors. This usually indicates either a large incisor liability or a substantial shortage of lower arch perimeter.

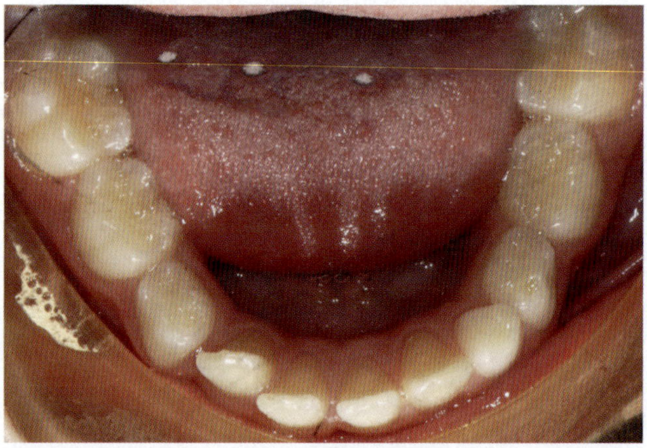

• **Fig. 11.39** This patient lost one primary canine when the lower incisors erupted and had a shift of the midline to the right. Shifts of this magnitude are, on average, rare.

of other teeth. As we have noted previously, osteoclasts above the crown of an erupting tooth resorb tooth roots as readily as bone.

Any permanent tooth can erupt ectopically, and examples are shown in several locations in this book, starting with the discussion in Chapter 6. Three patterns of deviant eruption, however, are both reasonably frequent and clinically significant, and deserve consideration during the mixed dentition: lateral incisors in both arches, maxillary first molars, and maxillary canines.

Lateral Incisors

When the permanent lateral incisors erupt in both arches, some degree of root resorption of the primary canines is common, and less frequently, one or both these teeth are lost. In some patients, this is just a symptom of the temporary incisor crowding (incisor liability—the difference in the size of the primary and permanent incisors) that is normal in the early mixed dentition (see Chapter 4) and not an indication of long-term crowding. More often, loss of one or both primary canines indicates a significant lack of enough space for all the permanent teeth. Space analysis, including an assessment of the anteroposterior incisor position and the facial profile, is needed to determine whether space maintenance, space management of the leeway space, space regaining, or more complex treatment involving arch expansion or extraction will be required.

Early loss of one or both primary *maxillary* canines almost never requires immediate treatment; indeed, as you will see later, early extraction of primary maxillary canines is important in preventing impaction of the permanent canines, but closure of the space rarely occurs.

In contrast, early loss of one or both primary *mandibular* canines can be a more complex problem that is best managed in specialty practice but is discussed here.

When both primary mandibular canines are lost as the lateral incisors erupt, either there is a substantial "incisor liability" that can still be accommodated by space management of the available leeway space with a lingual arch during the transition (see later in this chapter) or there is a true arch length shortage (Fig. 11.38). If there is a moderate shortage and the incisor position can tolerate expansion, that is an option. If the crowding is more severe, extraction of permanent teeth is a more reasonable option (see Chapter 12 for details on both these topics). Guidance for these decisions comes from doing a space analysis and assessing the incisor position.

An early decision as to how to manage patients with early loss of one mandibular primary canine also is required (Fig. 11.39). In that situation, the predominant thinking has been that the remaining retained primary canine should be extracted to prevent a shift of the midline, a lingual arch placed to keep the incisors from tipping lingually, and a fixed appliance used to correct a developing midline asymmetry if that was occurring. This has recently been shown not to be the usual result of the loss of one primary canine more than a year before the loss of the contralateral primary canine. Using data from the Iowa and Burlington growth studies, Christensen et al.[17] showed that the prevalence of a clinically significant midline shift after premature loss of one primary canine was not statistically or clinically greater than what was seen in patients with normal eruption (1.3 and 1.0 mm, respectively).

With this in mind, the clinician faced with early loss of one mandibular primary canine now can choose among several approaches. A passive lingual arch to prevent lingual tipping only could still be used, but the new data suggest that it is not necessary to hold the midline or extract the contralateral tooth in addition to the lingual arch. An early phase of 2 × 4 or 2 × 6 treatment to correct minor midline changes also could be deferred until nearer the time of mandibular canine eruption if the problem persists.

Maxillary First Molars

Ectopic eruption of a permanent first molar presents an interesting problem that is usually diagnosed from routine bitewing radiographs rather than clinically because it is painless. When only small amounts of resorption of the distal root of the primary maxillary second molar (<1 to 1.5 mm) are observed (Fig. 11.40), a period of watchful waiting is indicated because self-correction is possible and occurs in about two-thirds of the cases. If the blockage of eruption persists for 6 months or if resorption continues to increase, treatment is indicated. Lack of timely intervention may cause loss of the primary second molar and space loss as the permanent molar erupts mesially and rotates mesiolingually.

Several methods can be helpful when intervention is necessary.[18] The basic approach is to move the ectopically erupting tooth away from the primary molar it is resorbing. If a limited amount of movement is needed but little or none of the permanent first molar is visible clinically, a 28-mil brass wire looped and tightened around the contact between the primary second molar and the permanent molar is suggested (Fig. 11.41). It may be necessary to anesthetize the soft tissue to place the brass wire, and depending on the tooth position and depth of the contact between the permanent and primary molars, it can be difficult to successfully direct the brass wire subgingivally. If no subgingival space is seen on the radiograph, fishing the wire between the teeth is pointless. The brass wire should be tightened at each adjustment visit,

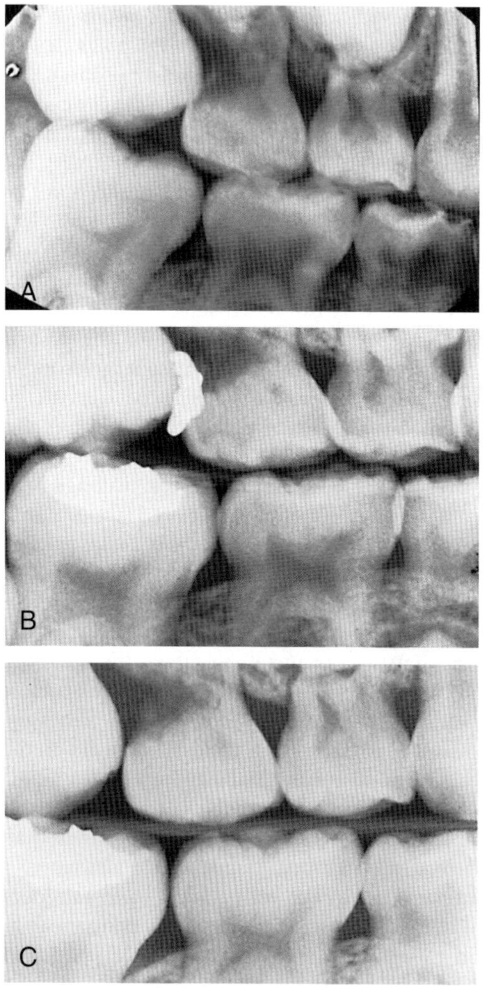

• **Fig. 11.41** Moderately advanced resorption from ectopic eruption of the permanent maxillary first molar requires active intervention. (A) This distal root of the primary maxillary second molar shows enough resorption that self-correction is highly unlikely. (B) A 28-mil dead soft brass wire is guided under the contact (starting from either the facial or lingual surface) and then looped around the contact between the teeth and tightened at approximately 2-week intervals; (C) the permanent tooth is dislodged distally and erupts past the primary tooth that is retained.

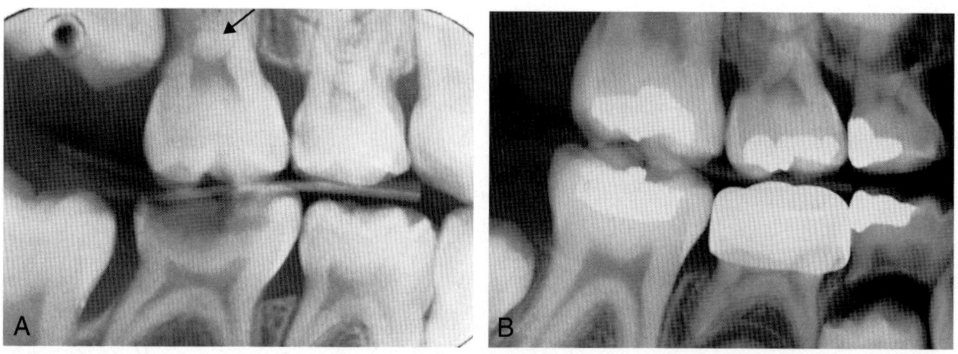

• **Fig. 11.40** Ectopic eruption of the permanent first molar is usually diagnosed from routine bitewing radiographs. If the resorption is limited, immediate treatment is not required. (A) The distal root of the primary maxillary second molar shows minor resorption from ectopic eruption. (B) This radiograph taken approximately 18 months later illustrates that the permanent molar was able to erupt without treatment.

approximately every 2 weeks, so that it will not move in relation to the teeth. If the wire is not tightened to the point that the patient feels some discomfort, it has not been appropriately adjusted. Treatment is slow but reliable when used with limited resorption.

A steel spring clip separator, available commercially, may work if only a small amount of resorption of the primary molar roots exists. These clips are difficult to place if the point of contact between the permanent and primary molars is much below the cementoenamel junction of the primary molar, although some are available that have greater vertical dimensions for just these situations (Fig. 11.42). They can be activated on a biweekly basis.

Elastomeric separators wedged mesial to the permanent first molar also can be used to push it distally so it can erupt but are not recommended. The current elastomeric separators are large. They are well retained for normally positioned teeth, but they require substantial force to place them below the contact of an impacted molar. They have the potential to become dislodged in an apical direction and cause periodontal irritation. If this occurs, the separators are hard to locate and retrieve, especially if the material is not radiopaque.

If resorption on the distal roots of the primary second molars is severe and more distal movement is required than can be provided by the brass wire or metal separators, the situation becomes more complicated. If access can be gained to the occlusal surface of the molar, a simple fixed appliance can be fabricated to move the molar distally. The appliance consists of a band on the primary molar (which can be further stabilized with a transpalatal arch) with a soldered spring that is bonded to the permanent molar (Fig. 11.43). In lieu of using a soldered appliance that must be fabricated in the laboratory, a similar but alternative appliance can be fabricated intraorally with either a band and looped spring (Fig. 11.44A) or two bonded brackets (a permanent first molar bracket on the primary second molar and a permanent second molar bracket on the permanent first molar) and a looped spring (Fig. 11.44B). With either appliance, if the movement is not sufficient in 2 weeks, the loop can be reactivated.

If the permanent molar has caused extensive resorption of the primary molar, there may be no choice but to extract the primary

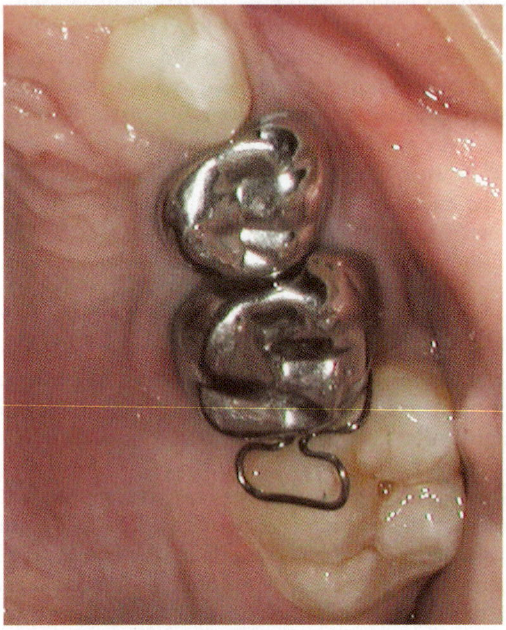

• **Fig. 11.42** An Arkansas spring (Arkansas Dental Products Co, West Plains, MO), a scissors-like spring that extends below the contact point, can be effective in tipping a permanent first molar distally so that it can erupt. The posterior bow is crimped to bring the subgingival legs together and apply pressure to separate the teeth.

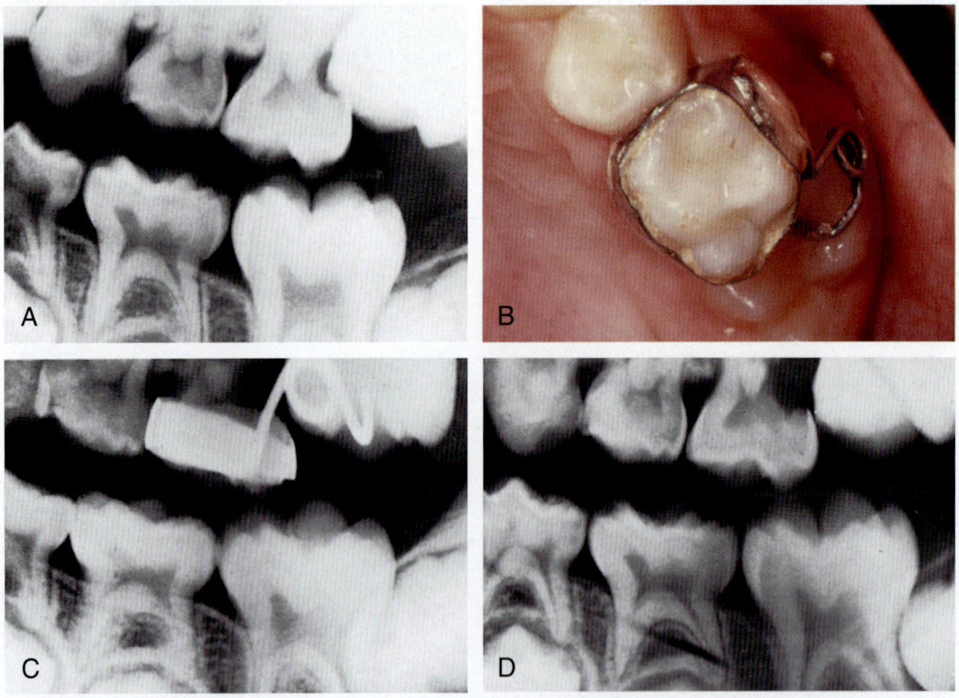

• **Fig. 11.43** Ectopic eruption with severe resorption may require appliance therapy. (A) This primary maxillary second molar shows severe resorption. (B) If the occlusal surface of the permanent molar is accessible, the primary molar can be banded and a 20-mil spring soldered to the band. (C) The permanent molar is tipped distally out of the resorption defect and (D) once disengaged, is free to erupt.

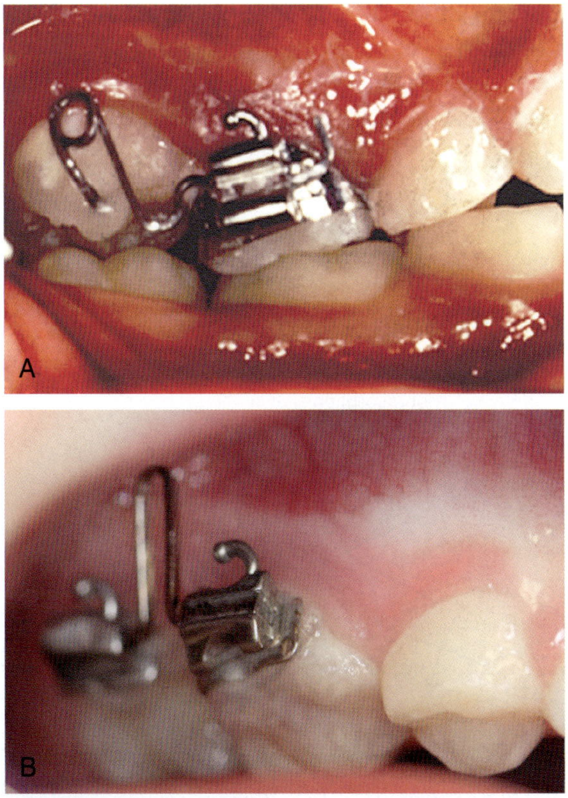

• **Fig. 11.44** (A) A band and spring appliance can be fabricated intraorally with a savings of time and laboratory expense. A band with an attachment having a buccal tube is cemented on the primary second molar. Next a large omega-shaped loop and a helical loop are bent distal to the primary molar. The spring is activated, and the wire is inserted into the primary molar tube from the distal surface and secured with a bend anterior to the molar tube. The helical loop is compressed during bonding to the occlusal surface of the permanent first molar. The appliance is reactivated intraorally by opening the omega loop with loop-forming pliers with the round beak positioned superior to the wire. (B) Another option for repositioning an ectopically erupting first molar is to bond archwire tubes on both the primary second molar and the permanent first molar. Then, bend an opening loop or loops from either rectangular beta-titanium or stainless steel wire, and compress it to seat from the distal into the primary molar tube and from the mesial into the permanent molar tube. The force from the activated loop will retain the rectangular wire, which can be carefully positioned adjacent to the soft tissue. This avoids banding and laboratory procedures.

tooth, which allows the permanent molar to continue to move mesially and shorten the arch length. Unless the second premolar is missing and the arch length is purposefully being reduced or unless considerable mesial molar movement is tolerable and later premolar extraction is planned, a distal shoe that guides the erupting molar should be placed after the extraction (see later in this chapter). Even if this technique is used, some space has already been lost and the permanent molar will have to be repositioned distally after it fully erupts using another type of space-regaining appliance described in this chapter or Chapter 12.

A flowchart summarizes the decision-making for ectopic eruption of permanent first molars (Fig. 11.45).

Maxillary Canines

At approximately age 10, if a maxillary primary canine is not mobile and there is no observable or palpable facial canine bulge, ectopic eruption of maxillary canines should be considered. Canine ectopic eruption is a relatively frequent occurrence (the incidence of ectopic eruption and impaction of canines is in the 1%–2% range).[19] This can lead to either or both of two problems: (1) impaction of the canine and/or (2) resorption of permanent lateral and/or central incisor roots.[20] There appears to be a genetic basis for this eruption phenomenon, and in some cases it is related to small or missing maxillary lateral incisors and missing second premolars.[21] Root resorption of the permanent incisors is significantly more likely to occur when no space is available for the canine.[22]

Although multiple studies now have shown that cone beam computed tomography (CBCT) images are superior to two-dimensional (2D) images for both localization of impacted canines and evaluation of resorption of roots of other teeth,[23] it is probably better to get a full view of the status of the patient first with a digital panoramic radiograph because dental anomalies are genetically related, and other anomalies may well be present (peg or missing lateral incisors, missing premolars, and transposed teeth). Then, depending on the findings, it is sensible to obtain detailed information on root resorption and position of the canine eruption from a small field-of-view (FOV) CBCT (Fig. 11.46). These views can be supplemented with a traditional cephalometric digital image if required for limited or comprehensive orthodontic care. This is less radiation than to initially obtain a full-field CBCT (see Table 6.10).

Given the potential complications of continued ectopic canine eruption, early diagnosis and intervention are warranted to either prevent or limit root resorption. When a mesial position of the erupting permanent canine is detected and incisor root resorption is threatened but has not yet occurred, extraction of the primary canine is indicated (Fig. 11.47). Ericson and Kurol found that if the permanent canine crown was overlapping less than half of the root of the lateral incisor as seen in a panoramic radiograph, there was an excellent chance (91%) of normalization of the path of eruption. When more than half of the lateral incisor root was overlapped, early extraction of the primary tooth resulted in a 64% chance of normal eruption and likely improvement in the position of the canine even if it was not totally corrected.[24] A systematic review confirms this effect.[25] Extraction of the primary canine with maxillary expansion appears to encourage improved permanent canine eruption even more.[26]

Supernumerary Teeth

Supernumerary teeth can disrupt the normal eruption of other teeth and cause crowding or spacing. Treatment is aimed at extracting the supernumeraries before problems arise or at minimizing the effects if other teeth have already been displaced.

The most common location for supernumerary teeth is the anterior maxilla. These teeth are often discovered on a panoramic or occlusal radiograph when a child is about 6 to 7 years of age, either during a routine examination or when permanent incisors fail to erupt. The simple cases are those in which a single supernumerary tooth is present and superficially located. If the tooth is not inverted, it will often erupt before or along with the normal tooth and can be extracted before it interferes with the adjacent teeth.

The choice of which tooth to retain and which one is the supernumerary can be difficult, but it really makes no difference. The tooth that should be retained is the one with the best size, color, morphologic characteristics, and position related to the other teeth. All other things being equal, the tooth that is nearest to the

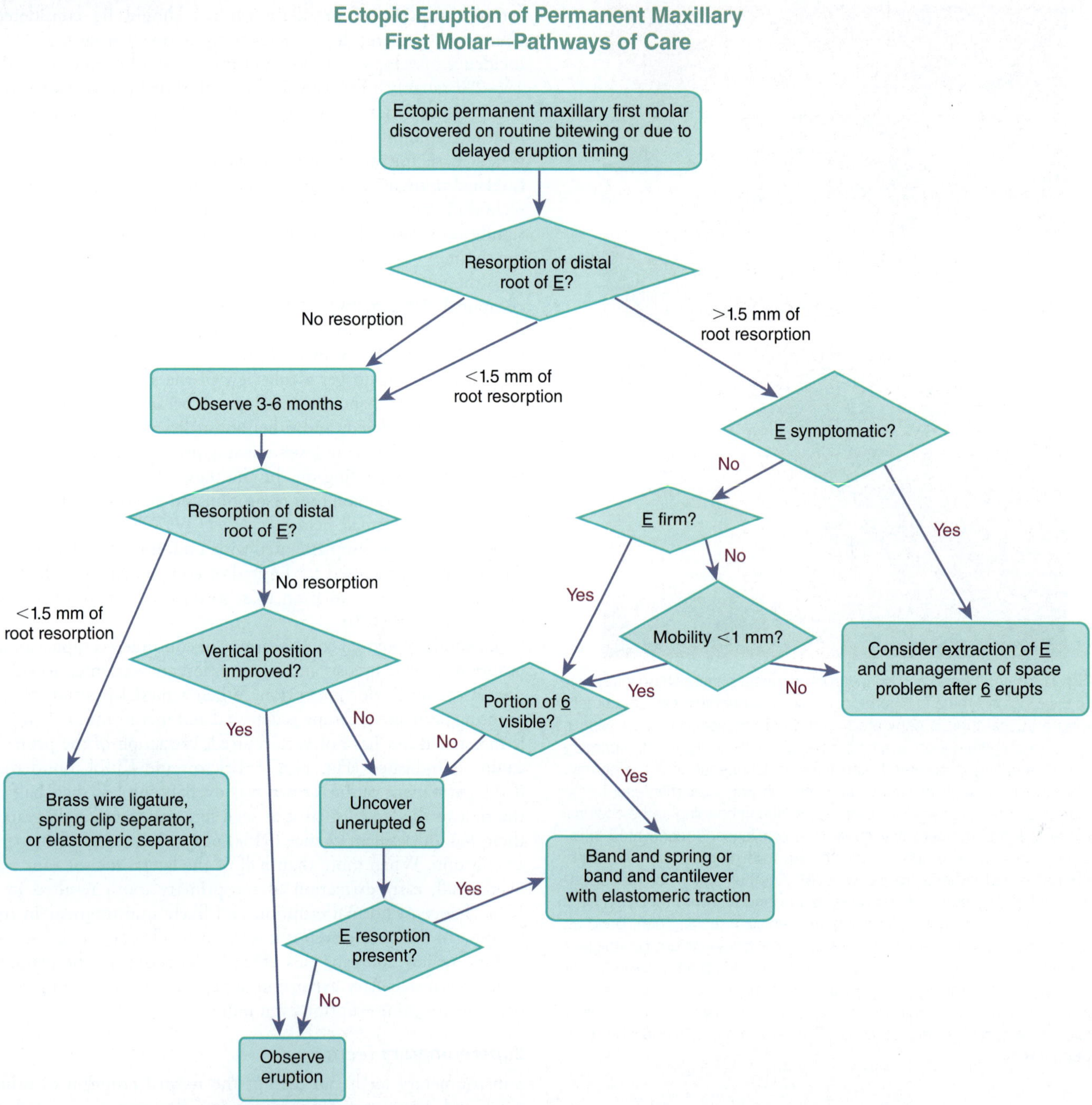

• **Fig. 11.45** This flowchart can be used to aid decision-making regarding possible options when a permanent molar is ectopically erupting during the mixed dentition. Answers to the questions posed in the chart should lead to successful treatment pathways. E, The primary maxillary second molar; 6, the permanent maxillary first molar. (Modified from Kennedy D, Turley P. The clinical management of ectopically erupting first permanent molars. *Am J Orthod Dentofac Orthop*. 1987;92:336–345.)

ultimate final position should be retained (Fig. 11.48). These decisions are difficult to make from conventional radiographs when the teeth are unerupted, and supernumerary teeth can be missed or continue to develop. Small-FOV CBCT can be helpful and is indicated now for evaluation of most of these patients.

When multiple supernumerary teeth are discovered or suspected, the difficulty of diagnosis and treatment is amplified. This is covered in Chapter 12.

Delayed Incisor Eruption

When an incisor has failed to erupt more than 6 months to a year past the normal eruption time and adjacent teeth have erupted, there is no excuse for delaying treatment. The esthetic and social consequences along with the impact on ultimate eruption and development of the dentition are bound to be significant. A retained primary tooth, supernumerary tooth, or some type of pathologic condition is most commonly associated with delayed

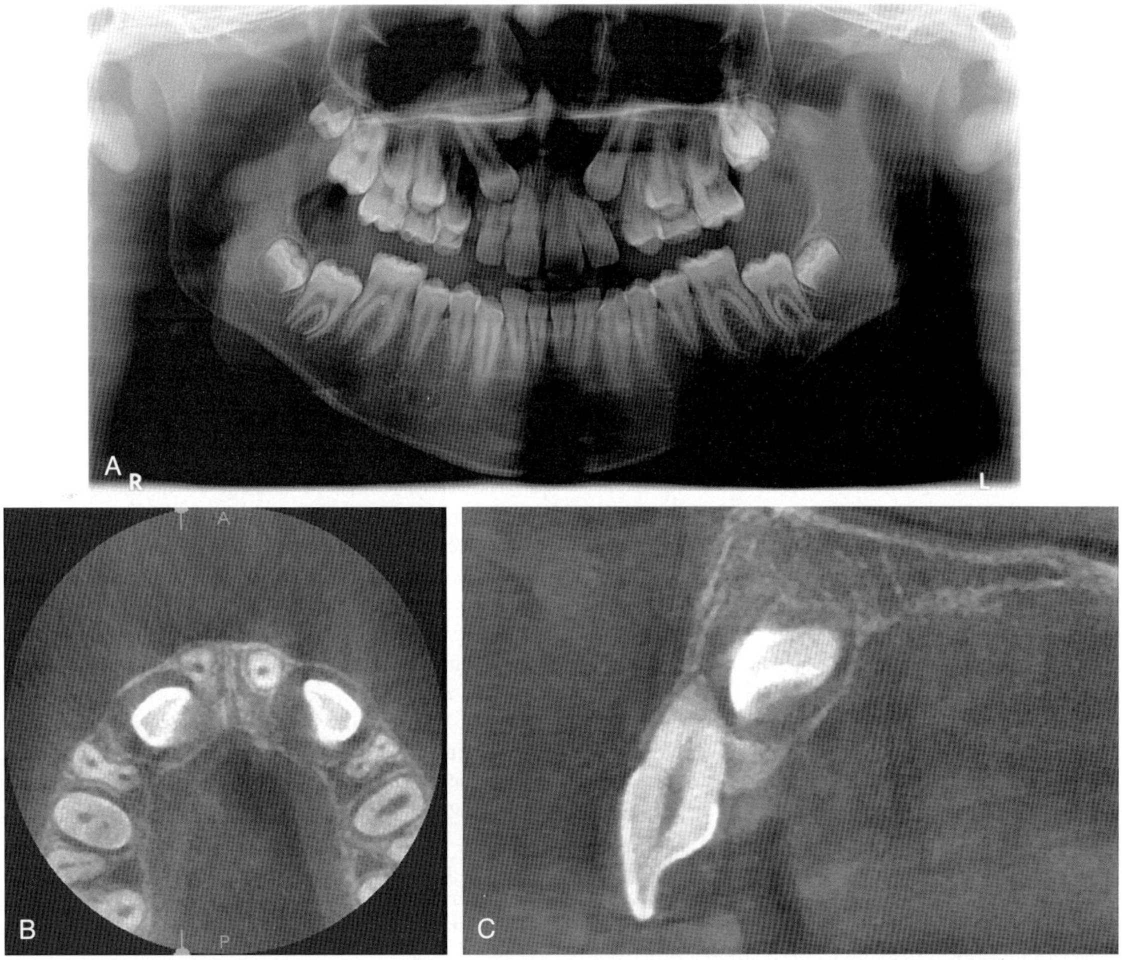

• **Fig. 11.46** (A) Panoramic radiograph showing damage to the maxillary lateral incisor roots from ectopically erupting canines. (B and C) Three-dimensional images from small–field-of-view cone beam computed tomography (CBCT), which clarify the position of the unerupted canines and establish the initial direction of movement of the canines that will be needed to prevent further damage to the laterals. The radiation exposure for a CBCT of this type is about the same as with a digital panoramic radiograph, and the CBCT is needed because of its potential to change the treatment plan.

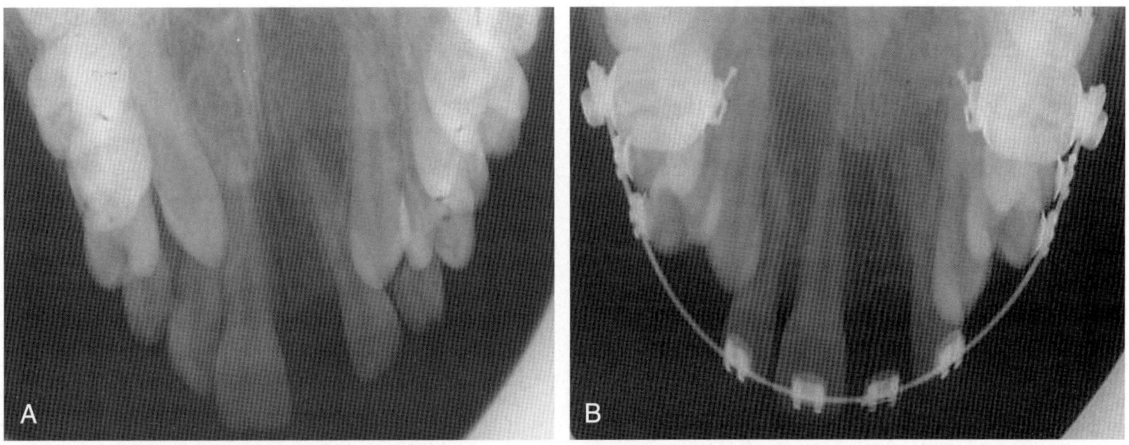

• **Fig. 11.47** (A) This patient has a maxillary right canine positioned over the root of the maxillary right lateral incisor with more than 50% overlap. The left permanent canine overlapped less than 50% of the permanent lateral incisor root. This positioning is associated with an increased risk of resorption of the incisor roots. The adjacent primary canines were extracted and (B) improvement was observed as the right canine nearly totally corrected while the left one made only minor changes in lateral position. These changes probably would not have occurred without the intervention.

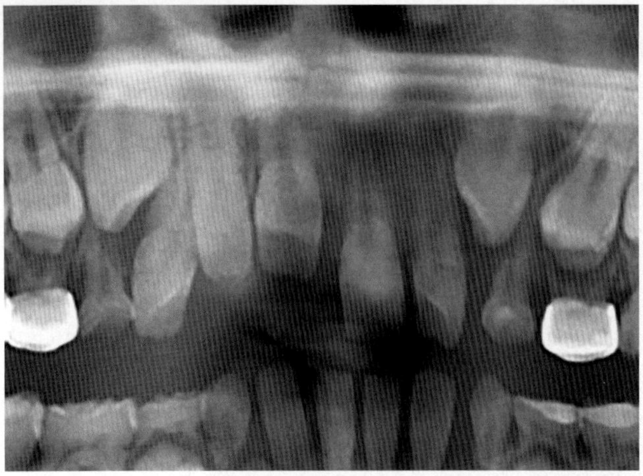

• **Fig. 11.48** When patients have supernumary teeth, and in this patient it was a maxillary lateral incisor that was the most distal of the two teeth, a decision needs to be made which one to keep and which to extract. Generally speaking, the tooth nearest to the final position of the teeth is maintained. That reduces the orthodontic movement. In this case, due to the tooth form and size, the most mesial tooth was extracted.

incisor eruption. The best advice is to count the teeth and pay close attention to departures from normal eruption timing.

The first consideration in evaluating this situation is the morphologic features (usability) of the unerupted tooth and its position. If the tooth is not malformed and is located superficially under the keratinized tissue, it can be exposed with a simple soft tissue excision and usually will erupt rapidly (Fig. 11.49). If the tooth is more deeply positioned or associated with pathology that has disrupted its orientation, it is likely to need surgical uncovering, removal of the pathology and fixed appliance treatment to bring it into proper position. This is discussed in Chapter 12.

Ankylosed Primary Teeth

Ankylosed primary teeth with permanent successors, especially ankylosed primary molars, constitute a potential alignment problem for the permanent teeth. Although these teeth usually resorb without creating long-term problems, occasionally they fail to resorb or are retained by a bony attachment in the cervical region. This delays the erupting permanent tooth and can deflect it from the normal eruption path. Appropriate management of an ankylosed primary molar consists of maintaining it until an interference with eruption or drift of other teeth begins to occur (Fig. 11.50), then extracting it and placing a lingual arch or other appropriate fixed appliance if needed. If adjacent teeth have tipped over the ankylosed tooth, they will need to be repositioned to regain space. Vertical bony discrepancies will be eradicated when the permanent tooth brings bone with it during eruption.

The situation is completely different when an ankylosed primary tooth has no permanent successor. Then, to avoid long-term periodontal problems, there are two approaches. Either the ankylosed primary molar should be extracted before a large vertical occlusal discrepancy develops and with it a large vertical periodontal bony defect (Fig. 11.51)[27] or the tooth can be decoronated. This procedure is more complex and is described in Chapter 12.

Because erupting teeth bring alveolar bone with them, early extraction of the primary molar without a successor and space maintenance will not solve the problem of continued ridge resorption in the edentulous area. The longer the ankylosed primary tooth is left in place, the greater the chance of a long-term defect because alveolar bone has not formed in that area. Although extraction of the primary tooth without a successor will result in some loss of alveolar bone, this is preferable to a long-term periodontal problem due to reduced attachment and exposed cementum on the adjacent teeth. This plan will require later bone grafting.

It is advisable to have an experienced clinician remove these teeth. Unless the extraction is managed carefully, an even worse periodontal defect may occur.

Space Analysis: Quantification of Space Problems

Space problems must be considered from the viewpoint of the space available, which is quantified by the space analysis. The space analysis results must be considered in the context of the profile because reducing protrusion reduces the amount of available space. Conversely, when teeth are retroclined and then moved facially to the correct position, more space is available. The vertical dimension also has an impact on space. It is generally contraindicated to expand when there is limited overbite because tipping teeth facially usually moves them vertically as well and an anterior open bite may develop. In a child with a deep overbite and an accentuated curve of Spee, leveling the arch will make teeth more protrusive.

It is important to quantify the amount of crowding within the arches because treatment varies, depending on the severity of the crowding. Space analysis, using the dental casts, is required for this purpose. Such an analysis is particularly valuable in evaluating the likely degree of crowding for a child in the mixed dentition when the permanent teeth are erupting and real or transitional crowding is evident, because it predicts the size of unerupted permanent teeth.

Principles of Space Analysis

Space analysis requires a comparison between the amount of *space available* for the alignment of the teeth and the amount of *space required* to align them properly in the dental arches (Fig. 11.52). The analysis can be done either manually on plaster or printed dental casts or with a computer system using virtual digital casts.

Whether the space analysis is done manually or virtually, the first step is calculation of space available. This is accomplished by measuring arch perimeter from the mesial of one permanent first molar to the other, over the contact points of posterior teeth and the incisal edges of the anterior teeth. There are two basic ways to accomplish this manually: (1) by dividing the dental arch into segments that can be measured as straight-line approximations of the arch (Figs. 11.53A) or (2) by contouring a piece of wire (or a curved line on the computer screen) to the line of occlusion and then straightening it out for measurement. The first method is preferred for manual calculation because of its greater reliability. Either method can be used with an appropriate computer program.

The second step is to calculate the amount of space required for alignment of the teeth. This is done by measuring the mesiodistal width of each erupted tooth from contact point to contact point, estimating the size of unerupted permanent teeth (if necessary), and then summing the widths of the individual teeth (see Fig. 11.53B). If the sum of the widths of the permanent teeth is greater than the amount of space available, there is a space deficiency and crowding will occur. If available space is larger than the space required (excess space), gaps between some teeth will be expected.

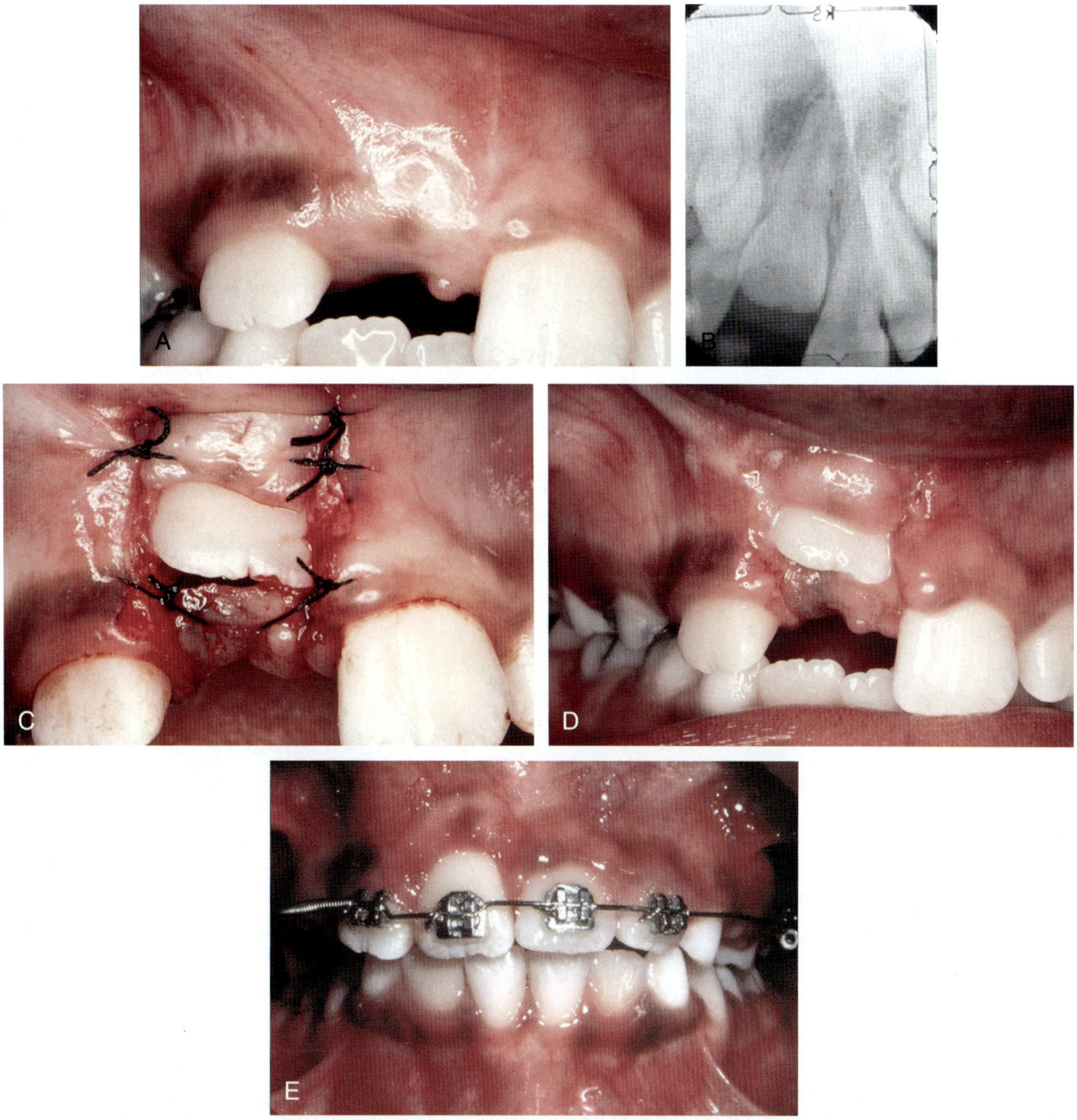

• **Fig. 11.49** (A) This patient had a superficially positioned permanent maxillary right central incisor that was unerupted and substantially delayed. (B) The radiograph shows the tooth at the crestal bone level. (C) The flap has been released on both sides, repositioned apically, and sutured in place with adequate exposed tooth structure. (D) One week after surgery, the tissue is healing well. (E) Appliances in place for the final positioning. Note the uneven gingival borders of the two central incisors, which will become more similar with age as the left central incisor's attachment migrates apically. Or, later the margins can be modified with a diode laser.

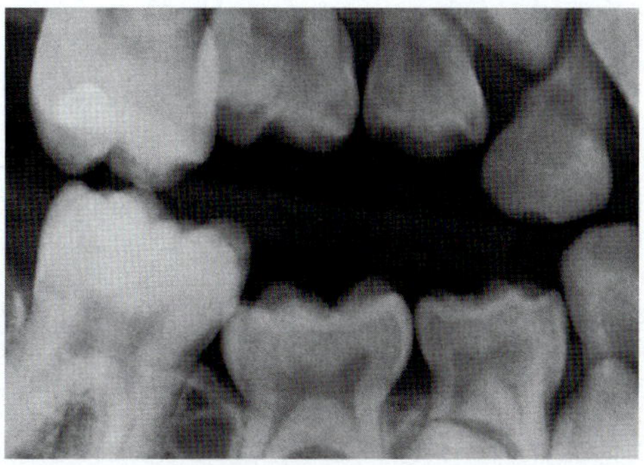

• **Fig. 11.50** This radiograph demonstrates both anterior and posterior teeth tipping over adjacent ankylosed primary molars. The ankylosed teeth should be removed if significant tipping and space loss are occurring.

Space analysis carried out in this way is based on three important assumptions: (1) the anteroposterior position of the incisors is correct (i.e., the incisors are neither excessively protrusive nor retrusive), (2) the space available will not change because of growth and dental compensatory tipping, and (3) all the teeth are present and reasonably normal in size. None of these assumptions can be taken for granted. All of them must be kept in mind when space analysis is done.

With regard to the first assumption, it must be remembered that incisor protrusion is relatively common and that retrusion, though uncommon, does occur. There is an interaction between crowding of the teeth and their protrusion or retrusion: if the incisors are positioned lingually (retruded), this accentuates any crowding; but if the incisors protrude, the potential crowding

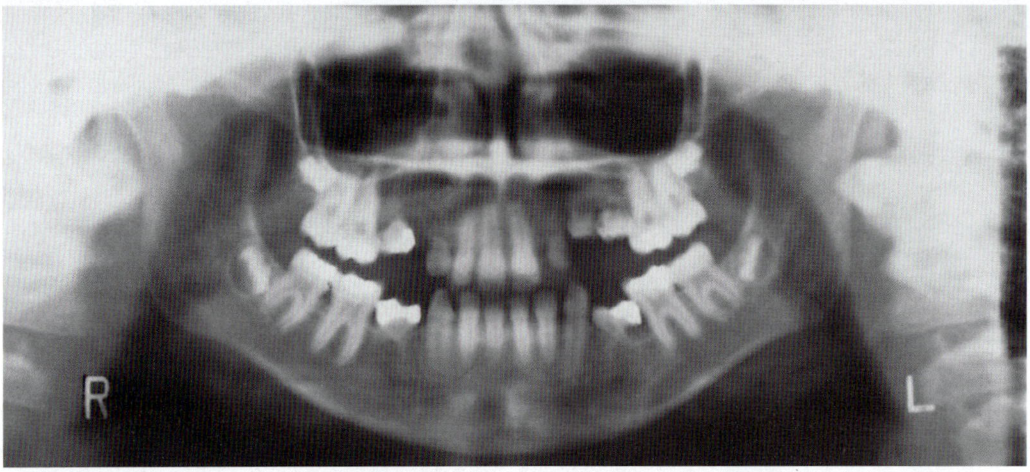

• **Fig. 11.51** If they have no successors, ankylosed primary teeth can be carefully removed when vertical discrepancies begin to develop. It is better to allow permanent teeth to drift into the edentulous space and bring bone with them, and then reposition the teeth before implant or prosthetic replacement, so that large periodontal defects such as those adjacent to the primary molars in this patient do not develop. Another approach is to decoronate the primary molar.

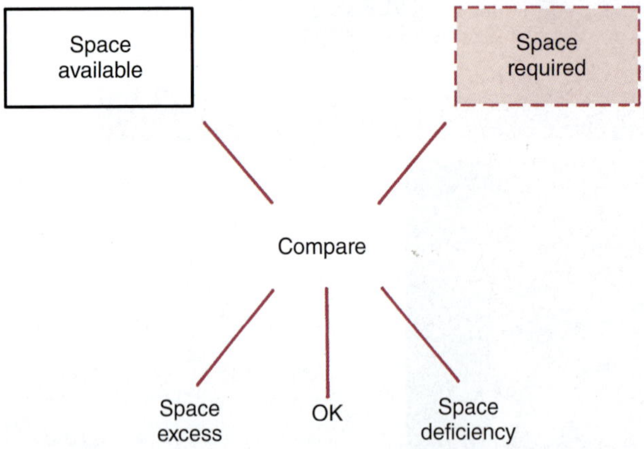

• **Fig. 11.52** A comparison of space available versus space required establishes whether a deficiency of space within the arch will ultimately lead to crowding, whether the correct amount of room is available to accommodate the teeth, or whether excess space will result in gaps between the teeth.

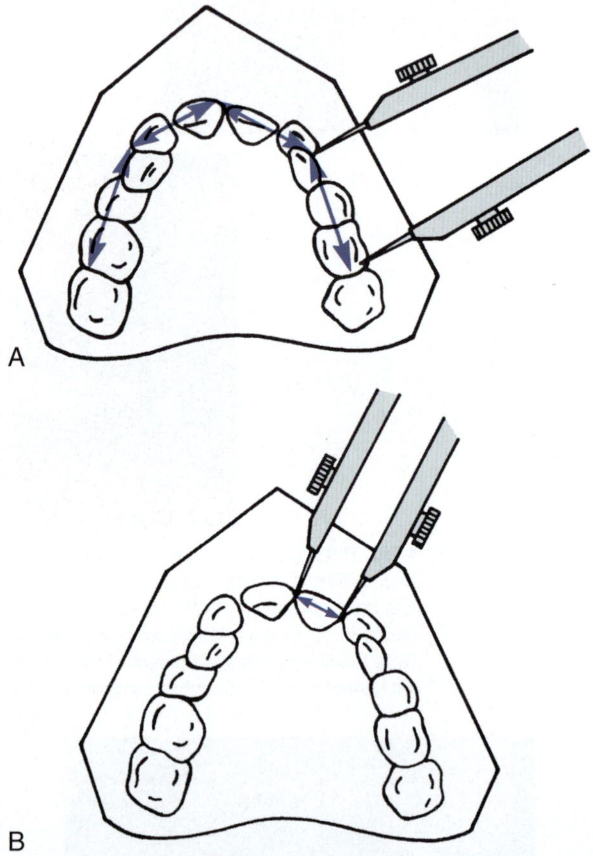

• **Fig. 11.53** (A) Space available can be measured most easily by dividing the dental arch into four straight segments as shown. Each segment is measured individually with a divider or sharpened Boley gauge. (B) Space required is the measured sum of the mesiodistal widths of all individual erupted permanent teeth plus the estimated sizes of the unerupted permanent teeth.

will not be fully expressed. Crowding and protrusion are really different aspects of the same phenomenon. If there is not enough room to properly align the teeth, the result can be crowding, protrusion, or (most likely) some combination of the two. For this reason, information about how much the incisors protrude must be available from clinical examination to evaluate the results of space analysis. This information comes from facial form analysis or from cephalometric analysis (see Chapter 6).

The second assumption, that space available will not change during growth, is valid for most but not all children. In a child with a well-proportioned face, there is little or no tendency for the dentition to be displaced during jaw growth, but the teeth often shift anteriorly or posteriorly in a child with a jaw discrepancy. For this reason, space analysis is less accurate for children with skeletal problems (Class II, Class III, long face, short face) than in those with good facial proportions.

Even for children with well-proportioned faces, the position of the permanent molars changes when they erupt and when primary molars are replaced by the premolars (see Chapter 3 for a detailed review). If space analysis is completed in the mixed dentition, it may be necessary to adjust the space available measurement to reflect the shift in permanent first molar position that can be anticipated when the primary second molars are lost during the late mesial shift.

The third assumption can (and must) be checked by clinical and radiographic examination. All permanent teeth must be present and of normal size and shape. Missing teeth make the projections of space requirements invalid. Anomalies in tooth size have significant implications for space in the dental arches (see Fig. 5.22).

Estimating the Size of Unerupted Permanent Teeth

Estimation is useful in the permanent dentition when a few permanent teeth are unerupted and crowding or spacing are suspected. More often estimation is helpful in the early mixed dentition when space issues are suspected and the direction of treatment for different situations needs to be determined. Taking periapical radiographs to measure the size of the unerupted permanent teeth includes a radiation burden and getting adequate canine images in the lower arch is difficult and uncomfortable for young patients. For these situations, the space analysis was created. There are two basic approaches to doing this:

1. *Measurement of the teeth on radiographs.* This requires an undistorted radiographic image, which is achieved with multiple periapical radiographs. Even with this method, it is often difficult to obtain an undistorted view of the canines, and this inevitably reduces the accuracy. With any type of radiograph, it is necessary to compensate for enlargement of the radiographic image. This can be done by measuring an object that can be seen both in the radiograph and on the casts, usually a primary molar tooth. A simple proportional relationship can then be set up. Accuracy is fair to good, depending on the quality of the radiographs, rotated unerupted teeth, and their position in the arch. The technique can be used in maxillary and mandibular arches for all ethnic groups, but the radiation burden is justified only in unusual cases.
2. *Estimation from proportionality tables.* There is a reasonably good correlation between the size of the erupted permanent lower incisors and the unerupted canines and premolars. By using the mesiodistal width of the *lower* incisors, the size of *both* the lower and upper unerupted canines and premolars can be predicted. The size of the lower incisors correlates better with the size of the upper canines and premolars than does the size of the upper incisors because upper lateral incisors are extremely variable teeth. No radiographs are required, and it can be used for the upper or lower arch.

Tanaka and Johnston developed a simple variation of the proportionality method, using a single equation and the width of the lower incisors to predict the size of unerupted canines and premolars (Box 11.1).[28] For children from a European population group, the method has good accuracy despite a small bias toward overestimating the unerupted tooth sizes. It requires neither radiographs nor reference tables (once the equation is memorized), which makes it very convenient, but two specific problems now are recognized: It tends to overestimate the required space for Caucasian females in both arches and underestimate the space required in the lower arch for African-American males.

• BOX 11.1 Tanaka and Johnston Prediction Values

One-half of the mesiodistal width of the four lower incisors	+10.5 mm = estimated width of mandibular canine and premolars in one quadrant
	+11.0 mm = estimated width of maxillary canine and premolars in one quadrant

Most computer algorithms for space analysis are based on correlations of tooth sizes and should be used with caution if the radiographs show anything unusual (unless the computer program allows for introduction of radiographic information).

Which of these methods is best for an individual patient depends on the circumstances. The prediction tables work surprisingly well when applied to the population group from which they were developed: white schoolchildren of northern European descent. On balance, the Tanaka-Johnston method probably is most practical for manual calculation because no radiographs are required and the simple ratio can be printed right on the space analysis form or memorized, so no reference tables must be consulted.

Remember that the potential mesial shift of the molars is not included in the Tanaka-Johnston analysis, so if the mesial shift is essential, it should be included in your thinking and will shorten the available space. This can be ignored if the goal is simply to calculate the space present and to consider how to use it during treatment planning. Also, the results of the facial form analysis must be factored in to the results of the space analysis to determine if the current incisor and lip positions are appropriate or if the incisor and lip positions needs to be proclined or retroclined for esthetics which will increase or decrease, respectively, the space in the arch. The space must reside within the face!

A screen capture from a commercial computer analysis is shown in Fig. 11.54. Computer analysis is faster and easier, but it is important to remember that its accuracy will depend on the accuracy of the digitized input and how well the patient meets the assumptions that underlie a correlation approach.

Treatment of Space Problems

In the section of the chapter that follows, you will recognize that the problems become increasingly more complex but are still within reach of many general practitioners. Other space problems, more complex still, usually will be addressed in a specialty practice and are discussed in Chapter 12.

Premature Tooth Loss With Adequate Space: Space Maintenance

Early loss of a primary tooth presents a potential alignment problem because drift of permanent or other primary teeth is likely unless it is prevented. Space maintenance is appropriate only when adequate space is available, and when all unerupted teeth are present and at the normal stage of development. Space maintenance is also inappropriate if the child is judged or proven to be noncompliant with appliance wear. Poor oral hygiene and a history of high caries susceptibility also preclude space maintenance. If a permanent successor will erupt within 6 months (i.e., if more than one-half to two-thirds of its root has formed), a space maintainer is unnecessary. If there is not enough space for the permanent tooth or if it is missing, space maintenance alone is inadequate or inappropriate, and the other treatment approaches discussed here will be needed.

Several treatment techniques can be used successfully for space maintenance, depending on the specific situation. Because

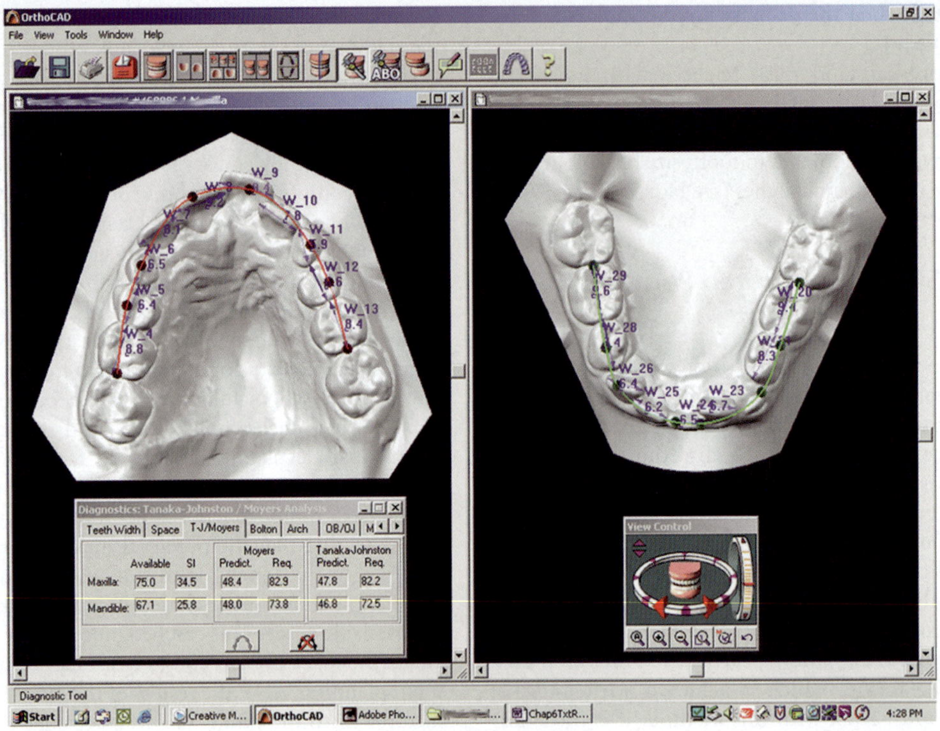

• **Fig. 11.54** Space analysis can be accomplished by a computer algorithm. The data for the arch dimensions and tooth widths can be entered by digitizing the already present digital casts. Then the computer does the calculations.

these appliances are at risk for breakage and loss, they must be monitored carefully, probably at 3- to 6-month intervals, to be successful.

Band-and-Loop Space Maintainers

The band and loop is a unilateral fixed appliance indicated for space maintenance in the posterior segments. The simple cantilever design makes it ideal for isolated segmental space maintenance (Fig. 11.55). Because the loop has limited strength, this appliance must be restricted to holding the space of one tooth and is not expected to accept functional forces of chewing. Although bonding a rigid or flexible wire across the edentulous space has been advocated as an alternative, this has not proved satisfactory clinically. It is also no longer considered advisable to solder the loop portion to a stainless steel crown because this precludes simple appliance removal and replacement. Teeth with stainless steel crowns should be banded like natural teeth.

If a primary second molar has been lost, the band can be placed on either the primary first molar or the erupted permanent first molar. Some clinicians prefer to band the primary tooth in this situation because of the risk of decalcification around any band, but primary first molars are challenging to band because of their morphologic features, which converge occlusally and make band retention difficult. A more important consideration is the eruption sequence of the succedaneous teeth. The primary first molar should not be banded if the first premolar is developing more rapidly than the second premolar because loss of the banded abutment tooth would require replacement of the appliance.

Before eruption of the permanent incisors, if a single primary molar has been lost bilaterally, a pair of band-and-loop space maintainers is recommended instead of the lingual arch that would be used if the patient were older. This is advisable because the permanent incisor tooth buds are lingual to the primary incisors and often erupt lingually. The bilateral band and loops enable the permanent incisors to erupt without interference from a lingual wire. At a later time, the two band-and-loop appliances can be replaced with a single lingual arch if necessary.

The survival of band and loops is not impressive. It has been judged to be approximately 18 months, with cement failure cited as the most frequent problem.[29] This speaks to the need to evaluate these space maintainers at routine recall visits or more frequently.

Partial Denture Space Maintainers

A partial denture is most useful for bilateral posterior space maintenance when more than one tooth has been lost per segment and the permanent incisors have not yet erupted. In these cases, because of the length of the edentulous space, band-and-loop space maintainers are contraindicated, and the likely lingual position of the permanent incisors at initial eruption makes the lingual arch a poor choice. The partial denture also has the advantage of replacing some occlusal function.

Another indication for this appliance is posterior space maintenance in conjunction with replacement of a missing primary incisor or delayed permanent incisor eruption (Fig. 11.56). Anterior space maintenance is unnecessary because arch circumference generally is not lost even if the teeth drift and redistribute the space. Primary anterior teeth are not required for nutrition or speech development, and children adapt readily to missing teeth in most cases, so replacement of missing anterior teeth is done solely to improve appearance. This may have social advantages, however, even for young children.

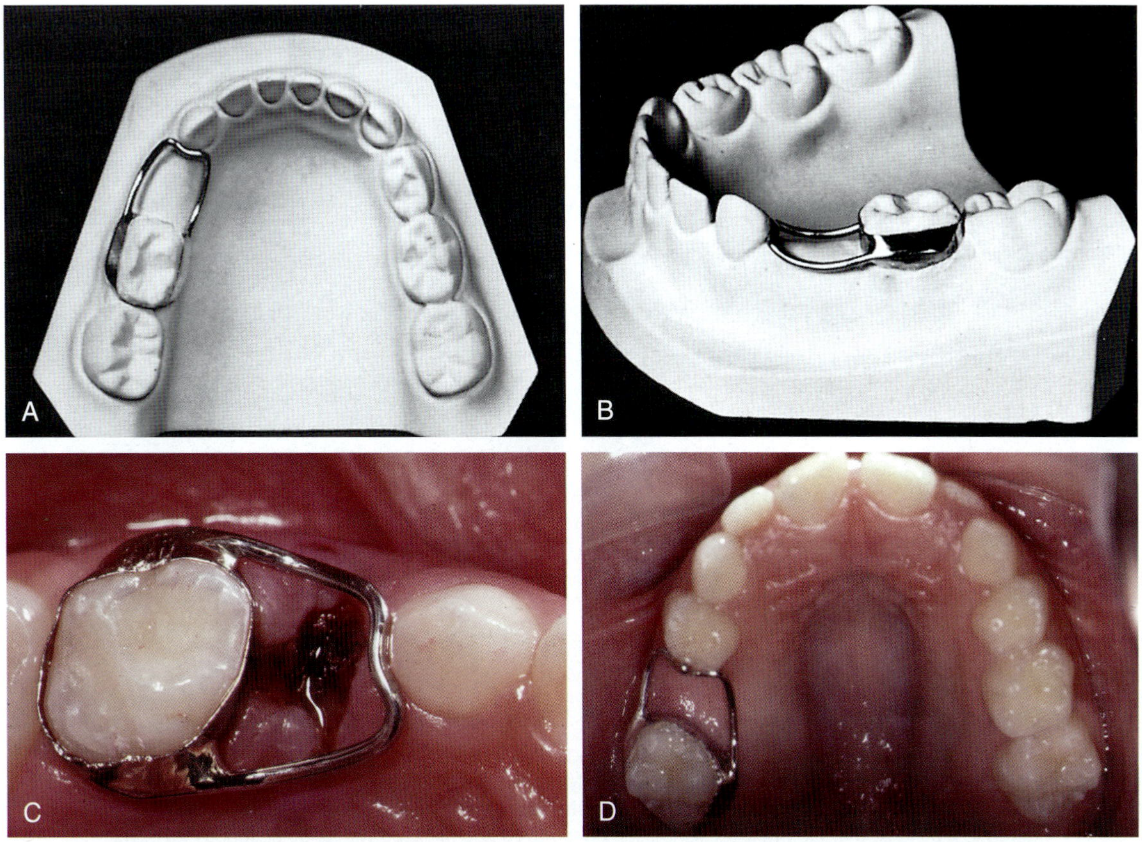

• **Fig. 11.55** A band-and-loop space maintainer is typically used in mixed dentition to save the space of a single prematurely lost primary molar. It consists of a band on either a primary or permanent molar and a wire loop to maintain space. (A) The loop portion made from 36-mil wire is carefully contoured to the abutment tooth without restricting lateral movement of the primary canine, and (B) the loop is also contoured to within 1.5 mm of the alveolar ridge. The solder joints should fill the angle between the band and wire to avoid food and debris accumulation. (C) A completed band and loop maintainer in place after extraction of a primary first molar; (D) an occlusal rest, shown here on the primary first molar, can be added to the loop portion to prevent the banded teeth from tipping mesially.

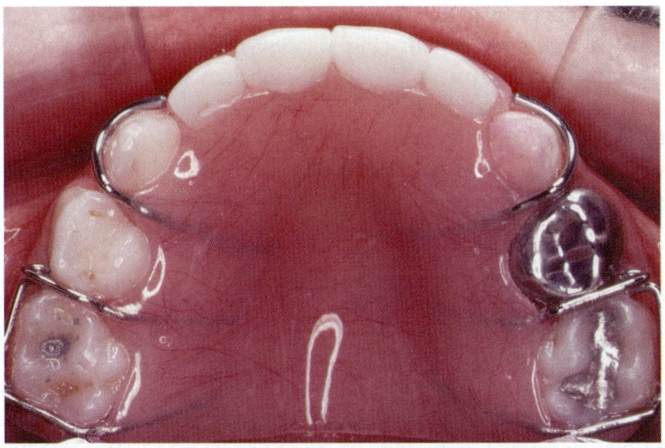

• **Fig. 11.56** In a young child, a removable partial denture is used to replace anterior teeth for esthetics. At the same time, it can maintain the space of one or more prematurely lost primary molars. For this patient, the four incisors are replaced by the partial denture. Multiple clasps, preferably Adams clasps, are necessary for good retention. Both the clasps and the acrylic need frequent adjustment to prevent interference with physiologic adjustment of primary teeth during eruption of permanent teeth. The C-clasps on the primary canines provide limited retention and are good examples of clasps that need continued careful attention.

Distal Shoe Space Maintainers

The distal shoe has a unique application and is the appliance of choice when a primary second molar is lost before eruption of the permanent first molar. This appliance consists of a metal or plastic guide plane along which the permanent molar erupts. The guide plane is attached to a fixed or removable retaining device (Fig. 11.57). When fixed, the distal shoe is usually retained with a band instead of a stainless steel crown so that it can be replaced by another type of space maintainer after the permanent first molar erupts. Unfortunately, this design limits the strength of the appliance and provides no functional replacement for the missing tooth. If primary first and second molars are missing, the appliance must be removable and the guide plane is incorporated into a partial denture because of the length of the edentulous span. This type of appliance can provide some occlusal function.

To be effective, the guide plane must extend into the alveolar process so that it is located approximately 1 mm below the mesial marginal ridge of the permanent first molar, at or before its emergence from the bone. An appliance of this type is tolerated well by most children but is contraindicated in patients who are at risk for subacute bacterial endocarditis or are immunocompromised because complete epithelialization around the

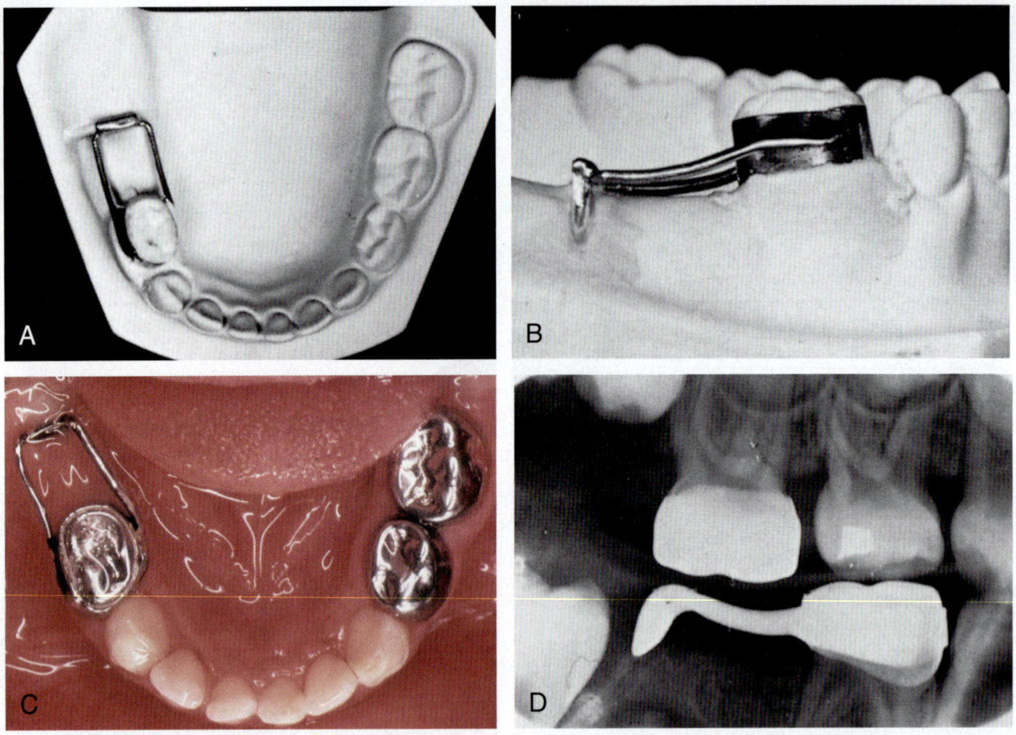

• **Fig. 11.57** The distal shoe space maintainer is indicated when a primary second molar is lost before eruption of the permanent first molar and is usually placed at or very soon after the extraction of the primary molar. (A) The loop portion, made of 36-mil stainless steel wire, and the intraalveolar blade are soldered to a band so that the whole appliance can be removed and replaced with another space maintainer after the permanent molar erupts. (B) The loop portion must be contoured closely to the ridge because the appliance cannot resist excessive occlusal forces from the opposing teeth. (C) This distal shoe space maintainer was placed at the time of extraction of the primary second molar. (D) The blade portion must be positioned so that it extends approximately 1 mm below the mesial marginal ridge of the erupting permanent tooth to guide its eruption. This position can be measured from pretreatment radiographs and verified by a radiograph taken at try-in or after cementation. An additional occlusal radiograph can be obtained if the faciolingual position is in doubt.

intraalveolar portion has not been demonstrated.[30] Careful measurement and positioning are necessary to ensure that the blade will ultimately guide the permanent molar. Faulty positioning and loss of the appliance are the most common problems with this appliance.

Lingual Arch Space Maintainers

A lingual arch is indicated for space maintenance when single or multiple primary posterior teeth are missing and the permanent incisors have erupted (Fig. 11.58A and B). A conventional lingual arch, attached to bands on the permanent first molars and contacting the maxillary or mandibular incisors, prevents anterior movement of the posterior teeth and posterior movement of the anterior teeth.

A lingual arch space maintainer is usually soldered to the molar bands but can be fabricated to be removable. Removable lingual arches (e.g., those that fit into attachments welded onto the bands) are more prone to breakage and loss. Regardless of whether it is removable, the lingual arch should be positioned to rest on the cingula of the incisors, approximately 1 to 1.5 mm off the soft tissue. It should be stepped to the lingual in the mid-canine region to support the canine and remain away from the primary molars and unerupted premolars so that there is no interference with their eruption. Incorporating a U loops mesial to the permanent first molars insures the arch can be adjusted for a good and passive fit. The loops also enable activation of the arch for tooth movement (Fig. 11.58C). Lingual arches should have ideal arch form so the teeth can align if they have space. Making the arch conform to dental irregularities is not appropriate. Approximately 25% to 30% of lingual arch-type appliances fail, usually because of cement loss and solder joint breakage. Their survival time is estimated at less than 24 months.[31] Careful instructions to parents and patients can reduce these problems, but regular recall is advisable.

Maxillary lingual arches as space maintainers are not familiar to many clinicians but are contraindicated only in patients whose bite depth causes the lower incisors to contact the archwire on the lingual aspect of the maxillary incisors (Fig. 11.58D). When bite depth does not allow use of a conventional design, either the Nance lingual arch (Fig. 11.58E) or a transpalatal arch (Fig. 11.58F) can be considered. The Nance arch is an effective space maintainer or anchorage device and not an active appliance, but palatal soft tissue irritation can be a problem. The best indication for a transpalatal arch is when one side of the arch is intact and more than one primary tooth is missing on the other side. In this situation, the rigid attachment to the intact side usually provides adequate stability for space maintenance. When primary molars have been lost bilaterally, however, both permanent molars can tip

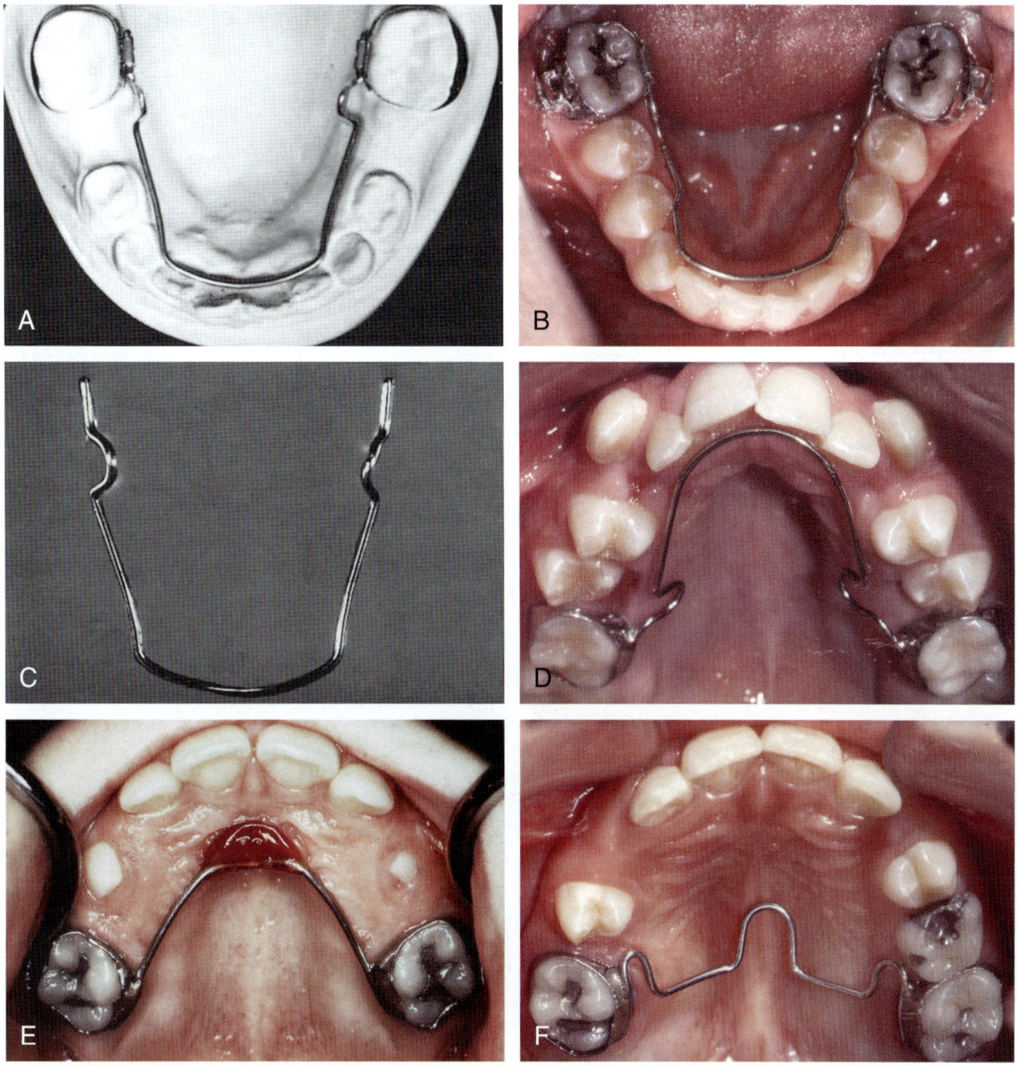

• **Fig. 11.58** A lingual holding arch usually is the best choice to maintain space for premolars after premature loss of the primary molars when the permanent incisors have erupted. (A) The lingual arch is made of 36-mil wire with adjustment loops mesial to the permanent first molars. (B) This soldered lingual arch successfully maintained the space for the premolars. (C) The lingual arch is stepped away from the premolars starting in the canine area to allow their eruption without interference, which results in a keyhole design. The wire is also 1.5 mm away from the soft tissue at all points. (D) A maxillary lingual arch is used when the overbite is not excessive, or (E) a Nance arch with an acrylic button in the palatal vault is indicated if the overbite is excessive. The palatal button must be monitored because it may cause soft tissue irritation. (F) The transpalatal arch prevents a molar from rotating mesially into a primary molar extraction space, and this largely prevents its mesial migration. Several adjacent teeth should be present on at least one side of the arch when a transpalatal design is employed as a sole space maintainer to resist drift of the teeth.

mesially despite the transpalatal arch, and a conventional lingual arch or Nance arch is preferred.

A flowchart is provided to help guide decision-making for space maintenance (Fig. 11.59).

Localized Space Loss (3 mm or Less): Space Regaining

Potential space problems can be created by drift of permanent incisors or molars after early extraction of primary canines or molars, which usually begins during the first 6 months after extraction. Teeth usually move when space is available from the posterior and the anterior, but predominantly from the posterior in the maxilla and anterior in the mandible. Then, repositioning the teeth to regain space and reduce the space discrepancy to zero, followed by a space maintainer, is necessary to prevent further drift and space loss until the succedaneous teeth have erupted. A space maintainer alone is not adequate treatment for a space deficiency.

Up to 3 mm of space in a quadrant can be reestablished in a localized area with relatively simple appliances and a good prognosis. Space loss greater than that constitutes a complex problem and usually requires comprehensive treatment to achieve acceptable results. The methods to regain major space loss are considered in Chapter 12. The treatment necessary to regain the space during

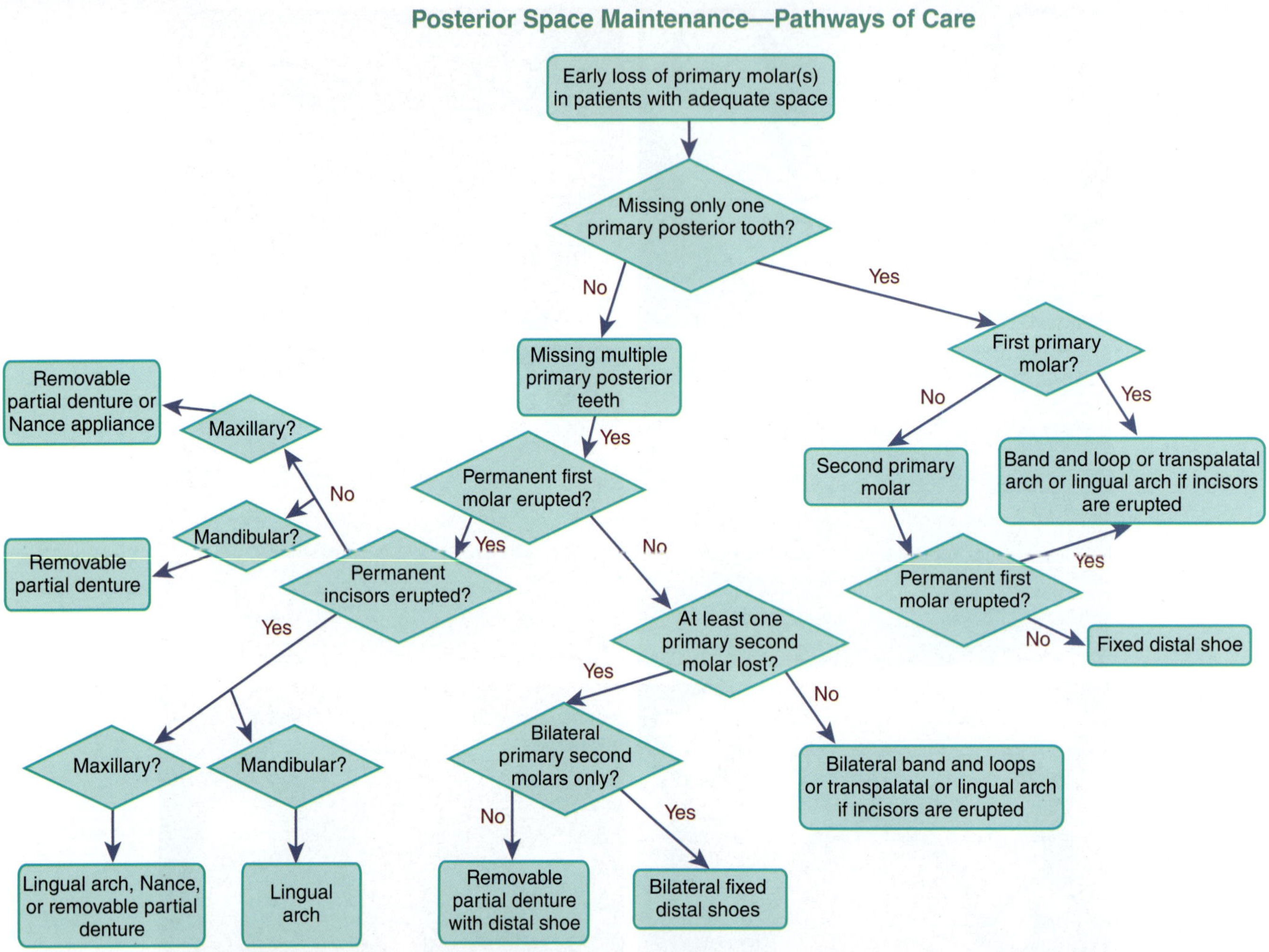

• **Fig. 11.59** This flowchart can be used to aid decision-making regarding possible options for space maintenance in the primary and mixed dentitions.

the mixed dentition, especially if a second stage of treatment will be required in any event, may be more than is reasonable when one analyzes the cost–benefit ratio. Extraction with drift and then space closure often is a better choice. In other circumstance, the crowding can be accepted during the mixed dentition so that the ultimate space closure occurs under control when complete fixed appliances are present.

Maxillary Space Regaining

In general, space is easier to regain in the maxillary than in the mandibular arch because of the increased anchorage for removable appliances afforded by the palatal vault and the possibility of using extraoral force (headgear). Permanent maxillary first molars can be tipped distally to regain space with either a fixed or removable appliance, but bodily movement requires a fixed appliance. Because the molars tend to tip forward and rotate mesiolingually, distal tipping and de-rotation are often satisfactory to regain 2 to 3 mm.

A removable appliance retained with Adams clasps and incorporating a helical fingerspring adjacent to the tooth to be moved is very effective. This appliance is the ideal design for distally tipping one molar (Fig. 11.60). One posterior tooth can be moved up to 3 mm distally during 3 to 4 months of full-time appliance wear. The spring is activated approximately 2 to 3 mm to produce 1 mm of movement per month. The molar typically will derotate spontaneously as it is tipped distally.

For unilateral space regaining with bodily movement of the permanent first molar, a fixed appliance is preferred. The anchorage provided by the remaining teeth can support the forces generated by a coil spring on a segmental archwire, with good success (Fig. 11.61), but to be effective, the support of a modified Nance arch usually is needed.

Regardless of the method used to regain space, a space maintainer is required when adequate space has been restored. A fixed space maintainer is recommended, rather than trying to maintain the space with the removable appliance that was used for space regaining, because it may become distorted and allow inadvertent space loss.

Regaining bilateral localized space loss of any amount is more complex and is discussed in Chapter 12.

Mandibular Space Regaining

For moderate amounts of space regaining, removable appliances can be used in the mandibular arch just as they are in the maxillary arch, but as a rule they are less satisfactory because they are more fragile and prone to breakage. They do not fit as well and

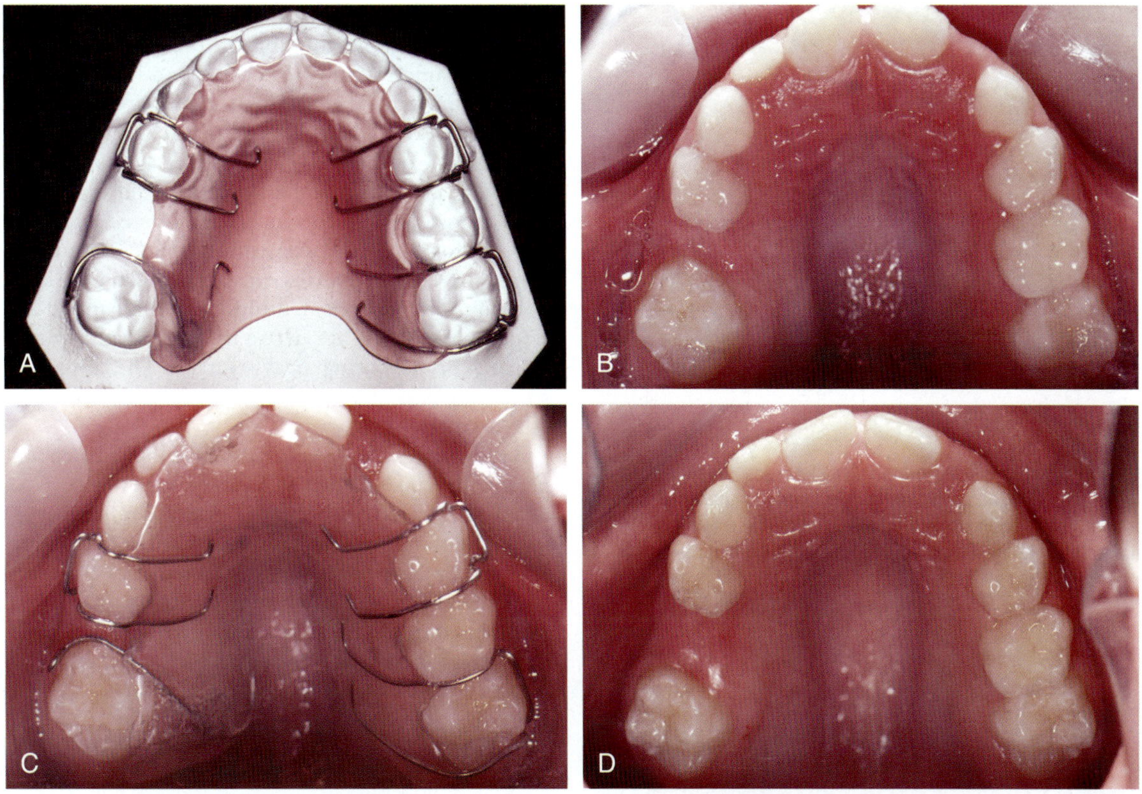

• **Fig. 11.60** A removable appliance with a fingerspring can be used to regain space by tipping a permanent first molar distally. (A) The appliance incorporates multiple Adams clasps and a 28-mil helical spring that is activated 2–3 mm per month. (B) Premature loss of the primary second molar has led to mesial drift and rotation of the permanent first molar. (C) This removable appliance can be used to regain up to 3 mm of space. (D) After space regaining, the space should be maintained with a band and loop or lingual arch if the permanent incisors have erupted.

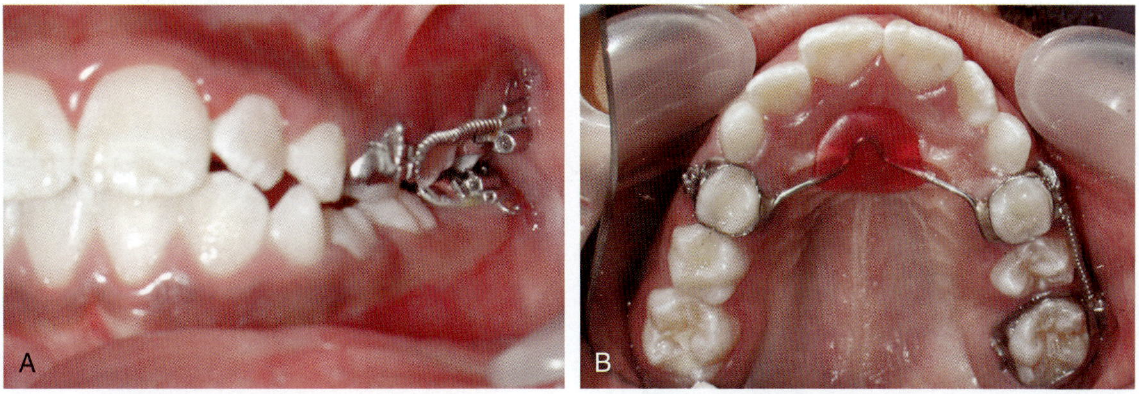

• **Fig. 11.61** (A) A fixed appliance also can be used to regain space in the maxillary posterior regions, with a coil spring generating the distalizing force. (B) Palatal anchorage was gained using a Nance arch and the erupted teeth.

lack the palatal anchorage support. Problems with tissue irritation frequently are encountered, and patient acceptance tends to be poorer than with maxillary removable appliances.

For unilateral mandibular space regaining, the best choice is a fixed appliance. A lingual arch can be used to support the tooth movement and provide anchorage when used in conjunction with a segmental archwire and coil spring (Fig. 11.62).

If space has been lost bilaterally because of lingual incisor tipping, there are two choices short of bands and brackets: a lip bumper or an adjustable lingual arch. With the lip bumper, which is a labial appliance fitted to tubes on the molar teeth (Fig. 11.63), the idea is that the appliance presses against the lip, which creates a distal force to tip the molars posteriorly without affecting the incisors. Although some posterior movement of the

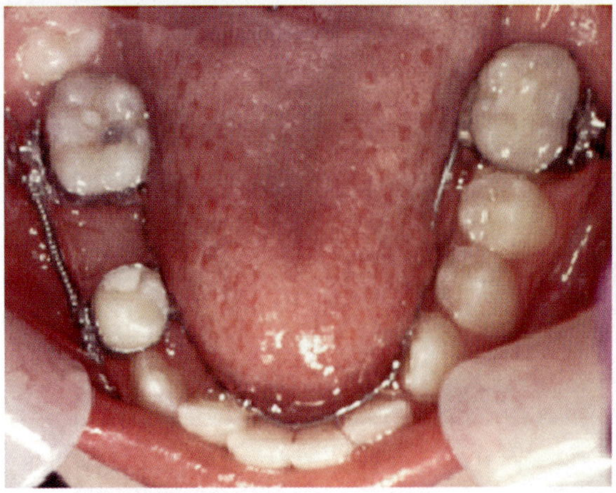

• **Fig. 11.62** Moving molars distally in the mandibular arch, especially unilaterally, is quite challenging and requires support from a number of teeth. Use of a lingual arch, to incorporate anchorage from the permanent and primary molars as well as the incisors, and force from a coil spring on a segmental archwire can be effective.

molars can be observed when a lip bumper is used, the appliance also alters the equilibrium of forces against the incisors, removing any restraint from the lip on these teeth. The result is forward movement of the incisors.[32] Depending on the type of lip bumper used and its clinical manipulation, transverse widening also may occur.

When an active lingual arch pits posterior movement of both molars against the anchorage offered by the incisors, significant forward displacement of the incisors must be expected (Fig. 11.64). The expansion can be accomplished by slightly opening the loops located mesial to the banded molars. Small steps in activation are necessary because the wire is large and capable of delivering heavy forces. The appliance can then serve as a passive retainer or be replaced with a soldered lingual arch.

On balance, the effects of an active lingual arch and a lip bumper are similar. A lingual arch can be left in place as a space maintainer after space has been regained. A lip bumper is not a good space maintainer and should be replaced with a lingual arch when long-term maintenance of the regained space is needed.

Bilateral molar distalization to regain space or moving the mandibular midline to resolve an asymmetry are both considered complex problems and are addressed in Chapter 12.

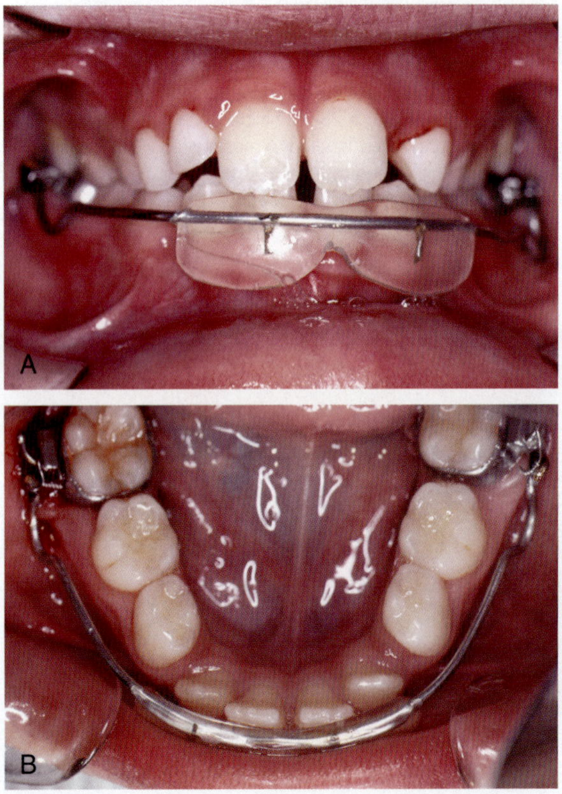

• **Fig. 11.63** (A) A lip bumper constructed of a 36-mil wire bow with an acrylic pad, which fits into tubes on the permanent first molars, is sometimes used to increase arch length. This occurs when the appliance stretches the lower lip and transmits force to move the molars back. The appliance also disrupts the equilibrium between the lip and tongue and allows the anterior teeth to move facially. The result is nearly equal molar and incisor change. This appliance can be used for either minor space regaining or for moderate arch expansion. (B) The lip bumper is ligated in place so that it remains in the proper position during treatment and to increase compliance. Periodically, it needs to be advanced a couple of millimeters facial to the incisors so they can migrate facially.

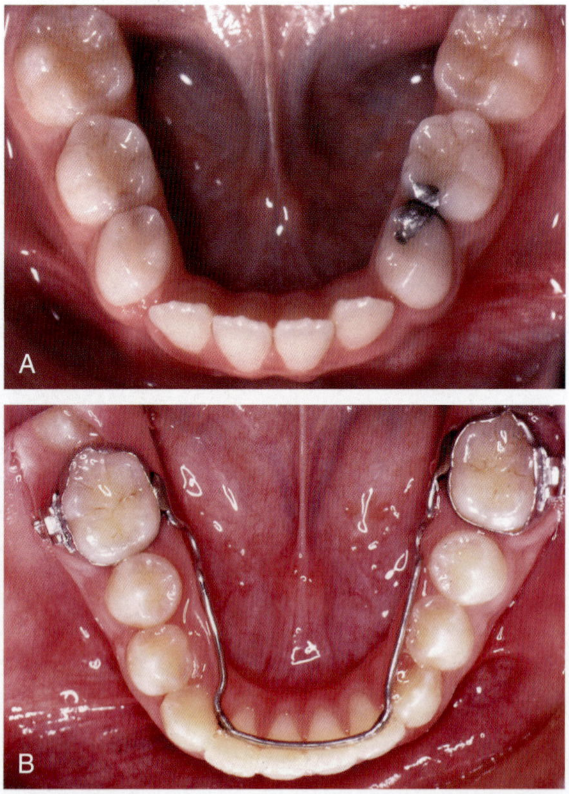

• **Fig. 11.64** (A) Limited space regaining or moderate lower arch expansion can be accomplished by using a lingual arch when the incisors have good alignment and little spacing, as in this patient who requires additional arch length to accommodate the unerupted premolars and canines. (B) When the lingual arch is in place and active, it will rest high on the lingual surface of the incisors and should exert a downward tipping force. Two or three 1- to 1.5-mm activations at 4- to 6-week intervals will achieve the desired movement.

Mild Crowding of Incisors With Adequate Space

Irregular Incisors, Minimal Space Discrepancy

In some children, space analysis shows that enough space for all the permanent teeth ultimately will be available, but relatively large permanent incisors and the clinical reality of the "incisor liability" (see Chapter 4) cause transient crowding of the permanent incisors. This crowding is usually expressed as mild faciolingual displacement or rotation of individual anterior teeth.

Studies of children with normal occlusion indicate that when they go through the transition from the primary to the mixed dentition, up to 2 mm of incisor crowding may resolve spontaneously without treatment. From this perspective, there is no need for treatment when mild incisor crowding is observed during the mixed dentition. Not only is correction of this small amount of crowding probably not warranted, but also there is no evidence that long-term stability will be greater. The only reason for treatment may be temporary esthetic improvement.

If exaggerated parental concern makes mild crowding a problem, one could consider disking the interproximal enamel surfaces of the remaining *primary* canines and first primary molars (Fig. 11.65) as the anterior teeth erupt. This can help with faciolingual discrepancies but not rotations. It is possible to gain as much as 3 to 4 mm of anterior space through this procedure, but the teeth may align in a more lingual position and actually make the space problem worse in the long run when the other permanent teeth are erupted. Remember, at this point in the transitional dentition no disking or interproximal stripping should be attempted on *permanent* teeth. This could create a tooth-size discrepancy that later will be difficult to resolve. Permanent tooth stripping should not be undertaken until all the permanent teeth have erupted and their interarch size relationships can be evaluated.

Correction of incisor rotations caused by this transitional crowding requires space and controlled movement to align and derotate them, using an archwire and bonded attachments on the incisors. It is rare that a child who needs this type of treatment in the mixed dentition does not require further treatment after all permanent teeth have erupted, so extensive early treatment is usually not indicated.

Moderate Transitional Incisor Crowding With Adequate Space: Space Management

In some children, more severe transitional crowding occurs when the incisors erupt. Space analysis often shows that the space available is adequate or nearly so. The goal is to use and control all the space between the mesial of the permanent first molars. When the mesial movement of the permanent molars to a Class I occurs (into the leeway space or the E space) as the primary second molars are lost, there will be a space deficiency. For these patients, if the loss of leeway space or E space (see Chapter 5 to review those concepts) could be prevented, there would be little or no space deficiency. Gianelly reported that in patients seeking treatment at Boston University, 75% would have approximately enough space to align the teeth if molar drift were prevented.[33] This group does not need much treatment, it should be relatively easy to provide, and there is always the possibility that if early treatment is done, later treatment might not be necessary.

If it is possible to delay beginning treatment in the early mixed dentition, children with moderate crowding but little or no space discrepancy can begin intervention with a lingual arch in the late mixed dentition, just before the second primary molars exfoliate. The transitional incisor crowding would simply be tolerated up to that time, on the theory that it could be corrected along with other crowding in the arch when the space occupied by the large second primary molars became available. In these patients, beginning comprehensive treatment earlier is judged not to be cost-effective—it takes longer for both patient and doctor, without producing a better long-term result.

A primary indication does exist, however, for starting treatment earlier in some of these patients who have overall adequate space but various amounts of transitional crowding. Loss of both primary canines or delayed eruption of either canines or premolars due to transitional crowding is an indication for earlier space management with a lingual arch. Placement of a lingual arch will prevent distal movement of the incisors and mesial movement of the permanent first molar—both shorten arch length (Fig. 11.66).[34] The lingual arch should be left in position until the second premolars erupt, so the start of comprehensive treatment can be delayed.

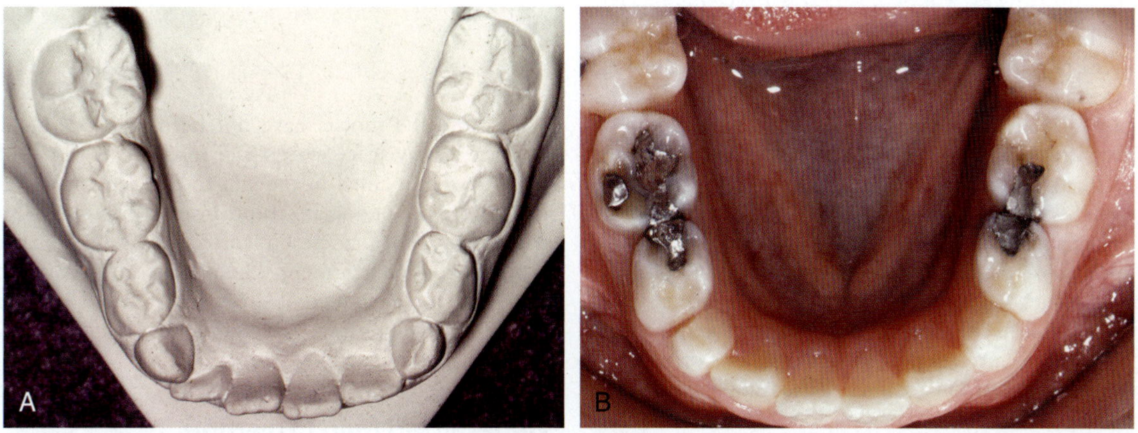

• **Fig. 11.65** Disking can be used on multiple surfaces of primary teeth—especially the primary canines—when limited transitional crowding is apparent. (A) This pretreatment cast shows minor anterior crowding. (B) Disking of the mesial and distal surfaces of the primary canines allowed spontaneous alignment to occur without appliance therapy.

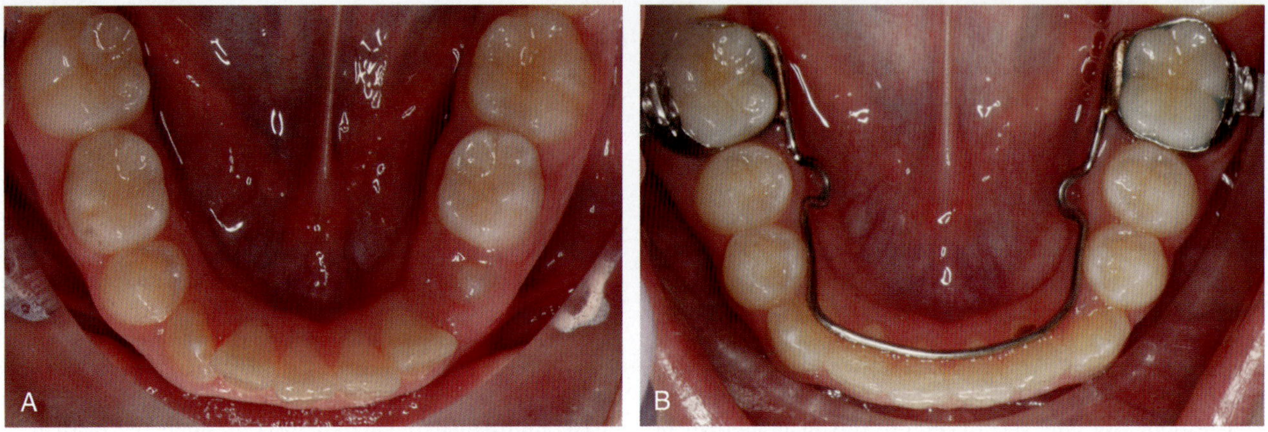

• **Fig. 11.66** A lingual arch in conjunction with primary tooth extraction or exfoliation can be an effective way to take advantage of the leeway space and reduce crowding. (A) The primary second molars are in place, and there is some anterior crowding that is within the range of the leeway space—really the "E space," because all other primary teeth have exfoliated. (B) With the lingual arch in place to take advantage of the leeway space, the second premolars erupted and incisor and canine alignment improved spontaneously.

With this approach to space management, there is also some evidence for better long-term stability.[35]

In the absence of early loss of primary teeth, the other major reason for early intervention in a child who has transitional crowding is esthetic concern because of the obvious crowding. Parents may want treatment for this sooner rather than later.

In either case, interference with tooth eruption or esthetic concerns, a combination of early extraction of primary canines and possibly molars, along with disking to reduce the width of primary molars can provide space to allow the permanent incisors and canines to erupt and align. This can be carried further posteriorly in the arch as more teeth erupt (Fig. 11.67). The minimum orthodontic appliance therapy is a lingual arch that will support the incisor teeth and control the molar position and arch perimeter by preventing any mesial shift. Midlines can also be corrected at this time, if necessary for canine eruption, but this is a more complex problem (see Chapter 12). If necessary, the lingual arch can be activated slightly to tip molars distally and incisors facially to obtain a modest, but potentially unstable, increase in arch length (see Fig. 11.64). A lip bumper also can be used in the lower arch to maintain the position of the molars or perhaps tip them slightly distally, while removing lip pressure and allowing the incisors to move facially.

When space is created in this way, the incisors often align spontaneously if the irregularity is from faciolingual tipping, but rotations are less likely to resolve. An exception is the child whose incisor segment is straight, without anterior arch curvature. In these children, extraction of primary canines usually leads to spacing of the incisors or maintenance of essentially the same arch form. Alignment does not improve even when the space is available and a lingual arch is in place to serve as a template for tooth position (Fig. 11.68). Correction of incisor rotations or residual irregularity in incisor position requires a fixed appliance, using an archwire and bonded attachments on the incisors. Accepting some incisor crowding and deferring treatment until as late as possible—when the premolars are erupting—is usually the best judgment.

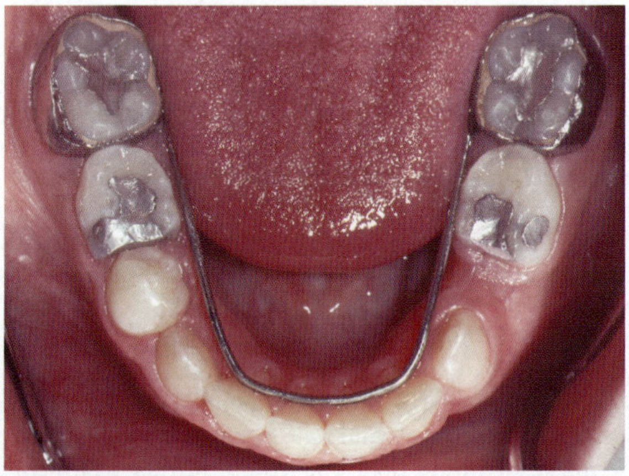

• **Fig. 11.67** Disking primary posterior teeth in conjunction with space maintenance is an effective method to use the leeway space and all available arch length. Note that the disking must be completed perpendicular to the occlusal plane so that the height of contour of the tooth is reduced. Occlusally convergent slices that do not reduce the mesiodistal width of the tooth are not helpful.

Because the molars have not been allowed to shift forward into the leeway space when space management is employed, they often are maintained in the end-to-end relationship that is normal before the premolars erupt, instead of moving into a Class I relationship. For that reason, correction of the molar relationship is also a goal of treatment. Doing this during the second phase of treatment, when a complete fixed appliance is available, is the most efficient approach. The techniques used for molar correction are discussed in detail in Chapter 15.

Generalized Mild Crowding

A child with a generalized arch length discrepancy of up to 4 mm and no prematurely missing primary teeth can be expected to have

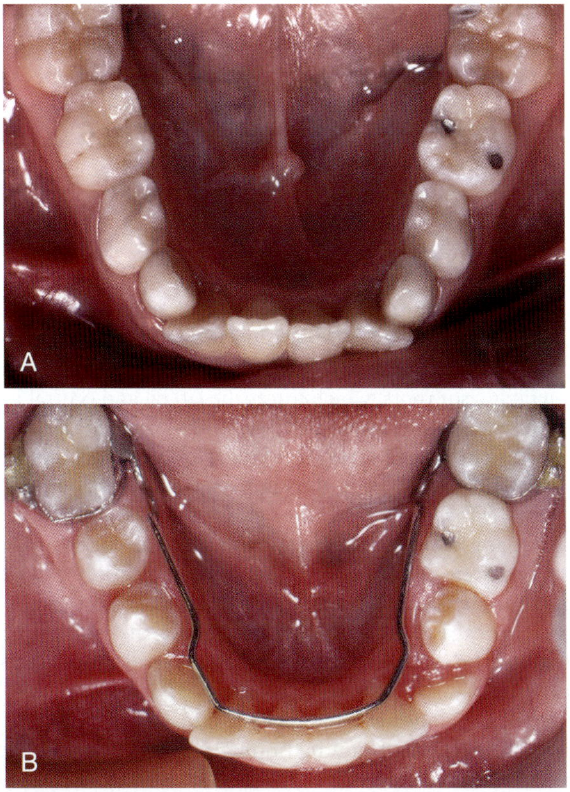

• **Fig. 11.68** (A) Anterior crowding combined with a straight anterior incisor segment. (B) Straight incisor segments with lateral incisors that overlap the mesial surface of the primary canine usually do not align into the ideal arch form when the primary canines are extracted, even if a lingual arch is used as a template for alignment.

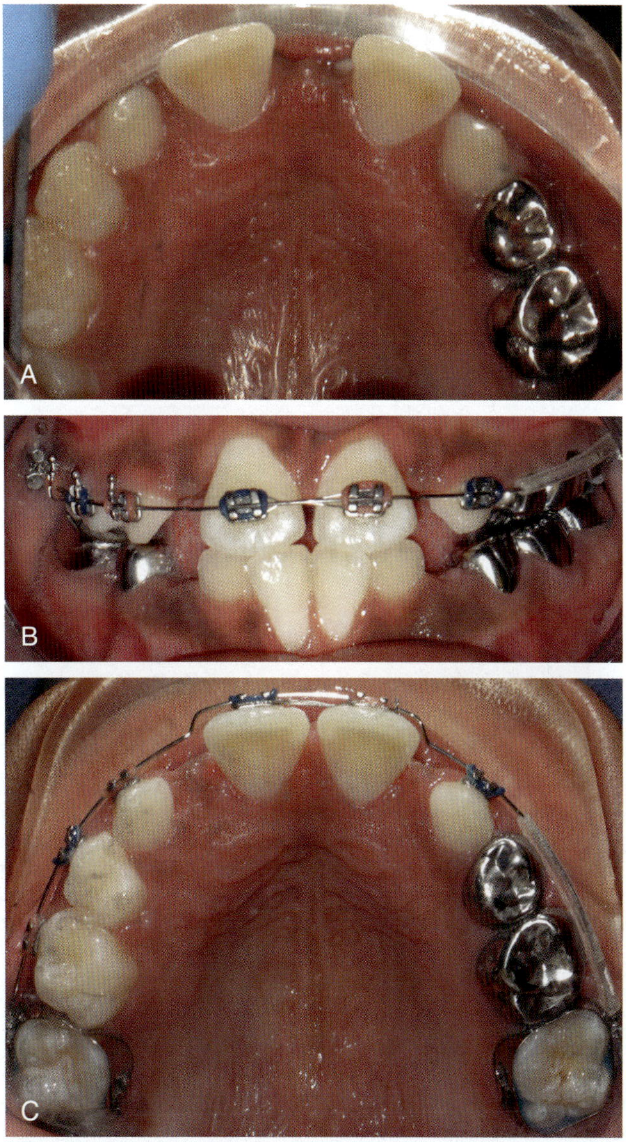

• **Fig. 11.69** Limited maxillary appliances can be used in the mixed dentition to align teeth and distribute space. (A) This patient had unerupted maxillary lateral incisors as a result of the large midline diastema. (B and C) The teeth were aligned and the diastema closed. Even after space closure, it appears the primary canines may need to be disked on the mesial or the incisors advanced to allow permanent lateral incisor eruption Note the tubing that protects the patient's lip from the expanse of continuous wire on the patient's left side.

mildly crowded incisors. This occurs in about 25% of each ethnic group in the United States (see Fig. 1.11). Unless the incisors are severely protrusive, the long-term plan would be a generalized expansion of the arch to align the teeth. The major advantage of doing this in the mixed dentition is improved dentofacial esthetics, and the benefit is largely for the parents, not the child.

If the parents strongly desire early treatment for mild crowding, an adjustable lingual arch is the appliance of choice in the mandibular arch for simple expansion by tipping tooth movement. In the maxilla, either a removable or fixed appliance can be employed (Fig. 11.69). Keep in mind that rotated incisors will not usually correct spontaneously even if space is provided, so early correction would require bonded attachments for these teeth. Mild crowding corrected this early will need continuous supervision with retention and can be unstable in the long run. Moderate to severe localized and generalized crowding are addressed in Chapter 12.

Other Tooth Displacements

Spaced and Flared Maxillary Incisors

In children with spaced and flared maxillary incisors who have Class I molar relationships and good facial proportions, space analysis should show that the space available is excessive rather than deficient. If the spacing is minor, it may not require treatment. Parents and children may seek treatment for esthetics. Unless the overjet is significantly increased and the lips are protusive and incompetent, the risk of trauma is probably not imminent (see Chapter 12). Moderate incisor spacing and flaring are often found in the mixed dentition after prolonged thumb-sucking and frequently occur in connection with some narrowing of the maxillary arch. A thumb or finger habit should be eliminated before attempts are made to retract the incisors. Physiologic adaptation to the space between the anterior teeth requires placing the tongue in this area to seal off the gap for successful swallowing and speech. This "tongue thrust" is not the cause of the protrusion or open bite

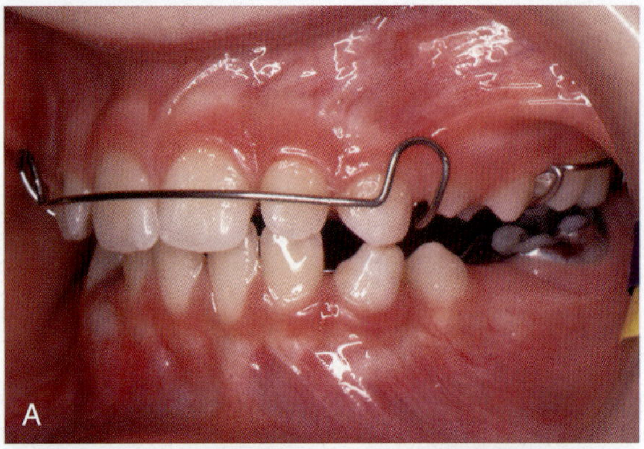

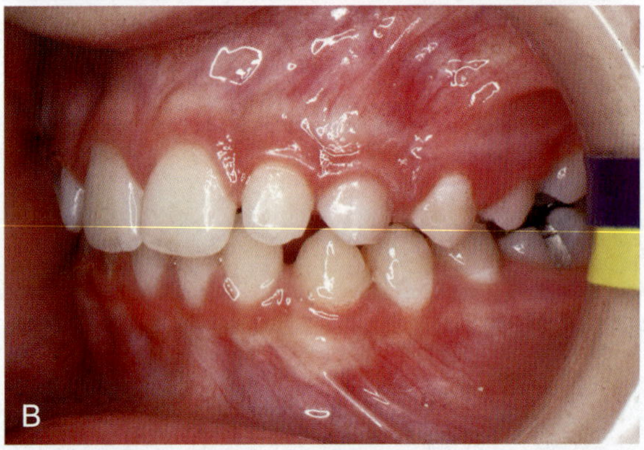

• **Fig. 11.70** A removable appliance can be used in the mixed dentition to retract spaced and protruding anterior teeth. (A) The labial bow is activated 1.5–2 mm and will achieve approximately 1 mm of retraction per month as the maxillary anterior teeth tip lingually. At each appointment, the labial bow should be adjusted and lingual acrylic removed to provide space for the tooth movement and gingival buildup. (B) A near-normal occlusion in the late mixed dentition.

and should not be the focus of therapy. If the teeth are retracted, the tongue thrust will disappear as the tongue adapts to the new morphologic characteristics.

If the upper incisors are flared forward and there is no contact with the lower incisors, the protruding upper incisors can be retracted quite satisfactorily with a removable appliance. A Hawley-type appliance using multiple clasps and a labial bow can be effective for this purpose (Fig. 11.70). Of course, the patient must be cooperative in wearing the appliance, and it must be constructed with adequate retention and a flexible labial bow (28-mil wire). Incorporating loops in the bow can aid the flexibility. During the course of treatment, the appliance is adjusted approximately 2 mm per month to achieve 1 mm of lingual tipping of the incisors and space closure. The palate-covering plastic lingual to the incisors must be removed to provide space for posterior movement of the teeth and gingiva. After space closure, the teeth need to be retained with the existing removable appliance.

On the other hand, if there is a deep overbite, protruding upper incisor teeth cannot be retracted until the overbite is corrected. The lower incisors biting against the lingual of the upper incisors prevent the upper teeth from being moved lingually. Even if anteroposterior jaw relationships are Class I, a skeletal vertical problem may be present, and complex treatment is likely to be required.

Teeth that are flared and rotated or that require bodily movement during retraction are more difficult to move and control. This is a complex problem and discussed in Chapter 12.

Maxillary Midline Diastema

A small maxillary midline diastema, which is present in many children, is not necessarily an indication for orthodontic treatment. The unerupted permanent canines often lie superior and distal to the lateral incisor roots, which forces the lateral and central incisor roots toward the midline while their crowns diverge distally (Fig. 11.71). In its extreme form, this condition of flared and spaced incisors is called the "ugly duckling" stage of development (see Chapter 4). These spaces tend to close spontaneously or at least reduce in size when the canines erupt and the incisor root and crown positions change—the prevalence of a midline diastema drops from about 25% in the early mixed dentition to approximately 7% at ages 12 to 17.[1] Until the permanent canines erupt, it is difficult to be certain whether the diastema will close completely or only partially.

A small but unesthetic diastema (2 mm or less) can be closed in the early mixed dentition by tipping the central incisor crowns together. A maxillary removable appliance with clasps, finger springs, and possibly an anterior bow can successfully complete this type of treatment (Fig. 11.72). Under no circumstances should an unsupported rubber band be looped around the central incisors; there is a high probability that it will slip apically and destroy the periodontal attachment. The elastic can become an effective way to extract both teeth.

When a larger diastema (>2 mm) is present, a tooth-size problem, midline supernumerary tooth or intrabony lesion must always be suspected in that order (Fig. 11.73), and complete spontaneous closure is unlikely. A diastema this large is disproportionately prevalent in the African-American population. Depending on what radiographs are already available, one of several images may be appropriate—a panoramic radiograph, a maxillary occlusal radiograph, or a maxillary anterior CBCT image with a small FOV. Missing permanent lateral incisors also can lead to a large space between the central incisors because the permanent central incisors frequently move distally into the available space. Some digit-sucking habits can lead to diastemas and spacing.

Whatever its cause, a diastema greater than 2 mm is unlikely to close spontaneously[36] and may inhibit eruption of the lateral incisors. Closure of a large midline diastema will usually require bodily tooth movement and retention[37] and is addressed in Chapter 12.

Sometimes the soft tissue of the midline frenum attachment is blamed for the space between the central incisors, but it is hard to be sure whether this is the case. Usually it is advisable to proceed with the tooth movement and determine if there are further problems with retention. If there are, then a frenectomy can be considered if there is excessive tissue bunched up in the midline. Early frenectomy should be avoided.

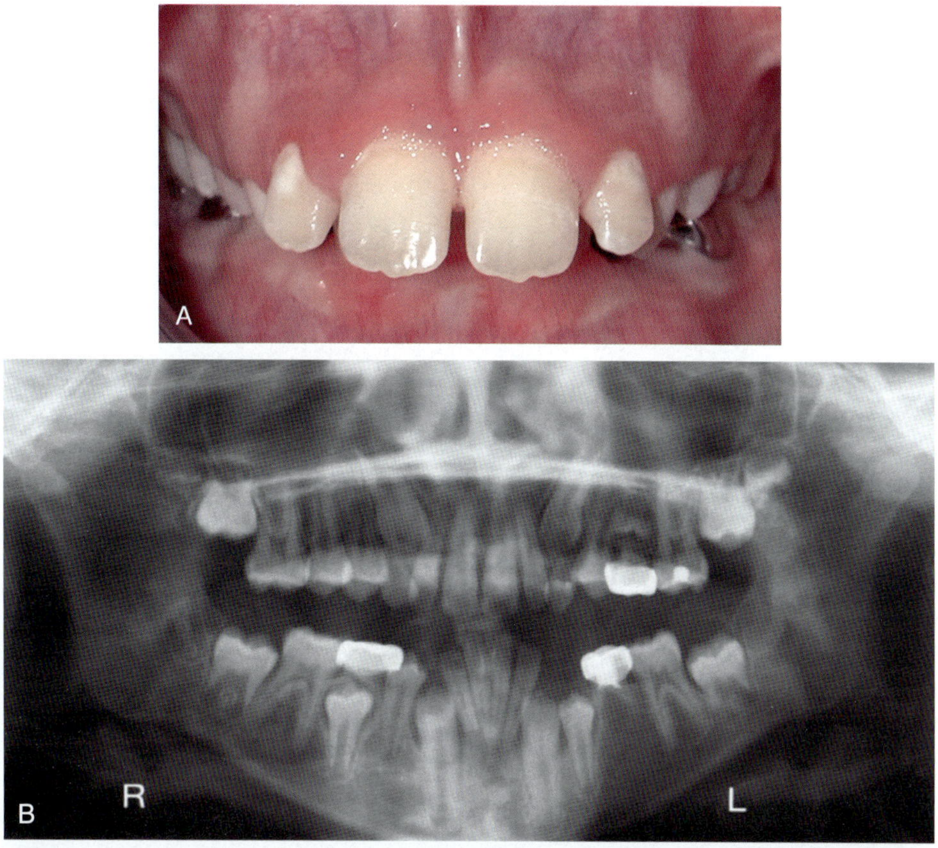

• **Fig. 11.71** The "ugly duckling" phase of dental development. (A) Spacing and mesial root position of the maxillary incisors result from the position of the unerupted permanent canines. (B) This panoramic radiograph shows that the canines are erupting and in close proximity to the roots of the lateral incisors. The spaces between the incisors, including the midline diastema, decrease and often completely disappear when the canines erupt.

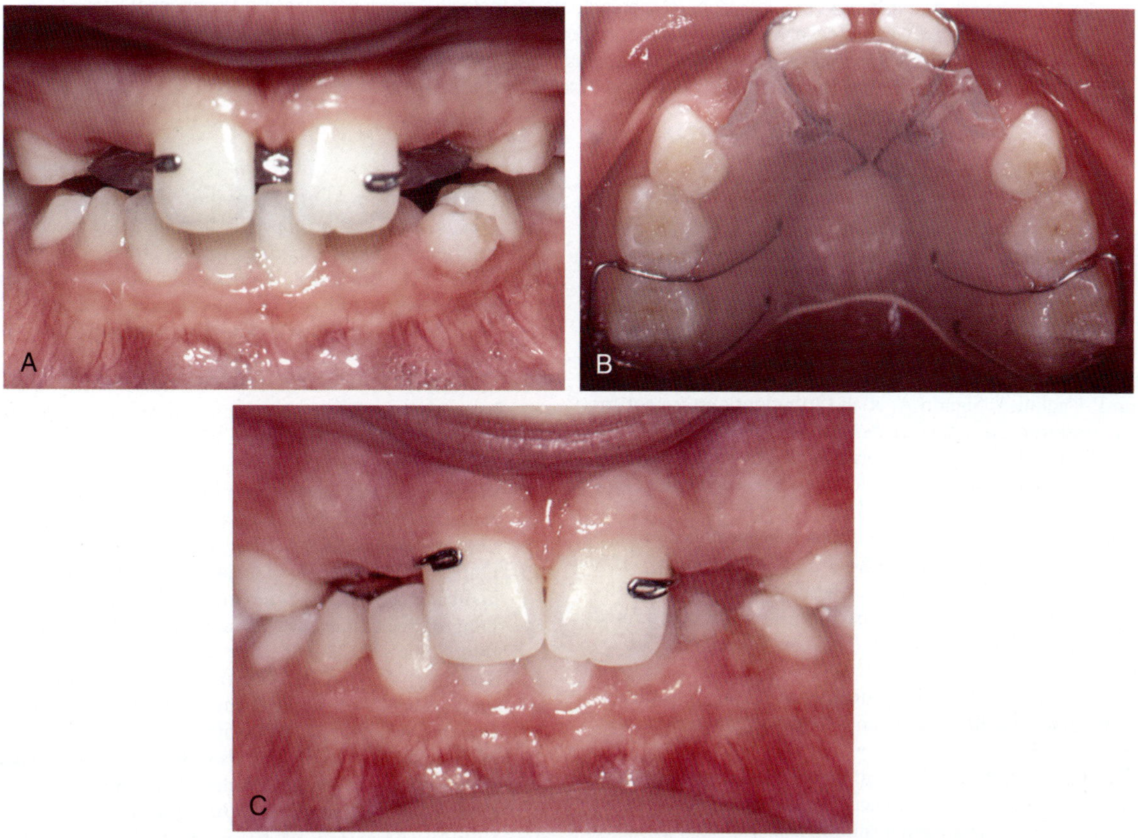

• **Fig. 11.72** (A) Closure of a midline diastema can be accomplished with a removable appliance and fingersprings to tip the teeth mesially. (B) The 28-mil helical fingersprings are activated to tip the incisors together. (C) The final position can be maintained with the same appliance or a bonded central to central lingual light wire.

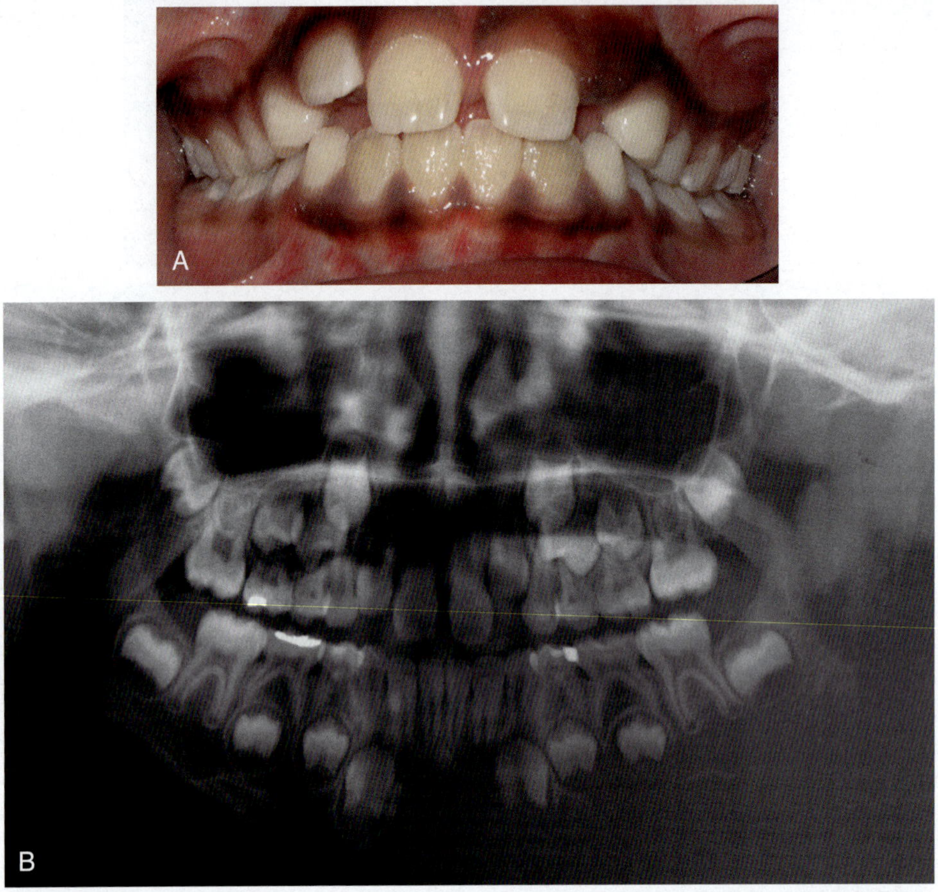

• **Fig. 11.73** In the mixed dentition, sizable diastemas should be investigated to determine if they are the result of a tooth-size problem, supernumerary tooth, pathologic conditions, or missing permanent lateral incisors. (A) In this case, at least one lateral incisor is present along with the diastema, but (B) the accompanying radiograph shows that a midline supernumerary near the apex of the maxillary left central incisor is present. Clearly, the cause of the diastema dictates the treatment response.

References

1. Brunelle JA, Bhat M, Lipton JA. Prevalence and distribution of selected occlusal characteristics in the US population, 1988-91. *J Dent Res*. 1996;75:706–713.
2. Adkins MD, Nanda RS, Currier GF. Arch perimeter changes on rapid palatal expansion. *Am J Orthod*. 1990;97:10–19.
3. Agostino P, Ugolini A, Signori A, et al. Orthodontic treatment for posterior crossbites. *Cochrane Database Syst Rev*. 2014:CD000979.
4. Godoy F, Godoy-Bezerra J, Rosenblatt A. Treatment of posterior crossbite comparing 2 appliances: a community-based trial. *Am J Orthod Dentofac Orthop*. 2011;139:e45–e52.
5. Corbridge JK, et al. Transverse dentoalveolar changes after slow maxillary expansion. *Am J Orthod Dentofac Orthop*. 2011;140:317–325.
6. Petrén S, Bjerklin K, Bondemark L. Stability of unilateral posterior crossbite correction in the mixed dentition: a randomized clinical trial with a 3-year follow-up. *Am J Orthod Dentofac Orthop*. 2011;139:e73–e81.
7. Ngan P, Hu AM, Fields HW. Treatment of Class III problems begins with differential diagnosis of anterior crossbites. *Pediatr Dent*. 1997;19:386–395.
8. Schott TC, Ludwig B. Microelectronic wear-time documentation of removable orthodontic devices detects heterogeneous wear behavior and individualizes treatment planning. *Am J Orthod Dentofac Orthop*. 2014;146:155–160.
9. Lentini-Oliveira DA, Carvalho FR, Rodrigues CG, et al. Orthodontic and orthopaedic treatment for anterior open bite in children. *Cochrane Database Syst Rev*. 2014:CD005515.
10. Abreu LG, Paiva SM, Pordeus IA, Martins CC. Breastfeeding, bottle feeding and risk of malocclusion in mixed and permanent dentitions: a systematic review. *Braz Oral Res*. 2016;30 [Epub 2016 Mar 28].
11. Scavone Jr H, Guimarães Jr CH, Ferreira RI, et al. Association between breastfeeding duration and non-nutritive sucking habits. *Am J Orthod Dentofac Orthop*. 2010;137:54–58.
12. Melink S, Vagner MV, Hocevar-Boltezar I, et al. Posterior crossbite in the deciduous dentition period: its relation with sucking habits, irregular orofacial functions, and otolaryngological findings. *Am J Orthod Dentofac Orthop*. 2010;138:32–40.
13. Duncan K, McNamara C, Ireland AJ, et al. Sucking habits in childhood and the effects on the primary dentition: findings of the Avon Longitudinal Study of Pregnancy and Childhood. *Int J Paediatr Dent*. 2006;18:178–188.
14. Warren JJ, Slayton RL, Bishara SE, et al. Effects of non-nutritive sucking habits on occlusal characteristics in the mixed dentition. *Pediatr Dent*. 2005;27:445–450.
15. Haryett R, Hansen R, Davidson P, et al. Chronic thumbsucking: the psychological effects and the relative effectiveness of the various methods of treatment. *Am J Orthod*. 1967;53:559–585.
16. Villa NL, Cisneros GJ. Changes in the dentition secondary to palatal crib therapy In digit-suckers. *Pediatr Dent*. 1997;19:323–326.

17. Christensen RT, Fields HW, Christensen JR, Beck FM, Casamassimo PS, McTigue DJ. The effects of primary canine loss on permanent lower dental midline stability. *Pediatr Dent.* 2018;40(4): 279–284.
18. Kennedy DB, Turley PK. The clinical management of ectopically erupting first permanent molars. *Am J Orthod Dentofac Orthop.* 1987;92:336–345.
19. Aydin U, Yilmaz HH, Yildirim D. Incidence of canine impaction and transmigration in a patient population. *Dentomaxillofac Radiol.* 2004;33:164–169.
20. Naoumova J, Kurol J, Kjellbert H. A systematic review of the interceptive treatment of palatally displaced maxillary canines. *Eur J Orthod.* 2011;33:143–149.
21. Garib DG, Alencar BM, Lauris JR, et al. Agenesis of maxillary lateral incisors and associated dental anomalies. *Am J Orthod Dentofac Orthop.* 2010;137(732):e1–e6.
22. Cernochova P, Krupa P, Izakovicova-Holla LA. Root resorption associated with ectopically erupting maxillary permanent canines: a computed tomography study. *Eur J Orthod.* 2011;33:483–491.
23. Alqerban A, Jacobs R, Fieuws S, et al. Comparison of two cone-beam computed tomographic systems versus panoramic imaging for localization of impacted maxillary canines and detection of root resorption. *Eur J Orthod.* 2011;33:93–102.
24. Ericson S, Kurol J. Early treatment of palatally erupting maxillary canines by extraction of the primary canines. *Eur J Orthod.* 1988;10:283–295.
25. Almasoud NN. Extraction of primary canines for interceptive orthodontic treatment of palatally displaced permanent canines: a systematic review. *Angle Orthod.* 2017;87:878–885.
26. Sigler LM, Baccetti T, McNamara Jr. JA. Effect of rapid maxillary expansion and transpalatal arch treatment associated with deciduous canine extraction on the eruption of palatally displaced canines: a 2-center prospective study. *Am J Orthod Dentofac Orthop.* 2011;139:e235–e244.
27. Kurol J, Thilander B. Infraocclusion of primary molars with aplasia of the permanent successor: a longitudinal study. *Angle Orthod.* 1984;54:283–294.
28. Tanaka MM, Johnston LE. The prediction of the size of unerupted canines and premolars in a contemporary orthodontic population. *J Am Dent Assoc.* 1974;88:798–801.
29. Tunc ES, Bayrak S, Tuloglu N, et al. Evaluation of survival of 3 different fixed space maintainers. *Pediatr Dent.* 2012;34:e97–e102.
30. Mayhew M, Dilley G, Dilley D, et al. Tissue response to intragingival appliances in monkeys. *Pediatr Dent.* 1984;6:148–152.
31. Moore TR, Kennedy DB. Bilateral space maintainers: a 7-year retrospective study from private practice. *Pediatr Dent.* 2006;28:499–505.
32. Hashish DI, Mostafa YA. Effect of lip bumpers on mandibular arch dimensions. *Am J Orthod Dentofac Orthop.* 2009;135:106–109.
33. Gianelly AA. Crowding: timing of treatment. *Angle Orthod.* 1994;64:415–418.
34. Brennan M, Gianelly AA. The use of the lingual arch in the mixed dentition to resolve crowding. *Am J Orthod Dentofac Orthop.* 2000;117:81–85.
35. Little RM. Stability and relapse: early treatment of arch length deficiency. *Am J Orthod Dentofac Orthop.* 2002;121(6):578–581.
36. Huang WJ, Creath CJ. The midline diastema: a review of its etiology and treatment. *Pediatr Dent.* 1995;17:171–179.
37. Moffitt AH, Raina J. Long-term bonded retention after closure of maxillary midline diastema. *Am J Orthod Dentofac Orthop.* 2015;148:238–244.

12 Complex Nonskeletal Problems in Preadolescent Children: Preventive and Interceptive Treatment

HENRY W. FIELDS AND WILLIAM R. PROFFIT

CHAPTER OUTLINE

Eruption Problems

Complex Delayed Incisor Eruption

When an incisor has delayed eruption and there is no impediment such as a supernumerary tooth or other pathology, simple excision of the overlying soft tissue is recommended (see Chapter 11). This usually leads to normal eruption.

If there is *any* doubt regarding the potential for eruption, whether there has been adequate exposure of the crown, the tooth is deeper in the alveolus or when it has a nonideal orientation due to tip or rotation, the tooth should have an attachment bonded to it (a bracket or button, depending on access). A metal chain (*not* a wire ligature around the cervical portion of the tooth) is attached to the bracket or button and extended out of the tissue so traction can be applied using a fixed appliance if necessary (Fig. 12.1). If space is not adequate, preoperative space opening should be accomplished so the sequence of treatment is seamless.

In general, the force against the unerupted tooth is applied by using either elastomeric chain or (better) a nickel-titanium (NiTi) overlay wire supported by a heavy base wire with bonded brackets on several teeth for anchorage. The chain is adequate for initial movement because it is not as irritating to the soft tissue. The overlay NiTi wire has advantages over a continuous NiTi wire because with the continuous wire the reciprocal forces on the adjacent teeth may lead to their intrusion. As the tooth erupts, the bracket initially placed often requires repositioning because the initial bonding during the surgical procedure was less than ideal. Final root positioning can be left until a second stage of treatment during the permanent dentition if one is anticipated.

Complicated Ectopic Eruption

If resorption of a permanent tooth root occurs due to an adjacent ectopically erupting tooth, it is usually necessary to surgically expose the erupting permanent tooth and use orthodontic traction to bring it away from the affected tooth, to correct its position (Fig. 12.2). This will stop the resorption caused by the ectopic tooth, but some continued resorption and blunting of the roots may continue when further tooth movement of the affected tooth occurs. A common scenario for this to occur is when an ectopic canine is erupting. This comprehensive treatment will extend into the early permanent dentition period (see Chapter 15).

Transposition

Transposition is a rare positional interchange of two adjacent teeth. It occurs with a prevalence of approximately 0.3% and equally affects

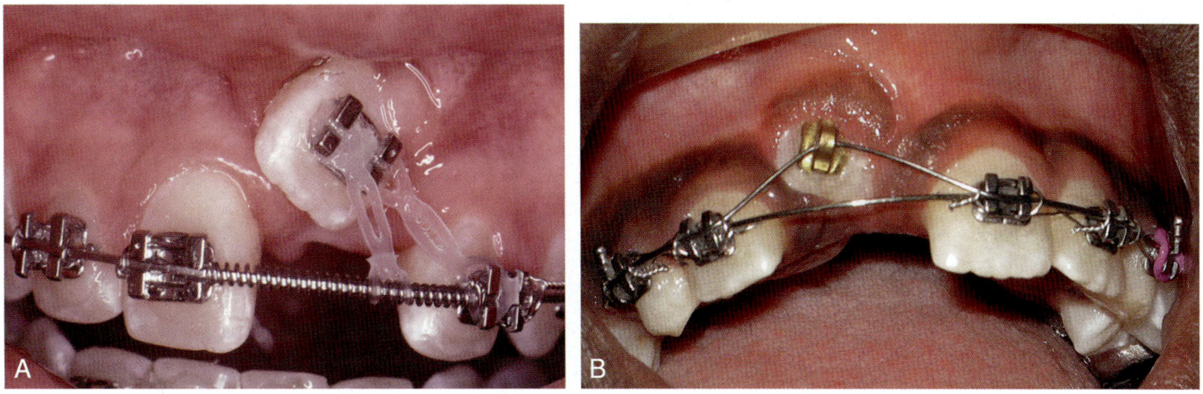

• **Fig. 12.1** (A) For initial traction to an unerupted incisor, it is acceptable to use a heavy base archwire and elastomeric chain to the teeth. Although this places relatively heavy forces on the teeth and has limited range, the limited invasiveness and bulk make it a sensible starting method. (B) A simple and more efficient option is to use the flexibility of a superelastic auxiliary archwire (austenitic nickel-titanium [A-NiTi]) while stabilizing with another stiffer wire to control the reciprocal forces. This is accomplished by tying the superelastic wire over the base archwire at one or two brackets on either side of the unerupted tooth to keep friction low, and deflecting it gingivally to provide the traction. The overlay wire should be tied loosely with steel ligatures to further reduce friction and released at adjustment appointments so the wire regains its superelastic properties. As the tooth erupts, it can be incorporated in a continuous flexible wire or the base wire will have to be offset to allow for the bracket to pass it.

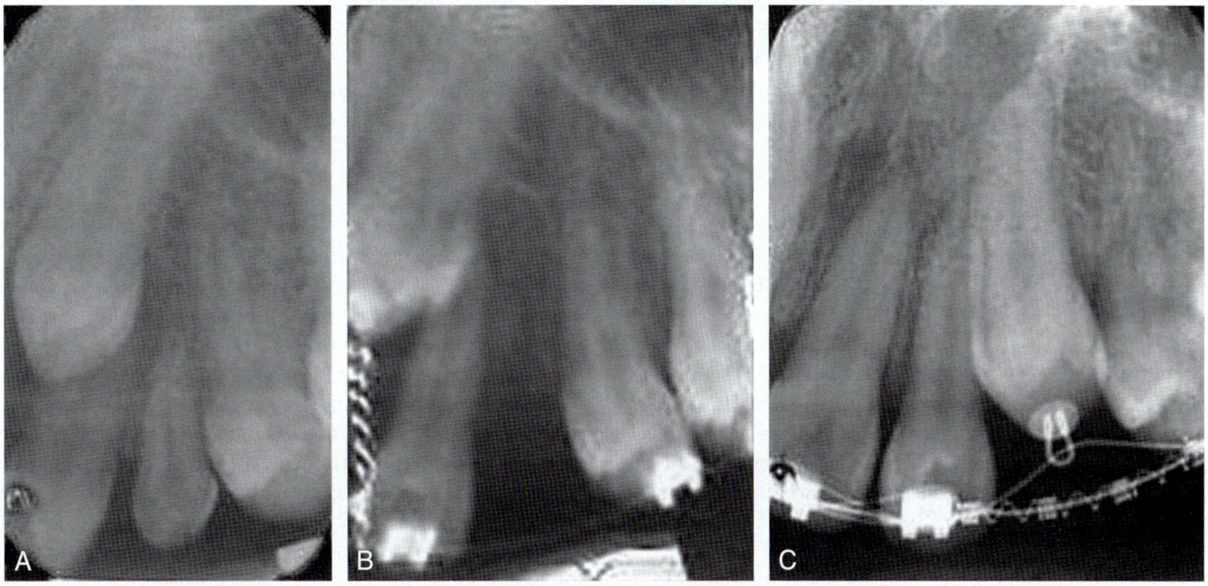

• **Fig. 12.2** (A) The maxillary left canine is positioned over the root of the adjacent lateral incisor and causing some initial root resorption. (B) Because of the resorption, the permanent canine was exposed surgically, the primary canine was extracted, and an attachment and metal chain were bonded to the crown of the permanent canine and ligated to the archwire. Attachments are sometimes difficult to bond because of contamination of the tooth surface by saliva and hemorrhage, but the alternative approach of looping a wire around the cervical part of the crown is no longer recommended. That approach requires more extensive bone removal and increases the risk of ankylosis and potential reduced gingival attachment. Using an acid etch as opposed to a combination etch/sealant usually will stop hemorrhage for a short time to enable the bonding. (C) Subsequently, the canine was repositioned distally away from the lateral incisor and into its correct position. This limited the continued resorption of the lateral incisor.

males and females.[1] The teeth most likely to be transposed are mandibular incisors and maxillary premolars, and this usually occurs as a consequence of ectopic eruption (discussed in Chapter 11). There appears to be a genetic component to this problem.[2]

In the early mixed dentition years, transposition can develop when distally directed eruption of the permanent mandibular lateral incisor leads to loss of the primary mandibular canine and primary first molar (Fig. 12.3). Interceptive treatment requires repositioning the lateral incisor mesially (Fig. 12.3C), which eliminates the possibility of the complete transposition with the canine. This means either bonding the tooth or gaining surgical access to the tooth and applying traction to tip the tooth back to its natural position. In addition to a labial fixed appliance, a lingual arch is usually required for supplemental anchorage. The benefit of this type of early

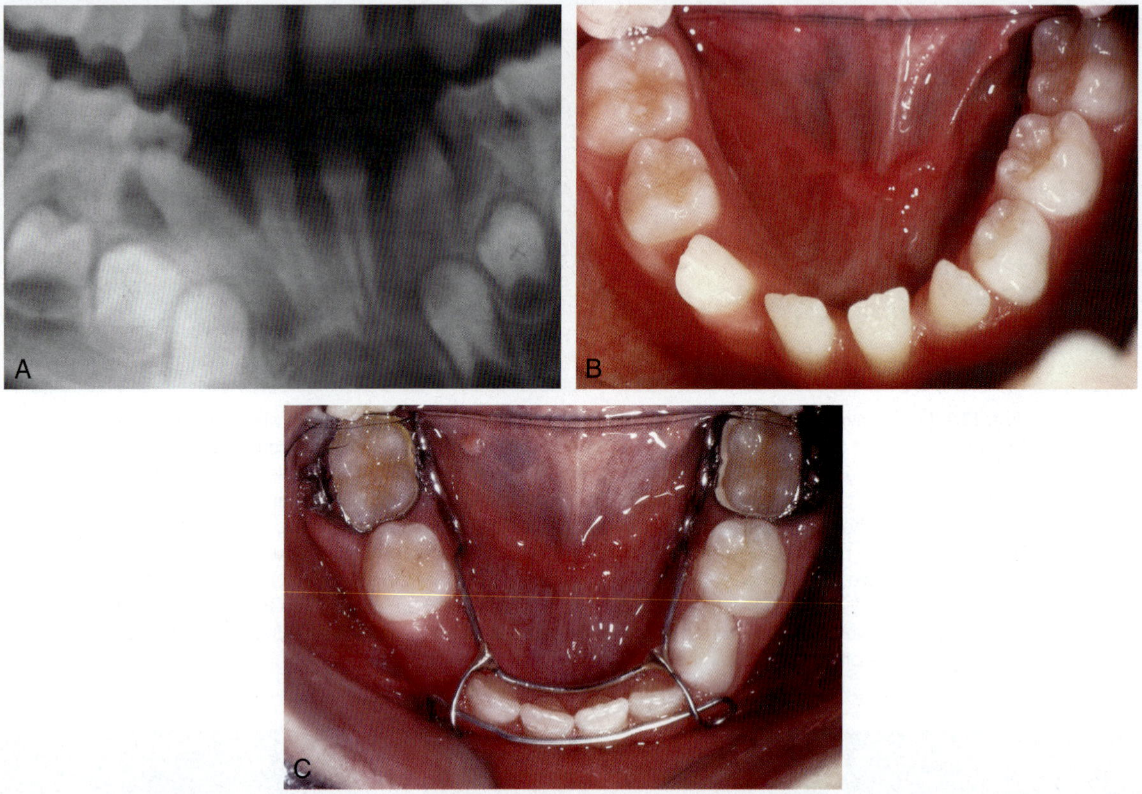

• **Fig. 12.3** (A) This radiograph shows that the right mandibular lateral incisor is erupting ectopically and has resorbed the roots of the primary canine and first molar. (B) Failure to reposition the right lateral incisor will lead to true transposition of the permanent lateral and canine. (C) The lateral incisors have been repositioned with fixed appliances and are now retained.

intervention is that a simple tipping movement can usually reposition the tooth. Left until later, bodily movement of the erupted teeth is required. One adverse consequence of this early repositioning is potential resorption of the lateral incisor root because it may be brought into contact with the unerupted canine. This is unlikely because of the usual facial position of the unerupted canine, but this should be discussed with the patient and parents before treatment. Beginning treatment before the canine is actively erupting is important. If left untreated, this can result in a true transposition of the permanent lateral incisor and canine (Fig. 12.4) This results in more extensive and lengthy treatment.

Later in the mixed dentition, the more prevalent transposition is of the maxillary canine and first premolar or maxillary canine and lateral incisor.[3] Treatment of transpositions involving the maxillary canine if not addressed early is quite challenging. Moving the teeth to their natural positions can be difficult because this requires bodily repositioning, translating the canine facially or lingually past the other tooth. Careful consideration of alveolar width and the integrity of the attached supporting tissue is required. Often, the best approach is to move a partially transposed tooth to a total transposed position or to leave fully transposed teeth in that position (Fig. 12.5). This requires careful finishing with reshaping of the transposed tooth both to improve its appearance and fit it within the dental arch. Although this can be difficult, the time and difficulty in correcting the transposition make it even more challenging.

Primary Failure of Eruption

Primary failure of eruption (PFE) is characterized by these five clinical and radiographic signs in almost all patients who have the PTH1R genetic variant (see Chapter 3)[4]: involvement of posterior teeth, involvement of the teeth distal to the most mesial affected, nothing obstructing the path of eruption, altered vertical growth of the alveolar process, and posterior open-bite.[5] The condition has a prevalence less than 0.06%, and due to a lack of complete data, possibly more common in females.[6] The average age of onset is also vague—PFE is usually noted in the late mixed dentition when some or all the permanent first molars have still not erupted and eruption of other posterior teeth anterior to the affected teeth appears normal[7] (Fig. 12.6). The affected teeth are not ankylosed but do not erupt and do not respond normally to orthodontic force, so they cannot be moved into occlusion. If tooth movement is attempted, usually the affected teeth will ankylose after little or no movement in any direction, and only what were supposed to be the anchor teeth will move.

Table 12.1 contrasts the diagnostic characteristics of PFE with the much more frequent situation of mechanical obstruction.[8] Obtaining a genetic analysis to confirm the diagnosis (which can be done using just a saliva sample) can help guide the patient and parents in accepting the reality of the problem, and circumvent treatment attempts that will not be successful. As the table points out, the most difficult diagnosis is whether a single unerupted molar is due to isolated ankylosis or PFE, and the table explains why doing nothing is not appropriate treatment.

Because this is the unusual case in which orthodontics simply doesn't work, acceptance of premolar occlusion in affected quadrants usually is the best long-term option. Prosthetic replacement of the teeth that failed to erupt, or possibly segmental osteotomies or distraction osteogenesis, is almost the only treatment possibility—and such treatments are indicated only in mild cases. It is somewhat

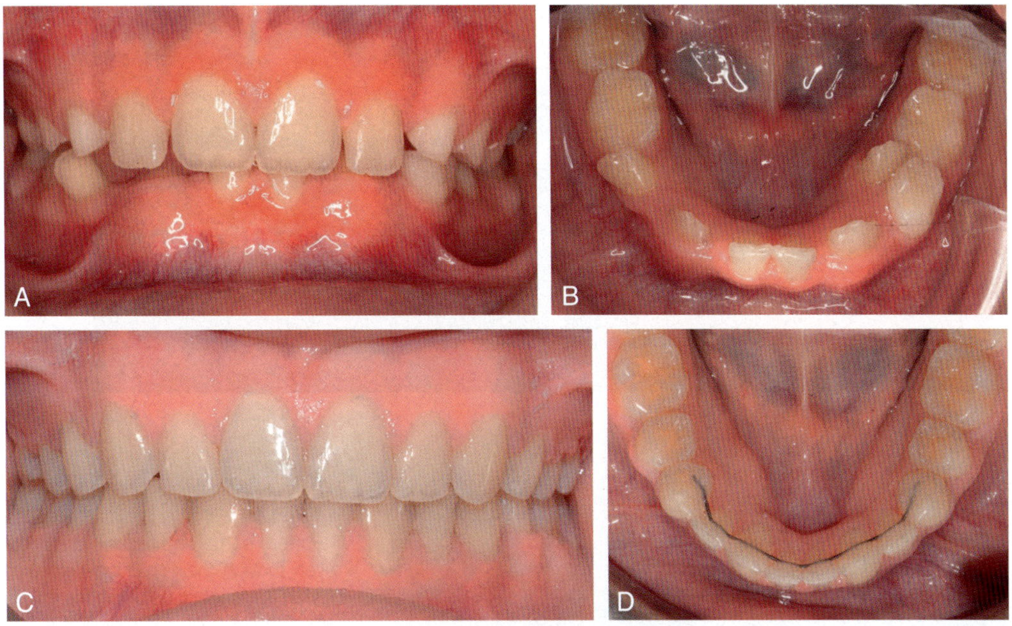

• **Fig. 12.4** (A and B) When the transposition of the mandibular lateral incisors and canines is complete, the choice is to reposition the teeth to either their natural positions or accept the transposition and align the teeth, which requires much less tooth movement. (C and D) The transposition was accepted and the teeth aligned and proper root positioning obtained for a functional and esthetic result. (Courtesy Dr. Tim Shaughnessy.)

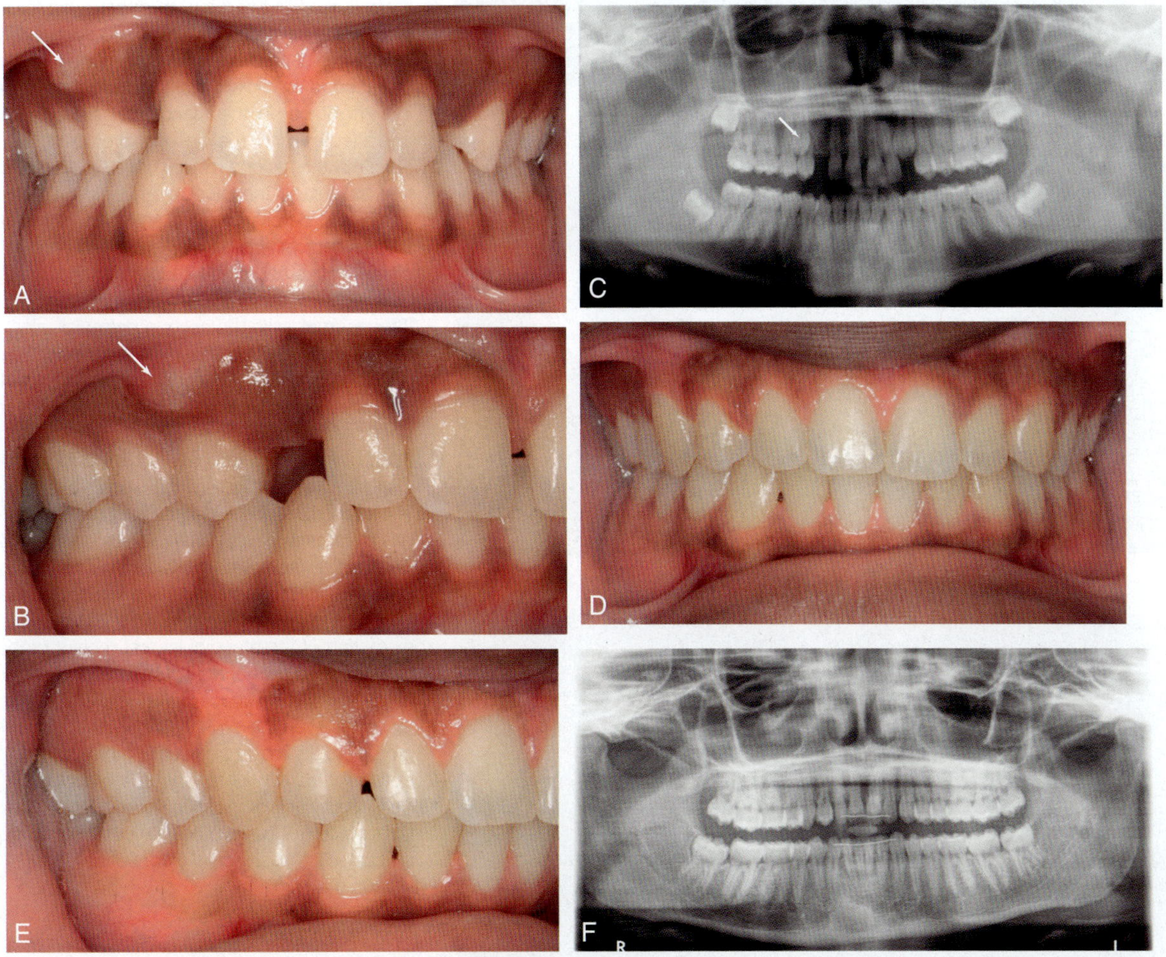

• **Fig. 12.5** (A and B) This patient has a transposed permanent maxillary canine in the mixed dentition that is visible under the tissue between the first and second premolars. (C) This preoperative radiograph confirms its position. (D and E) The canine was left in the transposed position and brought into the arch between the premolars. (F) This postoperative radiograph confirms its position.

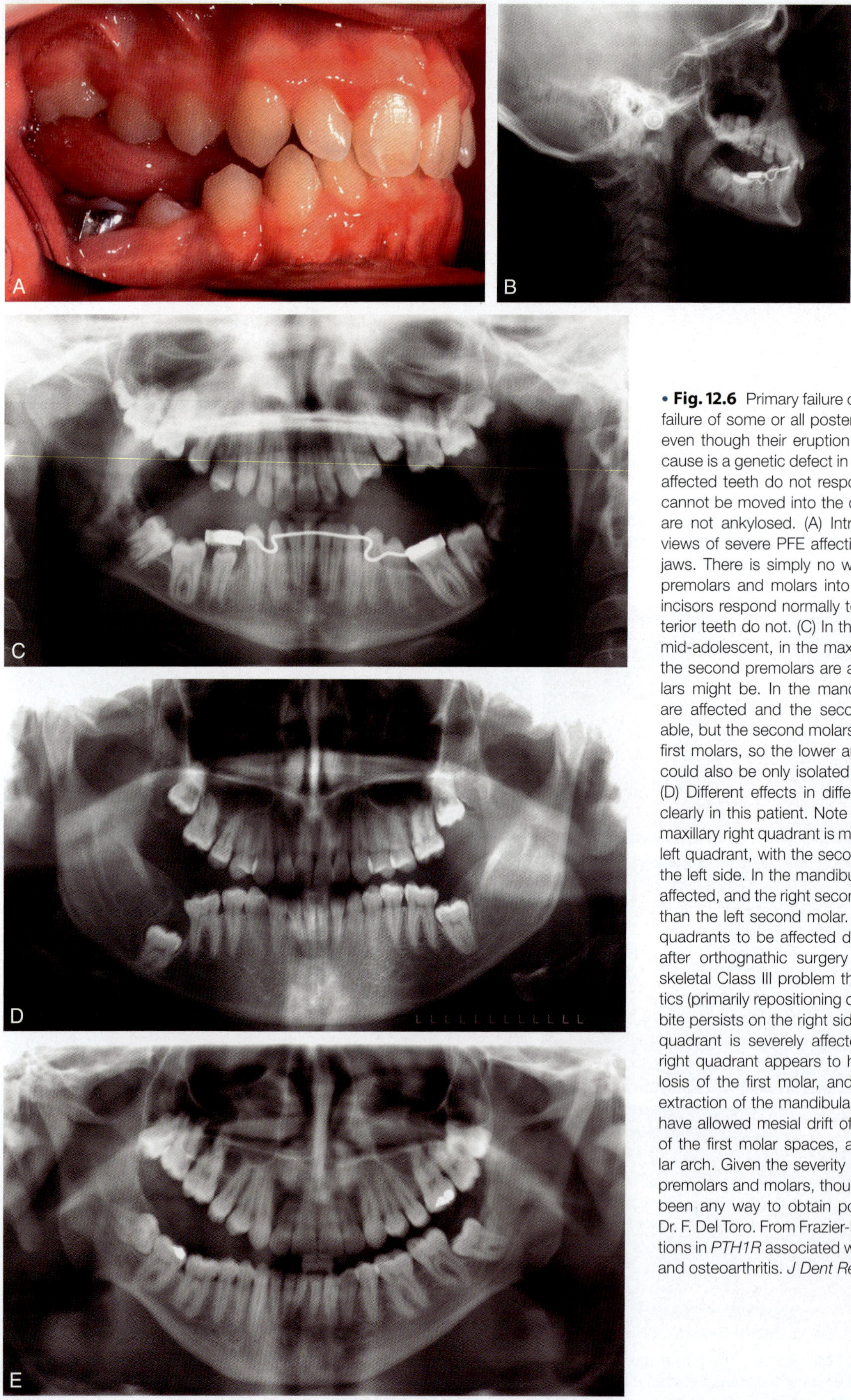

• **Fig. 12.6** Primary failure of eruption is characterized by failure of some or all posterior permanent teeth to erupt even though their eruption path has been cleared. The cause is a genetic defect in the eruption mechanism. The affected teeth do not respond to orthodontic force and cannot be moved into the dental arch even though they are not ankylosed. (A) Intraoral and (B) cephalometric views of severe PFE affecting all posterior teeth in both jaws. There is simply no way to bring these unerupted premolars and molars into occlusion. The canines and incisors respond normally to orthodontic force; the posterior teeth do not. (C) In this panoramic radiograph of a mid-adolescent, in the maxillary arch, it is apparent that the second premolars are affected, and the first premolars might be. In the mandibular arch, the first molars are affected and the second premolars are questionable, but the second molars have erupted more than the first molars, so the lower arch could be type 2 PFE but could also be only isolated ankylosis of the first molars. (D) Different effects in different quadrants can be seen clearly in this patient. Note in the maxillary arch that the maxillary right quadrant is more severely affected than the left quadrant, with the second premolar affected only on the left side. In the mandibular arch, only the molars are affected, and the right second molar was affected sooner than the left second molar. It is not unusual for different quadrants to be affected differently. (E) For this patient, after orthognathic surgery to improve an asymmetric skeletal Class III problem that included some orthodontics (primarily repositioning of the incisors), a severe open bite persists on the right side because the maxillary right quadrant is severely affected by PFE. The mandibular right quadrant appears to have had only isolated ankylosis of the first molar, and with 20/20 hindsight, early extraction of the mandibular first molars probably would have allowed mesial drift of the second molars, closure of the first molar spaces, and leveling of the mandibular arch. Given the severity of the effect on the maxillary premolars and molars, though, there still would not have been any way to obtain posterior occlusion. (Courtesy Dr. F. Del Toro. From Frazier-Bowers SA et al. Novel mutations in *PTH1R* associated with primary failure of eruption and osteoarthritis. *J Dent Res*. 2014;93:134–139.)

TABLE 12.1 Distinguishing Primary Failure of Eruption (PFE) From Other Eruption Disorders

PFE	Other Disorder
Affects posterior teeth only	Affects some or all anterior teeth also
Molars: always	Canines
Second premolars: sometimes	Lateral incisors
First premolars: rarely	Central incisors
Eruption pathway clear (no mechanical obstruction)	Mechanical obstruction of eruption (ankylosis, eruption pathway blocked)
Affected teeth do not respond to orthodontic force	Teeth respond normally after eruption path is cleared (ankylosis is permanent)
Family history (some, not all)	History of pathologic condition or trauma
PTHR1 mutation is diagnostic (but not all have this)	No or unknown genetic cause

The biggest diagnostic problem: One affected first molar (usually mandibular)—is it isolated ankylosis or PFE?

- If it's PFE, the second molar also will be affected and will not erupt normally.
- If it's isolated ankylosis, the second molar will erupt normally (including mesial drift).

What do you do? *Extract the unerupted first molar as early as possible.*

- If it was isolated ankylosis, the second molar will drift forward, bringing bone with it.
- And if it was PFE, the second molar will be abnormal and also a candidate for extraction.

Bottom line: You have nothing to lose with early extraction, and often something to gain.

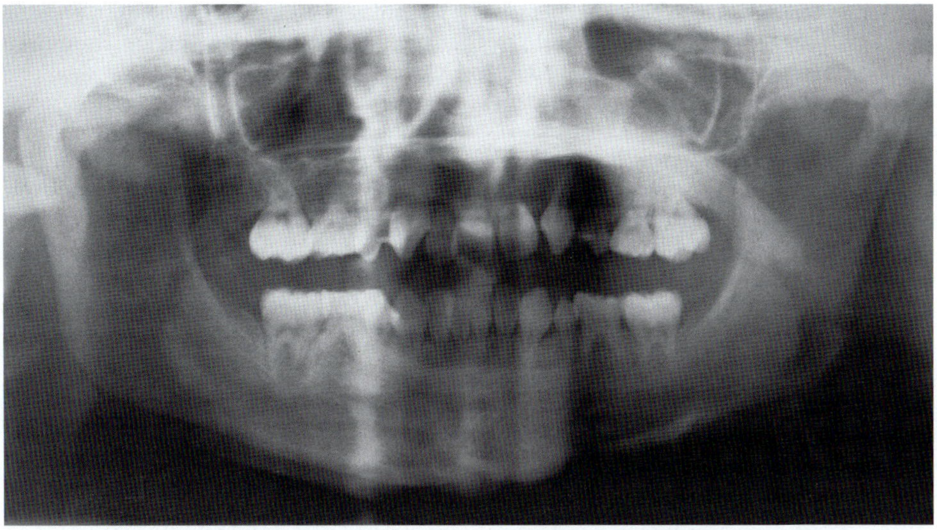

• **Fig. 12.7** This patient's panoramic radiograph shows shortening of the roots of multiple permanent teeth following radiation therapy. These teeth can be moved orthodontically, if necessary, with limited objectives and light forces. (Courtesy Dr. D. Grosshandler.)

distressing, but very useful, to know what you can't do as well as what you can.

Impact of Radiation Therapy and Bisphosphonates

Because of the increased prevalence of successful stem cell transplantation (SCT) and total body irradiation (TBI) for treatment of childhood cancers, more patients with missing teeth and altered tooth morphology are being observed. Early age at SCT (younger than 5 years old) is more of a risk factor than TBI.[9] Shortened roots are the result of high-dose chemotherapy and TBI, especially when treatment is in the 3- to 5-year age group.[10] Because these patients have high survival rates, they now seek orthodontic treatment. Some of the irradiated teeth fail to develop, others fail to erupt, and some may erupt even though they have extremely limited root development. Although the roots are short, light forces can be used to reposition these teeth and achieve better occlusion without fear of tooth loss (Fig. 12.7).

Children are increasingly receiving bisphosphonates in conjunction with other therapies, especially for steroid-induced osteoporosis or osteogenesis imperfecta. This drug class has known implications for dentistry and makes orthodontic tooth movement almost impossible (see Chapter 8).[11,12] Orthodontic treatment should not be attempted while bisphosphonates are actively being used. Currently, as children who previously underwent bisphosphonate treatment reach the age at which orthodontic tooth movement will be a possibility, it is important to assess the impact of this therapy. Intravenous treatments appear to produce more long-term impact than oral medication, as does the length of treatment and the number of intervening years since treatment.

Traumatic Displacement of Teeth

Treating traumatically injured teeth is complicated, and recommendations continue to change and evolve. Here we will provide a summary of the current (2022) knowledge in selected areas. In order to remain current, clinicians are encouraged to consult The Dental Trauma Guide (https://dentaltraumaguide.org/)[13] which is continuously updated.

Immediately after a traumatic injury, teeth that have not been irreparably damaged usually are repositioned with finger pressure to a near-normal position and out of occlusal interference. They are then stabilized (with a light wire or nylon filament) for 4 weeks. At this point, the teeth usually exhibit physiologic mobility. If the alveolus has been fractured (usually determined by mobility of several teeth as a group), then the teeth should be stabilized with a heavy wire for 4 weeks.

Following either of these initial treatments, if the teeth are not in ideal positions, orthodontic treatment to reposition them is indicated. For most patients it is advised to wait 3 to 4 months to begin active treatment, but for more severe periodontal-type injuries (luxation, intrusion, extrusion, or avulsion), some clinicians recommend longer waiting times (of up to 1 year).[14]

On the other hand, if after an injury, treatment has not been sought until the teeth have consolidated in a position that causes an occlusal interference, tooth movement should be started earlier to remove the interference (although final positioning of the teeth should be delayed after that). In either scenario, light force should be used. In orthodontic treatment that begins after significant trauma, even tipping forces can lead to loss of vitality and root resorption for previously traumatized teeth,[15] and patients who had partial obliteration of the pulp as a result of trauma are at particular risk.[16]

This increased risk of devitalization also applies to patients injured during orthodontic treatment, even though the orthodontic appliance often prevents extreme displacement of the teeth. Devitalization is still quite likely for those who have severe periodontal trauma.[17]

Until recently, traumatized teeth were evaluated initially with multiple radiographs at numerous vertical and horizontal angulations to rule out vertical and horizontal root fractures that could make it impossible to save the tooth or teeth (Fig. 12.8). Now cone beam computed tomography (CBCT) with a small field of view is an option to obtain more detail when root or crown fractures are suspected (see Fig. 6-84). During orthodontic treatment, it is reasonable to follow the teeth clinically by observing clinical mobility, sensitivity to percussion and cold, and electric pulp testing. The patients should immediately report tooth discoloration, pain, swelling, and any discharge from the surrounding tissues. Radiographically, periapical radiographs at 8 and 12 weeks, 6 months, and 1 year are indicated to determine periapical pathology.

If the apex is complete at the time of the injury, it is more likely that the tooth will become nonvital from luxation injuries. If that happens, pulpal extirpation and treatment are recommended, possibly even during the splinting time. External root resorption can jeopardize the tooth quite rapidly. When this is observed, immediate pulpal extirpation and antiresorptive treatment are recommended as the best approach.

Traumatic vertical displacement of teeth has a more guarded prognosis. For intruded immature teeth, a 4-week period allowing for reeruption is merited for any amount of displacement. If after that, no eruption is noted, orthodontic traction can be initiated using light traction. Monitoring the teeth for pulpal degeneration both clinically and radiographically is important.

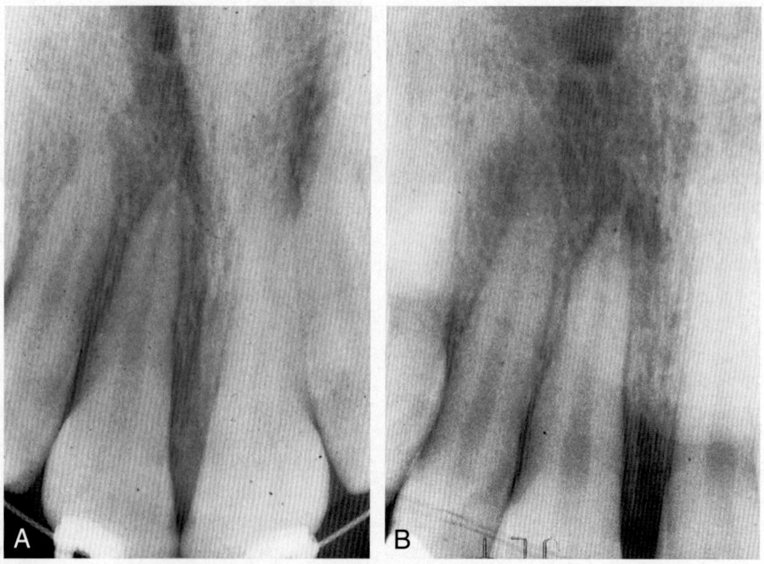

• **Fig. 12.8** Multiple vertically positioned radiographs are required to adequately diagnose previously traumatized teeth. (A) This radiograph displays no periapical pathology 2 weeks post injury to the central incisor, but (B) another radiograph obtained at the same time from a different vertical position shows a periapical radiolucency at the apex of the maxillary right central incisor.

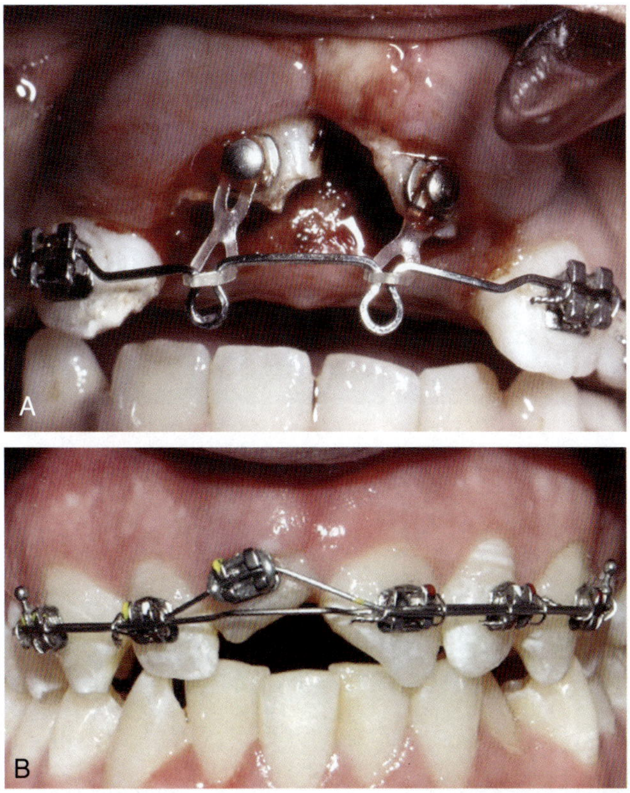

• **Fig. 12.9** (A) Following intrusion of permanent teeth without open apices, a potentially short waiting period for reeruption can be followed by orthododontic traction to ensure adequate endodontic access, if necessary. To begin, elastomeric chain can be used. (B) A more efficient method is to use a heavy base archwire complemented by a nickel-titanium (NiTi) overlay wire for rapid tooth movement. Note that the base archwire has been stepped facially to allow the bracketed tooth to pass on its lingual side.

For intruded teeth with mature roots, the prognosis is more guarded. If the intrusion is 3 mm or less, then allowing for reeruption for 4 weeks is recommended. Endodontic treatment can be started during this period depending on clinical and radiographic indications. If there is no change in 4 weeks, orthodontic traction with light forces can begin. Mature teeth with 3 to 7 mm of intrusion can have orthodontic treatment beginning immediately to extrude the tooth, but this may be impractical in terms of treatment time and appointments required (Fig. 12.9). If orthodontic extrusion is successful, 4 to 8 weeks of retention is recommended. For greater than 7 mm of intrusion, immediate surgical repositioning is recommended. For teeth with less severe intrusion, orthodontics provides better supporting tissue outcomes than surgical repositioning.[18] Remember, periodontal injury can lead to ankylosis that makes orthodontics impossible, but although nearly all severely displaced teeth with complete roots will have pulpal necrosis that requires endodontics,[19] nonvital teeth can be moved orthodontically after endodontic treatment. Even though the goal is to preserve pulpal vitality with intruded teeth and this is enhanced by reeruption, repositioning is critical to improve access for endodontics and to complete the diagnosis. Crown and root fractures can remain undiagnosed even with extensive radiographs. If reeruption does not occur in 4 weeks, there is no way to ensure endodontic access to reduce the possibility and extent of resorption. Practically, the approach is to wait the 4 weeks only if the teeth with immature or mature apices are actively reerupting. Otherwise, intervene with orthodontics or surgical repositioning sooner. If access still cannot be obtained, a gingivectomy should be performed to facilitate access. Fortunately, an endodontically treated tooth that will need orthodontics can be successfully moved without much fear of resorption.[20]

Even in the mixed or early permanent dentition, teeth that have been traumatically injured with resulting extensive crown fractures often need extrusion so interim restorations can be placed for esthetics and to maintain the integrity of the tooth. For these patients, the previous overlay wire technique can be employed or a continuous wire can be used with several adjacent teeth included as anchorage (Fig. 12.10). With careful bonding, the predetermined amount of tooth extrusion can be planned so that when the wire is straight, the extrusion is complete. Then periodontal crown lengthening can be completed and the tooth restored. This appears to be more predictable than rapid forced eruption as described in Chapter 20, that usually requires periodontal surgery at some point as well.

Traumatically extruded teeth also are at increased risk for losing pulp vitality. Those that were not immediately repositioned with finger pressure and have stabilized in their posttrauma position pose a difficult problem after complete healing. These teeth have reduced bony support and a poor crown-root ratio. Attempts to intrude them result in bony defects between the teeth, and loss of pulp vitality is a major risk (especially for lateral incisors), so orthodontic intrusion is not a good plan.[21] When the discrepancy is minor to moderate, reshaping the elongated tooth by crown reduction may be the best plan (Fig. 12.11). On the other hand, tramatically extruded teeth or avulsed teeth, that were not completely seated in the socket during initial injury treatment and are extruded as a result, can be successfully orthodontically repositioned if treatment begins immediately (Fig. 12.12).

Another consideration for patients with traumatically injured anterior teeth that cannot be restored is decoronation, removing the clinical crown of the compromised tooth and root structure to below the soft tissue level and removing vital pulp tissue. If this is accomplished before the growth spurt, bone will be maintained and even deposited in the area without substantial vertical resorption. Even if the patient is nongrowing, bone can be held in the edentulous area until vertical growth is completed and then an implant can be placed.[22] This adjunctive procedure reduces the chance of ridge resorption and the need for later bone grafting. If the tooth is compromised and can still be moved orthodontically, it can be repositioned and the root buried at the optimal place. The root can subsequently be removed or the implant placed through it (Fig. 12.13).

Ankylosed Primary Molars Without Successors

Ankylosed primary molars are common and most have successors and will exfoliate in reasonable time. If the premolar is blocked by the retained crown of an ankylosed primary molar, the remainder of the crown should be extracted. The teeth that are problematic are ankylosed primary second molars without successors (remember, the succedaneous second premolars are frequent congenitally missing) that are *not* planned for extraction and drift or space closure (addressed later in this chapter). As other teeth erupt and the ankylosed ones do not, large vertical occlusal discrepancies and vertical periodontal defects with the adjacent permanent teeth can develop. If this occurs and the ankylosed teeth are extracted, a great deal of bone will be lost and the cementum of the adjacent permanent teeth will be exposed—compromising these teeth.

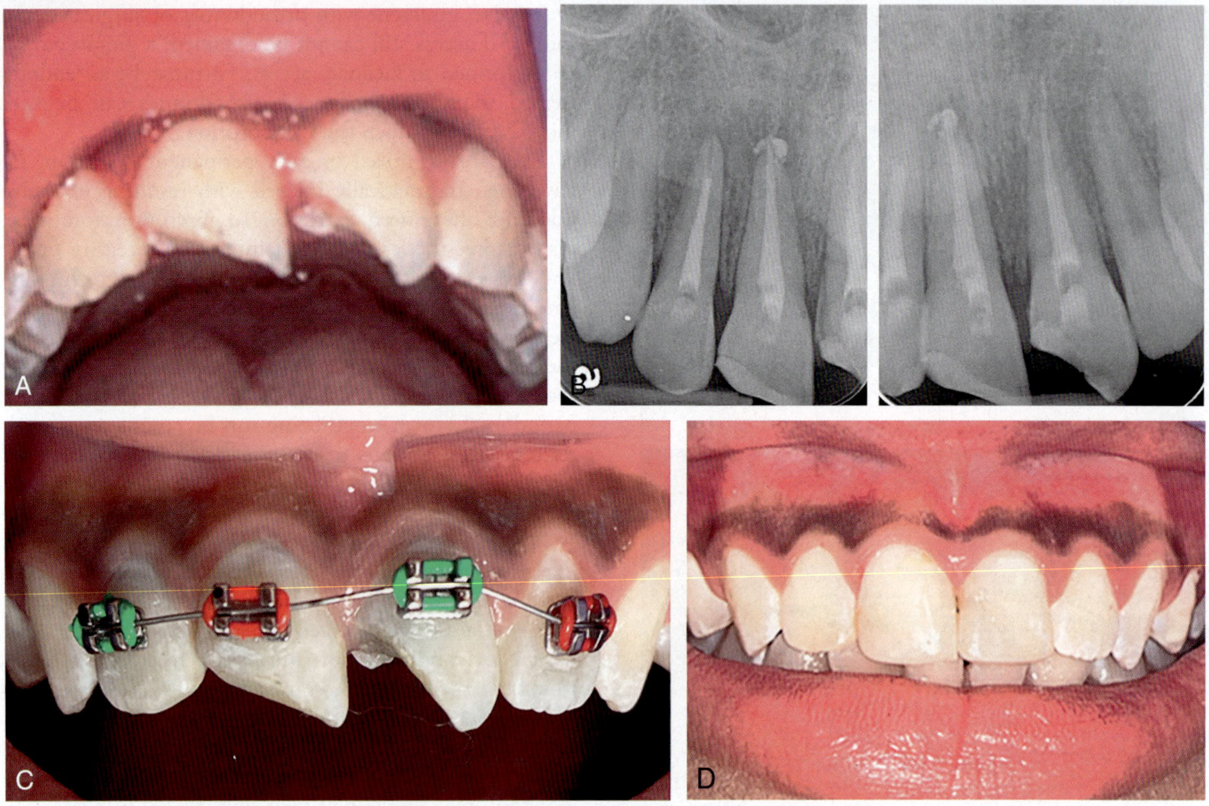

• **Fig. 12.10** (A) These teeth with complete root formation have been fractured and luxated. The goal is to stabilize the pulpal status of the teeth, determine the extent of the dental fracture, extrude and crown lengthen some teeth for restorations and retain. (B) A small field CBCT revealed pulpal necrosis on teeth #8 and 9 and a vertical shear fracture on the lingual of tooth #9. These periapical views show tooth #7 had definitive pulpectomy, while #8 and 9, have CaOH treatment due to necrotic pulps. (C) Appliances have been place to align and extrude teeth 8 and 9 approximately 2–3 mm. (D) The interim restorations. The extrusion was followed by crown lengthening for better restorative access and retention and bony and gingival contouring.

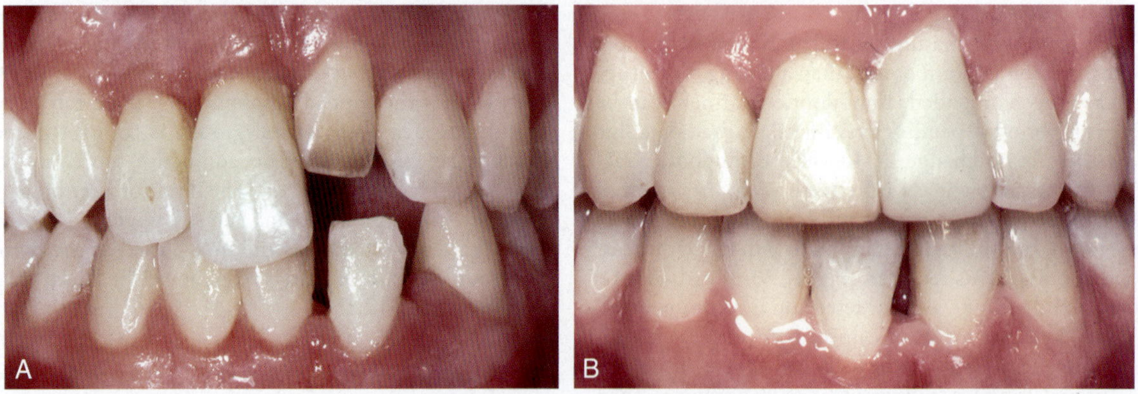

• **Fig. 12.11** (A) This patient had extrusive displacement injuries to the maxillary permanent right incisors. (Also note that the permanent mandibular left central incisor was reimplanted as the lost permanent maxillary left central incisor.) (B) Because it is difficult to intrude these maxillary incisors and there is a risk of a subsequent bony defect, the crowns of these teeth were reduced to provide a better crown-root ratio and improve the appearance.

One solution is early extraction of the ankylosed primary second molar before any vertical defect advances too far, and *not* placing a space maintainer. Letting the permanent first molar drift mesially is desirable for two reasons: It reduces the size of the implant to closer to the size of a second premolar, and the first molar brings bone with it as it moves forward. Certainly, after the extraction, the bony ridge will deteriorate, but the periodontal attachments will have limited compromise.

The other possibility is decoronation, as described earlier, which is increasingly indicated for patients who still have the growth spurt remaining but for some reason (potentially unsupported posterior teeth, incisor retrusion or other spacing in the arch) are not going to have space closure but later implants for the missing teeth (Fig. 12.14). For these patients, the vertical defect at the time of implant placement is reduced and bone grafting may not be necessary. It is possible that new bone will form coronal

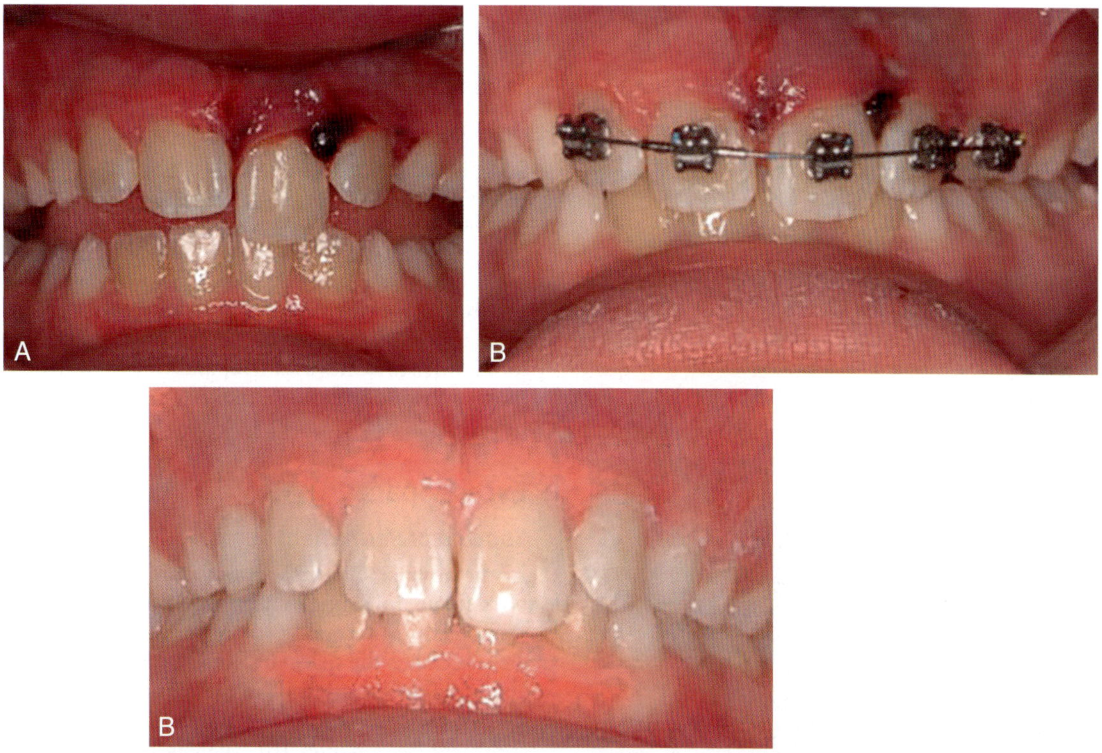

• **Fig. 12.12** (A) This patient had traumatic extrusion of #9, but no root fracture. (B) Two days after intrusion was begun immediately with a segmental superelastic archwire and light force. (C) The improved tooth position 10 weeks later and continued pulp vitality. (Courtesy Dr. John Christensen.)

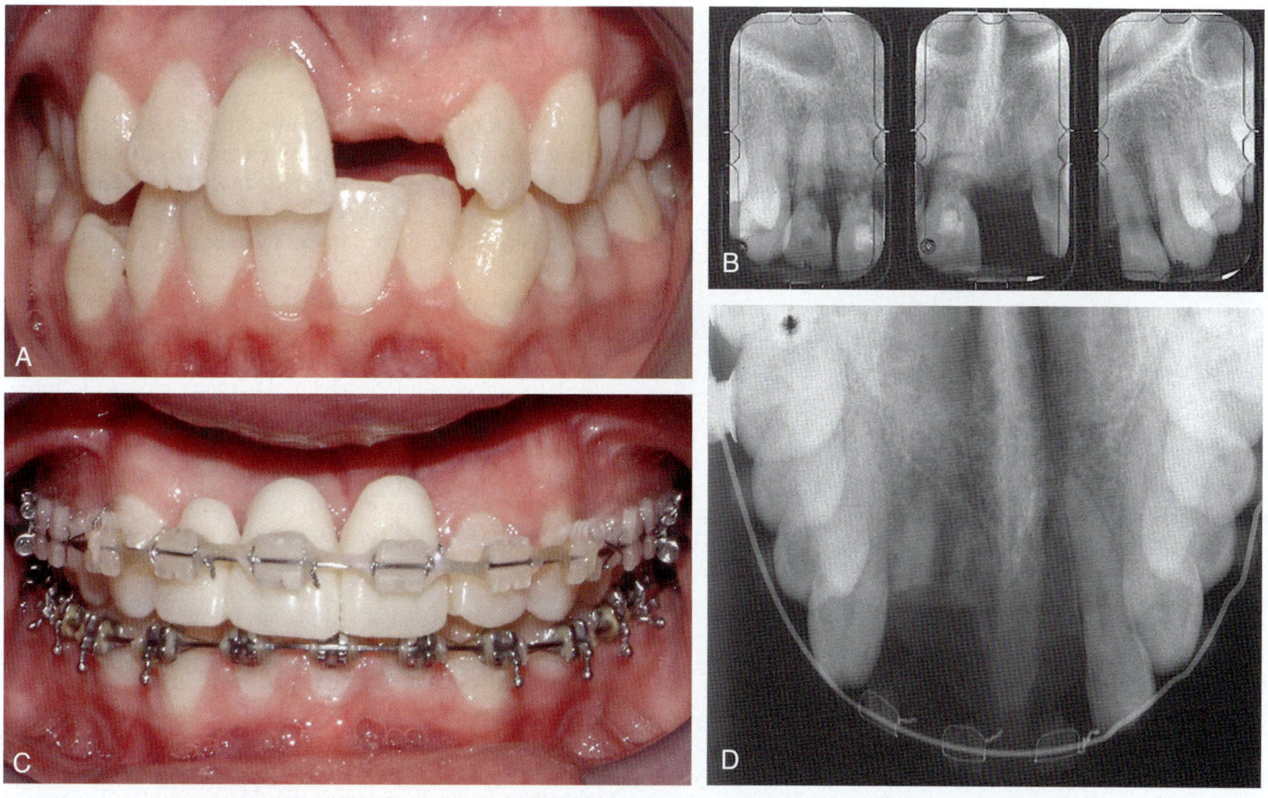

• **Fig. 12.13** This patient had root burial to retain the maxillary anterior alveolar bone. (A) The maxillary left central incisor was avulsed. (B) The maxillary radiograph shows severe resorption of the roots of the maxillary right central and lateral incisors. Instead of extracting these two teeth, they were decoronated (crowns removed, pulps extirpated, and roots covered with soft tissue) to maintain the ridge. (C) The pontics are in place during orthodontic treatment for space control and esthetics; the roots maintain the ridge as seen on the radiograph (D).

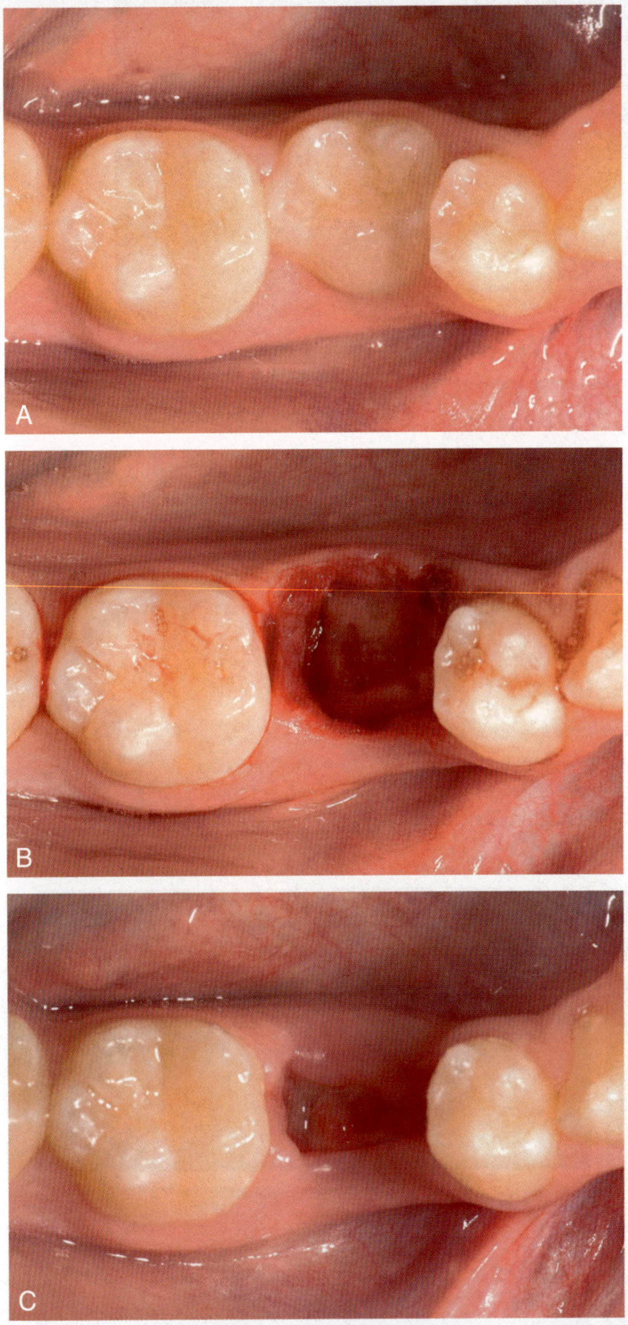

• **Fig. 12.14** When an ankylosed tooth without a successor, like this second primary molar, is retained and the aim is to maintain bone for a later implant, decoronation of the primary molar is a treatment option. (A) The primary molar before decoronation with a developing vertical discrepancy. (B) The crown removed 2 mm below the gingival level with all pulpal vital tissue removed, and (C) the tooth 1 week postoperatively.

to the buried root structure (Fig. 12.15), and an implant in late adolescence with good bony support should be possible.

Space-Related Problems

The most frequent cause of irregular and malaligned teeth in the early mixed dentition is a lack of adequate space for the alignment of permanent incisors. The loss of space due to mesial drift of permanent molars after the early loss of primary second molars is the major indication for treatment in the early mixed dentition beyond the interferences with eruption that we have discussed. Early treatment to align crowded incisors may or may not be indicated. The decision as to whether this should be done in the mixed dentition and how it will be accomplished depends on the impact on esthetics as judged by the child and parents, as well as the location and magnitude of the problem.

The goal should be to keep as many sensible options open as possible but to refrain from treatment when either the problem is too minor or later treatment will obviously be needed. The following section focuses on more complex space problems that require more expertise in diagnosis, treatment planning, and biomechanics in order to achieve a useful and timely treatment. These treatments must be truly beneficial to the patient in the long run to be justified.

Excess Space

Spacing of Permanent Teeth

In the absence of incisor protrusion, generalized excess space is not a frequent finding in mixed dentition. It can result from either small teeth in normal-sized arches or normal-sized teeth in large arches. Unless the space presents an esthetic problem, it is reasonable to allow eruption of the remaining permanent teeth before closing the space with fixed appliances as part of comprehensive treatment (see Chapter 16). There is little or no advantage to early treatment unless it is for compelling esthetic reasons.[23]

A midline diastema is often a localized excess space problem (if not complicated by pathologic conditions, supernumerary teeth, a tooth size problem or missing adjacent teeth). Tipping anterior teeth to close a small diastema was addressed in Chapter 11, but closing a large, unesthetic diastema that may also be inhibiting eruption of adjacent teeth requires bodily repositioning of the central incisors to maintain proper inclinations of the teeth. Mesial crown and root movement provides more space for the eruption of the lateral incisors and canines. When the situation demands bodily mesiodistal movement and no retraction of the teeth, an anterior segmental archwire from central to central incisor or a segmental archwire including more anterior teeth is needed. Initial alignment of the incisors with a flexible wire is required. Then a stiffer archwire can be employed as the teeth slide together (with 22-slot brackets, 18-mil round or 16 × 22-mil rectangular steel is a good choice; Fig. 12.16). The force to move the incisors together can be provided by an elastomeric chain. Diastema closure is more predictable if only mesiodistal movement is required. If protruding incisors are part of the problem and need to be retracted to close the space, then careful attention to the posterior anchorage, overbite, and type of incisor tooth movement (tipping versus bodily retraction) is required (see later).

In a few instances, multiple supernumerary teeth are located superficially, and uncomplicated extractions can be performed without interfering appreciably with the normal teeth. The guideline is that the more supernumeraries there are, the more abnormal their shape, and the higher their position, the harder it will be to manage the situation. Multiple abnormal supernumeraries are likely to have disturbed the position and eruption timing of the normal teeth before their discovery, and tubercle teeth are unlikely to erupt. Extractions should be completed as soon as the supernumerary teeth can be removed without harming the developing normal teeth (Fig. 12.17). The surgeon may wish to delay extraction until continued growth has improved both access and the child's ability to tolerate surgery. Further root development

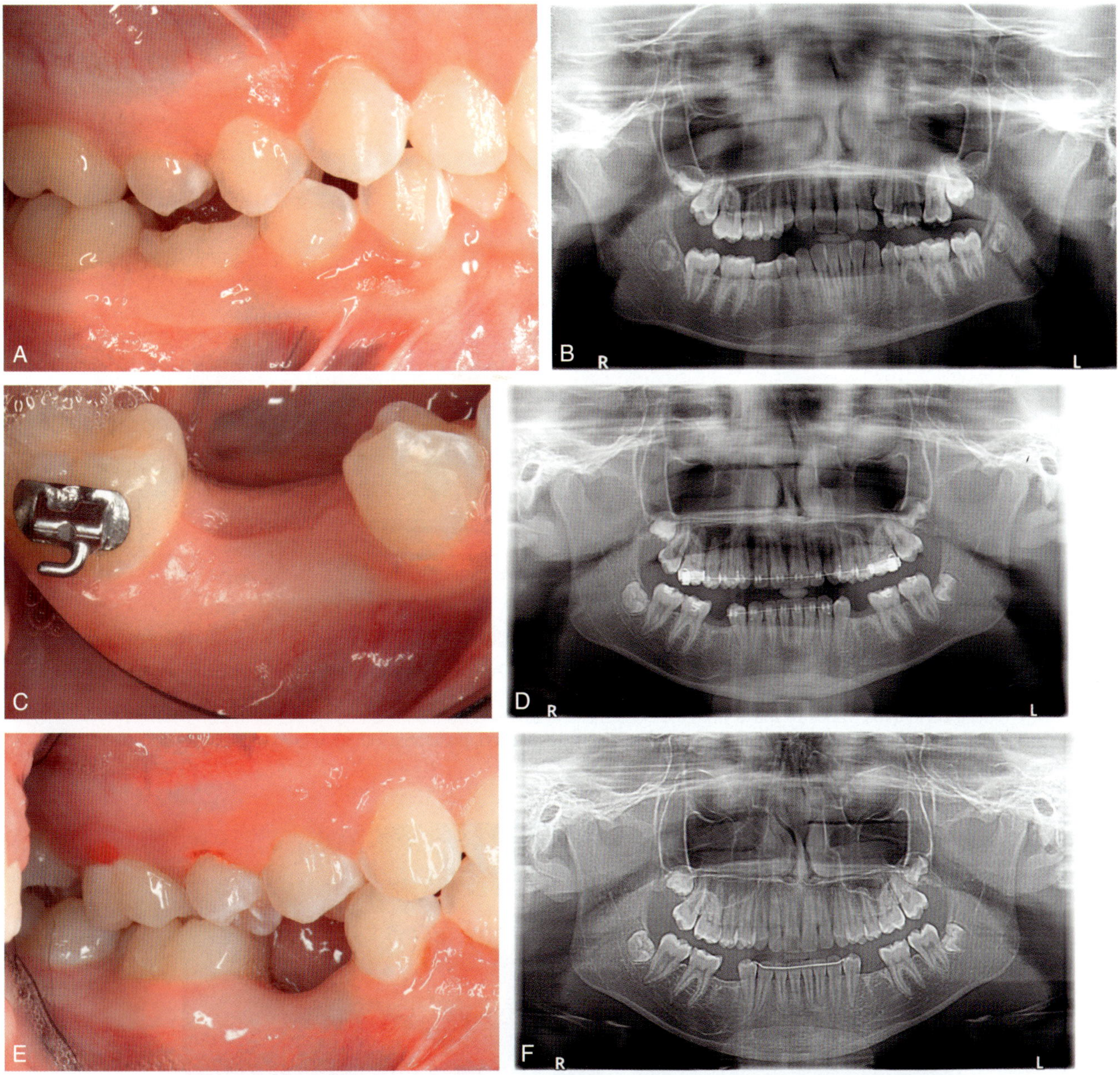

• **Fig. 12.15** Preop and postop images of decoronation patient from Fig 12.14 with a vertical discrepancy developing with the ankylosed primary second molars without successors. (A) The preoperative intraoral and (B) panoramic radiographs. (C) The healed primary second molar decoronation site and (D) panoramic radiograph showing the extent of crown removal and retained root structure. (E) The postorthodontic intraoral view with the healed decoronation site and space for an implant. (F) Postorthodontic panoramic radiograph showing the maintained bone levels and root structure that will serve as the ultimate implant sites.

will improved the prognosis for the teeth that remain. This is reasonable, but the earlier the supernumeraries can be removed, the more likely that the normal teeth will erupt without further intervention. Conversely, the later the extractions, the more likely it is that the remaining unerupted normal teeth will need surgical exposure, orthodontic traction, or both to bring them into the arch. Usually banding and bonding multiple primary and permanent teeth will be required to close spaces and bodily reposition the permanent teeth so that the adjacent teeth can erupt in normal positions. This can involve more advanced biomechanics and rectangular wires for root torquing movements.

The experienced clinician's desire to close diastemas at an early age is tempered by knowledge of how difficult it can be to keep the space closed as the other permanent teeth erupt. If the lateral incisors and canines have not erupted when the diastema is closed, a removable retainer will allow the central incisors to adjust to the erupting teeth, but will require constant modification. If the overbite is not prohibitively deep, an alternative approach for retention is to bond a 17.5-mil multistrand archwire to the linguocervical portion of the central incisors (Fig. 12.18). This provides excellent retention with less maintenance. If the centrals and laterals have erupted, a removable appliance instead of a lingual bonded retainer is best. The removable appliance will allow the adjustment of the lateral incisal roots when the canines erupt along their distal root surfaces. A bonded retainer will not allow that adjustment and may potentially contribute to lateral incisor root resorption.

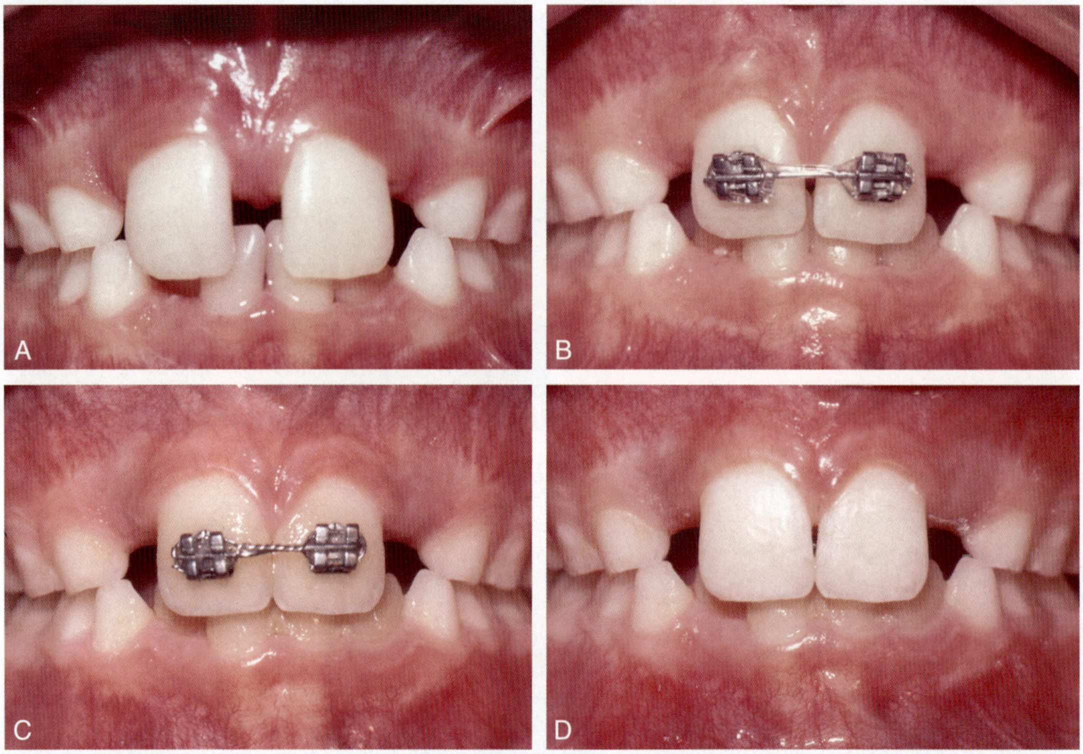

• **Fig. 12.16** Closure of a diastema with a fixed appliance. (A) This diastema requires closure by moving the crowns and roots of the central incisors. (B) The bonded attachments and rectangular wire control the teeth in three planes of space while the elastomeric chain provides the force to slide the teeth along the wire. (C) Immediately after space closure, the teeth are retained, preferably with (D) a fixed lingual retainer (see Fig. 18.12), at least until the permanent canines erupt.

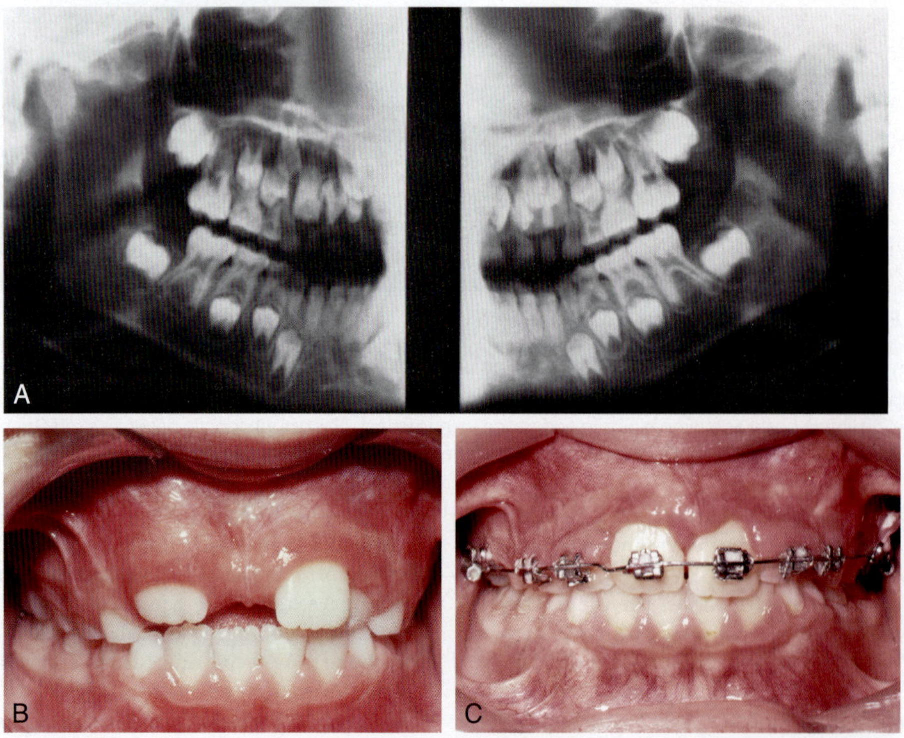

• **Fig. 12.17** Multiple supernumerary teeth in the anterior maxilla are often the cause of spacing and delayed eruption of anterior teeth. (A) This patient has an exceptionally wide diastema and delayed eruption of the maxillary lateral incisors. (B) The panoramic radiograph reveals three supernumeraries of various shapes and orientations. Conical and noninverted supernumeraries usually erupt, whereas tubercle-shaped and inverted ones do not. (C) The supernumeraries were removed, the diastema was closed, and the incisors were aligned with fixed appliances after they erupted.

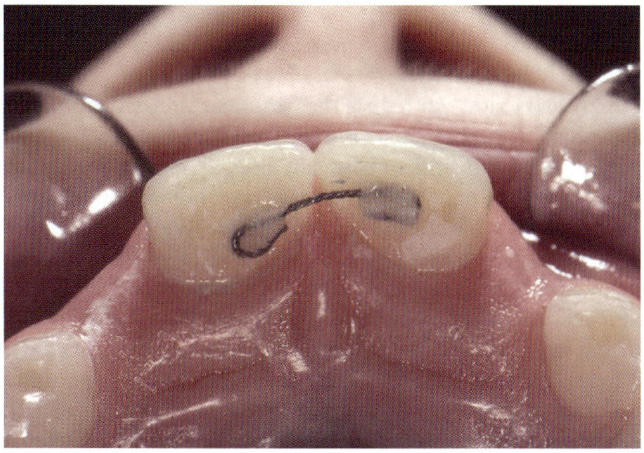

• **Fig. 12.18** A fixed retainer to maintain diastema closure. A bonded 17.5-mil multistrand wire with loops bent into the ends is bonded to the lingual surfaces of anterior teeth to serve as a permanent retainer. This flexible wire allows physiologic mobility of the teeth and reduces bond failure but can be used only when the overbite is not excessive.

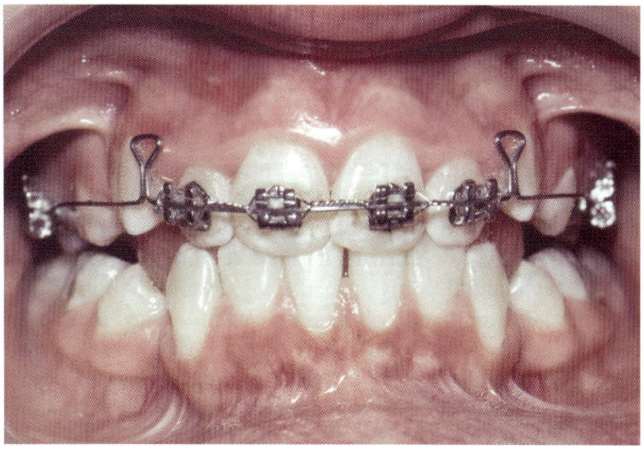

• **Fig. 12.19** This closing loop archwire was used to retract protrusive maxillary incisors and close space. Each loop was activated approximately 1 mm/month, and the posterior anchorage was reinforced with headgear.

The difficulty in keeping a midline diastema closed is due primarily to failure of the gingival elastic fibers to cross the midline when a large diastema is present, but may be aggravated by the presence of a large or inferiorly attached labial frenum. A frenectomy after space closure and retention may be necessary in some cases, but it is difficult to determine the potential contribution of the frenum to retention problems from its pretreatment morphology. Therefore a frenectomy before treatment is contraindicated, and a posttreatment frenectomy should be done only if unresolved bunching of tissue between the teeth shows that it is necessary.

Maxillary Dental Protrusion and Spacing

Treatment for maxillary dental protrusion during the early mixed dentition is indicated only when the maxillary incisors protrude with spaces between them and are esthetically objectionable or in danger of traumatic dental injury (TDI). When this occurs in a child who has no skeletal discrepancies, it is often a sequel to a prolonged finger-sucking habit. Eliminating the finger habit before tooth movement is necessary (see Chapter 11). The more common cause for maxillary incisor protrusion is a Class II malocclusion that often has a skeletal component, and, in that case, treatment must address the larger problem (see Chapter 14).

There are relationships between malocclusion and TDI. It is clear that children with protruding teeth, increased overjet, incompetent lips, and a history of previous dental injury in the primary dentition or before age 9 are at risk for dental trauma.[24–26] Although it might seem this is a reason to treat many patients with Class II malocclusion early, this is not supported by longitudinal data and the benefits of early treatment.[27] This is especially true if we recognize that most TDIs are enamel and dentin fractures with moderate long-term sequelae, not periodontal injuries that have significant long-term consequences. Predicting who is most at risk for significant injury is not easy. Risk-taking behavior may play a role.[28]

Early orthodontic treatment for those who have increased overjet, incompetent lips, and a history of permanent dentition TDI before age 9 years makes some sense if the treatment is limited to retraction of the incisors (not early Class II growth modification). This, combined with a good mouth guard for sports, can greatly reduce TDIs.

If there is adequate vertical clearance (not a deep bite) and space within the arch, maxillary incisors that are proclined or have been tipped facially by a sucking habit can be tipped lingually with a removable appliance as described in Chapter 11. When the teeth require bodily movement or correction of rotations, a fixed appliance is required (Fig. 12.19). In these cases, an archwire should be used with bands on permanent first molars and bonded brackets on incisors. This appliance must provide a retracting and space-closing force, which can be obtained from closing loops incorporated into the archwire or from a section of elastomeric chain. To ensure bodily movement, a rectangular archwire must be used so that the crown and root movement are controlled (as described in Chapter 9), and undue tipping does not occur and leave the patient with upright or "rabbited" teeth. Bodily incisor retraction places a large strain on the posterior teeth, which tends to pull them forward. Depending on the amount of incisor retraction and space closure, a headgear or Nance appliance, with consideration for vertical facial and dental characteristics, may be necessary for supplemental anchorage support.

If the overbite is deep, it will bring the upper and lower incisors into vertical contact before the upper incisors can be retracted enough to close spaces between them and eliminate the excess overjet. In some properly selected patients this can be addressed with a biteplate that allows eruption of posterior teeth and reduces the overbite, but it is rare that skeletal Class II malocclusion is not part of the total picture when excessive overjet and overbite are both present. This presents a much more complex treatment problem that requires skeletal change and most likely comprehensive orthodontic treatment.

Missing Permanent Teeth

When permanent teeth are congenitally missing, a thorough evaluation of the patient must be performed to determine the correct treatment. The diagnostic variables of profile, incisor position, tooth color and shape, skeletal and dental development or position, and space availability or deficiency can be crucial in treatment planning. The most commonly missing permanent teeth are second premolars (especially mandibular) and maxillary lateral incisors. These two conditions pose different problems.

Missing Second Premolars

Second premolars have a tendency to form late and may be thought to be missing, only to be discovered to be forming at a subsequent visit. A premolar that begins formation very late is likely to be very late in erupting, and may be abnormal in other ways, so careful observation and caution are required. Good premolars seldom form after the child is 8 years of age.

If the patient has an acceptable occlusion, maintaining the primary second molars is a reasonable plan, because many can be retained at least until the patient reaches the early 20s or beyond (Fig. 12.20). Many reports exist of primary molars surviving until the patient is 40 to 60 years of age. Some reduction of their mesiodistal width may be needed to improve the interdigitation of the posterior teeth, but if this is done, there is a risk of resorption of the mesiodistal diverging roots of the primary molar when they contact the adjacent permanent tooth roots. Even if eventual replacement of the primary molar with an implant or bridge is required, keeping the primary molar as long as possible is an excellent way to maintain alveolar bone in that area.

If the space, profile, and jaw relationships are good or somewhat protrusive, it can be advantageous to extract primary second molars that have no successor at age 7 to 9 and allow the first molars to drift mesially (Fig. 12.21). This can produce partial or even complete space closure. Unfortunately, the amount of mesial drift varies (Fig. 12.22). And, first premolars may drift distally. Unless the second premolars are missing in all quadrants, it may be necessary to extract teeth in the opposing arch to reach a near-ideal Class I occlusion. Otherwise, space closure will result in a class II or class III molar relationship. The molar relationship itself is not a problem, but later overeruption of unopposed second molars may become one.

Early extraction can reduce the treatment time when the space of missing second premolars is to be closed, but later comprehensive orthodontic treatment is usually needed. If only one primary molar is missing, unless there has been true unilateral space loss or there is considerable crowding on the contralateral side, restorative rather than conventional orthodontic resolution of the problem is usually indicated. It is nearly impossible to close space unilaterally in mixed dentition without affecting the midlines and other anterior interarch relationships. Remember that temporary anchorage devices (TADs) to facilitate unilateral space closure are not indicated before about 12 years of age because of bone density, so unilateral space closure would have to be reserved for a later time.

Another solution to missing second premolars is to combine hemisectioning of the primary tooth and pulp therapy so that the first permanent molar is protracted into the primary molar space without loss of alveolar bone from a more long-standing extraction. This treatment is described in more detail in Chapter 16.

Missing Maxillary Lateral Incisors

Long-term retention of primary laterals, in contrast to primary molars, is almost never an acceptable plan. When the lateral

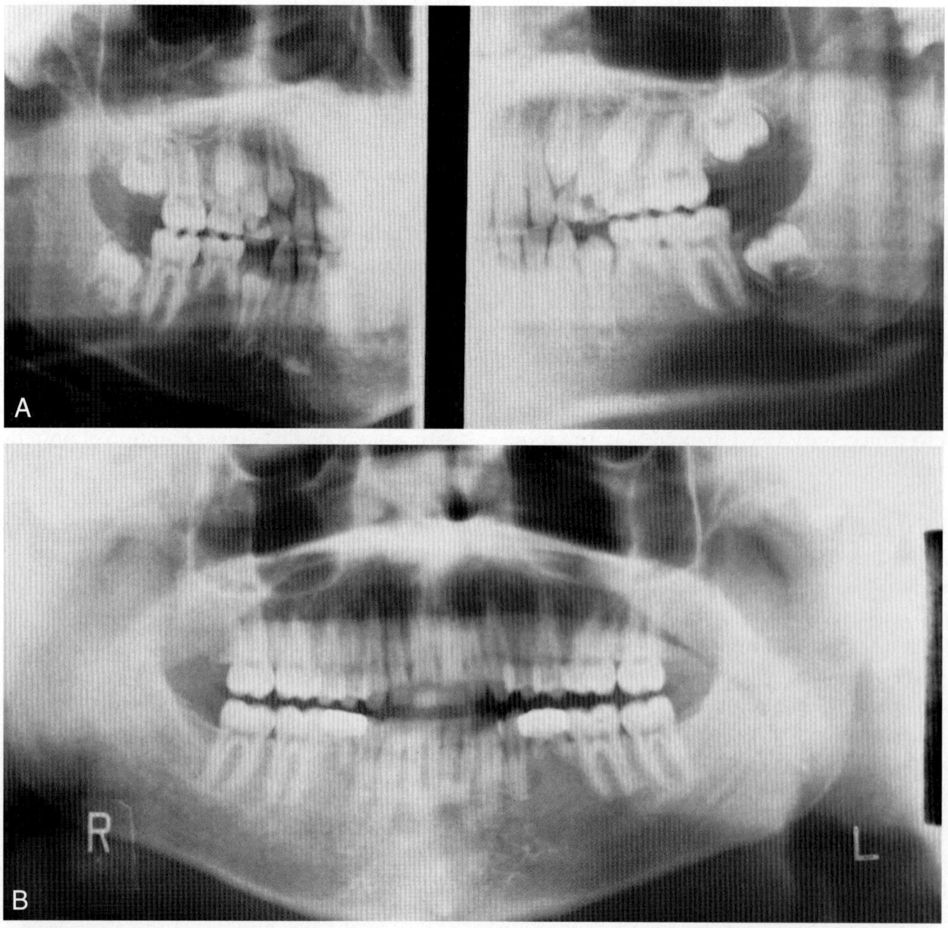

• **Fig. 12.20** Primary mandibular second molars can be retained when the second premolars are missing. (A) This patient was identified before orthodontic treatment as having missing mandibular second premolars. (B) The decision was to retain the primary mandibular second molars because of the lack of crowding in the mandibular arch and their excellent root structure. These teeth were reduced mesiodistally and restored with stainless steel crowns during the finishing stages of orthodontic treatment to provide good occlusion.

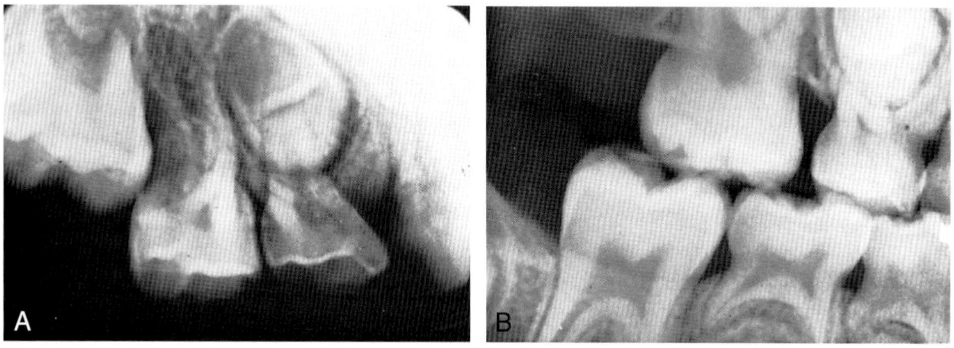

• **Fig. 12.21** Missing second premolars can be treated by extraction of primary second molars to allow drifting of the permanent teeth and spontaneous space closure. (A) This patient has ectopic eruption of the permanent maxillary first molar and a missing permanent maxillary second premolar. Since there was no other evidence of a malocclusion, the primary molar was extracted and (B) the permanent molar drifted anteriorly and closed the space during eruption. This eliminates the need for a prosthesis at a later date.

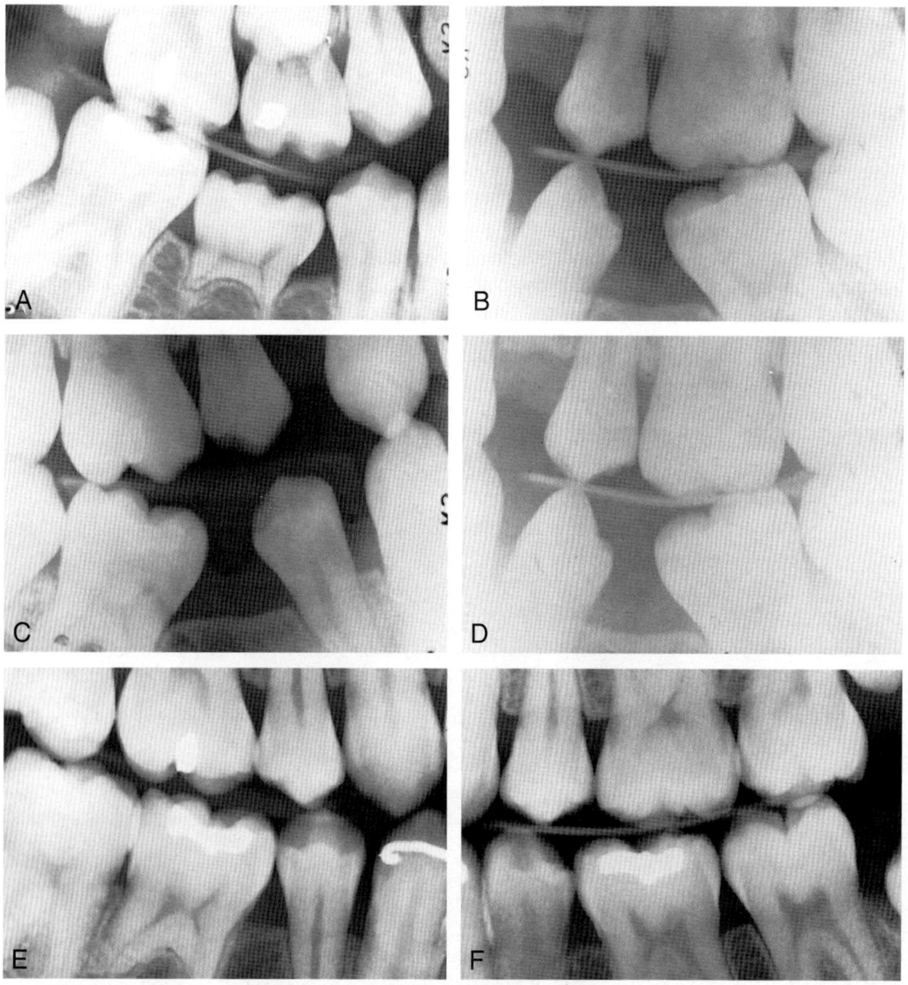

• **Fig. 12.22** (A and B) In this patient with bilaterally missing permanent mandibular second premolars, the decision was made to extract the retained primary molars to allow as much spontaneous drift and space closure as possible before full appliance therapy. (C and D) Although posterior teeth did drift anteriorly and the anterior teeth distally, the space did not completely close. The pattern of drift to close the space of congenitally missing mandibular second premolars is highly variable and unpredictable. (E and F) The residual space was closed and the roots paralleled with full appliances.

incisors are missing, there are two possible sequelae. In some patients, the erupting permanent canine resorbs the primary lateral incisor and spontaneously substitutes for the missing lateral incisor, which means that the primary canine has no successor and is sometimes retained (Fig. 12.23). This is seen occasionally in adults, but most primary canines are lost by the end of adolescence even if they were retained after their successors erupted mesially into the lateral incisor space. Less often, the primary lateral is retained when the permanent canine erupts in its normal position. This usually means the lateral incisor space is reduced to the size of the primary lateral incisor and the remaining primary incisor is unesthetic.

Having the permanent canine erupt in the position of a congenitally missing lateral incisor is advantageous, whether or not the ultimate treatment is substitution of the canine for the lateral or opening space for a prosthetic lateral replacement, because its eruption in that area generates the formation of alveolar bone. In addition, the canine shape and color can be determined, which may have some influence on whether they are retracted and implants placed or substituted for the lateral incisors. Both

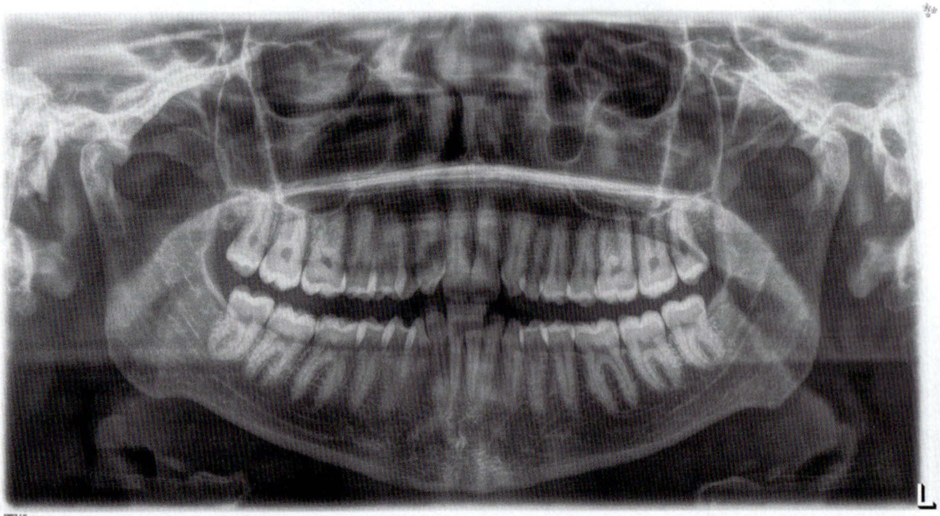

• **Fig. 12.23** Missing permanent maxillary lateral incisors are often replaced spontaneously by permanent canines. This phenomenon occurs without intervention, but the resorption noted on the retained primary canines probably will continue to progress. If implants to eventually replace the missing laterals are planned, it is desirable for the canines to erupt mesially so that alveolar bone forms in the area of the future implant. The canines can be moved into their final position just before the implant surgery. (Courtesy Dr. M. Larson.)

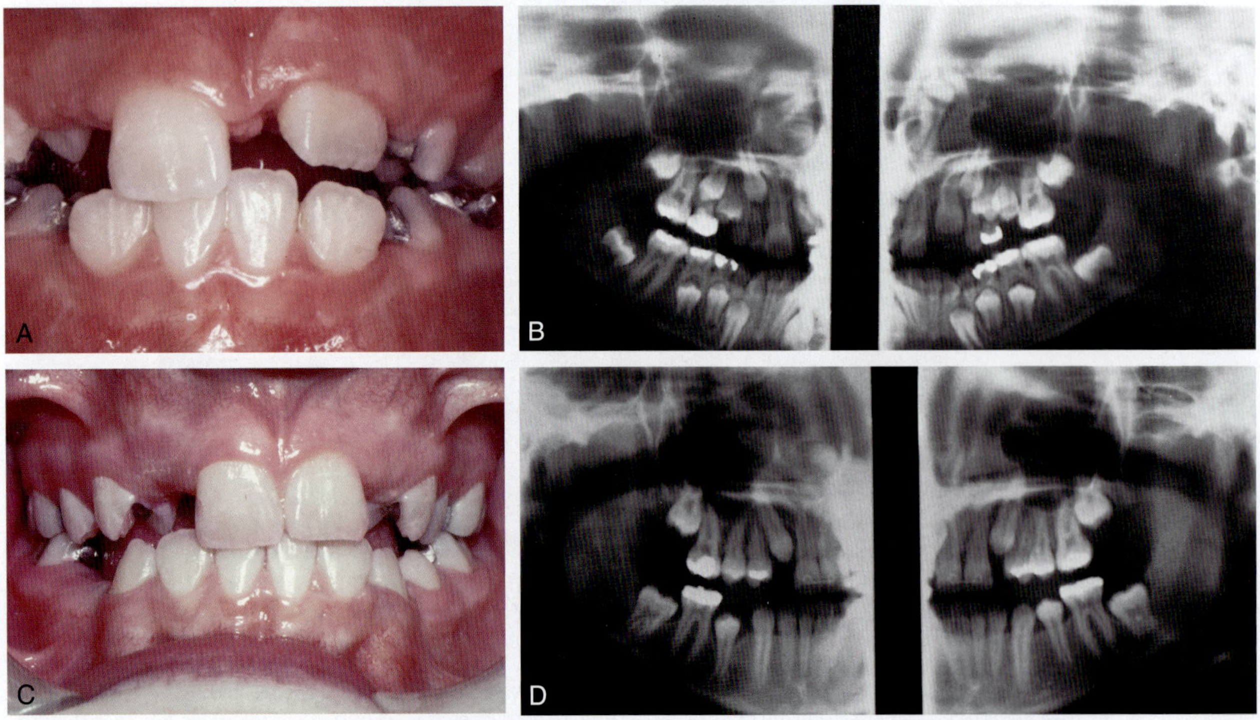

• **Fig. 12.24** When permanent lateral incisors are congenitally missing, often a large diastema develops between the permanent central incisors. (A) This patient has that type of diastema, and the unerupted permanent canines will be substituted for the missing lateral incisors. (B) This radiograph shows the unerupted canines in an excellent position for substitution for the lateral incisors. (C) The diastema has been closed to obtain maximum mesial drift of the canines. (D) This technique enables the canines to erupt closer to their final position and eliminates unnecessary tooth movement during full appliance therapy.

solutions require comprehensive orthodontic treatment in adolescence, and this also is discussed in more detail in Chapter 16.

If space closure is the goal and the primary lateral incisors are replaced by the permanent canines as they erupt, little immediate attention in the mixed dentition is necessary. Sometimes the absence of lateral incisors causes a large diastema to develop between the permanent central incisors. To maximize mesial drift of the erupting permanent canines, this diastema can be closed and retained (Fig. 12.24). Later in the transition to the permanent dentition, the primary canines should be extracted if they are not resorbing, so that some spontaneous closure of the canine space can occur (Fig. 12.25). This space closure option is best when the incisors are slightly protrusive and the molars are tending toward class II in the posterior so that reciprocal space closure can be employed between the anterior and posterior teeth. Space closure is usually avoided when the patients have a class III tendency, because of the possibility of inadvertently creating an anterior crossbite. Once again, TADs can help in these less-than-ideal situations. These are intricacies of comprehensive treatment.

Autotransplantation

In patients with a congenitally missing tooth or teeth lost to TDI, autotransplantation is a possible solution. This is especially indicated if there is crowding in one area and missing teeth in another. Teeth can be transplanted from one position to another in the same mouth, if this is done when the transplanted tooth has approximately two-thirds to three-fourths of its root formed.[29] This means that the decision for autotransplantation must be made during mixed dentition (Fig. 12.26).

Transplantation is most commonly used to move premolars into the location of missing maxillary incisors. For replacement of incisors, especially maxillary lateral incisors, the mandibular

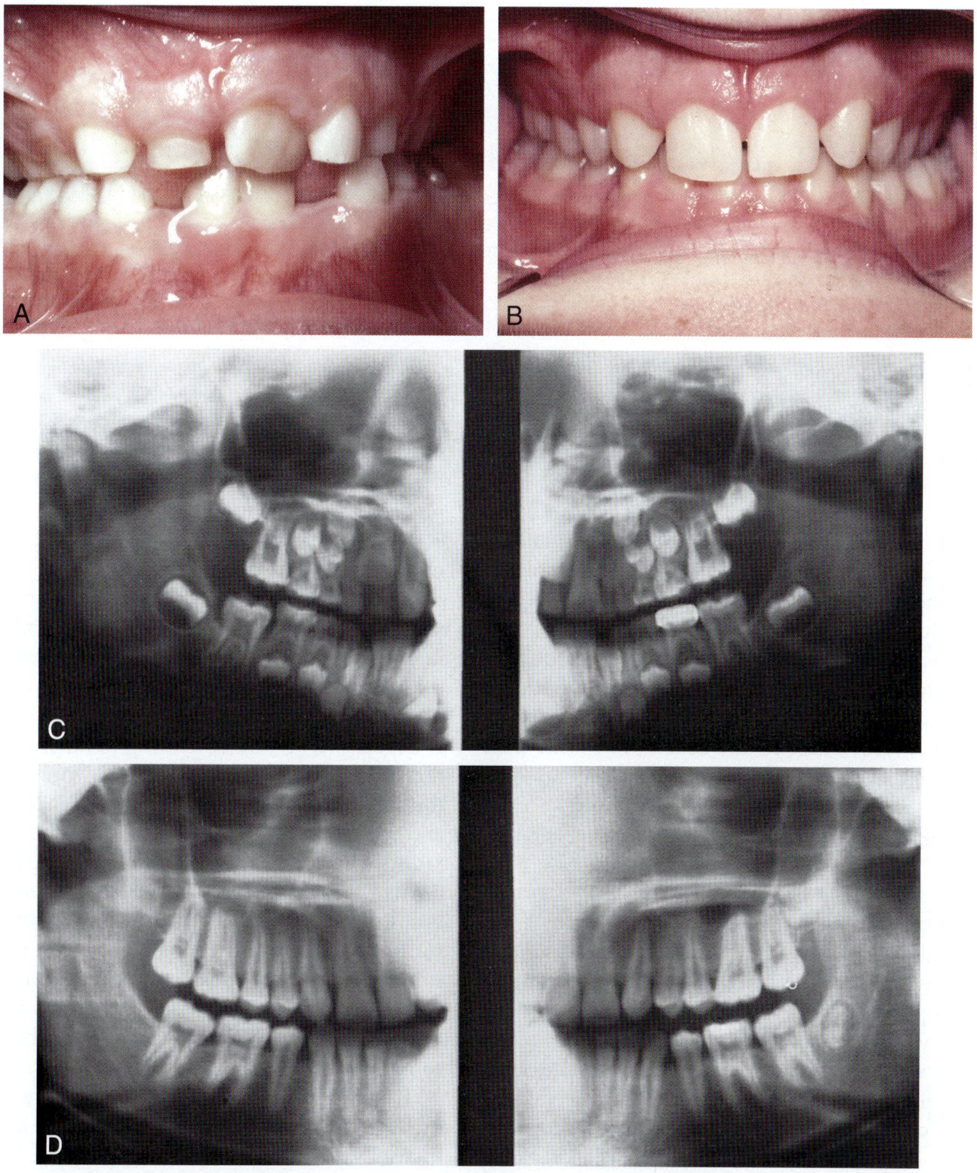

• **Fig. 12.25** Selective removal of primary teeth when permanent maxillary lateral incisors are missing can lead to a shortened second phase of fully banded treatment. (A and B) This patient had primary canines and primary first molars extracted to maximize the mesial drift of the permanent posterior teeth. (C and D) This intervention resulted in good tooth position that will require little fixed appliance therapy to complete.

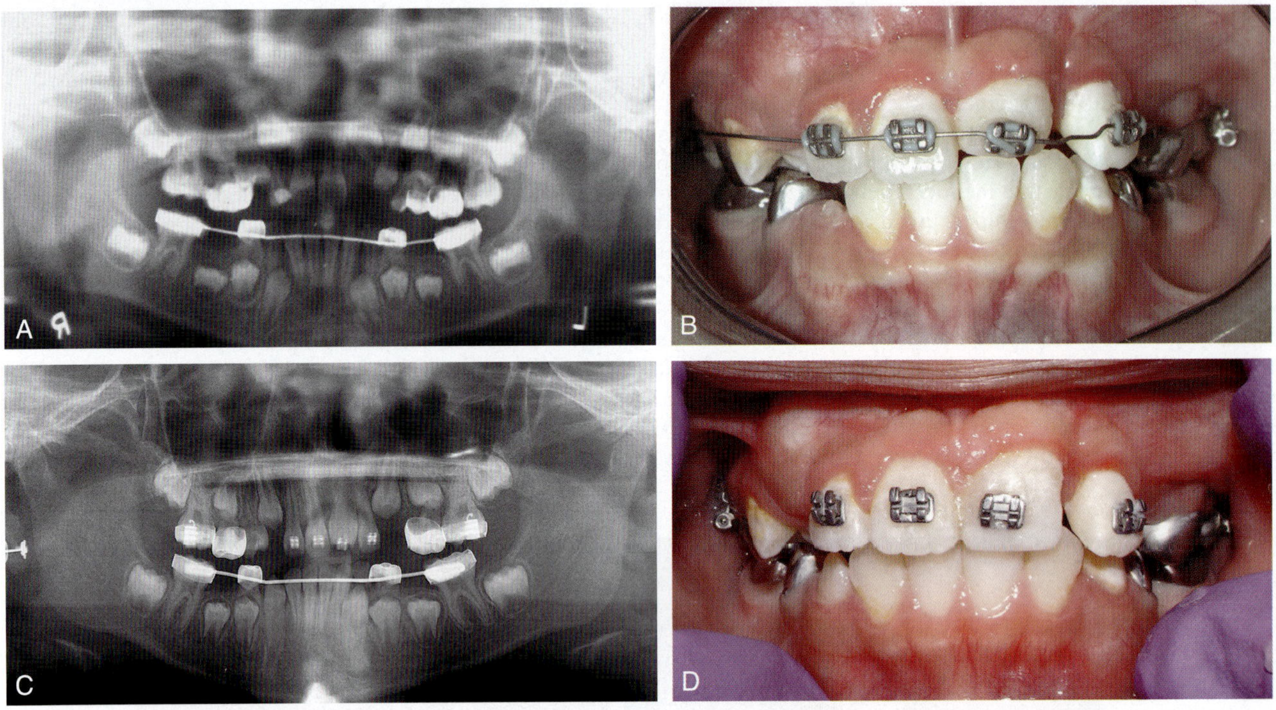

• **Fig. 12.26** (A) This patient has an unerupted permanent maxillary left central incisor with a dilacerated root, possibly due to previous trauma. It was determined that it could not be repositioned surgically or moved orthodontically. (B) To relieve crowding, premolar extraction was indicated, and the maxillary left first premolar was transplanted to the maxillary left central incisor position and moved after a short healing period. (C) Root development and healing have continued and indicate a vital tooth. (D) The tooth will continue to be recontoured and restored with resin before definitive restorative treatment.

first premolar has the best crown and root form and often is preferred if it is available.[30] It is unreasonable to require the extraction of multiple additional teeth, just to transplant mandibular first premolars, since other teeth can suffice if the root morphology (divergent premolar roots) are not a problem. Autotransplantation can also be used to replace missing first molars with third molars, a decision that can be made a little later (Fig. 12.27).[31] A combination of careful surgical intervention and positioning of the transplant, 3 months of healing, followed by light orthodontic forces will achieve final tooth position. Restorative treatment to recontour the crown of the transplanted tooth can result in long-term functional and esthetic success. The success rate with this type of treatment is high (>90%) and predictable.

Localized Moderate-to-Severe Crowding

In some children, there is moderate-to-severe localized crowding (>3 mm). In a posterior quadrant of the dental arches, this is most likely the result of severe space loss after early loss of a primary molar or ectopic eruption. Typically this prevents eruption of a succedaneous tooth, usually a second premolar.

If there is enough space in other areas of the dental arches and no indication that comprehensive orthodontics will be needed in the near future, it is often sensible to extract the impacted tooth and close the space. This typically takes less time than regaining space and encouraging eruption of the impacted tooth or teeth. If space regaining is the goal after careful weighing of the options, the biomechanical issues are sizable and include unilateral space opening without disruption of the rest of the arch or occlusion. Sometimes the space loss may be bilateral. Distal molar movement is often part of the equations for correction of the problem. Reciprocal forces, which are the easiest and most predicable for orthodontics, cannot be employed. These types of treatment are covered later in this chapter under distal molar movement.

In the anterior portion of the arch, the most common localized problem of this type is a shift of the mandibular dental midline. Tooth movement is more often used to solve this problem than simple single tooth extraction. If the midline has moved and no permanent teeth will be extracted, midline correction is needed before the remaining permanent teeth erupt in asymmetric positions and localized crowding becomes worse. If the midline has moved and the space is inadequate, both the space and midline problems need to be addressed before the canines erupt. This is most successfully accomplished by using a supportive lingual arch to maintain molar symmetry and control, bonding of the incisors, and correction of the midline and incisor position with differential length coil springs (Fig. 12.28). In some cases, disking or extraction of a primary canine or molar will be required to provide the necessary room to reestablish the midlines and space. A lingual arch can then be used as a retainer to maintain the correction.

If both mandibular primary canines are lost and the permanent incisors tip lingually, which reduces the arch circumference and increases the apparent crowding, an active lingual arch to tip them facially or a banded and bonded appliance may be indicated. In some of these children, however, space analysis will reveal that the crowding would still be severe enough after the incisors are repositioned to require comprehensive treatment later.

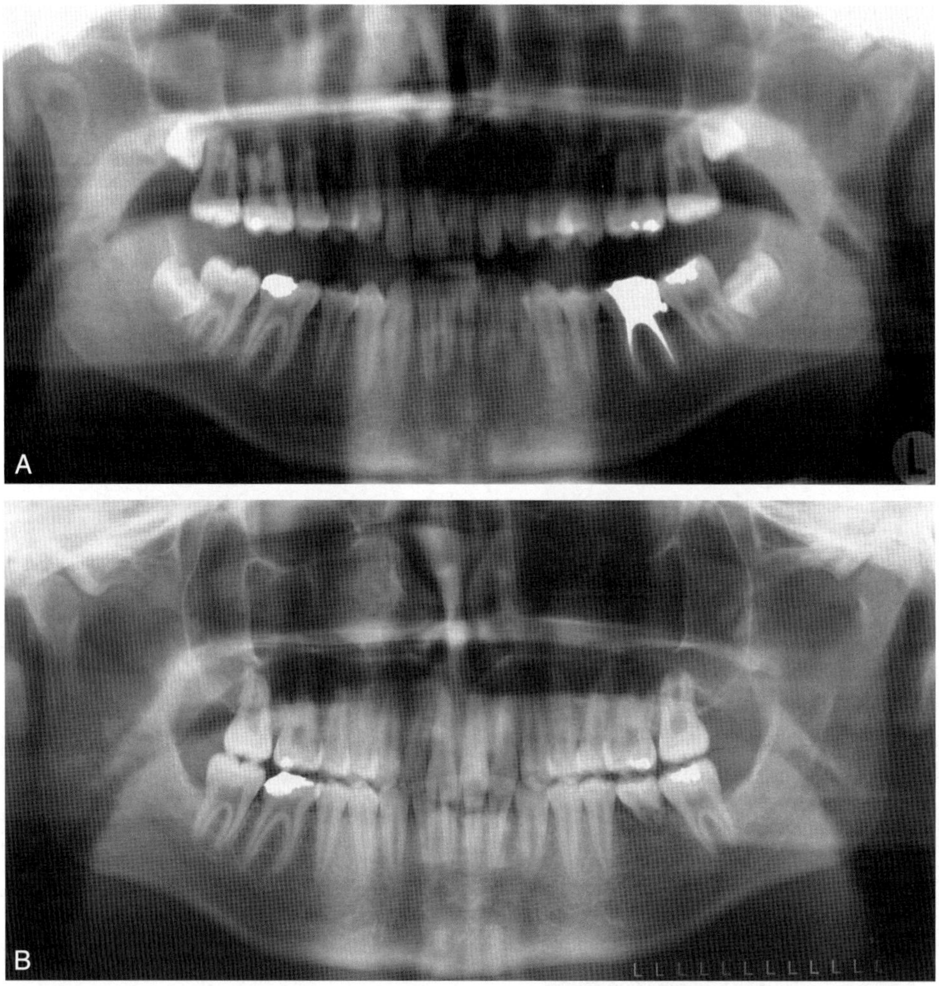

• **Fig. 12.27** (A) The mandibular permanent first molar was restoratively compromised. With the developing third molar in the maxillary left quadrant available (B), it was decided to transplant it into the first molar position when the root development was appropriate, rather than plan a restoration for the first molar. The transplanted third molar was subsequently repositioned during orthodontic treatment and served well as a replacement.

Generalized Moderate and Severe Crowding

Expansion Versus Extraction in Mixed Dentition Treatment

For children with a moderate space deficiency, usually there is generalized but not severe crowding of the incisors, but sometimes the primary canines are lost as the lateral incisors erupt, and the severe crowding that will develop goes largely unrecognized. Children with the largest arch-length discrepancies often have reasonably well-aligned incisors in the early mixed dentition because both primary canines were lost when the lateral incisors erupted.

Potentially severe crowding is usually obvious in primary dentition, even before a space analysis can be completed. These children have little developmental spacing between primary incisors and occasionally some crowding in the primary dentition. The two major symptoms of severe crowding in the early mixed dentition are severe irregularity of the erupting permanent incisors and early loss of primary canines caused by eruption of the permanent lateral incisors. After a definitive analysis of the profile and incisor position, these patients face the same decisions as those with moderate crowding: whether to expand the arches or extract permanent teeth and when this should be done (see Chapter 7 for a review of factors influencing this decision). In the presence of severe crowding, limited mixed dentition treatment will not be sufficient and extraction has to be considered.

Expansion for Treatment of Crowding in the Early Mixed Dentition

For most children with crowding and inadequate space in the early mixed dentition, some facial movement of the incisors and expansion can be accommodated, especially if:

- The lower incisor position is normal or somewhat retrusive.
- Lips are normal or retrusive.
- Overjet is adequate.
- Overbite is not excessive.
- There is good keratinized tissue facial to the lower incisors.

If facial movement is anticipated and the amount and quality of gingival tissue is questionable, a periodontal consultation regarding a gingival graft is appropriate. Surgical or nonsurgical management of the soft tissue may be required before or following tooth movement.

A key question is whether early expansion of the arches (before all permanent teeth erupt) gives more stable results than later

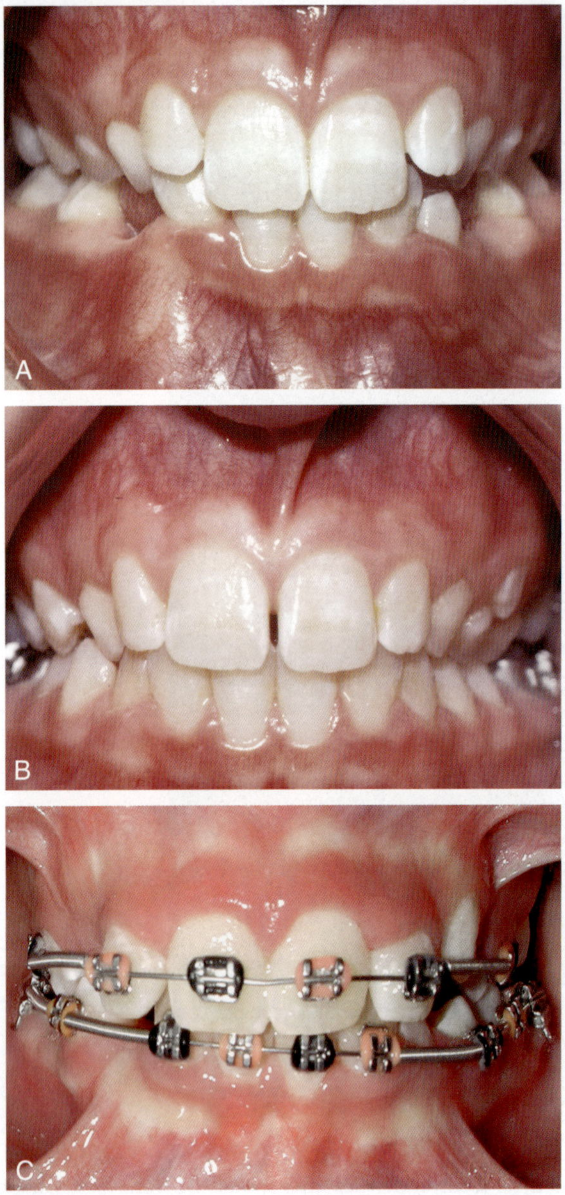

• **Fig. 12.28** Some midline shifts require bodily tooth movement. (A) The midline of the mandibular arch has bodily shifted to the patient's right because of premature loss of a primary canine. (B) The teeth were moved back to their proper position by using a fixed appliance and are supported until eruption of the canines with a lingual holding arch. (C) This type of movement is best achieved with an archwire and coil springs to generate the tooth moving forces. Active coil springs can be replaced with passive coils to gain stability prior to retention.

expansion (in the early permanent dentition). Partly in response to the realization that recurrent crowding occurs in many patients who were treated with premolar extractions (see Chapter 7), early arch expansion has recently gained some popularity in spite of a lack of data to document its effectiveness. This early expansion can involve any combination of several possibilities:

- Maxillary dental or skeletal expansion, moving the teeth facially and/or opening the midpalatal suture
- Mandibular buccal segment expansion by facial movement of the teeth
- Advancement of the incisors and distal movement of the molars in either arch

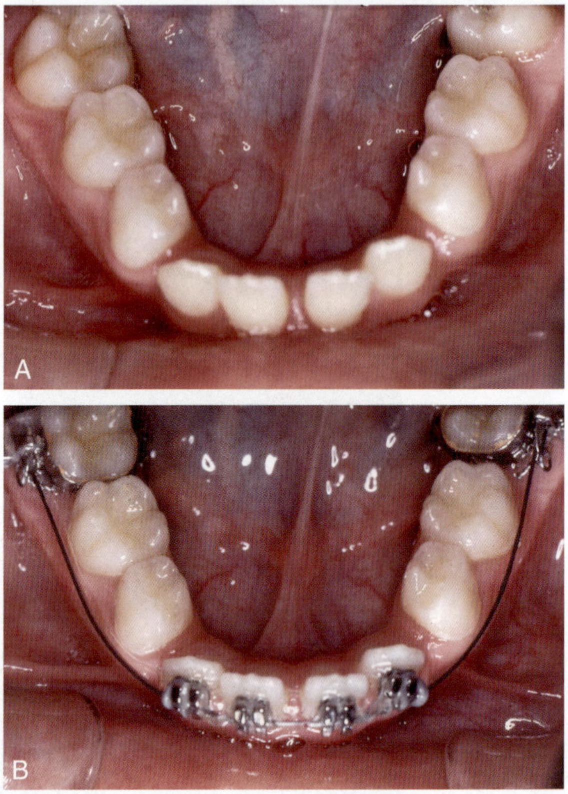

• **Fig. 12.29** (A) In this patient who had lower anterior teeth that were lingually tipped and spaced, lower arch expansion with a fixed appliance was required because the spacing could not be adequately controlled with a lingual arch or lip bumper. (B) The fixed appliance in place during alignment and before space closure in the incisor area. After space closure, the incisors can be further proclined if necessary.

The most aggressive approach to early expansion, in terms of timing, uses maxillary and mandibular lingual arches in the complete primary dentition. This produces an increase in both arch perimeter and width, which must be maintained for variable periods during the mixed dentition years. The ability of expansion in the primary dentition to meet the challenge of anterior crowding is highly questionable and unsubstantiated.[32]

A sensible approach to moderate crowding in the early mixed dentition is to perform a space analysis when the incisors erupt and then begin to work toward arch expansion or extraction with the eruption of the remaining permanent teeth (canines and premolars). Long-term holding of inadequate space is hard on the teeth and soft tissues and is not merited.

To execute the expansion decision, placing a lingual arch after the extraction of the primary canines and ultimately using the lingual arch or another appliance to increase the arch length is a solution. Alternatively, timely extractions can be done.

Clinical experience indicates that a considerable degree of faciolingual irregularity will resolve if space is available, but rotational irregularity will not. If the incisors are rotated, severely irregular, or spaced, and early correction is felt to be important, a fixed appliance will be needed for treatment, either in the mixed or early permanent dentition (Fig. 12.29).

Lower incisor teeth usually can be tipped 1 to 2 mm facially without much difficulty, which creates up to 4 mm of additional arch length, but only if overbite is not excessive and overjet is adequate. To create substantial space and control tooth movement, it is best to band the permanent molars, bond brackets on the incisors, and use

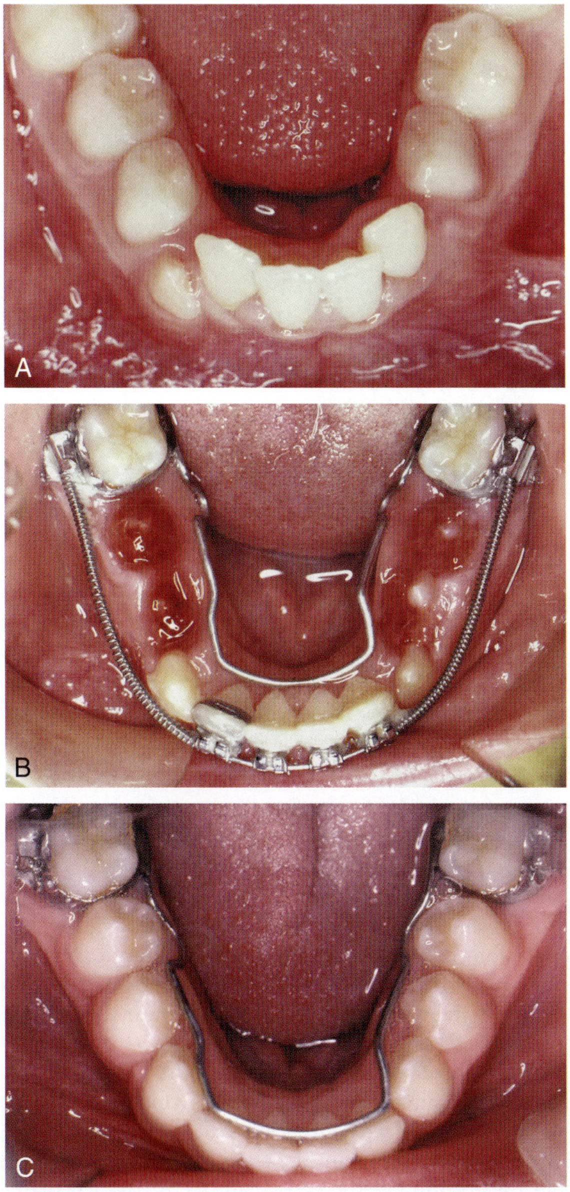

• **Fig. 12.30** Moderate arch-length increases can be accomplished by using a multiple bonded and banded appliance and a mechanism for expansion. (A) This patient has moderate lower arch irregularity and space shortage. (B) The appliance is in place with the tooth movement completed. In this case, coil springs served to generate the tooth moving force, but other methods using loops and flexible archwires are available. Note the lingual arch used to control transverse molar dimensions. (C) The lingual arch is adjusted by opening the loops and advancing the arch so it can serve as a retainer following removal of the archwire and bonded brackets.

a compressed open coil spring on a labial archwire to gain additional space (Fig. 12.30). Alternatively, advanced archwires can be used that tip the incisors facially (see Chapter 11). The multiple band and bond technique is usually followed with a lingual arch for retention. The advantage of the bonded and banded appliance is to provide rotational and mesiodistal space control and bodily movement if necessary. Some expansion of the buccal segments can be included in addition to incisor movement. The long-term stability of these expansion approaches indicates long-term retention is advisable.

A somewhat more aggressive approach is to expand the upper arch transversely in the early mixed dentition, not to correct

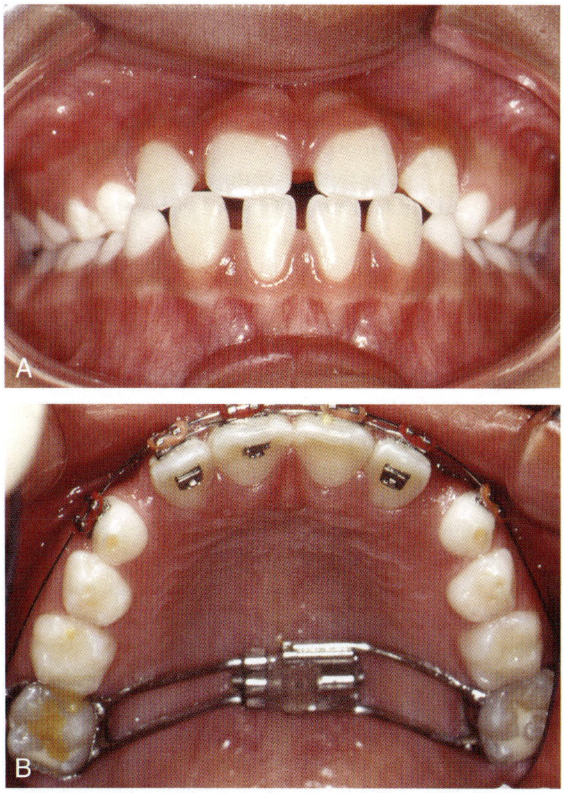

• **Fig. 12.31** (A and B) Some practitioners advocate early expansion by opening the midpalatal suture, usually using a jackscrew-type appliance as in this patient, even in the absence of a posterior crossbite or an apparent arch-length shortage, on the theory that this will improve the long-term stability of arch expansion. Little or no data exist to support this contention.

posterior crossbite but specifically to gain more space in the dental arch. This is accomplished by using a lingual arch or jackscrew expander to produce dental and skeletal changes (Fig. 12.31), but jackscrew expansion must be done carefully and slowly if it is used in early mixed dentition. The theory is that this would ensure more space at a later time.[33] To date, there is no credible long-term post-retention evidence that early intervention to "prepare," "develop," "balance," or expand arches by any other name has any efficacy in providing a less crowded permanent dentition later. Unfortunately, even in children who had mild crowding initially, incisor irregularity can recur soon after early treatment if retention is not managed carefully. Parents and patients should know the issues and uncertainties associated with this type of treatment.

It has been suggested that this type of early expansion not only provides more space and better esthetics, but can also reduce occlusal disharmonies between the arches that are present in Class II malocclusions.[34] Data supporting the long-term effectiveness of this technique are unavailable. It seems unlikely that the soft tissues, which establish the limits for arch expansion, would react quite differently to transverse expansion at different ages (see the discussion of equilibrium influences in Chapter 5) or that jaw growth in other planes of space would be greatly affected by transverse expansion.

Expansion for Crowding in the Late Mixed Dentition: Molar Distalization

Transverse expansion to gain additional space can be used in the late as well as the early mixed dentition, and the previous comments also apply to the late mixed dentition. An additional approach in the late mixed dentition is to obtain additional space by repositioning molars distally. Unless TADs are used, which is not recommended before age 12 because of inadequate bone density, intraoral appliances for distal molar movement will be accompanied by facial incisor movement. With this knowledge, there are some indications for this type of treatment:

- Less than 4 to 5 mm of space per side, with some tipping of the molars acceptable.
- Erupted maxillary anterior teeth and ideally, first premolars for anchorage.
- Normal or retrusive lip and maxillary dental position, because about one-third of the movement will be experienced as facial incisor movement (even with Nance Arch support).
- Likewise, overjet should be limited.
- The vertical facial dimensions should be normal or with a short-face tendency because the distal movement of the molars can open the bite.
- Similarly, the overbite should be somewhat greater than normal owing to the bite opening mechanics.

Until relatively recently, headgear to move maxillary molars distally was the preferred approach. It has the advantage of simplicity and the major disadvantage that good patient compliance is needed. To tip or bodily move molars distally, extraoral force via a facebow to the molars is a straightforward method. The force is directed specifically to the teeth that need to be moved, and reciprocal forces are not distributed on the other teeth (the incisors) that are in the correct positions. The force should be as nearly constant as possible to provide effective tooth movement and should be moderate because it is concentrated against only two teeth. The more the child wears the headgear, the better; 12 to 14 h/day is minimal. Approximately 400 g of force per side is appropriate but not particularly friendly to the teeth. The teeth should move at the rate of 1 mm/month, so a cooperative child would need to wear the appliance for 3 to 5 months to obtain the 3 mm of correction that would be a typical requirement in this type of treatment with good cooperation (see Chapter 14 for headgear management details)

For the short-term duration of this type of treatment, either cervical or high-pull headgear can be chosen, but high-pull headgear is an excellent option (Fig. 12.32). Baumrind et al. reported that this approach is particularly effective in producing distal molar movement.[35]

When bodily distal movement of one or both permanent maxillary first molars is needed to adjust molar relationships and gain space there are several other options. There must be adequate anterior teeth for anchorage—tolerance for some anterior incisor movement and adequate overbite. All are built around the use of a heavy lingual arch, usually with a Nance acrylic pad against the anterior palate to provide anchorage (Fig. 12.33). Often, the anterior teeth also are bonded and stabilized with an archwire. The force can be generated by coil springs on a segmental wire or a stopped superelastic long wire. Often a palate-covering appliance (incorporating a Nance-type button) using either helical springs (the pendulum appliance) or a steel or superelastic coil springs (distal jet) is used.[36]

In the mandibular arch, appliances that change arch dimensions (not passive lingual holding arches to hold the dimensions) can cause problems with lower second molar eruption.[37] Erupted upper second molars make distalization of the first molars even more difficult, and use of a fixed appliance to bring the lower incisors forward may be more acceptable if there is available overjet and adequate keratinized facial tissue (Fig. 12.34).

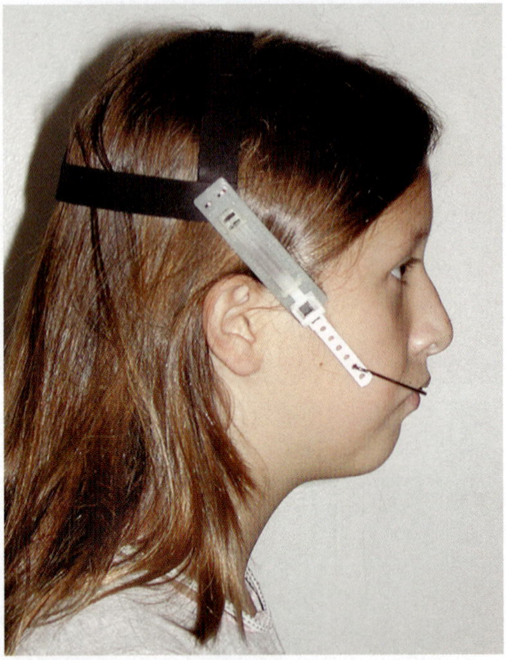

• **Fig. 12.32** A high-pull headgear has been demonstrated to be the most effective extraoral appliance to move molars distally. Of course, compliance is required, but no reciprocal incisor protrusion occurs.

The primary method now for distalization of molars, which can be used with children 12 years of age and older, is the use of TAD-supported molar-distalizing appliances (Fig. 12.35).[38] These appliances can distalize molars in both arches without creating forward movement of the incisors because of the nearly absolute anchorage, but the TADs can tip anteriorly without consequence. It is more likely that TADs placed in the palate lingual or lingual and slightly distal to the first premolars and near the midline will be more stable.[39]

There are three major limitations to this approach: (1) the surgery to place and remove the TADs, which is quite acceptable to patients can have complications, (2) the long duration of treatment to move and retain the teeth from the mixed dentition through the eruption of the permanent teeth, and (3) the uncertain stability of the long-term result. The question is not whether the tooth movement is possible—it is. Rather, the question is the wisdom of major expansion of the arches or distal movement, especially in the mixed dentition.

No matter how molars were moved distally, if the time before eruption of the premolars will be longer than a few months, it will be necessary to hold them back after they are repositioned. Maxillary and mandibular lingual arch space maintainers (see Fig. 11.58) are the best insurance to guard against space loss. Remember, too, that this new posterior molar position has to be maintained if incisors are to be retracted. This is a difficult task without TADs to reinforce the anchorage, most likely palatal TADs in the maxilla.

Early (Serial) Extraction

In many children with severe crowding, a decision can be made during the early mixed dentition period that expansion is not advisable and that some permanent teeth will have to be extracted to make room for the others. A planned sequence of tooth removal can reduce crowding and irregularity during the transition from

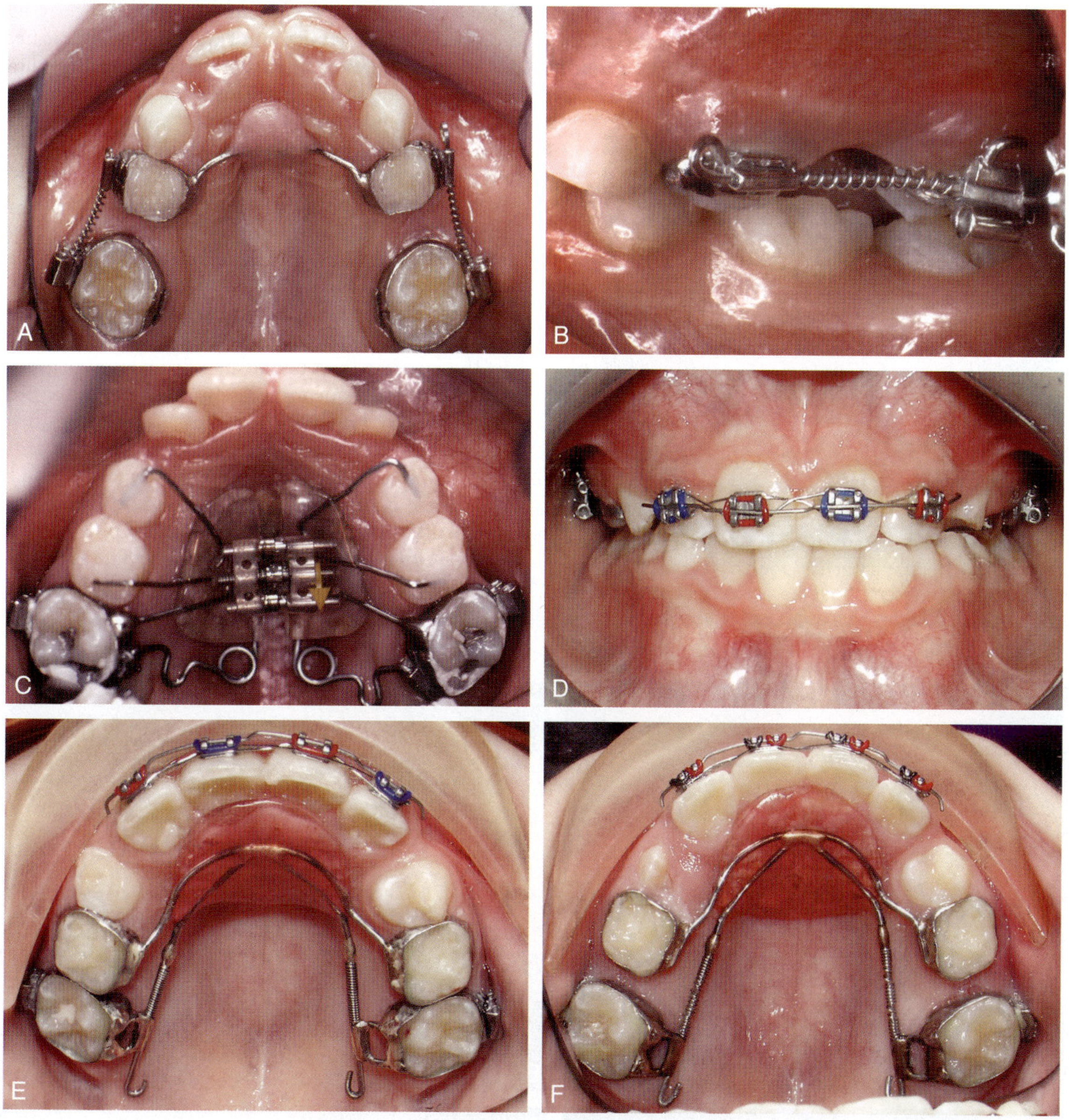

• **Fig. 12.33** Several approaches can be taken to increasing arch circumference by distalizing molars, if the correct diagnosis is made and the incisor protrusion that usually results can be accepted. (A and B) Bilateral coil springs provide the force that is resisted by the anchorage of the primary molars and the palate using a Nance arch. (C) Alternatively, a pendulum appliance can be used that also gains anchorage from the palate but uses helical springs to supply the force. (D–F) This fixed appliance also uses palatal and dental anchorage and nickel-titanium (NiTi) coil springs to slide the molars along heavy lingual wires. Once placed, the appliance can be monitored until the desired tooth movement is achieved and then it can be modified to serve as a retainer. (A–C, Courtesy Dr. M. Mayhew.)

the primary to the permanent dentition.[40] It will also allow the teeth to erupt over the alveolus and through keratinized tissue, rather than being displaced buccally or lingually. This sequence, often termed *serial extraction*, simply involves the timed extraction of primary and, ultimately, permanent teeth to relieve severe crowding. It was advocated originally as a method to treat severe crowding without or with only minimal use of appliance therapy. Now it is viewed as an adjunct to later comprehensive treatment instead of a substitute for it.

Although serial extraction makes later comprehensive treatment easier and often quicker, by itself it almost never results in ideal tooth position or closure of excess space. Serial extraction is directed toward severe dental crowding. For this reason, it is best used when no skeletal problem exists and the space discrepancy is large—greater than 10 mm/arch. If the crowding is severe, little space will remain after the teeth are aligned, which means there will be little tipping and uncontrolled movement of the adjacent teeth into the extraction sites. If the initial space discrepancy is smaller, more residual space must be anticipated. Although it is possible to use serial extraction to compensate for minor and moderate skeletal Class II and Class III problems (with a usual extraction sequence of only upper teeth in Class II and only lower teeth in Class III problems),[40] this type of treatment is much more complex. The residual space closure probably needs to be selectively directional (i.e., all from the front or all from the back) and requires a much better command of biomechanics than most nonspecialists have.

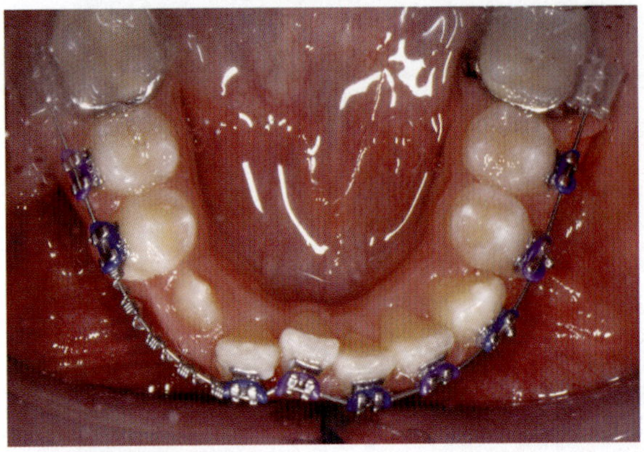

• **Fig. 12.34** For mixed dentition treatment of significant lower crowding and irregularity, banded and bonded attachments and an archwire provide the most efficient approach. This patient has crowding and irregularity that indicates fixed appliance treatment. Note the use of a superelastic coil spring to create space for the erupting mandibular right canine.

Serial extraction treatment begins in the early mixed dentition period with extraction of primary incisors if necessary, followed by extraction of the primary canines to allow eruption and alignment of the permanent incisors (Fig. 12.36). As the permanent teeth align without any appliances in place, there is usually some lingual tipping of the lower incisors, and overbite often increases during this stage. Labiolingual displacements resolve better than rotational irregularity. After extraction of the primary canines, crowding problems are usually under control for 1 to 2 years, but foresight is necessary. The goal is to influence the permanent first premolars to erupt ahead of the canines so that they can be extracted and the canines can erupt and move distally into this space.

The maxillary first premolars usually erupt before the canines, so the eruption sequence is rarely a problem in the upper arch. In the lower arch, however, the canines usually erupt before the first premolars, which causes the canines to be displaced facially. To avoid this result, the primary lower first molar should be extracted when there is one-half to two-thirds root formation of the first premolar. This will usually speed up the premolar eruption and cause it to enter the arch before the canine (Fig. 12.36C). The result is easy access for extraction of the first premolar before the canine erupts (Fig. 12.36D).

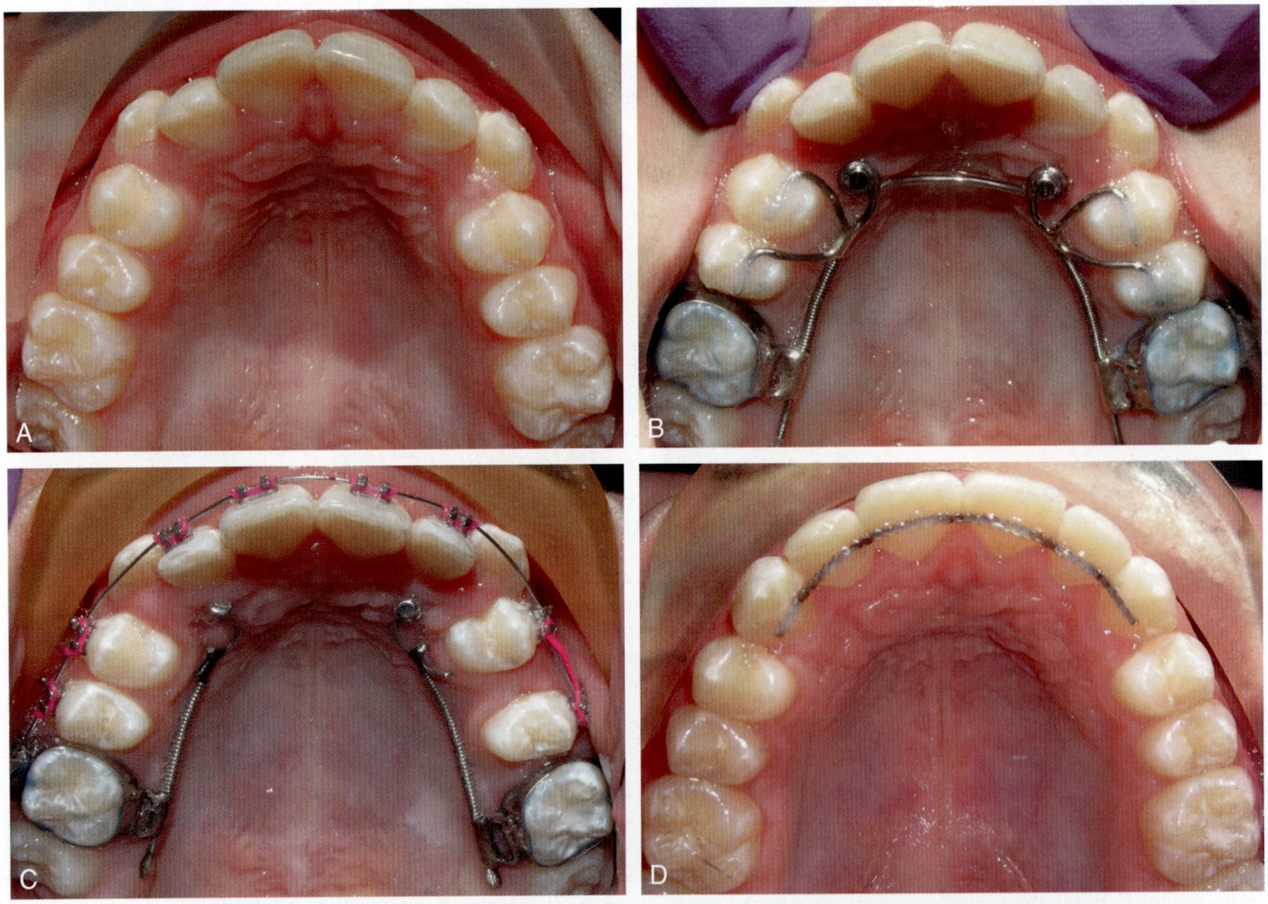

• **Fig. 12.35** (A) This patient had temporary anchorage device (TAD)-supported molar distalization in the late mixed dentition to accommodate the initial crowding and a nonextraction treatment plan. This is not recommended for patients much younger than 12 years because of inadequate bone density and resulting TAD instability. (B) The wire framework supports the TADs in the anterior palate with the distal force provided by the coil springs. No anchorage is provided by the anterior teeth. (C) Good tooth movement with intact TADs at the end of active distalization, even with the second molars erupted. (D) The final arch in retention.

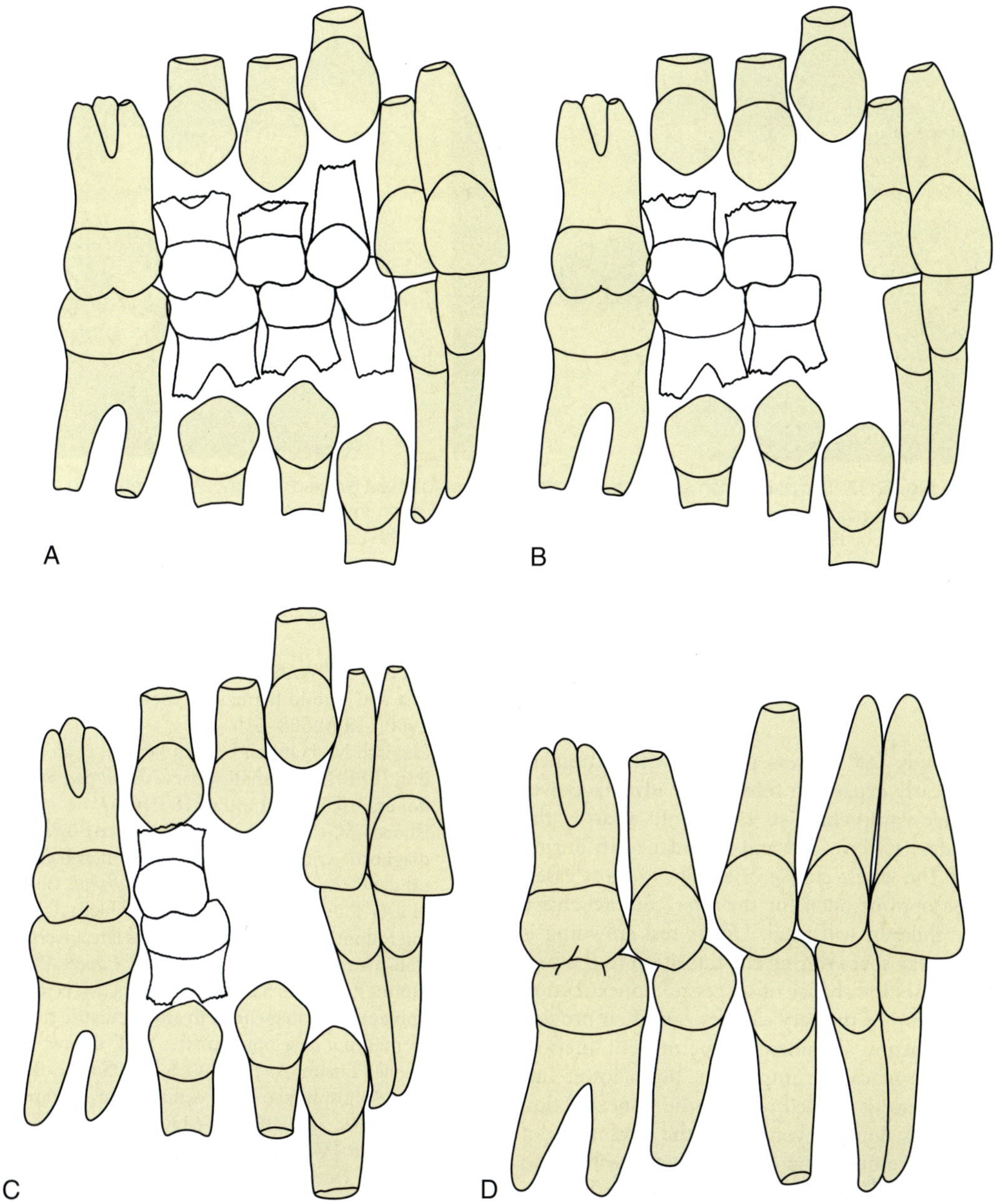

• **Fig. 12.36** Serial extraction is used to relieve severe arch-length discrepancies. (A) The initial diagnosis is made when a severe space deficiency is documented and there is marked incisor crowding. (B) The primary canines are extracted to provide space for alignment of the incisors. (C) The primary first molars are extracted when one-half to two-thirds of the first premolar root is formed, to speed eruption of the first premolars. (D) When the first premolars have erupted they are extracted and the canines erupt into the remaining extraction space. The residual space is closed by drifting and tipping of the posterior teeth unless full appliance therapy is implemented.

A complication can occur if the primary first molar is extracted early and the first premolar still does not erupt before the canine. This can lead to impaction of the premolar that requires later surgical removal. When the primary first molar is being removed, it may be obvious that the canine will erupt before the premolar. In this case the underlying premolar can also be extracted at the same time—a procedure termed *enucleation*. If possible, however, enucleation should be avoided because the erupting premolar brings alveolar bone with it. Early enucleation can leave a bone defect that persists.

After the first premolar has been extracted, the second primary molars should exfoliate normally. The premolar extraction spaces close partially by mesial drift of the second premolars and permanent first molars but largely by distal eruption of the canines. If serial extraction is not followed by mechanotherapy, ideal alignment, root positioning, correct rather than deep overbite, and space closure usually are not achieved (Fig. 12.37).

Serial extraction was used much more frequently 25 to 30 years ago than now. It was overused then and perhaps is underused now. It can be a useful adjunct to treatment, shortening the time of comprehensive treatment if it is used correctly, but the patients must be chosen and supervised carefully as they develop. It is far from a panacea for treatment of crowding.

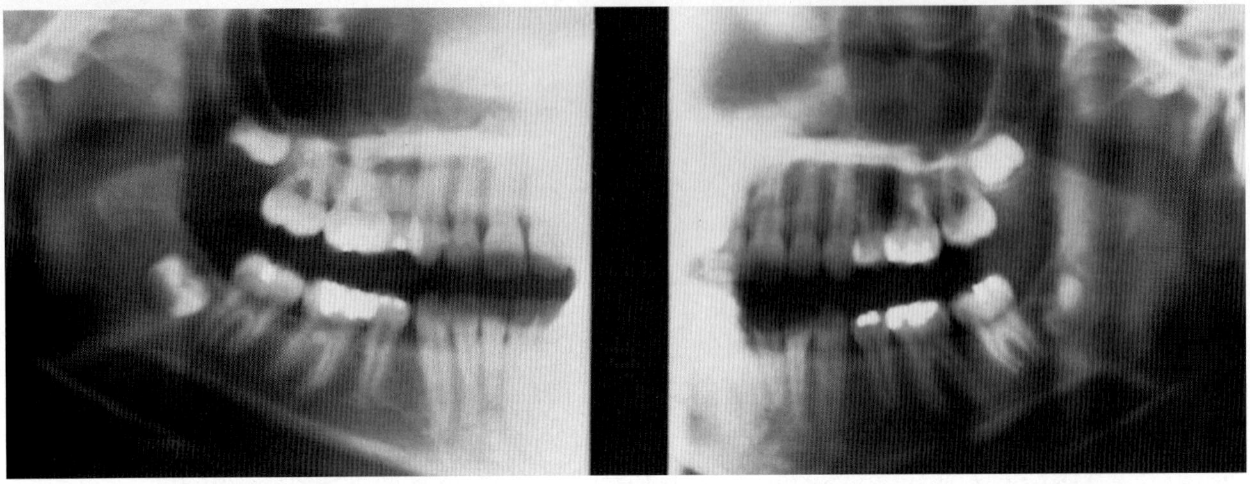

• **Fig. 12.37** This patient had serial extraction that was not followed by fixed appliance treatment, with an excellent result. Properly timed serial extraction usually results in incomplete space closure. Teeth drift together by tipping, which results in nonparallel roots between the canine and second premolar. Lack of root parallelism, residual space, and other irregularities can be addressed with subsequent fixed appliance therapy.

The Borderline Crowding Case: What Do You Do?

If early extraction is only for the few patients with extremely severe crowding, and early expansion offers little advantage over expansion during later comprehensive treatment, what is the best approach to moderately crowded and irregular teeth during the mixed dentition? The wisest course of action, in most cases, is simply to keep the options open for the later comprehensive treatment that these children will need. Unless real crowding is severe, maintaining leeway space during the transition to the permanent dentition increases the chance of successful nonextraction treatment. Early extraction of primary canines can often provide space for some spontaneous alignment of permanent incisors and decrease the chance of canine impaction, but a lower lingual arch to maintain space is needed to keep the nonextraction option open when this is done. Beyond that, the advantages of early appliance therapy are questionable and must be viewed in the context of an increased burden of treatment versus little or no additional benefit.

References

1. Papadopoulos MA, Chatzoudi M, Kaklamanos EG. Prevalence of tooth transposition. A meta-analysis. *Angle Orthod*. 2010;80: 275–285.
2. Garib DG, Peck S, Gomes SC. Increased occurrence of dental anomalies associated with second-premolar agenesis. *Angle Orthod*. 2009;79:436–441.
3. Peck S, Peck L. Classification of maxillary tooth transpositions. *Am J Orthod Dent Orthop*. 1995;107:505–517.
4. Frazier-Bowers SA, Simmons D, Wright JT, et al. Primary failure of eruption and PTH1R: the importance of a genetic diagnosis for orthodontic treatment planning. *Am J Orthod Dentofacial Orthop*. 2010;137:160.e1–160.e7. discussion 160-1.
5. Pilz P, Meyer-Marcotty P, Eigenthaler M, Roth H, Weber BHF, Stellzig- EA. Differential diagnosis of primary failure of eruption (PFE) with and without evidence of pathogenic mutations in the PTHR1 gene. *J Orofac Orthop*. 2014;75:226–239.
6. Baccetti T. Tooth anomalies associated with failure of eruption of first and second permanent molars. *Am J Orthod Dentofac Orthop*. 2000;118(6):608–610.
7. Hanisch M, Hanisch L, Kleinheinz J, et al. Primary failure of eruption (PFE): a systematic review. *Head Face Med*. 2018;14:5. https://doi.org/10.1186/s13005-018-0163-7.
8. Rhoads SG, Hendricks HM, Frazier-Bowers SA. Establishing the diagnostic criteria for eruption disorders based on genetic and clinical data. *Am J Orthod Dentofacial Orthop*. 2013;144:194–202.
9. Hölttä P, Alaluusua S, Saarinen-Pihkala UM, et al. Agenesis and microdontia of permanent teeth as late adverse effects after stem cell transplantation in young children. *Cancer*. 2005;103:181–190.
10. Hölttä P, Hovi L, Saarinen-Pihkala UM, et al. Disturbed root development of permanent teeth after pediatric stem cell transplantation. Dental root development after SCT. *Cancer*. 2005;103:1484–1493.
11. Iglesias-Linares A, Yáñez-Vico RM, Solano-Reina E, et al. Influence of bisphosphonates in orthodontic therapy: systematic review. *J Dent Res*. 2010;38:603–611.
12. Hellstein JW, Adler RA, Edwards B, et al. Managing the care of patients receiving antiresorptive therapy for prevention and treatment of osteoporosis. Recommendations from the American Dental Association Council on Scientific Affairs. *J Am Dent Assoc*. 2011;142:1243–1251.
13. International Association of Dental Traumatology. *The Dental Trauma Guide* https://dentaltraumaguide.org/.
14. Kindelan SA, Day PF, Kindelan JD, et al. Dental trauma: an overview of its influence on the management of orthodontic treatment; part 1. *J Orthod*. 2008;35:68–78.
15. Brin I, Ben-Bassat Y, Heling I, Engelberg A. The influence of orthodontic treatment on previously traumatized permanent incisors. *Eur J Orthod*. 1991;13:372–377.
16. Bauss O, Röhling J, Meyer K, Kiliaridis S. Pulp vitality in teeth suffering trauma during orthodontic therapy. *Angle Orthod*. 2009;79:166–171.
17. Bauss O, Röhling J, Rahman A, Kiliaridis S. The effect of pulp obliteration on pulpal vitality of orthodontically intruded traumatized teeth. *J Endodont*. 2008;34:417–420.
18. Diangelis AJ, Andreasen JO, Ebeleseder KA, et al. International Association of Dental Traumatology guidelines for the management of traumatic dental injuries: 1. Fractures and luxations of permanent teeth. *Dent Traumatol*. 2012;28:2–12.

19. Tsilingaridis G, Malmgren B, Andreasen JO, et al. Scandinavian multicenter study on the treatment of 168 patients with 230 intruded permanent teeth—a retrospective cohort study. *Dent Traumatol.* 2016;32:353–360.
20. Esteves T, Ramos AL, Pereira CM, Hidalgo MM. Orthodontic root resorption of endodontically treated teeth. *J Endodont.* 2007;33:119–122.
21. Bauss O, Röhling J, Sadat-Khonsari R, Kiliaridis S. Influence of orthodontic intrusion on pulpal vitality of previously traumatized maxillary permanent incisors. *Am J Orthod Dentofac Orthop.* 2008;134:12–17.
22. Malmgren B, Tsilingaridis G, Malmgren O. Long-term follow up of 103 ankylosed permanent incisors surgically treated with decoronation—a retrospective cohort study. *Dent Traumatol.* 2015;31:184–189.
23. Little R, Riedel R. Postretention evaluation of stability and relapse—mandibular arches with generalized spacing. *Am J Orthod.* 1989;95:37–41.
24. Bauss O, Freitag S, Rohling J, Rahman A. Influence of overjet and lip coverage on the prevalence and severity of incisor trauma. *J Orofac Orthop.* 2008;69:402–410.
25. Goettems ML, Brancher LC, da Coasta CT, et al. Does dental trauma in the primary dentition increases the likelihood of trauma in the permanent dentition? A longitudinal study. *Clin Oral Investig.* 2017;21:2415–2420.
26. Glendor U, Koucheki B, Halling A. Risk evaluation and type of treatment of multiple dental trauma episodes to permanent teeth. *Endod Dent Traumatol.* 2000;16:205–210.
27. Thiruvenkatachari B, Harrison JE, Worthington HV, O'Brien KD. Orthodontic treatment for prominent upper front teeth (Class II malocclusion) in children. *Cochrane Database Syst Rev.* 2013;(11):Art. No. CD003452.
28. Huang B. *Determinants of Traumatic Dental Injuries in Fifteen-to-eighteen Year Old Students in Taiwan. Diss.* University of London; 2004.
29. Paulsen HU, Andreasen JO, Schwartz O. Tooth loss treatment in the anterior region: autotransplantation of premolars and cryopreservation. *World J Orthod.* 2006;7:27–34.
30. Zachrisson BU, Stenvik A, Haanaes HR. Management of missing maxillary anterior teeth with emphasis on autotransplantation. *Am J Orthod Dent Orthop.* 2004;126:284–288.
31. Bauss O, Sadat-Khonsari R, Engelke W, Kahl-Nieke B. Results of transplanting developing third molars as part of orthodontics space management. Part 2: results following the orthodontic treatment of transplanted developing third molars in cases of aplasia and premature loss of teeth with atrophy of the alveolar process. *J Orofac Orthop.* 2003;64:40–47.
32. Lutz HD, Poulton D. Stability of dental arch expansion in the deciduous dentition. *Angle Orthod.* 1985;55:299–315.
33. O'Grady PW, McNamara Jr JA, Baccetti T, Franchi LA. Long-term evaluation of the mandibular Schwarz appliance and the acrylic splint expander in early mixed dentition patients. *Am J Orthod Dentofac Orthop.* 2006;130:202–213.
34. McNamara Jr JA, Sigler LM, Franchi L, et al. Changes in occlusal relationships in mixed dentition patients treated with rapid maxillary expansion. A prospective clinical study. *Angle Orthod.* 2010;80:230–238.
35. Baumrind S, Korn EL, Isaacson RJ, et al. Quantitative analysis of orthodontic and orthopedic effects of maxillary traction. *Am J Orthod.* 1983;84:384–398.
36. Fontana M, Cozzani M, Caprioglio A. Non-compliance maxillary molar distalizing appliances: an overview of the last decade. *Prog Orthod.* 2012;13:173–184.
37. Rubin RL, Baccetti T, McNamara Jr. JA. Mandibular second molar eruption difficulties related to the maintenance of arch perimeter in the mixed dentition. *Am J Orthod Dentofacial Orthop.* 2012;141:146–152.
38. Grec RH, Janson G, Branco NC, et al. Intraoral distalizer effects with conventional and skeletal anchorage: a meta-analysis. *Am J Orthod Dentofac Orthop.* 2013;143:602–615.
39. Wilmes B, Ludwig B, Vasudavan S, Nienkemper M, Drescher D. The T-Zone: Median vs. Paramedian Insertion of Palatal Mini-Implants. *J Clin Orthod.* 2016 Sep;50(9):543–551. PMID: 27809213.
40. Hotz RP. Guidance of eruption versus serial extraction. *Am J Orthod.* 1970;58:1–20.

SECTION 5

Growth Modification

If it were possible, the best way to correct a jaw discrepancy would be to get the patient to grow out of it. That requires inducing differential growth of one jaw relative to the other, either stimulating one to grow faster or restraining it so the other jaw can catch up. Because the pattern of facial growth is established early in life and rarely changes significantly (see Chapter 2), this is unlikely without treatment.

Three important principles must be kept in mind when growth modification is considered for a preadolescent or adolescent child: (1) if you start growth modification too late, it doesn't work, but if you start too soon, treatment is extremely long because it requires long active retention until growth is nearly complete; (2) growth occurs on a different timetable for the three planes of space; and (3) children's compliance with treatment is affected by both their stage of maturation and the difficulty in doing what the doctor wants.

Timing in Relation to the Amount of Growth Remaining

This section of the book appropriately fits between the discussion of treatment for preadolescent children and adolescents, because some growth modification procedures must be done before adolescence whereas others are much more effective and efficient if done in adolescents. Whatever the type of appliance that is used or the kind of growth effect that is desired, if growth is to be modified, the patient must be growing. That means growth modification has to be done before the adolescent growth spurt ends. In theory, it could be done at any point up to that time.

Because of the rapid growth exhibited by children during the primary dentition years, one might think that treatment of jaw discrepancies by growth modification should be successful at a very early age. The rationale for very early treatment at ages 4 to 6 would be that because of the rapid rate of growth and the smaller and more plastic skeletal components, significant amounts of skeletal discrepancy could be overcome in a short time. This has been tested and does occur. The further rationale is that once discrepancies in jaw relationships have been corrected, proper function will cause harmonious growth thereafter without further treatment.

If this were the case, very early treatment in the primary dentition would be indicated for many skeletal discrepancies. Unfortunately, that is not correct. Although most anteroposterior and vertical jaw discrepancies can be corrected during the primary dentition years, relapse occurs because of continued growth in the original disproportionate pattern. If children are treated very early, they will need further treatment during the mixed dentition and again in the early permanent dentition periods to maintain the correction. For all practical purposes, early orthodontic treatment for skeletal problems now is restricted to the mixed dentition years, with a second phase of treatment required during adolescence.

The opposite point of view would be that because treatment in the permanent dentition will be required anyway, there is no point in starting treatment until then. Delaying treatment that long has two potential problems: (1) by the time the canines, premolars, and second molars erupt, there may not be enough growth remaining for effective modification, especially in girls, and (2) some children who would benefit from early treatment would be denied the psychosocial and trauma reduction benefits of treatment during an important period of development.

This particularly applies to children with a skeletal class II problem, which—as we will discuss in detail later—is otherwise better delayed until the adolescent growth spurt. Some of these children suffer from the psychosocial impact of ridicule or bullying because of their dentofacial appearance. This is most often associated with maxillary skeletal or dental protrusion many times including dental spacing. This is an indication for early intervention. Another indication for preadolescent class II treatment is a dental and skeletal profile highly susceptible to trauma, such as increased overjet, incompetent lips, and protrusive incisors that often accompany class

II relationships. The data are clear that these individuals encounter more dental trauma (see Chapter 1 and Fig. 1.18). The type and extent of trauma are highly variable. It makes the most sense to treat the psychosocially susceptible and trauma-prone class II children (those who experienced trauma to the incisors before 9 years of age) by only retracting the protruding incisors instead of performing early growth modification, which would be more productive and stable during the growth spurt. More generally, for each patient the benefits of early treatment must be considered against the risk and cost of prolonging the total treatment period.

Different Timing for Different Planes of Space

The timing of maturation and the potential to effect a change in the different facial planes of space are not uniform. Maxillary growth in the transverse plane of space, the first to cease growing, stops when the first bridging of the midpalatal suture begins, not at final complete fusion. This means that for most children, palatal width increases would normally end by mid adolescence, and to alter this later with appliance therapy would require heavier force to open the midpalatal suture. Transverse maxillary expansion is therefore more physiologic if done before adolescence.

Anteroposterior facial growth is most obvious in class II and III malocclusions as the maxilla and mandible both move forward. For class III maxillary deficiencies, skeletal protraction by stretching the open facial sutures using the dentition as anchorage is easiest before age 11, but with TAD-supported skeletal anchorage it is also possible during adolescence. Using skeletal plates and intraoral elastics provides even some later options. In the mandible, compressive forces against the condyle have not demonstrated long-term potential to restrict growth. But compressive force at the sutures above and behind the maxilla during adolescence can redirect and restrain maxillary growth while the mandible grows forward. It also means that anteroposterior growth modification treatment must be continued until growth is essentially complete, to prevent uncontrolled late growth from ruining retention of what was thought to be completed treatment.

Vertical facial growth is the last to stop. It often continues into the late teens in girls and early 20s in boys, and prolonged retention is needed for both long- and short-face patients. Recurrence of deep overbite can be controlled relatively easily, but starting early requires prolonged retention. Excessive vertical growth is difficult to control, and early attempts to do this would have to extend for inordinately long periods to outlast growth.

So, different timing for different problems is important. Palatal expansion and maxillary protraction are seemingly more urgent in earlier years, anteroposterior mandibular growth modification is more a midgrowth activity, and vertical control requires a later approach if it can be accomplished.

Because of the limited magnitude and control of growth modification, tooth movement always accompanies growth modification. This really means that growth modification as skeletal structures is modest and includes a form of camouflage from tooth movement as well.

Timing in Relation to Patient Compliance

Patient compliance is affected by both the patient's relative maturity and the burden of treatment from the patient's perspective. Timing of treatment interventions must be viewed relative to their effectiveness and the practical weighing of likely patient tolerance and compliance. This evaluation is not one of whether a change can be made, but whether the change is worth it in terms of time, financial and behavioral impact, and alternative treatment approaches such as surgery.

In the discussion of growth modification treatment techniques that follows, we will review the evidence that supports the timing that is advocated for different methods, along with management of the treatment procedures.

13

Treatment of Skeletal Transverse and Class III Problems

HENRY W. FIELDS, WILLIAM R. PROFFIT, AND KAITRIN KRAMER

CHAPTER OUTLINE

Growth Modification in the Transverse Plane of Space

It is appropriate to address maxillary transverse deficiency at the beginning of this discussion of skeletal problems because this is the first dentofacial dimension to cease growing. Like all craniofacial sutures, the midpalatal suture becomes more tortuous and interdigitated with increasing age, so there is some demand to be timely with treatment.

Patients with maxillary transverse deficiency usually have a narrow palate and a posterior crossbite (see Fig. 6.94). If the maxilla is narrow relative to the rest of the face, a diagnosis of transverse maxillary deficiency is justified. As we have emphasized in Chapter 6, the appropriate comparison of maxillary width should be to other transverse proportions in the same patient (e.g., bizygomatic width), not to population averages. Remember, a narrow maxilla accompanied by a narrow mandible and normal occlusion should not be considered a problem just because the jaw widths are below the population mean. Finally, transverse deficiencies or excesses can be mistakenly diagnosed because there is really an anteroposterior mandibular protrusion/maxillary retrusion or maxillary protrusion/mandibular retrusion problem, and not really a transverse problem (Fig. 13.1). Accurate diagnoses can avoid unnecessary treatment.

A narrow maxillary arch is related to the extraction-nonextraction decision because a child with crowded teeth and deficient maxillary width can have transverse expansion to provide space to align the teeth.[1] Many of these patients have some distortion of the arches, tooth abrasion from interferences of anterior teeth, and either anterior or lateral mandibular shifts that can lead to the possibility of mandibular skeletal asymmetry.[2] Customarily, treatment occurs by opening the midpalatal suture, which widens the roof of the mouth and the floor of the nose (Fig. 13.2). The maxilla generally opens as if on a hinge superiorly at the bridge of the nose (i.e., opens more inferiorly than superiorly) and also opens more anteriorly than posteriorly. This transverse expansion corrects the posterior crossbite that almost always is present. The expansion sometimes moves the maxilla forward a little (but is about as likely to lead to backward movement),[3] increases space in the arch, and repositions underlying permanent tooth buds as they move along with the bone in which they are embedded. Adequate expansion that coordinates the arches will also eliminate mandibular shifts and interferences.

Because of maturation of the palatal suture, palatal expansion can be done relatively easily at any time before the end of the adolescent growth spurt, but the response varies with continued maturation and the type of appliance used.

Midpalatal Suture Maturation

From histologic studies, we know that the midpalatal suture matures slowly and fusion begins as a posterior to anterior change at approximately 15 years of age.[4] Sutural fusion advances with age from the oral surface to the nasal surface.[5] Using CBCT images, it was found that midpalatal suture maturation could be divided into five classifications—A to E. Stages D and E indicated partial or complete sutural fusion. This study also indicated that any sutural fusion was infrequent in boys or girls prior to age 14.[6]

To help gauge the midpalatal suture maturation, correlating palatal suture maturation to cervical vertebra maturation staging was proposed as a clinical tool.[7] Also, the "midpalatal suture density ratio" (MSDR) appeared to have potential as an indicator of midpalatal maturation.[8] Unfortunately, further study indicated

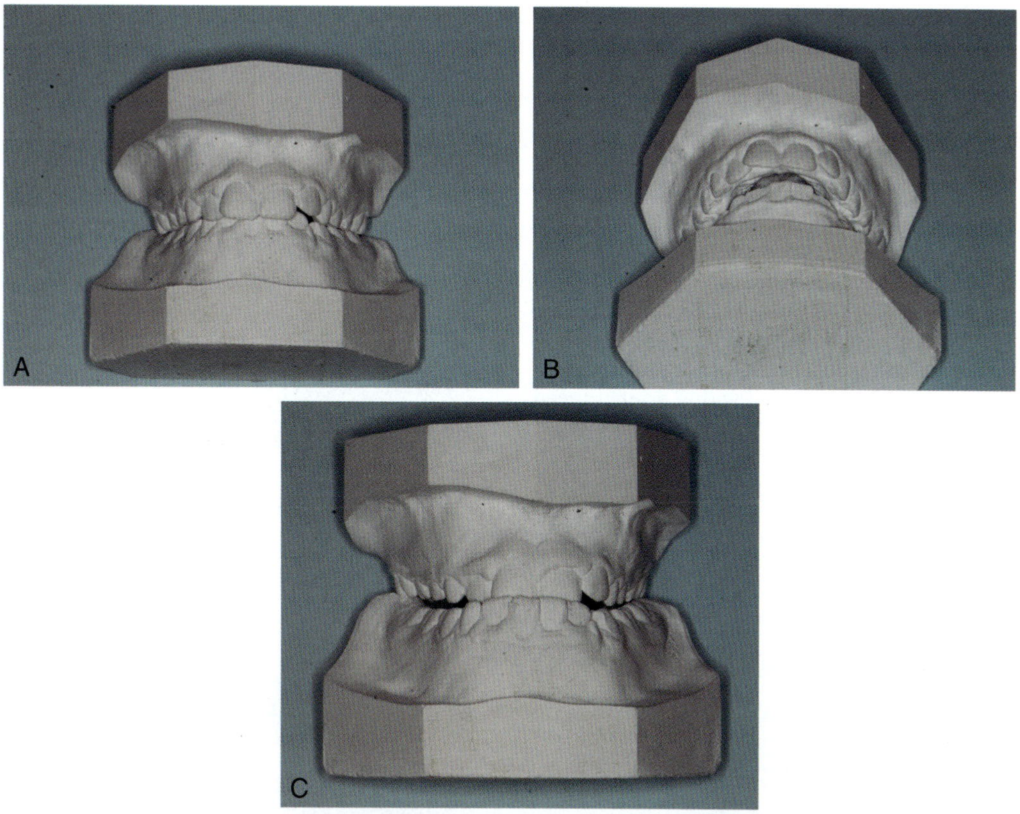

• **Fig. 13.1** There is an interaction between the transverse dimension and the anteroposterior dimension. The same demonstration casts were used for each simulated occlusion, but different perspectives were used to show the posterior transverse relationships. (A) A class I posterior occlusion shows coordinated arches with an appropriate buccal overjet and no crossbites. (B) A class II posterior occlusion, increased overjet and a maxillary posterior buccal crossbite. (C) A class III posterior occlusion and an anterior crossbite combined with a maxillary posterior lingual crossbite.

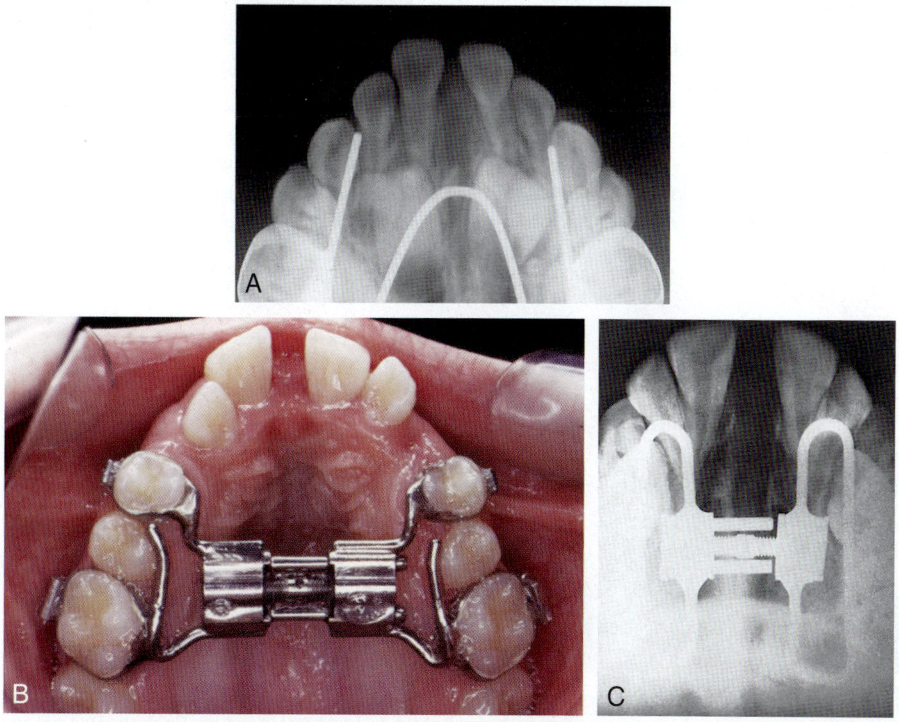

• **Fig. 13.2** (A) Before adolescence, the midpalatal suture can be opened during maxillary expansion by using a number of methods. This occlusal radiograph taken during the primary dentition years illustrates sutural opening in response to the W-arch appliance. (B) Transverse force across the maxilla in children and adolescents can open the midpalatal suture. The expansion force is usually delivered with a jackscrew mechanism fixed to maxillary teeth, as in this Hyrax expander with metal framework, seen at the end of rapid expansion (0.5 mm/day). The maxilla opens as if on a hinge, with its apex at the bridge of the nose. (C) The suture also opens on a hinge anteroposteriorly, separating more anteriorly than posteriorly, as shown in this radiograph of a patient after rapid expansion.

these maturity indicators did not show correlation that were clinically useful for predict skeletal expansion effects.[9]

Potential Maxillary Expansion Devices

As noted above, not only the timing, but the appliance type is a critical feature of successful palatal expansion. The most common appliances are: (1) a split removable plate with a jackscrew or heavy midline spring often included in a functional appliance design (Fig. 13.3); (2) a lingual arch type, often of the W-arch or quad-helix design (see Fig 11.17 and 11.18); (3) a palatal expander with a jackscrew (commonly called an RPE for Rapid Palatal Expander), which is either attached to bands, incorporated into a bonded appliance (Fig. 13.4) or used with a printed metal framework (Fig. 13.5). Note that some also have palatal acrylic shelves to apply force to the palate (Haas type, Fig. 13.6); (4) a spring loaded expander using either a steel (Fig.13.7) or NiTi calibrated spring (Fig. 13.8) attached to bands; and (5) jackscrew or calibrated spring expanders attached to TADS and bands known

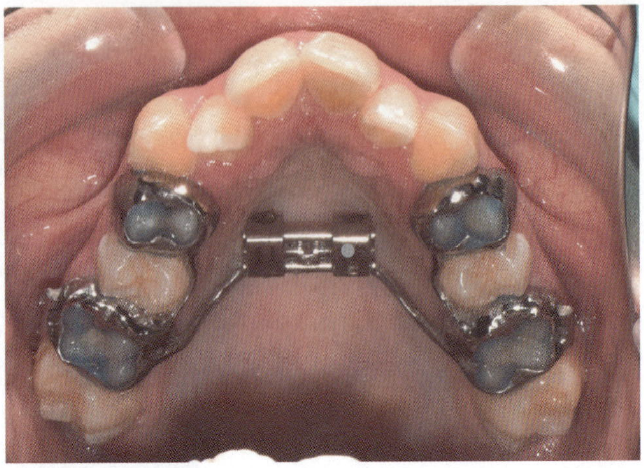

• **Fig. 13.5** This printed metal palatal expander can be designed to attach to a number of teeth in unconventional configurations that can alter anchorage. It also has the advantage of not requiring separation before seating.

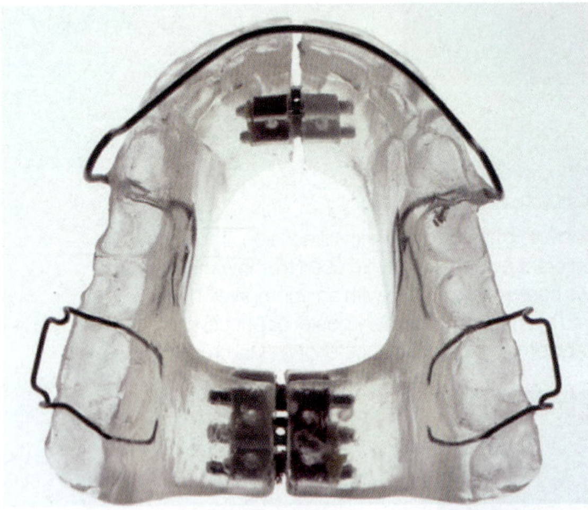

• **Fig. 13.3** This removable maxillary expander has two transverse expansion screws, but all it can do is produce a small amount of tooth movement, and it has to be activated very slowly in order to do that. The split plate is part of a class II functional appliance intended to advance the mandible.

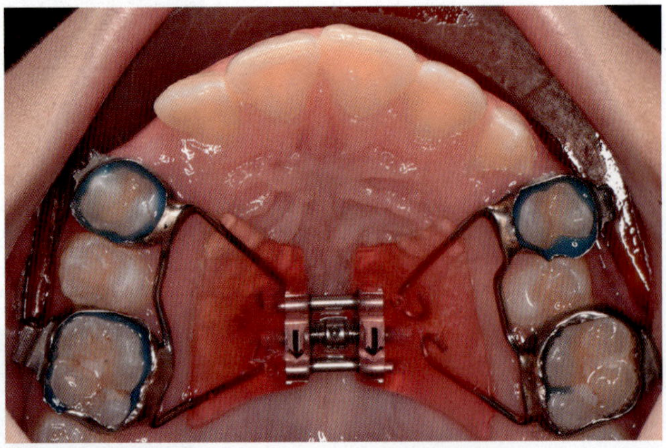

• **Fig. 13.6** This Haas-type rapid palatal expander has a jackscrew to transmit the force to the teeth and acrylic palatal shelves to also apply support and force to the palatal vault in an effort to enhance skeletal expansion. (Courtesy Dr. Ian Segall.)

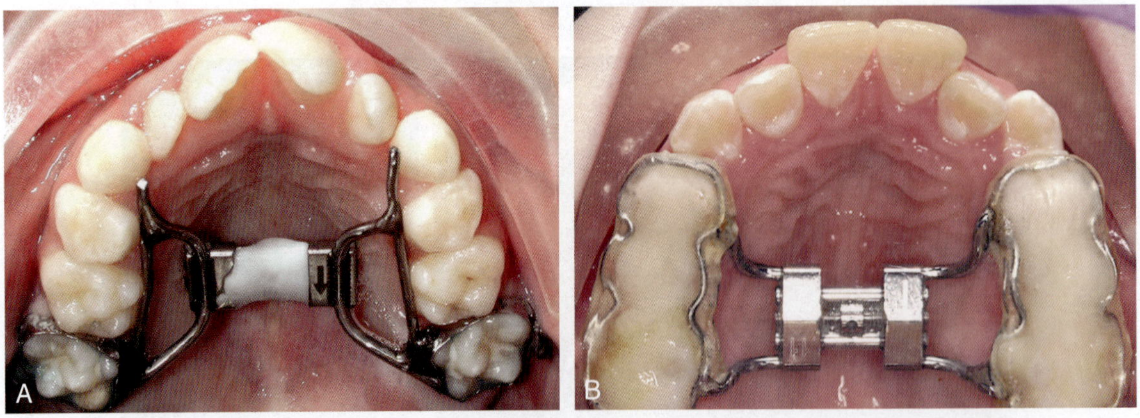

• **Fig. 13.4** (A) This banded palatal expander, attached only to the first molars in a patient in the mid mixed dentition, has been stabilized after expansion by using cold-cure acrylic so it will not relapse. This will remain in place for 3 months. (B) For a bonded palatal expander, during fabrication the plastic base is extended over the occlusal, facial, and lingual surfaces of the posterior teeth. In general, a composite bonding agent is used to retain the appliance, with only the facial and lingual surfaces of the posterior teeth etched. Etching the occlusal surface is not recommended; bonding there is unnecessary for retention and can greatly complicate appliance removal.

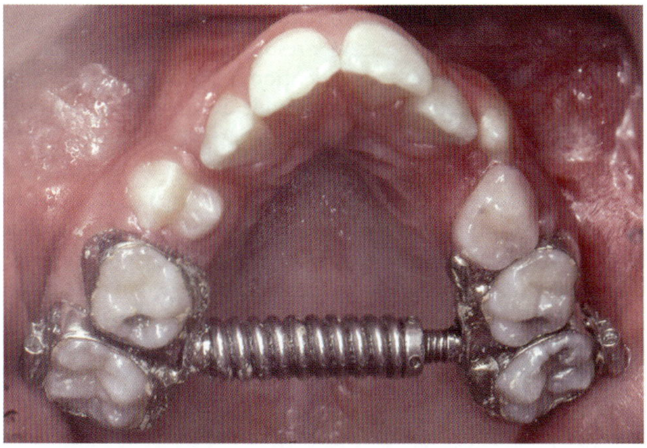

• **Fig. 13.7** This expander uses a coil spring to provide the force as the stop on the threaded connector is turned to compress the spring. It can be calibrated to determine and monitor the force that is active. This prevents delivery of either low or excessive forces during the expansion.

as Mini-implant Assisted RPE (MARPE) or Tooth Bone Borne (TBB) expanders (Fig. 13.9).

These appliances can be used for slow 0.25 mm/day or 0.25 mm every other day (one-quarter turn of the jackscrew) or rapid ≥0.5 mm/day expansion (two-quarter turns of the jackscrew). The split plate is usually considered a slow palatal expander, because it is retained by clasps and easily dislodged by heavy forces.

Rapid and Slow Palatal Expansion—The Details

The major goal of growth modification always is to maximize the skeletal changes and minimize the dental changes produced by treatment. The object of maxillary expansion is to widen the maxilla, not just expand the dental arch by moving the teeth relative to the bone. Originally, rapid palatal expansion (RPE) was recommended to help meet this goal. The theory was that with rapid, heavy force application to the posterior teeth there would not be enough time for tooth movement via frontal resorption because the force would be transferred to the suture, and the suture would

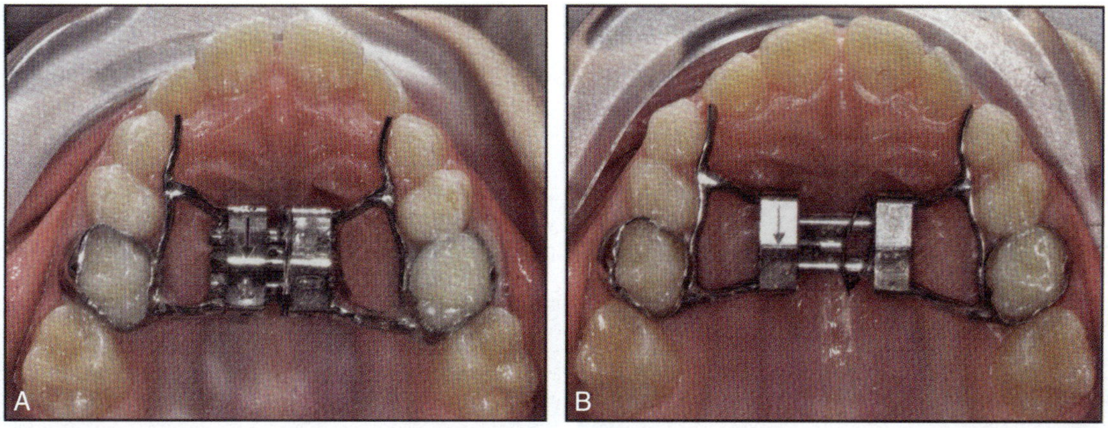

• **Fig. 13.8** (A) Pretreatment two banded expander using a calibrated NiTi compressed leaf spring. (B) Following expansion note the open left spring (elliptical appearance). Due to the range of the spring and consistent forces, it needs infrequent adjustment by the practitioner, eliminating parental compliance. (From Lanteri C, Beretta M, Lanteri V, et al. The leaf expander for non-compliance treatment in the mixed dentition. *J Clin Orthod*. 2016;50(9):552–560.)

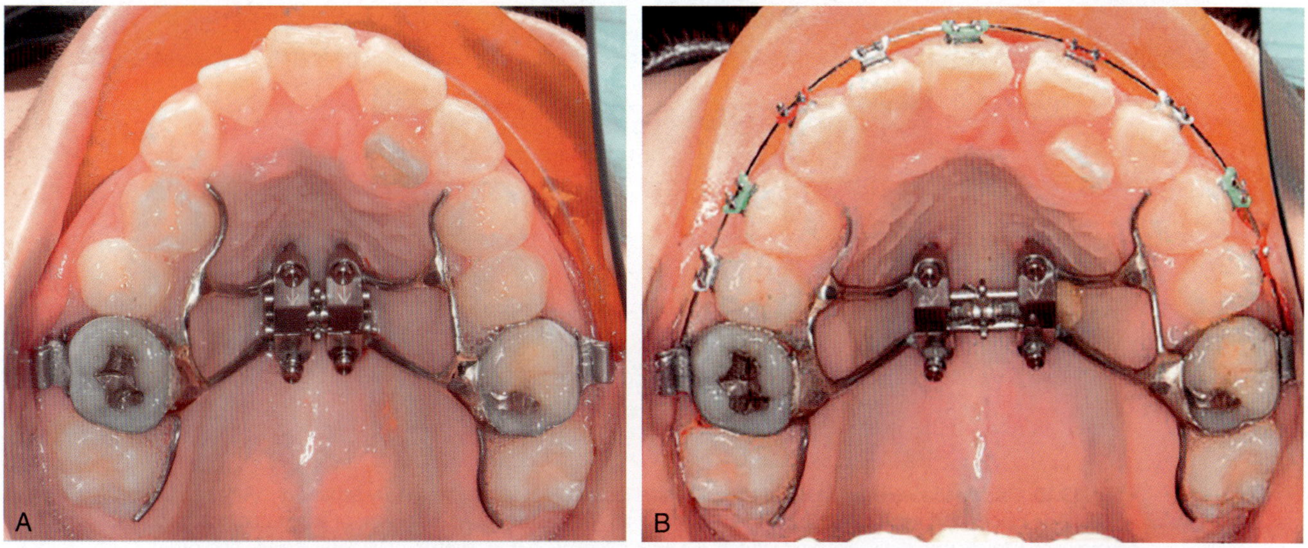

• **Fig. 13.9** (A) The preferred configuration now for bone and tooth-borne expanders, particularly with the MARPE technique that uses rapid and then slow expansion is a pair of linked bone screws at the base of the palate. (B) End of expansion for this patient, with opening of space between the central incisors. Closing the midline diastema should provide space to bring the lingually positioned lateral incisor into the arch. (Courtesy Drs. D. Grauer and G.Sameshima.)

open up while the teeth moved only minimally relative to their supporting bone. In other words, rapid activation was conceived as a way to maximize skeletal change and minimize dental change. That is true in the first couple of weeks, but not thereafter.

With RPE at a rate of 0.5 mm/day (two-quarter turns of the screw with 1 turn in the am and 1 in the pm), a centimeter or more of expansion can be obtained in 2 to 3 weeks, with 10 to 20 lb of pressure across the suture. Most of the movement is separation of the two halves of the maxilla, but force also is transmitted to adjacent posterior structures.[10] A space between the central incisors develops because the midpalatal suture opens wider and faster anteriorly and suture maturation begins in the posterior area (Fig. 13.10).

The space created at the midpalatal suture is filled initially by tissue fluids and hemorrhage, and at this point the expansion is highly unstable. The expansion device must be stabilized so that it cannot screw itself back shut and is left in place for 3 to 4 months. By then, new bone has filled in the space at the suture, and the skeletal expansion is stable. The midline diastema decreases and may disappear during this time. The diastema closes from a combination of skeletal relapse and tooth movement created by stretched gingival fibers.

The aspect of rapid expansion that was not appreciated initially was that orthodontic tooth movement continues after the expansion is completed, until bone stability is achieved. In most orthodontic treatment, the teeth move relative to a stable bony base. It is possible, of course, for tooth movement to allow bony segments to reposition themselves while the teeth are held in the same relationship to each other, and this is what occurs during the approximately 3 months required for bony fill-in at the suture after rapid expansion. During this time, the dental expansion is maintained by the appliance but the two halves of the maxilla move back toward each other as a result of soft tissue forces.

After the 3- to 4-month retention period, the fixed appliance can be removed, but a removable retainer that covers the palate is often needed as further insurance against early relapse (Fig. 13.11). A relatively heavy, expanded maxillary archwire provides retention and support if further treatment is being accomplished immediately. If not, a transpalatal lingual arch or a large expanded labial auxiliary wire (36 or 40 mil) in the headgear tubes will help maintain expansion while a more flexible wire is used in the brackets.

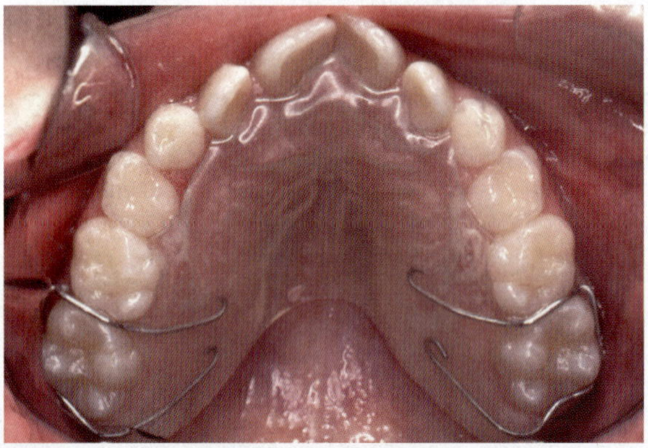

• **Fig. 13.11** Following palatal expansion, even after 3 months of retention with the passive expander, an acrylic retainer that covers the palate is advisable to control relapse and stabilize the skeletal components.

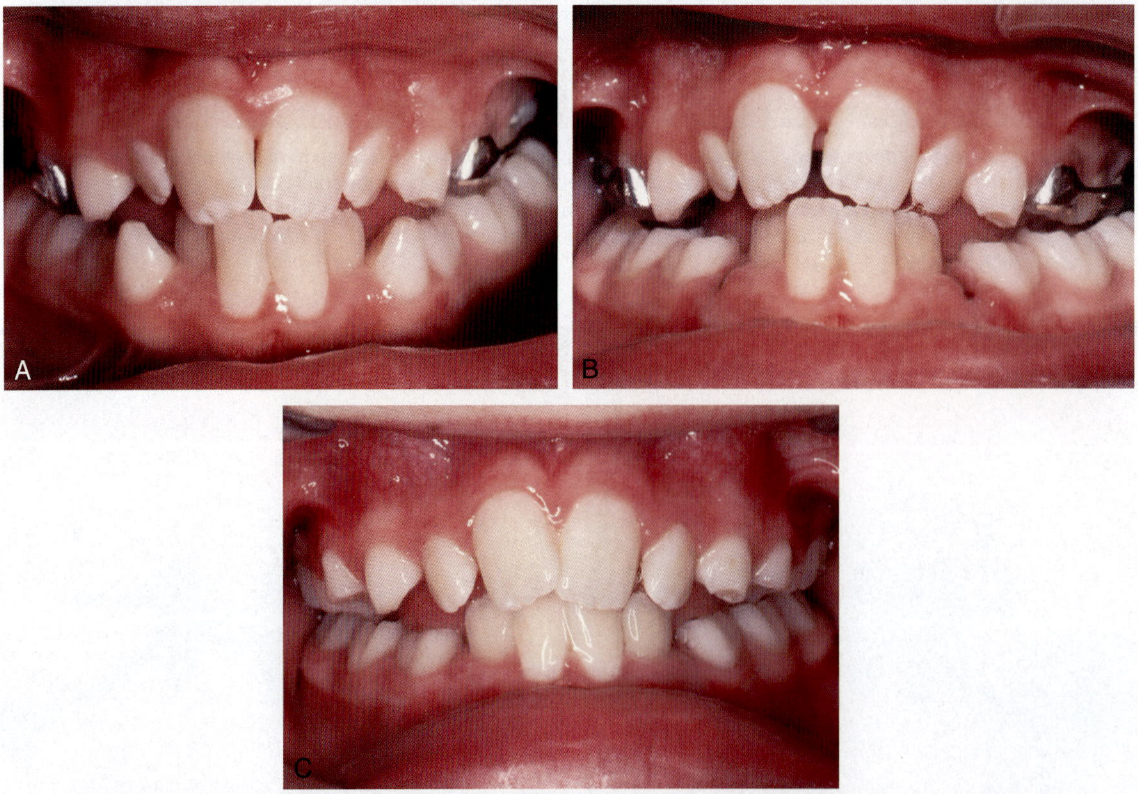

• **Fig. 13.10** Usually spaces develop between the central incisors during rapid maxillary expansion. (A) When the appliance is placed and treatment begins, there is only a tiny diastema. (B) After 1 week of expansion, the teeth have moved laterally with the skeletal structures. (C) After retention, a combination of skeletal relapse and pull of the gingival fibers has brought the incisors together and closed the diastema. Note that the expansion was continued until the maxillary lingual cusps occlude with the lingual inclines of the buccal cusps of the mandibular molars.

Slow Palatal Expansion (SPE) using low activation of the expansion appliance at the rate of 0.25 mm/day or every other day, which produces about 2 lb of pressure in a child with a mixed dentition, opens the suture at a rate that is close to the maximum speed of bone formation. The suture can show some opening on radiographs, but no midline diastema appears. Even so, it has been stated that both skeletal and dental changes occur together with less stress on the skeletal, dental, and periodontal structures.

The question is what method (rapid or slow) expansion should be used at different levels of palatal suture maturation.

Expansion Methods Related to Palatal Suture Maturation

Although this is not an exact science, conclusions for the various stages of maturation seem to be supported by the data.

In the primary, early and late mixed dentitions skeletal expansion is easiest because the midpalatal suture has not fused so that heavy force and extensive microfracturing are not needed to separate the palatal halves. Almost any expansion device will tend to separate the midpalatal suture in addition to moving the molar teeth in a child up to age 9 or 10.

In this age group, three methods can be used for palatal expansion: (1) a split removable plate with a jackscrew or heavy midline spring, (2) a lingual arch, often of the W-arch or quad-helix design, or (3) a fixed palatal expander with a jackscrew or calibrated spring, which can be either attached to bands or incorporated into a bonded appliance.

With a split removable plate, the rate of expansion and the force employed during the process must be low because faster expansion produces higher forces that create problems with retention of the appliance. Multiple clasps that are well adjusted are mandatory. Because of the instability of the teeth during the expansion process, failure to wear the appliance for even 1 day requires adjustment of the jackscrew, usually by the practitioner, to constrict the appliance until it again fits and expansion can be resumed. Compliance in activation and wear time are always issues with these appliances. Successful expansion with a removable appliance can take considerable time, which makes it less cost effective.

Lingual arches of W-arch and quad-helix designs have been demonstrated to open the midpalatal suture in young patients (Fig. 13.2A). These appliances generally deliver a few hundred grams of force and provide slow expansion. They are relatively clean and reasonably effective, producing a mix of dental and skeletal change that approximates 6 to 1 dental to skeletal change.[3] There is some evidence that these appliances are more effective than removable appliances[11] as well as more comfortable for the patient and more efficient.

Fixed jackscrew appliances attached to bands or bonded splints also can be used in the early treatment of maxillary constriction (Fig. 13.2B and C). The appliances show a 2.5 to 1 dental to skeletal change. When comparing jackscrew RPE to an expansion lingual arch, there are two major differences. First, a jackscrew appliance is bulky and more difficult to place and remove. The patient inevitably has problems cleaning it, which leads to soft tissue irritation, and either the patient or parent must activate the appliance, so there are compliance issues. Banding permanent molars and primary second molars is relatively simple, but banding primary first molars can be challenging. Use of a bonded jackscrew appliance in the mixed dentition is relatively straightforward, but it can be difficult to remove if conventional bonding techniques are used. Using a calibrated spring with bands requires less compliance because it is activated only periodically by the clinician.

Second, jackscrew appliances can be activated rapidly, which in young children is a disadvantage, not an advantage, and can cause facial distortion (Fig. 13.12). There is no evidence of any advantage of rapid movement and high forces in children, and ample evidence that this can be dangerous. The calibrated spring appliance can help control exaggerated forces.

When comparing lingual arch-type appliances to removable RPE appliances the changes at 3 years post op were comparable. Although the crossbites were corrected, the transverse dental dimensions never reached those of the normal control groups.[12] It also appears that anteroposterior dental changes in terms of overjet are not consistently correlated with early maxillary expansion.[12,13] There is no convincing evidence that a removable plate or a quad helix (both as SPE) or RPE is better in skeletal or dental expansion terms.[14] In patient and clinician terms, the quad helix reduces compliance requirements and ease of clinical manipulation. A systematic review showed no difference in periodontal health between quad helix (SPE) and RPE appliances.[15]

In the preadolescent late mixed dentition, the midpalatal suture still is not fused. A fixed jackscrew appliance (either banded or bonded) can be used, but high force is not required. With the printed metal expanders that are cemented in place (Fig. 13.5) unique designs can be developed to alter anchorage with as many teeth as possible included in the anchorage unit. Printed appliances need no separation of teeth prior to appliance placement. In the late mixed dentition, root resorption of primary molars may have reached the point at which these teeth offer little resistance, and it may be wise to wait for eruption of the first premolars before beginning expansion.

Many functional appliances for class II treatment (discussed in Chapter 14), which may be occurring during the mixed dentiton, especially in females, incorporate some components to expand the maxillary arch (Fig. 13.3), either intrinsic force-generating mechanisms such as springs and jackscrews or buccal shields that reduce cheek pressure against the dentition. When arch expansion occurs during functional appliance treatment, it is possible that some opening of the midpalatal suture contributes to it, but the precise mix of skeletal and dental change is not well documented. SPE using the expanded inner bow of a headgear for class II correction also has been used to expand the arches during this time period.

Although some studies have reported increases in vertical facial height with maxillary expansion mainly due to dental tipping and maxillary lingual cusp interferences, long-term evidence indicates this change is transitory.[13] A bonded appliance that covers the occlusal surface of the posterior teeth has been proposed for a preadolescent child with a long-face tendency because it produces less clockwise mandibular rotation than a banded appliance. In the long term, evidence does not support a clear difference in these appliances.[16] Perhaps the best summary is that the older the patient when maxillary expansion is done, the less likely it is that vertical changes will be recovered by subsequent growth.

An important consideration in skeletal expansion is the rate of activation of the expander, so that rapid or slow expansion is obtained. This really brings us to the question of early slower expansion or later rapid expansion as choices, but both in the preadolescent period. Two studies that demonstrate age-appropriate approaches are instructive. One, with patients who averaged 8 years 10 months of age at the start, used a bonded acrylic splint and a slow approach of 0.25 mm of expansion per day.[17] The other, with patients averaging 12 years 2 months of age at the start, used a Haas-type RPE (jackscrew RPE with palatal shelves) device turned twice for

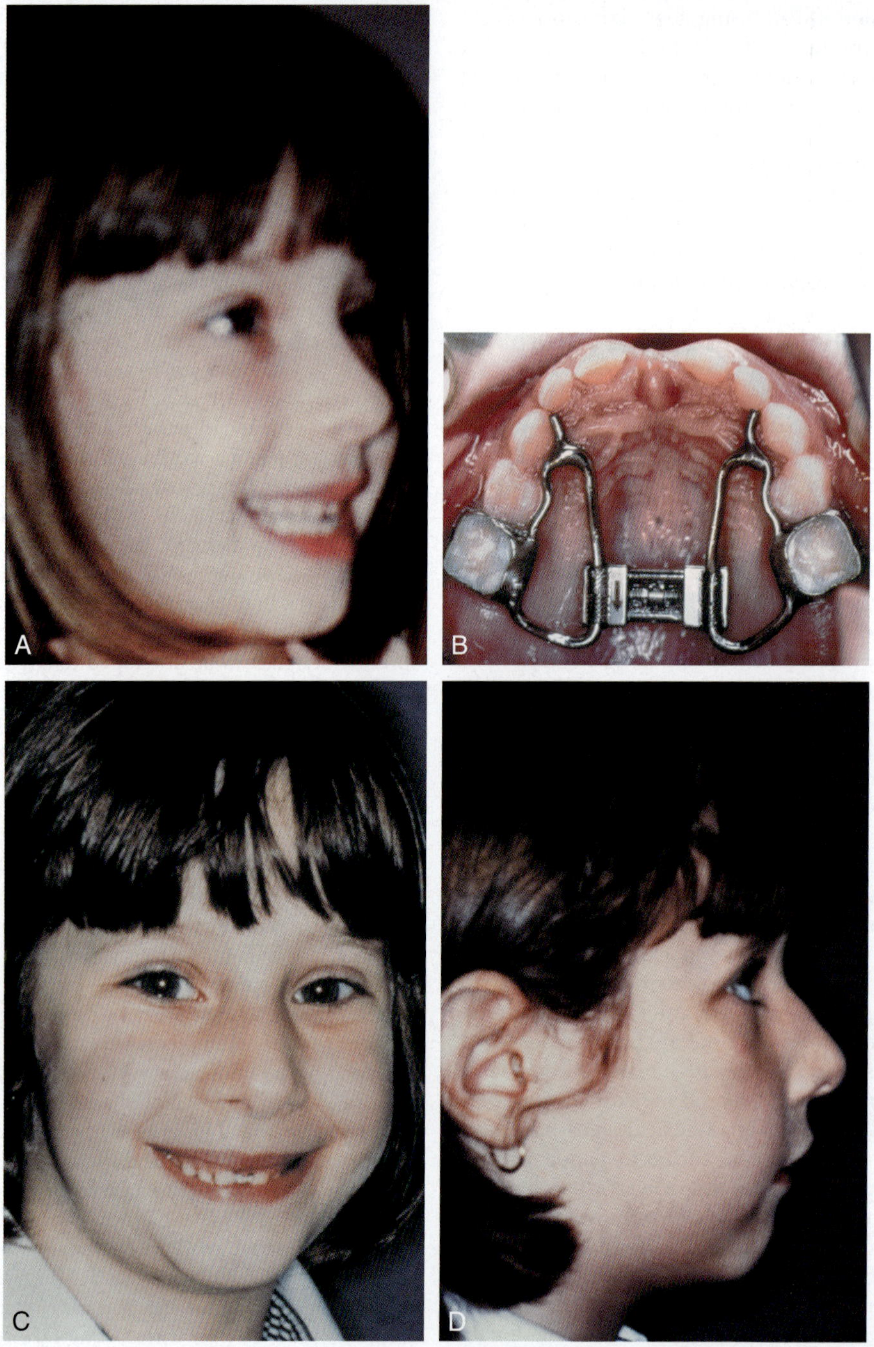

• **Fig. 13.12** Rapid palatal expansion in young children can lead to undesirable changes in the nose, as in this 5-year-old who had expansion at the rate of 0.5 mm/day (two-quarter turns of the jackscrew per day). (A) Nasal contours before treatment. (B) Jackscrew appliance after activation over a 10-day period. (C and D) Nasal hump and paranasal swelling, which developed after the child complained of discomfort related to the expansion. (Courtesy Dr. D. Patti.)

0.5 mm of expansion per day of treatment.[18] Both followed the expansion with retention, and ultimately the patients underwent full treatment without further purposeful expansion. At the long-term evaluation points (19 years 9 months and 20 years 5 months, respectively), the expansion across the molars and canines and the increase in arch perimeter were quite similar, which indicates equivalent long-term results.

There are other data for preadolescents that more directly examined slow and rapid expansion. One study found that for the maxillary dimensions, there was only a significantly greater expansion (~2 mm) at the end of active treatment and retention periods for the intercanine dimension in the RME group. The arch perimeter in the RME group in retention was greater, but by less than a millimeter.[19] A randomized study showed no differences between rapid and slow expansion for dental dimensions and no clinical differences for skeletal changes.[20]

When TB (Tooth Borne) vs TBB (Tooth Bone Borne) expansion were evaluated at the level of the base of the nose and the dental arch, the dimensions were equivalent 5 years after treatment for late mixed dentition patients. This probably indicates that the density of the bone was not sufficient to justify BB (Bone Borne) anchorage in this age group.[21]

When SPE using a calibrated spring and RPE in the early and late mixed dentitions were compared for difference in pain, difficulty speaking, hypersalivation, or patient or parent satisfaction, there were few differences.[22]

These data, taken together, appear to show equivalent results for slow and rapid maxillary expansion in dimensional and patient centered terms. In the late mixed dentition, either rapid or slow expansion is clinically acceptable, but simplicity and consideration for tissue irritation probably favors slow expansion. So, a lingual arch-type appliance, a calibrated spring or fixed jackscrew appliance, if activated carefully and slowly are probably acceptable options.

In Adolescents (Early Permanent Dentition) there is greater need to actually open a partially or greater fused midpalatal suture. This is best accomplished with a banded or bonded expansion device. Studies have compared adolescents 12 to 13 years of age using TB, BB and TBB appliances by evaluating digital casts and CBCTs. The assessment was that the amount of skeletal and dental changes were similar with dental tipping in all groups.[23] When assessing 13 to 14 year olds with TB and TBB appliances using CBCTs, the skeletal width and dental molar expansion changes were similar between groups. but there was greater expansion in the TB premolar region in one study. Generally, dental tipping was similar in the groups, as was buccal bone thickness decreased except in the TB premolar region.[24,25] So, in the mid adolescent group, there is little need for bone borne appliances for maxillary expansion. When including a slightly older age group, a systematic review concluded it appears MARPE with both tooth or bone support provides more predictability and fewer side effects than traditional RPE for patients 11 to 16.[26] There is greater expansion, less tipping,[27] and less root resorption[28] with MARPE expansion.

In Post Adolescents, fusion of the suture reaches the point that opening it may no longer be possible. When guidance for decision making regarding the state of the midpalatal suture is required it is probably best obtained from CBCT images staged for suture maturity.[6] This method also provides the opportunity to determine the areas of greatest bone density and bicortical anchorage for potential TAD placement.

For older (more mature) adolescents and adults, heavier force is needed to fracture the suture. The chance that opening of the suture will occur with moderate force declines with increasing bone maturity, and the chance increases that even with heavier force, tooth-supported expanders will just move teeth rather than open the suture.

Traditionally a therapeutic diagnosis was followed. Try RPE and see what happens. Initially rapid activation quickly led to one of two possible responses: The desired fracture of sutural bridging occurs, or the patient experienced significant pain. At that point, RPE was abandoned and other options were considered—surgical-assisted or implant-supported expanders. From the perspective of patient management, it would be better to consider a skeletally anchored expander from the beginning for the mature patient.

More information on implant-supported RPE (MARPE) continues to emerge. The location of the skeletal anchors for palatal expansion is important. A randomized clinical trial at the University of Alberta in 2009 and 2010 compared the percentage of skeletal versus dental change with bone screws at the base of the alveolar process versus conventional expansion. The surprising and discouraging result was no significant difference between the two groups, because the alveolar process bent outward in the skeletal anchorage group.[29] Since then, research has shown that bone screws in the palate provide better anchorage and significantly less tooth movement, when compared with tooth-borne expanders.[30,31] It must be kept in mind, however, the teeth do move apart as the suture expands, and that the possibility of tooth movement allowing skeletal relapse still exists—so the implant anchorage needs to remain in place for 3 to 4 months after the expansion is completed.

At this point, the goal of treatment with skeletally anchored expanders is not so much to provide heavy force as to apply the force directly against the bone so that there is reduced pressure against the teeth (Fig. 13.9). This provides a way to expand the maxilla and minimize tooth movement in patients with a normal dentition. There are a number of designs for expanders, including hinged ones that expand more anteriorly than posteriorly, and these can be adapted for skeletal anchorage if desired (Fig. 13.13),

Bone screws in the palate now are routinely used for expansion in mature patients. Most commonly 10–12 mm TADs that are 1.8 mm in diameter are used. Bicortical engagement of the palate and nasal floor appears advantageous. More precise and greater bone thickness locations have been documented by some from the mid first premolar area to the second premolar- first molar contact at the midline and 3 to 6 mm parasagatally as well as midsagitally from the second premolar to the second molar area. This has been referred to as the T-Zone because of the shape of the desirable implant area. (Fig. 13.14).[32] Generally speaking, palatal bone is thinner farther laterally and posteriorly.

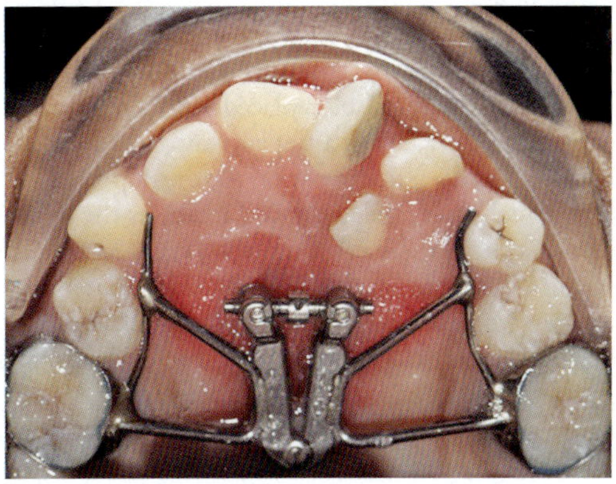

• **Fig. 13.13** Many configurations of maxillary expanders are available. This one has a hinge in the posterior and the expansion screw in the anterior. This design holds the posterior teeth and their transverse dimension stable and expands only the anterior part of the arch.

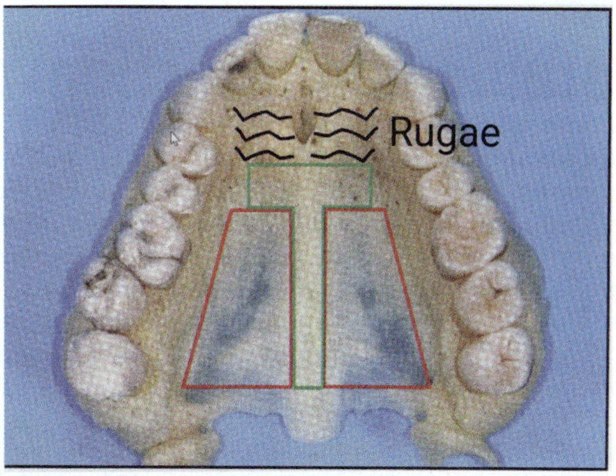

• **Fig. 13.14** The T-zone (in green) where the anchorage for TAD support of MARPE expanders is expected to be most advantageous due to bone thickness and density. The zone extends from mid maxillary first premolar to the second premolar-molar contact and otherwise near the midpalatal suture. (From Wilmes B, Ludwig B, Vasudavan S, Nienkemper M, Drescher D. The T-zone: median vs. paramedian insertion of palatal mini-implants. *J Clin Orthod*. 2016;50(9):543–551. PMID: 27809213.)

Based on a meta analysis, for patients older than 16, MARPE can provide skeletal and dental arch increases with a high (>90%) success rate. The mean skeletal increase was 2+ mm and the dental width change was 6+ mm with a skeletal component of 36%. There was dental buccal tipping accompanied by a significant decrease in the mean buccal bone thickness and in buccal alveolar height.[33] Unfortunately, the evidence was not high quality.

In a somewhat older sample of patients comparing BB and TBB appliances, both appliances showed greater skeletal to dental changes and forward and downward maxillary movement, but skeletal changes above the nasal cavity were greater in the BB group. The midpalatal suture opened more anteriorly in the BB group. Both groups had 50% asymmetric expansion.[34]

Based on a systematic review and meta analysis[35] for adolescent and adult patients, where the majority of appliances were hybrid (using bone and dental anchorage-TBB) and used a rapid palatal expansion activation method, it appeared that the skeletal expansion effects were less at the zygomatic area than inferiorly at the molar alveolus. Expansion was also greater in the anterior palate than the posterior palate, but greater in the molar than in the canine area. All changes were nonparallel. The percentage of skeletal expansion at PNS was 55.76%, molar alveolar expansion was 24.37%, and dental expansion at the molars was 19.87%.

As mentioned earlier, with RPE and SPE, the consensus is that a tooth-supported expansion appliance should remain in place for 3 to 4 months and then can be replaced with a removable retainer or other retention device. With implant-supported expansion, the guideline is about the same as with tooth-supported expansion. With skeletal anchorage, the expansion increases the light but constant pressure against the teeth from the stretched palatal mucosa and soft tissues of the cheeks. Placing a blocking material to prevent the screw from turning (see Fig. 13.4A) helps to retain the skeletal expansion, but dental relapse still can occur. With no retention at all, both skeletal and dental relapse would be expected.

MARPE, along with surgically assisted palatal expansion (SARPE) and segmental osteotomy of the maxilla are the possibilities for the more mature patients in whom tooth-supported expanders will not work. These techniques are discussed in more detail in Chapters 20 and 22.

Clinical Management of Palatal Expansion Devices

Most traditional palatal expansion devices use bands for retention on permanent first molars and first premolars, if possible. During the late mixed dentition years, the first premolars often are not fully erupted and are difficult to band. If the primary second molars are firm, they can be banded along with the permanent first molars. Alternatively, only the permanent first molars can be banded and the supporting framework extended anteriorly, contacting the other posterior primary and erupting permanent teeth near their gingival margins (see Fig. 13.4A). A comparison of four-band (see Fig. 13.2B) versus two-band devices showed that the four-band devices provided more transverse expansion and arch perimeter increase, especially after 12 years of age when the suture was more calcified.[36] If first premolars are available, they should be banded.

Banding is a balance between a retentive fit and enough band circumference to allow a path of insertion and removal of all the bands simultaneously. Also, the teeth can be sensitive at the time of expander removal. In those patients, sectioning the bands is appropriate. Prefittting bands for continued treatment after expander removal, so there is less impact on sensitive teeth, certainly can improve patient comfort.

An alternative approach is to use a bonded palatal expander covering the occlusal surfaces of the maxillary teeth (see Fig. 13.4B). Because there is no band fitting, the appliance is easier to place for both the patient and doctor, and during treatment it is manipulated like any other RPE appliance. But, removal of this appliance can be difficult. It is accomplished with a band remover engaged under a facial or lingual margin to flex the appliance and break the bond. In addition, if a portion of the occlusal surface is not covered by the plastic splint, the appliance usually needs to be sectioned or portions of the occlusal plastic removed for a direct purchase on the teeth so the band remover can effectively lift and separate the plastic from the teeth. Complete removal of the bonding agent (typically a filled resin that will adhere to etched tooth surfaces and to the appliance) can be laborious, so use of only an adequate amount is crucial, but insufficient resin will lead to excessive leakage onto the nonbonded surfaces, which can result in decalcification or appliance loss. For these reasons, some clinicians use a resin-modified glass ionomer cement that will bond to both the plastic appliance and the teeth for retention. The strength of the material usually is adequate, and the short-term fluoride release may be beneficial (see Chapter 10).

A factor in the decision between an occlusal bonded and banded expander is the vertical effect of maxillary expansion. As mentioned earlier, expansion creates dental interferences as soon as the posterior teeth begin to move laterally, and the effect is to rotate the mandible downward and backward. This is largely transient but may be more problematic in nongrowing patients.

For a patient who had a deep bite as well as a posterior crossbite, this is good. For one who had an open bite, this makes the open bite worse. In theory, the splint between the teeth with a bonded expander would interfere with eruption of the posterior teeth in both arches, and there is some (weak) evidence that this is the case in the short term. It may be reasonable to use a bonded expander in long-face or open-bite patients who need expansion rather than a banded one, but because simply by placing brackets and bands plus an archwire on a patient, there is an extrusive force, any reduced dental extrusion is mitigated by the subsequent fixed appliances. For patients with a deep bite, it seems to make no difference in the vertical effects of expansion which type of expander is used.

Alternative Expansion Approaches

Another expansion protocol with alternate rapid maxillary expansion and constriction (Alt-RAMEC) was initially devised by Liou for treatment of patients with class III cleft palate with maxillary transverse and anteroposterior deficiency. It requires the patient to alternatively expand and constrict the maxilla on a weekly basis by 1 mm/day (two turns in the morning and two turns in the evening for a weekly total of 7 mm) using a double-hinged expander. This is done for 7 to 9 weeks,[37] then the patient wears a facemask for maxillary protraction. The goal is to disrupt not only the midpalatal suture but also the lateral and posterior sutures. As we point out in the discussion of maxillary protraction later in this chapter, ALT-RAMEC for protraction cannot be recommended now.

What makes this of interest in our discussion of maxillary expansion is whether this protocol has any application to expansion without protraction. It appears from data obtained using the Alt-RAMEC protocol with noncleft children over a 9-week period that there were statistically significant transverse changes to the maxilla, adjacent sutures, and soft tissues, along with approximately 1 mm of forward and downward movement at A point, but not clinically different transverse changes from what one would see with routine maxillary expansion.[38] So, as a singular approach to maxillary expansion treatment alone, this is a much more aggressive approach than is necessary, and it carries with it the risks that are described later in the discussion of maxillary protraction.

Maxillary Expansion and Sleep-Disordered Breathing

There is little doubt that nasal airway and nasopharynx volume are increased by RPE. The problem remains that the methods used to evaluate the space do not inform us of the physiologic benefits. Chapters 5 and 6 detail the etiology of breathing issues as well as the history, screening, examination and record based evidence. More studies are emerging that are incorporating control groups and appropriate measures related to sleep-disordered breathing.

According to the white paper provided by the American Association of Orthodontists, at this point the evidence is lacking for maxillary expansion performed for the sole purpose of attempting to improve sleep-disordered breathing, especially in the absence of posterior crossbite or maxillary deficiency.[39] Chapter 7 discusses appropriate treatment planning for care related to sleep apnea and Chapters 20 and 22 address nonsurgical and surgical options, respectively.

Treatment of Transverse Mandibular Constriction

Unlike the maxilla, the mandible has no midline suture. It started as two halves, but they fused during the first year of life, and the midline is solid bone. Although removable appliances that look like midpalatal expanders can be used (Fig. 13.15), they can only move the teeth (and do not do that very well). Mandibular transverse expansion was impossible until distraction osteogenesis became available. The first step in distraction, of course, is to cut through the bone; then it is possible to manipulate the healing callus and generate new bone (Fig. 13.16). There still is a limitation: The expansion is much greater anteriorly than in the molar

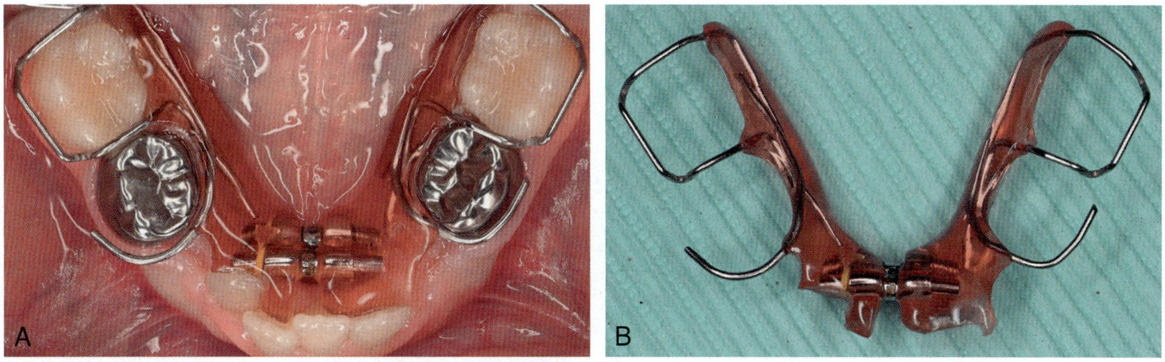

• **Fig. 13.15** The Schwarz appliance is a mandibular dental expander that is designed to move teeth laterally, since there is no suture to open. (A) The anterior jackscrew must be activated slowly so the appliance continues to fit, be retained and can tip the teeth. (B) The active screw component and clasps are more evident in this extraoral image.

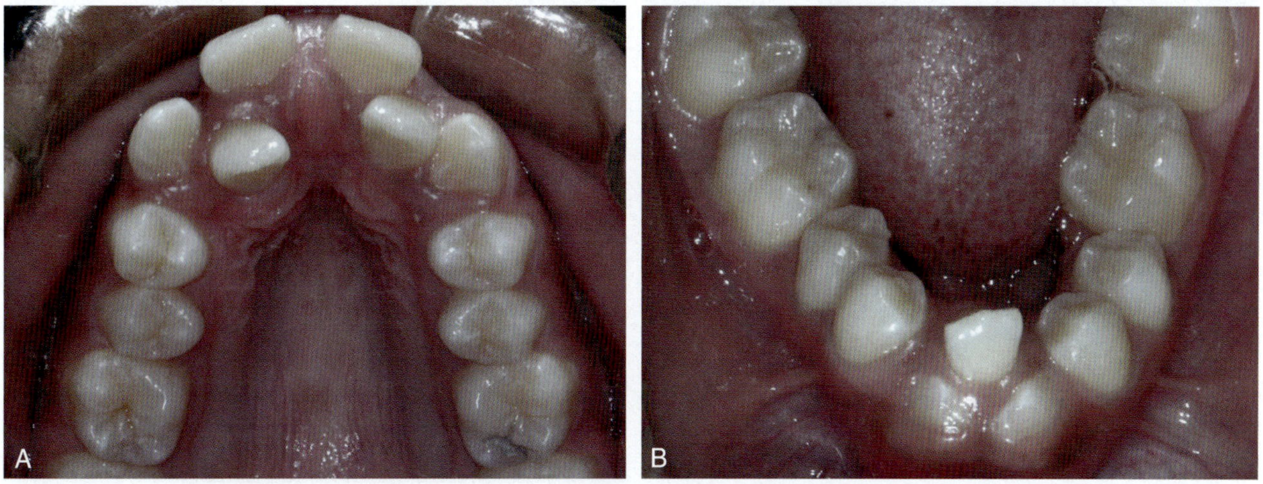

• **Fig. 13.16** (A and B) This patient had both a narrow maxillary arch with crowded-out lateral incisors and the unusual condition of a mandible with an imperfect alignment of the two halves of the mandible early in fetal life. Note that the mandibular canines were almost in contact in the midline. Three lower incisors were congenitally missing; one was only in soft tissue in the midline. (C) The maxillary arch was expanded at the rate of 1 mm/day with a banded jackscrew device. At the time of the photo the expansion was complete and was being retained (note the wire ligature to prevent further movement of the jackscrew). (D and E) The screw-retained expander for mandibular symphysis distraction osteogenesis, after removal of the lone incisor, immediately after cuts through the cortical bone. Expansion at the rate of 1 mm/day was done after a 7-day latency period. (F and G) The expander was stabilized when the desired expansion had been obtained and left in place for 4 months for maturation and remodeling of the new bone. (H) Nearly 1 year later, with orthodontic alignment of both arches completed and a temporary retainer in place. (I) Panoramic radiograph at the time distractor was removed. Note the fill in mature bone in the distraction area. Symphysis distraction is the only way to deal with problems created by missing areas of the anterior mandible. (Courtesy Drs. D. Grauer and D. Hall.)

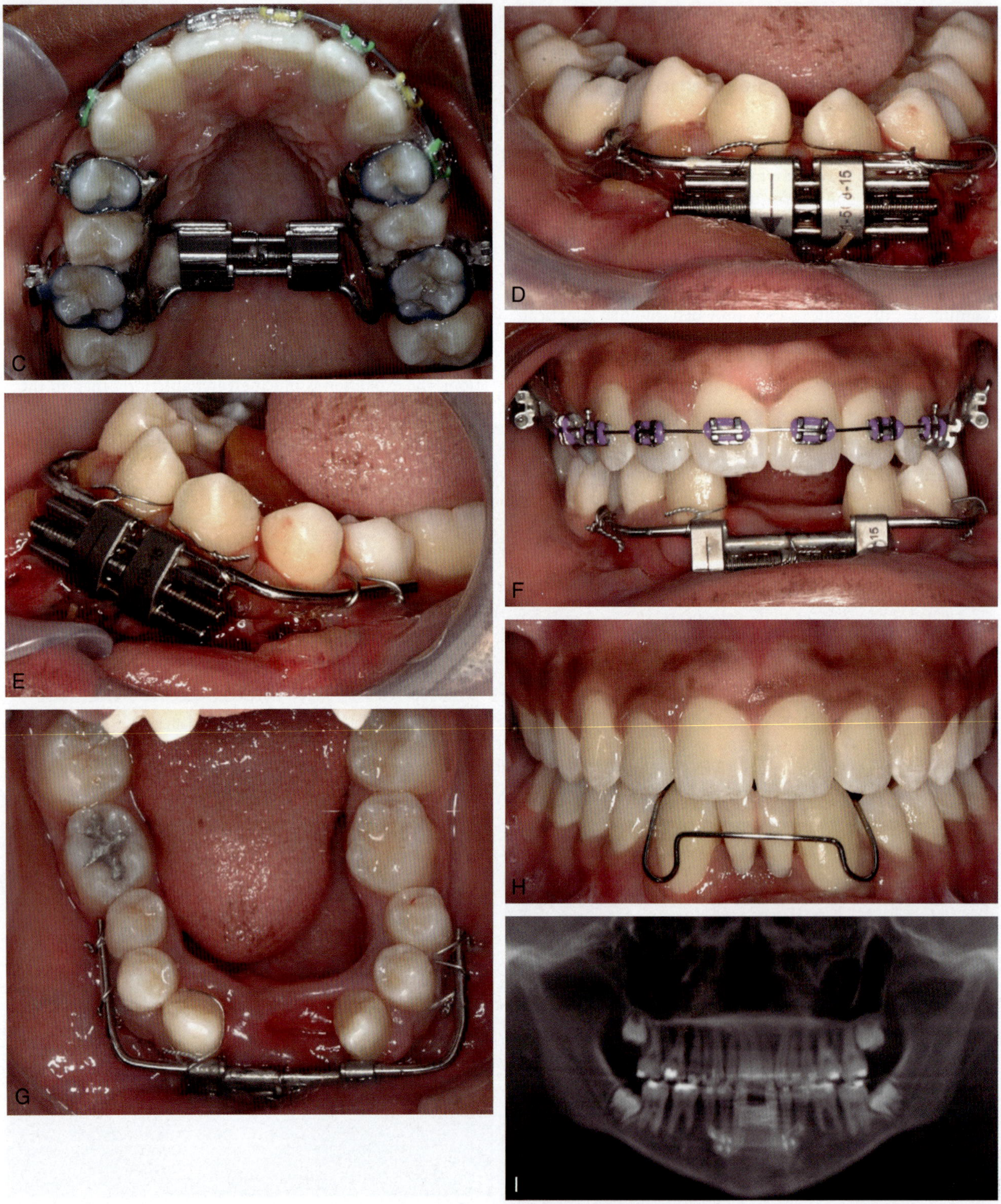

• **Fig. 13.16, cont'd**

region, and the condyles rotate slightly but do not move laterally. Fortunately, this amount of condylar rotation is tolerated without creating any problems.

Restriction of Excessive Transverse Growth

Restriction of transverse growth in both jaws is exceptionally difficult, almost impossible. In the maxillary arch a transpalatal lingual arch during the preadolescent period would maintain molar width but does not affect skeletal growth or arch width across the premolars and canines. In the mandibular arch the length of a lingual arch makes it flexible enough that some increase in intermolar width probably would occur despite its presence, and there would be the same lack of effect on both jaw width and the other teeth.

The major problem this creates is posterior crossbite in a patient with normal maxillary arch width and very large mandibular arch width. Patients of that type usually have a wide tongue. Even heroic efforts to decrease the mandibular intermolar width (for instance, wearing an elastic across the arch, running it over the top of the tongue), rarely succeed, and immediate relapse is likely. That leaves the orthodontist with two options: expand the maxillary arch to match the wide lower arch, or tolerate the crossbite.

As we have illustrated earlier, sutural expansion increases maxillary width more anteriorly than posteriorly, just the reverse of what is needed to match a mandibular arch that widens posteriorly, and dental expansion risks fenestration of the molar roots. Patients with posterior crossbite have a problem only when it forces a mandibular shift on closure, and without that, there are neither functional nor esthetic reasons for correcting it. A segmental maxillary osteotomy (see Chapter 22) can provide more expansion posteriorly than anteriorly. That is simply not indicated for a condition that really is not a problem for the patient. The best option: Take that type of posterior crossbite off the problem list and tolerate it.

Class III Growth Modification

Concepts of Class III Treatment

We have emphasized in the diagnosis and treatment planning chapters that it is critically important to recognize the skeletal versus dental components of problems in all three planes of space. The focus of the following discussion is on treatment of class III jaw discrepancies, due to some combination of deficient growth of the maxilla and/or excessive growth of the mandible. Treatment of the milder and largely dental class III problems that can be managed by altering the dental occlusion in adolescents and adults is discussed in Chapters 15–17 and 20.

This distinction between dental and skeletal problems, of course, was not made by the pioneers of orthodontics. Edward Angle's concept was that class III malocclusion was due almost exclusively to excessive mandibular growth and that class III elastics could control this excessive growth in all but the most severely prognathic patients. This was shown to be incorrect in the first studies using cephalometric radiographs. In fact, almost any combination of deficient maxillary growth and excessive mandibular growth can be found in patients with class III malocclusion, and in a broad view maxillary deficiency and mandibular excess are about equally likely.

The realization that maxillary deficiency is so frequently a component of skeletal class III malocclusion, and the discovery over 50 years ago that extraoral force could pull the growing maxilla forward if done in the early mixed dentition period, led to a great increase in treatment aimed at promoting maxillary growth. Fortunately, although some data from randomized clinical trials exist, data from well-documented retrospective studies now provide a clearer picture of both the best time for facemask protraction and the amount of short- and long-term change that can be expected.

In contrast, extraoral force via a chin cup anchored against the cranium has been shown to produce more transient downward and backward rotation of the mandible than true growth restraint. A large mandible cannot be rotated to decrease chin prominence without creating a long-face deformity except in patients who also have short anterior face height. That class III phenotype is most prevalent in those of Asian descent but is less frequent in Caucasians. Not surprisingly, this has led to a great decrease in chin-cup therapy, especially in Europe and the Americas.

A more recent discovery is that class III elastics between bone anchors above the posterior maxilla and in the anterior mandible are effective in bringing the maxilla forward and that alterations in mandibular growth also occur. This is now an effective growth-modifying method that requires surgical intervention for placement and removal of bone anchors but there are still many unanswered questions.

In evaluating current growth modification possibilities for skeletal class III problems, we begin with maxillary deficiency.

Anteroposterior and Vertical Maxillary Deficiency

Both anteroposterior and vertical maxillary deficiency can contribute to class III malocclusion. If the maxilla is small or positioned posteriorly there is a direct effect on class III malocclusion. If the maxilla does not grow vertically, there is an indirect effect on the mandible, which then rotates upward and forward as it grows, producing an appearance of mandibular prognathism that may be due more to the vertical position of the mandible than its actual size.

In order of increasing effectiveness, there are four possible approaches to growth modification to correct maxillary deficiency: Frankel's FR-III functional appliance, reverse-pull headgear (facemask) to the dentition, reverse-pull headgear to skeletal anchors, and class III elastics to skeletal anchors.

FR-III Functional Appliance

The FR-III appliance (Fig. 13.17) is made with the mandible positioned posteriorly and rotated open and with pads to stretch the upper lip forward. In theory, the lip pads stretch the periosteum in a way that stimulates forward growth of the maxilla. In a review of cases selected from Frankel's archives, Levin et al. reported that in patients with class III skeletal and dental relationships and good compliance who wore the FR-III appliance full-time for an average of 2.5 years and then part-time in retention for 3 years, there was significantly enhanced change over controls in maxillary size and position. There was improved mandibular position combined with more lingual lower incisor bodily position, so the patients had more overjet. This held up at the long-term follow-up over 6 years after active treatment.[40]

The available data from most other studies, however, indicate little true forward movement of the upper jaw.[41] Instead, most of the improvement is from dental changes. The appliance allows the maxillary molars to erupt and move mesially while holding the lower molars in place vertically and anteroposteriorly. The appliance tips the maxillary anterior teeth facially and retracts the mandibular anterior teeth (Fig. 13.18). Rotation of the occlusal plane as the upper molars erupt more than the lowers also contributes to a change from a class III to a class I molar relationship (Fig. 13.19).

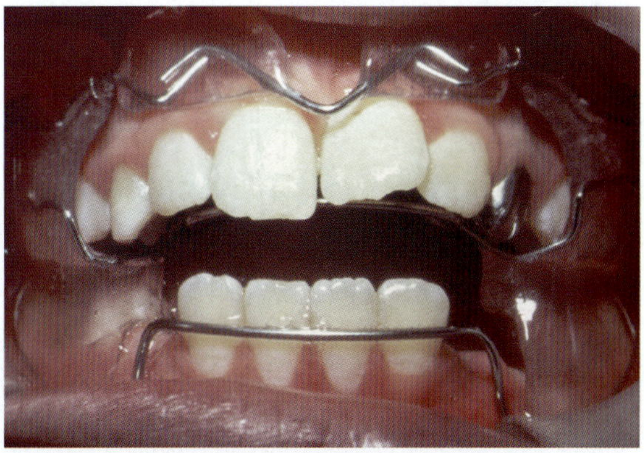

• **Fig. 13.17** The FR-III appliance stretches the soft tissue at the base of the upper lip, attempting to stimulate forward growth of the maxilla by stretching the maxillary periosteum while maintaining the mandible in its most retruded position. The vertical opening is used to enhance downward and forward eruption of maxillary posterior teeth.

In addition, if a functional appliance of any type rotates the chin down and back, the class III relationship will improve because of the mandibular rotation, not an effect on the maxilla, and the face will lengthen. In short, functional appliance treatment, even with the use of upper lip pads, has little or no effect on maxillary deficiency and, if considered, should be used only in mild cases. If this appliance is used, there are long treatment and retention periods that require excellent compliance to maintain limited changes.

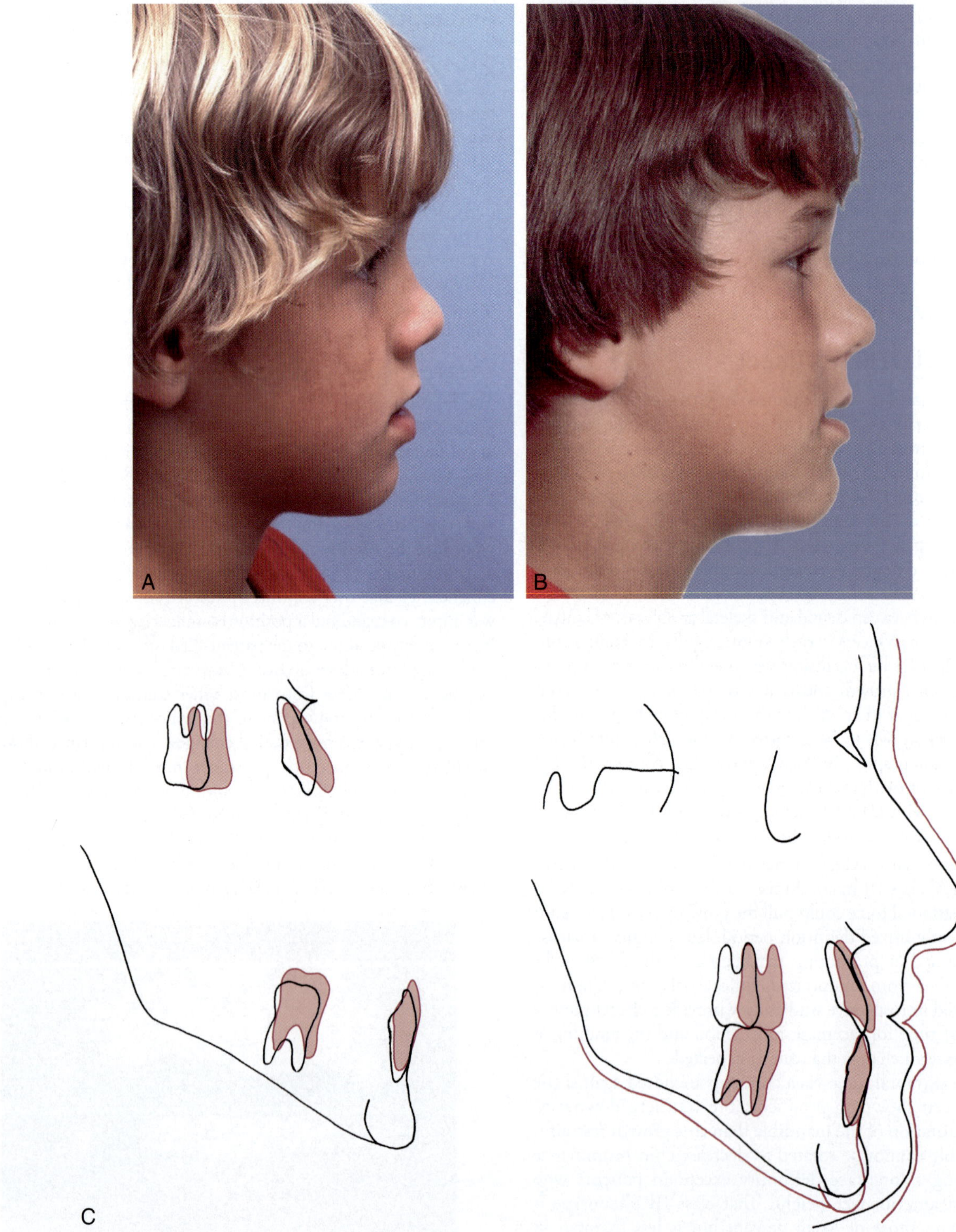

• **Fig. 13.18** Response to a FR-III functional appliance. (A) Pretreatment profile. (B) Posttreatment profile. (C) Cephalometric superimpositions. Note in the cranial base superimposition that the mandible rotated inferiorly and posteriorly to a less prominent position. The maxillary incisors moved facially while there was lower incisor eruption, but there was little if any differential forward growth of the maxilla. In essence, the treatment traded increased face height for decreased chin prominence.

Reverse-Pull Headgear (Facemask)

Dental Anchorage

After Delaire's demonstration that at an early age, a facemask attached to a maxillary splint could move the maxilla forward by inducing growth at the maxillary sutures, this approach to maxillary deficiency became popular in the late 20th century (Fig. 13.20). The age of the patient is a critical variable. It is easier and more effective to move the maxilla forward at younger ages. Although some recent reports indicate that anteroposterior changes can be produced up to the beginning of adolescence, the chance of true skeletal change appears to decline beyond age 8, but this is the youngest practical age to begin this treatment (see more below). The chance of clinical success begins to decline at ages 10 to 11.[42]

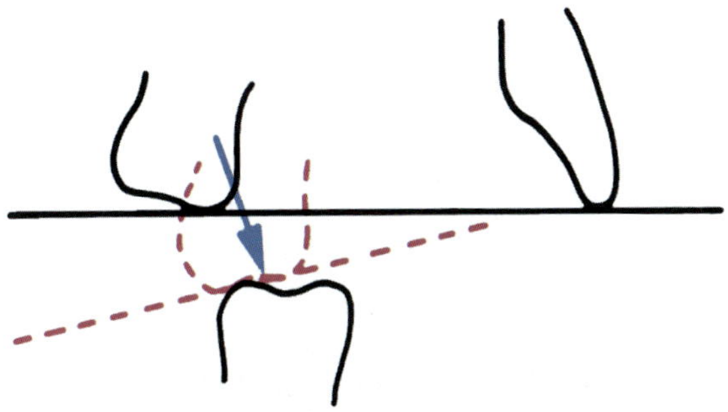

• **Fig. 13.19** To facilitate class III correction, the mesial and vertical eruption of the maxillary molar can be emphasized so that the occlusal plane rotates down posteriorly. This facilitates normal interdigitation of the molars in a class III patient.

When force is applied to the teeth for transmission to the sutures, tooth movement in addition to skeletal change is inevitable. Whatever the method of attachment to the teeth (Fig. 13.21), the appliance must have hooks for attachment to the facemask that are located in the canine-primary molar area above the occlusal plane. This places the force vector nearer the purported center of resistance of the maxilla and limits maxillary rotation (Fig. 13.22).

Facemask treatment is most suited for children with minor-to-moderate skeletal problems, so that the negative overjet is small when the incisors have the correct axial inclination and the patient is biting in centric relation. This type of treatment also is best used in children who have true maxillary deficiency.

In general, it is better to defer maxillary protraction until the permanent first molars and incisors have erupted. The molars can be included in the anchorage unit and the inclination of the incisors can be controlled to affect the overjet and overbite. Many clinicians use protraction with a facemask following or simultaneously with palatal expansion, on the theory that this increases the responsiveness of the sutures above and behind the maxilla to the protraction force—but that is not correct. A randomized clinical trial showed that simultaneous palatal expansion made no difference in the amount of anteroposterior skeletal change,[43] and this has also been shown by a recent retrospective study.[44] If the maxilla is narrow, palatal expansion is quite compatible with maxillary protraction and the expansion device is an effective splint; there is no benefit, however, from expanding the maxilla just to improve the protraction.

It is claimed by some clinicians that aggressive maxillary expansion (Alt-RAMEC previously discussed for maxillary expansion in this chapter) to create greater maxillary mobility significantly facilitates forward movement with traction from a facemask. This

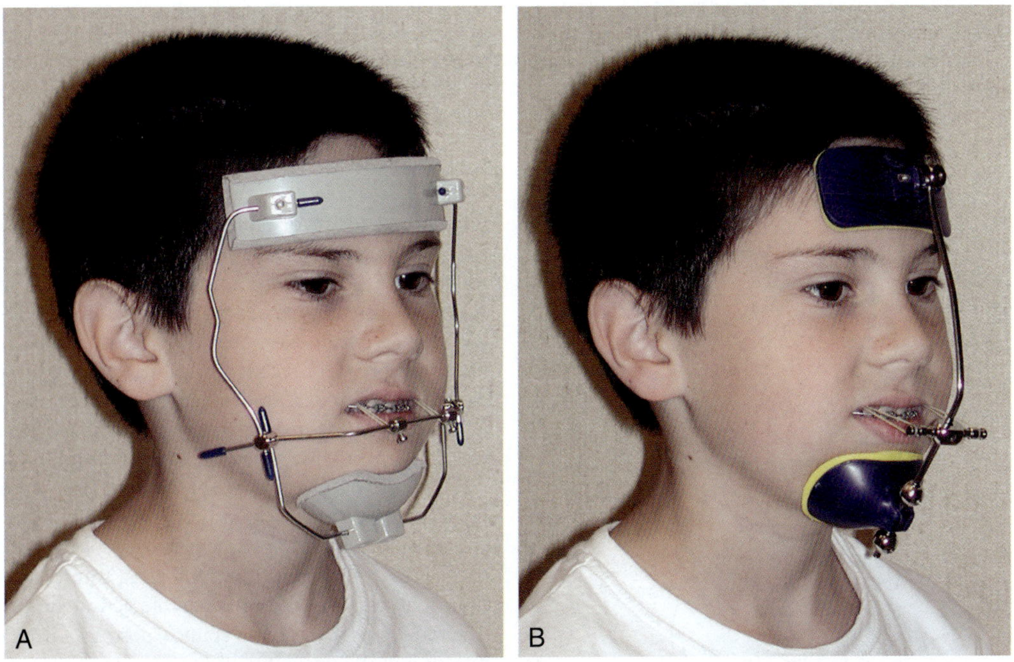

• **Fig. 13.20** (A) This Delaire-type facemask (sometimes called *reverse headgear*) offers good stability when used for maxillary protraction. It is rather bulky and can cause problems with sleeping and wearing eyeglasses. With even modest facial asymmetry, it can appear to be ill-fitted on the face. Note the downward and forward direction of the pull of the elastics. (B) This rail-style facemask provides more comfort during sleeping and is less difficult to adjust. It also can be adjusted to accommodate some vertical mandibular movement. Both types can lead to skin irritation caused by the plastic forehead and chin pads. These occasionally require relining with an adhesive-backed fabric lining for an ideal fit or to reduce soft tissue irritation. Clinical experience indicates that some children will prefer one type over the other, and changing to the other type of facemask can improve cooperation if the child complains.

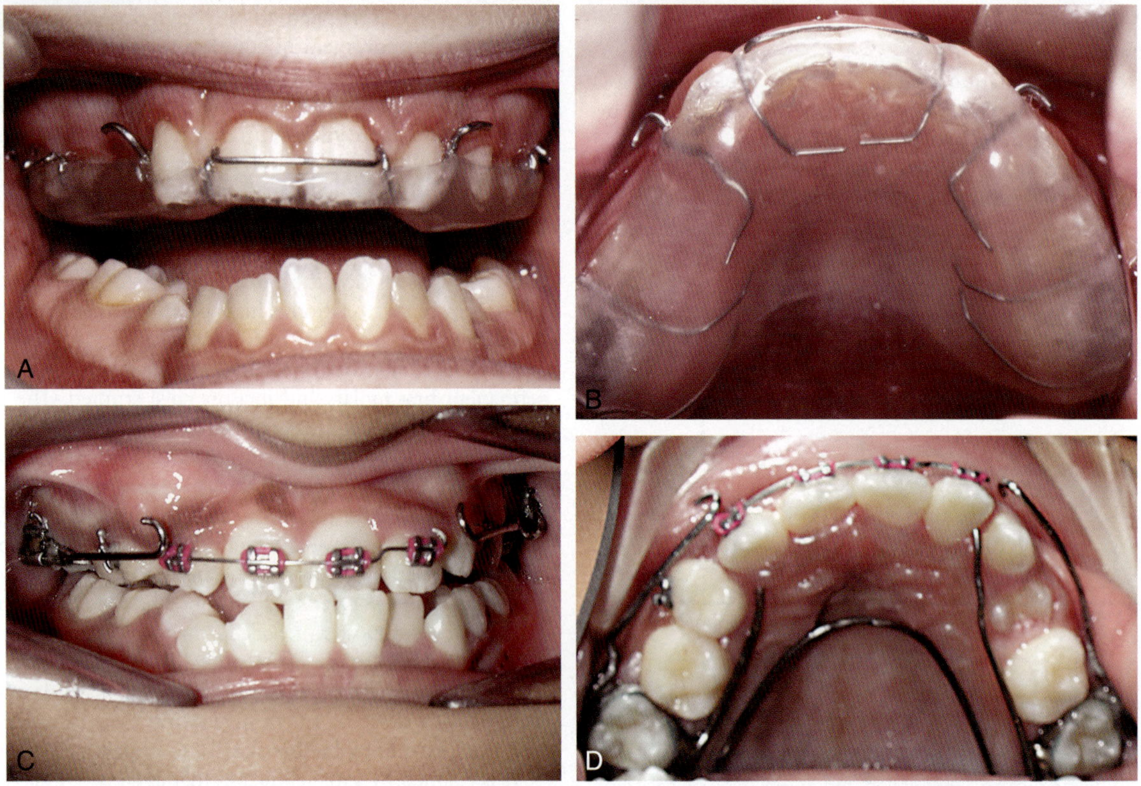

• **Fig. 13.21** A maxillary removable splint is sometimes used to make the upper arch a single unit for maxillary protraction. (A) The splint incorporates hooks in the canine and premolar region for attachment of elastics and should cover the anterior and posterior teeth and occlusal surfaces for best retention (B). Note that the hooks extend gingivally, so the line of force comes closer to the center of resistance of the maxilla. Multiple clasps also aid in retention. If necessary, the splint can be bonded in place, but this causes hygiene problems and should be avoided if possible for long-term use. (C) and (D) A banded expander or wire splint also can be used for delivery of protraction force. It consists of bands on primary and permanent molars or just permanent molars connected by a palatal wire for expansion or transverse stability and hooks on the facial aspect for facemask attachments.

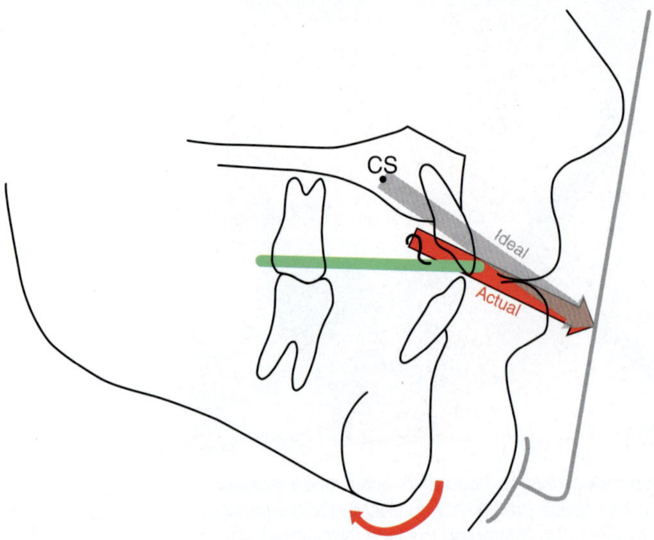

• **Fig. 13.22** With the splint attached to the maxillary arch, the ideal line of force would be directed at the center of resistance (CS) of the maxilla, so the hooks on the splint should be above the occlusal plane. Even so, the actual line of force is likely to be below the center of resistance, so some downward movement of the posterior maxilla and opening of the bite anteriorly can be anticipated.

procedure consists of rapid expansion for a week at 1 mm/day, followed by turning the screw in the opposite direction to constrict for another week, and continuing this over a 7- or 9-week period. It certainly creates maxillary mobility, sometimes extreme mobility, and there seems to have been little consideration of possible adverse effects and risks. A recent clinical trial showed a statistically significant further forward movement with facemask therapy after Alt-RAMEC, but the investigators noted that the greater change was so small (1 mm) that it probably was not clinically significant.[45]

There also are concerns about the effects of compression of the facial sutures during back-and-forth opening and closure of the suture, which are particularly pertinent in view of the recent demonstration that Gli1+ cells within the craniofacial sutures are critical for formation of all craniofacial bones and are activated during injury repair.[46] Their loss is associated with craniosynostosis. Given the minimal if any benefit and the possibility of injury to multiple sutures (which, given the excessive mobility that sometimes occurs, may not be trivial), Alt-RAMEC cannot be recommended.

For most young children, a facemask is as acceptable as conventional headgear. Contouring an adjustable facemask for a comfortable fit on the forehead is not difficult for most children, with either of the primary designs (see Fig. 13.20). Minor facial asymmetry may make the mask-type appliance appear more uneven on the face and cause parental concern. This is easier to overcome with the rail-style facemask. Approximately, 350 to 450 g of force per side is applied for 12 to 14 h/day. Most children with maxillary deficiency are deficient vertically, as well as anteroposteriorly, which means that a slight downward direction of elastic traction between the intraoral attachment and the facemask frame often is desirable, and some downward and backward mandibular rotation improves the jaw relationship. A downward pull would be contraindicated if lower face height is already disproportionately large.

A maxillary-deficient child who cooperates with facemask treatment usually shows a noticeable improvement in facial esthetics as the maxilla moves forward (SNA ~2° and A point 2 mm)[47,48] (Fig. 13.23). Cephalometric superimposition tracings

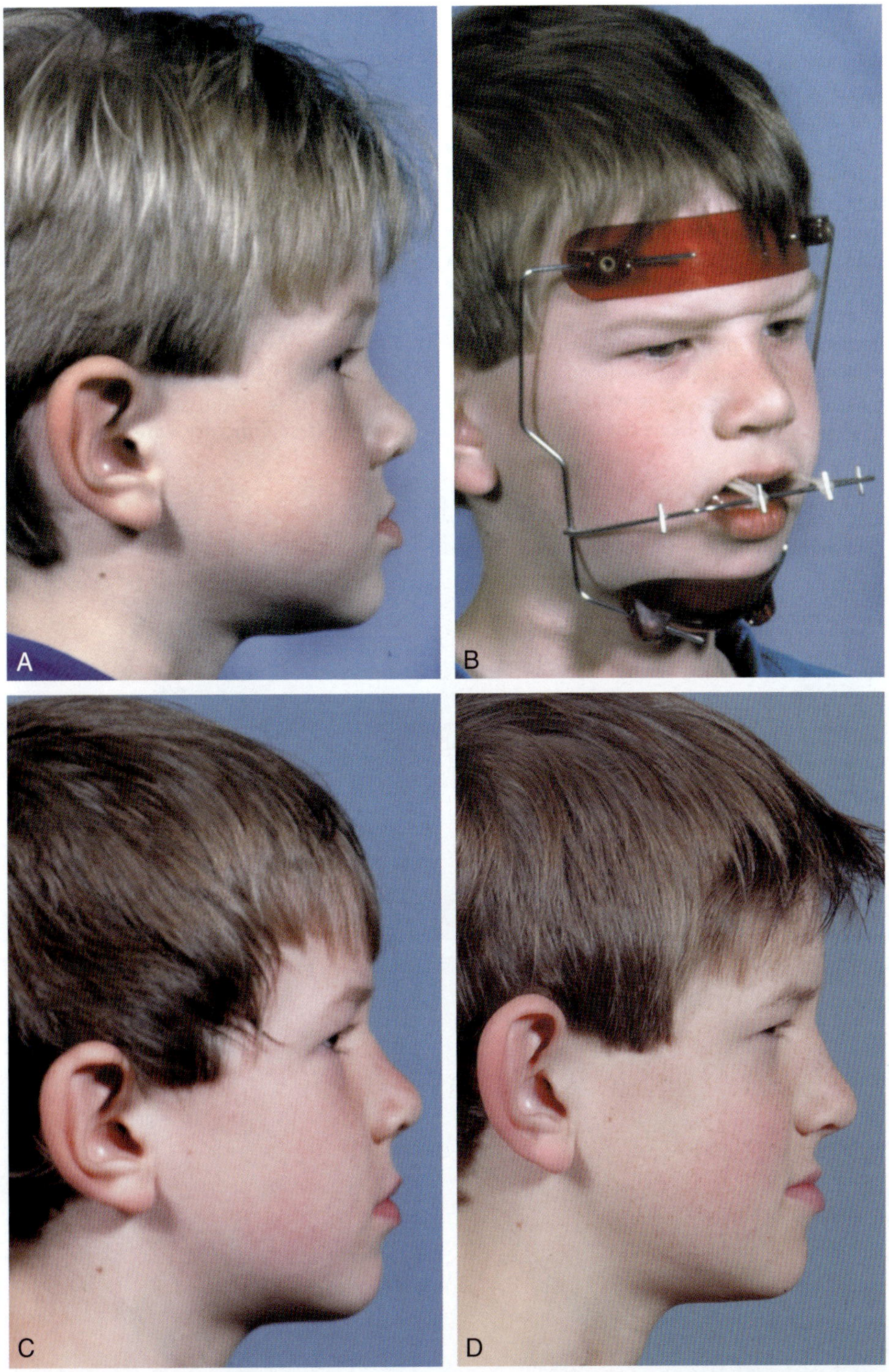

• **Fig. 13.23** If forward traction is applied at an early age, it is possible to produce forward displacement of the maxilla rather than just displacement of teeth. (A) Age 5 years, 2 months before treatment. (B) Age 5 years, 2 months, wearing a Delaire-type facemask. (C) Age 7 years, 10 months, at the time facemask treatment was discontinued. Note the increased fullness of the midface. (D) Age 11 years, 3 months, at the beginning of phase 2 treatment. When facemask treatment is discontinued, there is usually a rebound of mandibular growth similar to what occurred for this patient. Whether surgery eventually will be required will be determined by mandibular growth during and after adolescence. (From Proffit WR, White RP, Sarver DM. *Contemporary Treatment of Dentofacial Deformity*. Mosby; 2003.)

show that backward displacement of the mandibular incisors and forward displacement of the maxillary teeth also typically occur in response to this type of treatment. Following treatment the maxilla may change minimally while the mandible appears to show catch-up growth. Usually some of the class III correction is lost as the mandible outgrows the maxilla. As children come closer to adolescence, mandibular rotation and displacement of maxillary teeth—not forward movement of the maxilla—are the major components of the treatment result.

A key question is how much of the effect is retained after the adolescent growth spurt. If the mandible grows forward during adolescence and the maxilla doesn't keep pace, orthognathic surgery might still be necessary although the jaw discrepancy was largely corrected before adolescence. Several studies have looked at long-term outcomes of facemask therapy to dental anchorage, and most came to a remarkably similar conclusion: In patients who initially responded well, there is a 25% to 33% chance 8 years later of recurrence of anterior crossbite because of excessive mandibular growth, not because the maxilla relapsed, and most of the patients who experienced this needed orthognathic surgery.[42] Knowing that, how do you deal with informed consent for preadolescent facemask therapy? The message is straightforward: "If we do this treatment, your child is very likely to have a short-term improvement, and there is about a 75% chance of long-term success; but that also means there is about one chance in four that surgery still will be needed later." The parents need to understand that fact to have a full picture when signing informed consent.

Facemask Traction to Skeletal Anchorage

Clearly, a major negative side effect of conventional maxillary protraction is tooth movement, or dental side effects that detracts from the skeletal change. Mini-implants (TADs) and miniplates with bone screws are now readily available as temporary skeletal anchorage for maxillary protraction. Single alveolar bone screws are not adequate, but TADs or bone screws can support other appliances such as maxillary expanders or miniplates.

In 9 to 10 year olds, when TAD-supported RPE devices were compared to tooth-borne RPE both with facemasks, the movement of A point was similar at 1.5 mm, but the maxillary incisor changes and vertical skeletal and dental changes were decreased in the TAD-supported patients.[49] TAD-anchored facemasks appear to have less dentoalveolar effect. When miniplates were used in 11 to 12 years old with a facemask, a time when the bone is more dense and able to retain the screws better, the change at A point is likely to be 3 mm to 5 mm of anterior change (Fig. 13.24). The greatest difficulty with this approach is that miniplates on

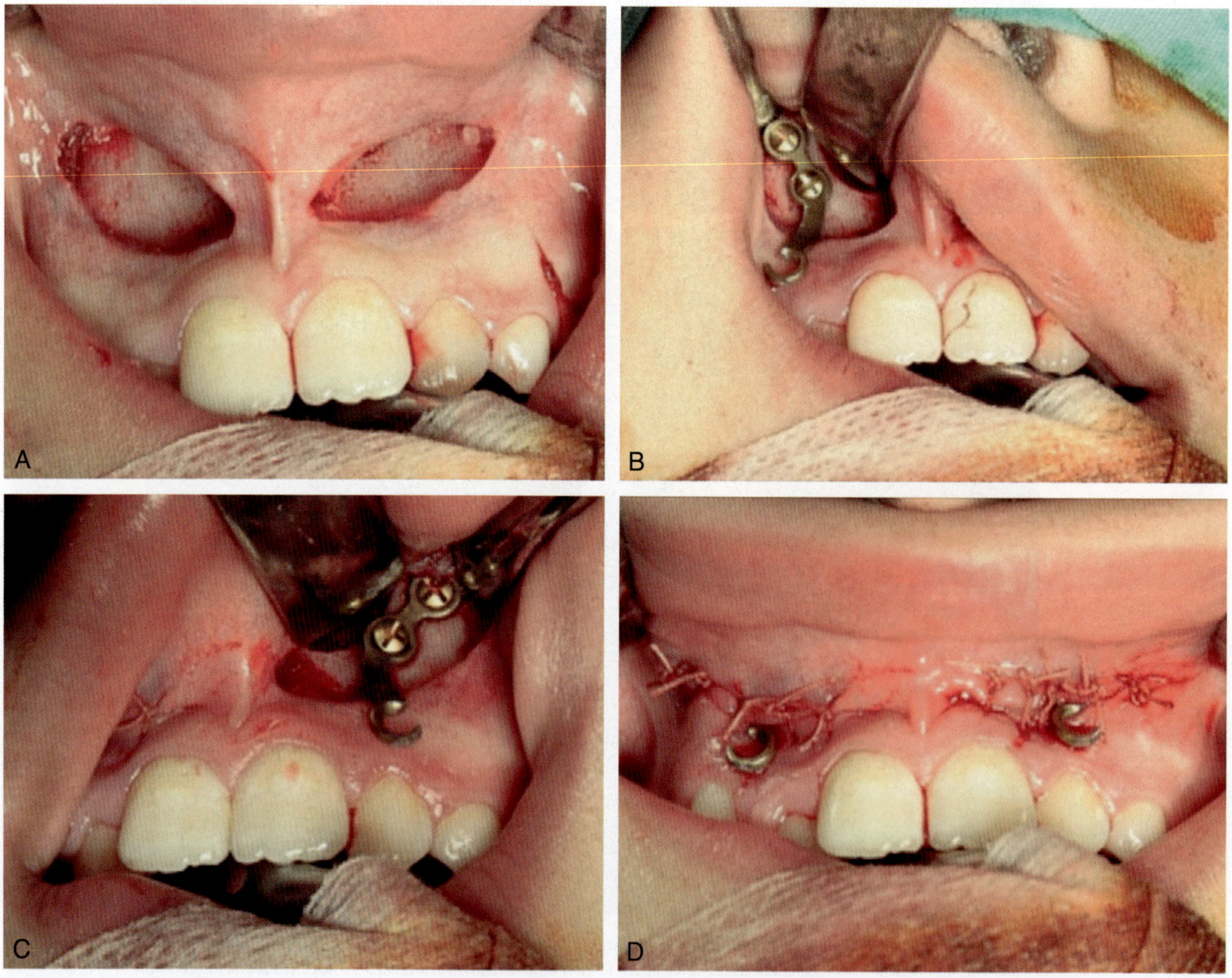

• **Fig. 13.24** Skeletal anchorage for attachment of a facemask for maxillary protraction. (A) Exposure of the anterior surface of the maxilla. (B and C) Placement of a miniplate held by with two screws. (D) Attachments for the facemask extending into the anterior vestibule. (From Sar C, Sahinoğlu Z, Özçirpici AA, Uçkan S. Dentofacial effects of skeletal anchored treatment modalities for the correction of maxillary retrognathia. *Am J Orthod Dentofacial Orthop*. 2014;145:41–54.)

the anterior surface of the maxilla require surgery for placement and removal. Results show a positive change at A point and that dental changes are reduced compared to tooth-borne appliances.

Class III Elastics to Maxillary and Mandibular Miniplates

The most effective approach to protraction of the maxilla is class III elastics between bone-supported miniplates at the base of the zygoma above the maxillary molars and the anterolateral surface of the mandible, so that light force is delivered to the jaws rather than the teeth. This method was introduced by De Clerck and coworkers in 2010[50] and has been studied extensively since then.

Sequence and Timing of Treatment

The first step is placement of the bone anchors, with a three-screw plate at the base of the zygomatic arch and a two-screw plate on the anterolateral surface of the mandible (Fig. 13.25). This requires reflection of a flap and placement of the miniplate to follow the curving surface of the bone. It is technique-sensitive and is best done by a surgeon with training and experience in doing this.[51] To reduce the risk of infection at the implant site, it is important that the emergence of the intraoral connector into the mouth is just below the upper extent of attached gingiva rather than through mucosa, and the connector should be both smooth and round to minimize soft tissue irritation, if possible.

In the timing of treatment, two related factors are important. First, adequate bone density to retain the screws does not develop until approximately age 11; second, the mandibular bone plates should not be inserted until the permanent mandibular canines have erupted, which should not be a problem because they usually erupt at approximately 9 years of age. This means treatment with this method cannot begin until the patient is already too old for a good response to facemask therapy—but it also means that now there is a way to obtain excellent maxillary protraction for patients who are too old for facemask therapy. With the skeletally anchored class III elastics, a favorable growth response can be obtained throughout the adolescent growth spurt, so treatment for about 1 year between the ages 12 and 14 is the best plan.

It was once thought that higher force would be needed for moving bones than for moving teeth, but with the nearly continuous class III elastics, this is not correct. Only light force is needed to obtain the desired growth modification (initial force of 100 g with a final force of 175 g; maximum force level is 200 g). With the miniplate anchorage, stability is better if elastic wear begins within 2 weeks of placement of miniplates. Steady force against the anchors is tolerated better than heavier discontinuous force, so patients should avoid intermittent finger or tongue pressure against the miniplates.

In typical treatment with this method, intermaxillary traction is maintained for about 12 months, which is almost always enough time to correct the jaw discrepancy. This is demonstrated by an average maxillary A point anterior movement of 3.7 mm and mandibular retraction of 2.7 mm accompanied by mandibular bending. The bending occurred by backward movement of the condyles and ramus along with a smaller gonial angle. A second phase of treatment with a fixed orthodontic appliance follows. In these maxillary-deficient patients, often there is insufficient space for the maxillary canines, and because of the forward growth of the maxilla, a class III or class I molar occlusion is likely to be transformed into a near-class II or class II relationship. The same zygomatic anchors used for growth modification can be used to distalize the maxillary posterior teeth, opening space for the canines and completing nonextraction treatment (Fig. 13.26).[52] It is possible that after debonding, even if this is toward the end of adolescence, some additional growth in the class III pattern can occur. For that reason, it is wise not to remove the miniplates for another 6 to 12 months (or longer if mandibular growth continues) so that additional elastic wear can be used if needed. Often, elastic wear can be continued at night time for retention through growth, with removal of the plates at the same time as wisdom tooth removal at an older age.

Comparison With Facemask and Dental Anchorage

How do these results compare with facemask treatment? In a comparison of facemask patients treated at the University of Michigan using dental anchorage with a group treated with class

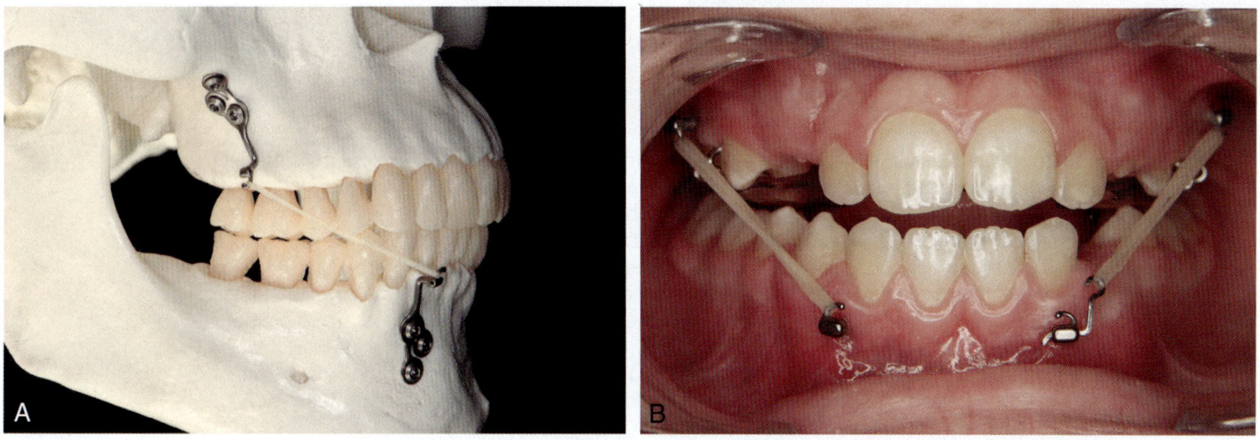

• **Fig. 13.25** (A) Y-shaped miniplates on a skull, to show where they are placed high on the posterior maxilla at the base of the zygomatic arch and on the mandible mesial to the mandibular canines. (B) A maxillary-deficient child wearing class III elastics to an earlier version of the mandibular miniplates that did not have an upward projection for the elastic hook. An auxiliary 21 × 25 archwire in the tube that penetrated the gingiva allowed adjustment of the position of the attachment for the elastic on the left side so that it did not press against the soft tissue. Being able to move the point to which force is applied, of course, is one of the advantages of miniplates.

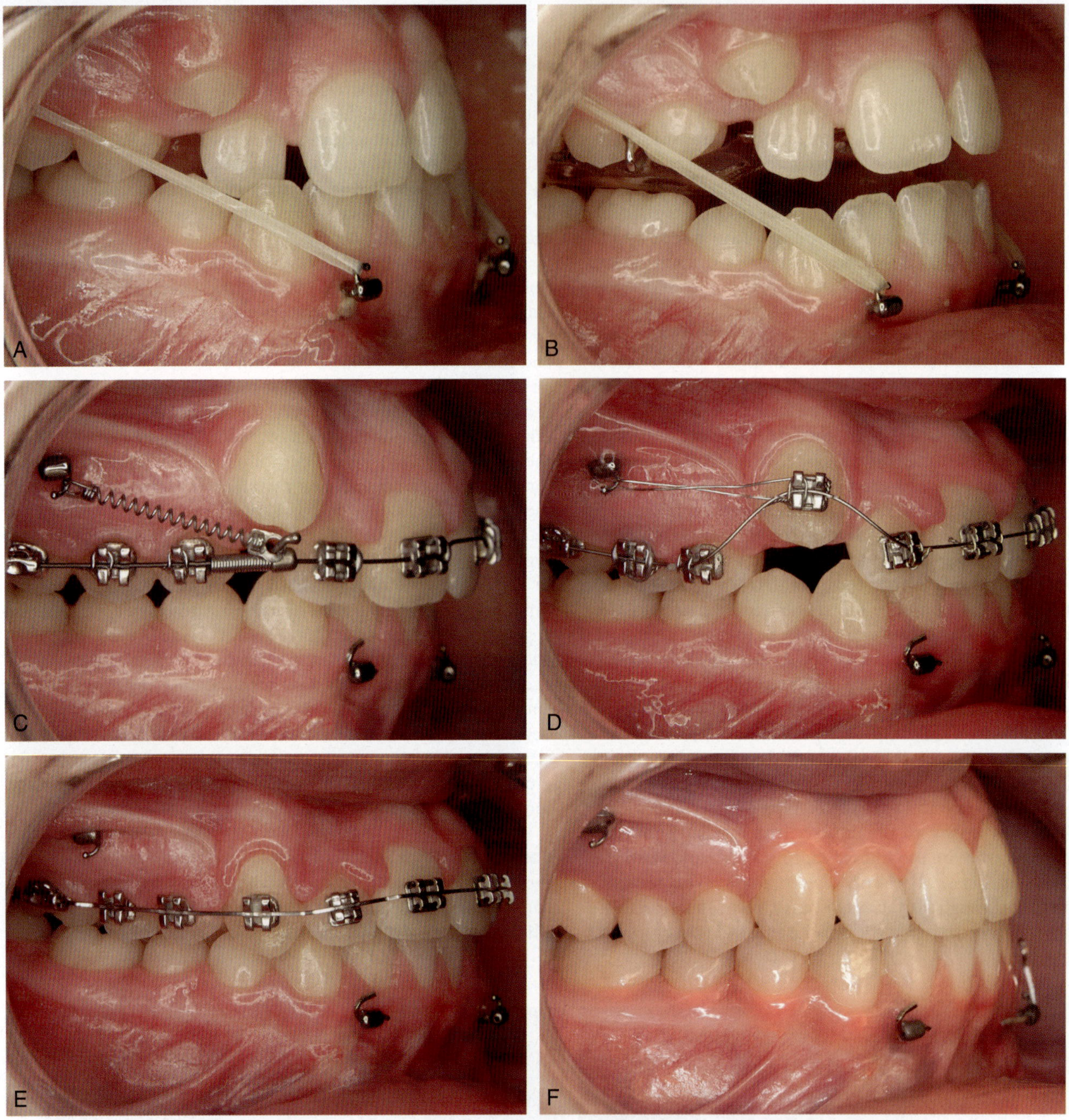

• **Fig. 13.26** In typical treatment of class III problems with a major component of skeletal maxillary deficiency, anterior crossbite is likely to be present initially, even in children in whom some compensatory lingual tipping of mandibular incisors has occurred, and blocked-out maxillary canines also are present. (A) Start of treatment: Note the lateral incisor in crossbite and position of the maxillary canine. (B) Use of a biteplate to unlock the incisors, with use of about 6 ounces (180 g) of elastic force full-time. (C) to (F) Force from the maxillary implant being used for distalization of the maxillary posterior teeth, making room for the canine and bringing it posteriorly into the occlusion, and end of treatment. This method avoids premolar extraction and places the first molars in normal occlusion but requires extraction of the maxillary third (or sometimes) second molars. (From De Clerck H, Proffit WR. Growth modification of the face: a current perspective with emphasis on Class III treatment. *Am J Orthod Dentofacial Orthop*. 2015;148:37–46.)

III elastics and miniplates in Brussels and at the University of North Carolina,[53] the data were as follows:

- Facemask patients were younger; mean age at start of treatment was 8 years 3 months versus 11 years 10 months for class III elastics and miniplates.
- Force with facemask was twice as large: 300 to 500 versus 150 to 200 g.
- On average, there was 2 to 3 mm more movement of the maxilla with class III elastics and miniplates.
- Midface changes were not seen with facemask treatment but occurred in 32% of the elastics group (discussed in detail later).

In a comparison of skeletally anchored facemask treatment (data from Sar et al.)[54] versus the same group of patients with class III elastics and miniplates:

- The facemask patients were younger, but the mean age at start of treatment was 10 years 9 months, more than a year older than the Michigan group who had dental anchorage. That reflects the necessity to wait for adequate bone density before beginning traction against the maxillary anterior bone plates, and more recent patients from the same group were 11 years 9 months at the beginning.
- The data showed that on average there was about 2.3 mm of maxillary anterior movement in the skeletally anchored facemask group or 40% more change with the elastics, and about the same amount of change with the skeletally anchored facemask as with the dentally anchored Michigan group.

In a later report,[55] the Sar group reported about 3.1 mm of advancement with facemask to skeletal anchorage, so the miniplates and elastics provided 20% more anterior change.

Facial Outcomes

The facial changes that accompany this treatment skeletal anchorage and intraoral elastics were greater in magnitude and extended into the midface—but there was considerable variation in the response. The best way to appreciate this is to view Fig. 13.27, with three-dimensional (3D) superimpositions showing the treatment change in 25 consecutive patients treated by De Clerck in Brussels.[56]

In Fig. 13.27, the direction of change is shown by the color of various areas, and the amount of change is shown by the intensity of the color. Begin your examination of this figure by looking at the maxillary and midface changes. Thirty-two percent showed more than 4 mm of forward movement of the midface as well as maxillary change. This appears to occur because sutures above and behind the maxilla are affected by the light consistent force (Fig. 13.28) with opening of the zygomaticomaxillary and zygomaticofrontal sutures. These sutures were affected in all the patients who showed midface advancement.

Forty-eight percent of the patients had smaller amounts of movement of the maxilla and midface, some of just the maxilla but others with a smaller amount of midface change as well. Eighty percent of this group of patients had a favorable response, and 32% had a highly favorable response.

Finally, note the patients whose mandible grew forward during treatment. These are growing children, and you would expect at least some forward mandibular growth along with the enhanced maxillary growth. But forward movement of the chin happened in only 20% of the patients. In short, what did not happen to the position of the chin in most of those with maxillary growth also is significant.

One thing that is not seen in the 3D aforementioned superimpositions is likely to be noted clinically: When the maxilla is moved forward, a wider part of the maxillary arch comes into occlusion with the mandibular arch, so just the change in the jaw relationship reduces the magnitude of a posterior crossbite. This increases the chance that a posterior crossbite can be managed with archwire expansion. If the crossbite is severe enough that skeletal expansion by opening the midpalatal suture will be required, this should be deferred until the A-P jaw relationship is corrected.

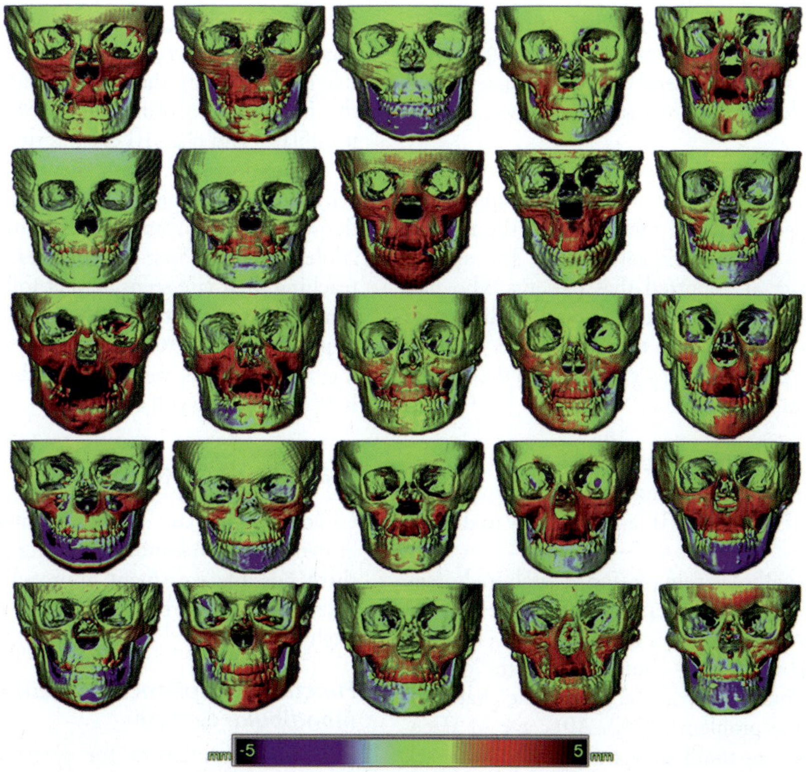

• **Fig. 13.27** Color map cranial base superimposition of 25 consecutive patients treated in Brussels by De Clerck and analyzed at the University of North Carolina by using the method developed by Cevidanes. The red and blue colors show the direction of movement (*red* = forward, out of the screen toward you; *blue* = backward), and the intensity of the color indicates the amount of movement (*dark red or blue* = >4 mm, *lighter red or blue* = 2–4 mm).

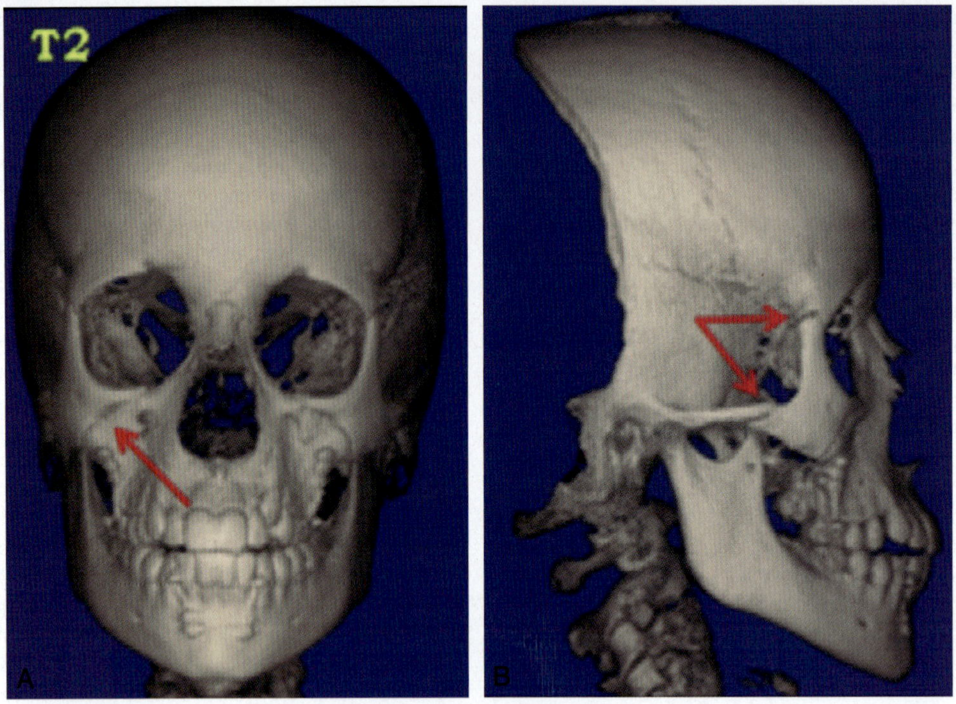

• **Fig. 13.28** Forward movement of the midface had not been seen previously with class III traction. The mechanism is opening of the zygomaticomaxillary (A) and zygomaticofrontal (B) sutures, which occurs in about one-third of patients with class III elastics to miniplates.

Several other reports of growth changes with posterior maxillary miniplates to mandibular anterior miniplates have appeared, many of which used a lower attachment to the maxilla. With a similar protocol to De Clerck's, the reported outcomes also are similar.[57]

Given the current emphasis on a possible role for orthodontics in prevention or management of obstructive sleep apnea (see Chapter 7), could orthopedic forward movement of the maxilla facilitate air flow through the pharyngeal airway? The answer seems to be *no*. Nguyen et al. reported that patients who had responded to miniplates and class III elastics showed no difference in airway diameter at the "choke point" that determines air flow. The conclusion: Maxillary protraction does no harm to the airway, but sleep apnea is not an indication for it.[58]

Summary of Maxillary Protraction Experience

The only class III functional appliance that attempts to overcome maxillary deficiency is the Frankel FR-III, and its ability to do that is limited.

Maxillary protraction with a facemask and dental anchorage at an early age (8–10, after first molars and incisors have erupted but before adolescence) usually produces clinical improvement in a patient with class III malocclusion—but the more the growth pattern is excessive mandibular growth, the greater the chance of long-term recurrence of the problem (25%). After age 11, facemask therapy largely produces tooth movement and down-back mandibular rotation unless skeletal anchorage is used. In the 11- to 12-year-old period, facemasks and skeletal anchorage can produce good forward and limited dental and vertical changes, but unless it is attached to a maxillary appliance supported by TADS, surgery will be required to attach to miniplates.

Class III elastics between bone anchors at the base of the zygoma and the anterior surface of the mandible are more effective in protracting the maxilla than facemask therapy, even when the facemask traction is to bone anchors on the maxilla. The miniplates and class III elastics treatment cannot be done as early as conventional facemask therapy but is effective during adolescent growth. That is a disadvantage if preadolescent treatment is desired, but an advantage if treatment was not sought until early adolescence. The first patients treated during adolescence now are reaching their late teens, and at follow up it appears the maxillary change is stable with some anterior mandibular change, resulting in potentially a 10% to 15% failure rate. These data are encouraging, and with this method mandibular as well as maxillary growth is affected, as we will see later.

Mandibular Excess

Children who have class III malocclusion because of excessive growth of the mandible are extremely difficult to treat. There are three possible treatment approaches: class III functional appliances, extraoral force to a chin cup, and class III elastics to skeletal anchors.

Functional Appliances in Treatment of Excessive Mandibular Growth

Functional appliances for patients with excessive mandibular growth make no pretense of restraining mandibular growth. They are designed to rotate the mandible down and back and guide the eruption of the teeth so that the upper posterior teeth erupt down and forward while eruption of lower teeth is restrained. This rotates the occlusal plane in the direction that favors correction of a class III molar relationship (see Fig. 13.19). These appliances also tip the mandibular incisors lingually and the maxillary incisors facially, introducing an element of dental camouflage for the skeletal discrepancy.

To produce the working bite for a class III functional appliance, the steps in preparation of the wax bite, practice for the patient, and use of a guide to determine the correct vertical position are identical to the procedure for patients with class II problems (discussed in detail in Chapter 14). However, the working bite itself is significantly different: The mandible is rotated open on its hinge axis but is not advanced. This type of bite is easy to obtain because light force can be placed on each side of the mandible to guide the mandible and retrude it.

How far the mandible is rotated open depends on the type of appliance and the need to interpose bite blocks and occlusal stops between the teeth to limit eruption. The general guideline is that the mandible should be rotated at least 3 and not more than 5 to 6 mm beyond its postural rest position. If this is not enough or would produce excessive anterior face height, the problem is too severe for functional appliance treatment. As we have noted previously, class III functional appliance treatment is applicable only to patients in whom a large and prominent mandible is combined with vertical maxillary deficiency, so that they have both mandibular excess and short anterior face height.

Chin-Cup Appliances: Restraint of Mandibular Growth?

In theory, extraoral force directed against the mandibular condyle would restrain growth at that location, but there is little evidence that this occurs in humans (see Chapter 7). What chin-cup therapy does accomplish is a change in the direction of mandibular growth, rotating the chin down and back, which makes it less prominent but increases anterior face height. The data seem to indicate a transitory restraint of growth that is likely to be overwhelmed by subsequent growth. In essence, the treatment becomes a trade-off between decreasing the anteroposterior prominence of the chin and increasing face height. In addition, lingual tipping of the lower incisors often occurs because the appliance presses on the lower lip and dentition (Fig. 13.29), which often is undesirable.

For chin-cup treatment, a hard plastic cup fitted to a cast of the patient's chin or a soft cup made from an athletic helmet chinstrap can be used. The more the chin cup or strap migrates up toward the lower lip during appliance wear, the more lingual movement of the lower incisors will be produced, so soft cups produce more incisor uprighting than hard ones. The headcap that includes the spring mechanism can be the same one used for high-pull headgear. It is adjusted in the same manner as the headgear. A persistent recommendation through the years has been a force of approximately 16 ounces/side aimed directly at the head of the condyle, on the theory that this would reduce growth. Once it is accepted that mandibular rotation, not growth inhibition, is the major treatment effect, lighter force oriented to produce greater rotation makes more sense (Fig. 13.30). One concern about chin-cup treatment always has been the possibility that it could create temporomandibular dysfunction problems. A recent systematic review of the literature indicates that this is not a problem, especially if very heavy force is avoided.[59]

In essence, chin-cup therapy does the same thing as a class III functional appliance, but offers at least a slim chance of some growth inhibition. For children with a large mandible, chin-cup treatment is essentially transient camouflage. For that reason, it has limited application.

Class III Elastics to Skeletal Anchors

The use of class III elastics to skeletal anchors as an effective way of producing maxillary protraction was discussed earlier—but this force system also affects the mandible and may eventually provide a way to restrain mandibular growth.[60] Let's begin our evaluation of the mandibular effects by again examining the consecutive cases shown in Fig. 13.26. Four striking effects on the mandible can be observed:

- In 12% of the patients, the chin moved backward 4 to 5 mm. At first that seems anatomically impossible, but it can (and did)

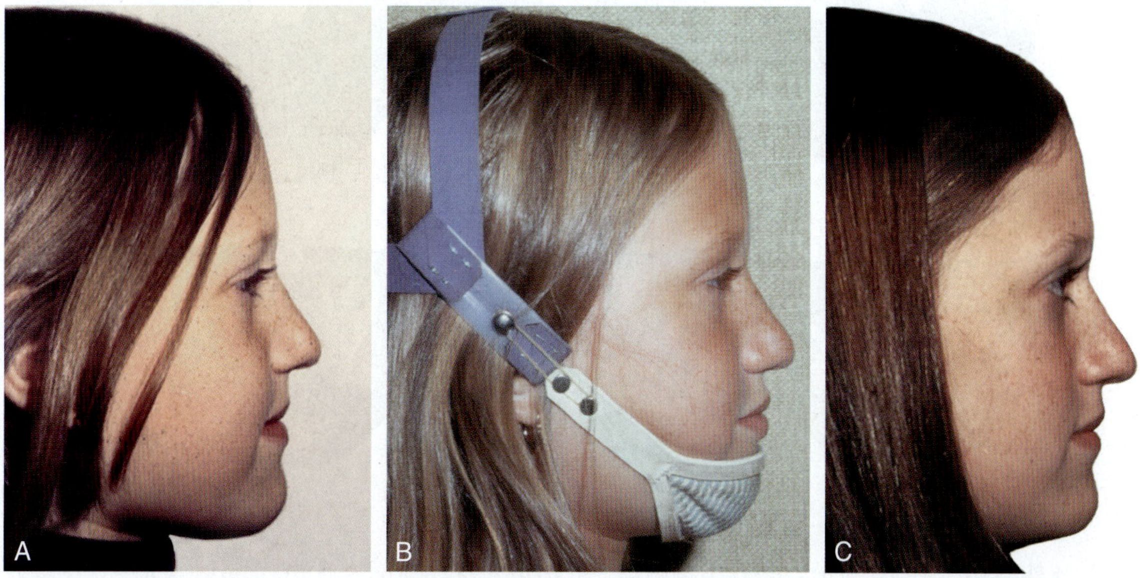

• **Fig. 13.29** A typical response to chin-cup treatment. (A) Pretreatment profile, (B) chin-cup placement, (C) posttreatment profile. This treatment reduces mandibular protrusion primarily by increasing anterior face height, very similar to the effect of class III functional appliances.

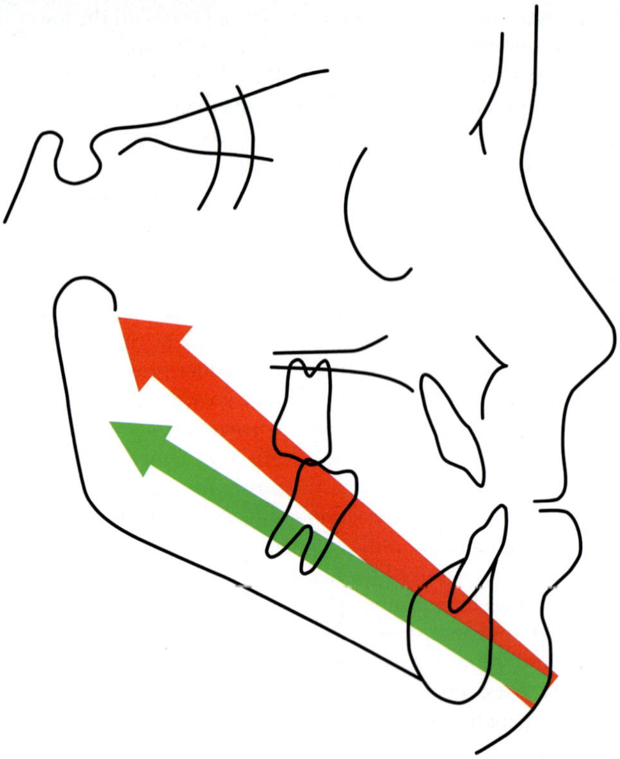

• **Fig. 13.30** The traditional view of chin-cup treatment was that heavy force aimed directly at the condyles *(red line)* would correct excessive mandibular growth by inhibiting condylar growth. Now that downward and backward rotation of the mandible is the usual treatment objective, directing a lighter force below the condyles *(green line)* is more tolerable to patients and equally effective. Heavy force with chin cups is no longer recommended.

happen by a combination of two things: redirection of vertical growth at the condylar fossa and modeling of both the fossa and condylar head.

- It is important to remember that the point of articulation of the mandible with the temporal bone does grow downward relative to the cranial base. Usually the direction of growth is straight down, and growth in length of the mandible results in projection of the chin. Sometimes the direction of growth has a backward component. This is terribly frustrating when it happens in a skeletal class II patient because the chin is projected down and not forward (see Fig. 4.10), but it compensates for growth in length of the mandible in a class III patient.
- With the 3D superimpositions, it is possible to remove the other structures and view the jaws from the rear (Fig. 13.31). You can visualize backward movement of the condyles in two of these patients and see that in one the chin moved back, and in the other it stayed in the same place. Backward repositioning of the joint contributed to this.
- Modeling of the condyles goes on throughout life, is part of the response to orthognathic surgery, and occurs during growth modification. Modeling on the interior surface of the condylar fossa also occurs in some patients.
- Significant forward movement of the mandible, which would have been expected in this adolescent group, did not occur in 80% of these patients. What did occur in most of them was what you see in more detail in Fig. 13.32: an increase in mandibular length, with the chin staying where it was (green) and mandibular growth expressed as backward movement of the condyles (red). In short, there was a component of inhibition of mandibular growth in far more patients than those who showed backward movement of the chin.
- An unusual pattern of mandibular modeling, with slight backward movement of the condyles and ramus and a decrease

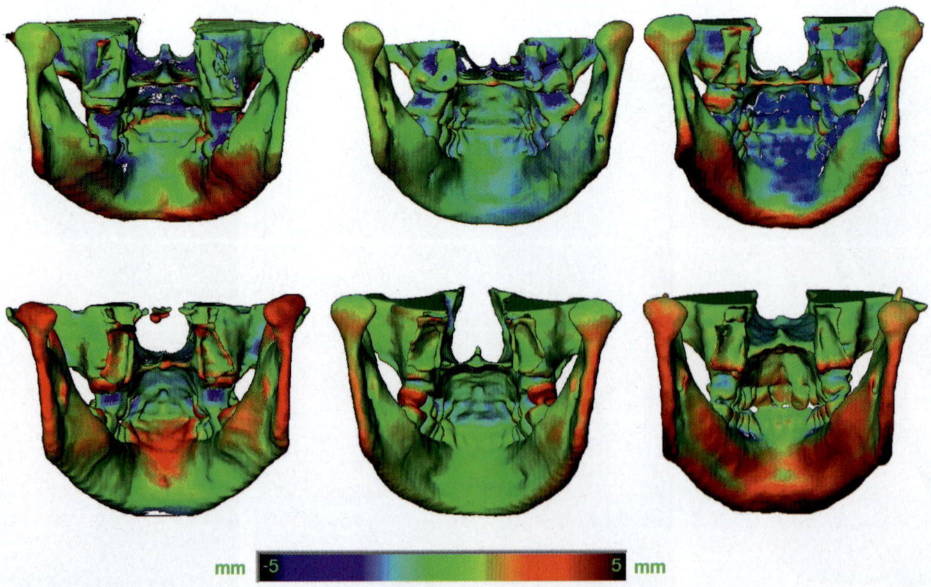

• **Fig. 13.31** With the three-dimensional cranial base superimpositions, it is possible to remove the structures behind the mandibular condyles and observe their direction of change. The red color again indicates movement out of the screen toward you—and what you see is that in one of these six patients, the condyles moved backward more than 4 mm, and in another there was 2–4 mm of backward movement.

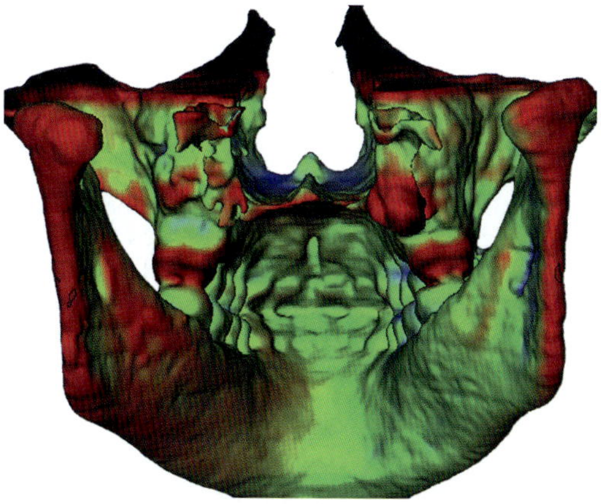

• **Fig. 13.32** In this patient you see another unexpected finding with the three-dimensional superimpositions, a lack of forward growth of the chin in a patient in whom forward growth of the mandible would be expected. As you see here, the chin remained in its previous position (*green* = no growth) while the ramus and condylar processes moved back. A lack of forward projection of the chin was seen in more than 80% of these patients.

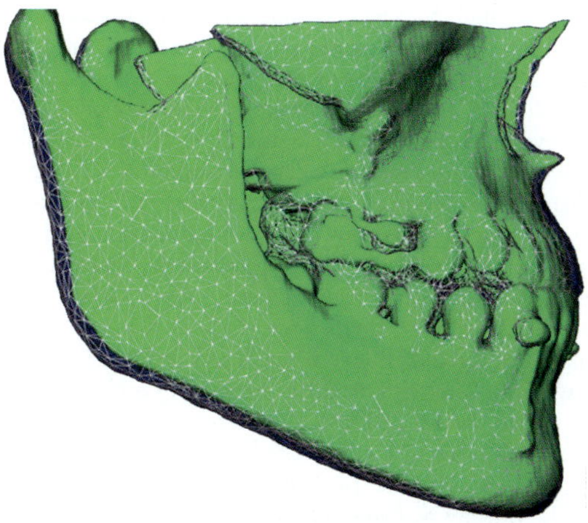

• **Fig. 13.33** This detailed superimposition of the mandibular change in a typical patient is still another unexpected finding: what amounts to a bending of the mandible at the gonial angle, so the chin is not projected forward as much as it would have been if the inclination of the ramus to the mandibular body had not been changed by the pattern of modeling with the consistent class III elastic force.

in the gonial angle and mandibular plane angle (Fig. 13.33), also occurred in the majority of the patients—a bending of the mandible that would limit forward movement of the chin although growth was occurring.[61]

Does this pattern of change mean that the De Clerck method could be used as much to inhibit mandibular growth as facilitate maxillary growth? Perhaps—but it remains true that the most likely and largest change in treatment was stimulation of forward growth of the maxilla, and that would not be desired in treatment of true mandibular prognathism. As more data for outcomes in relation to patient characteristics become available, it should be possible to better predict whether treatment of an individual will have a greater or lesser effect on mandibular growth.

Summary

Transverse deficiencies can be treated in the mixed dentition until early adult years. Different appliances and different force levels are required moving from the tooth-supported lingual arch to the tooth-supported RPE and finally to the Mini-implant (TAD)-supported expander.

Correction of maxillary A-P deficiency also follows a similar pattern. In the mixed dentition, functional appliances offer little help, but tooth-supported facemasks can be effective. Near 11 years of age, skeletal anchorage and facemasks can be effective. Later, skeletal anchorage and light class III elastics can make changes.

Controlling excessive mandibular growth remains one of the greatest challenge in orthodontics. Mandibular functional appliances offer no possibility of inhibiting the excessive growth. They are capable only of downward-backward rotation of the mandible, which risks creating a long-face problem.

Backward heavy force against the mandible via chin cups attached to high-pull headgear also offers little beyond downward-backward mandibular rotation.

Class III elastics from miniplates at the base of the zygoma to the anterior surface of the mandible now have been shown to significantly change the pattern of mandibular growth. This includes a lack of forward growth, the possibility of backward movement of the chin, and a reshaping of the mandible with an decrease in the gonial angle—that is, an uprighting of the ramus relative to the body of the mandible. Because most skeletal Class III patients have a component of both maxillary deficiency and mandibular excess, the effect on both jaws is an improvement over changing the growth of just one.

For patients whose problem is primarily excessive mandibular growth, camouflage and orthognathic surgery remain the most helpful treatments, with camouflage having limitations with esthetics and vertical excesses.

References

1. Adkins MD, Nanda RS, Currier GF. Arch perimeter changes on rapid palatal expansion. *Am J Orthod*. 1990;97:10–19.
2. Kilic N, Kiki A, Oktay H. Condylar asymmetry in unilateral posterior crossbite patients. *Am J Orthod Dentofacial Orthop*. 2008;133:382–387.
3. Sandikcioglu M, Hazar S. Skeletal and dental changes after maxillary expansion in the mixed dentition. *Am J Orthod Dentofacial Orthop*. 1997;111:321–327.
4. Melsen B. A histological study of the influence of sutural morphology and skeletal maturation on rapid palatal expansion in children. *Trans Eur Orthod Soc*. 1972;48:499–507.
5. Persson M, Thilander B. Palatal suture closure in man from 15 to 35 years of age. *Am J Orthod*. 1977;72:42–52.
6. Angelieri F, Cevidanes LH, Franchi L, Gonçalves JR, Benavides E, McNamara JA. Jr. Midpalatal suture maturation: classification method for individual assessment before rapid maxillary expansion. *Am J Orthod Dentofacial Orthop*. 2013;144(5):759–769. https://doi.org/10.1016/j.ajodo.2013.04.022.
7. Baccetti T, Franchi L, Cameron CG, McNamara JA. Jr. Treatment timing for rapid maxillary expansion. *Angle Orthod*. 2001;71:343–350.
8. Grünheid T, Larson CE, Larson BE. Midpalatal suture density ratio: a novel predictor of skeletal response to rapid maxillary expansion. *Am J Orthod Dentofacial Orthop*. 2017;151:267–276.
9. Acar YB, Abuhan E. Evaluation of the relationship between midpalatal suture maturation indicators as predictors for surgically-assisted and conventional rapid maxillary expansion. *J*

Craniofac Surg. 2021;32(2):678–681. https://doi.org/10.1097/SCS.0000000000007323.
10. Leonardi R, Sicurezza E, Cutrera A. et al. Changes of circumaxillary sutures in young patients treated with rapid maxillary expansion. *Angle Orthod.* 2011;81:36–41.
11. Agostino P, Ugolini A, Signori A, et al. Orthodontic treatment for posterior crossbites. *Cochrane Database Syst Rev.* 2014;8 Art. No.: CD000979.
12. Petrén S, Bjerklin K, Bondemark L. Stability of unilateral posterior crossbite correction in the mixed dentition: a randomized clinical trial with a 3-year follow-up. *Am J Orthod Dentofacial Orthop.* 2011;139:e73–e81.
13. Chang JY, McNamara Jr JA, Herberger TA. A longitudinal study of skeletal side effects induced by rapid maxillary expansion. *Am J Orthod Dentofacial Orthop.* 1997;112:330–337.
14. Petrén S, Bondemark L, Söderfeldt B. A systematic review concerning early orthodontic treatment of unilateral posterior crossbite. *Angle Orthod.* 2003 Oct;73(5):588–596. https://doi.org/10.1043/0003-.
15. Travassos da Rosa Moreira Bastos R, Nassar Blagitz M, Santos de Castro Aragón M, et al. Periodontal side effects of rapid and slow maxillary expansion: *A systematic review. Angle Orthod.* 2019;89(4):651–660. https://doi.org/10.2319/060218-419.1.
16. Reed N, Ghosh J, Nanda RS. Comparison of treatment outcomes with banded and bonded RPE appliances. *Am J Orthod Dentofacial Orthop.* 1999;116:31–40.
17. Geran RG, McNamara JA, Baccetti T, et al. A prospective long-term study on the effects of rapid maxillary expansion in the early mixed dentition. *Am J Orthod Dentofacial Orthop.* 2006;129:631–640.
18. McNamara JA, Baccetti T, Franchi L, et al. Rapid maxillary expansion followed by fixed appliances: a long-term evaluation of changes in arch dimensions. *Angle Orthod.* 2003;73:344–353.
19. Akkaya S, Lorenzon S, Uçem TT. Comparison of dental arch and arch perimeter changes between bonded rapid and slow maxillary expansion procedures. *Eur J Orthod.* 1998 Jun;20(3):255–261. https://doi.org/10.1093/ejo/20.3.255.
20. Martina R, Cioffi I, Farella M, et al. Transverse changes determined by rapid and slow maxillary expansion--a low-dose CT-based randomized controlled trial. *Orthod Craniofac Res.* 2012 Aug;15(3):159–168. https://doi.org/10.1111/j.1601-6343.2012.01543.
21. Bazargani F, Knode V, Plaksin A, et al. Three-dimensional comparison of tooth-borne and tooth-bone-borne RME appliances: a randomized controlled trial with 5-year follow-up. *Eur J Orthod.* 2023 https://doi.org/10.1093/ejo/cjad024. cjad024.
22. Rutili V, Nieri M, Franceschi D, Pierleoni F, Giuntini V, Franchi L. Comparison of rapid versus slow maxillary expansion on patient-reported outcome measures in growing patients: a systematic review and meta-analysis. *Prog Orthod.* 2022 Dec 12;23(1):47. https://doi.org/10.1186/s40510-022-00440-5.
23. Canan S, Şenışık NE. Comparison of the treatment effects of different rapid maxillary expansion devices on the maxilla and the mandible. Part 1: evaluation of dentoalveolar changes. *Am J Orthod.* 2017;151(6):1125–1138.
24. Lagravère MO, Carey J, Heo G, et al. Transverse, vertical, and anteroposterior changes from bone-anchored maxillary expansion vs traditional rapid maxillary expansion: a randomized clinical trial. *Am J Orthod Dentofacial Orthop.* 2010;137:304.e1–304.e12.
25. Toklu MG, Germec-Cakan D, Tozlu M. Periodontal, dentoalveolar, and skeletal effects of tooth-borne and tooth-bone-borne expansion appliances. *Am J Orthod.* 2015;148(1):97–109.
26. Inchingolo AD, Ferrara I, Viapiano F, et al. Rapid maxillary expansion on the adolescent patient: systematic review and case report. *Children (Basel).* 2022;9(7):1046. https://doi.org/10.3390/children9071046.
27. Jia H, Zhuang L, Zhang N, et al. Comparison of skeletal maxillary transverse deficiency treated by microimplant-assisted rapid palatal expansion and tooth-borne expansion during the post-pubertal growth spurt stage. *Angle Orthod.* 2021;91:36–45. https://doi.org/10.2319/041920-332.1.
28. Yildirim M, Akin M. Comparison of root resorption after bone-borne and tooth-borne rapid maxillary expansion evaluated with the use of microtomography. *Am J Orthod Dentofac. Orthop.* 2019;155:182–190. https://doi.org/10.1016/j.ajodo.2018.03.021.
29. Lagravère MO, Carey J, Heo G, et al. Transverse, vertical, and anteroposterior changes from bone-anchored maxillary expansion vs traditional rapid maxillary expansion: a randomized clinical trial. *Am J Orthod Dentofacial Orthop.* 2010;137:304.e1–304.e12.
30. Hourfar J, Kinzinger GS, Ludwig B, et al. Differential treatment effects of two anchorage systems for rapid maxillary expansion: a retrospective cephalometric study. *J Orofac Orthop.* 2016;77:314–324.
31. Lin L, Ahn HW, Kim SJ, et al. Tooth-borne vs bone-borne rapid maxillary expanders in late adolescence. *Angle Orthod.* 2015;85:253–262.
32. Wilmes B, Ludwig B, Vasudavan S, Nienkemper M, Drescher D. The T-zone: median vs. paramedian insertion of palatal mini-implants. *J Clin Orthod.* 2016;50(9):543–551. PMID: 27809213.
33. Kapetanović A, Theodorou CI, Bergé SJ, et al. Efficacy of miniscrew-assisted rapid palatal expansion (MARPE) in late adolescents and adults: a systematic review and meta-analysis. *Eur J Orthod.* 2021;43:313–323. https://doi.org/10.1093/ejo/cjab005.
34. Bazzani M, Cevidanes LHS, Najla N, et al. Three-dimensional comparison of bone-borne and tooth-bone borne maxillary expansion in young adults with maxillary skeletal deficiency. *Orthod Cranfac Res.* 2022;26:151–162. https://doi.org/10.1111/ocr.12595.
35. Siddhisaributr P, Khlongwanitchakul K, Anuwongnukroh N, Manopatanakul S, Viwattanatipa N. Effectiveness of miniscrew assisted rapid palatal expansion using cone beam computed tomography: a systematic review and metaanalysis. *Korean J Orthod.* 2022;52(3):182–200. https://doi.org/10.4041/kjod21.256.
36. Davidovitch M, Efstathiou S, Sarne O, Vardimon AD. Skeletal and dental response to rapid maxillary expansion with 2- versus 4-band appliances. *Am J Orthod Dentofacial Orthop.* 2005;127:483–492.
37. Liou EJ, Tsai WC. A new protocol for maxillary protraction in cleft patients: repetitive weekly protocol of alternate rapid maxillary expansions and constrictions. *Cleft Palate Craniofac J.* 2005;42:121–127.
38. Yilmaza BS, Kucukkeles N. Skeletal, soft tissue, and airway changes following the alternate maxillary expansions and constrictions protocol. *Angle Orthod.* 2015;85:117–126.
39. Behrents RG, Shelgikar AV, Conley RS, Flores-Mir C, Hans M, Levine M, McNamara JA, Palomo JM, Pliska B, Stockstill JW, Wise J, Murphy S, Nagel NJ, Hittner J. Obstructive sleep apnea and orthodontics: an American Association of Orthodontists White Paper. *Am J Orthod Dentofacial Orthop.* 2019 Jul;156(1):13–28.e1. https://doi.org/10.1016/j.ajodo.2019.04.009. PMID: 31256826.
40. Levin AS, McNamara Jr JA, Franchi L, et al. Short-term and long-term treatment outcomes with the FR-3 appliance of Fränkel. *Am J Orthod Dentofacial Orthop.* 2008;134:513–524.
41. Baik HS, Jee SH, Lee KJ, Oh TK. Treatment effects of Fränkel functional regulator III in children with class III malocclusions. *American Journal of Orthodontics and Dentofacial Orthopedics.* 2004;125(3):294–301.
42. Wells AW, Sarver DM, Proffit WR. Long-term efficacy of reverse-pull headgear therapy. *Angle Orthod.* 2006;76:915–922.
43. Vaughn GA, Mason B, Moon HB, et al. The effects of maxillary protraction therapy with or without rapid palatal expansion: a prospective, randomized clinical trial. *Am J Orthod Dentofacial Orthop.* 2005;128:299–309.
44. Halicioglu K, Yavuz I, Ceylan I, Erdem A. Effects of face mask treatment with and without rapid maxillary expansion in young adult subjects. *Angle Orthod.* 2014;84:853–861.
45. Liu W, Zhou Y, Wang X, Liu D, Zhou S. Effect of maxillary protraction with alternating rapid palatal expansion and constriction vs expansion alone in maxillary retrusive patients: a single-center, randomized controlled trial. *Am J Orthod Dentofacial Orthop.* 2015;148:641–651.

46. Zhao H, Feng J, Ho TV, Grimes W, et al. The suture provides a niche for mesenchymal stem cells of craniofacial bones. *Nat Cell Biol*. 2015;17:386–396.
47. Woon SC, Thiruvenkatachari B. Early orthodontic treatment for Class III malocclusion: A systematic review and meta-analysis. *Am J Orthodontics Dentofacial Orthop*. 2017;151(1):28–52.
48. Cordasco G, Matarese G, Rustico L, et al. Efficacy of orthopedic treatment with protraction facemask on skeletal Class III malocclusion: a systematic review and meta-analysis. *Orthod Craniofac Res*. 2014;17:133–143.
49. Ngan P, Wilmes B, Drescher D, Martin C, Weaver B, Gunel E. Comparison of two maxillary protraction protocols: tooth-borne versus bone-anchored protraction facemask treatment. *Prog Orthod*. 2015;16:26.
50. De Clerck H, Cevidanes L, Baccetti T. Dentofacial effects of bone-anchored maxillary protraction: a controlled study of consecutively-treated Class III patients. *Am J Orthod Dentofacial Orthop*. 2010;138:577–581.
51. Cornelis MA, Scheffler NR, Mahy P, et al. Modified miniplates for temporary skeletal anchorage in orthodontics: placement and removal surgeries. *J Oral Maxillofac Surg*. 2008;66:1349–1445.
52. De Clerck H, Proffit WR. Growth modification of the face: a current perspective with emphasis on Class III treatment. *Am J Orthod Dentofacial Orthop*. 2015;148:37–46.
53. Cevidanes L, Baccetti T, Franchi L, et al. Comparison of two protocols for maxillary protraction: bone anchors versus face mask with rapid maxillary expansion. *Angle Orthod*. 2010;80:799–806.
54. Sar C, Arman-Özçırpıcı A, Uçkan S, et al. Comparative evaluation of maxillary protraction with or without skeletal anchorage. *Am J Orthod Dentofacial Orthop*. 2011;139:636–649.
55. Sar C, Sahinoğlu Z, Özçirpici AA, Uçkan S. Dentofacial effects of skeletal anchored treatment modalities for the correction of maxillary retrognathia. *Am J Orthod Dentofacial Orthop*. 2014;145:41–54.
56. Nguyen T, Cevidanes L, Cornelis MA, et al. 3D assessment of maxillary changes associated with bone anchored maxillary protraction. *Am J Orthod Dentofacial Orthop*. 2011;140:790–798.
57. Elnagar MH, Elshourbagy E, Ghobashy S, et al. Comparative evaluation of 2 skeletally anchored maxillary protraction protocols. *Am J Orthod Dentofacial Orthop*. 2016;150:751–762.
58. Nguyen T, De Clerck H, Wilson M, Golden B. Effect of Class III bone anchor treatment on airway. *Angle Orthod*. 2015;85:591–596.
59. Zurfluh MA, Kloukos D, Patcas R, Eliades T. Effect of chin-cup treatment on the temporomandibular joint: a systematic review. *Eur J Orthod*. 2015;37:314–324.
60. De Clerck HJ, Nguyen T, de Paula LK, Cevidanes L. Three-dimensional assessment of mandibular and glenoid fossa changes after bone-anchored Class III intermaxillary traction. *Am J Orthod Dentofacial Orthop*. 2012;142:25–32.
61. Nguyen T, Cevidanes L, Paniagua B, et al. Use of shape correspondence analysis to quantify skeletal changes associated with bone-anchored Class III correction. *Angle Orthod*. 2014;84:329–336.

14

Growth Modification in Class II, Open Bite/Deep Bite, and Multidimensional Problems

HENRY W. FIELDS AND WILLIAM R. PROFFIT

CHAPTER OUTLINE

Class II Growth Modification

Patients with a class II growth pattern have some combination of deficient forward mandibular growth and excessive maxillary growth that is more likely to be downward than forward. For growing patients, stimulation of forward mandibular growth or restraint of maxillary growth would be ideal treatment. Alternatively, if the facial appearance is acceptable except for protruding maxillary incisors, mild or moderate class II skeletal relationships can be accepted and the teeth moved with or without extraction to fit together (camouflage). This is a solution more often chosen in slow or nongrowing adolescent or postadolescent patients and, although outlined here, is discussed in detail in Chapter 16.

Evolution of Class II Growth Modification Treatment Strategies

In the early years of the 20th century, it was all but taken for granted that pressure against the growing face could change the way it grew. Extraoral force to the maxilla (headgear) was used by the pioneer American orthodontists (Fig. 14.1), who found it reasonably effective. This method of treatment was later abandoned, not because it did not work, but because Angle and his contemporaries thought that class II elastics (from the lower molars to the upper incisors) would cause the mandible to grow forward and that this would produce an easier and better correction. If intraoral elastics could produce a true stimulation of mandibular growth while simultaneously restraining the maxilla, there would be no need to ask a patient to wear an extraoral appliance, nor would there be any reason to begin treatment until the permanent teeth were available.

With the advent of cephalometric analysis, it became clear that interarch elastics corrected class II malocclusion much more by displacing the mandibular teeth mesially than by stimulating mandibular growth. Even if the lack of desired change in jaw relationships is overlooked, correcting a skeletal class II problem in this way is undesirable because the protruding lower incisors tend to upright after treatment, and then lower incisor crowding and overjet return. Because of this, these methods, and with them the idea of mandibular growth stimulation, fell into disrepute in the United States.

Perspectives on Growth Modification

Growth stimulation versus restraint can be viewed in two ways: (1) as the attainment of a final size larger than would have occurred

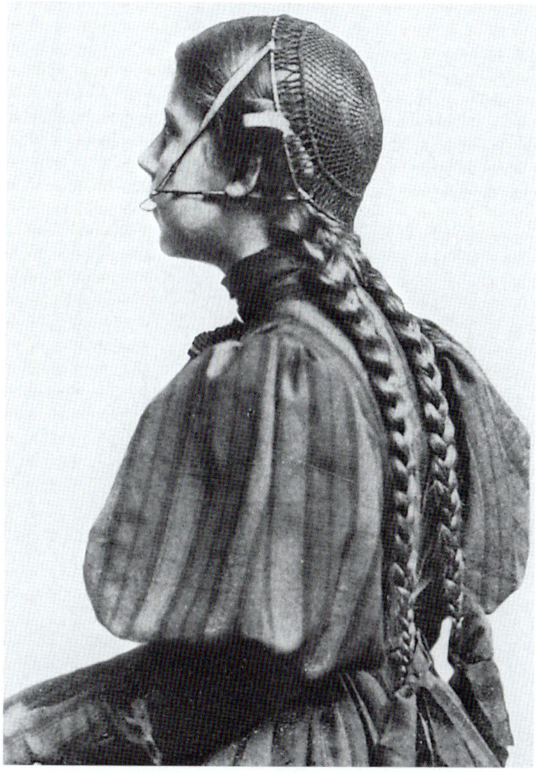

• **Fig. 14.1** Extraoral force to the maxilla was used for class II correction in the late 1800s and then abandoned, not because it was ineffective, but because the pioneer orthodontists thought that intraoral elastics produced the same effect. (From Angle EH. *Treatment of Malocclusion of the Teeth*. 7th ed. SS White Manufacturing Co; 1907.)

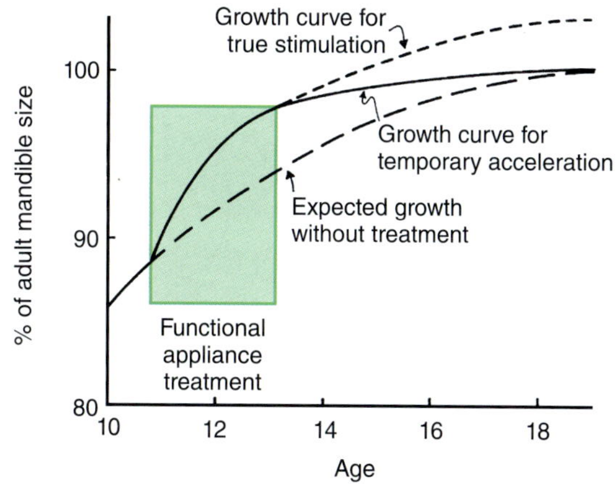

• **Fig. 14.2** The difference between growth acceleration in response to a functional appliance and true growth stimulation can be represented on a growth chart. If growth occurs at a faster-than-expected rate while a functional appliance is being worn and then continues at the expected rate thereafter so the ultimate size of the jaw is larger, true stimulation has occurred. If faster growth occurs while the appliance is being worn, but slower growth thereafter ultimately brings the patient back to the line of expected growth, there has been an acceleration, not a true stimulation. Although there is a great deal of individual variation, the response to a functional appliance most often is similar to the solid line in this graph, although some claim stimulation when treatment is performed in conjunction with the adolescent growth spurt.

without treatment or (2) as the occurrence of more growth during a given period than would have been expected without treatment. Fig. 14.2 is a hypothetical plot of the response to functional appliance treatment, illustrating the difference between absolute stimulation (larger as an adult) and temporal stimulation (acceleration o f growth). The more you believe in absolute stimulation, the more enthusiastic you are likely to be about "growing mandibles," and vice versa.

As the figure suggests, an acceleration of growth often occurs when a functional appliance is used to treat mandibular deficiency, but the final size of the mandible is little if at all larger than it would have been without the treatment.[1] Cephalometric superimposition often shows more mandibular growth in the first months of functional appliance treatment than would have been expected (Fig. 14.3). This is likely to be followed by a decrease in growth later, so although the mandible grew faster than normal for a while, later growth was slower than would have been expected and the ultimate size of the mandible in treated and untreated patients is similar.

Some published data suggest that timing mandibular growth modification to coincide with the mandibular growth spurt can provide growth change beyond what usually occurs.[2] These data are usually tied to determining the growth spurt timing from the level of maturation of the cervical vertebrae, a method that has supporters, detractors and questionable validity.[3,4]

Functional Appliances

By definition, a functional appliance is one that changes the posture of the mandible and causes the patient to hold it open and/or forward for class II correction or back or open for class III correction. In fact, these appliances also can affect the maxilla and the teeth in both arches. When the mandible is held forward, the elastic stretch of soft tissues produces a reactive effect on appliances that hold it forward. If the appliance contacts the teeth, this reactive force produces an effect like that of class II elastics, moving the lower teeth forward and the upper teeth back, and rotating the occlusal plane (Fig. 14.4). In addition, even if contact with the teeth is minimized, soft tissue elasticity can create a restraining force on forward growth of the maxilla, so that a "headgear effect" is observed. Any combination of these effects can be observed after functional appliance treatment.

The monobloc developed by Robin in the early 1900s is generally considered the forerunner of all functional appliances, but the activator developed in Norway by Andresen in the 1920s was the first functional appliance to be widely accepted (Fig. 14.5C and D). Both the appliance system and its theoretical underpinnings were improved and extended elsewhere in Europe, particularly by the German school led by Haupl.

Functional appliances were introduced into American orthodontics in the 1960s through the influence of orthodontic faculty members with a background in Europe (of whom Egil Harvold was prominent) and later from personal contact by a number of American orthodontists with their European counterparts. The most popular were the Bionator (Fig. 14.5A and B) and the Frankel appliance (Fig. 14.6). A major boost to functional appliance treatment in the United States came from the publication of animal experiment results in the 1970s, which showed that skeletal changes really could be produced by posturing the mandible to a new position and held out the possibility that true stimulation of mandibular growth could be achieved.

With functional appliances, additional growth is supposed to occur in response to the movement of the mandibular condyle out

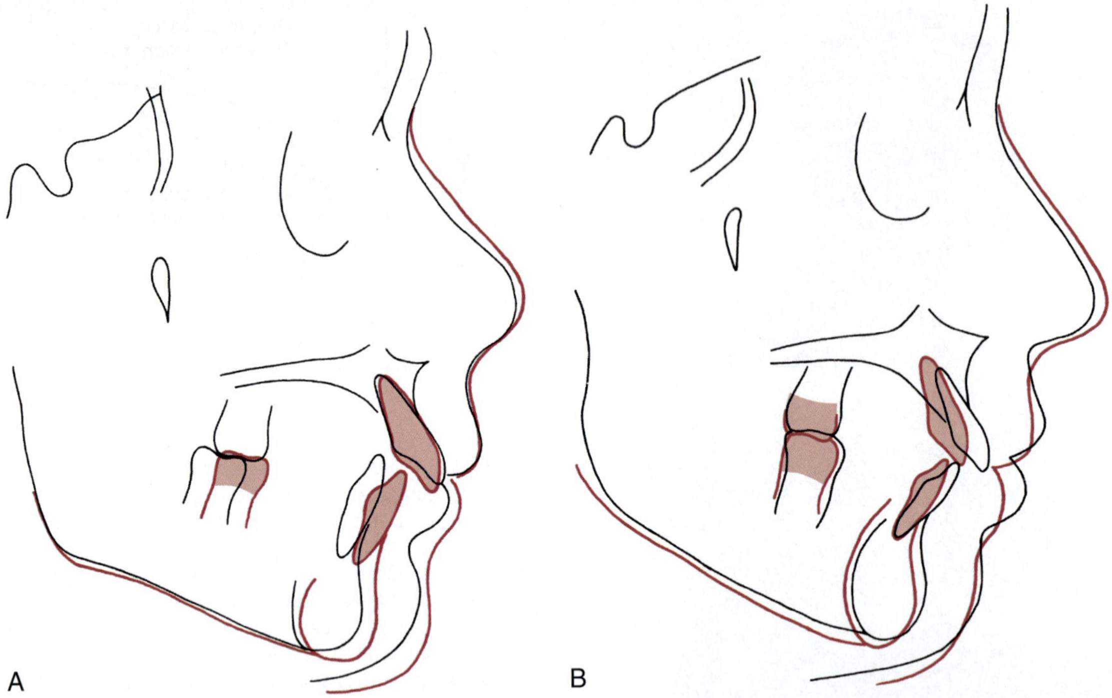

• **Fig. 14.3** (A) Cephalometric superimposition during treatment with a functional appliance (activator), showing excellent downward and forward mandibular growth between ages 11 and 13. (B) Cephalometric superimpositions for same patient between ages 13 and 15, during fixed appliance therapy for final positioning of teeth. For this patient, the growth response to the activator was much more an acceleration than a true stimulation, as revealed by more growth than expected at first, and less growth later; yet the activator phase of treatment was quite successful in improving the jaw relationship.

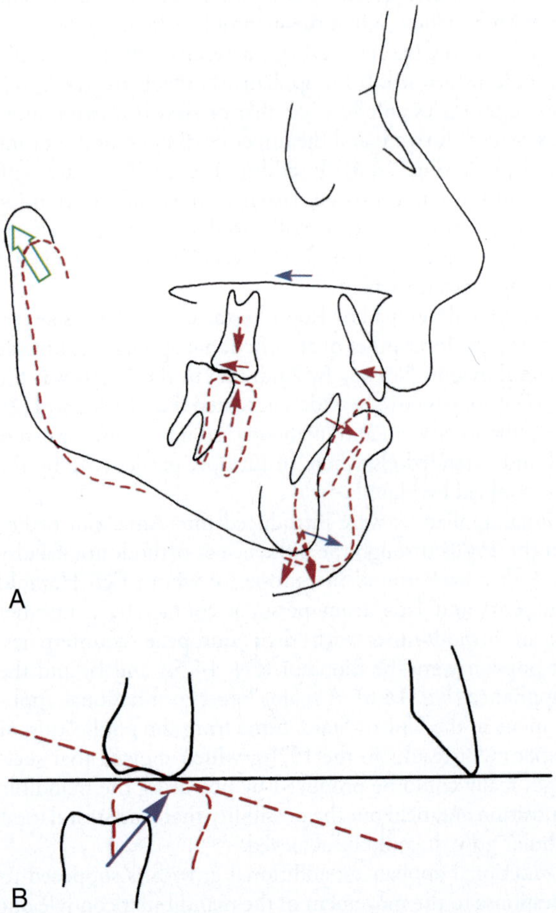

• **Fig. 14.4** (A) The potential effects of functional appliance therapy for correction of a class II skeletal malocclusion are illustrated here. The most desirable and variable effect is for the mandible to increase in length by growth at the condyles (*green arrow*), which may be accompanied by repositioning the articular fossa by apposition of bone on its posterior wall. The "headgear effect" (*blue arrow*) restrains the maxilla and the maxillary teeth, and holding the mandible forward often creates forces against the lower teeth that cause anterior movement of the mandibular dentition. The direction in which mandibular growth is expressed, forward (*blue arrow*) and/or inferiorly, is most related to the eruption of the molars. If the molars erupt more than the ramus grows in height (*dashed lines*), the forward mandibular change will be negated and the class II malocclusion will not improve. (B) To facilitate class II correction, the mesial and vertical eruption of the mandibular molar can be used advantageously. Rotating the occlusal plane upward posteriorly will in itself improve the molar relationship.

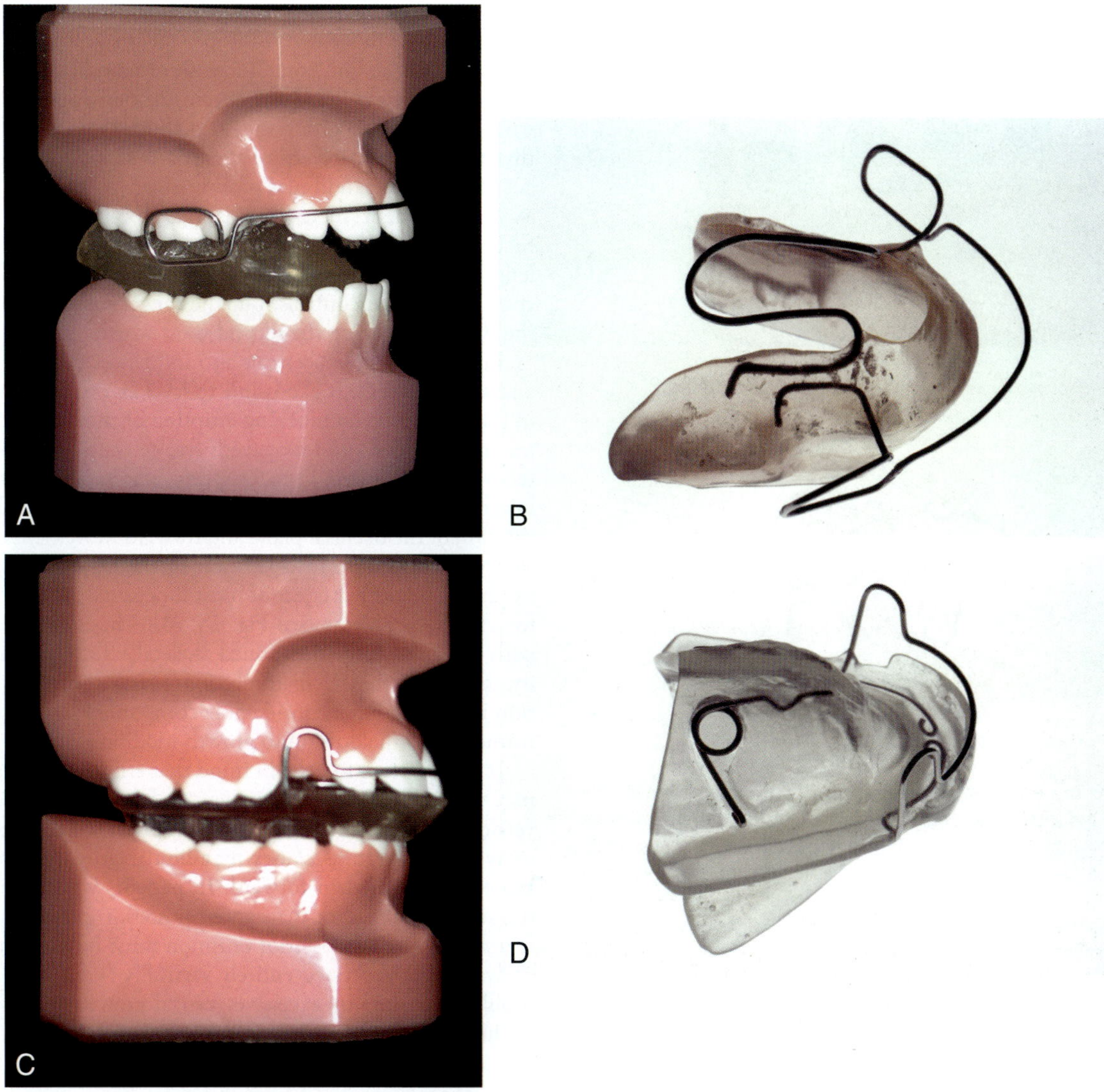

• **Fig. 14.5** (A) The Bionator is tooth-borne and induces mandibular advancement with contact of lingual flanges with the lingual mucosa. It usually has a buccal wire to maintain the lips off the teeth and can incorporate bite blocks between the posterior teeth and a tongue shield as this one does. (B) The Bionator also incorporates a major palatal connector to stabilize the posterior segments, but the appliance is limited in bulk and relatively easy for the patient to accommodate. (C) The activator is also used to actively advance the mandible and can incorporate anterior and posterior bite blocks and a labial bow. (D) The activator's lingual shields usually extend deeper along the mandibular alveolus than other functional appliances, and sometimes the appliance incorporates a displacing spring so that the patient has to close down and advance the mandible to retain the appliance in place. The theory is that activating the mandibular musculature is important in obtaining a growth effect (thus the activator name), but this theory has not been supported by data and has largely been discarded.

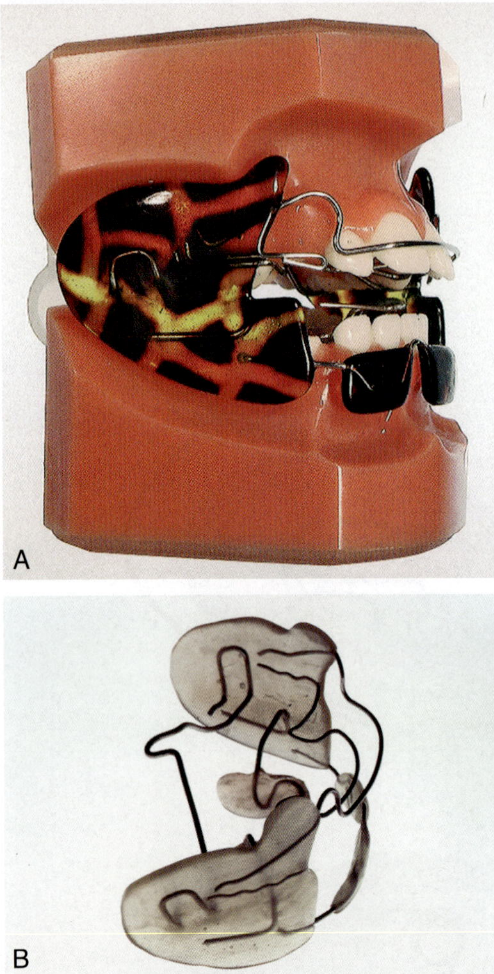

• **Fig. 14.6** (A) The Frankel-II appliance actively advances the mandible via contact of the lingual pad behind the lower incisors with the mucosa in that area and fosters expansion of the arches with the buccal shields. The lower lip pad also moves the lower lip facially. The appliance is largely tissue-borne and potentially causes more soft tissue irritation than other functional appliances, but a patient can talk normally with it in place, which makes full-time wear feasible. (B) Because of the wire framework, it is more susceptible to distortion than functional appliances made largely with plastic. (A, Courtesy Allesee Orthodontic Appliances [AOA], Sturtevant, WI.)

of the fossa, mediated by reduced pressure on the condylar tissues or by altered muscle tension on the condyle (Fig. 14.7). Although an acceleration of mandibular growth can occur and has been demonstrated now in several clinical trials,[5] a long-term increase in size is difficult to demonstrate. What does happen for patients with class II relationships is (1) a modest change in the size of the mandible's overall length, which, taken over several types of appliances, averaged 0.16 mm/month (range, 0.09–0.24 mm per month),[6] and (2) often a reorientation of the maxilla and the mandible, usually facilitated by a clockwise tipping of the occlusal plane (Fig. 14.4B) and a rotation of the maxilla, the mandible, or both. A reduction in forward growth of the maxilla also occurs with class II functional appliances (the "headgear effect"). This is typically less than 1 mm/year.[7] Although the Twin-Block appliance is reputed to be quite successful in stimulating mandibular growth in preadolescents, published data show that it is equally successful at the peak of the growth spurt as when used early,[8] and the changes it produces are a combination of skeletal (40%) and dental (60%). The dental change is largely a strong class II elastics-like effect—that is, forward movement of the lower arch and distal tipping of the upper incisors (25%). Meta-analysis of short-term twin-block treatment showed the classic combination of class II changes—proclination of lower incisors, retroclination of upper incisors, distal movement of upper molars and mesial movement of lower molars, and some increase in mandibular length. There was limited, if any, headgear effect. Although none of the changes were dramatic, as a group they had clinical impact. It was obvious that the mandibular vertical versus a-p changes were a balancing act to produce mandibular prominence.[9]

A subsequent meta-analysis that took a longer term view focused on removable functional appliances and mandibular length. On average they produced ~1.5 mm mandibular change compared to the controls, but the range was up to 3.4 mm with the twin block being the second most worthy performer.[10]

Functional appliances can also influence eruption of posterior and anterior teeth. It is possible to level an excessive curve of Spee in the lower arch by blocking eruption of the lower incisors while leaving the lower posterior teeth free to erupt. If upper posterior teeth are prohibited from erupting and moving forward while lower posterior teeth are erupting up and forward, the resulting rotation of the occlusal plane and forward movement of the dentition will contribute to correction of the class II dental relationship. This is another effect of most functional appliance treatment for class II problems (see Fig. 14.4B). These changes combined with the previously mentioned skeletal effects provide the ability to correct class II malocclusions—and show that the correction inevitably has a considerable component of tooth movement (camouflage) in addition to growth modification.

It is important to keep in mind that eruption of posterior teeth in a mandibular-deficient patient is beneficial only when good vertical growth is occurring. More eruption of posterior teeth than growth of the ramus causes mandibular growth to be projected more downward than forward. In patients who have a tendency toward vertical rather than anteroposterior growth even without treatment, further posterior eruption must be prevented to avoid growth being expressed entirely vertically (Fig. 14.8). The special problems created by excessive vertical growth are discussed later in this chapter.

Headgear

The other possible treatment for mandibular deficiency is to restrain growth of the maxilla with extraoral force (Fig. 14.9) and let the mandible continue to grow more or less normally so that it catches up with the maxilla (Fig. 14.10). After a period in which this method was largely abandoned, an influential 1936 paper by Oppenheim revived the idea that headgear would serve as a valuable adjunct to treatment.[11] However, it was not until the 1940s when Silas Kloehn's impressive results with headgear treatment of class II malocclusion became widely known[12] and extraoral force to the maxilla again became an important part of US orthodontics.

Cephalometric studies of patients treated with Kloehn-type headgear, which used a neckstrap and relatively light (300–400 g) force, showed that skeletal change in the form of a reorientation of jaw relationships did occur.[13] Experience soon revealed that although greater skeletal effects might be produced by higher levels of force than Kloehn had advocated, this required an upward

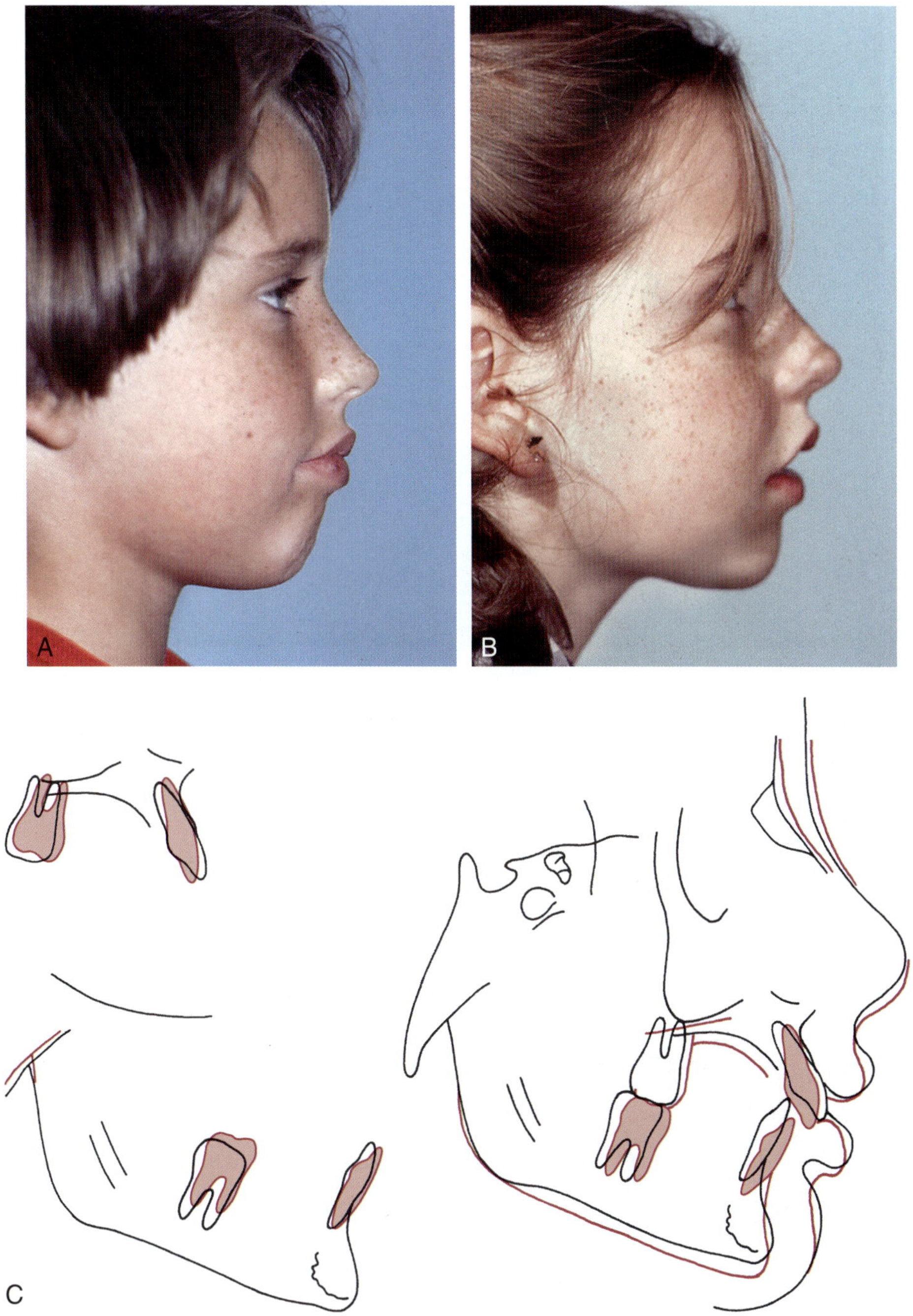

• **Fig. 14.7** This child was treated with a functional appliance in an effort to correct her class II malocclusion by changing the skeletal relationships. (A) Pretreatment profile. (B) Posttreatment profile. (C) Cephalometric superimposition. Note that the major skeletal change seen in the cranial base superimposition is restriction of forward growth of the maxilla. This "headgear effect" is observed in most functional appliance treatment that anteriorly positions the mandible, presumably because the soft tissues are stretched when the mandible is advanced and this force is transferred to the maxilla. Note also the differential eruption of the lower molars and forward movement of the lower teeth.

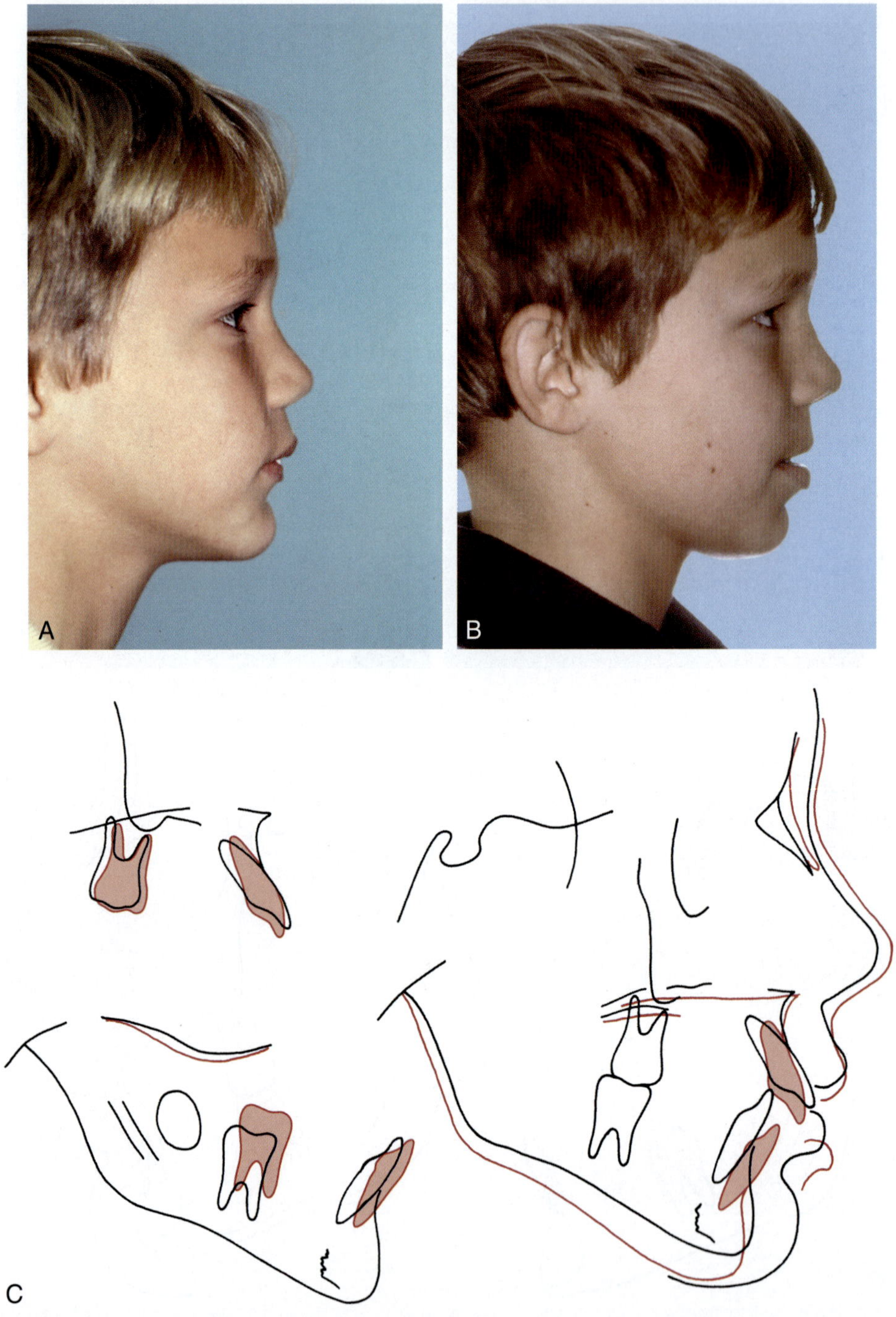

• **Fig. 14.8** A poor response to class II functional appliance treatment. (A) Pretreatment profile. (B) Posttreatment profile. (C) Cephalometric superimpositions. Note that before treatment the child had a tendency toward increased lower face height and a convex profile. The cranial base superimposition indicates that the mandible rotated inferiorly and backward because of excessive eruption of the lower molar, which further increased the lower face height and facial convexity. Note in the mandibular and maxillary superimpositions the anterior movement of the lower incisors and retraction of the upper incisors, neither of which was desirable.

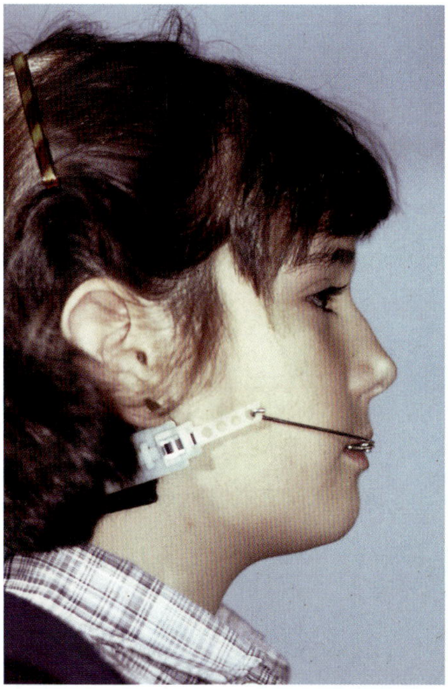

• **Fig. 14.9** A Kloehn-type or cervical headgear appliance. This appliance uses a cervical neckstrap and a facebow to produce distal force on the maxillary teeth and maxilla. Its goal is to control forward growth of the maxilla while allowing the mandible to grow forward.

direction of pull from a headcap to prevent excessive downward movement of the maxilla and a subsequent downward and backward rotation of the mandible.[14]

No effect on the mandible would be expected, but restraint of mandibular growth along with restraint of maxillary growth is never observed, and some studies have found improvement in mandibular growth and chin prominence during headgear treatment when used with a posterior biteplate.[15]

Beyond the skeletal effects, functional appliances and headgear also differ in their effects on the dentition. Removable functional appliances, especially those that rest against the teeth (i.e., tooth-borne ones with a labial bow and a lingual pad), often tip the upper incisors lingually and the lower incisors facially. Headgear force against the maxillary molar teeth often tips them distally. This often is accompanied by some distal movement of the maxillary premolars as force is transmitted to them by the supercrestal gingival fibers. There also is a vertical effect on the posterior teeth, extrusive with cervical headgear, possibly intrusive with high-pull headgear (true intrusion rarely occurs, but downward movement of the maxilla and posterior teeth is impeded). Remember that the mere fact that the teeth are moving distally will tend to open the bite anteriorly.[16]

Functional Appliances Versus Headgear: Some Clarity From Randomized Clinical Trials

In the 1990s, two major projects using randomized clinical trial methodology were carried out at the University of North Carolina (UNC) and University of Florida to compare the effects of functional appliances and headgear versus growth in untreated patients.[5,15] Another major trial at the University of Manchester in the United Kingdom was completed more recently,[17] and several additional smaller trials also have been completed. The results provide by far the best data that have ever been available for the response to early class II treatment. The data from all the trials show that on average, children treated with either headgear or a functional appliance had a small but statistically significant improvement in their jaw relationship during the treatment period (late preadolescence and early adolescence), whereas the untreated children did not. There is no question now that growth modification in children with class II problems is effective—it works in the majority of the patients.

A more important question relative to the timing of treatment is "Did early treatment with headgear or a functional appliance produce a long-term difference when early treatment outcomes are compared with the outcome of later (adolescent) treatment?" The UNC trial was extended into a second phase of treatment for all the subjects in the study, to compare early two-stage with later one-stage treatment more completely; long-term data from the Florida trial are also available. Both the former controls and the two groups of patients who underwent preadolescent growth modification treatment received comprehensive fixed appliance orthodontics (phase 2) when their permanent teeth erupted, during adolescence.

These data show that changes in skeletal relationships created during early treatment were at least partially reversed by later compensatory growth in both the headgear and functional appliance groups. By the end of phase 2, the skeletal relationships between the former controls and the early treatment groups were similar. Peer Assessment Rating (PAR) scores, which reflect the alignment and occlusion of the teeth, also were not different at the end of phase 2 between the children who had undergone early treatment and those who had not. The groups were also similar for extractions and eventual surgical treatment, although functional appliance treatment tended to increase the need for extractions.

From these studies, what can be concluded about the success of attempts to modify growth in children with class II relationships and the benefits of early treatment for class II problems? It appears that:

- Skeletal changes are likely to be produced by early treatment with headgear or a functional appliance but tend to be diminished or eliminated by subsequent growth and later treatment.
- Skeletal changes account for only a portion of the treatment effect, even when an effort is made to minimize tooth movement.
- After later comprehensive treatment, alignment and occlusion are very similar in children who did and did not undergo early treatment.
- Early treatment does not reduce the number of children who require extractions during a second phase of treatment or the number who eventually require orthognathic surgery.
- The duration of phase 2 treatment is quite similar in those with and without a first phase of early treatment aimed at growth modification.

Based on these results, it seems clear that for most children with class II problems, early treatment is no more effective than later treatment, and it is more efficient to modify growth during the adolescent growth spurt than before adolescence.

If early treatment is pursued, when the maxillary skeletal and dental effects that go along with any enhancement of mandibular growth are considered, functional appliances are usually preferred.

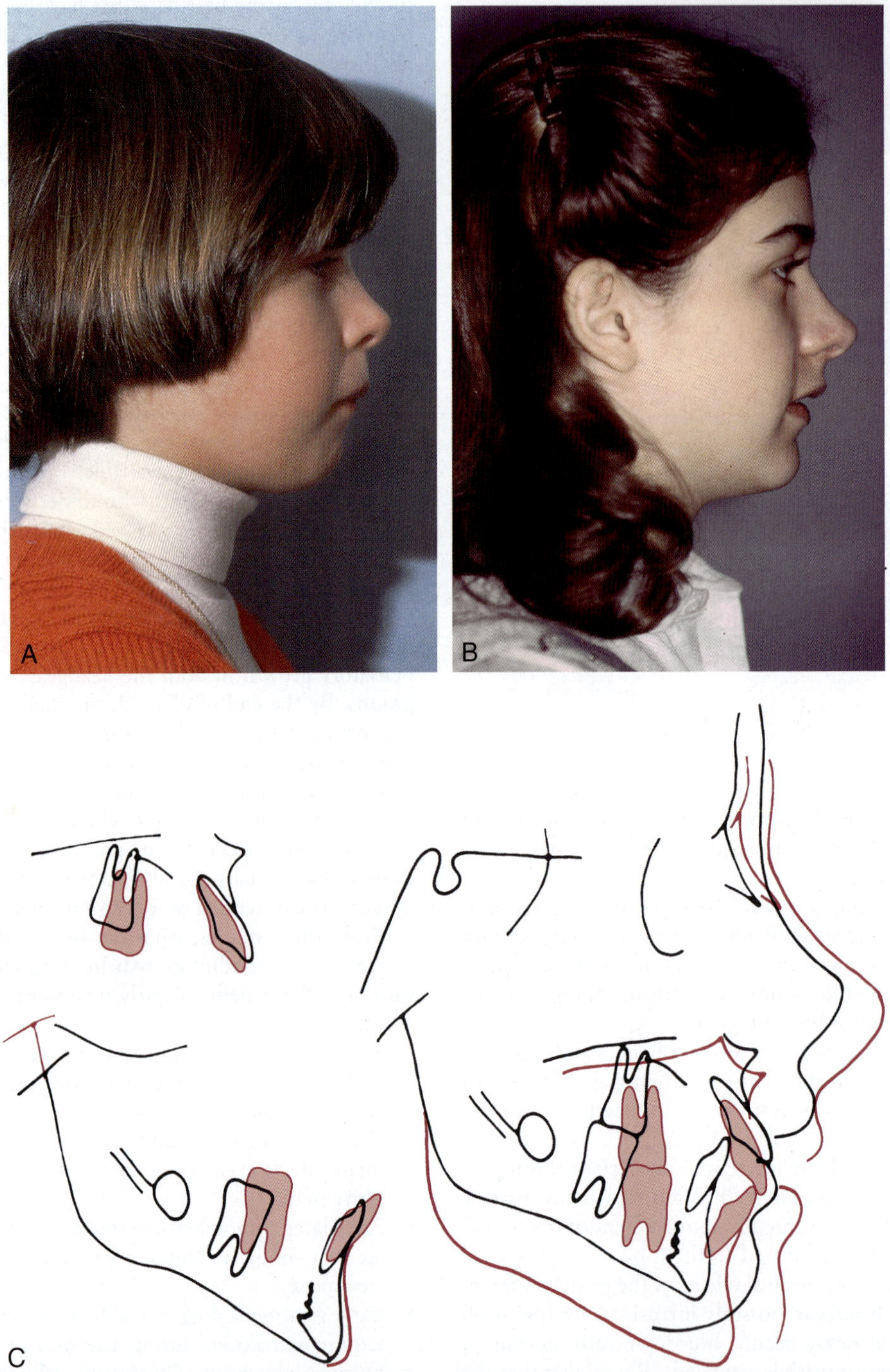

• **Fig. 14.10** Headgear can be effective treatment for patients with mandibular deficiencies if the mandible grows while they are wearing it. Facial appearance before (A) and after (B) treatment using headgear and class II elastics. (C) Pretreatment and posttreatment cephalometric superimpositions. This patient showed restriction of anterior maxillary growth and some impressive mandibular growth, combined with distal movement of the upper anterior teeth and mesial movement of the lower teeth, which were accompanied by posterior eruption.

For many patients who do not have a definitive maxillary excess or mandibular deficiency as part of the class II problem, either a functional appliance or headgear can be used with some degree of success, and allowing these patients to choose which one they prefer may improve compliance. Headgear probably is a better choice for a patient with frank maxillary excess.

Another finding from the early treatment studies was that among the treated and control groups, both of which had reasonably high self-concepts to begin with, the early treatment group reported less anxiety, higher self-concepts, and better physical appearance, popularity, happiness, and satisfaction than the controls at the end of phase 1. The treated patients also believed the benefits of treatment were general well-being, confidence, health of teeth, and mouth function.[18] This difference, however, disappeared by the end of phase 2 when both groups finished comprehensive treatment, so psychosocial benefits appear to be equally likely with early or later class II growth modification.

What the clinical trials did not say was that early treatment for increased overjet should never be attempted. For those with esthetic concerns or psychosocial problems related to dental and facial appearance some intervention appears reasonable, if only retracting or aligning the anterior teeth. In the clinical trials, those who had early treatment had fewer incidents of incisor trauma, especially with functional appliances.[19] For those with protruded front teeth, spacing problems, and a history of trauma, retraction of the front teeth and later growth modification make sense.[20,21] What this means is that early class II treatment of some type is indicated for some, but by no means all children.

Class II treatment commonly involves extractions and headgear. The impact of extractions or headgear on obstructive sleep apnea were not examined until recently. Two newer studies and a white paper have failed to find connections between headgear wear or extractions related to obstructive sleep apnea.[22–24]

Fixed Class II Correctors: Another Class II Treatment Approach

Fixed class II correctors (Herbst), the mandibular anterior repositioning appliance (MARA), cemented Twin-Block and Forsus devices (Figs. 14.11–14.13) are historically newer developments that have recently become quite popular for use in the mixed and early permanent dentitions. The major attraction of these appliances is that they require less patient cooperation than inserting and wearing a removable functional appliance or headgear.

Herbst created his appliance in the early 1900s and reported on it in the 1930s, but then it was largely forgotten until Pancherz rediscovered and popularized it in the 1970s. It forces the patient to maintain an advanced mandibular position and can generate both skeletal and dental changes. In long-term studies of the outcome of treatment with the Herbst appliance, Pancherz noted substantial rebound in the immediate posttreatment period. He now recommends the Herbst appliance for the early permanent dentition when the changes are more localized to the protrusion of the mandible but not for use in the mixed dentition.[25] Because the Herbst appliance can produce maxillary posterior

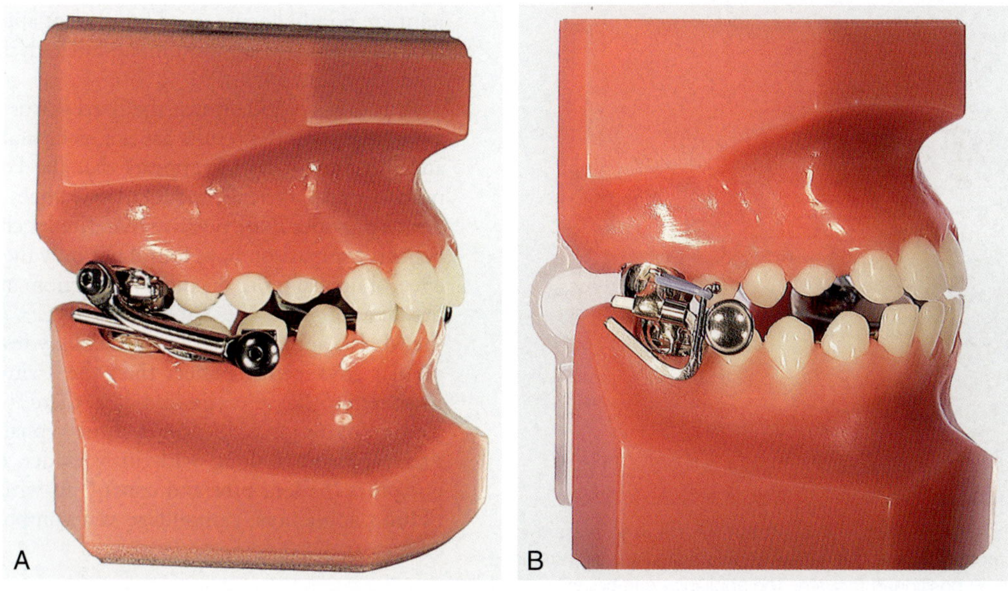

• **Fig. 14.11** (A) The Herbst appliance is probably most successful at the end of the mixed dentition. The most popular design currently uses crowns on the upper first molars and lower molars supported by lingual arch–type connectors for stability. The mandible is forced anteriorly in a passive manner by the plunger and tube that is anchored on the maxillary molars and cantilevered off the lower molar. (More recently, a telescopic design has been used). Spacers can be added to the plunger to advance the mandible farther. This appliance does not require compliance for wear, because it is cemented, but it does require compliance to prevent breakage. (B) The mandibular anterior repositioning appliance (MARA) requires the patient to advance the mandible in order to close. Otherwise, the upper elbow interferes with the lower fixed arm. The appliance, which uses crowns on the molars connected by lingual arches, is durable and stable. Patients find it less bulky than the Herbst appliance and tend to prefer it over the Herbst. To increase the advancement, shims are added to the horizontal portion of the elbow and the elbow is tied back with an elastomeric tie. (Courtesy Allesee Orthodontic Appliances [AOA], Sturtevant, WI.)

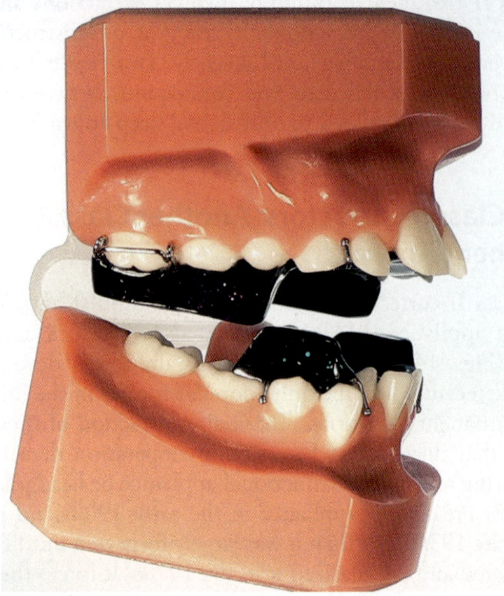

• **Fig. 14.12** The Twin-Block functional appliance is retained on the teeth with conventional clasps (but can be cemented in place). The complementary inclines on the upper and lower portions are relatively steep, forcing the patient to advance the mandible in order to close. The plastic blocks also can be used to control posterior eruption. (Courtesy Allesee Orthodontic Appliances [AOA], Sturtevant, WI.)

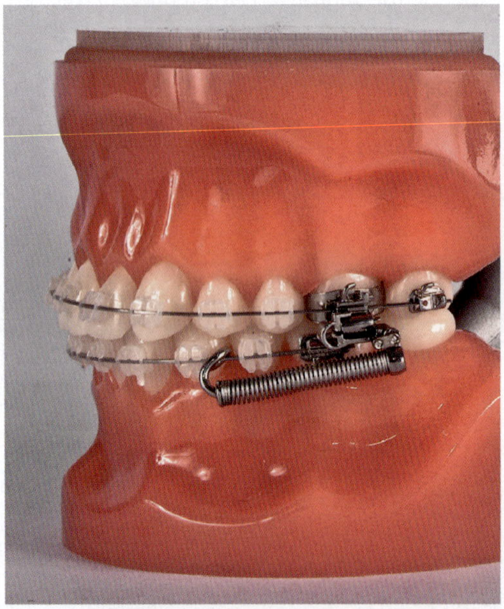

• **Fig. 14.13** The Forsus appliance is another of the fixed class II correctors. It has moderate bulk but is flexible and adjustable as it causes the mandible to be positioned forward. The appliance can be assembled intraorally by attaching it to the headgear tube and heavy archwires. It is adjusted by adding shims to one or both sides for more mandibular advancement. Clearly, and similar to other fixed correctors, there are upper distal and intrusive and lower mesial dental movements.

dental intrusion, it provides better results when used in patients with normal or slightly long anterior face height.[26] Although less patient compliance is an advantage, breakage has long been recognized as a significant disadvantage.

In the 1990s, Toll and Eckhart jointly developed the MARA as a more durable and less bulky alternative to the Herbst appliance, but with the same fixed properties and anterior bite guidance. The MARA appears to have a significant if temporary headgear effect and affects the mandible. As measured by change in the SNB angle, it affects the mandible less than the Twin-Block and Herbst appliances.[27]

When looked at as a group, fixed functional appliances offer ~1 degree of SNA reduction per year, 1 degree of SNB increase per year and <2 degrees of ANB change per year.[28] Most fixed functionals tip teeth and have predominantly dentoalveolar effects when used in adolescents.[28,29] The amount of tipping depends on which anterior and posterior teeth are included in the anchorage units through supplementary bonding or banding. In addition, they exert a protrusive effect on the mandibular dentition because the appliance contacts the lower teeth, and some of the reaction force from forward posturing of the mandible is transmitted to them continuously from full-time wear.[30] Although this type of dental change can be reduced with skeletal anchorage, this supplemental anchorage has small clinical effects on the skeletal relationships (SNB < 1 degree, ANB ~ 1 degree).[31]

The combination of maxillary dental retraction and mandibular dental protrusion that all functional appliances (fixed and removable) create is similar to the effect of interarch elastics.[32] This "class II elastics effect" can be quite helpful in children who have maxillary dental protrusion and mandibular dental retrusion in conjunction with a class II skeletal problem, but is deleterious in patients who exhibit maxillary dental retrusion or mandibular dental protrusion. Mandibular dental protrusion usually contraindicates functional appliance treatment. Finally, at present the effects of fixed functional appliances on the temporomandibular joint are poorly documented but do not appear to differ from the low prevalence of temporomandibular dysfunction problems in removable functionals.[33]

It is possible to contrast the fixed versus removable functional appliances, and the results are not as favorable to the fixed appliances as anticipated. It appears that the Forsus device produces more vertical skeletal and dental changes and the Twin-Block device provides more positive mandibular changes.[34] Others making this comparison have found not only the different mandibular effects but also more maxillary restriction and mandibular incisor proclination with the Forsus appliance.[35] As mentioned earlier, the MARA appliance has more maxillary restriction but less mandibular advancement effect than the Twin-Block device, in the short term.[27] Based on limited data, there is little difference in the amount of overjet reduction or other cephalometric changes with these appliances along with little evidence of patient-centered outcomes (patient pros and cons).[36] As with other growth modification appliances, camouflage is a component of fixed class II correctors.

Components of Removable and Fixed Class II Functional Appliances

The changes observed with functional appliances, especially the effects on the teeth, are the result of the appliance design. This section will briefly illustrate how the components of the appliances can be used to produce wanted effects and possibly mitigate unwanted effects. An appropriate appliance prescription specifies the appliance components that would be most effective in solving the patient's specific problems. It is important to have the

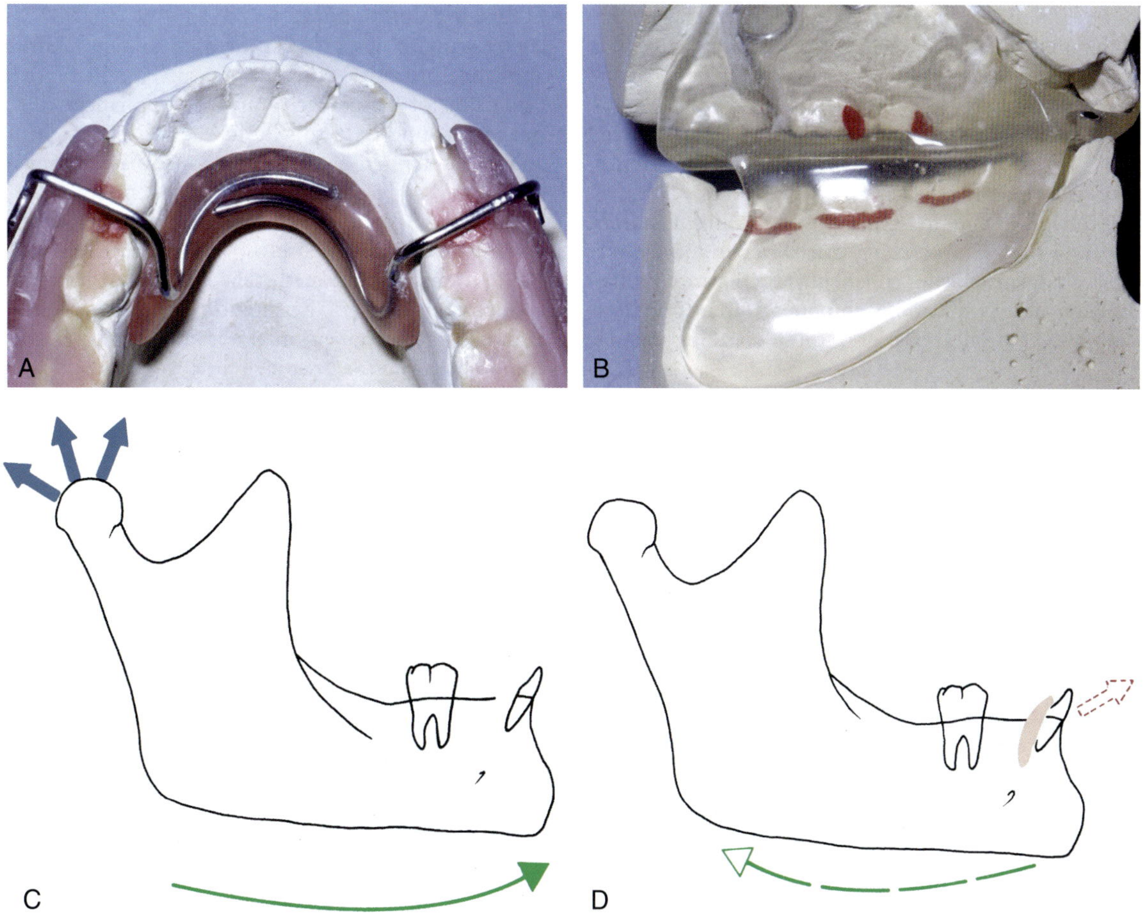

• **Fig. 14.14** The lingual pad or flange determines the anteroposterior and vertical mandibular posture for most functional appliances. (A) The small lingual pad from a Frankel appliance. (B) The extensive lingual flange from a modified activator. (C) The lingual components not only position the mandible forward but also exert a protrusive effect (D) on the mandibular incisors when the mandible attempts to return to its original position, especially if some component of the appliance contacts these teeth.

appliance design in mind before the impressions and bite registration because the impression technique is affected by what appliance components are selected, where they will be placed, and the intra-arch space required for them.

Components to Advance the Mandible

Components to advance the mandible are often classified as active or passive. If the patient has to voluntarily move the mandible to avoid an interference, the appliance is active. If it allows only a restricted path of movement or closure, it is passive. By that definition, appliances such as the Bionator, Activator, Frankel, Twin-Block, and MARA are active appliances, and the Herbst and Forsus are passive appliances.

For most mandibular-deficient patients, a Bionator or Activator-type appliance (see Fig. 14.5) is the simplest, most durable, and most readily accepted appliance. Flanges, either against the mandibular alveolar mucosa below the mandibular molars or lingual pads contacting the tissue behind the lower incisors, provide the stimulus to posture the mandible to a new more anterior position (Fig. 14.14). The Frankel appliance uses lingual pads against the gingiva below the lower incisors to stimulate forward posturing of the mandible (Fig. 14.14A). Ramps supported by the teeth, as in the Twin-Block appliance (see Fig. 14.12), are another mechanism for posturing the mandible forward. So is the elbow in the MARA appliance (see Fig. 14.11). With all these appliances, the concept is that growth modification is the result of the patient using his or her own musculature to posture the mandible forward (active), as opposed to the mandible being held forward passively by the appliance, which produces external pressure on the teeth while the patient relaxes.

All the fixed Herbst and Forsus appliances have the advantage of full-time wear and permanent postural change. The disadvantage is that pressure against the teeth, which produces compensatory incisor and molar movements, cannot be avoided—the patient simply cannot actively hold the mandible forward all the time. The point may be not whether the appliance is active or passive, but where and how the forces are applied to the teeth and how much dental compensation is built into the treatment. The more dental change, the less room there is for skeletal change by whatever means.

Other Possible Components

Vertical Control Components

When acrylic or wire is placed in contact with a tooth's occlusal or incisal surface it cannot erupt. If the vertical dimension is opened past the normal postural position, the stretch of the soft tissues will exert an intrusive force on the teeth (Fig. 14.15). Intrusion usually does not occur, probably because the force is not constant, but eruption is usually impeded. These methods including bite blocks, control the vertical position of anterior or posterior teeth. If no such control is placed, teeth will erupt. This is key to determining whether any mandibular growth is expressed anteriorly or vertically.

The same principle applies to tongue position. Lingual shields prevent the resting tongue from being placed between the teeth (Fig. 14.16). This has the effect of enhancing anterior tooth eruption. One caution here is that this component often limits the patient's acceptance of the appliance because speaking can be difficult.

Stabilizing Components

An assortment of clasps can be used to help retain a functional appliance in position in the mouth (Fig. 14.17A) (see also the discussion of clasps for removable appliances in Chapter 10) but in the long-term this limits the active element of the appliance. Clasps often help the first-time wearer adapt to the appliance. They can be used initially and then removed, deactivated, or allowed to gradually loosen with wear if desired, when the patient has learned to use the appliance. The labial bow across the maxillary incisor teeth that is included in many functional appliances (Fig. 14.17B) should be considered and managed as a stabilizing component in almost all instances and not an active component to retract teeth.

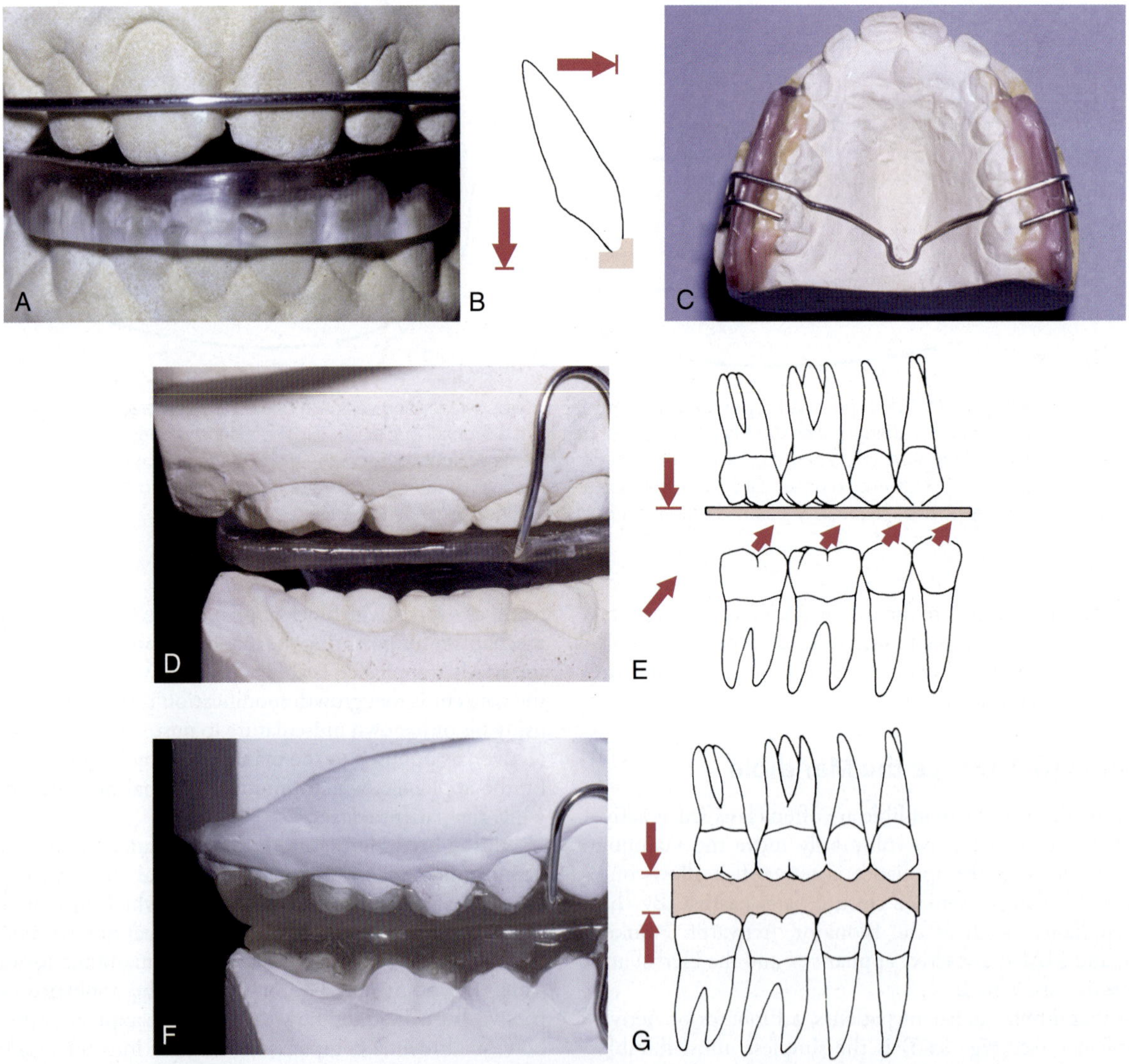

• **Fig. 14.15** Incisal and occlusal stops control eruption of anterior and posterior teeth, respectively. (A) The acrylic caps the lower incisors and serves as a stop for the upper incisors, which prohibits eruption of these incisors. (B) Incisal stops can extend to the facial surface and control the anteroposterior incisor position, as shown for the upper arch in this diagram. (C) Posterior stops can be constructed of wire or acrylic (D) and (E) This positioning of the occlusal stops inhibits maxillary eruption but allows mandibular teeth to erupt. (F) A complete acrylic posterior bite block impedes both maxillary and mandibular eruption (G) and is useful in controlling the amount of increase in anterior face height.

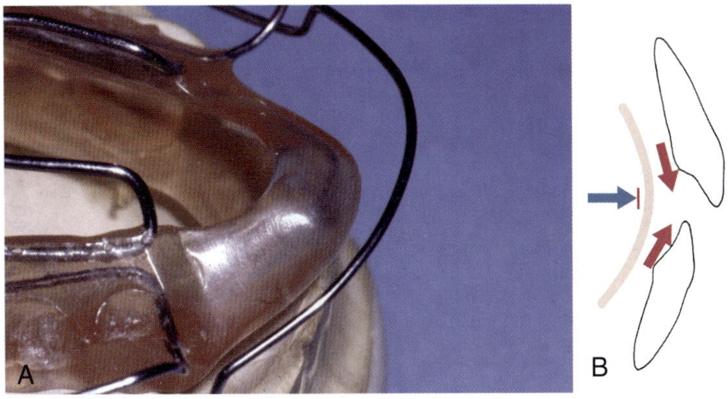

• **Fig. 14.16** (A) A lingual shield restricts the resting tongue (and thumbs, fingers, and other objects) from being positioned between the teeth. (B) The acrylic shield is placed behind the anterior teeth, leaving the anterior teeth free to erupt while (typically) the posterior teeth are blocked.

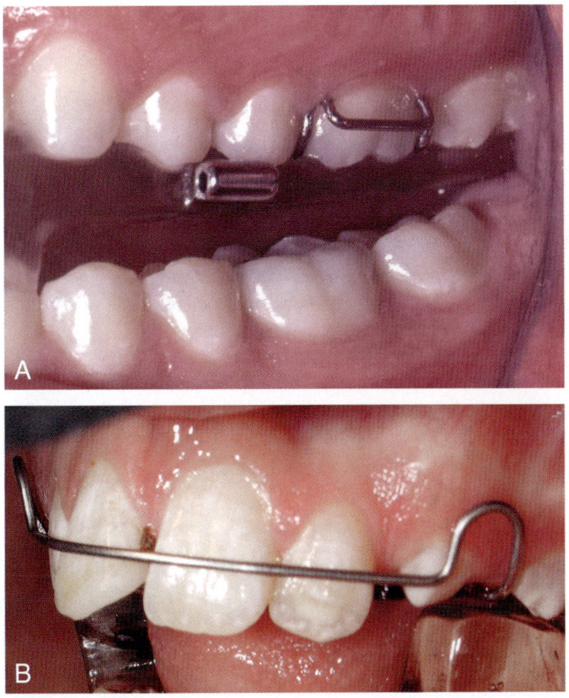

• **Fig. 14.17** Clasps add retention, which is needed to help maintain some types of appliances with active components such as springs and expansion screws in position. The clasps also can serve as a training device when patients are learning to accommodate to a functional appliance that repositions their jaws. (A) Note the headgear tube, for high-pull headgear that can stabilize the appliance and provide an extraoral distal force to the maxilla. (B) The purpose of a labial bow on a functional appliance is to help guide the appliance into proper position, not to tip the upper incisors lingually. For this reason, the bow is adjusted so that it does not touch the teeth when the appliance is seated in position. Even then it often contacts them during movement or displacement of the appliance. Undesirable lingual tipping of incisors during functional appliance wear therefore usually reflects a failure of the child to keep the mandible positioned forward while wearing the appliance.

Passive Components

Plastic buccal shields and lip pads, both of which are incorporated into the Frankel appliance (Fig. 14.18), hold the soft tissues away from the teeth. The effect is to disrupt the tongue-lip/cheek equilibrium, and this in turn leads to both facial movement of the teeth and arch expansion that results in an increase in arch circumference.

Buccal shields and lip pads can be added to any appliance to facilitate arch expansion. Their disadvantage is that they add to the potential for soft tissue irritation that can inhibit patient compliance.

Active Expansion and Alignment Components

In theory, there is no reason that growth guidance with a functional removable appliance cannot be combined with active tooth movement produced by springs or screws. The original activators did not use any springs or screws, but later, modified activators added the elements of active plates to an activator framework so that teeth could be moved while jaw growth was being manipulated (Fig. 14.19).

But, incorporating active elements into a functional removable appliance is a decidedly mixed blessing. There are three problems. The first is that correcting the occlusal relationships by actively moving teeth is not the goal of functional appliance therapy, and, in fact, the more tooth movement, the less skeletal change can be used or achieved (Fig. 14.20). Next, precise tooth positions cannot be achieved with springs or screws in removable appliances. Finally, the tooth movement will be only from tipping, which is less stable and more susceptible to relapse.

Treatment Procedures With Functional Appliances

Pretreatment Alignment

After treatment goals have been established and the decision has been made to use a functional appliance, the incisor position should be carefully examined. Because functional appliances for the treatment of mandibular deficiency require the mandible to be held in a protruded position to have a treatment effect, the patient's ability to posture forward at least 4 to 6 mm is critical. Most mandibular-deficient children have a large overjet and can do this readily, but in some patients incisor interferences prevent the mandible from being advanced to the correct position for the bite registration. The problem can be either lingual displacement of the upper incisors (a class II division 2 incisor pattern) or flared lower incisors. Functional appliance treatment will move lower incisors facially, so aligning crowded lower incisor will move them even further facially and reduce ultimate mandibular advancement.

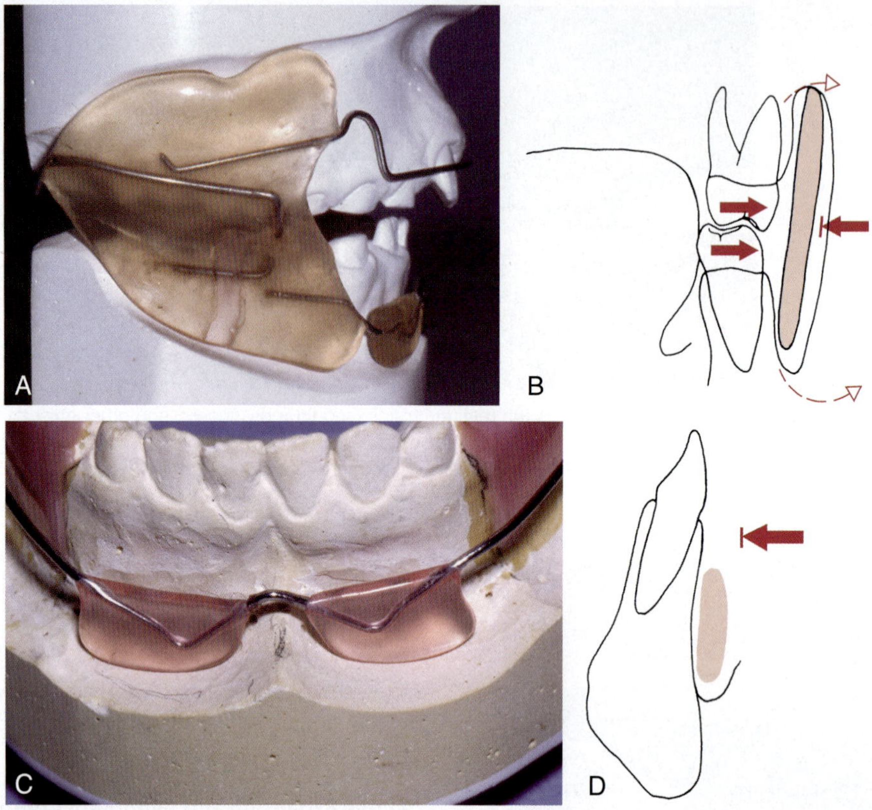

• **Fig. 14.18** (A) A buccal shield holds the cheek away from the dentition and facilitates posterior dental expansion (B) by disrupting the tongue-cheek equilibrium. The shield is placed away from the teeth in areas where arch expansion is desired. If the shield is extended to the depth of the vestibule, there is the potential for periosteal stretching that facilitates deposition of bone *(dashed arrows)*. (C) The lip pad holds the lower lip (or upper lip with a Frankel FR-III appliance) away from the teeth and forces the lip to stretch to form a lip seal. (D) The pad must be carefully positioned at the base of the vestibule to avoid soft tissue irritation.

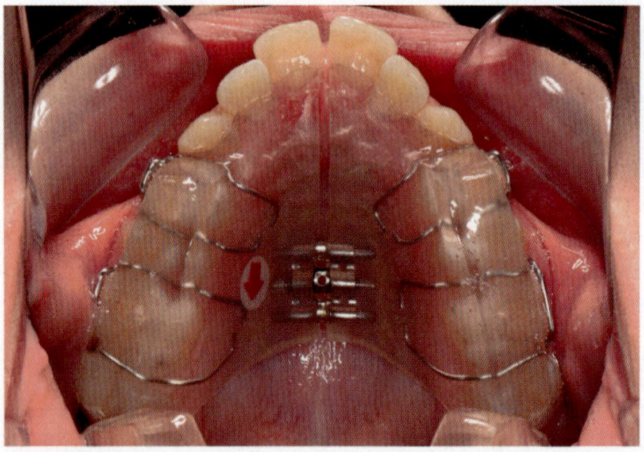

• **Fig. 14.19** Maxillary occlusal view of a twin-block functional appliance, which has an expansion screw to widen the maxillary arch. As the mandible moves forward relative to the maxilla during treatment, some maxillary expansion is likely to be needed to prevent the development of a posterior crossbite. The jackscrew and midline split of the appliance are a tooth-moving adjunct to allow maxillary arch expansion. Activation of a screw like this must be done slowly and in small increments. It is best managed with activation only by the orthodontist at recall visits. It is possible to add other tooth-moving components to functional appliances, such as wire springs to reposition the incisors, and that was popular in Europe when all the treatment was done with removable appliances. Now auxiliary springs and other adjuncts have largely disappeared, and the usual procedure is to follow the functional appliance with a second phase of fixed appliance treatment to obtain the final tooth positions because this is both more effective and more efficient. If a severe posterior crossbite is present and opening the midpalatal suture is needed, it is better to do this before or after the period of functional appliance treatment. (Courtesy Dr. R. Shah.)

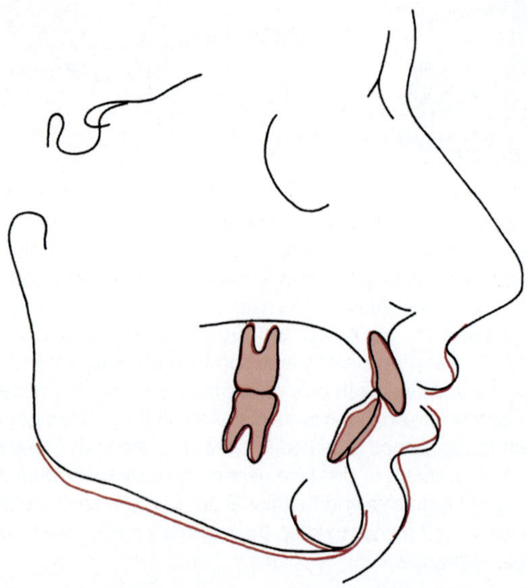

• **Fig. 14.20** Cephalometric superimposition showing an unsatisfactory response to a removable functional appliance for a skeletal class II malocclusion. Note the lack of skeletal response but dental changes, including forward movement of the lower incisors, slight retraction and elongation of the upper incisors, and downward and backward rotation of the mandible. Adding springs to a functional appliance, if it accentuates this pattern of tooth movement, makes the treatment response worse rather than better.

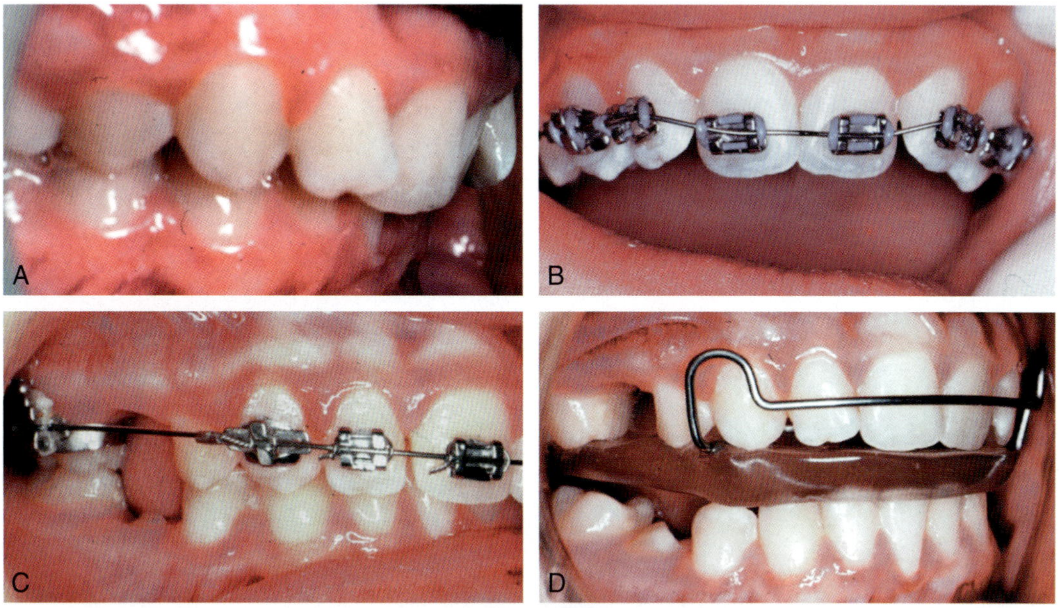

• **Fig. 14.21** (A) For this girl with a class II division 2 malocclusion, it was impossible to take the bite registration for a functional appliance until the maxillary incisors were tipped facially. (B) Although a change of this type was made with a removable maxillary appliance with fingersprings until recently, the prefunctional alignment can often now be accomplished more efficiently with a partial fixed appliance. In this case, the molars were banded, the canines and incisors were bonded, and a superelastic nickel–titanium (NiTi) wire was placed. (C) The same patient 2 months later, with alignment accomplished and overjet established. (D) Same patient 4 months later, with a deep bite Bionator in place. (From Proffit WR, White RP, Sarver DM. *Contemporary Treatment of Dentofacial Deformity*. Mosby; 2003.)

For both the class II division 2 patient with limited overjet and the class II division 1 patient with crowded upper incisors, the first step in treatment is to tip the upper incisors forward and/or align them (Fig. 14.21). Either fixed or removable appliances can be used for this purpose, depending on the type and magnitude of tooth movement required. In general, a short period of treatment with limited banding and bonding of the maxillary teeth accomplishes the necessary alignment and overjet. To control the tendency of the repositioned incisors to relapse lingually, they should be held in place for several months after being repositioned. Then, the appropriate working bite can be obtained with the mandible positioned anteriorly and inferiorly to correct the horizontal and vertical deficiency.

Impressions and Working Bite

The next step is to make impressions of the upper and lower arches and register the desired mandibular position—the "working bite."

The impression technique for a removable functional appliance depends on the appliance components that will be used. Good reproduction of the teeth and an accurate representation of the area where the lingual pads or flanges will be placed are mandatory. If buccal shields or lip pads are to be used, it is important not to overextend the impressions so that tissue is displaced because this makes it difficult or impossible to accurately locate the appliance components in the vestibule. Improper location of the components leads to long-term soft tissue irritation, discomfort, difficulty in appliance adjustment, and poor patient compliance.

For a cemented, bonded, or partially fixed functional appliance, accurate impressions of the teeth are essential, but extension of the impressions into the vestibules is not important. If bands or steel crowns are used to retain a Herbst appliance, they can be fabricated indirectly by a laboratory on the cast by disking the teeth to create space, and many clinicians prefer this time-saving method. If the clinician supplies the bands or crowns on casts or in impressions, separation is required before the bands are fit and at appliance delivery. If laboratory bands or crowns are used, then separation is required only before appliance delivery. Most clinicians have deserted bands for retention of fixed functional appliances because they have proved to be easily distorted and broken. Metal crowns, which are fit without reducing the teeth; cast or printed splints that can be bonded; or bonded acrylic splints are more satisfactory. These appliances avoid the separation step and save time. The crowns should have holes, not for the release of cement but for access to the occlusal surface during appliance removal. This provides a point of leverage on tooth structure.

The working bite, the jaw position to which the appliance is assembled, is the same for fixed and removable functional appliances. It is obtained by advancing the mandible to move the condyles out of the fossa and establishing the desired vertical opening (Fig. 14.22).

Unless an asymmetry is to be corrected, the mandible should be advanced symmetrically so that the pretreatment midline relationships do not change appreciably. We recommend a 4- to 6-mm advancement and a 3- to 4-mm vertical opening, but always one that is comfortable for the patient and does not move the incisors past an edge-to-edge incisor relationship. The practical reason for recommending this modest advancement is better patient comfort, facial esthetics, and patient compliance than with large advancements. Small advancements lead to more appliance adjustments. The claim that small advancements are more effective

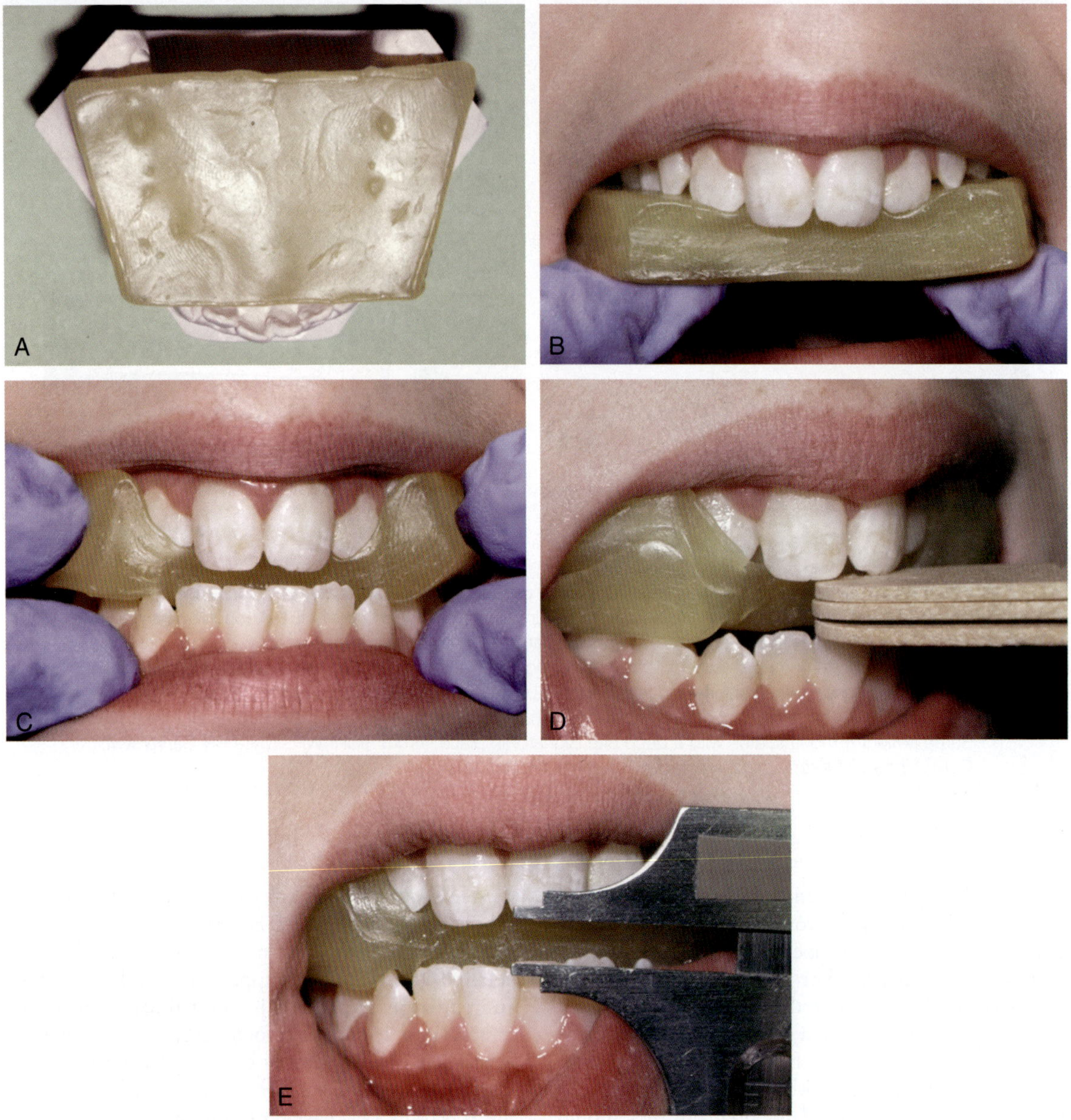

• **Fig. 14.22** Steps for obtaining a "working bite" for functional appliance construction. (A) Multiple layers of hard wax are luted together and cut to the size of the mandibular arch. The patient's preliminary record casts can be used to trim the wax to a size that will register all posterior teeth, without covering the anterior teeth or contacting the retromolar areas. It is important to avoid interferences from retromolar soft tissues. If such an interference is not detected, the finished appliance will not seat correctly. At best, this will require reduction of the posterior plastic stops if they were integrated into the design. At worst, a new bite registration and appliance will be necessary. (B) In preparation for obtaining the working bite, the wax is softened in hot water and the child is directed to practice the working bite position. Some children can easily reproduce working bites after only a few practice tries, but others need more opportunities and perhaps some help. The softened wax is seated on the maxillary posterior teeth and pressed into place to ensure good indexing of the teeth. (C) With the anterior teeth exposed, the position of the mandible can easily be judged while the bite is being taken. The mandible is guided to the correct anteroposterior and vertical position by watching the midline relationships and the incisal separation. There must be enough space for the laboratory technician to place wire and plastic between the teeth to connect major components of the appliance and construct occlusal and incisor stops. The minimal posterior opening to achieve the vertical space is 3–4 mm. Interocclusal stops or facets to guide eruption, as in most activators and Bionators, usually require 4–5 mm of posterior separation to be effective. (D) Either stacked tongue blades or (E) a Boley gauge can be used to control the amount of closure and help the patient reproduce the correct bite. If a vertical stop made of tongue blades is used, it must remain in the proper orientation (parallel to the true horizontal). Otherwise, as the tongue blades incline either inferiorly or superiorly, the mandible will either be closed and retruded or opened, respectively, to an incorrect position. When the correct bite has been obtained, the wax should be cooled and removed from the mouth. The bite should be examined for adequate dental registration and soft tissue interferences and rechecked for accuracy. Definite registration of both maxillary and mandibular teeth is required for proper appliance construction.

because muscle adaptation is better has not been supported by evidence. From a scientific perspective, it appears that quite large, modest, or relatively small advancements all can produce growth modification and that there is little difference in the results.[37]

If eruption of upper and lower posterior teeth is to be limited, as in a child with excessive vertical face height (see further discussion later in this chapter), the working bite should be taken with the patient open 2 to 3 mm past the resting vertical dimension (i.e., 5- to 6-mm total opening in the molar region) so that the soft tissue stretch against the bite blocks will produce a continuous force opposing eruption.

The Forsus appliance does not require a pretreatment working bite but is adjusted clinically to produce the same mandibular advancement as other appliances. Incisor position can be an issue, but anterior teeth can be aligned as with any other functional appliance to allow mandibular advancement, and it is good to have coordinated arches so that the transverse dimensions avoid upper and lower arch interferences. Also, enough alignment should be accomplished so that in a 22-mil appliance, a 19 × 25 steel wire can be inserted and secured with either a wire tied underneath the archwire to connect the teeth to prevent space opening or cinch-back bends to consolidate the arch.

Clinical Management of Functional Appliances

Removable Functional Appliances

When a removable functional appliance is returned from the laboratory, it should be checked for correct construction and fit on the working cast. The best technique for delivery is to adjust the appliance and work with the child to master insertion and removal before any discussion with the parent. This enables the child to be the full focus of attention initially and forestalls the effect of comments by the parents such as "That will be a mouthful!"

With any functional appliance, a break-in period is helpful. Having the child wear the appliance for only a short time per day to begin with and increasing this time gradually over the first few weeks is a useful introductory method. The child should be informed that speaking may be difficult for a while but that comfort and speaking facility will increase. Problems with speech are greatest when there is a bulk of acrylic behind or between the anterior teeth.

To be effective, functional appliances should be worn when growth is occurring and when teeth are erupting. If the appliance is in place during these hours, one can take advantage of skeletal growth and either use or inhibit tooth eruption. It is known now that skeletal growth has a circadian rhythm. Most growth occurs during the evening hours when growth hormone is being secreted; active eruption of teeth occurs during the same time period, typically between 8:00 and midnight or 1:00 a.m. To take practical advantage of this time period, it is suggested that children wear functional appliances from after the evening meal until they awake in the morning, which should be approximately 12 h/day. Waiting until bedtime to insert the appliance misses part of the period of active growth. Wearing the appliance during the day may add a small advantage, but this is difficult to achieve because it begins to impinge on school hours and can increase the negative social impact of the appliance, as well as appliance loss and breakage.

A good appointment schedule is to recall the child at 1 and 2 weeks after insertion for inspection of the tissues and the appliance. If the patient does not call about a problem during the first week, the 1-week appointment can be cancelled. Charts for children to record their "wearing time" are helpful, both for the data they provide and because the chart serves as a reinforcement for the desired behavior. Unfortunately, the time reported by patients and actual compliance often do not coincide. It is not unusual for patients to achieve half the requested wear time for orthodontic appliances.

If a sore spot develops, the child should be encouraged to wear the appliance a few hours each day for 2 days before the appointment so that the source of the problem can be determined accurately. Usually, smoothing the plastic components can be accomplished quickly. Gross adjustments should be avoided because jaw posture can be greatly altered. For example, heavy reduction of the lingual flanges will allow the patient to position the mandible in a more posterior position.

Because the initial mandibular advancement is limited to a modest 4 to 6 mm and many children require more anteroposterior correction, a new appliance may be needed after 6 to 12 months of wear and a favorable response. It is a good idea to reevaluate progress at 8 to 10 months after delivery with new records or at least a progress cephalometric radiograph. If little or no change has occurred in that time, then compliance is poor, the design is improper, or the patient is not responding to the appliance. In any case, a new treatment plan is needed.

Fixed Functional Appliances

At the insertion of a Herbst appliance, MARA, or cemented Twin-Block, discussion should focus on the care of the appliance and acceptable mandibular movements. Because these appliances are fixed, a wear schedule is not required, but some patients initially have problems adapting to the appliance and the forward mandibular position. It is good to warn the patient and parents of this and assure them that accommodation increases rapidly after several days. Soft tissue irritation is not a major problem with the Herbst, Twin-Block, or later versions of the Forsus, but the teeth may be more sensitive than with removable functional appliances. Patients should be instructed that the appliance is meant to remind them to posture the mandible forward and not to force the mandible forward with heavy pressure on the teeth. In this sense, sore teeth for an extended amount of time may indicate poor cooperation. Avoiding hard and sticky foods, large mouthfuls, and exaggerated mandibular movements (like wide opening and yawning) can greatly reduce the need for repair of a fixed functional appliance.

The Herbst appliance and the newer variations can produce good results (Figs. 14.23 and 14.24). The appliance must be carefully inspected for breakage at each visit. With the Herbst, after a positive treatment response is noted, changes in the pin and tube length can be made during treatment to increase the amount of advancement simply by adding sleeves to the pin to restrict its travel into the tube (Fig. 14.25). With the MARA, advancement is achieved with shims on the elbow wire to advance it (Fig. 14.26). A fixed (or removable) Twin-Block appliance can have plastic resin added to the inclines to increase the advancement without totally remaking the appliance. Plastic also can be removed adjacent to the teeth to allow drift, especially on the occlusal surfaces to encourage eruption when that is desirable.

It is possible to make a Twin-Block appliance partially fixed and partially removable (Fig. 14.27). This typically involves a fixed upper and removable lower splint. In this case, the fixed and removable parts should be carefully explained so that the child does not remove or loosen the appliance because of a misunderstanding.

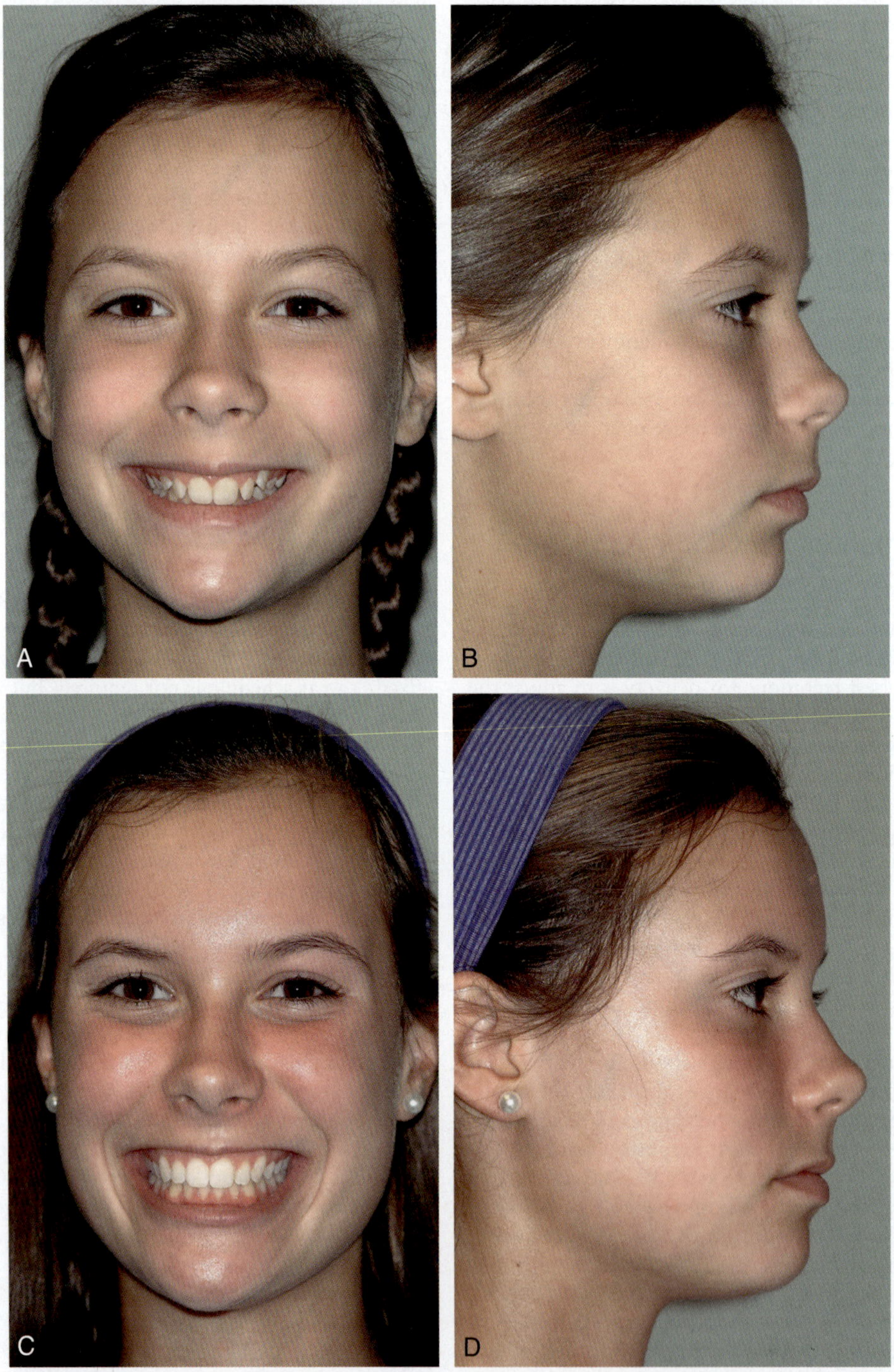

• **Fig. 14.23** (A) Pretreatment frontal and (B) lateral images of a patient treated with a Herbst appliance. The patient has mild class II skeletal and dental relationships and normal vertical facial proportions. (C and D) The posttreatment facial images show less facial convexity and, again, normal vertical proportions.

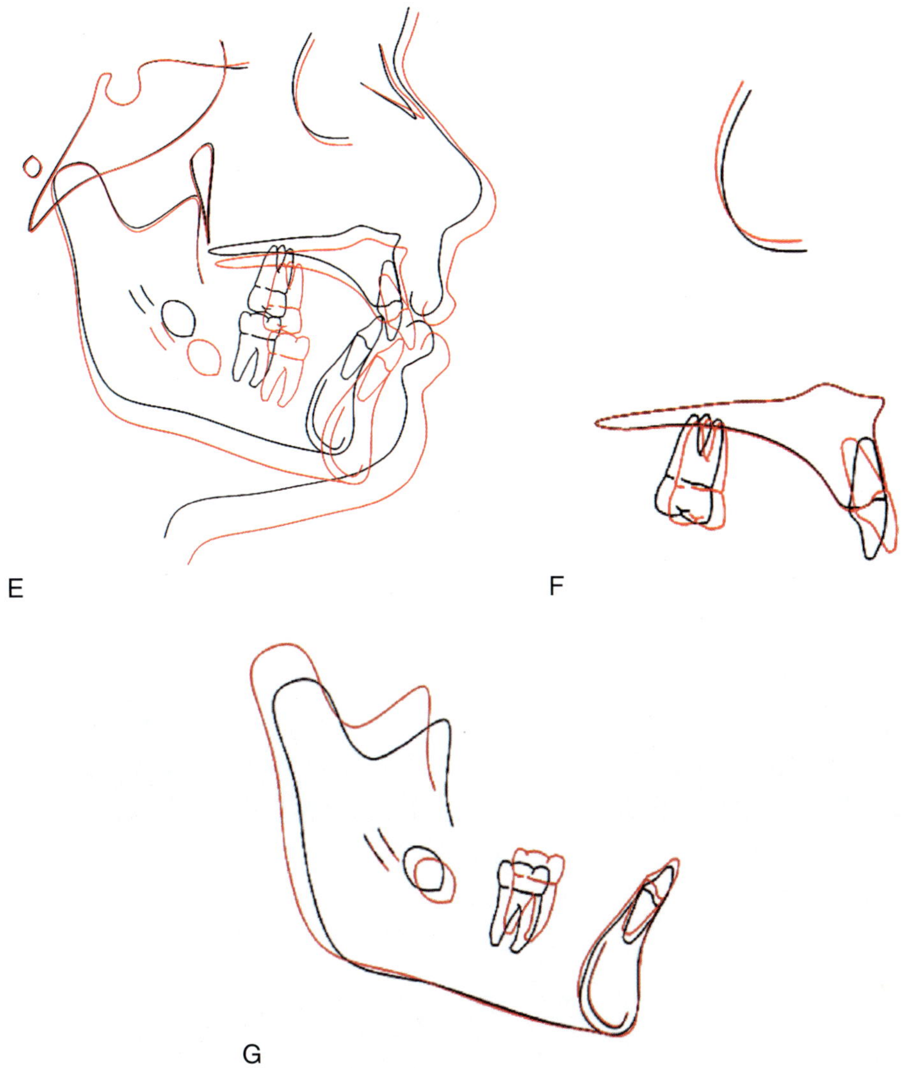

• **Fig. 14.23, cont'd** (E) The overall cranial base superimposition demonstrates some maxillary restraint (headgear effect) and mandibular downward and forward growth. (F) The maxillary superimposition shows the proclination of the upper incisors so the mandible could be advanced, and (G) the mandibular symposition shows lower molar eruption and mesial movement. These changes allowed and enhanced the class II correction. (Courtesy Dr. T. Shaughnessy.)

The Forsus appliance requires a different orientation because it is assembled from preformed parts chairside once the archwire sequence has advanced to the required stiffness after alignment of the teeth. It can be helpful to place buccal root torque in the incisors to combat proclination. The spring module is attached to the molar with use of the headgear tube. The Forsus measuring gauge is used to determine the correct size pushrod to insert into the spring module and to provide activation. The pushrod can be placed distal to either the lower canine or the first premolar by use of the loop closed around the archwire. This is determined by the direction of force desired and the amount of activation. The appliance can be reactivated for more advancement by either placement of a split spacer on the pushrod, moving from the distal aspect of the canine to the distal aspect of the premolar for pushrod placement, or use of a new, longer pushrod (Fig. 14.28). Usually a reasonable activation has 2 mm of space between the completely compressed spring and the pushrod stop when the patient is in centric relation. Different length pushrods on the right and left sides can be used to correct mild asymmetry.

When the desired advancement has been achieved with any of the fixed class II correctors and the patient is stable (anticipating 1–2 mm of relapse), then the appliance can be removed. A Herbst appliance usually is worn for 8 to 12 months, at which point the desired correction should have been obtained, and similar timing is expected with the other fixed functional appliances. In the case of the Herbst appliance or the MARA, a bur to cut the crowns, a crown or band slitter, or band-removing pliers inserted in the crown removal holes are possible removal methods.

For the Forsus, when the desired change has been accomplished after 6 to 8 months, the appliance is deactivated so that the spring is essentially passive for 4 to 6 weeks. Then the spring module is removed from the headgear tube and the pushrod is detached from the archwire by opening the loop with pliers, a cutter, or a scaler. For all the fixed functional appliances, adverse vertical

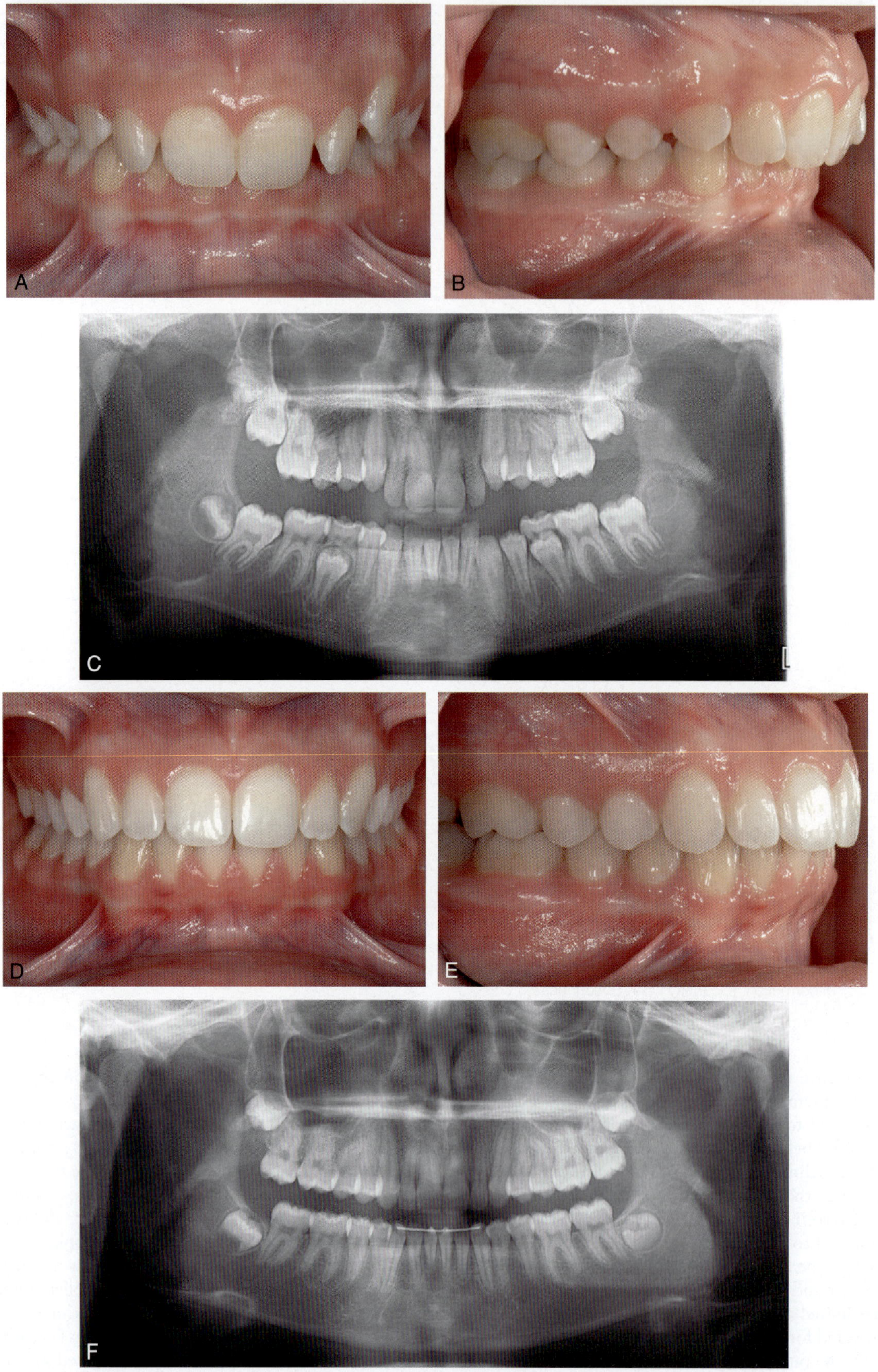

• **Fig. 14.24** (A and B) Prior to treatment, this patient had an anterior deep bite and a class II molar relationship but limited overjet due to the upright central incisors (really a class II division 2 incisor relationship). This made pre-Herbst appliance incisor proclamation necessary. (C) The panoramic radiograph shows all teeth present or erupting. (D and E) The posttreatment intraoral views show excellent molar, canine, and overjet relationships. (F) At the end of treatment, only third molars remain to erupt. (Courtesy Dr. T. Shaughnessy.)

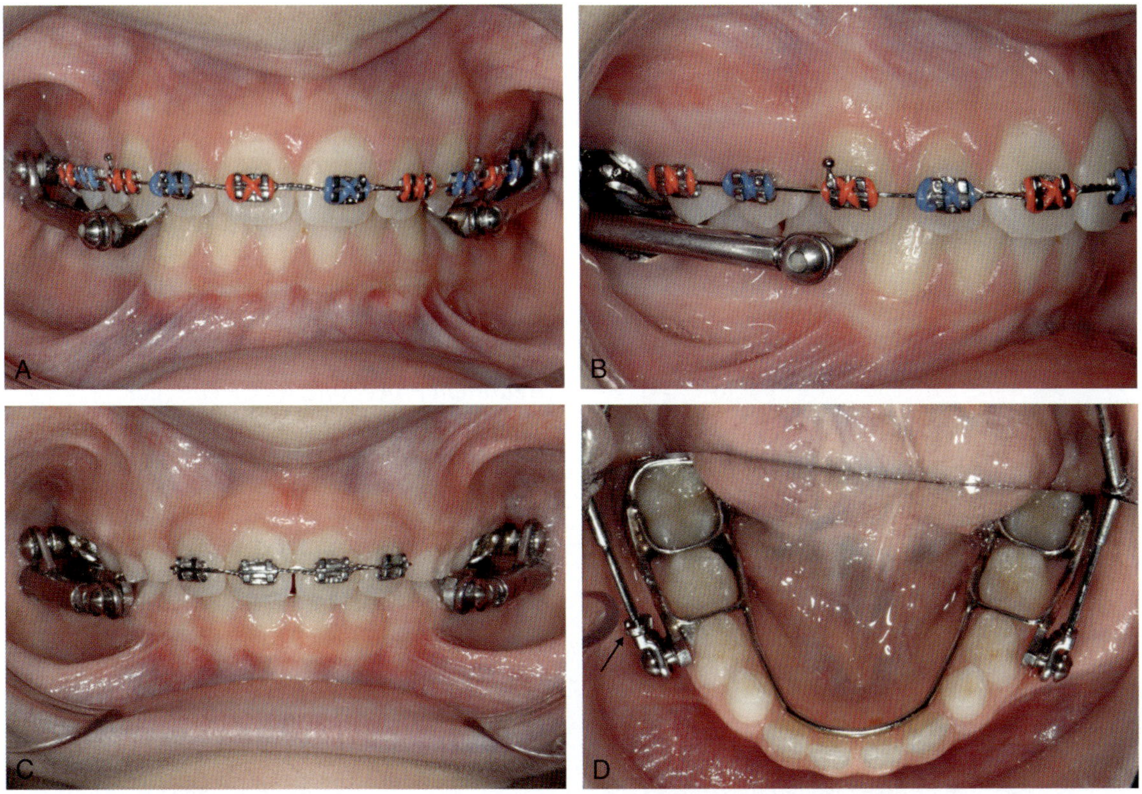

• **Fig. 14.25** (A and B) The Herbst appliance in place after upper incisor alignment. (C and D) Note the shim in place (*arrow* on mandibular right). This section of a split tube is placed over the plunger and crimped so that the tube is closed to further advance the mandible at an adjustment appointment. This banded appliance is cantilevered off the mandibular molars and supported with a lingual arch.

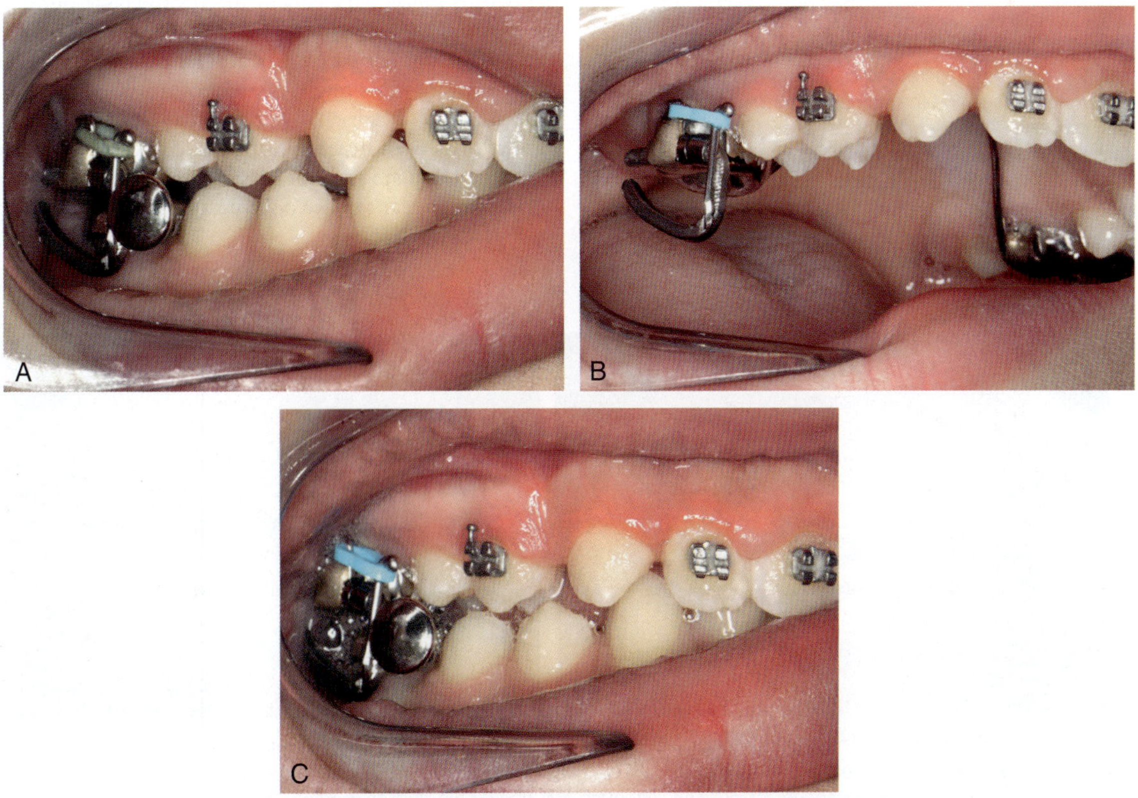

• **Fig. 14.26** (A) The mandibular anterior repositioning appliance (MARA) in place with the initial shim to advance the upper elbow and force the patient to advance the mandible forward to occlude. (B) A second and smaller shim in place to further advance the mandible. The elbow is secured with a new elastomeric module. (C) The patient in the occluded position after the adjustment.

effects (opening of the posterior bite) or adverse horizontal effects (class III over-correction or class II relapse) can occur. These can be countered with either a posterior box elastic, class III or class II elastics, respectively, if full appliances are in place.

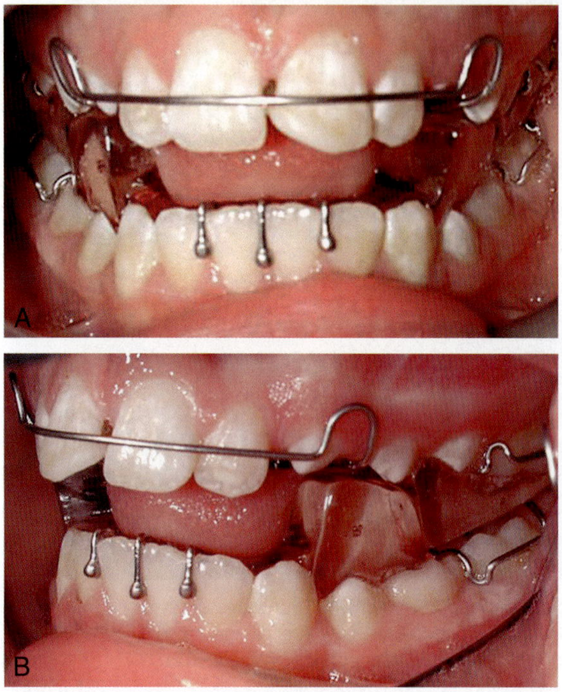

• **Fig. 14.27** The Twin-Block appliance can be used as a cemented (fixed) or removable appliance. (A) This patient had a class II malocclusion treated with a removable Twin-Block appliance that advanced the mandible (B). The ramps on the separate upper and lower units force the mandible to a more protruded and vertically increased position. Adjustments can be made to the occlusal coverage and the inclines to modify eruption and the amount of advancement. Cementing the upper section greatly increases the chance that both parts of the appliance will be worn because the patient then is more comfortable with the lower section in place. (Courtesy Dr. M. Mayhew.)

Records should be obtained at the end of phase 1 growth modification treatment to document the progress and plan the details and timing of the second phase of treatment. If the patient is still in the mixed dentition period when the desired correction is achieved, the Herbst appliance or MARA can be removed at that point, but it is important to consider use of a removable functional appliance of the activator or Bionator type as a retainer when this is done (see Chapter 18). This retainer should be worn approximately 12 h/day until the patient is ready for the second phase of fixed appliance treatment. Avoiding a prolonged retention period is a major reason for delaying fixed functional treatment until the adolescent growth spurt is beginning.

Treatment Procedures with Headgear

Components of Headgear

There are two major components of a headgear appliance: the facebow and the neckstrap or headcap. Facebows are fairly standard and simply apply the force to the teeth, although they come in varying sizes to accommodate the size of the arches. A facebow is usually applied to the permanent first molars but can be applied through splints and functional appliances. The anchorage component (headcap or neckstrap) is responsible for the direction of the force, either above the occlusal plane or below the occlusal plane, respectively (Fig. 14.29).

Effects of Extraoral Force on the Maxilla

Numerous studies, including recent clinical trials, have shown that headgear force can decrease the amount of forward and/or downward growth of the maxilla by changing the pattern of apposition of bone at the sutures. Class II correction is obtained as the mandible grows downward and forward normally while similar forward growth of the maxilla is restrained, so mandibular growth is a necessary part of the treatment response to headgear (Fig. 14.30). As noted earlier, there is some evidence of increased mandibular growth during treatment with headgear. Keeling et al. suggested that this might be due to the use of a biteplate in conjunction with headgear,[15] but a similar acceleration of mandibular growth has been noted in other studies of headgear outcomes in which a biteplate was not used. Whatever the mechanism, headgear does appear to have both maxillary and mandibular effects.

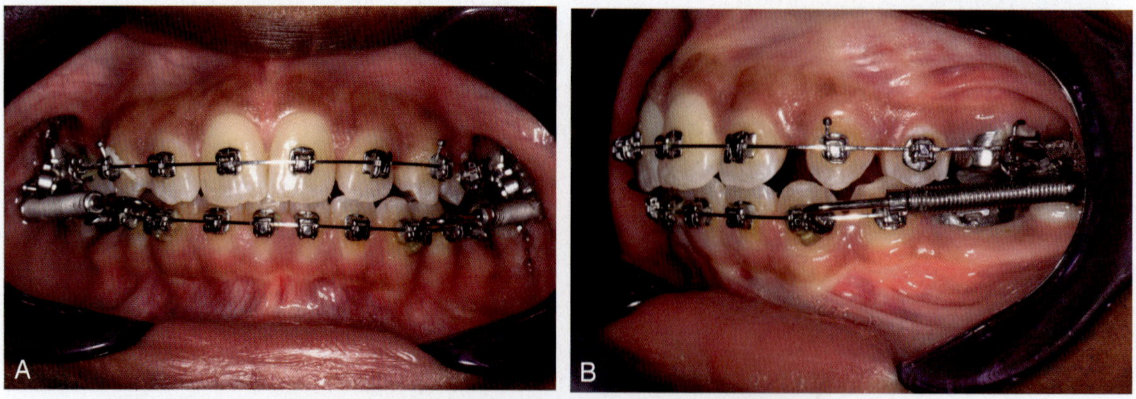

• **Fig. 14.28** (A) The Forsus appliance in place with heavy upper and lower archwires and the mandible advanced to near edge-to-edge incisors. (B) Note the crimped spacer adjacent to the spring that activates the mandibular advancement position. Although this shows the appliance from the upper molar to the distal of the canine, it can run from the upper molar to the distal aspect of the second premolar. This is less obtrusive to the patient but will have an increased vertical, intrusive component.

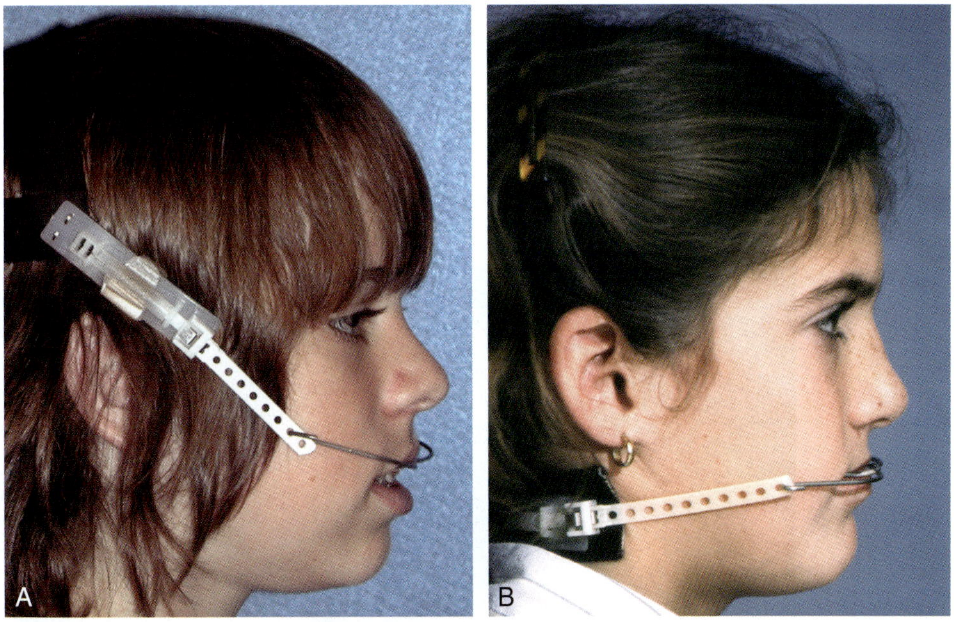

• **Fig. 14.29** Various types of headgear provide different directions of force for different clinical situations. (A) High-pull headgear consists of a headcap connected to a facebow. The appliance places a distal and upward force on the maxillary teeth and maxilla. (B) Cervical headgear is made up of a neckstrap connected to a facebow. This appliance produces a distal and downward force against the maxillary teeth and the maxilla.

In a growing patient, headgear must be worn regularly for at least 10 to 12 h/day to be effective in controlling growth. The growth hormone release that occurs in the early evening strongly suggests that, as with functional appliances, putting the headgear on right after dinner and wearing it until the next morning—not waiting until bedtime to put it on—is an ideal schedule. The current recommendation is a force of 12 to 16 ounces (350–450 g) per side. When teeth are used as the point of force application, some dental as well as skeletal effects must be expected. Extremely heavy forces (greater than 1000 g total) are unnecessarily traumatic to the teeth and their supporting structures; lighter force may produce dental but not skeletal changes.

To correct a class II malocclusion, the mandible needs to grow forward relative to the maxilla. For this reason it is important to control the vertical position of the maxilla and the maxillary posterior teeth. Downward movement of either the maxilla or the maxillary posterior teeth tends to project mandibular growth more vertically, which nullifies most of the forward mandibular growth that reduces the class II relationship (Fig. 14.31). The molars should not be elongated, and distal tipping of these teeth should be minimized when the objective is a change in skeletal relationships (Fig. 14.32). In addition, it is necessary to try to control vertical growth of the maxilla. For these reasons, high-pull headgear is usually preferred.

In theory, the movement of the maxilla can be controlled in the same way as a single tooth is controlled: by managing forces and moments relative to the center of resistance of the jaw. In practice, it is difficult to analyze exactly where the center of resistance and center of rotation of the maxilla might be, but they are above the teeth and most likely above the premolar teeth. Directing the line of force closer to the center of resistance is another major reason for including an upward direction of pull for most children who have headgear force to the maxilla.

Selection of Headgear Type

There are three major decisions to be made in the selection of headgear. First, the headgear anchorage location must be chosen to provide a preferred vertical component of force to the skeletal and dental structures. A high-pull headcap will place a superior and distal force on the teeth and maxilla, whereas a cervical neckstrap will place an inferior and distal force on the teeth and skeletal structures (see Fig. 14.29). A straighter distal pull can be produced by a combination of the two or a modified and lower headcap, but these methods are not commonly used. The initial choice of headgear configuration is usually based on the original facial pattern: the more signs of a vertically excessive growth pattern are present (see Chapter 6), the higher the direction of pull and vice versa. Reports of responses to headgear treatment show, however, that there is considerable variation and unpredictability in growth response. Cervical headgear does not always aggravate vertical problems, especially when there is good vertical mandibular growth[38] and minimal distal movement of maxillary molars, which is the best predictor of vertical opening.

The second decision is how the headgear is to be attached to the dentition. The usual arrangement is a facebow to the large headgear tubes on the permanent first molars. Alternatively, a removable maxillary splint or a functional appliance can be fitted to the maxillary teeth and the facebow attached to it. This may be indicated for children with excessive vertical growth (which is discussed further later in this chapter). Attaching headgear to an archwire anteriorly is possible but rarely practical in children with a mixed dentition and produces relatively heavy forces on anterior teeth.

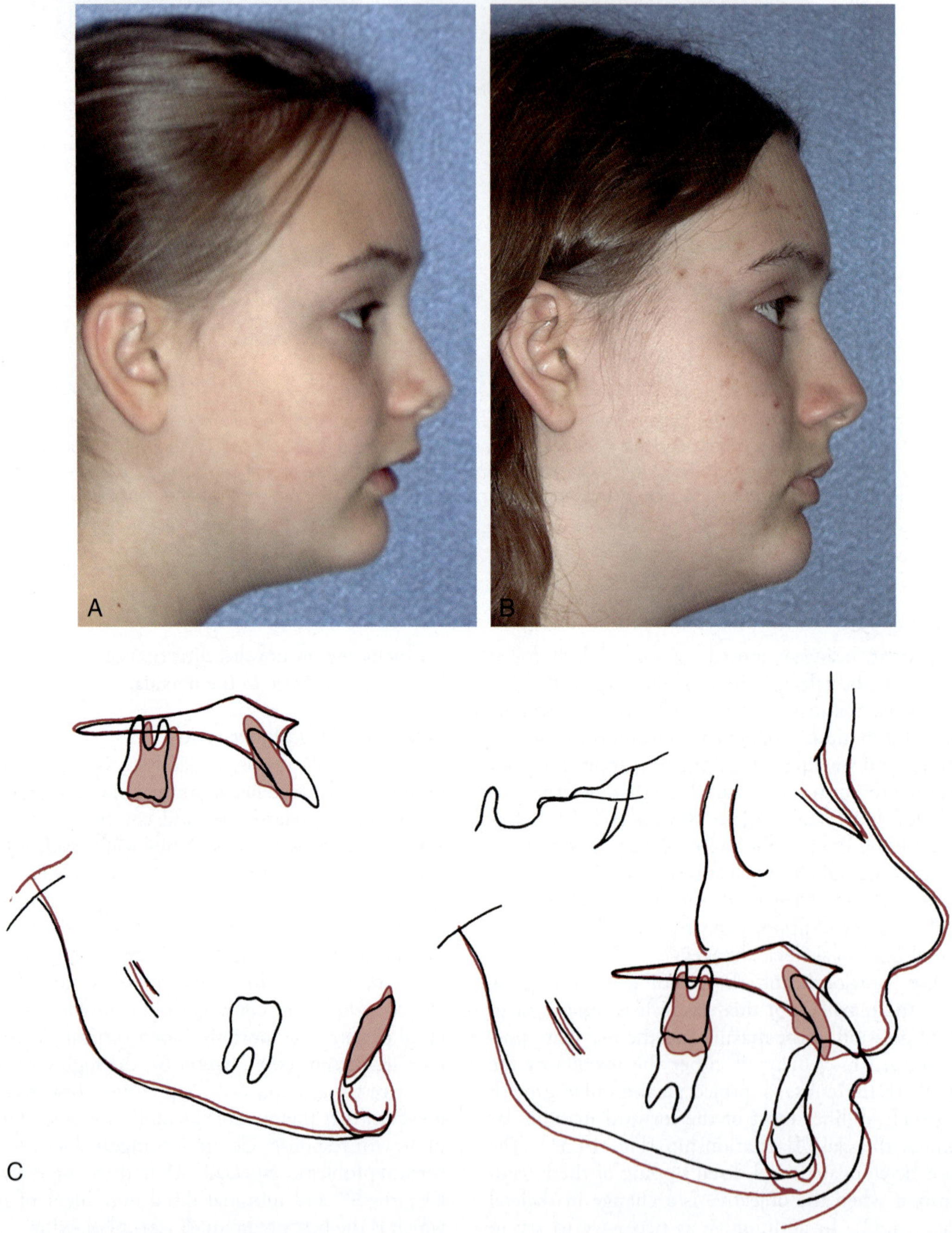

• **Fig. 14.30** A good response to headgear treatment. (A) Pretreatment. (B) Appearance after approximately 2 years of headgear treatment. (C) Cephalometric superimpositions. Note the favorable downward-forward mandibular growth with limited change in the maxillary position. There also were limited incisor changes other than some eruption and maxillary incisor retraction.

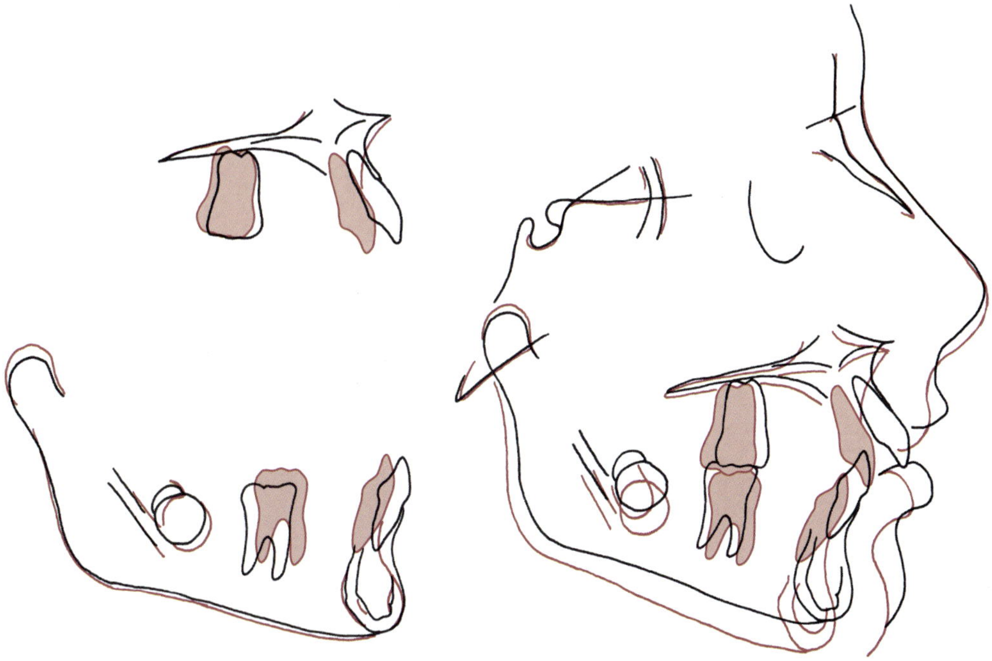

• **Fig. 14.31** This child had a poor response to headgear treatment for a class II malocclusion. The cranial base superimposition indicates that the lips were retracted and the maxilla did not grow anteriorly. The maxillary superimposition shows that the incisors were retracted and the molar movement and eruption were limited. All these effects were beneficial for class II correction, but the mandible rotated downward and backward because of the inferior movement of the maxilla and eruption of the lower molar. As a result, the profile is more convex than when treatment began, and the class II malocclusion is uncorrected.

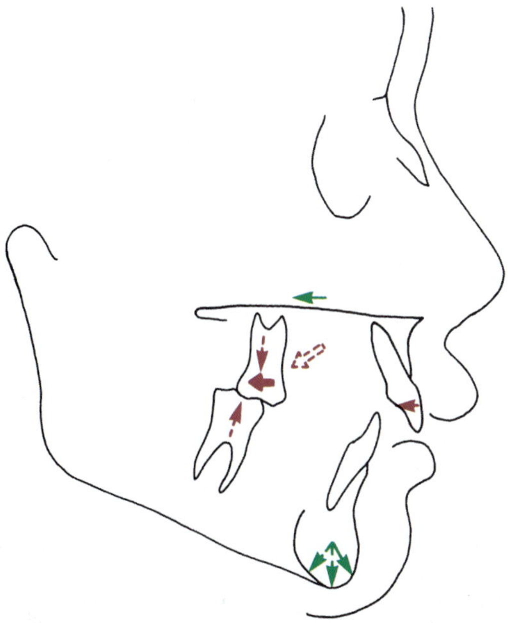

• **Fig. 14.32** Headgear treatment can have several side effects that complicate correction of class II malocclusion. If the child wears the appliance, maxillary skeletal and dental forward movement will be restricted. Although this helps in correction of the class II malocclusion, vertical control of the maxilla and maxillary teeth is important because this determines the extent to which the mandible is directed forward and/or inferiorly. Downward maxillary skeletal movement or maxillary and mandibular molar eruption (all shown in *dashed arrows*) can reduce or totally negate forward growth of the mandible.

Finally, a decision must be made as to whether bodily movement or tipping of the teeth is desired. Because the center of resistance for a molar is estimated to be in the midroot region, force vectors above this point should result in distal root movement. Forces through the center of resistance of the molar should cause bodily movement, and vectors below this point should cause distal crown tipping. The length and position of the outer headgear bow and the form of anchorage (i.e., headcap or neckstrap) determine the vector of force and its relationship to the center of resistance of the tooth. These factors determine the molar movement.

The various combinations of force direction (anchorage), length of outer bow, and position of outer bow are diagrammatically illustrated in Fig. 14.33. As in any growth modification treatment, tooth movement is usually an undesirable side effect, and with headgear, tooth movement is minimized because of the relatively heavy forces and the assumed need for undermining bone resorption.

Similar considerations apply to the maxilla: unless the line of force is through its center of resistance, rotation of the jaw (the skeletal equivalent of dental tipping) will occur. Control of the line of force relative to the maxilla is easier when a splint covering all the teeth is used to apply the headgear force. The facebow is usually attached to the splint in the premolar region so that the force can be directed through the center of resistance of the maxilla, which is estimated to be located above the premolar roots (see Fig. 14.33C). Distal tipping of the maxillary incisors is likely to occur, however, because the distal component of the force is delivered to these teeth.

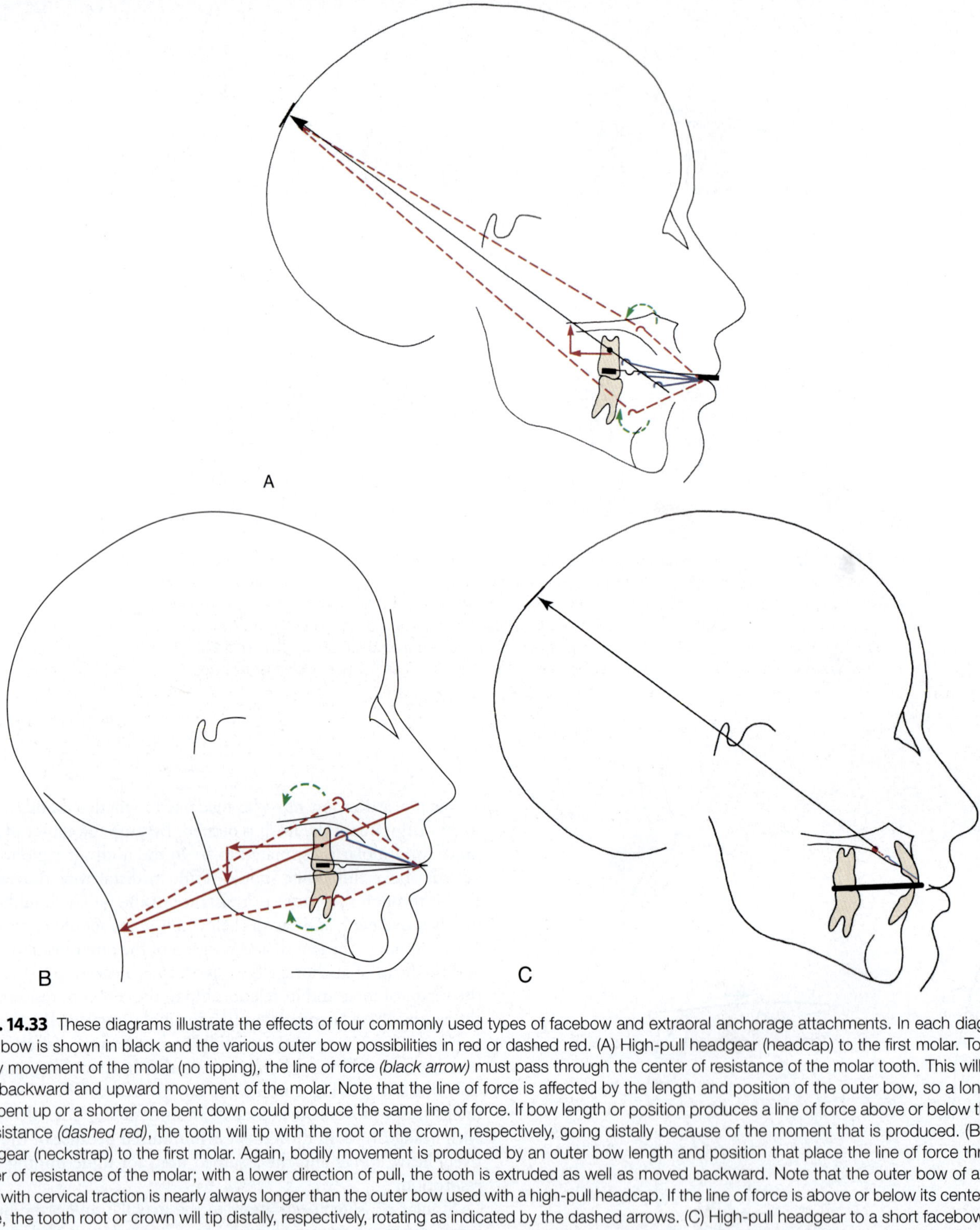

• **Fig. 14.33** These diagrams illustrate the effects of four commonly used types of facebow and extraoral anchorage attachments. In each diagram, the inner bow is shown in black and the various outer bow possibilities in red or dashed red. (A) High-pull headgear (headcap) to the first molar. To produce bodily movement of the molar (no tipping), the line of force *(black arrow)* must pass through the center of resistance of the molar tooth. This will produce both backward and upward movement of the molar. Note that the line of force is affected by the length and position of the outer bow, so a longer outer bow bent up or a shorter one bent down could produce the same line of force. If bow length or position produces a line of force above or below the center of resistance *(dashed red)*, the tooth will tip with the root or the crown, respectively, going distally because of the moment that is produced. (B) Cervical headgear (neckstrap) to the first molar. Again, bodily movement is produced by an outer bow length and position that place the line of force through the center of resistance of the molar; with a lower direction of pull, the tooth is extruded as well as moved backward. Note that the outer bow of a facebow used with cervical traction is nearly always longer than the outer bow used with a high-pull headcap. If the line of force is above or below its center of resistance, the tooth root or crown will tip distally, respectively, rotating as indicated by the dashed arrows. (C) High-pull headgear to a short facebow inserted into a maxillary splint. With all the teeth splinted, it is possible to consider the maxilla as a unit and to relate the line of force to the center of resistance of the maxilla. As with headgear force against the first molar, the relationship of the line of force to the center of resistance of the maxilla determines the rotational effect on the maxilla.

Clinical Management of Headgear

For headgear treatment, molar bands with headgear tubes (and any other attachments that might be needed later in treatment) are fitted and cemented. Bands, not bonded tubes, are necessary to accommodate the heavy forces, and tight-fitting bands, possibly crimped at the cervical margin, provide the best band retention. Fitting and adjustment of the preformed facebow, which must reflect the biomechanical goals of the treatment plan, are shown in Figs. 14.34 and 14.35.

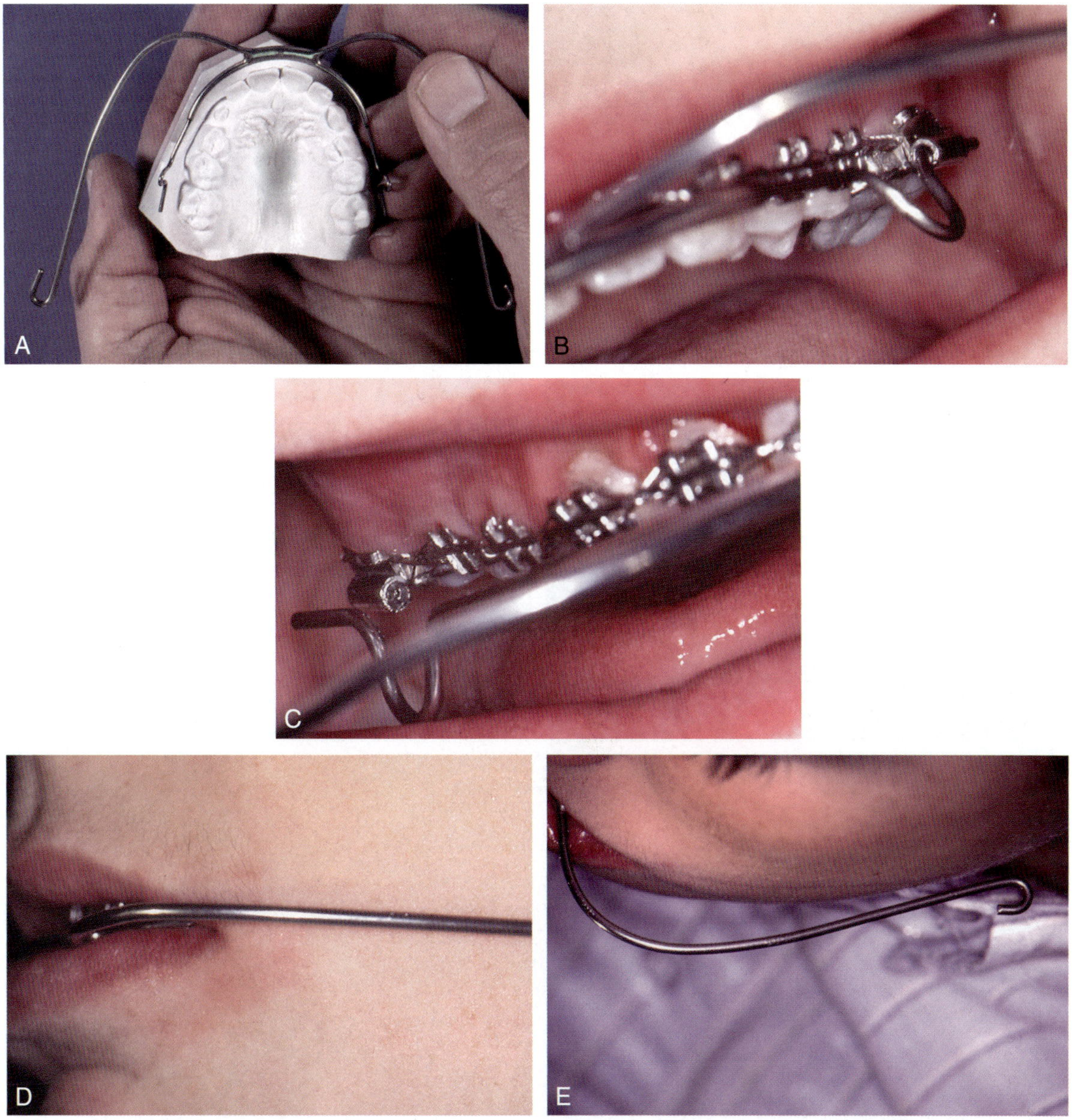

• **Fig. 14.34** The steps for fitting a facebow for a headgear. (A) Preformed facebows are supplied in a variety of inner bow sizes and usually also have an adjustment loop as part of the inner bow. The inner bow should fit closely around the upper arch without contacting the teeth except at the molar tubes (within 3–4 mm of the teeth at all points). A simple method for selecting the appropriate size is to fit the bow to the pretreatment maxillary cast. (B) After the bow has been placed in one molar headgear tube, the rest of the facebow is examined to see how it fits relative to the other molar tube and the teeth. (C) By adjusting the loops to expand or contract the inner bow and by bending the short portion of the bow that fits into the molar tubes and placing facial offsets, it is possible to make the bow passive and allow clearance from the teeth. It should be easy to insert and remove at this point. Then the inner bow must be expanded by 1–2 mm to keep the posterior teeth out of crossbite as anteroposterior changes are made. The extension of the inner bow out the end of the headgear tubes should be evaluated. Ideally the end of the inner bow would be flush with the end of the tube, but certainly there is no need for it to extend more than 1 mm past the end of the tube. This limited extension will reduce tissue irritation in the distal portion of the buccal vestibule and friction during application and removal. (D) The facebow should be adjusted so that the junction of the inner and outer bows rests passively and comfortably between the lips. (E) The outer bow should rest several millimeters from the soft tissue of the cheek. This adjustment must be checked both before and after the straps for the headcap or neckstrap are attached.

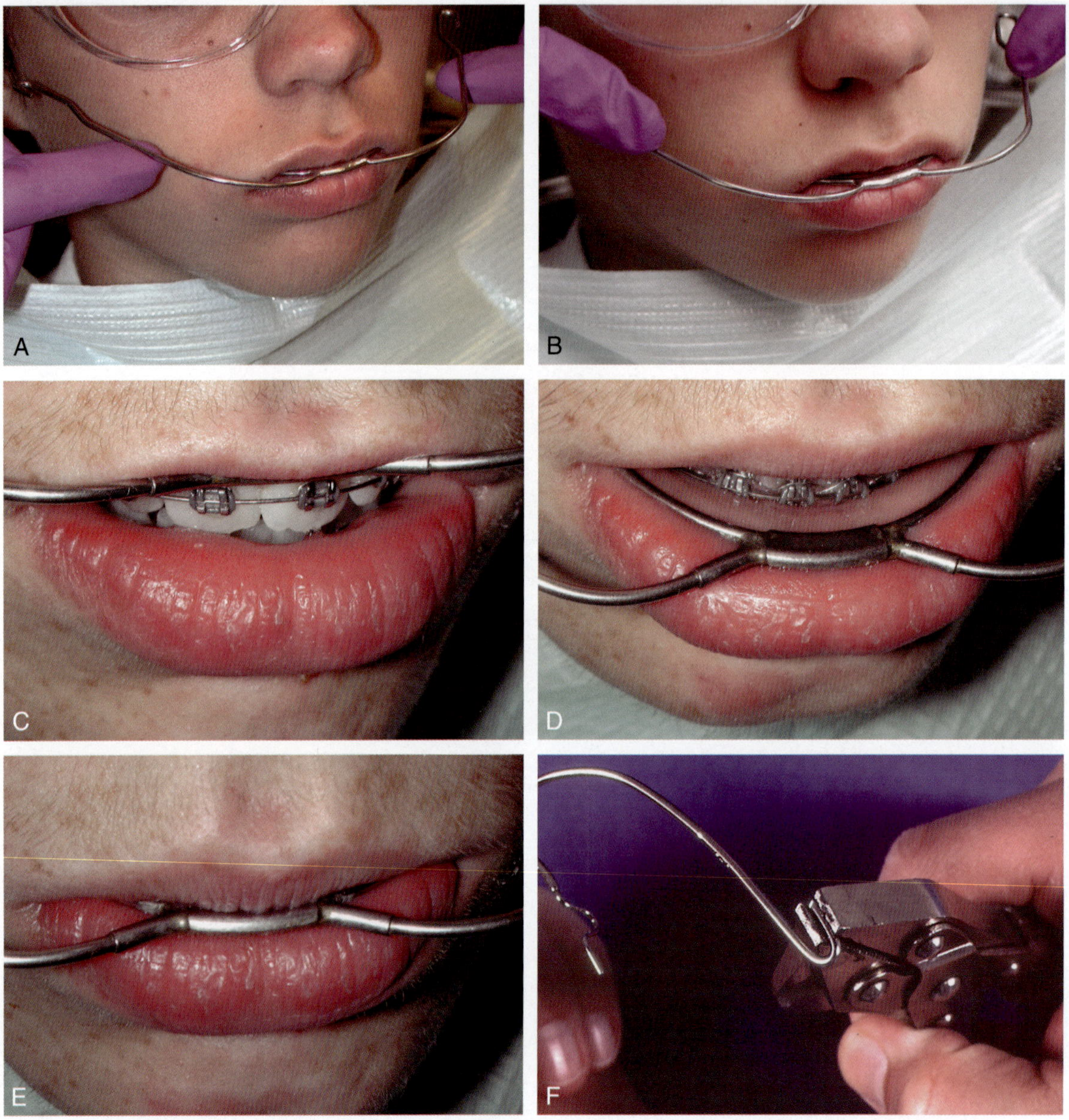

• **Fig. 14.35** To determine the proper length needed for the outer bow, use the index fingers to apply pressure in the direction of the headgear selected. (A) Pushing up and back in the direction of a high-pull headgear. (B) Pushing down and back in the direction of a cervical headgear. As the fingers are moved from the anterior portion of the outer bow to the posterior portion, the position of the bow between the lips will change. (C) If the bow moves up, the roots on the maxillary first molar will move distally. (D) If the bow moves down on the lower lip, the roots of the maxillary first molar will move mesially and the crown distally. (E) If the bow does not move, the force is through the center of resistance of the maxillary first molar and the molar will move bodily and not rotate. These rules hold true for both high-pull and cervical-pull headgears. (F) After the correct length is chosen and the outer bow cut with pliers, a hook is bent at the end with heavy pliers.

As a class II molar relationship is corrected, the relative forward movement of the lower arch will produce a crossbite tendency unless the upper arch width is expanded. This must be taken into account from the beginning of treatment. The inner bow should be expanded by 2 mm symmetrically so that when it is placed in one tube, it rests just outside the other tube. The patient will need to squeeze the inner bow as it is inserted to make it fit the tubes, thus providing the appropriate molar expansion.

The appropriate headcap or neckstrap is fitted by selecting the appropriate size. A spring mechanism or tension module—not elastic bands or straps—is strongly recommended to provide the force. The springs or module deliver consistent forces that can be documented and easily adjusted. The spring attachment is adjusted to provide the correct force with the patient sitting up or standing—not reclining in the dental chair (Figs. 14.29A and B and 14.36). It is usually a good idea to start with a low force level to acclimate the patient to the headgear and then gradually increase the force at subsequent appointments. Even if the correct force level is set at the first appointment, the forces will drop when the strap stretches slightly and contours to the patient's neck. Once the forces are correct, the bow position must be rechecked because the pull of the straps and any adjustments to the inner or outer

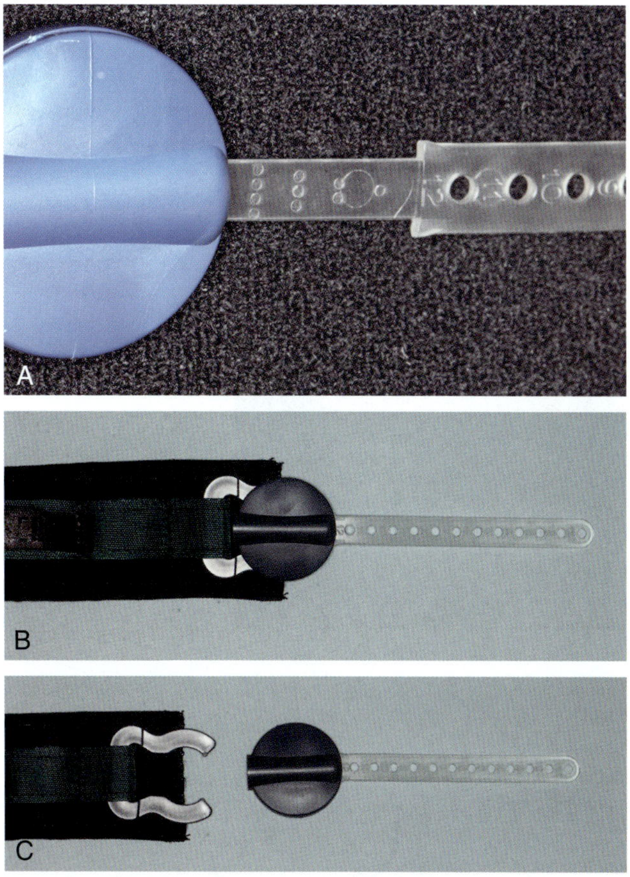

• **Fig. 14.36** Most headgear straps have some calibrated adjustment, either by a spring or a module. (A) This headgear module shows 4 levels of force as 1, 2, 3, or 4 dots equal to 4, 8, 12, or 16 ounces of force, respectively. (B) The module fully assembled on one side. When the clear portion with holes is extended, the calibrated marks are visible and the facebow hook can be placed in the proper hole. Usually the clear tab is cut leaving one extra hole for the patient to grasp when placing the headgear. (C) When excessive forward force is placed on the facebow as when someone grabbed it, the module breaks away to protect the patient from a spring back of the facebow and patient injury. Subsequently the module is reassembled.

bow to improve fit and patient comfort can alter the previous bow position so that it needs adjustment.

The patient should place and remove the headgear under supervision several times to be certain that they understand how to manipulate it and to ensure proper adjustment. Most headgear is worn after school, during relaxed evening hours, and during sleep. It is definitely not indicated during vigorous activity. Children should be instructed that if anyone grabs the outer bow, they should also grab the bow with their hands. This will prevent breakage and injury. The headgear straps must be equipped with a safety-release mechanism (Fig. 14.36C) to prevent the bow from springing back at the patient and injuring them if it is grabbed and pulled by a peer. Severe injuries, including loss of sight, have occurred from headgear accidents of this type.[39] In a review of commercially available headgear-release mechanisms that included 18 different designs, Stafford et al. noted that almost all released at 10 to 20 pounds of force and concluded that the amount of extension before release occurred and the consistency of release were the most important variables from a safety perspective.[40]

Some tooth movement inevitably accompanies efforts at class II growth modification, but that is not growth modification and, as we have noted, can be considered an undesirable side effect—except that it is often necessary to complete correction of the malocclusion. Of course, treatment with tooth movement alone can be successful if both the facial appearance and dental occlusion are satisfactory, as it can be for patients with less severe mandibular deficiency. This is discussed in Chapter 16, where the focus is on management of camouflage treatment.

Combined Vertical and Anteroposterior Problems

Skeletal vertical problems are so intertwined with excessive or deficient dental eruption that it can be difficult to determine the extent to which skeletal disproportions versus tooth eruption deviations are involved. The best way to think about this is to remember that as the mandible grows downward away from the maxilla, a space is created into which the teeth must erupt to remain in contact. From that perspective, it is apparent that a patient with deficient vertical growth would also have deficient eruption of the teeth, and vice versa. The situation is further confused, however, because the vertical position of the maxillary posterior teeth determines the vertical position of the mandible, and so if for some reason there is excessive eruption of those teeth, the mandible would be rotated downward and backward. That means that short-face problems are easier to manage with growth modification than long-face individuals.

Short Face/Deep Bite

Some children exhibit a skeletal vertical deficiency (short face), almost always in conjunction with an anterior deep bite and some degree of mandibular deficiency and often with a class II division 2 malocclusion. The reduced face height is often accompanied by everted and prominent lips that would be normal if the face height were normal.

Children with vertical deficiency can be identified at an early age. They tend to have a low mandibular plane angle (skeletal deep bite) and a long mandibular ramus. Growth is expressed in an anterior direction, with a tendency toward upward and forward rotation of the mandible. The challenge in correcting these problems is to increase eruption of posterior teeth and influence the mandible to rotate downward without decreasing chin prominence too much.

In a patient with class II malocclusion, one way to correct such problems is with cervical headgear, taking advantage of the extrusive tendency of extraoral force directed below the center of resistance of the teeth and the maxilla (Fig. 14.37). This extrudes the upper molars, and eruption of the lower molars can be accentuated by using a biteplate to open the bite along with the headgear. With no posterior occlusion, both upper and lower teeth can erupt.

The other way is to use a functional appliance (usually with mandibular advancement, depending on the anteroposterior jaw relationship) that inhibits eruption of maxillary posterior teeth with acrylic or wire posterior stops and allows free eruption of the mandibular posterior teeth (Fig. 14.38). Because many short-face children also have a class II malocclusion, it is important to remember that rotation of the occlusal plane down in front makes it easier to achieve a class I molar relationship. Cervical headgear

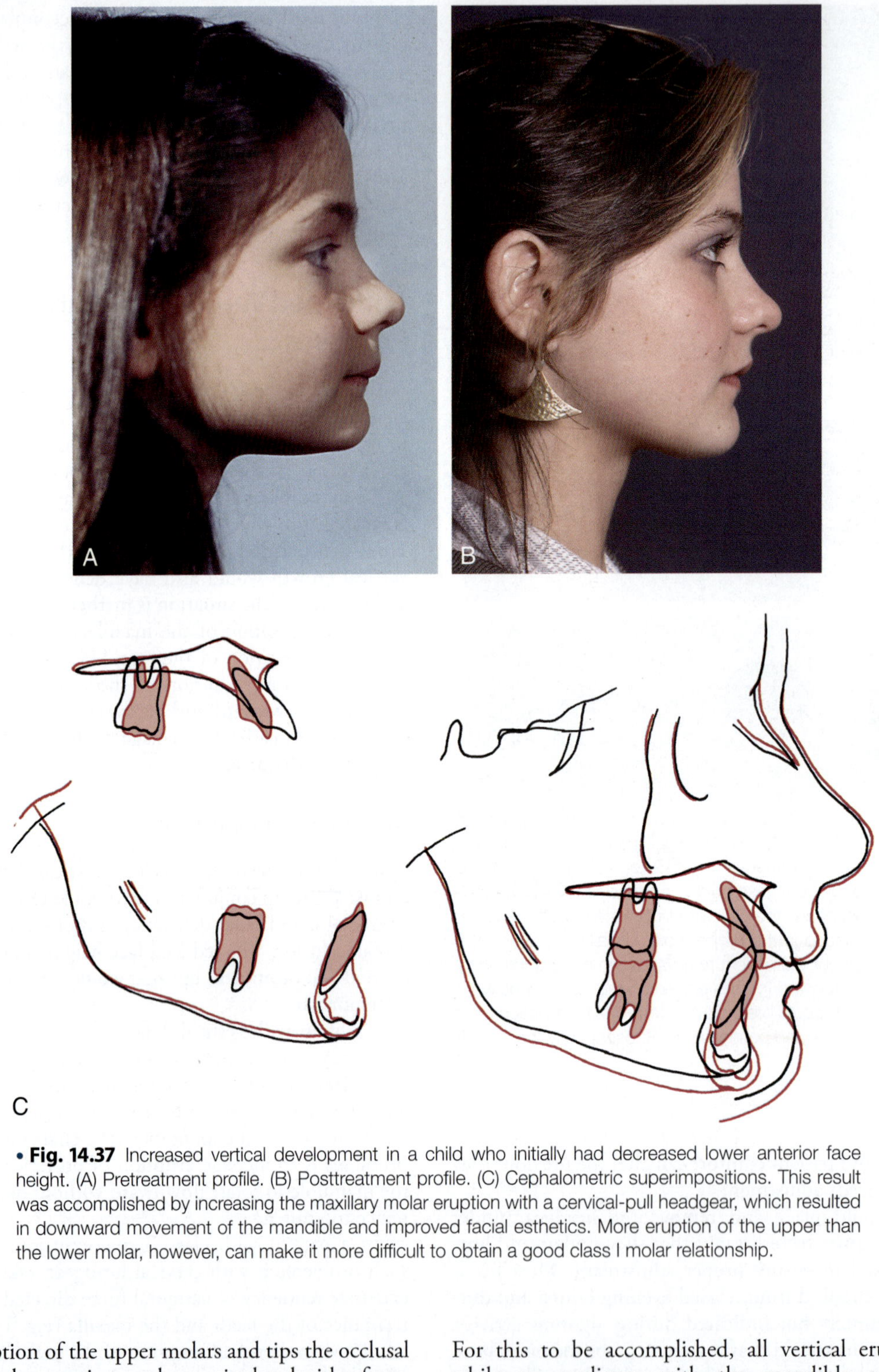

• **Fig. 14.37** Increased vertical development in a child who initially had decreased lower anterior face height. (A) Pretreatment profile. (B) Posttreatment profile. (C) Cephalometric superimpositions. This result was accomplished by increasing the maxillary molar eruption with a cervical-pull headgear, which resulted in downward movement of the mandible and improved facial esthetics. More eruption of the upper than the lower molar, however, can make it more difficult to obtain a good class I molar relationship.

produces more eruption of the upper molars and tips the occlusal plane down posteriorly; eruption can be manipulated with a functional appliance so that either the upper or lower molars erupt more. The desired rotation of the occlusal plane occurs when the lower molar erupts more than the upper, which means that, all other factors being equal, the functional appliance would be preferred.

The treatment of these short-face class II patients is a balance between the anteroposterior and the vertical reactions to treatment. One conservative option for a patient with a significant anteroposterior mandibular deficiency and reduced face height is to have growth expressed in an anterior direction first. For this to be accomplished, all vertical eruption is blocked while an appliance with the mandible advanced is used, which will create a posterior open bite when the appliance is not in place. When the class II jaw relationship is corrected, the posterior bite block gradually is cut away from the lower molars and premolars while correct overbite is maintained anteriorly, so that slow eruption of lower posterior teeth back into occlusion can occur. This type of treatment places into sharp focus the interaction between the anteroposterior and vertical planes of space that must be addressed during growth modification treatment. The priority is placed on the most severe problem, and then the accompanying problems are addressed.

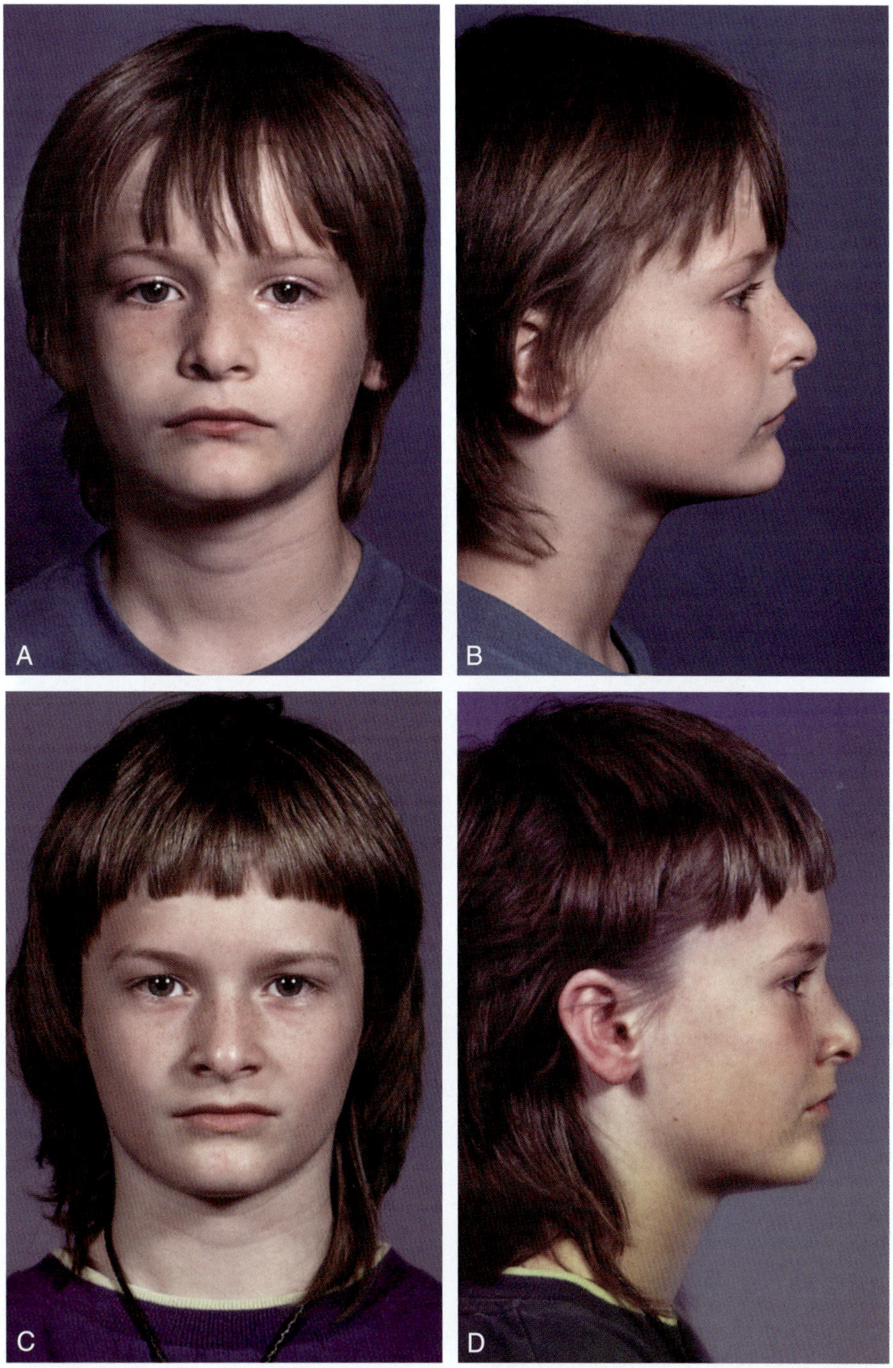

• **Fig. 14.38, cont'd** Facial changes produced by functional appliance treatment in a boy with a short face and skeletal deep bite malocclusion. (A and B) Age 10 before treatment. (C and D) Age 12 after 26 months of treatment. Note the increase in anterior face height and decrease in the labiomental fold.

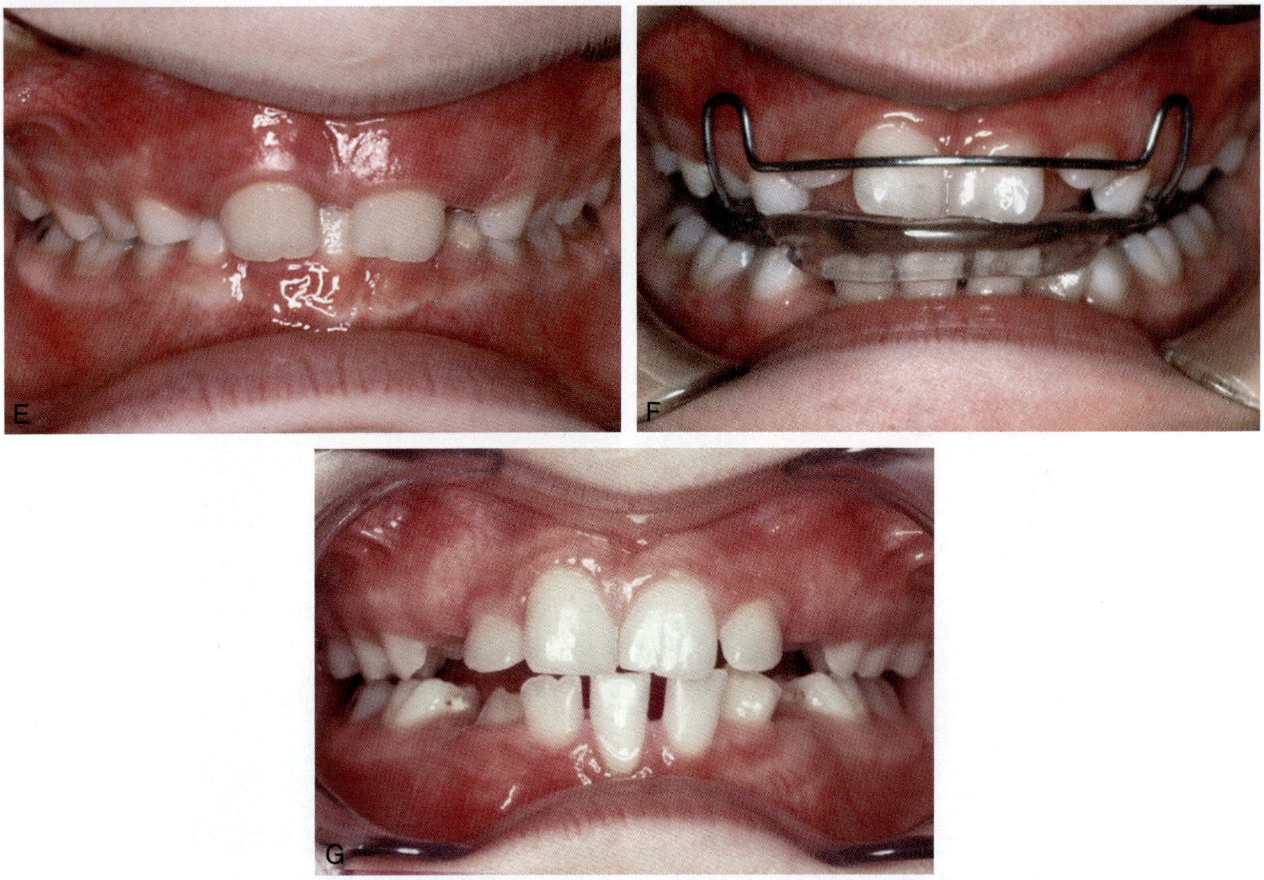

• **Fig. 14.38** (E) Before treatment. Note the gingival inflammation around the maxillary right central incisor resulting from palatal trauma from the deep bite. (F) Deep bite Bionator, constructed to allow eruption of lower posterior teeth and block eruption of incisors and upper posterior teeth. (G) Dental relationships at the conclusion of phase 1 treatment, age 12. A second stage of treatment will be needed when the remaining succedaneous teeth erupt.

Fixed functional appliances are not good choices in the treatment of short-face problems. Certainly, the Herbst, with its propensity to intrude the upper molars, is not an attractive option for younger patients needing increased vertical dimensions, even though the mandibular plane angle usually does not change very much in Herbst treatment.[41]

It is appropriate to remember that eruption occurs more rapidly in some patients than others, probably because it is affected by resting mandibular posture and freeway space as well as by the amount of appliance wear. Some short-face children show extremely rapid mandibular growth when the bite is opened and incisor overlap is removed, even with so simple an appliance as a biteplate. Unfortunately, this happens only occasionally, and except for the rare patients in whom there is no mandibular deficiency, posturing the mandible forward to allow the construction of a functional appliance is the better approach. Delivery and adjustment of a functional appliance for a vertically deficient patient are similar to the methods already discussed in the section on mandibular deficiency.

Long Face/Open Bite

Excessive growth of the maxilla in children with class II malocclusion has more of a vertical than an anteroposterior component (i.e., there is more excessive growth downward than forward), and if the maxilla moves downward, the mandible rotates downward and backward. The effect is to prevent mandibular growth from being expressed anteriorly. Fortunately, in many preadolescents and young adults, the open bite tendency reduces and may correct completely without treatment.[42] In others, the vertical growth pattern continues through adolescence and into the postadolescent years, and the open bite persists. This means that even successful treatment would need to be retained for a number of years, most likely into the late teens or early 20s. The ideal treatment for these patients would be to stop, or at least decrease, maxillary posterior vertical growth so that the mandible would rotate in an upward and forward direction (Fig. 14.39). This could be accomplished by controlling all tooth eruption if there were adequate mandibular vertical ramus growth.

Vertical facial growth continues through adolescence and into the postadolescent years in the same pattern that created a long-face problem to begin with, which means that even if growth can be modified successfully in the mixed dentition, active retention is likely to be necessary for a number of years. Whatever the appliance and whenever the treatment is started, retention would be critically important until vertical growth is essentially complete in the late teens or early 20s.[42]

The goal of growth modification treatment for long-face problems is to maintain the vertical position of the maxilla and inhibit

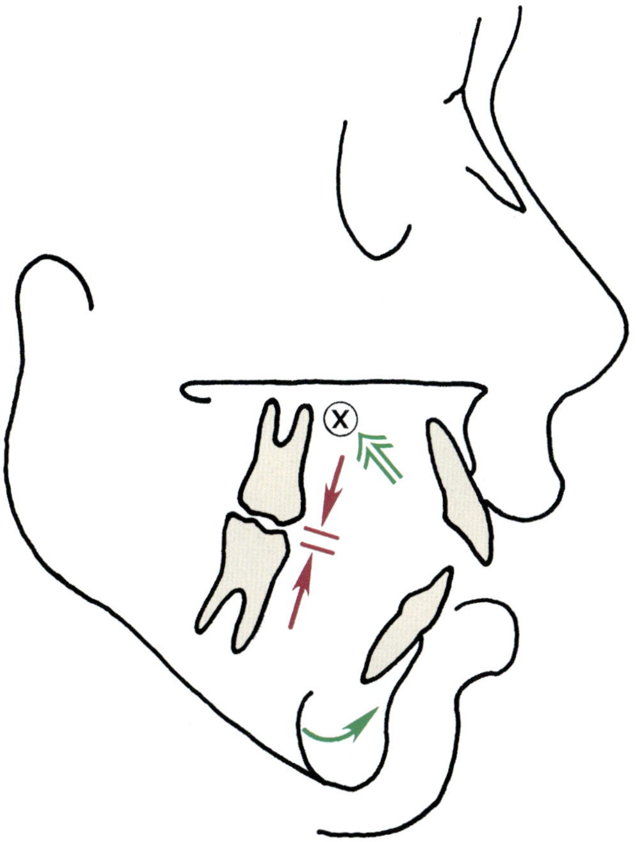

• **Fig. 14.39** Mandibular-deficient children with excessive lower face height need treatment with an appliance that restricts maxillary and mandibular posterior eruption and limits downward growth of the maxilla. This allows mandibular growth to be expressed anteriorly rather than vertically.

eruption of the maxillary and mandibular posterior teeth. There are several possible approaches to doing this during preadolescent and adolescent growth. In the order of increasing clinical effectiveness, they are as follows.

High-Pull Headgear to the Maxillary First Molars

High-pull headgear to the first molars can slow downward growth of the maxilla and stop the eruption of these teeth if it is consistently worn 14 hours a day. The most effective force is about 12 ounces per side (Fig. 14.40). This does not control eruption of the lower molars, which limits its effectiveness in some patients.

High-Pull Headgear to a Maxillary Splint

A more effective headgear approach for children with excessive vertical development is the use of a plastic occlusal splint to which the facebow is attached.[43] This allows vertical force to be directed against all the maxillary posterior teeth, not just the molars, and can be extended forward to contact the incisors if desired. An appliance of this type would be most useful in a child with excessive vertical development of the entire maxillary arch and too much exposure of the maxillary incisors from beneath the lip (i.e., a long-face child who does not have anterior open bite). To achieve both skeletal and dental correction, the patient must be compliant throughout what can be a very long treatment period.

Unfortunately, the maxillary splint still allows mandibular posterior teeth to erupt, and if this occurs, there may be neither redirection of growth nor favorable upward and forward rotation of the mandible.

Functional Appliance With Bite Blocks

A more effective alternative is the use of a functional appliance that includes posterior bite blocks. The retraction force of the headgear is replaced by the somewhat lesser "headgear effect" of the functional appliance. The primary purpose of the appliance is to inhibit vertical descent of the maxilla and eruption of posterior teeth in both arches. The appliance can be designed with or without positioning the mandible anteriorly, depending on how much mandibular deficiency is present.

Regardless of whether the mandible is brought forward in the working bite, the bite must be opened past the normal resting vertical dimension if molar eruption is to be affected. When the mandible is held in this position by the appliance, the stretch of the soft tissues (including but not limited to the muscles) exerts a vertical intrusive force on the posterior teeth. In children with anterior open bites, the anterior teeth are allowed to erupt, which reduces the open bite, whereas in children with the less common long-face problems without open bite, all teeth are held by the bite blocks. Because there is no compensatory posterior eruption, all mandibular growth should be directed more anteriorly, at least to the extent that the overbite allows.

In the short term, this type of functional appliance treatment can be effective in controlling maxillary vertical skeletal and dental growth,[44] and this helps to close anterior open bites (Fig. 14.41). In the long term, because of the continued vertical growth, if a functional appliance is used for a first phase of treatment during the adolescent growth spurt, posterior bite blocks or other components (such as bone screws for skeletal anchorage) will be needed to control vertical growth and tooth eruption during fixed appliance therapy and probably into retention. This is necessary because fixed appliances do not control eruption well and many biomechanical actions are extrusive.

High-Pull Headgear to a Functional Appliance With Bite Blocks

The most aggressive approach to maxillary vertical excess and a class II jaw relationship, which has been recommended as a way to treat the most severely affected long-face patients, is a combination of high-pull headgear and a functional appliance with posterior bite blocks to anteriorly reposition the mandible and control eruption (Fig. 14.42). The theory is that the extraoral force increases the control of maxillary growth and allows the force to be delivered to the whole maxilla rather than to simply the permanent first molars. The high-pull headgear improves retention of the functional appliance and produces a force direction near the estimated center of resistance of the maxilla (see Fig. 14.33C). The functional appliance provides the possibility of enhancing mandibular growth while controlling the eruption of the posterior and anterior teeth.

In reality, the addition of headgear appears to provide little if any more vertical skeletal and dental control and has only a modest anteroposterior maxillary skeletal impact. This benefit should be weighed against the effects of the simpler open bite functional appliance without headgear. A study with follow-up through a later stage of fixed appliance therapy concluded that there was so little skeletal impact of the headgear-functional appliance stage of treatment that it could no longer be recommended.[45] For severely affected children with the long-face pattern, the only successful treatment methods are intrusion of posterior teeth by means of skeletal anchorage and segmental

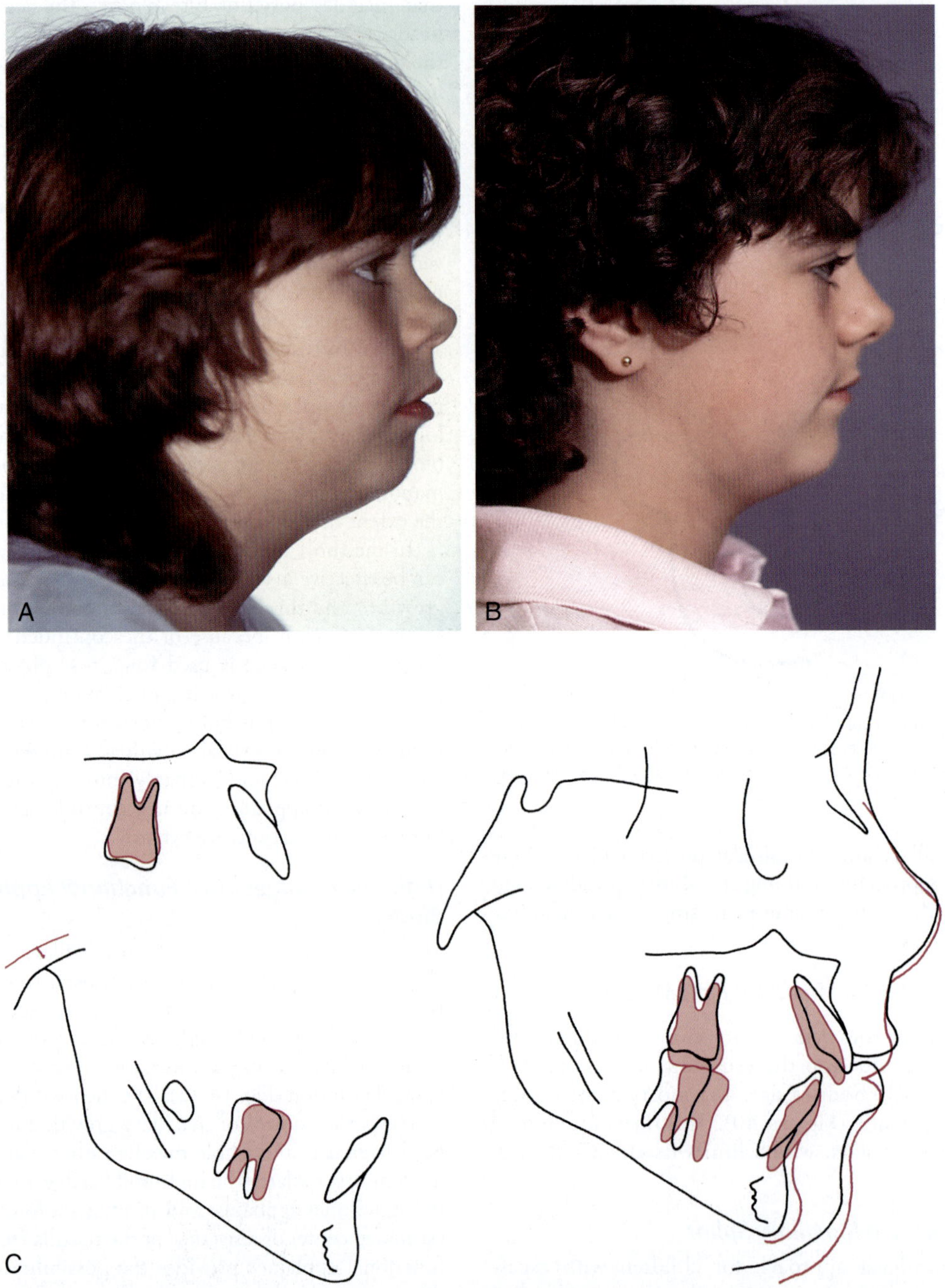

• **Fig. 14.40** These photos show an excellent response to high-pull headgear for a patient with excessive lower face height. (A) Pretreatment profile. (B) Posttreatment profile. (C) Cephalometric superimposition tracing. The cranial base superimposition shows that the maxilla and the maxillary teeth did not move inferiorly; as a result the mandible grew forward and not downward. The mandibular superimposition shows that the lower molar drifted forward into the leeway space. The incisor positions relative to the maxilla and mandible did not change.

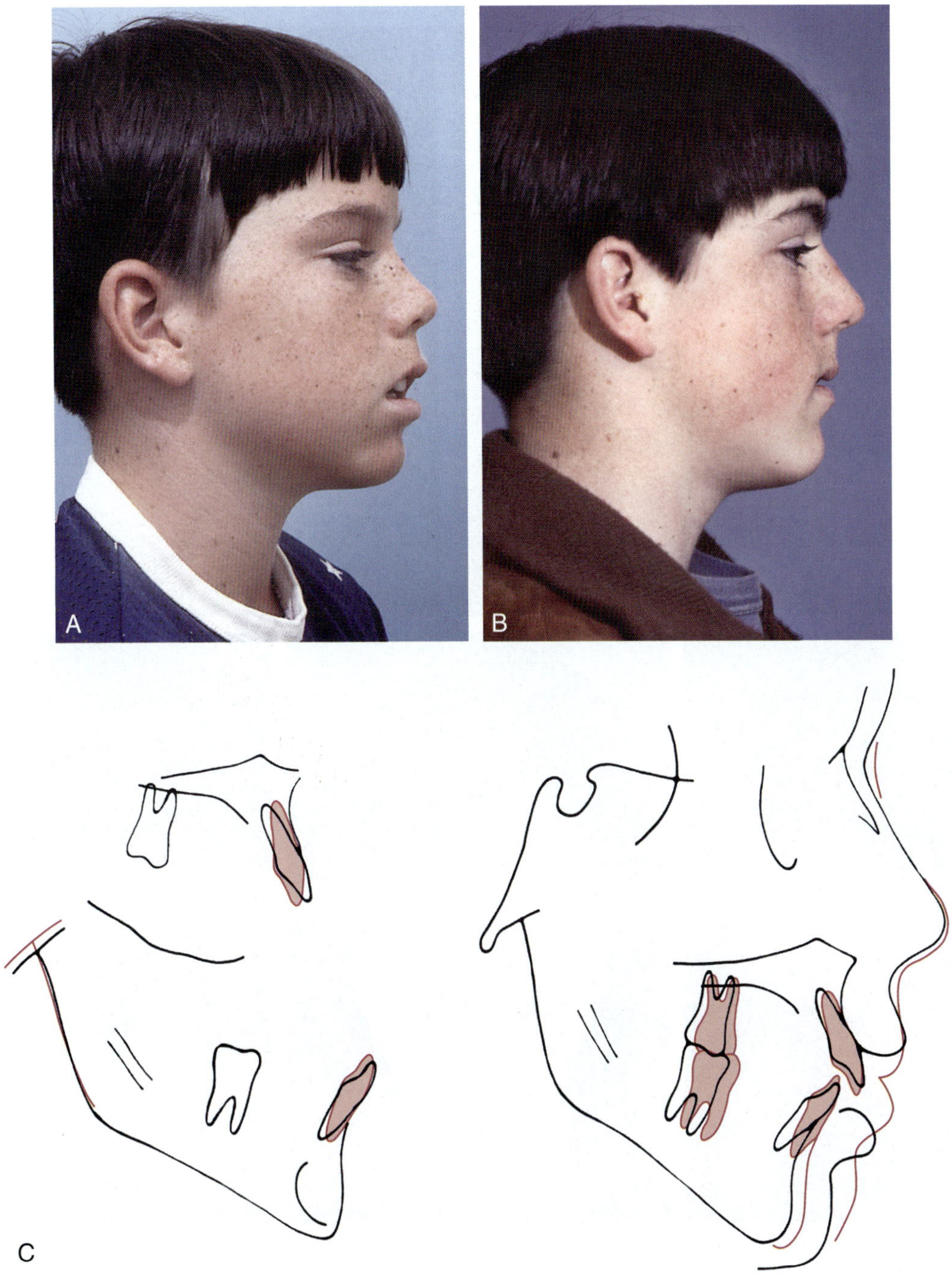

• **Fig. 14.41** This patient demonstrates a good response to functional appliance treatment designed to control vertical development with posterior bite blocks in a child with excessive lower face height. (A) Pretreatment profile. (B) Posttreatment profile. (C) Cephalometric superimposition tracing. Note that no posterior eruption occurred, and all mandibular growth was directed anteriorly. Face height was maintained, and anterior eruption closed the open bite. Maxillary and mandibular molar positions relative to their supporting bone were maintained.

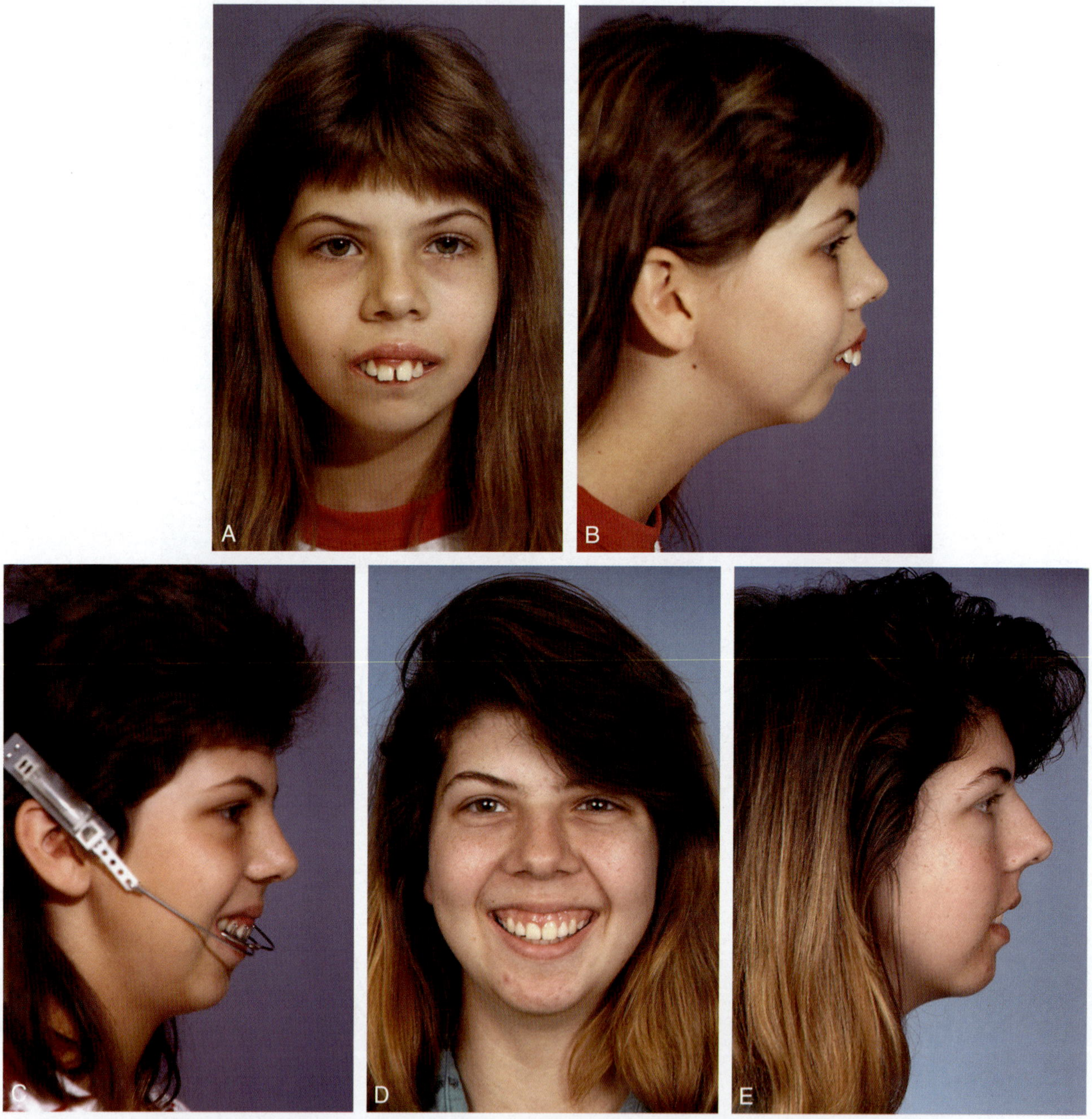

• **Fig. 14.42** The maximum growth-modification approach to a severe long-face, mandibular deficiency problem is high-pull headgear attached to a functional appliance with posterior bite blocks. (A and B) Facial appearance before treatment. (C) High-pull headgear with the facebow inserted into tubes in a functional appliance with bite blocks. (D and E) Posttreatment facial appearance is improved but not ideal. (F) Cephalometric superimposition showing continued downward and forward movement of the chin but no increase in the mandibular plane angle. The major effect of treatment was retraction of the protruding maxillary incisors into a premolar extraction space; little if any modification of the growth pattern occurred.

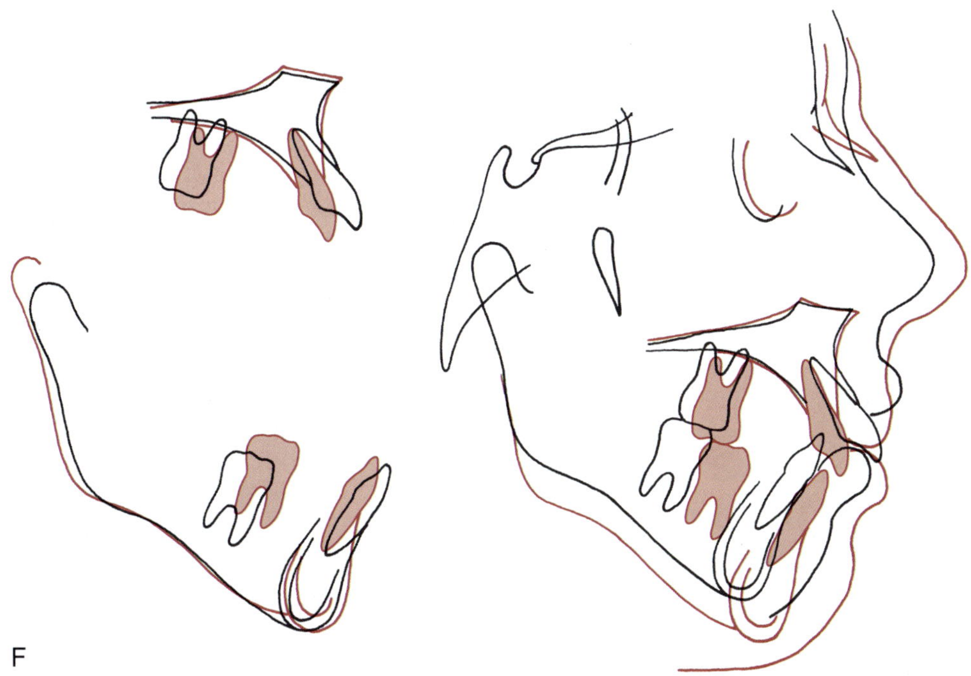

• **Fig. 14.42, cont'd**

maxillary osteotomy, which are discussed in Chapters 20 and 22, respectively.

Facial Asymmetry in Children

Although almost everyone has some facial asymmetry, asymmetric development of the jaws severe enough to cause a problem affects less than 0.5% of the US population. An asymmetry problem involving only the maxilla is quite rare and almost always is due to trauma to that part of the face. Asymmetry involving only the nose is more frequent and is also most likely to be the result of trauma if only the nose is affected. The mandible is involved in 85% to 90% of facial asymmetry cases because of a growth problem. However, asymmetric mandibular growth has secondary effects on the maxilla, and both jaws are likely to become involved as the asymmetry develops.

Asymmetric Mandibular Deficiency

Asymmetric mandibular deficiency in a child or adolescent can be due to hemifacial microsomia or occasionally another problem in prenatal growth. Most arise as a result of a fracture of the condylar process of the mandible (Fig. 14.43).[46] There are three aspects to the differential diagnosis between these two conditions:

1. A congenital anomaly of any severity is likely to be noticed at birth, and the later the asymmetric deficiency arises, the more likely it is to be due to a condylar fracture.
2. For a young patient with an asymmetry that was not noticed at birth, a mild form of hemifacial microsomia is part of the differential diagnosis. Because this condition usually affects the ear as well as the mandible, the key question is whether the ear on the affected side is small or malformed (see Fig. 5.6). Because there is a deficiency of soft tissue and muscle, growth modification is possible only in the least affected patients with this problem.
3. In contrast, the asymmetry after a condylar fracture is due to a restriction of growth in the condyle area caused by contraction of scar tissue created by the injury. Growth modification is possible for patients with less intensive restriction of growth.

When a condylar fracture is diagnosed in a child, maintaining function is the key to normal growth. Function does not mean simple opening and closing hinge movements but must also include translation of the mandibular condyles. Translation is necessary for regeneration and stretch of the associated soft tissues in the short term, and for normal growth in the long term. Fortunately, most jaw fractures in preadolescent children can be treated with little or no surgical manipulation of the segments and little immobilization of the jaws because the bony segments are self-retentive and the healing process is rapid. Treatment should involve short fixation times (usually maintained with intraoral intermaxillary elastics) and rapid return to function. Open reduction of the fracture should be avoided.[46]

A functional appliance during the postinjury period can be used to minimize any growth restriction. The appliance is a conventional activator or Bionator-type appliance that symmetrically advances the mandible to nearly an edge-to-edge incisor position. Using this appliance, the patient is forced to translate the mandible, and any remodeling can occur with the mandible in the unloaded and forward position.

Many condylar fractures are not diagnosed at the time of injury, so when a child with asymmetric mandibular deficiency is seen, trauma is the most likely cause even if a condylar injury was not noticed. The key to establishing the prognosis for growth modification is the extent to which the affected side can translate. Even if the mandible deviates to the affected side on opening, reasonably normal growth is possible if some

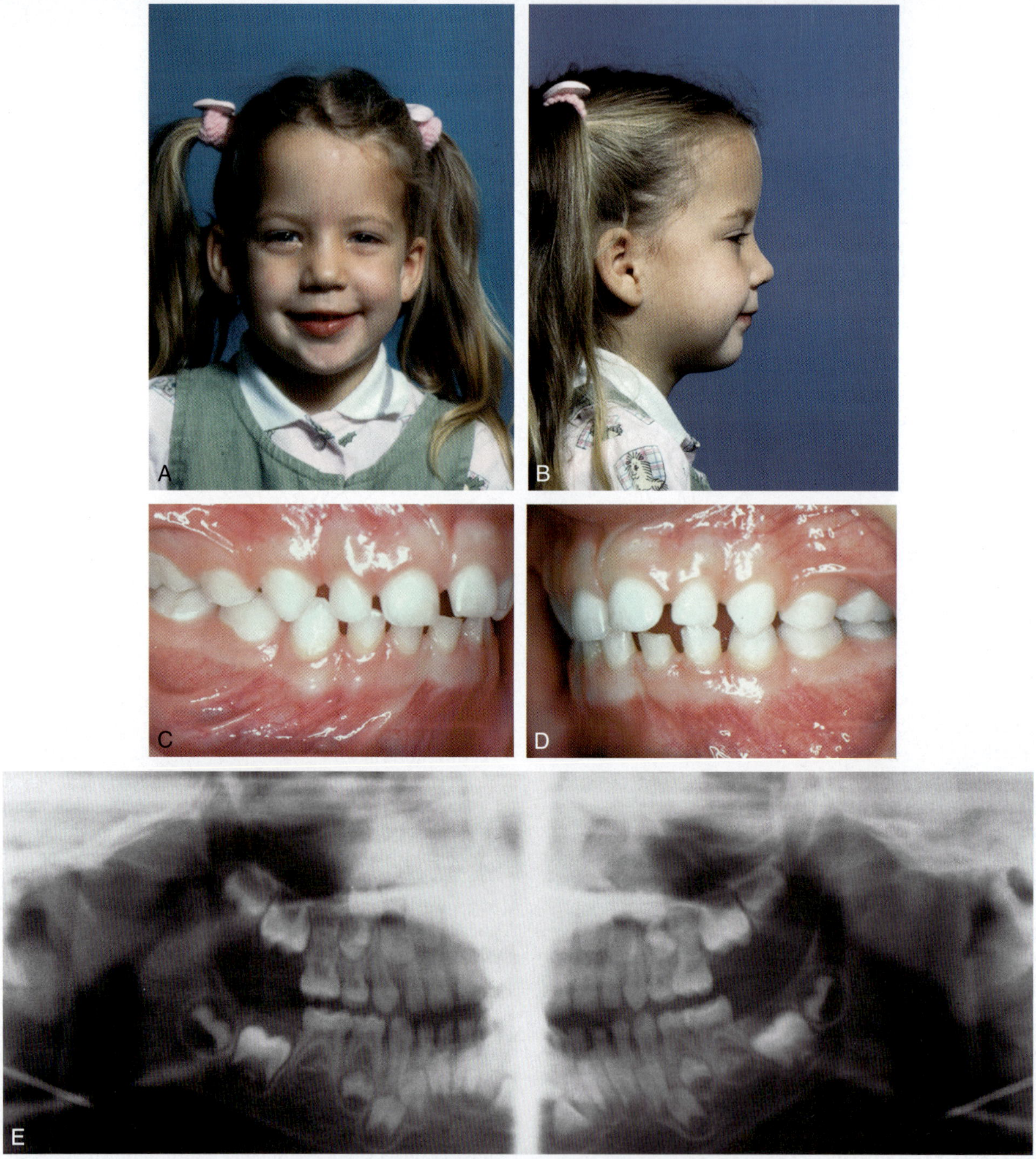

• **Fig. 14.43** (A and B) This 5-year-old girl's family dentist noted her facial asymmetry, with the chin off to the left (she deviated even more on opening) and referred her for further evaluation. (C and D) Her buccal occlusion was normal (class I) on the right and class II on the left. (E) The panoramic radiograph showed the classic appearance of a unilateral condylar fracture. Note the normal condyle on the right and only a condylar stub on the left. The injury almost surely occurred at age 2 when she fell but was not diagnosed at the time.

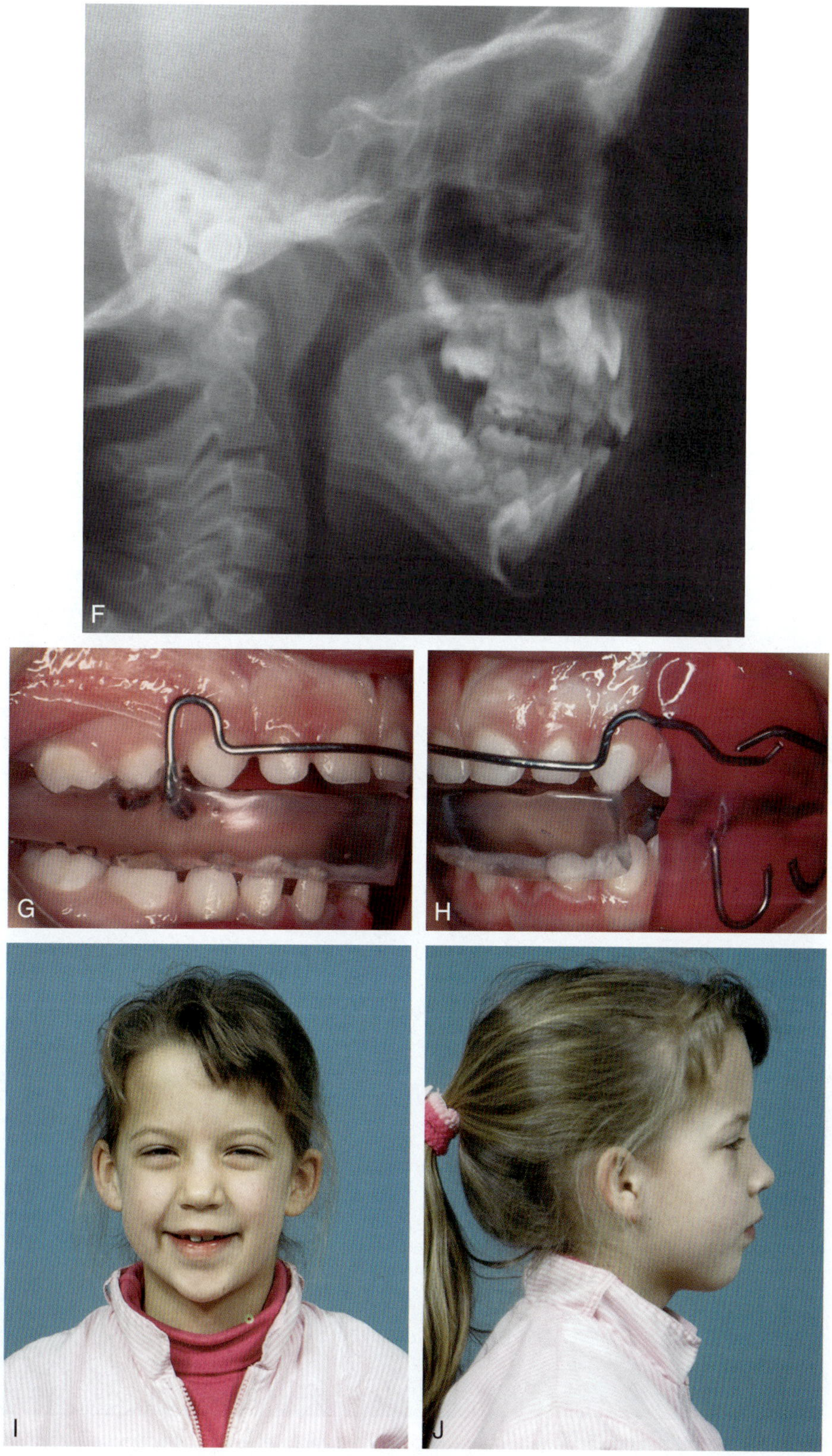

• **Fig. 14.43** (F) Note the two mandibular borders on the cephalometric radiograph resulting from the shorter ramus on the left. (G and H) She was treated with a series of hybrid functional appliances, with buccal and lingual shields on the left and a bite block anteriorly and on the right. The objective was to encourage mandibular growth and tooth eruption on the deficient left side and restrain eruption on the right. It is important to keep the tongue from between the teeth on the side where eruption is desired; therefore the lingual shield on the left side (cannot be seen in the photos) was a critically important part of the appliance. (I and J) Facial views 2 years later.

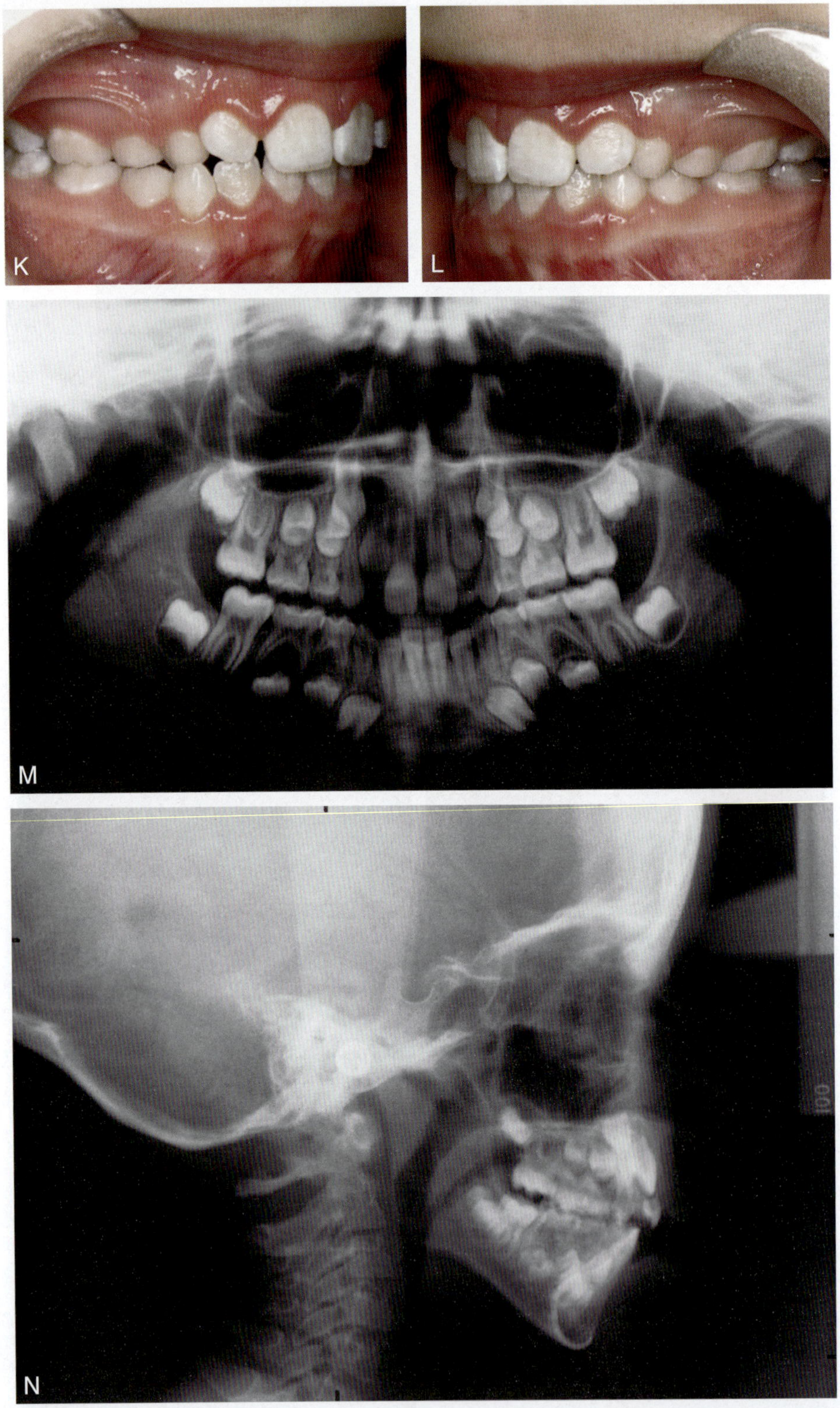

• **Fig. 14.43** (K and L) Intraoral views 2 years later. Note the improvement in both facial symmetry and occlusion. Treatment with hybrid functional appliances was continued. (M) Panoramic and (N) cephalometric progress views. Note the regeneration of the left condyle (seen clearly in the panoramic view) and reduction in the difference in height of the two mandibular rami, shown in the cephalometric radiograph.

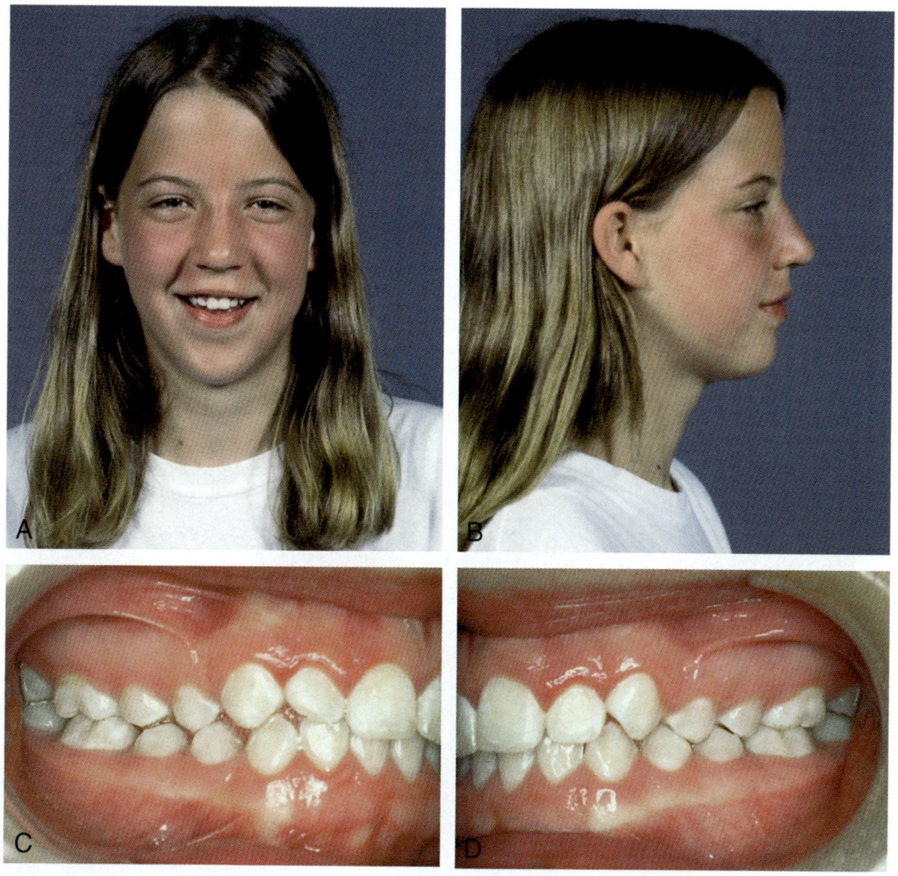

• **Fig. 14.44** (A and B) Facial and (C and D) intraoral views at age 13, with nearly complete resolution of the facial asymmetry, although the mandible still deviates to the left on wide opening. Functional appliance treatment was discontinued at age 10, and there was no further orthodontic therapy.

degree of translation occurs (see Fig. 14.44). Hybrid functional appliances (see Fig. 14.44G and H) offer a way to obtain more growth on one side than the other.[47] Although these appliances may appear confusing, they are simply various components logically combined to achieve specific purposes for individual patients. Progress over a 10-year period in management of this patient with a treatable restriction of growth is shown in Fig. 14.44. The surprising secondary adolescent growth spurt in this patient, and the return of some facial asymmetry when this growth was not controlled, demonstrate the difference with and without growth control.

Surgical intervention for a facial growth problem before adolescence has only one goal: to create an environment in which growth is possible. Therefore this is indicated only for patients with asymmetric deficiency in whom the abnormal growth is progressively making the problem worse, as in ankylosis that keeps one side from growing. The guideline is that a restriction of jaw opening of less than 15 mm is unlikely to respond to growth modification, whereas an opening of 20 mm or more usually makes nonsurgical growth guidance possible. For surgery patients, treatment with a hybrid functional appliance will be needed after surgery has made condylar translation possible, to correct the primary growth problem, decompensate the dental arches vertically, and guide function. Problems of this severity are usually better managed through a major health sciences center.

Asymmetric Mandibular Excess

Excessive growth of the mandible on one side is labeled now as hemimandibular hyperplasia because the ramus and body of the mandible are affected, although the old name of condylar hypertrophy was not totally wrong (see Chapter 7). This condition overwhelmingly affects females rather than males. It is a classic progressive condition, one that steadily gets worse (Fig. 14.45), and that makes the most severely affected patients candidates for early surgical intervention. Growth modification to stop the excessive growth is not possible. Surgical possibilities for these patients are discussed in Chapter 22.

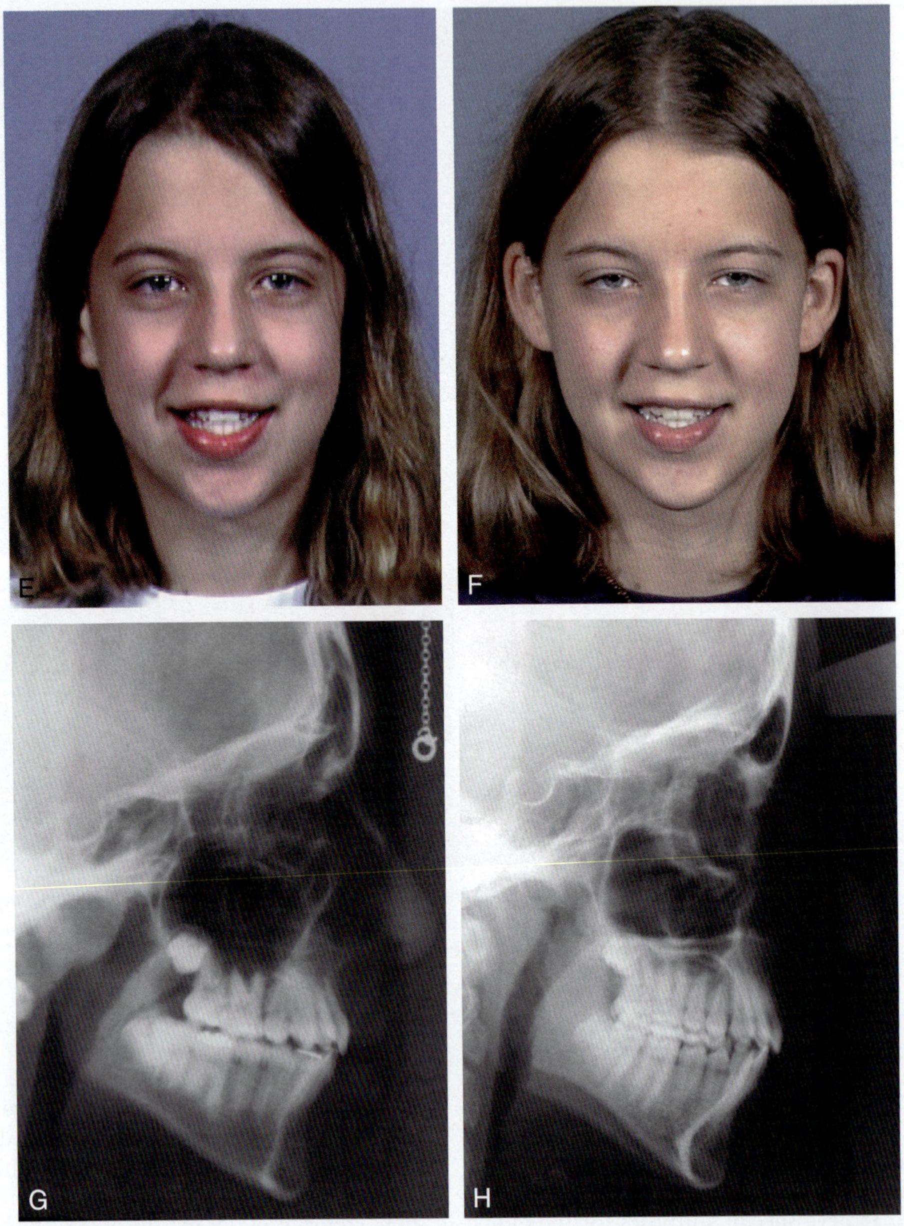

• **Fig. 14.44** (E and F) Facial and (G and H) intraoral views at age 15. The patient grew 3 inches taller between ages 13 and 15 in what amounted to a secondary adolescent growth spurt, although she was well beyond menarche at that time, and there was a mild return of the asymmetry when this growth was not controlled. Perhaps this unanticipated long-term effect is the best evidence that the series of appliances did control her symmetric growth during the initial stages of treatment.

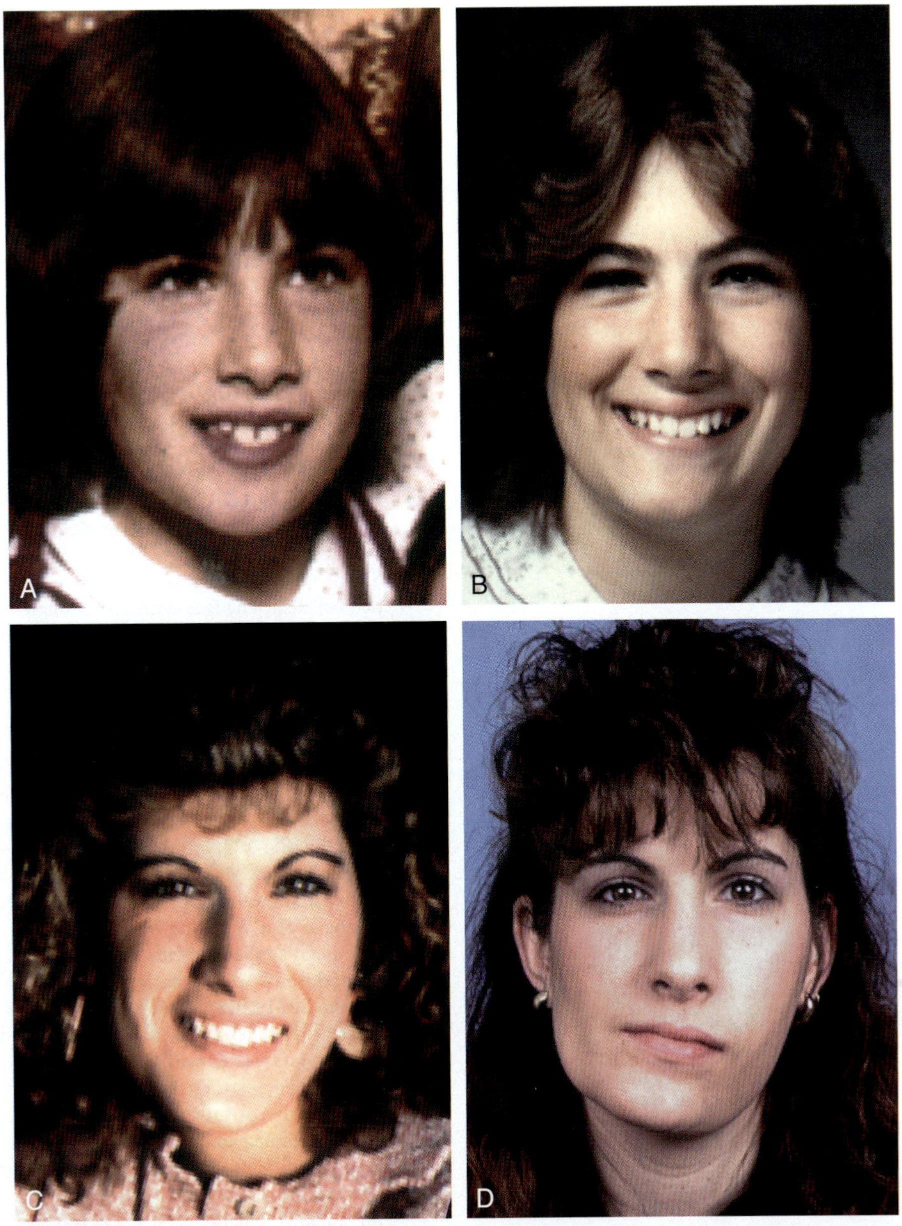

• **Fig. 14.45** Hemimandibular hypertrophy is the classic example of a progressive deformity: excessive growth of the condyle or lengthening of the condylar process starts with a mild mandibular asymmetry and slowly creates a major deformity if untreated. (A) Age 8, family photo. (B) Age 15. (C) Age 17, high school graduation photo. (D) Age 19, clinic photograph when she finally sought treatment. The age of onset for this patient was unusually early and the resulting deformity was unusually severe, but the gender and progressive course were typical.

References

1. Pancherz H, Fackel U. The skeletofacial growth pattern pre- and post-dentofacial orthopedics. *Eur J Orthod.* 1990;12:209–218.
2. Perinetti G, Primožič J, Franchi L, Contardo L. Treatment effects of removable functional appliances in pre-pubertal and pubertal class II patients: a systematic review and meta-analysis of controlled studies. *PLoS ONE.* 2015;10(10):e0141198.
3. Perinetti G, Primozic J, Sharma B, Cioffi I, Contardo L. Cervical vertebral maturation method and mandibular growth peak: a longitudinal study of diagnostic reliability. *Eur J Orthod.* 2018;40(6):666–672. https://doi.org/10.1093/ejo/cjy018. PMID: 29608692.
4. Morris KM, Fields HW, Beck FM, Kim DG. Diagnostic testing of cervical vertebral maturation staging: an independent assessment. *Am J Orthod Dentofac Orthop.* 2019;156:626–632.
5. Tulloch JF, Proffit WR, Phillips C. Outcomes in a 2-phase randomized clinical trial of early Class II treatment. *Am J Orthod Dentofac Orthop.* 2004;125:657–667.
6. Cozza P, Baccetti T, Franchi L, et al. Mandibular changes produced by functional appliances in Class II malocclusion: a systematic review. *Am J Orthod Dentofac Orthop.* 2006;129 599.e1–e12.
7. Nucera R, Lo GA, Rustico L, Matarese G, et al. Effectiveness of orthodontic treatment with functional appliances on maxillary growth in the short term: a systematic review and meta-analysis. *Am J Orthod Dentofac Orthop.* 2016;149:600–611. e3.
8. O'Brien K, Wright J, Conboy F, et al. Early treatment for Class II division 1 malocclusion with the Twin-Block appliance: a multi-center, randomized, controlled trial. *Am J Orthod Dentofac Orthop.* 2009;135:573–579.
9. Ehsani S, Nebbe B, Normando D, et al. Short-term treatment effects produced by the Twin-block appliance: a systematic review and meta-analysis. *Eur J Orthod.* 2015;Volume 37(Issue 2):170–176. https://doi.org/10.1093/ejo/cju030.
10. Santamaría-Villegas A, Manrique-Hernandez R, Alvarez-Varela E, et al. Effect of removable functional appliances on mandibular length in patients with class II with retrognathism: systematic review and meta-analysis. *BMC Oral Health.* 2017;17:52. https://doi.org/10.1186/s12903-017-0339-8.
11. Oppenheim A. Biologic orthodontic therapy and reality. *Angle Orthod.* 1936;6:69–79.
12. Kloehn S. Guiding alveolar growth and eruption of the teeth to reduce treatment time and produce a more balanced denture and face. *Am J Orthod.* 1947;17:10–33.
13. Wieslander L. The effects of orthodontic treatment on the concurrent development of the craniofacial complex. *Am J Orthod.* 1963;49:15–27.
14. Armstrong MM. Controlling the magnitude, direction and duration of extraoral force. *Am J Orthod.* 1971;59:217–243.
15. Keeling SD, Wheeler TT, King GJ, et al. Anteroposterior skeletal and dental changes after early Class II treatment with Bionators and headgear. *Am J Orthod Dentofac Orthop.* 1998;113:40–50.
16. Baumrind S, Molthen R, West EE, et al. Mandibular plane changes during maxillary retraction, part 2. *Am J Orthod.* 1978;74:603–621.
17. O'Brien K, Wright J, Conboy F, et al. Early treatment for Class II division 1 malocclusion with the Twin-Block appliance. *Am J Orthod Dentofac Orthop.* 2009;135:573–579.
18. O'Brien K, Wright J, Conboy F, et al. Effectiveness of early orthodontic treatment with the Twin-Block appliance: a multicenter, randomized, controlled trial. Part 2: psychosocial effects. *Am J Orthod Dentofac Orthop.* 2003;124:488–494.
19. Batista KB, Thiruvenkatachari B, Harrison JE, O'Brien KD. Orthodontic treatment for prominent upper front teeth (Class II malocclusion) in children and adolescents. *Cochrane Database Syst Rev.* 2018;3(3): CD003452.
20. Borzabadi-Farahani A, Borzabadi-Farahani A, Eslamipour F. An investigation into the association between facial profile and maxillary incisor trauma, a clinical non-radiographic study. *Dent Traumatol.* 2010;26:403–408.
21. Glendor U, Koucheki B, Halling A. Risk evaluation and type of treatment of multiple dental trauma episodes to permanent teeth. *Endod Dent Traumatol.* 2000;16:205–210.
22. Julku J, Pirilä-Parkkinen K, Pirttiniemi P. Airway and hard tissue dimensions in children treated with early and later timed cervical headgear-a randomized controlled trial. *Eur J Orthod.* 2018;40(3):285–295. https://doi.org/10.1093/ejo/cjx088.
23. Larsen AJ, Rindal DB, Hatch JP, et al. Evidence supports no relationship between obstructive sleep apnea and premolar extraction: an electronic health records review. *J Clin Sleep Med.* 2015;11(12):1443–1448. https://doi.org/10.5664/jcsm.5284.
24. Behrents RG, Shelgikar AV, Conley RS, et al. Obstructive sleep apnea and orthodontics: an American Association of Orthodontists White Paper. *Am J Orthod Dentofac Orthop.* 2019;156(1):13–28.e1. https://doi.org/10.1016/j.ajodo.2019.04.009.
25. Pancherz H. The effects, limitations, and long-term dentofacial adaptations to treatment with the Herbst appliance. *Semin Orthod.* 1997;3:232–243.
26. Franchi L, Baccetti T. Prediction of individual mandibular changes induced by functional jaw orthopedics followed by fixed appliances in Class II patients. *Angle Orthod.* 2006;76:950–954.
27. Siara-Olds NJ, Pangrazio-Kulbersh V, Berger J, et al. Long-term dentoskeletal changes with the Bionator, Herbst, Twin-Block and MARA functional appliances. *Angle Orthod.* 2012;80:18–29.
28. Zymperdikas VF, Koretsi V, Papageorgiou SN, Papadopoulos MA. Treatment effects of fixed functional appliances in patients with Class II malocclusion: a systematic review and meta-analysis. *Eur J Orthod.* 2016;38(2):113–126.
29. Perinetti G, Primozic J, Furlani G, et al. Treatment effects of fixed functional appliances alone or in combination with multibracket appliances: a systematic review and meta-analysis. *Angle Orthod.* 2014;85:480–492.
30. Pancherz H, Malmgren O, Hagg U, et al. Class II correction in Herbst and Bass therapy. *Eur J Orthod.* 1989;11:17–30.
31. Huang Y, Sun W, Xiong X, Zhang Z, Liu J, Wang J. Effects of fixed functional appliances with temporary anchorage devices on Class II malocclusion: A systematic review and meta-analysis. *J World Fed Orthod.* 2021;10(2):59–69.
32. Jones G, Buschang PH, Kim KB, Oliver DR. Class II non-extraction patients treated with the Forsus Fatigue Resistant Device versus intermaxillary elastics. *Angle Orthod.* 2008;78:332–338.
33. Al-Saleh MA, Alsufyani N, Flores-Mir C, et al. Changes in temporomandibular joint morphology in Class II patients treated with fixed mandibular repositioning and evaluated through 3D imaging: a systematic review. *Orthod Craniofac Res.* 2015;18:185–201.
34. Tarvade SM, Chaudhari CV, Daokar SG, et al. Dentoskeletal comparison of changes seen in Class II cases treated by Twin Block and Forsus. *J Int Oral Health.* 2014;6:27–31.
35. Giuntini V, Vangelisti A, Masucci C, et al. Treatment effects produced by the Twin-Block appliance vs the Forsus Fatigue Resistant Device in growing Class II patients. *Angle Orthod.* 2015;85:784–789.
36. Pacha MM, Fleming PS, Johal A. A comparison of the efficacy of fixed versus removable functional appliances in children with Class II malocclusion: a systematic review. *Eur J Orthod.* 2016;38(6):621–630.
37. Banks P, Wright J, O'Brien K. Incremental versus maximum bite advancement during Twin-Block therapy: a randomized controlled clinical trial. *Am J Orthod Dentofac Orthop.* 2004;126:583–588.
38. Haralabakis NB, Sifakakis IB. The effect of cervical headgear on patients with high or low mandibular plane angles and the "myth" of posterior mandibular rotation. *Am J Orthod Dentofac Orthop.* 2004;126:310–317.
39. Chaushu G, Chausu S, Weinberger T. Infraorbital abscess from orthodontic headgear. *Am J Orthod Dentofac Orthop.* 1997;112: 364–366.
40. Stafford GD, Caputo AA, Turley PK. Characteristics of headgear release mechanisms: safety implications. *Angle Orthod.* 1998;68:319–326.

41. Ruf S, Pancherz H. The effect of Herbst appliance treatment on the mandibular plane angle: a cephalometric roentgenographic study. *Am J Orthod Dentofac Orthop*. 1996;110:225–229.
42. Phelan A, Franchi L, Baccetti T, et al. Longitudinal growth changes in subjects with open-bite tendency: a retrospective study. *Am J Orthod Dentofac Orthop*. 2014;145:28–35.
43. Orton HS, Slattery DA, Orton S. The treatment of severe 'gummy' Class II division 1 malocclusion using the maxillary intrusion splint. *Eur J Orthod*. 1992;14:216–223.
44. Weinbach JR, Smith RJ. Cephalometric changes during treatment with the open bite Bionator. *Am J Orthod Dentofac Orthop*. 1992;101:367–374.
45. Freeman CS, McNamara Jr JA, Baccetti T, et al. Treatment effects of the Bionator and high-pull facebow combination followed by fixed appliances in patients with increased vertical dimensions. *Am J Orthod Dentofac Orthop*. 2007;131:184–195.
46. Proffit WR, Turvey TA, Vig KW. Early fracture of the mandibular condyles: frequently an unsuspected cause of growth disturbances. *Am J Orthod*. 1980;78:1–24.
47. Turvey TA, Ruiz R, Blakey GH, et al. Management of facial fractures in the growing patient. In: Fonseca RJ, Walker RV, Betts NJ, et al., eds. *Oral and Maxillofacial Trauma*. WB Saunders; 2005.

SECTION 6

Comprehensive Orthodontic Treatment in the Early Permanent Dentition

Comprehensive orthodontic treatment implies an effort to make the patient's occlusion as ideal as possible, repositioning all or nearly all the teeth in the process. From this perspective, the mixed dentition and growth modification treatment described in Chapters 11–14 is not comprehensive, despite its importance for some patients, because the final position of all the permanent teeth is not determined. A second phase of comprehensive treatment after the permanent teeth have erupted, during which the details of occlusal relationships are established, is almost always needed for children with moderate or severe malocclusion even if significant improvement occurred during a first phase of treatment in the mixed dentition.

Comprehensive treatment usually requires a complete fixed appliance or a series of well-designed and monitored clear aligners. In Chapters 15–17, the use of a contemporary edgewise appliance that incorporates offsets, angulation, and torque in the brackets (i.e., a straight-wire appliance) is assumed during much of the discussion. Chapter 18 focuses specifically on the use of clear aligners as a tool for comprehensive treatment. The ideal time for comprehensive treatment is during adolescence, when the succedaneous teeth have just erupted, some vertical and anteroposterior growth of the jaws remains, and social adjustment to orthodontic treatment is no great problem. Not all adolescent patients require comprehensive treatment, of course, and limited treatment to overcome specific problems can certainly be done at any age. Comprehensive treatment is also possible for adults, but it poses some special problems. These are discussed in Chapters 20 and 21.

The idea of dividing comprehensive orthodontic treatment into stages, which makes it easier to discuss technique, was introduced by Raymond Begg,[1] and the three major stages he proposed were the focus of his treatment planning. The stages were (1) alignment and leveling, (2) correction of molar relationship and space closure, and (3) finishing. These stages described edgewise treatment well at the time this book first appeared, when improvements in edgewise technique were pushing the Begg appliance into obsolescence. They still fit reasonably well with modern treatment, but three differences have led to modification of the chapters in this section.

First, Begg treatment was built around premolar extraction for most patients, and now extraction is much less frequent. Second, the sequence of treatment procedures in contemporary edgewise varies; you don't always start with alignment or complete leveling before correcting incisor protrusion, although finishing adjustments remain a final step for almost all patients. Third, with the availability of comprehensive treatment with clear aligners, the sequence of steps can be varied, and they may not be the same as what would be done with a fixed appliance.

What is still true of almost all fixed appliance treatment is that even with the most cleverly preadjusted edgewise appliance, change of archwires from round to rectangular will be needed before the finishing stage is reached, and some adjustments to rectangular archwires are quite likely to be necessary in completing the treatment. In this section, what is done primarily with round wires is the focus of Chapter 15. Chapter 16 describes the use of rectangular wires in retraction of protruding incisors and closure of extraction spaces, and Chapter 17 discusses the small but important adjustments that are routinely required in fixed appliance finishing. Chapter 18 is new to this edition of the book and focuses on the special considerations for planning and executing comprehensive treatment for adolescents with modern clear aligner treatment.

Whatever the orthodontic technique, treatment must be discontinued gradually, with some sort of retention appliance used for a time, and this important subject is covered in the last chapter of this section, Chapter 19.

Reference

1. Begg PR, Kesling PC. *Begg Orthodontic Theory and Technique*. WB Saunders; 1977.

15

Comprehensive Treatment in Adolescents: Alignment and Vertical Problems

BRENT E. LARSON, AND WILLIAM R. PROFFIT

CHAPTER OUTLINE

The overlap with growth modification and mixed dentition treatment has already been reviewed in Chapter 12. The equally important overlap with growth modification and adolescent treatment is discussed in Chapter 16, in which camouflage possibilities for skeletal problems, which revolve around repositioning incisors to help fit the dentition into an acceptable relationship with the face, are presented in detail. This chapter focuses on two things: correction of crowding of teeth in patients who have a normal jaw relationship, and problems in all three planes of space that are due more to displacement of teeth than discrepancies in jaw size and position.

At this point, we presume that the patient's problem list has been developed properly and that there is a treatment plan to maximize benefit for them. Now our discussion is not of what to do, but how to do it effectively and efficiently.

Class I Crowding/Protrusion

In almost all patients with malocclusion, at least some teeth are initially malaligned, so alignment is needed for patients with skeletal problems as well as those for whom crowding and/or protrusion is the major problem—but alignment techniques apply in the same way whether or not there also is a jaw discrepancy. For proper alignment, it is necessary not only to bring malposed teeth into the arch but also to specify and control the anteroposterior position of incisors, the width of the arches posteriorly, and the form of the dental arches. Even in the absence of a jaw discrepancy, patients are likely to have an excess overbite and an accentuated curve of Spee in the lower arch. It is necessary to determine and control whether the leveling should occur by elongation of posterior teeth, intrusion of incisors, or some specific combination of the two. In addition, it often is the case that the form of the upper arch is not compatible with that of the lower arch, and one or both must be changed if excellent occlusion is to be obtained.

Although the orthodontist has some latitude in changing arch form, more stable results are achieved when the patient's original lower arch form is preserved during orthodontic treatment (see Chapter 10 for a discussion of arch form and archwire shape). The light resilient archwires used in the first stage of treatment need not be shaped to the patient's arch form as carefully as the heavier archwires used later in treatment, but from the beginning, the archwires should reflect each individual's arch form. If preformed archwires are used for alignment (as is usually the case because superelastic austenitic nickel-titanium [A-NiTi] wires must be formed by the manufacturer), the appropriate arch form should be selected.

Because the orthodontic mechanotherapy will be different depending on exactly how alignment and leveling are to be accomplished, it is extremely important to clearly visualize the desired position of the teeth before beginning treatment. Technology now exists to make this easier (Fig. 15.1), but it is the thought process that counts. For instance, the best alignment procedures will result in incisors that are far too protrusive if the extractions necessary to prevent protrusion were not part of the plan. Similarly, unless leveling by intrusion is planned when it is needed, the appropriate mechanics are not likely to be selected. Orthodontic treatment without specific goals can be an excellent illustration of the old adage, "If you don't know where you're going, it doesn't matter which road you take."

Alignment

Properties of Alignment Archwires

The wires for initial alignment require a combination of excellent strength, excellent springiness, and a long range of action. Ideally, there would be an almost flat load-deflection curve, with the wire delivering about 50 g (the optimum force for tipping) at almost

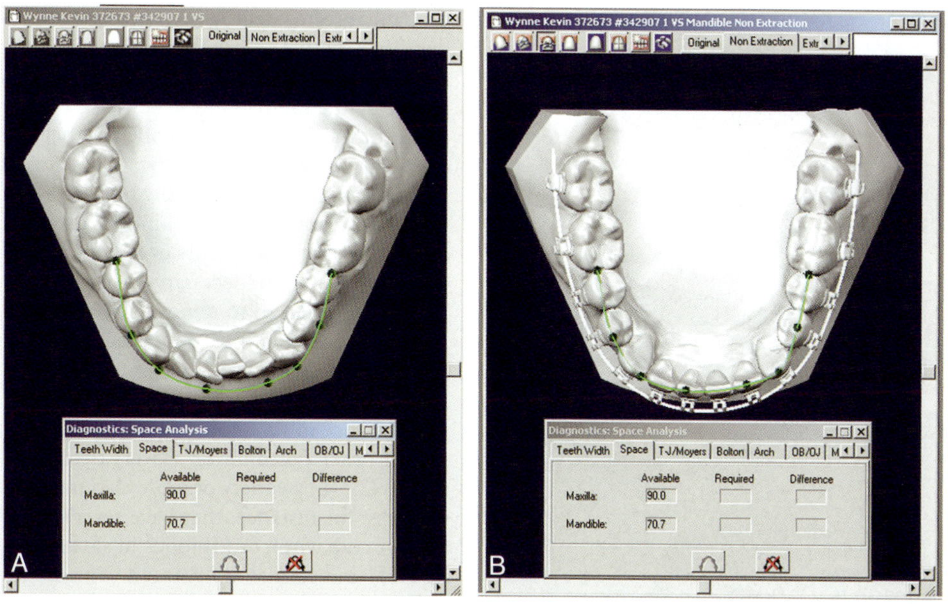

• **Fig. 15.1** Digitized dental casts (here in the Ortho-CAD system) can be used quite effectively to calculate the amount of space needed to align the teeth, show the probable outcome of alignment, and calculate the arch length needed. (A) Pretreatment occlusal view of the lower arch, with a line showing the amount of space required for alignment. (B) Virtual appliance in place. This setup can be used to generate the trays for indirect bonding.

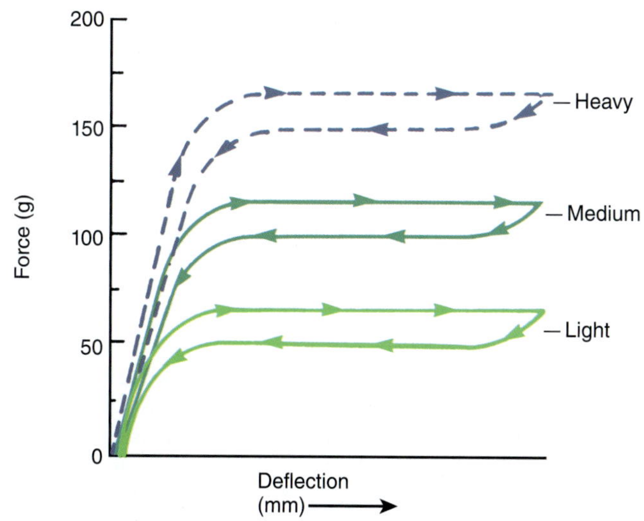

• **Fig. 15.2** Idealized force-deflection curves for 16-mil austenitic nickel-titanium (A-NiTi) wires (Sentinol, Dentsply Sirona, York, PA) prepared by the manufacturer to have different force delivery characteristics. For superelastic wires, the manufacturer's preparation, not the wire size, is the major factor in determining force delivery. Note that the light version of this wire delivers the desired 50 g for initial alignment. Data of this type should be available for all the archwires used in clinical practice.

any degree of deflection (Fig. 15.2). The variables in selecting appropriate archwires for alignment are the archwire material, its size (diameter or cross-section), and the distance between attachments (interbracket span; see Chapter 9).

At this point, superelastic A-NiTi wires are so much more effective and efficient for alignment than any alternative that there is almost no reason to discuss other possibilities. The key to their success is their ability to deliver light force over a long range. When superelastic wires were first introduced, fracture of the wire between appointments was a problem, but improved alloys and manufacturing techniques have largely eliminated this. Because the manufacturer's preparation of the material determines the clinical performance, wire size is a concern primarily with respect to clearance in the bracket slot.

It is possible now to obtain superelastic wires that are almost totally passive when cold but deliver the desired force when at mouth temperature. Placing a passive wire is much easier than placing a springy one, so chilling a segment of the wire to make it temporarily passive can be a significant advantage under some circumstances. On the other hand, once mouth temperature has been reached, there is no reason to expect such a thermally sensitive wire to perform better than one without this feature.

As discussed in Chapter 9, it is logical to use narrow (single) brackets with 18-slot edgewise and wider (twin) brackets with 22-slot appliances. Before the almost routine use of superelastic wires, bracket slot size and interbracket span were such strong influences on archwire choice that different initial wires were often used with the 18- and 22-slot appliances. This is no longer the case. But with superelastic wires, it is necessary to pay more attention to maintaining arch form during alignment, to the point that alignment when crowding is reasonably symmetric now must be viewed differently than alignment in highly asymmetric situations—an important point that is discussed later.

The flat load-deflection curve of superelastic nickel-titanium (NiTi; see Fig. 15.2) makes it ideal for initial alignment. The wire provides a remarkable range over which a tooth can be moved without generating excessive force (see Figs. 9.5–9.8). Under most circumstances, initial alignment can be accomplished simply by tying 14- or 16-mil A-NiTi that delivers about 50 g into the brackets of all the teeth. It must be kept in mind, however, that alignment requires opening space for teeth that are crowded out of the arch. There are two ways to do this: use a crimped stop on

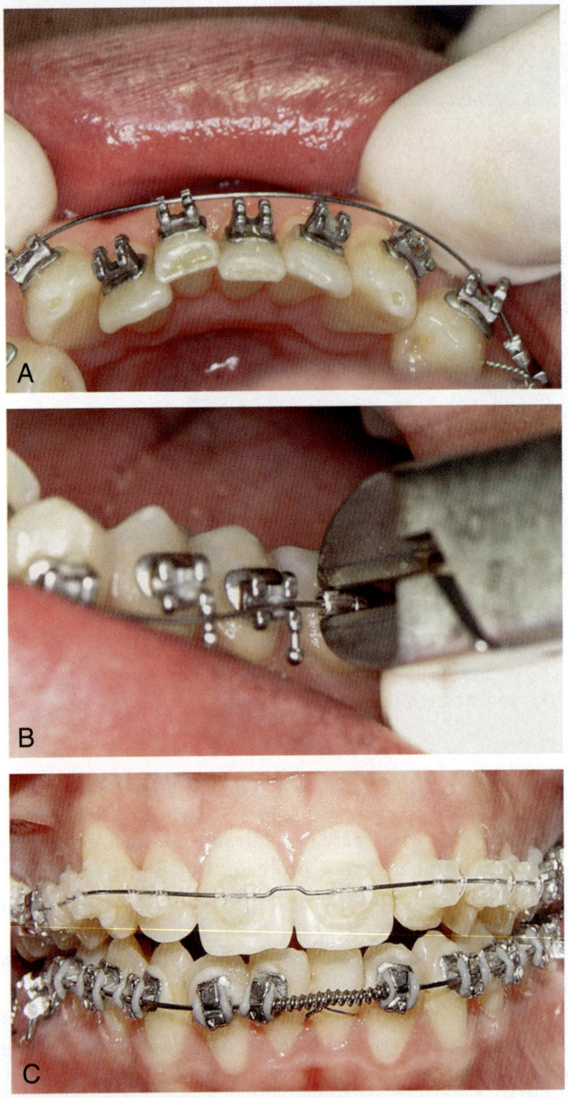

• **Fig. 15.3** When additional arch length is needed, advanced stops in the flexible initial archwire are useful. (A) Austenitic nickel-titanium (A-NiTi) archwire advanced relative to crowded incisors. Stops on the archwire are needed to hold it in a slightly advanced position. (B) Crimped split tube segments, such as those used to prevent travel, serve well as stops for superelastic initial wires. (C) An alternative for gaining arch length is compressed coil springs to open space for crowded-out incisors. The effect of the two methods is quite similar—incisor proclination occurs about equally.

the wire just in front of the molar tube so that the archwire is "proud" (slightly advanced from the crowded incisors) or use coil springs to open space (Fig. 15.3). If this is done, the springs must deliver only light force to prevent distortion of the arch form. The size of the superelastic wire is not a critical variable if it delivers the desired approximately 50 g of force, except that 18-mil wires should not be used in the 18-slot appliance.

When superelastic NiTi was first introduced, the major objection to it was its expense. If a large range is not necessary, a triple-strand 17.5-mil multistrand steel wire (3 × 8 mil) still offers good properties at a fraction of the cost. In theory, this size would be too large for effective use in 18-slot brackets. Clinical research has shown, however, that in both the 18- and 22-slot appliance, if these wires are recontoured monthly and retied with elastomeric ligatures, the time to alignment is equivalent to that with A-NiTi. Force levels are certainly more variable and patient discomfort is probably greater than with superelastic wires, but it is difficult to demonstrate that this makes a difference clinically.

The major reason for this surprisingly good clinical performance by the multistrand steel wire is that flexible archwires allow the teeth to move relative to one another during chewing, as alveolar bone bends under masticatory loads (see Chapter 8). This releases binding and allows the bracket to slide along the archwire to the next point at which binding occurs. But the lower cost of the steel archwire is quickly overshadowed by the cost of the additional clinical time necessary to retie it, especially if it must be taken out, reshaped to remove any areas of permanent distortion, and then re-ligated. In a busy practice, you can't afford to use the less expensive wire.

Laboratory data and clinical experience suggest that similar performance to the multistrand steel wire could be obtained with several other possibilities: (1) elastic martensitic nickel-titanium (M-NiTi), (2) a variety of more elaborate multistrand wires (coaxial wires, for instance, that have several smaller wires wound over a larger core wire), or (3) loops in small-diameter steel wires. Both M-NiTi and coaxial multistrand wires are expensive, and the time to bend loops in 14- or 16-mil steel wires also is expensive. These wires, although they were the standard of treatment for initial alignment not long ago, have little or no place in current therapy.

As one might expect, the extreme springiness of superelastic wires is not a totally unmixed blessing. When these wires are tied into a malaligned dental arch, they have a tendency to "travel" around the arch as the patient chews, especially if function is mostly on one side. Then the wire extends out the back of the molar tube on one side and is short out of the tube on the other side. Occasionally, this can be extreme enough to produce the kind of situation Mark Twain called "marvelous and dismaying" (Fig. 15.4A). Archwire travel can be prevented by crimping a stop tightly onto the archwire between any two brackets that are reasonably close together (see Fig. 15.4B) or by using a wire in which the manufacturer has placed a midline dimple in the wire to prevent travel (see Fig. 15.3C). A stop to prevent travel should be used routinely on initial superelastic wires.

Principles in the Choice of Alignment Arches

In nearly every patient with malaligned teeth, the root apices are closer to the normal position than the crowns because malalignment almost always develops as the eruption paths of teeth are deflected. Putting it another way, a tooth bud occasionally develops in the wrong place, but the root apices are likely to be reasonably close to their correct positions even though the crowns have been displaced as the teeth erupted. The major exceptions to this guideline are the displacement of all tissues in an area, most often seen as a result of cleft palate surgery, and the severe tipping from lip pressure that displaces maxillary central incisors in Class II division 2 malocclusion.

Bringing teeth into alignment requires a combination of labiolingual and mesiodistal tipping guided by an archwire, but usually not root movement. Several important consequences for orthodontic mechanotherapy follow from this:

- Initial archwires for alignment should provide light, continuous force of approximately 50 g to produce the most efficient tipping tooth movement. Heavy force, in contrast, is to be avoided.
- The archwires should be able to move freely within the brackets. For mesiodistal sliding along an archwire, at least 2 mil of clearance between the archwire and the bracket is needed, 4 mil of clearance is desirable, and more than that provides

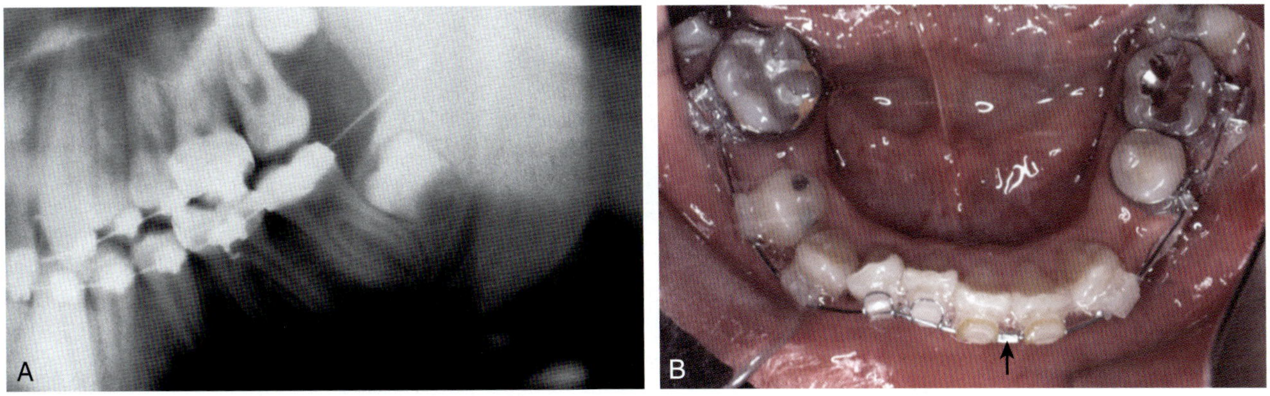

• **Fig. 15.4** One problem with superelastic wires for initial alignment is their tendency to "travel" so that the wire slips around to one side, protruding distally from the molar tube on one side and slipping out of the tube on the other. (A) This panoramic radiograph shows archwire travel to the point that on one side it penetrated into the ramus, almost to the depth of an inferior alveolar block injection (interestingly, the patient reported only mild discomfort). (B) The most effective way to prevent travel is to tightly crimp a split tube segment onto the wire between two adjacent brackets. The location of the crimped stop, here between the left central and lateral incisors, is not critical. Some preformed austenitic nickel-titanium (A-NiTi) wires now have a dimple in the midline to prevent the archwire from sliding excessively.

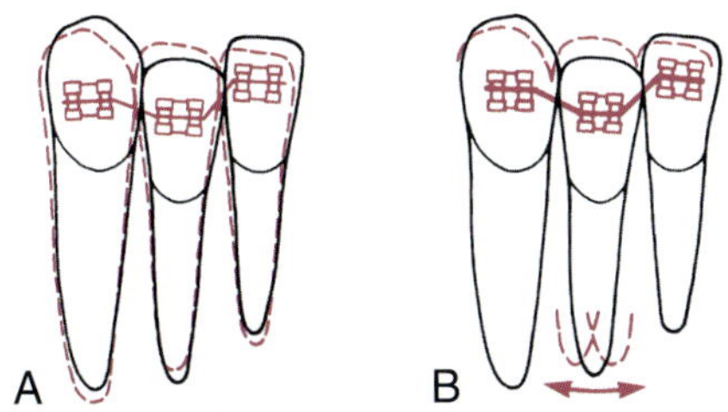

• **Fig. 15.5** A tightly fitting resilient rectangular archwire for initial alignment is almost always undesirable because not only is resistance to sliding likely to be problematic, but also the wire produces back-and-forth movement of the root apices as the teeth move into alignment. This occurs because the moments generated by the archwire change as the geometry of the system changes with alterations in tooth position. (A) Diagrammatic representation of the alignment of a malposed lateral incisor with a round wire and clearance in the bracket slot. With minimal moments created within the bracket slot, there is little displacement of the root apex. (B) With a rectangular archwire that has enough torsional stiffness to create root movement, back-and-forth movement of the apex occurs before the tooth ends up in essentially the same place as with a round wire. This has two disadvantages: it increases the possibility of root resorption, and it slows the alignment process.

no advantage. This means that the largest initial archwire that should be used with an 18-slot edgewise bracket is 16 mil, and 14 mil would be more satisfactory. With the 22-slot bracket, a 16- or 18-mil archwire would be satisfactory if it delivered the correct force. Whatever the archwire, it should be held loosely in the bracket; however, as we have pointed out in Chapter 9, friction is not the major component of resistance to sliding, and the claim that more rapid alignment is a major advantage of self-ligating brackets has been shown to be incorrect.

- Rectangular archwires, particularly those with a tight fit within the bracket slot so that the position of the root apex could be affected, should normally be avoided. The principle is that it is better to tip crowns to position during initial alignment rather than displacing the root apices; the corollary is that although a highly resilient rectangular archwire, such as 17 × 25 superelastic NiTi (A-NiTi), could be used in the alignment stage, this is not advantageous because the rectangular archwire can create unnecessary and undesirable root movement during alignment (Fig. 15.5). Superelastic NiTi wires have such low torsional stiffness that for all practical purposes they cannot torque roots,[1] so this complication is uncommon, but mesiodistal movement of the root apices can and does occur, and this tends to slow the tipping movements needed for alignment.

For that reason, round wires for alignment are preferred (Fig. 15.6). There is no reason to pay extra for a high-performance rectangular wire for initial alignment, when alignment with it will be predictably slower and possibly more damaging to the roots than a smaller round wire.

The more flexible the alignment archwire, the more important it is for the crowding to be at least reasonably symmetric. A frequent example of major asymmetry is when one incisor is completely blocked out of the arch but the rest of the arch is reasonably well aligned (Fig. 15.7). In that case, there is a danger that the arch form will be distorted if the crowding is resolved with a superelastic wire alone, because if it is tied into the teeth, all of them will experience a displacement force. What is needed is a rigid wire to maintain the arch form except where springiness is required and an auxiliary superelastic wire to reach the malaligned tooth and pull it into position after space for it has been opened.

The best way to manage severely asymmetric crowding is to open space for the displaced tooth (or teeth; the same system works with small segments of two teeth) by using a coil spring on a 16-mil steel wire to open space, and then adding a small-diameter superelastic wire as an auxiliary spring overlying the stiffer main wire (see Fig. 15.7). With this arrangement, the correct light force to bring the displaced tooth into alignment is provided by the NiTi wire, and the reciprocal force is distributed over all the rest of the teeth by the stiffer main wire. The result is efficient movement of the displaced tooth, with excellent preservation of arch form. When the displaced tooth is nearly into proper position, the steel base arch can be discarded and the NiTi auxiliary tied into the bracket slots.

Note that there are two advantages of using the superelastic wire as an auxiliary to a rigid steel wire: control of the tendency to distort arch form and light force against the tooth to be moved.

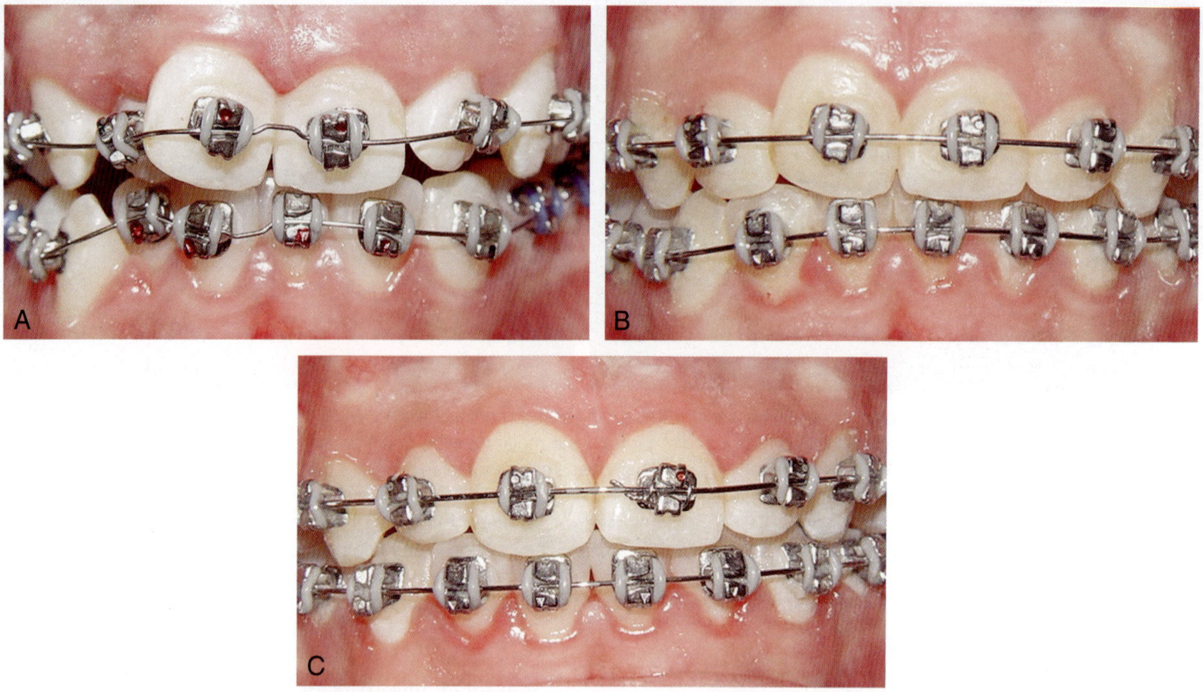

• **Fig. 15.6** The sequence of alignment with a fixed appliance, in this case with Tip-Edge brackets (see Chapter 10). (A) The initial superelastic round wire (16-mil austenitic nickel-titanium [A-NiTi]), which the manufacturer had formed with a midline dimple to prevent archwire travel. (B) Two months later, 16-mil steel for final alignment. (C) Alignment completed 3 months later.

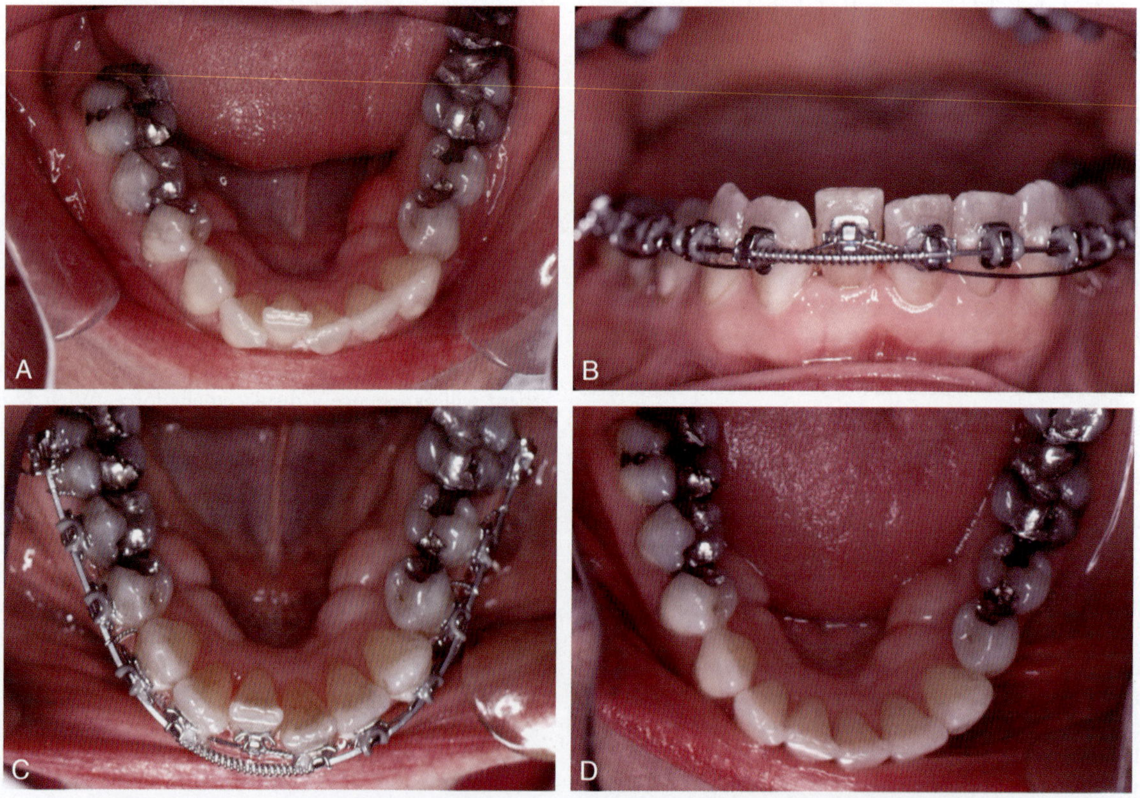

• **Fig. 15.7** Use of an auxiliary superelastic wire for incisor alignment in a patient with asymmetric crowding. (A) Crowding expressed largely as displacement of one lower lateral incisor in an adult with periodontal bone loss in whom light force was particularly important. (B and C) After space was opened for the right lateral incisor, a superelastic wire segment tied loosely beneath the brackets to reduce its slide friction was used to bring the lateral incisor into position, while arch form was maintained by a heavier archwire in the bracket slots. (D) Alignment completed. This approach allows use of optimal force on the tooth to be moved and distributes the reaction force over the rest of the teeth in the arch.

Although auxiliaries of this type are recommended routinely in modern orthodontics, it would be particularly important to use this method for adult patients with loss of alveolar bone and a reduced periodontal ligament area.

Arch Expansion for Alignment

Alignment in nonextraction cases requires increasing the arch length, moving the incisors farther from the molars. A key question, of course, is the amount of arch expansion that a given patient can tolerate without the creation of major esthetic and posttreatment stability problems. In the context of this discussion, that decision was made at the treatment planning stage, and the focus here is how to efficiently accomplish an appropriate amount of arch expansion.

For the alignment of crowded incisors, just tying a superelastic wire into the bracket slots is ineffective. Two objects cannot occupy the same space at the same time, so alignment cannot occur until space to allow it is created. The most straightforward way to accomplish this is to crimp a stop on a small round superelastic wire at the molar tube, so that it holds the wire just in front of the incisors (see Fig. 15.3). At subsequent appointments, if more arch length is needed, an additional stop or stops can be quickly slipped into position without removing the wire. When a broad arch form is used, transverse expansion across the premolars will occur. Even so, this type of arch expansion has the potential to carry the incisors facially, so it is not indicated in the presence of severe crowding unless incisor protrusion is desired.

An alternative is to bypass the brackets on teeth that are crowded lingually, and place coil springs over the A-NiTi archwire to generate space (see Fig. 15.3C). When this is done, the archwire must be free to slide forward through the molar tubes and must be slightly long initially so that it will not come completely out of the tubes. The coil spring force must be very light to prevent distortion of arch form, but it is a misconception that the force is so light the incisors will not be proclined. They will be, just as they are when advanced stops are used.

If incisor crowding is severe and arch expansion would produce unacceptable protrusion, premolar extraction is necessary. With the combination of a small superelastic wire in the bracket slots and NiTi springs to retract the canines (Fig. 15.8), efficient alignment without incisor protrusion can be obtained.

The methods just described gain space primarily by advancing the incisors. Another way to gain space for alignment is transverse expansion, which should be focused on expanding across the premolars and molars, not across the canines. Transverse expansion with broad archwires can increase posterior arch width by several millimeters. The limitation in doing this is primarily the risk of fenestration of roots through the labial alveolar bone (see Chapter 8), but it is also difficult to avoid undesirable canine expansion. In the absence of a posterior crossbite (see later), heavy force to open the midpalatal suture just to gain additional space for alignment is not recommended.

Missing or distorted maxillary lateral incisors can pose complex alignment problems, especially if the midline is off because one lateral is missing and the other is present but small (Figs. 15.9 and 15.10). A combination of appropriately stiff archwires and management of the space is required. Note the use of a bonded

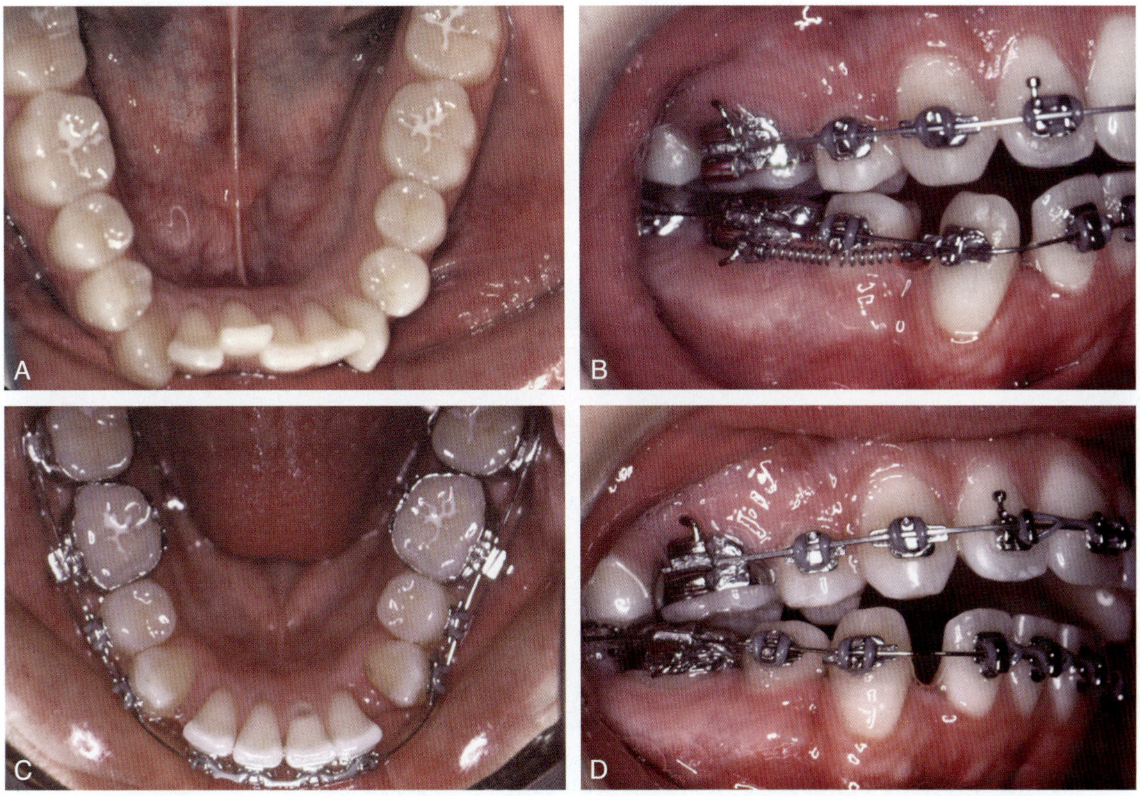

• **Fig. 15.8** Alignment of severely crowded lower incisors with simultaneous distal tipping of the canine into a first premolar extraction space with a nickel-titanium (NiTi) spring (the superelastic equivalent of the original "drag loop"). (A) Occlusal view before treatment. (B) Canine retraction with superelastic coil springs that provide 75 g of force, and alignment of incisors with a superelastic NiTi wire that incorporates an accentuated reverse curve of Spee and delivers 50 g. (C and D) Completion of canine retraction and incisor alignment after 5 months of treatment.

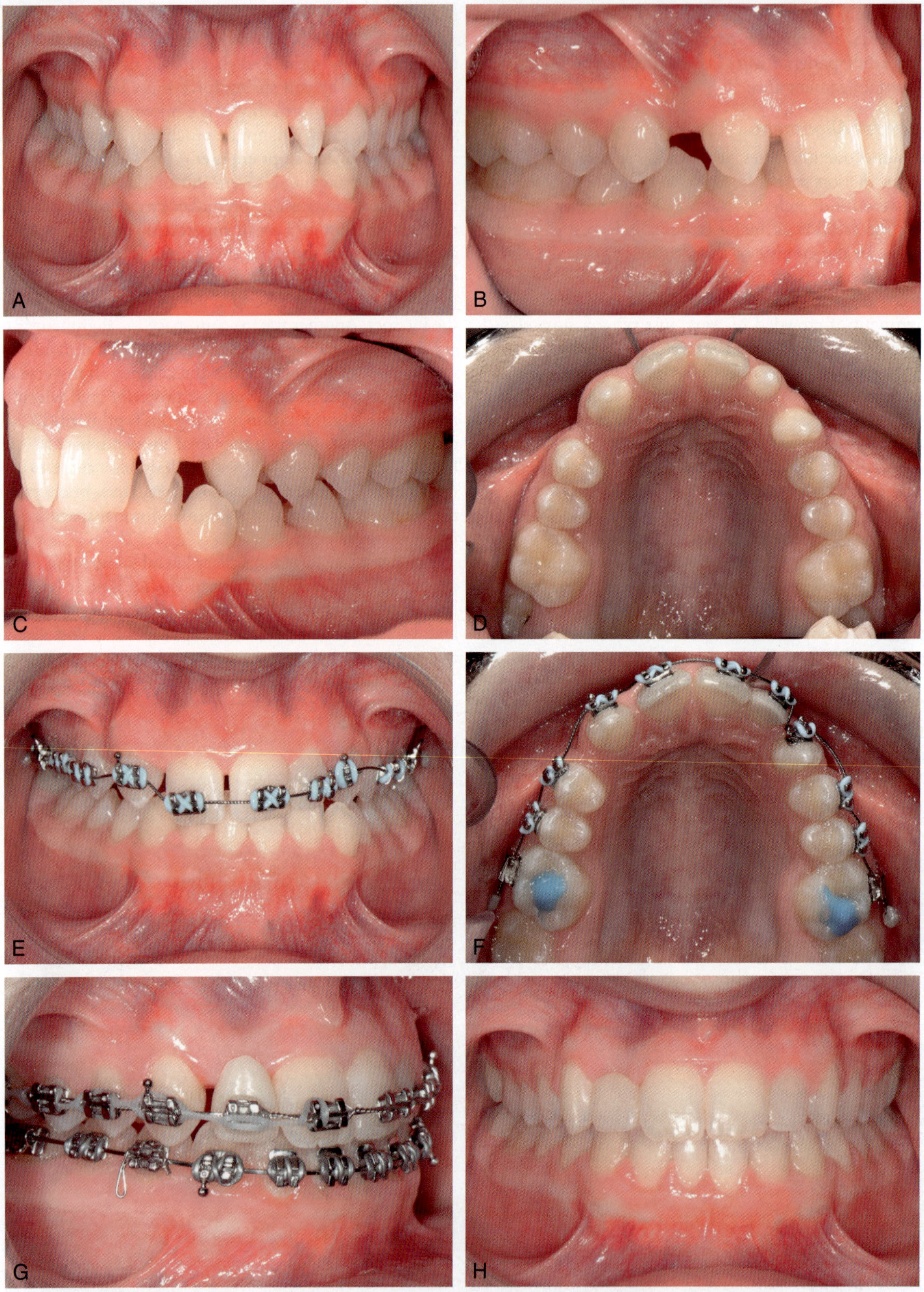

• **Fig. 15.9** A patient with a missing maxillary lateral incisor on one side and an abnormally small one on the other side poses a difficult treatment planning problem. (A–D) For this girl, the maxillary dental midline is well off to the right side, where the lateral incisor is missing; the small and misshapen lateral incisor on the other side is well mesial to the canine, which is rotated 90 degrees and in lingual crossbite with the lower canine but in a reasonably normal anteroposterior position. (E–G) The decision was to open space for an eventual implant to replace the missing lateral, which would facilitate correcting the maxillary incisor position relative to the midfacial line, and to do a prosthetic buildup on the small lateral. Bonded bite blocks were used to allow correction of the canine crossbite.

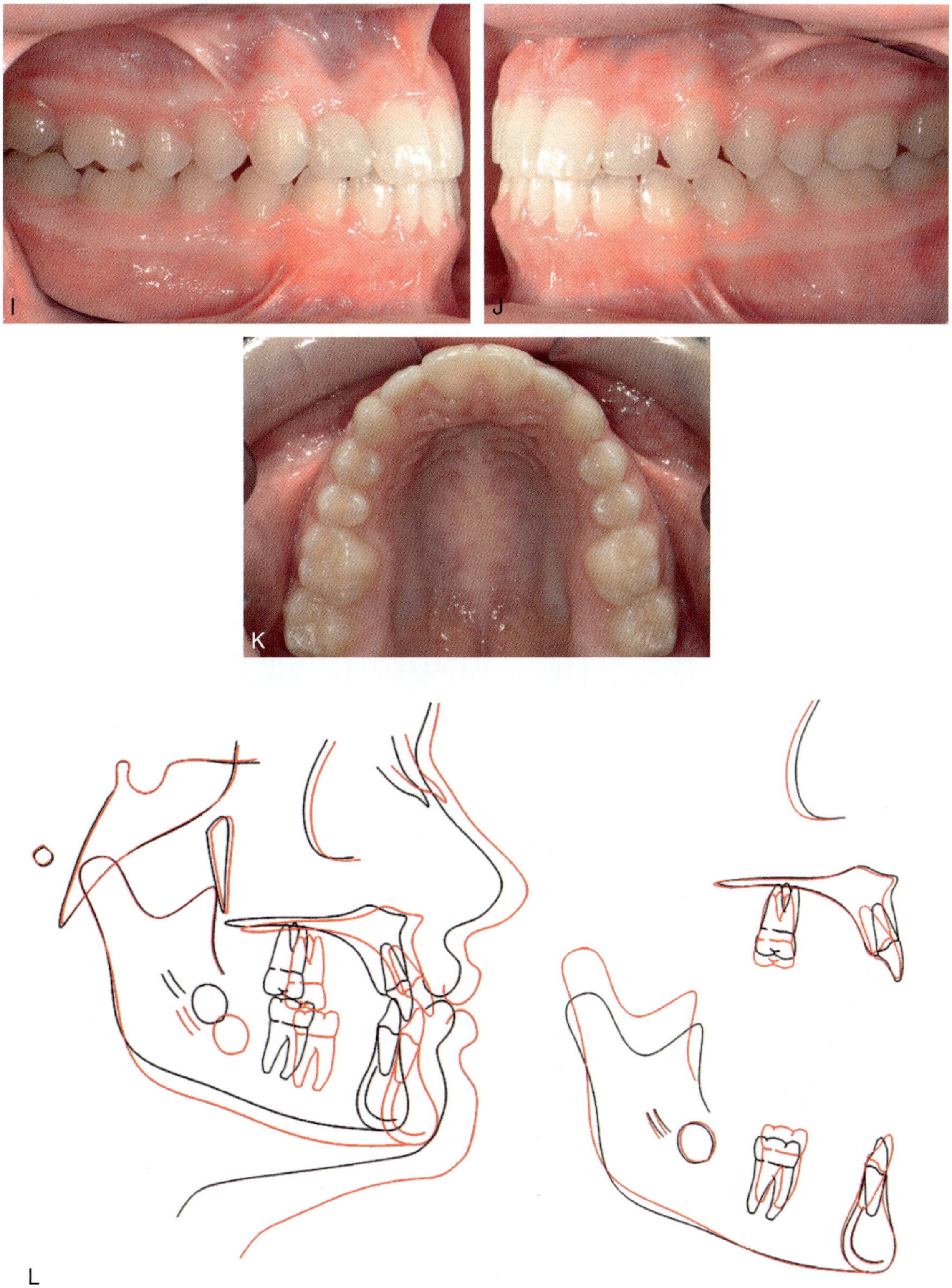

• **Fig. 15.9** (H–K) Note the use of a temporary bonded bridge consisting of a slightly oversize denture tooth, to be sure that enough space for the implant would be retained until the patient's late teens, when vertical growth was essentially complete, and the implant would not be left behind by continued eruption of the other teeth. This also stabilizes the rotated canine. A removable retainer is not indicated in this situation. (L) The cephalometric superimpositions show the considerable forward and vertical growth of both jaws during treatment. Note in the maxillary superimposition that the maxillary incisors required lingual root torque to obtain the proper inclination. (Courtesy Dr. T. Shaughnessy.)

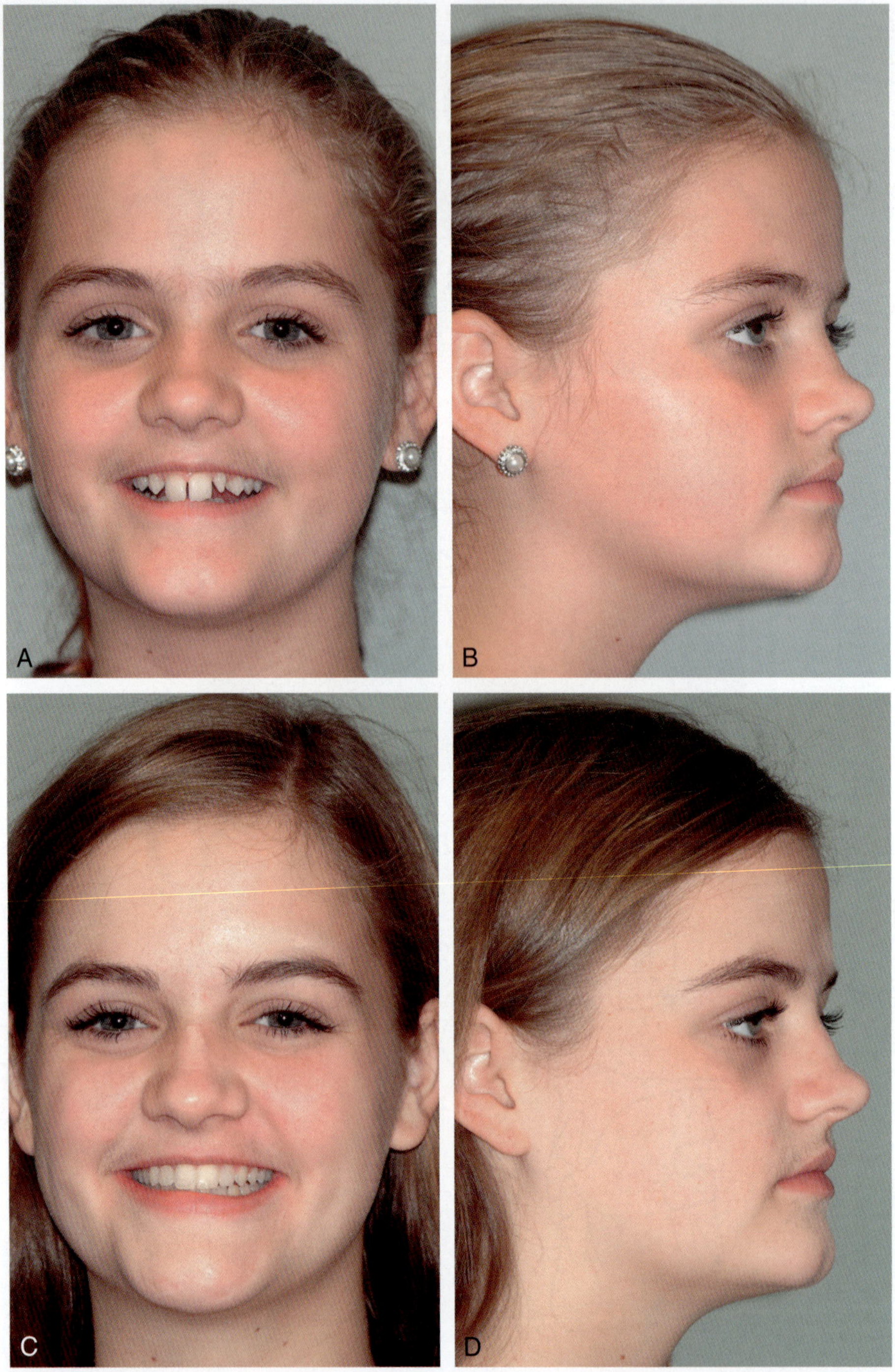

• **Fig. 15.10** Same patient as in Fig. 15.9. (A and B) Before treatment. The patient's chief concern was the appearance of the teeth on smile. (C and D) She was quite pleased with the improvement. (Courtesy Dr. T. Shaughnessy.)

denture tooth as a semipermanent retainer for the area where an implant eventually will be placed, with the pontic deliberately slightly oversize to ensure that there will be adequate space in the long term for the implant.

Crossbite Correction

Is crossbite correction really a part of alignment? That depends on the extent to which it is a largely a dental problem and on its severity. Skeletal crossbites have already been discussed in Chapter 13. The discussion here is of crossbites that are largely dental. Correcting them usually also provides more space for alignment.

Individual Teeth Displaced Into Anterior Crossbite

Anterior crossbite of one or two teeth almost always is an expression of severe crowding (Fig. 15.11). This is most likely to occur when maxillary lateral incisors that are somewhat lingually positioned to begin with are forced even more lingually by lack of space. Correction of the crossbite requires first opening enough space, then bringing the displaced tooth or teeth across the occlusion into proper position.

Occlusal interferences can make this difficult. The patient may tend to bite brackets off the displaced teeth, and as the teeth are moved "through the bite," occlusal force pushes them one way

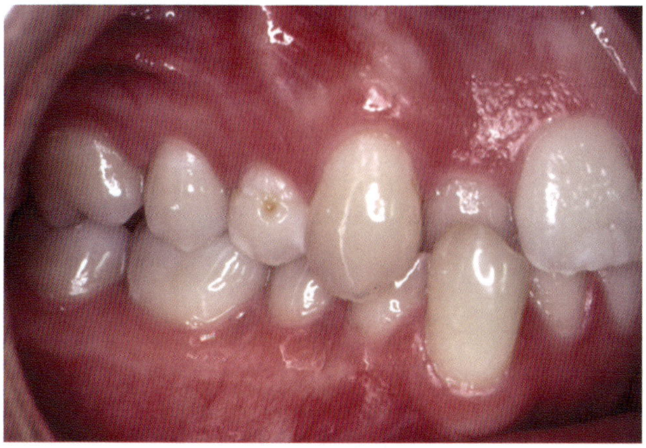

• **Fig. 15.11** Correction of a dental anterior crossbite, as in this patient in late adolescence, requires opening enough space for the lingually displaced maxillary incisor before attempting to move it facially into arch form. At that point, use of bonded bite blocks or a biteplate to obtain vertical clearance is often required.

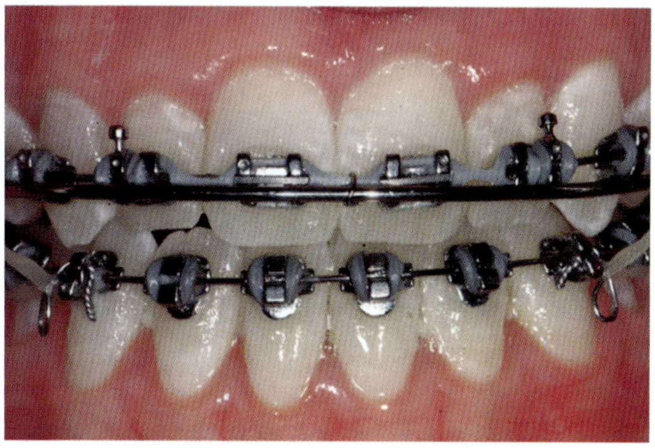

• **Fig. 15.12** A heavy labial archwire (usually 36- or 40-mil steel) placed in the headgear tubes on first molars can be used for a small amount of expansion and to maintain arch width after palatal suture opening while the teeth are being aligned. This is more compatible with fixed appliance treatment than a removable retainer and does not depend on patient cooperation. (From Proffit WR, White RP, Sarver DM. *Contemporary Treatment of Dentofacial Deformity*. Mosby; 2003.)

while the orthodontic appliance pulls them the other. It may be necessary to use bite blocks (usually bonding material on lower first molars) temporarily to separate the posterior teeth and create the vertical space needed to allow the teeth to move (see Fig. 15.9F). During rapid growth in early adolescence, incisors that were locked in anterior crossbite can often be corrected without temporarily opening the bite. After growth is largely completed, bite opening will probably be required.

Anterior crossbites of more than one or two teeth are usually due to a skeletal jaw discrepancy, and these patients are rarely candidates for tooth movement to correct malocclusion. That would be successful only if the patient met the criteria for Class III camouflage (discussed in Chapter 16). These patients may respond to growth modification treatment, especially if the problem is maxillary deficiency (see Chapter 13), but those with excessive mandibular growth probably will require surgery for correction (discussed in Chapter 22).

Correction of Dental Posterior Crossbites

Three approaches to correction of posterior crossbites due to lingual inclination of upper posterior teeth are feasible: a heavy labial expansion arch, as shown in Fig. 15.12; an expansion lingual arch; or cross-elastics. Removable appliances, although theoretically possible, are not compatible with comprehensive treatment and should be reserved for the mixed dentition or adjunctive treatment.

The inner bow of a facebow is also, of course, a heavy labial arch, and expansion of the inner bow is a convenient way to expand the upper molars in a patient who is wearing headgear (see Chapter 14). This expansion is nearly always needed for patients with a Class II molar relationship, whose upper arch is usually too narrow to accommodate the mandibular arch when it comes forward into the correct relationship because the upper molars are tipped lingually. The inner bow is simply adjusted at each appointment to be slightly wider than the headgear tubes and so it must be compressed by the patient when inserting the facebow. If the distal force of a headgear is not desired, a heavy labial auxiliary can provide the expansion effect alone. The effect of the round wire in the headgear tubes, however, is to tip the crowns outward, and so this method should be reserved for patients whose molars are tipped lingually.

A transpalatal lingual arch for expansion must have some springiness and range of action. As a general principle, the more flexible a lingual arch is, the better it is for tooth movement but the less it adds to anchorage (which becomes important in camouflage treatment, discussed in Chapter 16). This can be an important consideration in adolescent and adult patients. If anchorage is of no concern, a highly flexible lingual arch such as the quad-helix design (see Fig. 11.18) is an excellent choice for adolescents as well as children. When the lingual arch is needed for both expansion and anchorage, however, the choices are 30- or 36-mil steel wire with an adjustment loop or the newer lingual arch system that allows the use of 32 × 32 TMA wire, which is flexible enough to not need a loop (Fig. 15.13).

The third possibility for moderate maxillary dental expansion is the use of cross-elastics, typically running from the lingual aspect of the upper molar to the buccal aspect of the lower molar and used with a stabilizing lingual arch in the mandible to prevent tipping of the lower molars lingually (Fig. 15.14). These elastics are effective, but their strong extrusive component must be kept in mind. Adolescent patients can usually tolerate a short period of cross-elastic wear to correct a simple crossbite because any extrusion is compensated for by vertical growth of the ramus, but cross-elastics should be used with great caution, if at all, in adults. As any posterior crossbite is corrected, there is a tendency to rotate the mandible downward and backward, even if cross-elastics are avoided. The elastics accentuate this tendency.

If teeth are tightly locked into a posterior crossbite relationship, bite blocks or a biteplate to separate them vertically can make the correction easier and faster (Fig. 15.15). In children, this is rarely needed. In adolescents and adults, it can be quite helpful. Use of bite blocks during transverse expansion indicates that elongation of the posterior teeth and downward and backward rotation of the mandible is an acceptable outcome.

Maxillary expansion in adolescents by opening the midpalatal suture is a growth modification procedure and has been discussed in some detail in Chapter 13. As we noted there, opening the suture becomes more difficult after the end of the adolescent growth spurt, and skeletal anchorage for the expansion device becomes important. With the transition from late adolescence to early adult life, surgically assisted palatal expansion (SARPE) or

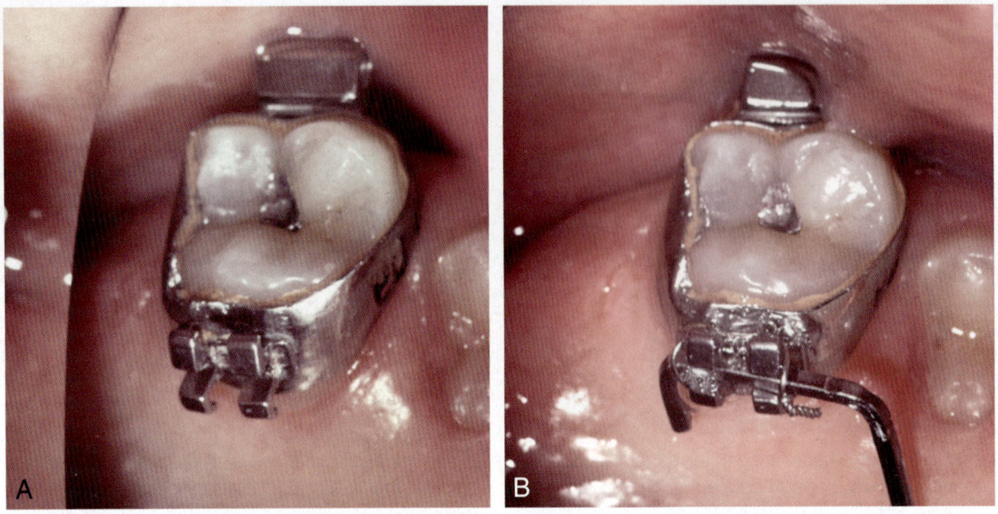

• **Fig. 15.13** A flexible transpalatal arch for expansion can be formed from rectangular 32 × 32 wire that fits into a horizontal tube or (A) into a special bracket on the lingual of upper first molars, as shown here. (B) Tying the wire into the bracket makes it easier to remove for adjustment and replace, but over time, gingival overgrowth can make re-ligation difficult.

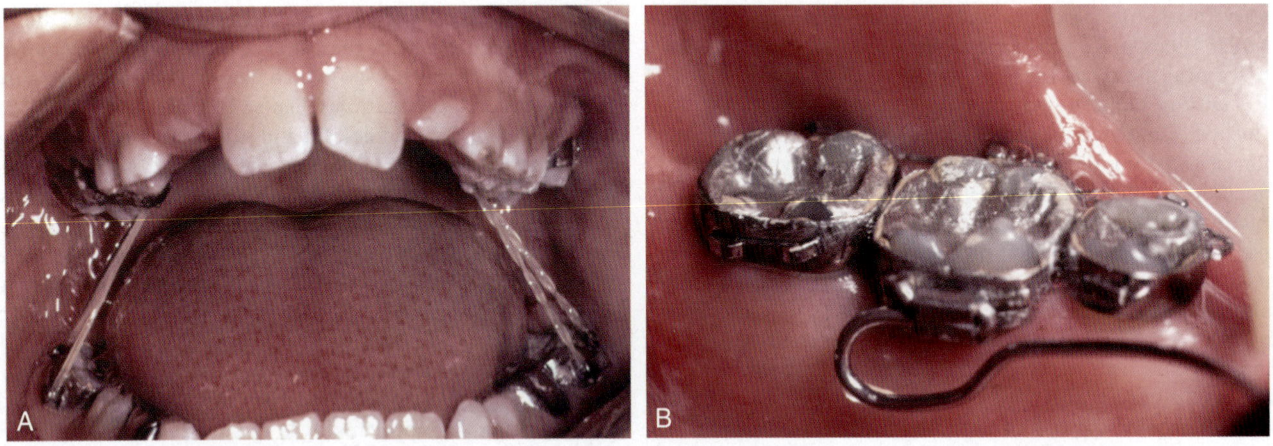

• **Fig. 15.14** (A) Cross-elastics to correct posterior crossbite, a method that also extrudes the teeth and therefore is not well suited to patients who no longer have vertical growth. (B) Cross-elastics often are used with a mandibular stabilizing lingual arch, like the one shown here, so that the major effect is buccal tipping of the upper molars rather than lingual tipping of the lower molars.

segmental maxillary osteotomy is the only way to generate more than 1 to 2 mm of skeletal expansion, and these methods are discussed in Chapter 20.

Other Space Problems

Impacted or Unerupted Teeth

Bringing an impacted or unerupted tooth into the arch creates a set of special problems during alignment. The most frequent impaction involves a maxillary canine or canines, but it is occasionally necessary to bring other unerupted teeth into the arch, and the same techniques apply for incisors, canines, and premolars. Impacted lower second molars pose a different problem and are discussed separately.

The problems in dealing with an unerupted tooth fall into three categories: (1) surgical exposure, (2) attachment to the tooth, and (3) orthodontic mechanics to bring the tooth into the arch.

Surgical Exposure

Before operation to expose an unerupted tooth, it is obviously important to know with some precision where it is. This is an indication for cone beam computed tomography (CBCT) with use of a unit with a small field of view (FOV) unless there is an indication for a large FOV (primarily, jaw asymmetry).[2] With a CBCT image, it is often apparent that before an impacted canine can be pulled downward toward its position in the dental arch, it will be necessary to move it away from the roots of the central or lateral incisor—information that changes treatment plans and was not available with previous radiographic methods.

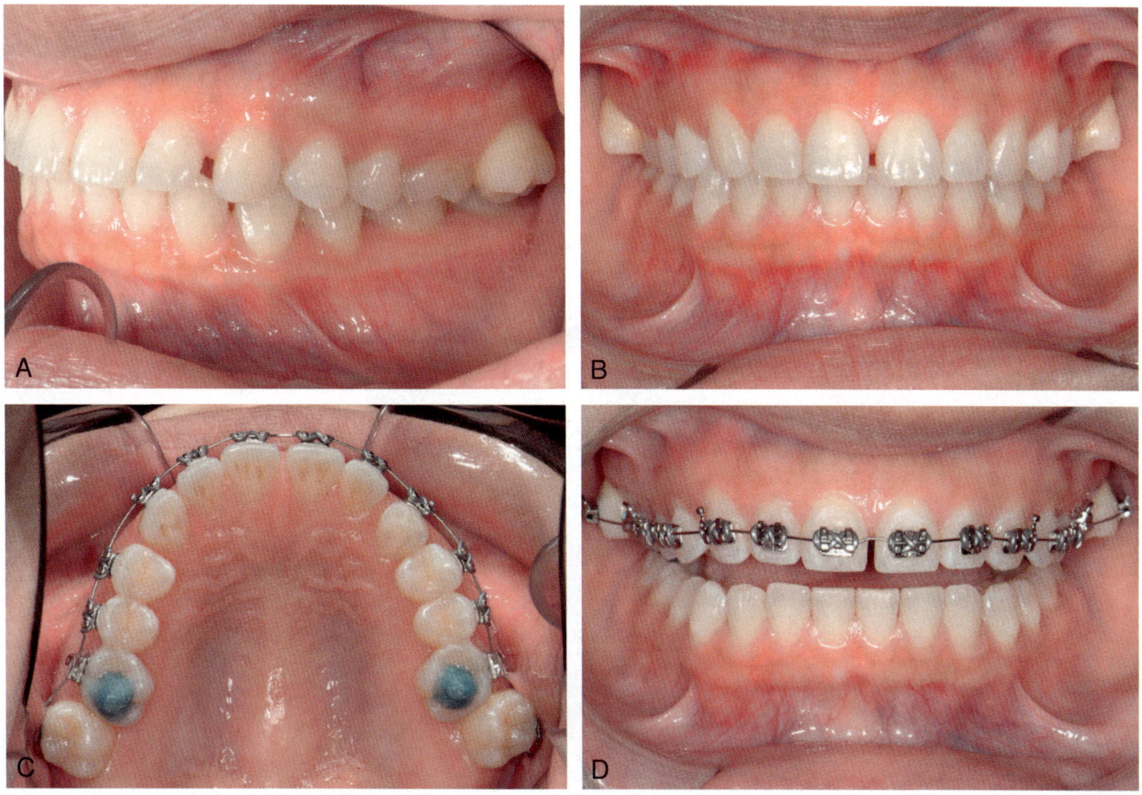

• **Fig. 15.15** For correction of a severe dental crossbite after growth is largely complete, temporary opening of the bite blocks to open the bite is needed. (A and B) This severe buccal crossbite of the second molars would be all but impossible to correct without use of either a removable bite plate or bonded bite blocks. (C) Bonded bite blocks are more effective because they are present full-time and also are more comfortable for the patient. Cross-elastics are extrusive and would not be indicated for a patient like this. (D) An extension of a flexible archwire to bring the second molars into occlusion is the preferred method.

It is important for a tooth to erupt through the attached gingiva, not through alveolar mucosa, and this must be considered when exposure of an unerupted tooth is planned. If the canine is labially positioned and has adequate attached tissue, the crown can be exposed with a laser (see Fig. 7.26). If the unerupted tooth is more apically positioned in the mandibular arch or on the labial side of the maxillary alveolar process, a flap should be reflected from the crest of the alveolus and sutured so that attached gingiva has been transferred to the region where the crown is exposed (see Fig. 11.49). If this is not done and the tooth is brought through alveolar mucosa, it is quite likely that tissue will strip away from the crown, leaving an unsightly and periodontally compromised gingival margin.[3] For a very high canine that is positioned labially, a tunnel method is an alternative to raising of a flap. If the unerupted tooth is on the palatal side, similar problems with the heavy palatal mucosa are unlikely, and an open exposure can be used.[4]

Occasionally a tooth will obligingly erupt into its correct position after obstacles to eruption have been removed by surgical exposure, and delaying orthodontic traction to palatally impacted canines with incomplete roots is now recommended, but favorable spontaneous movement rarely occurs after root formation is complete. At that stage, even a tooth that is aimed in the right direction usually requires orthodontic force to bring it into position.

Method of Attachment

The best contemporary approach is to directly bond an attachment of some type to an exposed area of the crown. In many instances, a button or eyelet is better than a standard bracket because it is smaller. Then, if the tooth will be covered when the flap is replaced, a piece of fine gold chain is tied to the attachment, and before the flap is repositioned and sutured into place, the chain is positioned so that it extends into the mouth. The chain is much easier to tie to than a wire ligature. Before the availability of direct bonding, a pin was sometimes placed in a hole prepared in the crown of an unerupted tooth, and this remains a possible but much more invasive alternative.

The least desirable way to obtain attachment is for the surgeon to place a wire ligature around the crown of the impacted tooth. This inevitably results in loss of periodontal attachment because bone that is destroyed when the wire is passed around the tooth does not regenerate when it is removed, and this increases the chance of ankylosis. At present, the use of wire ligatures around an unerupted tooth approaches malpractice and should be avoided.

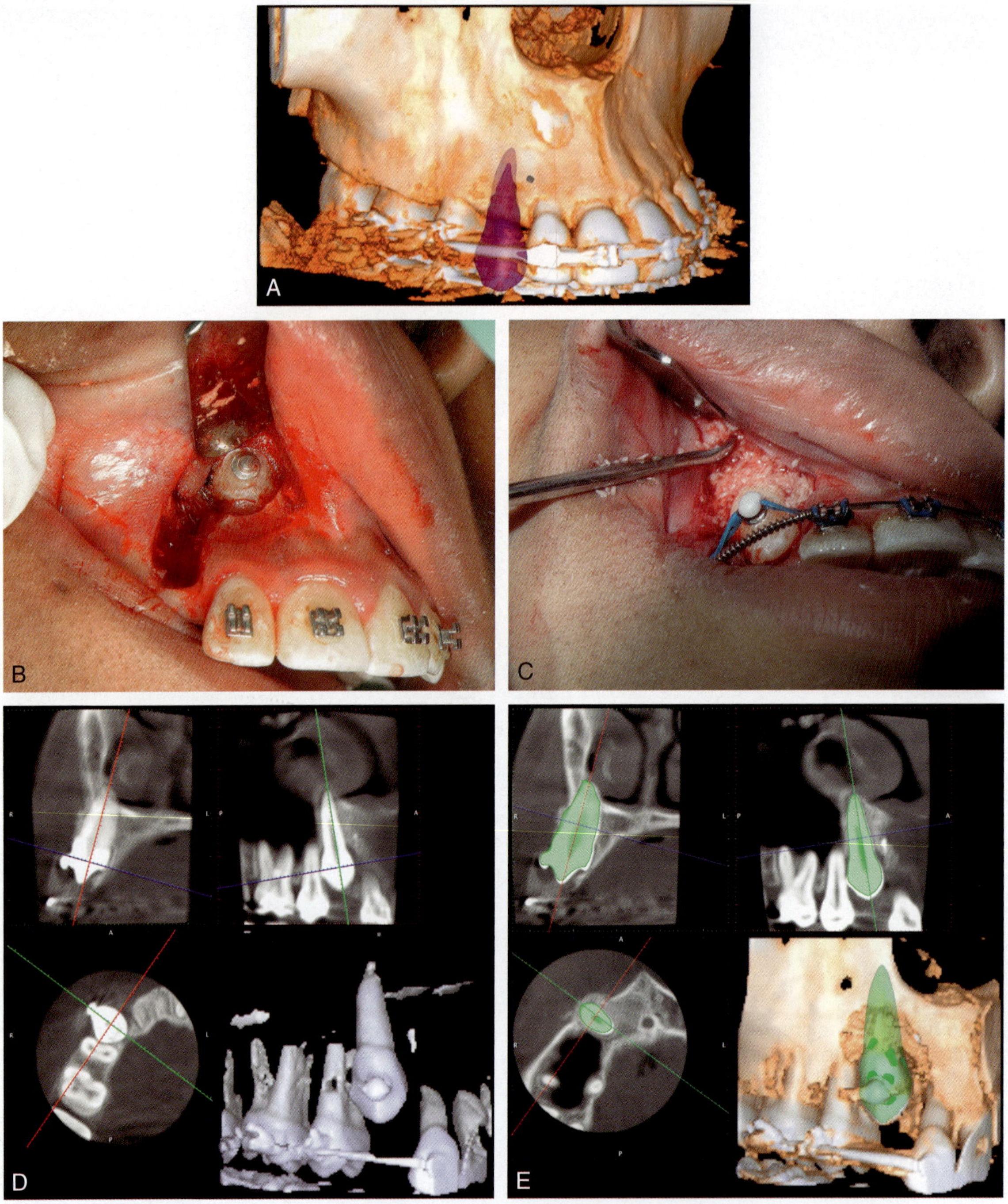

• **Fig. 15.16** In modern correction of impacted canines, three-dimensional (3D) images are necessary for more severe cases. (A) This 3D rendering shows the virtual projection of the impacted canine into the dental arch, which allows an evaluation of the amount of bone available in the area around the base of the crown of the tooth. Lack of bone in that area can be a long-term problem. (B) Surgical exposure of the tooth and the creation of an eruption path for it also are greatly facilitated by 3D images that allow creation of a path around the roots of other teeth. (C) The impacted tooth approaching the occlusal plane, with a bone slurry graft being placed over what otherwise would be a denuded root surface. (D and E) Views from the cone beam computed tomography image used in planning the exposure and eruption path. (Courtesy Dr. J. Fisher.)

It is critical for the surgeon performing the exposure procedure to be aware of the intended direction of orthodontic movement of the impacted tooth and that there is enough space for alveolar bone at the base of the crown when it comes into position (Fig. 15.16). CBCT views make this much more predictable and accurate and are now the standard of care for evaluating severely impacted teeth (Fig. 15.16).

Once the crown of the tooth has been exposed for bonding an attachment, the cells in the follicle that allow bone resorption around enamel are no longer present. This means that any bone left in the direction of the impacted crown movement will be difficult or impossible to resorb. The surgeon needs to remove adequate bone so that no enamel-to-bone contact is created as the tooth is brought into the mouth. Failure to do this can greatly reduce the speed of tooth movement and may make the impacted tooth appear to be ankylosed.

Mechanical Approaches for Aligning Unerupted Teeth

Orthodontic traction to move an unerupted tooth away from other permanent tooth roots, if necessary, and then toward its place in the dental arch should begin as soon as possible after the surgical procedure. Ideally, a fixed orthodontic appliance should already be in place before the unerupted tooth is exposed, so that orthodontic force can be applied immediately. If this is not practical, active orthodontic movement should begin no later than 2 or 3 weeks postoperatively.

This means that for a labially impacted canine, orthodontic treatment to open space for the unerupted tooth and allow stabilization of the rest of the dental arch must begin well before the surgical exposure. In this instance, the goals of the presurgical orthodontic treatment are to create enough space if it does not exist, as is often the case, and to align the other teeth so that a heavy stabilizing archwire (at least 18-mil round steel, preferably a rectangular steel wire) can be in position at the time of operation. This allows postsurgical orthodontic treatment to start immediately. For a palatally impacted canine, open exposure often leads to downward drift, so immediate active treatment can be deferred for many of these patients.

As we have noted previously, an unerupted tooth is an extreme example of an asymmetric alignment problem, with one tooth far from the line of occlusion. An auxiliary NiTi wire, overlaid on the stabilizing arch in the same way as recommended for other asymmetric alignment situations (see Fig. 15.7), is the most efficient way to bring an impacted tooth into position. The numerous alternatives include a special alignment spring, either soldered to a heavy base archwire or bent into a light archwire, or a cantilever spring from the auxiliary tube on the first molar.

Ankylosis of an unerupted tooth is always a potential problem. If an area of fusion to the adjacent bone develops, orthodontic movement of the unerupted tooth becomes impossible, and displacement of the anchor teeth will occur. Occasionally an unerupted tooth will start to move and will then become ankylosed, apparently held by only a small area of fusion. It can sometimes be freed to continue movement if the area is anesthetized and the tooth lightly luxated, breaking the area of ankylosis. If this procedure is done, it is critically important to apply orthodontic force immediately after the luxation, because it is only a matter of time until the tooth re-ankyloses. Nevertheless, this approach can sometimes allow a tooth to be brought into the arch that otherwise would have been impossible to move.

Canine impaction often accompanies a serious space discrepancy, so expanding the arch to make room for unerupted canines or extracting first premolars and using most of the extraction space becomes an important question at the treatment planning stage. Premolar extraction is a better choice than arch expansion that would create excessive incisor protrusion, especially if the canines are in a reasonably vertical position and only modest space closure would be needed (see Figs. 15.17 and 15.18).

Unerupted or Impacted Lower Second Molars

Unlike impaction of most other teeth, which is an obvious problem from the beginning of treatment, impaction of lower second molars usually develops during orthodontic treatment. This occurs when the mesial marginal ridge of the second molar catches against the distal surface of the first molar or on the edge of a first molar band so that the second molar progressively tips mesially instead of erupting. Moving the first molar posteriorly during the period of mixed dentition, or even preventing mesial movement to save space when second primary molars are lost, increases the chance that the second molar will become impacted. This possibility must be kept in mind when procedures to increase mandibular arch length are employed. Many clinicians now delay or avoid banding lower first molars because of this risk.

Correction of an impacted second molar requires tipping the tooth posteriorly and uprighting it (Fig. 15.19). In most cases, if the mesial marginal ridge can be unlocked, the tooth will erupt on its own. When the second molar is not severely tipped, the simplest solution is to place a separator between the two teeth. For more severe problems, an attachment must be bonded to the second molar. An auxiliary spring (Fig. 15.20) is often useful to bring both upper and lower second molars into alignment when they erupt late in orthodontic treatment. The easiest way to do this is to use a segment of NiTi wire from the auxiliary tube on the first molar to the tube on the second molar. A rectangular wire, usually 16 × 22 M-NiTi, is preferred. This provides a light force to align the second molars while a heavier and more rigid wire remains in place anteriorly, which is much better than going back to a light round wire for the entire arch just to align the second molars.

Another possibility in adolescents is surgical uprighting of the impacted second molar, taking advantage of the space that is created when the third molar is extracted. In carefully selected cases, this can work quite nicely. Vitality of the second molar is retained because it essentially is rotated around the root apex, and the defect on the mesial of the uprighted tooth fills in with bone in the same way that it does when orthodontic uprighting is done (Fig. 15.21).[5,6] The outcome is best when some vertical jaw growth remains so that the uprighted tooth does not remain elongated relative to the first molar.

Diastema Closure

A maxillary midline diastema is often complicated by the insertion of the labial frenum into a notch in the alveolar bone so that a band of heavy fibrous tissue lies between the central incisors. When this is the case, a stable correction of the diastema almost always requires surgery to remove the interdental fibrous tissue and reposition the frenum. The frenectomy must be carried out in a way that will produce a good esthetic result and must be properly coordinated with orthodontic treatment.

It is an error to surgically remove the frenum at an early age and then delay orthodontic treatment in the hope that the diastema will close spontaneously. If the frenum is removed while there is still a space between the central incisors, scar tissue forms between the teeth as healing progresses, and a long delay may result in a space that is more difficult to close than it was previously.

It is better to align the teeth before a frenectomy. Sliding them together along an archwire is usually better than using a closing loop because a loop with any vertical height will touch and irritate the frenum. If the diastema is relatively small, it is usually possible to bring the central incisors completely together before the surgical procedure (Fig. 15.22). If the space is large and the frenal attachment is thick, it may not be possible to completely close the space before surgical intervention. The space should be closed at least partially, and then orthodontic movement to bring the teeth together should be resumed immediately after the frenectomy so that the teeth are brought together quickly after the procedure. When this is done, healing occurs with the teeth together, and

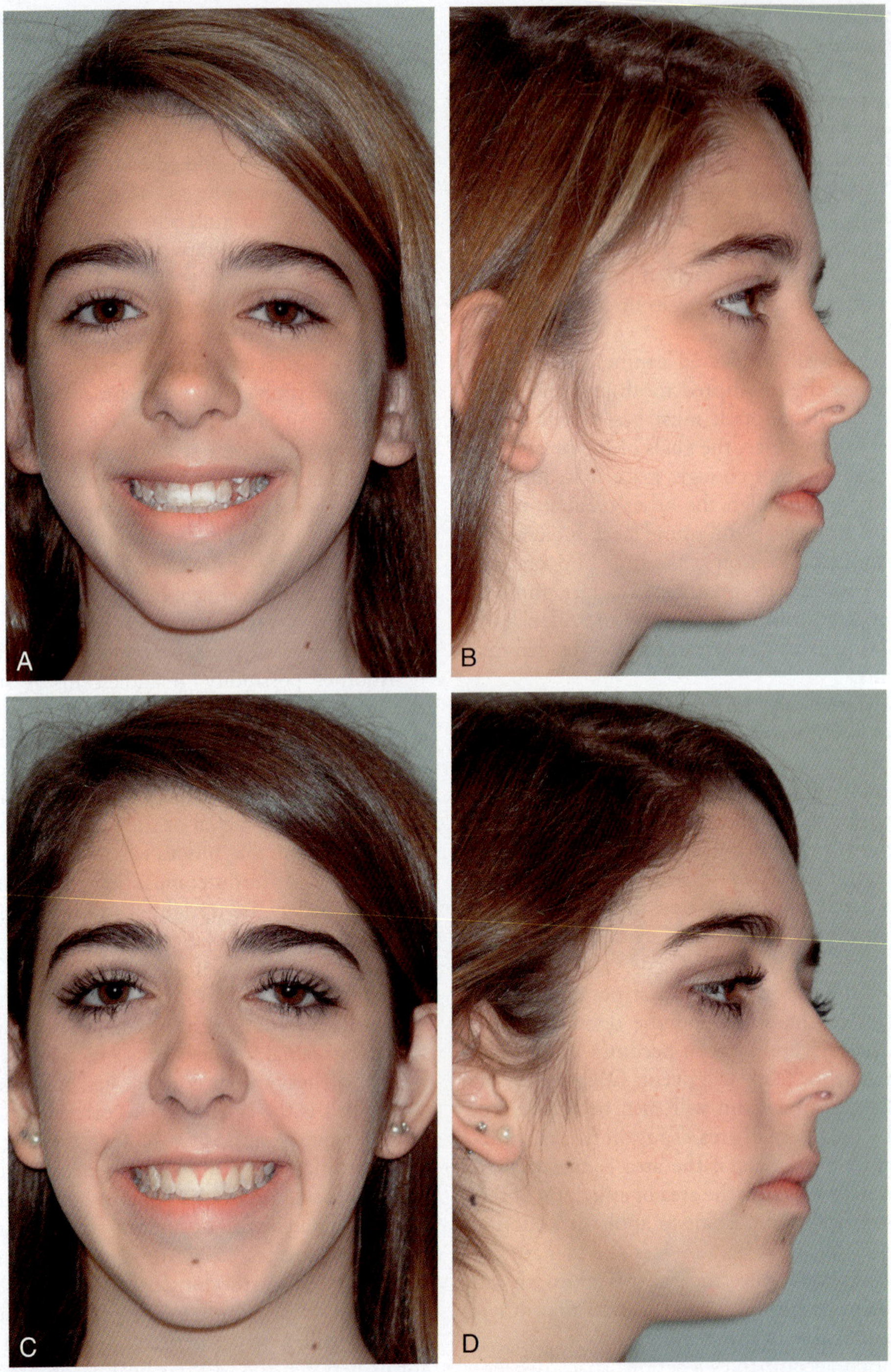

• **Fig. 15.17** (A and B) Pretreatment and (C and D) posttreatment facial appearance. Note the effect on the smile appearance of correcting both the maxillary incisor alignment and the relationship of the maxillary incisors to the lower lip on smile (the smile arc). (Courtesy Dr. T. Shaughnessy.)

the inevitable postsurgical scar tissue stabilizes the teeth instead of creating obstacles to final closure of the space.

The key to successful operation is removal of the interdental fibrous tissue. It is unnecessary and in fact undesirable to excise a large portion of the frenum itself. Instead, a simple incision is used to allow access to the interdental area, the fibrous connection to the bone is removed, and the frenum is then sutured at a higher level.[7]

A maxillary midline diastema tends to recur, no matter how carefully the space was managed initially. The elastic gingival fiber network typically did not cross the midline in these patients, and the operation interrupted any fibers that did cross. As a result, in this critical area the normal mechanism to keep teeth in contact is missing. A bonded fixed retainer is recommended (see Fig. 15.22G).

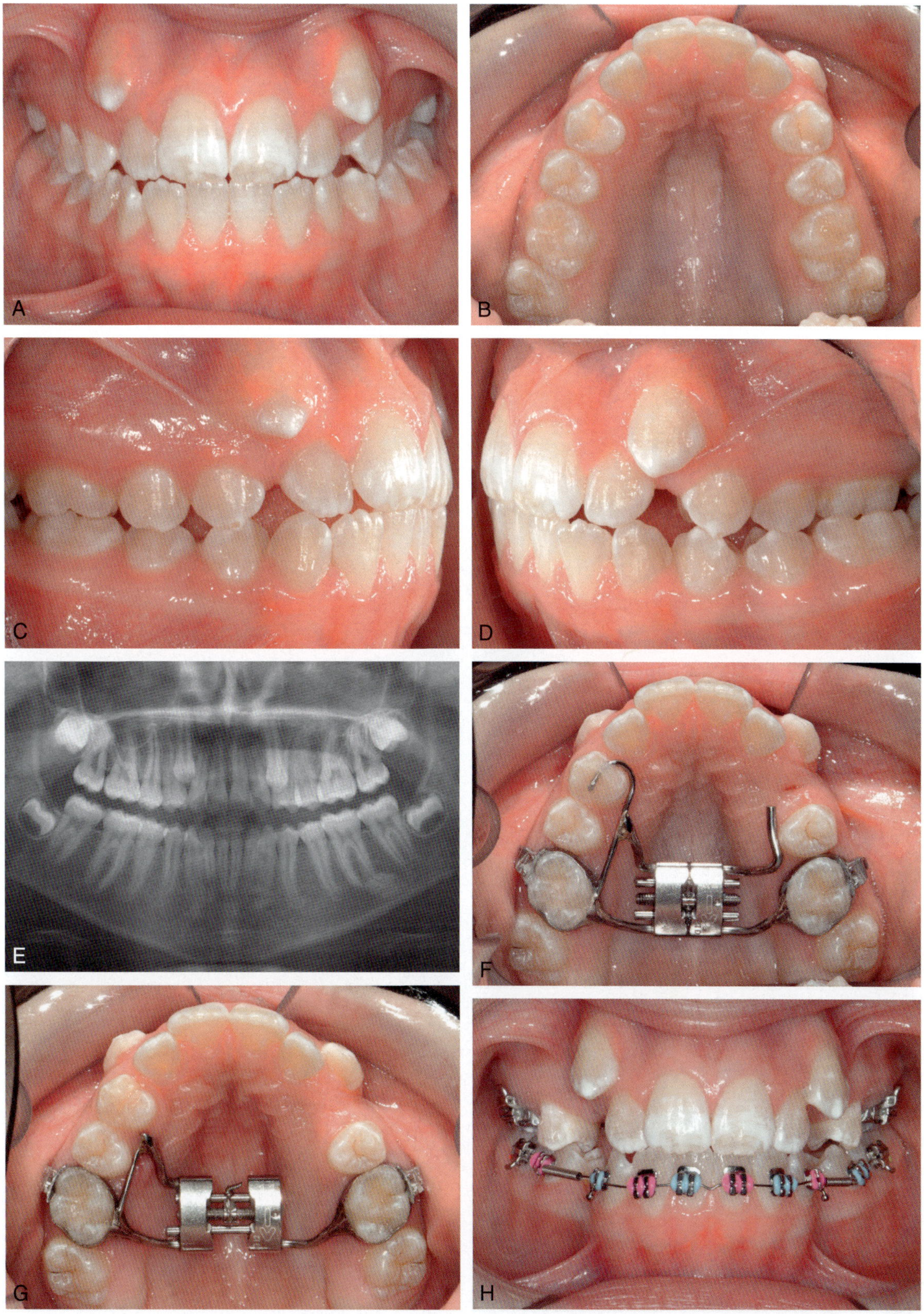

• **Fig. 15.18** Maxillary canines blocked out of the dental arch and erupting facially are a significant problem for a patient (same patient as in Fig. 15.17) who hears that he or she has "fangs." (A–D) This girl had not only facially projected canines but also a unilateral crossbite, with the maxillary arch constricted on the left side. (E) The panoramic radiograph showed that if space were opened, it should be straightforward to bring the canines into the arch. The key question was whether extractions would be necessary to keep the incisors from becoming too protrusive, and the answer for this patient was that extraction of four first premolars would be the best plan. (F–H)

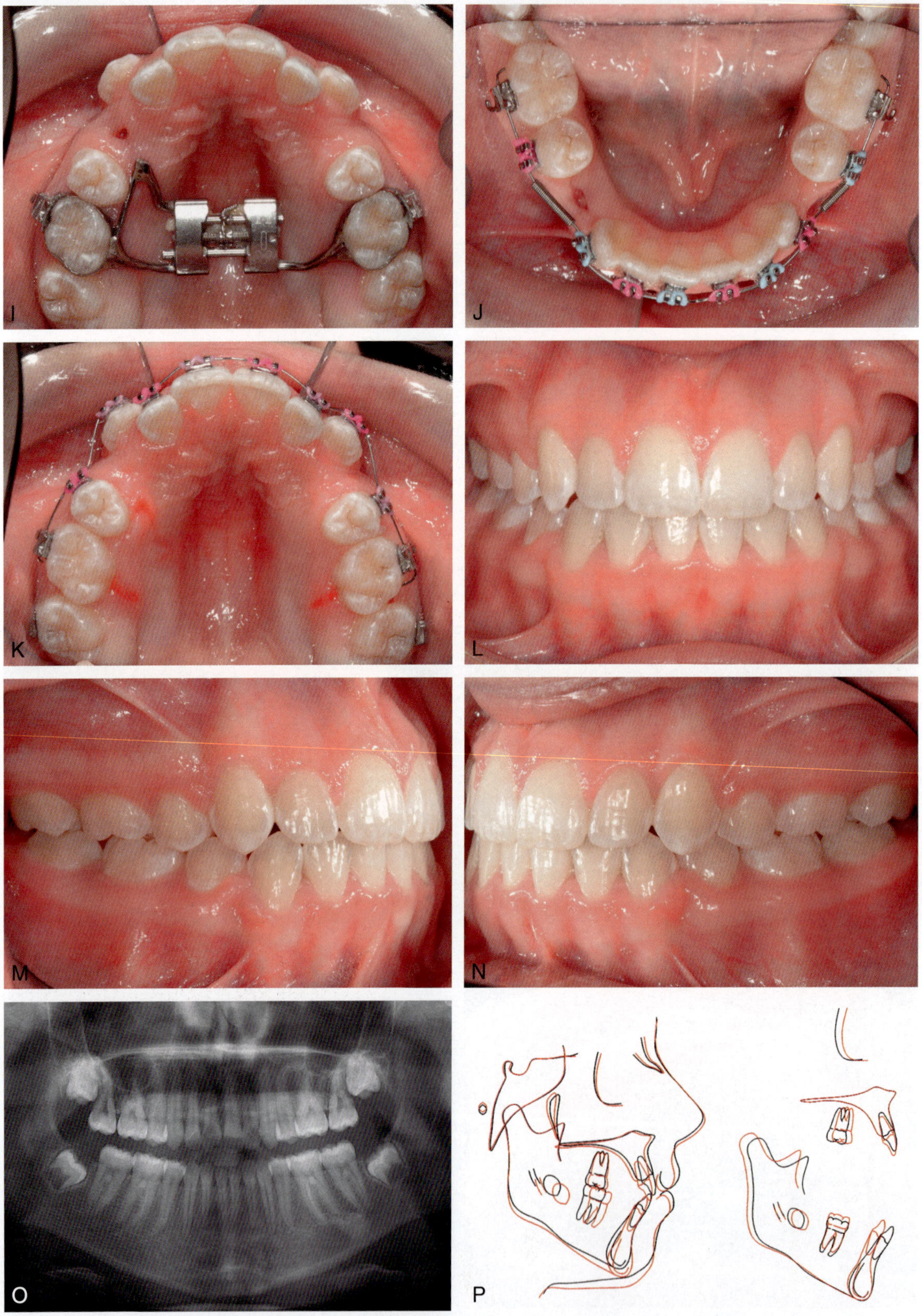

• **Fig. 15.18** Because unilateral expansion of the maxillary arch was needed, the first premolar on the maxillary right side was retained temporarily as additional anchorage, and this did result in the desired expansion on the constricted side. (I and J) Then the lower arch was leveled in preparation for space closure with moderate incisor retraction, and the maxillary canines were moved downward and backward into the premolar extraction site. (K–N) Satisfactory alignment, crossbite correction, and occlusion were obtained. (O) Panoramic radiograph at end of treatment. (P) The cephalometric superimposition shows normal position of the incisors posttreatment. For her, nonextraction treatment would have created excessive protrusion. (Courtesy Dr. T. Shaughnessy.)

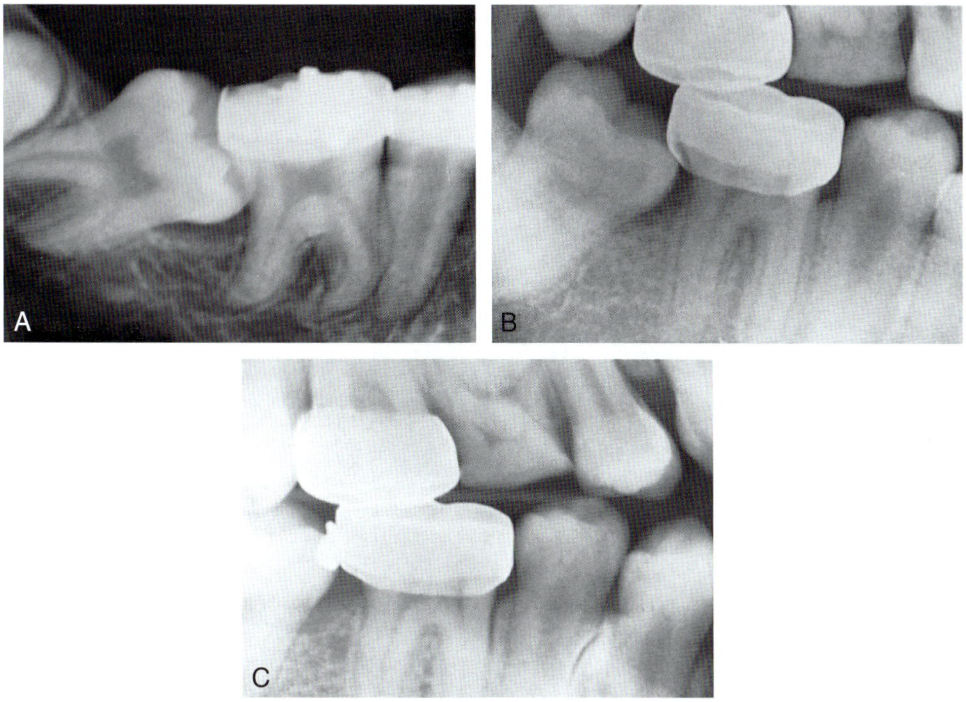

• **Fig. 15.19** (A) Radiographic view of an impacted mandibular second molar in a 16-year-old patient. Uprighting the tooth from this position requires surgical exposure of a portion of the facial surface of the crown and bonding an attachment (if possible, a tube) so that a spring can be used to tip the tooth distally and bring it into the arch. (B) For a second molar that is caught on the edge of a first molar band, a simpler approach is uprighting achieved with a 20-mil brass wire tightened around the contact. Usually it is necessary to anesthetize the area to place a separator of this type. (C) Uprighting and distal movement obtained with the brass wire separator (same patient as B). A spring clip (one type is sold as the Arkansas de-impaction spring) can be used in the same way, but both brass wire and spring clips are effective only for minimal molar uprighting. Neither would have worked for the situation shown in (A).

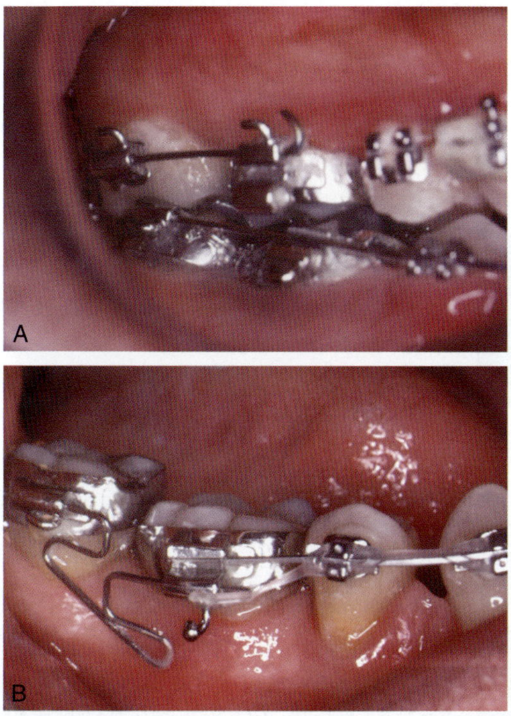

• **Fig. 15.20** When a second molar is banded or bonded relatively late in treatment, it is often desirable to align it with a flexible wire while retaining a heavier archwire in the remainder of the arch. (A) Repositioning a maxillary second molar by using a straight segment of rectangular austenitic nickel-titanium (A-NiTi) wire that fits into the auxiliary tube on the first molar and the tube for the main archwire on the second molar. (B) Repositioning a mandibular second molar by using a segment of steel wire with a loop that extends from the auxiliary tube on the first molar. In both arches, after the repositioning a continuous archwire can extend to the second molar.

Leveling

The archwire design for leveling the dental arch when there is an excessive curve of Spee depends on whether there is a need for absolute intrusion of incisors or whether relative intrusion is satisfactory. This important point is discussed in detail in Chapter 7, and the biomechanical considerations in obtaining intrusion are described in Chapters 8 and 9. As a general rule, relative intrusion is quite acceptable for adolescents; absolute intrusion is used for the most part in patients who are too old for relative intrusion to succeed. The following discussion assumes that an appropriate decision about the type of leveling has been made and focuses on the rather different techniques for leveling by relative intrusion (which is really differential elongation of premolars, for the most part) versus leveling by absolute intrusion of incisors (Fig. 15.23).

Leveling by Extrusion (Relative Intrusion)

Leveling by extrusion can be accomplished with continuous archwires simply by placing an exaggerated curve of Spee in the maxillary archwire and a reverse curve in the mandibular archwire. For most patients, it is necessary to replace the initial highly resilient alignment arch with a slightly stiffer one to complete the leveling. With both the 18- and 22-slot appliances, when preliminary alignment is completed, the second archwire is almost always 16-mil steel, with an exaggerated curve of Spee in the upper arch and a reverse curve in the lower arch. In most instances, this is sufficient to complete the leveling. A possible alternative is a 16-mil "potato chip" A-NiTi wire, preformed by the manufacturer with an extremely exaggerated curve. The extreme curve needed to generate enough force can lead to problems if patients miss

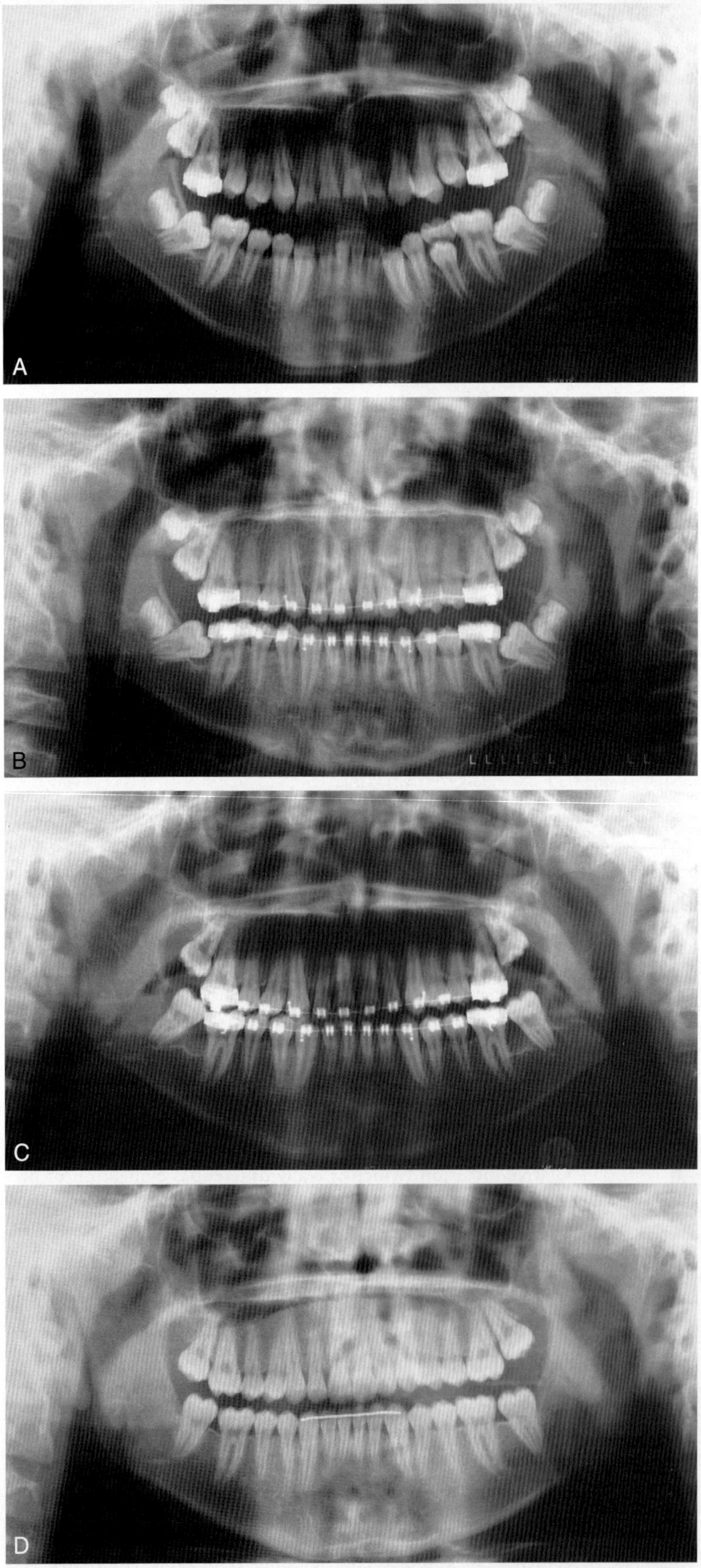

• **Fig. 15.21** Surgical uprighting of impacted mandibular second molars sometimes is the easiest way to deal with severe impactions. (A) Age 12, before loss of the second primary molars, with the permanent second molars tipped mesially against the first molars. Teeth in this position often upright spontaneously when the first molars drift mesially after the primary molars are lost. (B) Age 14, with severe impaction 1 year after the beginning of orthodontic treatment. (C) Age 14, after surgical uprighting of the second molar, which was rotated around its root apex into the space created by third molar extraction. Loss of pulp vitality usually does not occur when this is done. (D) Age 16, after completion of orthodontic treatment. Note the excellent fill-in of bone between the first and second molars.

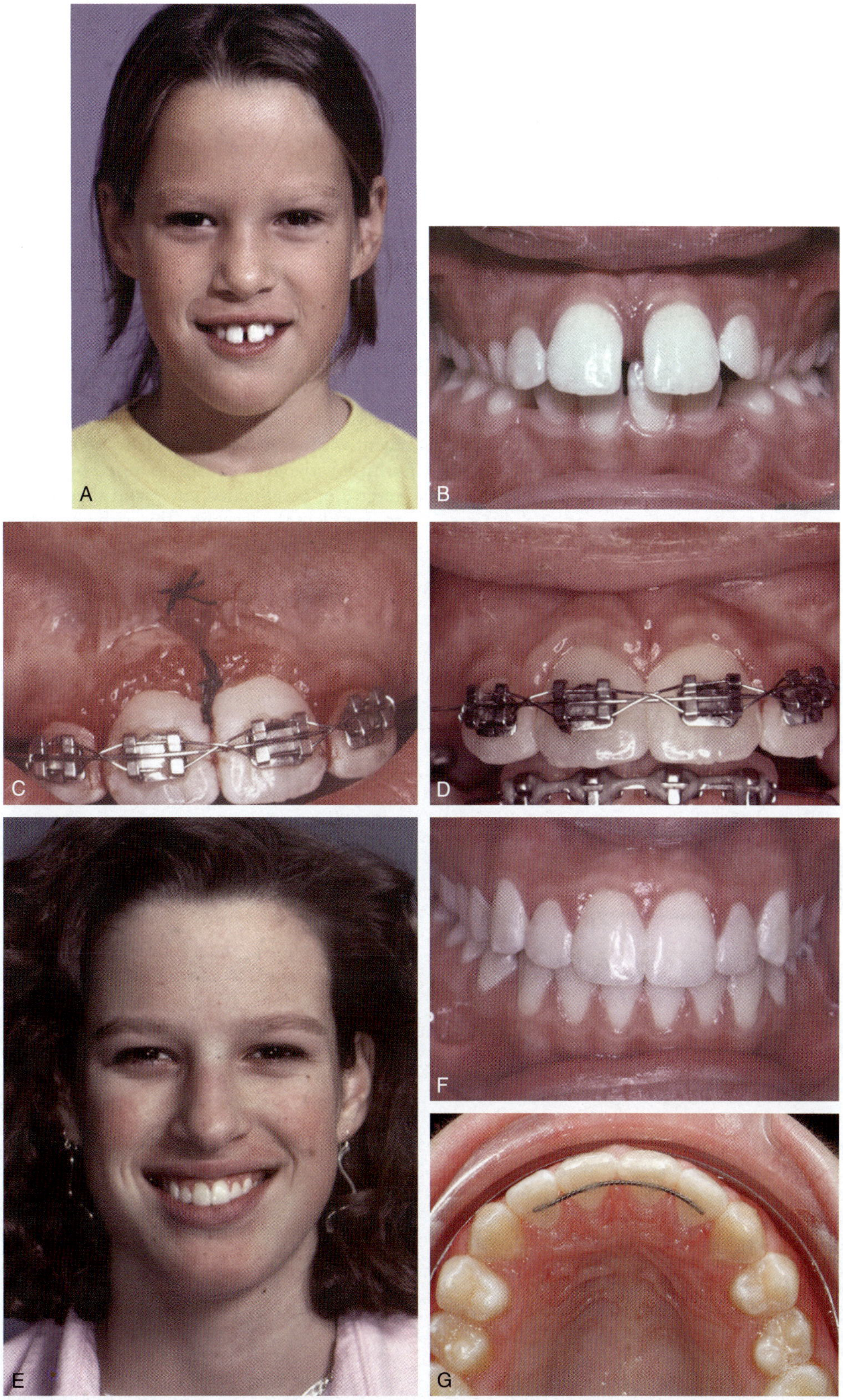

• **Fig. 15.22** Management of a maxillary midline diastema. (A) Facial appearance showing the protruding maxillary incisors caught on the lower lip. (B) Intraoral view before treatment. (C) Teeth aligned and held tightly together with a figure-of-eight wire ligature before frenectomy. (D) Appearance immediately after frenectomy with the conservative technique advocated by Edwards in which a simple incision is used to allow access to the interdental area, the fibrous connection to the bone is removed, and the frenal attachment is sutured at a higher level. (E) Facial appearance 2 years after completion of treatment. (F) Intraoral view 2 years after treatment. (G) Bonded retainer, made with 1.75-mil steel twist wire. It is important for the retainer wire to be flexible enough to allow some displacement of the incisors in function; a rigid wire is much more likely to break loose.

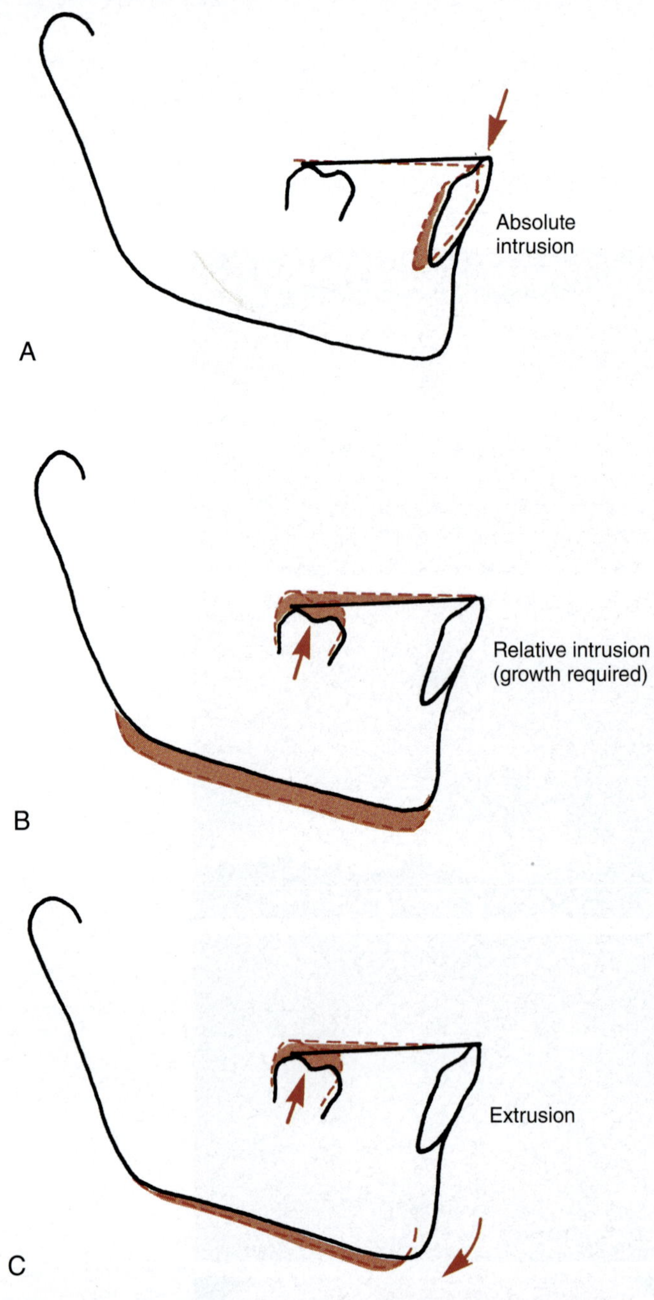

• **Fig. 15.23** There are three possible ways to level a lower arch with an excessive curve of Spee: (A) absolute intrusion; (B) relative intrusion, achieved by preventing eruption of the incisors while growth provides vertical space into which the posterior teeth erupt; and (C) extrusion of posterior teeth, which causes the mandible to rotate down and back in the absence of growth. Note that the difference between (B) and (C) is whether the mandible rotates downward. This is determined by whether the ramus grows longer while the tooth movement is occurring, not by the orthodontic mechanics.

appointments (i.e., the wire does not failsafe), so these wires are not recommended for routine use.

In some patients, particularly in those who have little if any remaining growth, an archwire heavier than 16-mil steel is needed to complete the leveling of the arches. With the 22-slot appliance, an 18-mil archwire is used almost routinely, as a step toward bracket engagement with a larger rectangular wire. With the 18-slot appliance, rather than using an 18-mil round wire, it is usually quicker and easier to leave the 16-mil wire in place and add an auxiliary leveling arch of 17 × 25 mil TMA or steel (Fig. 15.24A–B). This auxiliary wire inserts into the auxiliary tube on the molar and is tied anteriorly beneath the 16-mil base arch. In essence, this augments the curve in the base arch and results in efficient completion of the leveling by the same mechanism as a single continuous wire. Although the auxiliary leveling arch looks like an intrusion arch (Fig. 15.24C and D), it differs in two important ways: the presence of a continuous rather than segmented base arch and the higher amount of force. Leveling will occur almost totally by extrusion as long as a continuous rather than segmented wire is in the bracket slots, and segmenting the arch makes intrusion possible (Fig. 15.24E and F).

For a typical patient using the 22-slot appliance, initial alignment with an A-NiTi wire (delivery of light force, not size, is the critical variable) is usually followed by a 16-mil steel wire with a reverse or accentuated curve and then by an 18-mil round wire to complete the leveling. This archwire sequence is nearly always adequate for completion of leveling, and it is unusual that 20-mil wire or an auxiliary archwire is required.

With either slot size, it is an error to place a rectangular archwire with an exaggerated curve of Spee in the mandibular arch because the curve creates torque to move the incisor roots lingually. Almost always that is undesirable. Inadvertent torque of lower incisor roots is one of the commonest mistakes with the edgewise appliance. The arch should be level before a rectangular wire is placed, or step bends rather than a reverse curve of Spee should be placed in the rectangular wire, and torque in any rectangular wire should be monitored carefully. In the maxillary arch, however, a rectangular wire with an accentuated curve of Spee would be quite acceptable if lingual root torque of the upper incisors is needed, as it often is.

Clear Aligner Therapy

As we have noted, the most frequent problem in adolescent orthodontic patients is a combination of malaligned incisors and excessive overbite. For patients with this problem who want clear aligner therapy, the usual choice is arch expansion for alignment, and tipping the mandibular incisors facially can be enough to correct the overbite in mild cases. When more severe overbite is present, restraining further eruption of lower incisors and encouraging eruption of mandibular canines and premolars—relative intrusion—is needed. This can be managed reasonably well by leaving a space within the lower aligner above the canines and premolars while using attachments on the incisors and molars to stabilize the aligner. Detailed use of aligners in adolescents is demonstrated in Chapter 18.

Leveling by Intrusion

Leveling by intrusion with a fixed appliance requires a mechanical arrangement other than a continuous archwire attached to each tooth. The key to successful intrusion is light continuous force directed toward the tooth apex. It is necessary to avoid pitting intrusion of one tooth against extrusion of its neighbor because in that circumstance extrusion will dominate. This can be accomplished in three ways: (1) with continuous archwires that bypass the premolar (and frequently the canine) teeth, (2) with segmented archwires (so that there is no connection along the arch between the anterior and posterior segments) and an auxiliary depressing arch, and (3) with aligners that have attachments on the posterior teeth so that when an apical force is placed on the anterior teeth, the aligner does not dislodge.

Bypass Archwires

Use of the bypass arches approach to intrusion is most useful for patients who will have a lot of vertical growth (i.e., who are in either the mixed or early permanent dentition period). Three different mechanical arrangements are commonly used, each based on the same mechanical principle: uprighting and distal tipping of the molars, pitted against intrusion of the incisors.

A classic version of this approach to leveling was seen in the first stage of the Begg technique in which the premolar teeth were bypassed and only a loose tie was made to the canine. The same effect can be produced in exactly the same way by using the edgewise appliance, if the premolars and canines are bypassed with a 2 × 4 appliance (only two molars and four incisors included in the appliance setup)[8] (Fig. 15.25) or if brackets on premolars simply do not have the main archwire tied in (see Fig. 15.24E and F).

A more flexible variation of the same basic idea was developed as Ricketts' utility arch.[9] In most cases, a utility arch formed from rectangular wire was placed into the brackets with slight labial root torque to control the inclination of the teeth as the incisors move labially while they intrude. However, this results in a complex two-couple mechanical system that makes it impossible to predict exactly what the effect will be (see discussion in Chapter 9), and utility arches for intrusion have largely been replaced by the segmented arch approach described later because sometimes they work well and sometimes they do not.

Successful use of any type of bypass arch for leveling requires keeping the forces light. This is accomplished in two ways: by selecting a small-diameter archwire, and by using a long span between the first molar and the incisors. Wire heavier than 16-mil steel should not be used, and Ricketts recommended a relatively soft 16 × 16 cobalt-chromium wire for utility arches to prevent heavy forces from being developed. A more modern recommendation would be 16 × 22 beta-titanium (beta-Ti) wire. Whatever the wire choice, overactivation of the vertical bends can cause loss of control of the molars in all three planes of space.

In contrast to leveling with continuous fully engaged archwires, the size of the edgewise bracket slot is largely irrelevant when bypass arches for leveling are used. Whether an 18- or 22-slot appliance is used, the bypass arch should not be stiffer than 16-mil steel wire.

Two weaknesses of the bypass arch systems limit the amount of true intrusion that can be obtained. The first is that, except for some applications of the utility arch, only the first molar is available as posterior anchorage. This means that significant extrusion of that tooth may occur. In actively growing patients with a good facial pattern, this is not a major problem, but in nongrowing patients or those with a poor facial pattern in whom molar extrusion should be avoided, the lack of posterior anchorage compromises the ability to intrude incisors.

The second weakness is that the intrusive force against the incisors is applied anterior to the center of resistance, and therefore the incisors tend to tip forward as they intrude (Fig. 15.26). Without an extraction space, forward movement of the incisors is an inevitable consequence of leveling, but in extraction cases this becomes an undesirable side effect. An anchor bend at the molar in a bypass arch creates a space-closing effect that somewhat restrains forward incisor movement (Fig. 15.27), but this also tends to bring the molar forward, straining the posterior anchorage. A utility arch can be activated (like a closing loop) to keep the incisors from moving forward and has the additional benefit of a rectangular cross-section anteriorly so that tipping can be controlled, but the result is still a strain on posterior anchorage, and, more important, it results in an unknown intrusion force that may be too heavy or too light (see Fig. 9.39).

Segmented Archwires for Intrusion

The segmented arch approach developed by Burstone, which overcomes these limitations, is recommended for maximum control of the anterior and posterior segments of the dental arch. Data now exist to document equivalent long-term stability with leveling by continuous archwires versus sectional wires in the segmented arch technique.[10]

The segmented arch approach (see Figs. 15.24E and F and 15.26) allows attachments on all the teeth and so provides better control of anchorage. For intrusion of anterior teeth, it depends on establishing stabilized posterior segments and controlling the point of force application against an anterior segment. This technique requires auxiliary rectangular tubes on first molars in addition to the regular bracket or tube. After preliminary alignment, a full-dimension rectangular archwire is placed in the bracket slots of teeth in the buccal segment, which typically consists of the second premolar, first molar, and second molar. This connects these teeth into a solid unit. In addition, a heavy lingual arch (36-mil round or 32 × 32 rectangular steel wire) is used to connect the right and left posterior segments, further stabilizing them against undesired movement. A resilient anterior segmental wire is used to align the incisors while the posterior segments are being stabilized.

For intrusion, an auxiliary arch placed in the auxiliary tube on the first molar is used to apply intrusive force against the anterior segment. It should be made of rectangular wire that will not twist in the auxiliary tube. The auxiliary tube should be 18 × 25 whether the main appliance is an 18- or 22-slot appliance. In it, 17 × 25 steel wire with a 2½-turn helix or 17 × 25 TMA wire works well. If the auxiliary tube is 22 × 28, 19 × 25 TMA wire without a helix or a preformed M-NiTi intrusion arch is acceptable, but the range of light force is lower. This auxiliary arch is adjusted so that it lies gingival to the incisor teeth when passive and applies a light force (approximately 10 g per tooth, depending on root size) when it is brought up beneath the brackets of the incisors. It is tied underneath or in front of the incisor brackets but not into the bracket slots, which are occupied by the anterior segment wire.

Intrusion of maxillary incisors to level the arch is done more frequently than intrusion of mandibular incisors, but intruding these teeth is necessary for some patients. The technique is the same: an auxiliary intrusion arch is inserted into the auxiliary tubes on the mandibular first molars, and the base arch is segmented (see Fig. 15.30).

An auxiliary intrusion arch can be placed while a light resilient anterior segment is being used to align malposed incisors, but usually it is better to wait to add it until incisor alignment has been achieved and a heavier anterior segment wire has been installed. Full-dimension braided rectangular steel wire or a rectangular TMA wire is usually the best choice for the anterior segment while active intrusion with an auxiliary arch is being carried out.

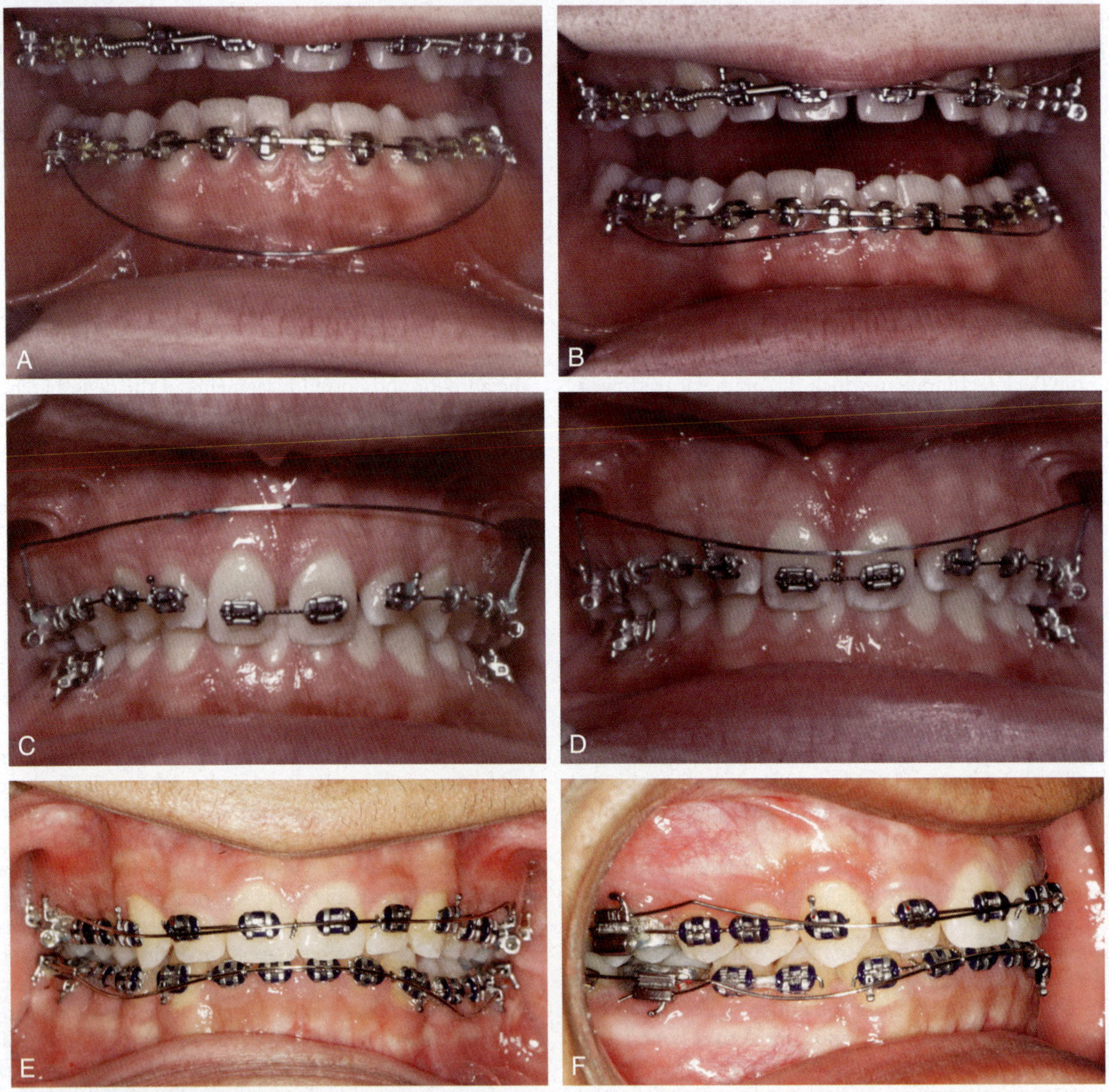

• **Fig. 15.24** With a continuous archwire in place, intrusion is essentially impossible, but an auxiliary leveling archwire can be useful in augmenting the leveling force from a wire tied into the brackets. (A) Auxiliary leveling wire before and after activation (B) by tying it beneath a continuous mandibular archwire. The appropriate force in this instance is approximately 150g, and the expected action is leveling by extruding the premolars rather than intruding the incisors. For absolute intrusion, light force (approximately 10g per tooth) is necessary. This requires the use of archwire segments and an auxiliary intrusion arch. (C) Intrusion arch before and after activation (D) by bending it downward and tying it to the segment to be intruded. The force delivered by the intrusion arch can be measured easily when it is brought down to the level at which it will be tied. (E) Auxiliary leveling arches for extrusion in the maxillary arch and (F) for incisor-canine intrusion in the mandibular arch. Note that the mandibular base arch is segmented, creating a separate incisor segment; a continuous archwire is in place in the maxillary arch and the auxiliary leveling arch is tied into the anterior brackets on top of it. Intrusion requires a segmented base arch and a light intrusive force (here, with six mandibular incisors in the anterior segment, approximately 50g would be used). Extrusion can be done with a segmented or continuous archwire by using about 50g per tooth in the segment to be extruded.

Two strategies can be used with segmented arches to prevent forward movement of the incisors as they are intruded. The first is the same as with bypass arches: a space-closing force can be created by tying the auxiliary arch back against the posterior segments. Even with stabilized posterior segments, this produces some strain on posterior anchorage.

The second and usually preferable strategy is to vary the point of force application against the incisor segment. If the anterior

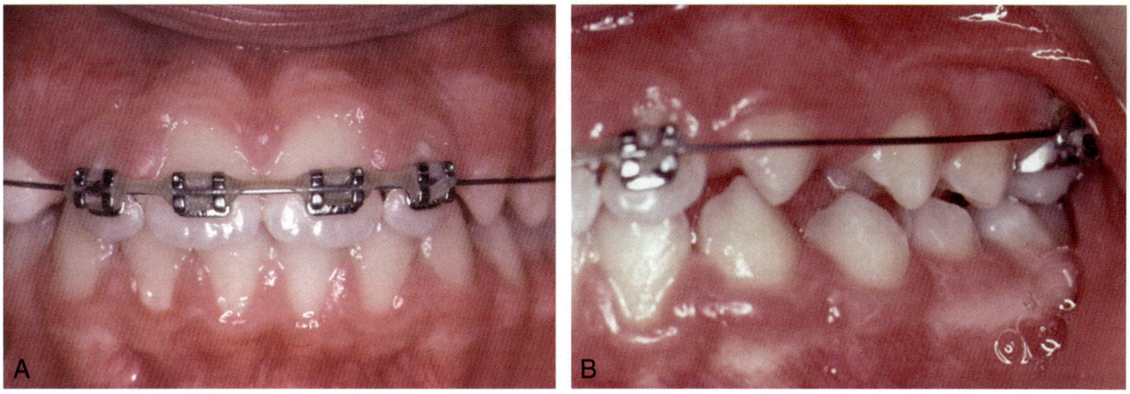

• **Fig. 15.25** (A and B) The long span of a 2 × 4 appliance makes it possible to create the light force necessary for incisor intrusion and also makes it possible to create unwanted side effects. This appliance is best described as deceptively simple. When incisor intrusion is desired before other permanent teeth can be incorporated into the appliance, a transpalatal lingual arch for additional anchorage is a good idea.

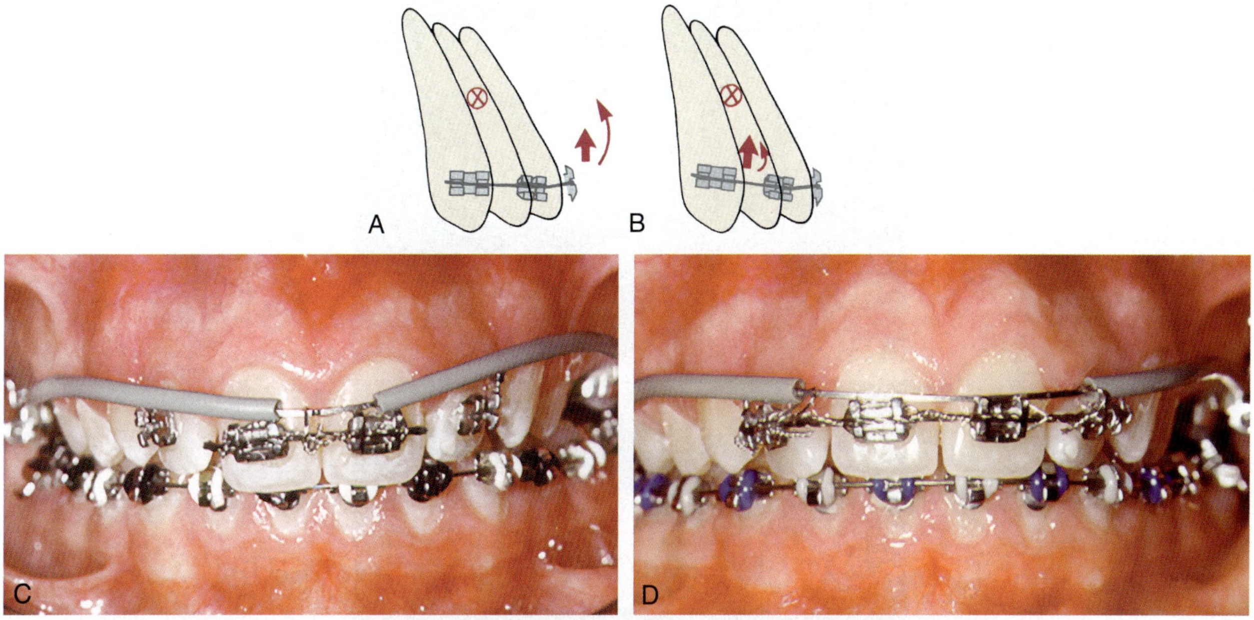

• **Fig. 15.26** (A) When the incisor segment is viewed from a lateral perspective, the center of resistance (X) is lingual to the point at which an archwire attaches to the teeth. For this reason, the incisors tend to tip forward when an intrusive force is placed at the central incisor brackets. (B) Tying an intrusion arch distal to the midline (for instance, between the lateral incisor and canine, as shown here) moves the line of force more posteriorly and therefore closer to the center of resistance. This diminishes or eliminates the moment that causes facial tipping of the teeth as they intrude. (C) Intrusion arch tied in the midline as only the central incisors are intruded, so that the incisors will tip facially as they intrude. (D) In the same patient later, an intrusion arch now is tied between the central and lateral incisors to intrude all four incisors while reducing the amount of facial tipping.

segment is considered a single unit (which is reasonable when a stiff archwire connects the teeth within the segment), the center of resistance is located as shown in Fig. 15.26. Tying the depressing arch distal to the midline, between the central and lateral incisors or distal to the laterals, also brings the point of force application more posterior so that the force is applied more nearly through the center of resistance. This prevents anterior tipping of the incisor segment without causing anchorage strain, but the auxiliary wire must be tied quite loosely at both points to avoid the risk of inadvertently creating a two-couple system.

Even with the control of posterior anchorage obtained by placing rectangular stabilizing segments and an anchorage lingual arch, the reaction to intrusion of incisors is extrusion and distal tipping of the posterior segments. A stabilizing transpalatal lingual arch is needed to augment anchorage. With careful attention to appropriate forces and moments with the segmented arch approach, it is possible to produce approximately four times as much incisor intrusion as molar extrusion in nongrowing adults. Although successful intrusion can be obtained with round bypass arches, the ratio of anterior intrusion to posterior extrusion is much less favorable.

It is quite feasible to intrude asymmetrically, which requires only adjusting the teeth that are placed in stabilizing and intrusion segments and tying the auxiliary intrusion arch in the area where

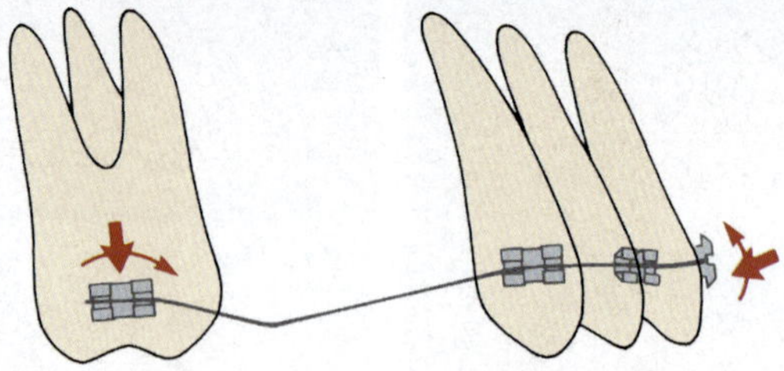

• **Fig. 15.27** Diagrammatic representation of the forces for a leveling arch that bypasses the premolars, with an anchor bend mesial to the molars. A force system is created that elongates the molars and intrudes the incisors. The wire tends to slide posteriorly through the molar tubes, tipping the incisors distally at the expense of bodily mesial movement of the molars. An archwire of this design was used in the first stage of Begg treatment but also can be used in edgewise systems. A long span from the molars to the incisors is essential.

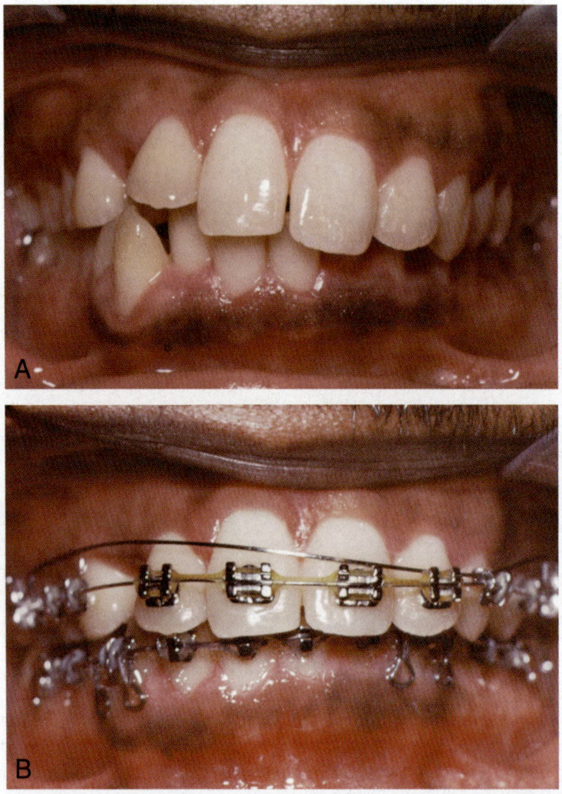

• **Fig. 15.28** (A) In this adult patient, the maxillary left central and lateral incisors and particularly the canine had supererupted. Asymmetric intrusion of those teeth was needed. (B) An auxiliary intrusion arch delivering about 30 g was tied to the elongated canine while preliminary alignment with an austenitic nickel-titanium (A-NiTi) wire was employed. The result was leveling of the maxillary arch with a component of intrusion on the elongated side. Asymmetric intrusion can be accomplished either by asymmetric activation of an intrusion arch that spans from one first molar to the other or by use of a cantilever intrusion arch on one side only.

intrusion is required (Fig. 15.28). If intrusion is desired on only one side, either a cantilevered auxiliary wire extending from one molar or a molar-to-molar auxiliary arch can be used. The key is tying the auxiliary arch at the point where intrusion is desired.

It also is possible to intrude posterior teeth to correct an anterior open bite. Frequently a major component of a skeletal open bite is a tipped palatal plane, and intrusion of maxillary posterior teeth (Fig. 15.29) can provide an acceptable dental compensation if the problem is not too severe. This requires skeletal anchorage. It should be deferred until after the adolescent growth spurt and for that reason is presented in detail in Chapter 20.

Correction of a severe Class II deep bite malocclusion, with leveling of the maxillary arch by labial tipping of the upper incisors and segmented arch intrusion of the elongated lower incisors, is shown in Fig. 15.30.

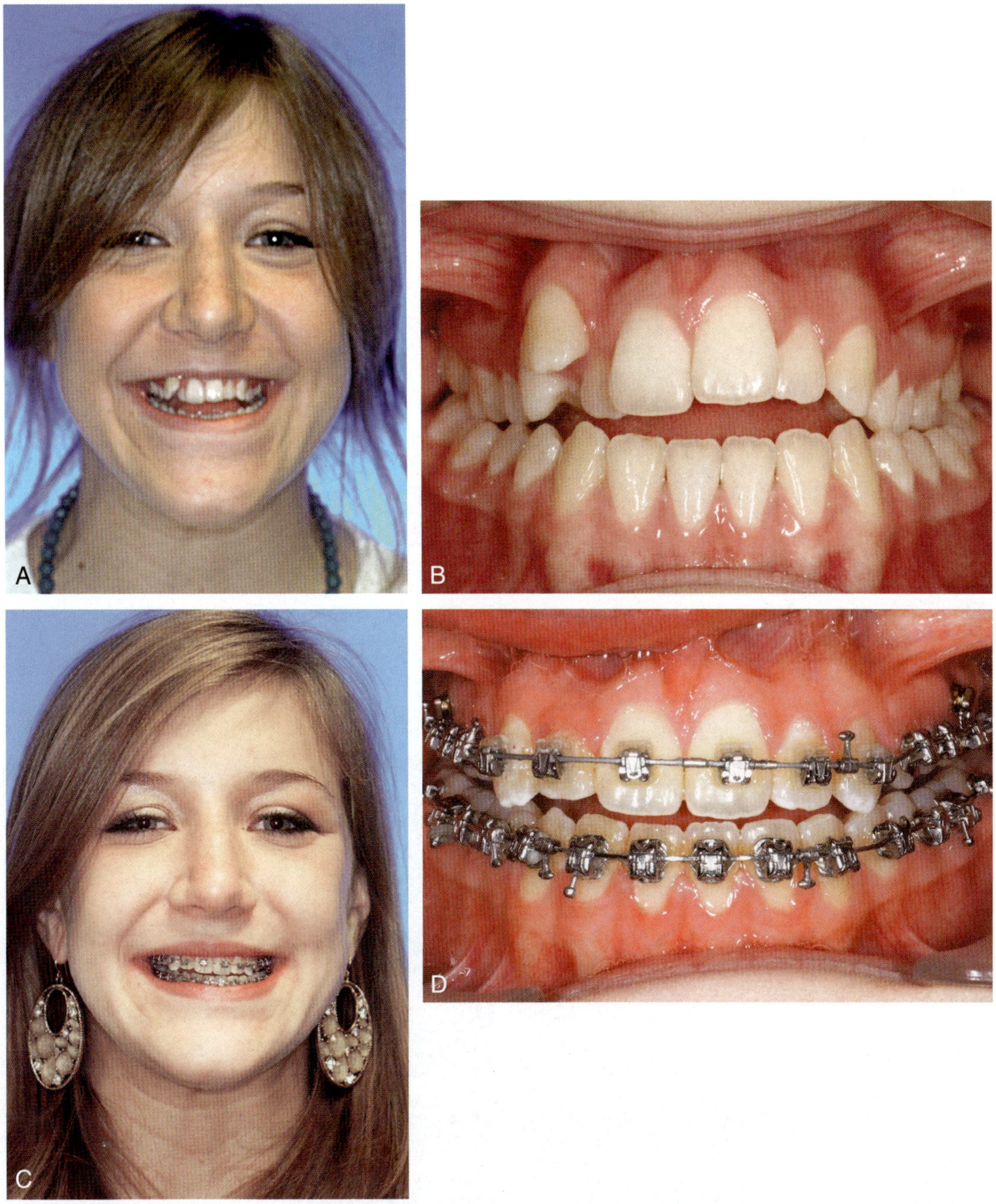

• **Fig. 15.29** (A and B) Prior to treatment, this 15-year-old girl had an unsightly maxillary left canine, anterior open bite, bilateral posterior crossbite, and an anterior crossbite. The treatment plan was to intrude the maxillary posterior teeth with 8-mm long alveolar bone screws bilaterally between the roots of the maxillary first molar and second premolar as anchorage and align the maxillary arch with transverse expansion. (C and D) Progress photos showing corrected alignment and decreased open bite. (E and F), Completion of treatment after 7 months of posterior intrusion (24 months total treatment). Note that the bone screws used for intrusion have been left in place so they can be used to control an open bite relapse tendency if needed (this can occur if vertical growth continues). (Courtesy Dr. N. Scheffler.)

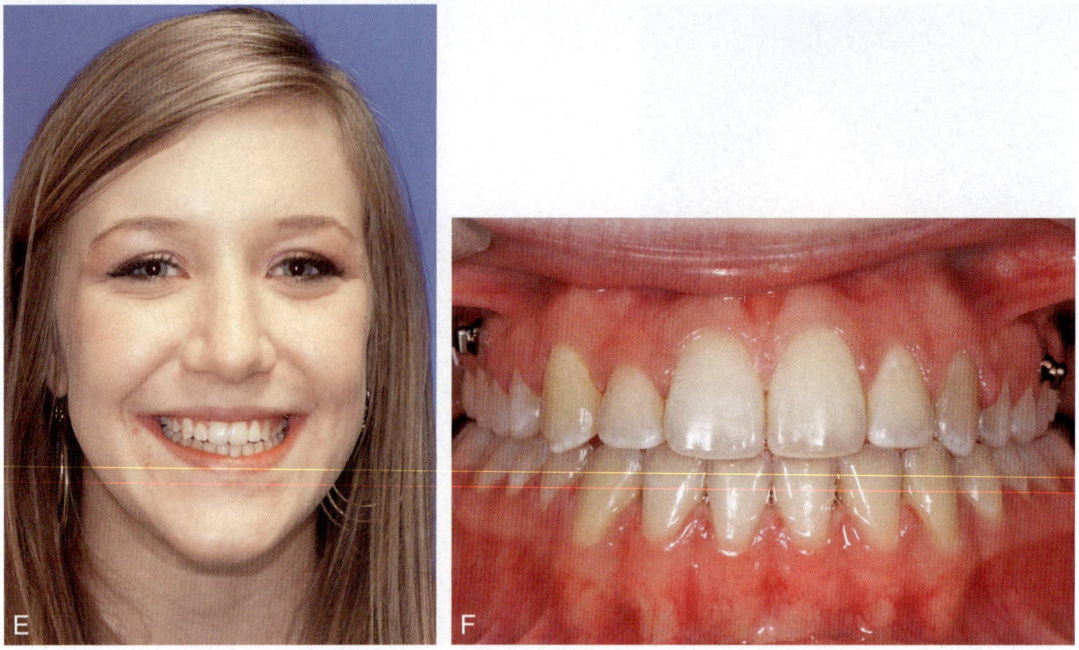

• **Fig. 15.29, cont'd**

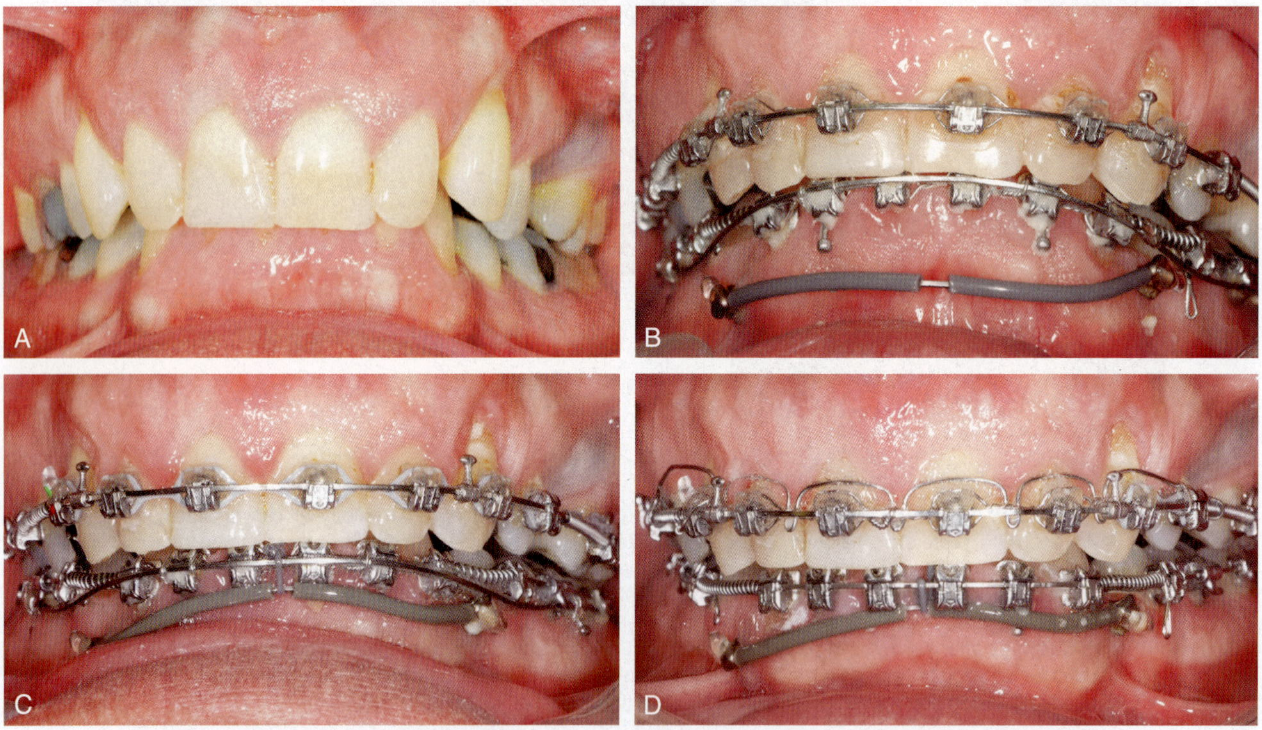

• **Fig. 15.30** (A) Extreme anterior deep bite in a 53-year-old male with short anterior face height, super-erupted lower incisors, previously extracted first premolars, and a Class II division 2 pattern of the maxillary incisors. The treatment plan included leveling the mandibular arch by extrusion of the posterior teeth and intrusion of the anteriors, advancement and torquing of the incisors in both arches, and opening spaces for the missing premolars, using a continuous rather than segmented main archwire. (B) The mandibular leveling auxiliary wire, anchored to 6-mm alveolar bone screws bilaterally, augments the leveling force provided by the main archwire. The tubing is to prevent lip and gingival irritation. (C) One-month progress. (D) Bite opening largely achieved after 4 months. Note the auxiliary maxillary torquing arch, which will tip the maxillary incisors anteriorly unless it is tied back posteriorly, allowing control of the amount of torque versus tipping. (Courtesy Dr. N. Scheffler.)

References

1. Bolender Y, Vernière A, Rapin C, et al. Torsional superelasticity of NiTi archwires. *Angle Orthod.* 2010;80:1100–1109.
2. Alqerban A, Willems G, Bernaerts C, et al. Orthodontic treatment planning for impacted maxillary canines using conventional records versus 3D CBCT. *Eur J Orthod.* 2014;36:698–707.
3. Incerti-Parenti S, Checchi V, Ippolito DR, et al. Periodontal status after surgical-orthodontic treatment of labially impacted canines with different surgical techniques. *Am J Orthod Dentofac Orthop.* 2016;149:463–472.
4. Parkin NA, Milner RS, Deery C, et al. Periodontal health of palatally displaced canines treated with open or closed surgical technique. *Am J Orthod Dentofac Orthop.* 2013;144:176–184.
5. Lau CK, Whang CZ, Bister D. Orthodontic uprighting of severely impacted mandibular second molars. *Am J Orthod Dentofac Orthop.* 2013;143:116–124.
6. Kravitz ND, Yanosky M, Cope JB, et al. Surgical uprighting of lower second molars. *J Clin Orthod.* 2016;50:33–40.
7. Edwards JG. Soft tissue surgery to alleviate orthodontic relapse. *Dent Clin North Am.* 1993;37:205–225.
8. Isaacson RJ, Lindauer SJ, Rubenstein LK. Activating a 2 × 4 appliance. *Angle Orthod.* 1993;63:17–24.
9. Ricketts RW, Bench RW, Gugino CF, et al. *Bioprogressive Therapy.* Rocky Mt Orthod; 1979.
10. Preston CB, Maggard MB, Lampasso J, et al. Long-term effectiveness of the continuous and the sectional archwire techniques in leveling the curve of Spee. *Am J Orthod Dentofac Orthop.* 2008;133:550–555.

16

Comprehensive Treatment in Adolescence: Space Closure and Class II/ Class III Correction

BRENT E. LARSON AND WILLIAM R. PROFFIT

CHAPTER OUTLINE

In Chapter 15 we covered alignment and related problems that would be corrected at or near the beginning of comprehensive treatment and that for the most part would be done with round rather than rectangular archwires. In this chapter, we move forward to treatment that involves bodily repositioning of teeth or root torque that is largely done with rectangular archwires.

Space Closure in Incisor Protrusion Problems

Excessive protrusion of incisors is a significant orthodontic problem in three conditions:

1. *Bimaxillary dentoalveolar protrusion*, is hereafter called just *bimaxillary protrusion* as in most of the orthodontic literature. To the orthodontist, this means that the anterior teeth in both arches are too far forward relative to the basal bone of the maxilla and mandible; to physical anthropologists, the same term describes protrusion of both jaws relative to the cranium.
2. *Class II malocclusion*, which is defined by the molar relationship but characterized by maxillary incisor protrusion creating excessive overjet. Epidemiologic studies have confirmed that the protruding maxillary incisors are the problem for the patient, who is not concerned about the molar relationship (see Chapter 1).
3. *Class III malocclusion*, also defined by the molar relationship but characterized by anterior crossbite and the protruding chin, which are the problems that patients perceive (even if the real problem is maxillary deficiency).

Bimaxillary protrusion is a dental problem in which the teeth are not properly positioned on both the maxilla and mandible. Growth modification for skeletal Class II and Class III problems has already been reviewed, and orthognathic surgery for the most severe of these problems is discussed in Chapter 20. The discussion here is on treatment to correct the malocclusion while creating acceptable dentofacial esthetics—that is, on methods to camouflage jaw discrepancies.

Sliding Versus Loop Mechanics in Space Closure

In the closure of an extraction space, it is necessary to generate both a force to move the teeth and a root-paralleling moment to move them bodily. With a fixed appliance, there are two major ways to do that: by sliding teeth along an archwire (sliding mechanics) or by tying the teeth tightly to archwire segments and moving the segments with a spring between them (closing loop mechanics). The differences are summarized in Table 16.1. Each of the methods has significant advantages and disadvantages. For sliding mechanics, there is significant resistance to sliding in the form of both binding and friction (big disadvantage), but there also is automatic generation of the root-paralleling moments at the extraction site (big advantage). For loop mechanics there is no frictional resistance (big advantage), but it is necessary to adjust the loop to generate a root-paralleling moment and keep it in proportion with the force to close the space (not necessarily a disadvantage, but extra work and complexity).

Let's explore those differences, starting with a brief review of the mechanical principles outlined in Chapter 9 and some additional clinical recommendations.

TABLE 16.1 Sliding Versus Loop Mechanics

Method	Sliding Teeth on an Archwire	Closing Loop between Segments
Generation of force	Alastic or NiTi spring to single tooth or group of teeth	Activate the loop
Net force desired	100 g per tooth	150 g per segment
Resistance to sliding	Approximately 100 g per tooth	None
Generation of moment	Automatic (bracket width)	Gable bend, approximately 45 degrees

NiTi, Nickel–titanium.

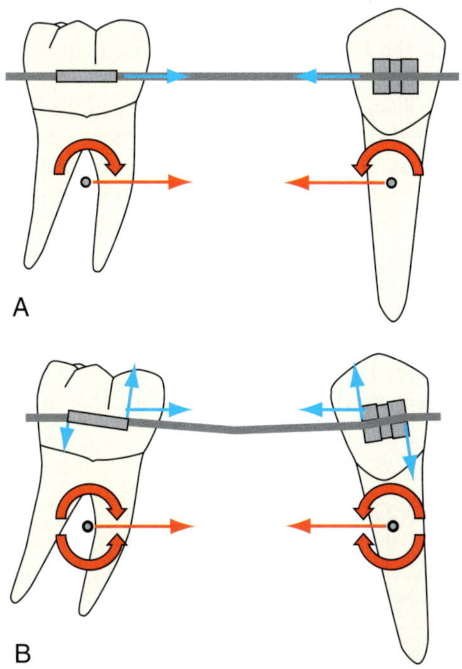

• **Fig. 16.1** (A) When a retraction force is placed across an extraction site *(blue arrows)*, the center of resistance of the adjacent teeth feels both a translational force and the moment of a force that initially causes tipping *(red arrows)*. (B) As the teeth tip, the wire engages at opposite edges of the bracket, creating a couple that resists tipping. After a certain level of tipping occurs, the moment of the couple and the moment of the force are in equilibrium and no further tipping occurs. This equilibrium point depends on the retraction force, wire stiffness, interbracket span, and bracket width.

Sliding Mechanics

For sliding closure of an extraction site, a rectangular archwire is needed to keep the tooth or teeth from rolling facially or lingually while being repositioned (although a small space can be closed on a round wire). The wire on which sliding occurs must have two properties: it must be undersized relative to the bracket and strong enough not to bend significantly when force is applied across the section that spans the extraction site.

The closer the contact between the wire and bracket, the greater the frictional resistance to sliding. Because almost all brackets have a slot size slightly larger than the nominal size and all archwires are slightly smaller than their nominal size, a full-dimension wire in a bracket still has some clearance, and sliding is possible. A 3-mil (0.03 in. = 0.5 mm) difference between bracket slot size and wire size is enough to largely eliminate friction, but of course resistance to sliding created by binding on the edges of the slot still is present (see Chapter 9). The usual combination of undersized wires and oversized bracket slots means that a nominal 2-mil clearance usually is adequate for sliding (for instance, 16 × 25 wire in an 18-slot bracket is acceptable, but 19 × 25 wire in a 22-slot is better). A 19 × 25 steel wire has excellent strength and rarely bends during sliding space closure, whereas smaller wires may distort.

To move a tooth bodily along the archwire, both a force to move the tooth and a moment to keep it from tipping are needed. In sliding the moment is generated automatically as the tooth begins to tip and the corners of the bracket contact the archwire. If the wire does not bend in response to the force, the result will be bodily movement; if it bends, tipping will occur (Fig. 16.1). The width of the bracket for sliding is important—wider is better to keep binding forces as low as possible and generate the root-paralleling moments—but if brackets are too wide, aligning the teeth is compromised. As noted in Chapter 9, the best compromise is specific brackets for each tooth that are half the width of the tooth.

Austenitic nickel–titanium (A-NiTi; superelastic) coil springs are an ideal source of force across the extraction site, because the approximate magnitude of the force is known and changes minimally as the space closes (Fig. 16.2). In contrast, elastomeric chains provide a rapidly decreasing force between appointments, which makes them less ideal for extraction space closure. In the minds of many orthodontists, the easier placement and better oral hygiene than with nickel–titanium (NiTi) springs tend to compensate for this.

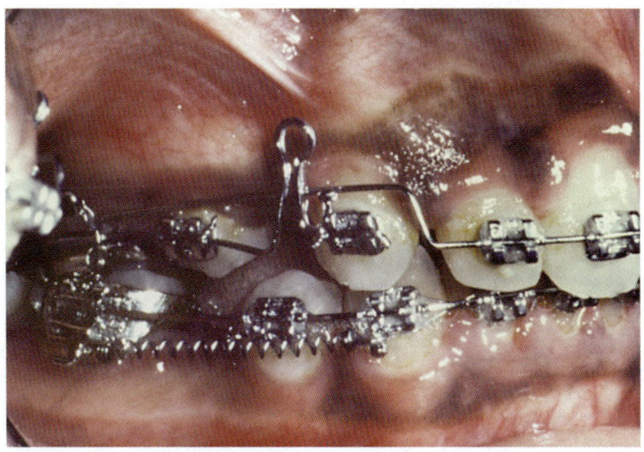

• **Fig. 16.2** In this patient with a 22-slot appliance, sliding space closure in the lower arch is being carried out with a nickel–titanium (NiTi) coil spring while a segmental closing loop is being used in the upper arch for retraction of the canine. Note that the maxillary base archwire bypasses the canine.

An important aspect of any orthodontic tooth movement is that it should failsafe. This means that the system should either do what it was designed to do or nothing, so that if it fails (or if the patient is lost to follow-up for a time), there are no major side effects. Sliding closure has excellent fail-safe characteristics. If the spring moving the teeth fails or the elastomeric chain breaks, tooth movement simply stops until the patient's next appointment, and in the meantime the heavy wire maintains the teeth where they were.

When maxillary incisors protrude, torque in the incisor brackets often is needed as the teeth are retracted, to keep them from becoming too upright. Sometimes it is forgotten that the reciprocal for incisor torque is a forward force on the posterior anchorage (Fig. 16.3). In patients with Class II malocclusion it is quite possible to see molars slipping toward a Class II relationship while active torque to the upper incisors is being used. The same effect, of course, could an advantage for patients with Class III malocclusion who would benefit from forward movement of the upper molars. The moral to the story: not all the moments generated during sliding space closure are so automatic that they require no thought.

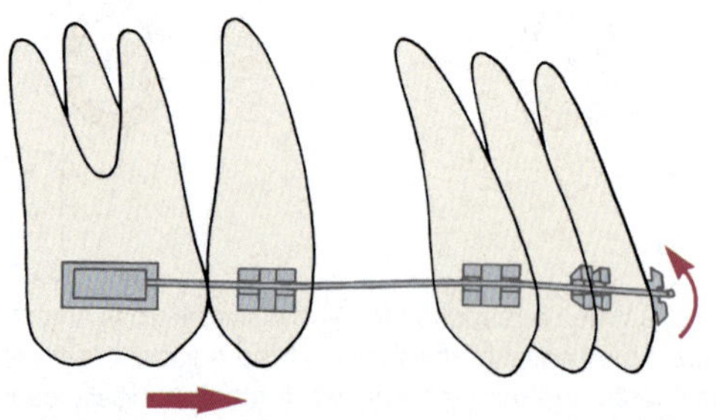

• **Fig. 16.3** Torque forces against the incisors create a crown-forward, as well as a root-backward, tendency. Preventing the incisor crowns from tipping forward tends to pull the posterior teeth forward. Because that would move them toward a Class II relationship, under most circumstances additional force against the molars to prevent this would be indicated—but it would be advantageous if closing space by bringing the posterior teeth forward were desired.

Closing Loop Mechanics

Closing loops also should be made with rectangular wire to prevent the wire from rolling in the bracket slots. The performance of a closing loop, from the perspective of engineering theory, is determined by three major characteristics: its spring properties (i.e., the amount of force it delivers and the way the force changes as the teeth move); the moment it generates, so that root position can be controlled; and its location relative to adjacent brackets (i.e., the extent to which it acts as a symmetric or asymmetric bend in the archwire). Other design principles also can affect clinical treatment. But the frictionless design of closing loops has the potential to reduce anchorage problems and decrease the time for space closure. Let's examine these performance considerations, starting with spring properties.

Spring Properties

The spring properties of a closing loop are determined almost totally by three things: the wire material (at present, either steel or TMA), the size of the wire, and the distance between points of attachment. This distance in turn is largely determined by the amount of wire incorporated into the loop but is affected also by the distance between brackets. Closing loops with equivalent properties can be produced from different types and sizes of wire by increasing the amount of wire incorporated into the loop as the size of the wire increases and vice versa. Wires of greater inherent springiness or smaller cross-sectional area allow the use of simpler loop designs.

Fig. 16.4, from the classic work of Booth,[1] illustrates the effects on the spring characteristics of a steel closing loop from changing wire size, the design of the loop, and the interbracket span. The combination of the last two parameters, of course, determines the amount of wire in the loop. Note that, as expected, changing the size of the wire produces the largest changes in characteristics, but the amount of wire incorporated in the loop is also important. The

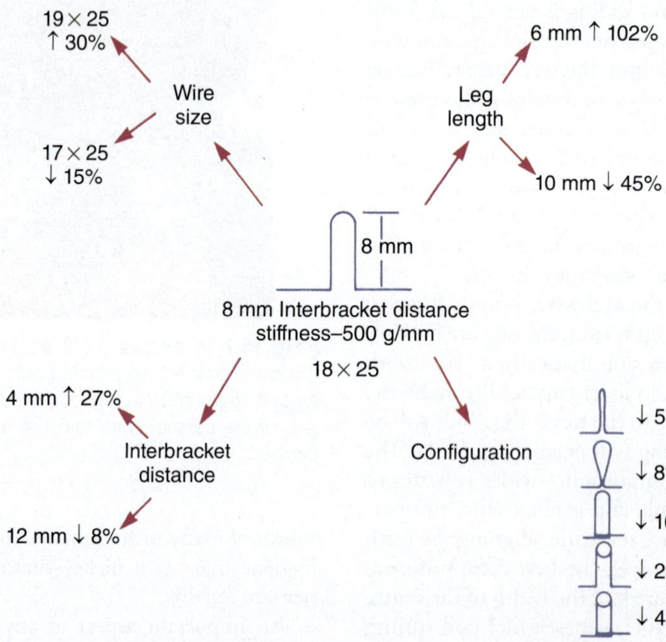

• **Fig. 16.4** The effect of changing various aspects of a closing loop in an archwire. Note that an 8-mm vertical loop in 18 x 25 SS wire produces twice as much force as the desired 250-g/mm activation. The major possibilities for producing clinically satisfactory loops are reducing wire size or incorporating additional wire by changing leg length, interbracket distance, and/or loop configuration. (Redrawn from Booth FA. *Optimum Forces With Orthodontic Loops* [MS thesis]. University of Texas Dental Branch; 1971.)

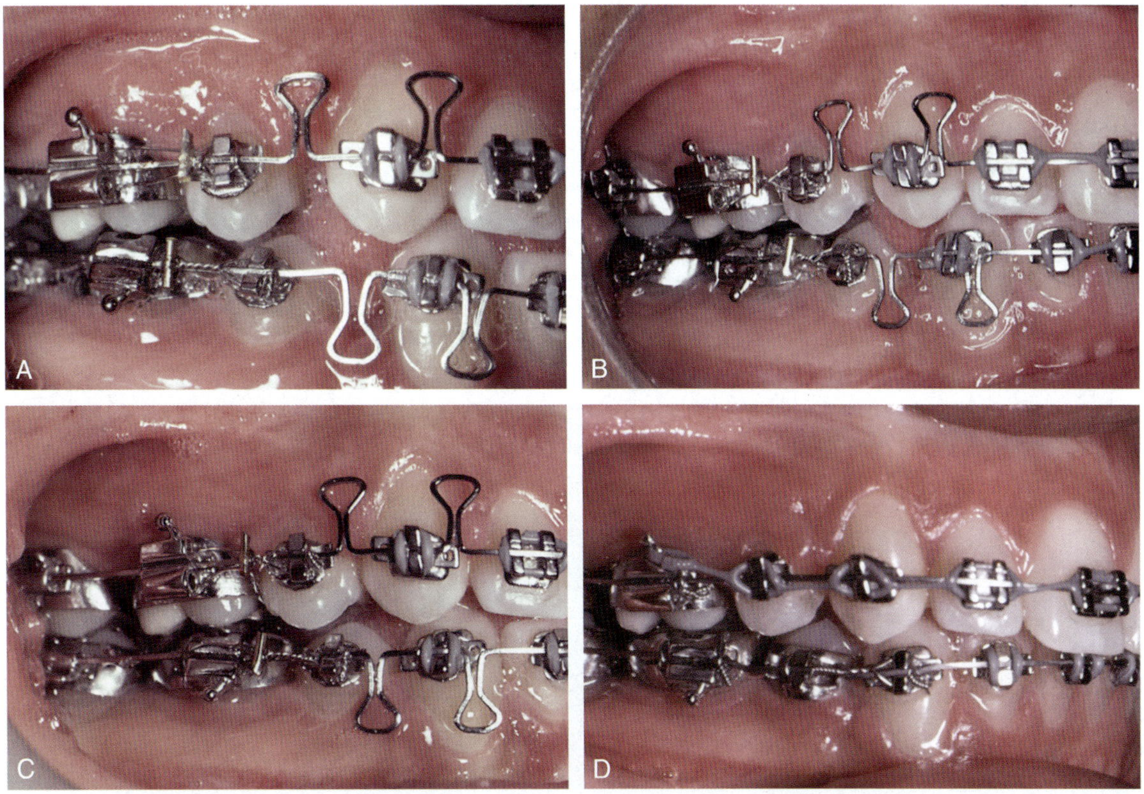

• **Fig. 16.5** Space closure with preformed closing loops in the 18-slot appliance. (A) Use of 16 × 22 closing loops at initial activation, after the completion of stage 1 alignment and leveling. Note the location of the closing loops and the soldered tiebacks for activation. (B) Three months later. (C) Spaces closed at 4 months. (D) Use of 17 × 25 beta-titanium (TMA) wire to begin the finishing phase of treatment.

force characteristics are determined by the center of the apical portion of the loop, regardless of the position of the loop legs.[2] TMA (beta-Ti) wire is a modern alternative to steel for closing loops, which for any size of wire or design of loop would produce about half the force of steel—but the same relative effects of changing these factors would be observed.

Root-Paralleling Moments

To close an extraction space while producing bodily tooth movement, a closing loop must generate not only a closing force but also appropriate moments to bring the root apices together at the extraction site. As we have discussed in Chapter 9, for bodily movement the moment of the force used to move the teeth must be balanced by the moment of a couple. If the center of resistance of the tooth is 10 mm from the bracket, a canine tooth being retracted with a 100-g force must also receive a 1000 g-mm moment if it is to move bodily. If the bracket is 1 mm wide, a vertical force of 1000 g must be produced by the archwire at each side of the bracket.

This requirement to generate a moment limits the amount of wire that can be incorporated to make a closing loop springier because if the loop becomes too flexible, it will be unable to generate the necessary moments even though the retraction force characteristics are satisfactory. Loop design is also affected. Placing some of the wire within the closing loop in a horizontal rather than a vertical direction improves its ability to deliver the moments needed to prevent tipping. Because of this and because a vertically tall loop can impinge on soft tissue, a closing loop that is only 7 to 8 mm tall while incorporating 10 to 12 mm or more of wire (e.g., a delta-, L-, or T-shaped loop) is preferred (Fig. 16.5).

If the legs of a closing loop were parallel before activation, opening the loop would place them at an angle that in itself would generate a moment in the desired direction. Calculations show that unacceptably tall loops would be required to generate appropriate moments in this manner,[3] so additional moments must be generated by gable bends (or their equivalent) before the loop is placed in the mouth (Fig. 16.6).

Location of the Loop

A final engineering factor in the performance of a closing loop is its location along the span of wire between adjacent brackets. Because of its gable bends, the closing loop functions as a V-bend in the archwire, and the effect of a V-bend is quite sensitive to its position. Only if it is in the center of the span does a V-bend produce equal forces and couples on the adjacent teeth (see Figs. 9.40 and 9.41). If it is one-third of the way between adjacent brackets, the tooth closer to the loop will be extruded and will feel a considerable moment to bring the root toward the V-bend, while the tooth farther away will receive an intrusive force but no moment.[3] If the V-bend or loop is closer to one bracket than one-third of the distance, the more distant tooth will not be intruded but will receive a moment to move the root away from the V-bend (which almost never is desirable).

For routine use with fail-safe closing loops (described later), the preferred location for a closing loop is at the spot that will be the center of the embrasure when the space is closed (Fig. 16.7). This means that in a first premolar extraction situation, the closing loop should be placed about 5 mm distal to the center of the canine tooth. The effect is to place the loop initially at the one-third position relative to the canine. The moment on the premolar

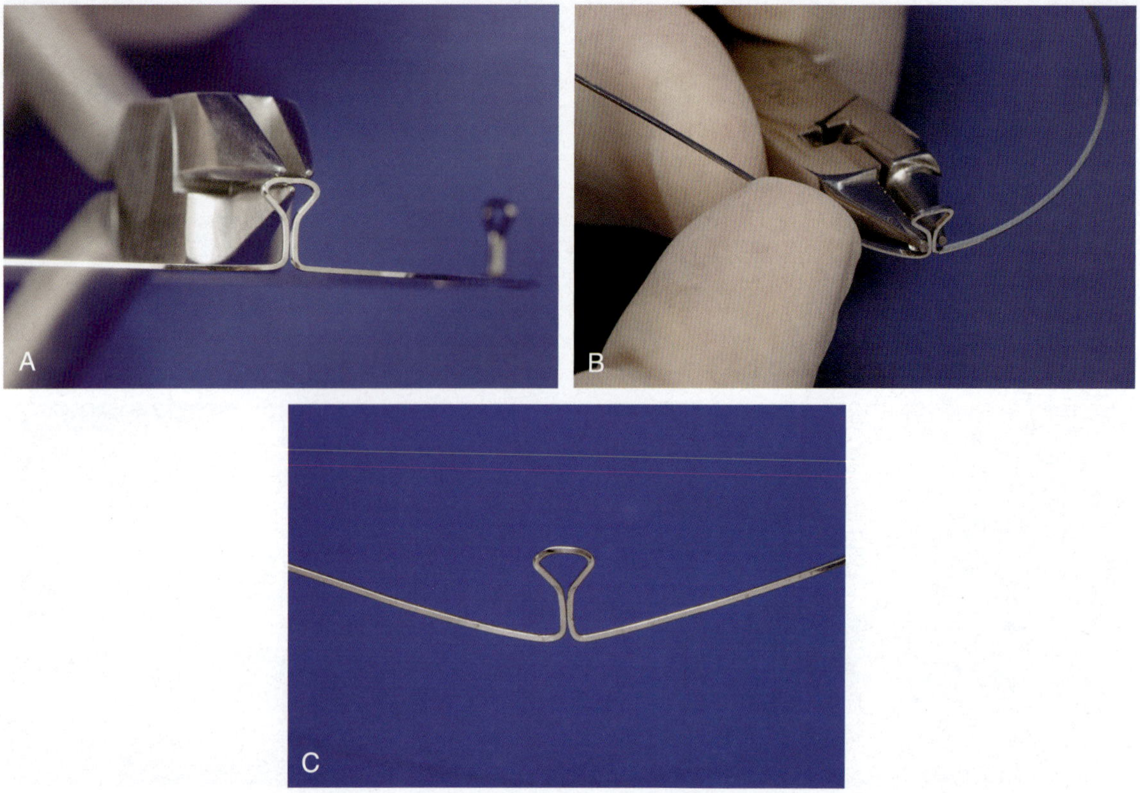

• **Fig. 16.6** Adjustment of the preformed closing loop before placing it in the mouth. (A) Three-prong pliers should be used to bring the vertical legs of a closing loop together if they are separated. The legs should touch lightly before the loop is activated by opening it. (B) Gable bends to create the root-paralleling moment are placed by bending the wire at the base of the loop. (C) Appropriate gable for a 16 × 22 closing loop (40–45 degrees total, half that on each side).

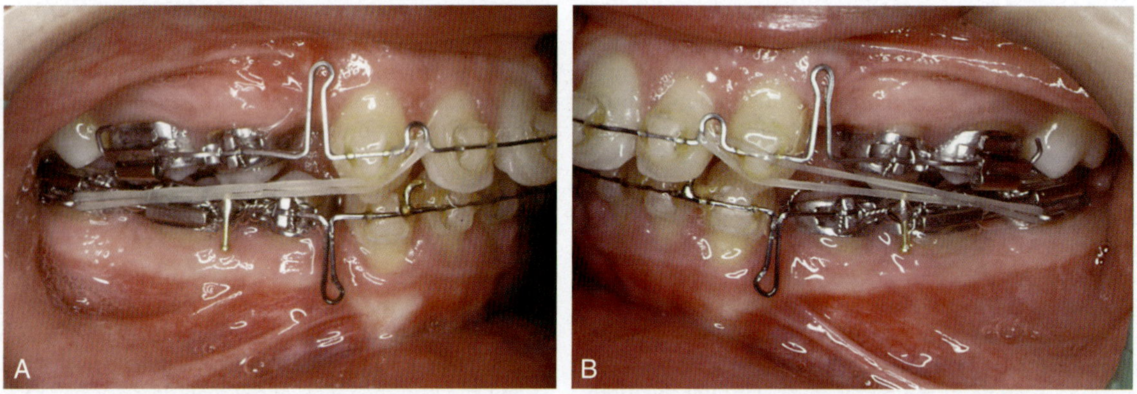

• **Fig. 16.7** (A and B) Closing loops in 16 × 22 wire of fail-safe design and 8-mm height, used with Class II elastics in this patient. Note that the maxillary loop has been activated by pulling the wire through the molar tube and bending it up. In the mandibular arch, the loop is not active at this time, and the approximation of the legs to create a rigid archwire is apparent. The lower archwire has a tieback mesial to the first molar so that this loop can be activated by tying a ligature from the posterior teeth to the wire rather than by bending over the end of the wire distal to the molar tube.

increases as space closure proceeds. This is not ideal for maximum anchorage but is unavoidable with a loop in a continuous archwire.

Additional Design Principles

As it was in sliding and other types of tooth movement, an important principle in closing loop design is that the loop should fail-safe. This means that, although a reasonable range of action is desired from each activation, tooth movement should stop after a prescribed range of movement. Too long a range of action with too much flexibility could produce disastrous effects if a distorted spring were combined with a series of broken appointments. The ideal loop design therefore would deliver a continuous, controlled force designed to produce tooth movement at a rate of approximately 1 mm/month but would not include more than 2 mm of range before it locked up. That would stop the movement if the patient missed a second consecutive monthly appointment. With

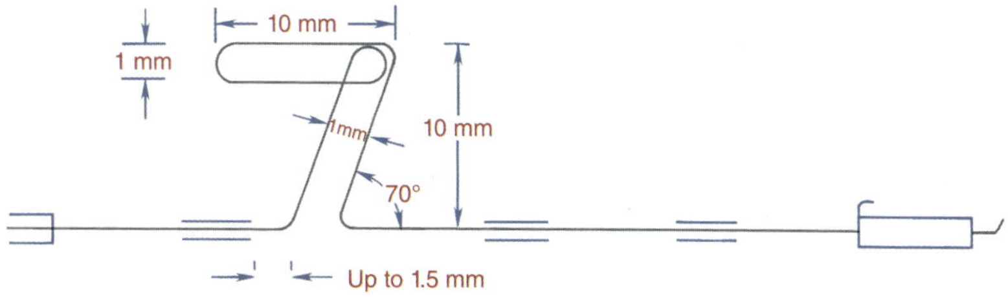

• **Fig. 16.8** The Opus closing loop designed by Siatkowski offers excellent control of forces and moments so that space can be closed under good control. The loop can be fabricated from 16 × 22 or 18 × 25 steel wire or from 17 × 25 TMA wire. It is activated by tightening it distally behind the molar tube and can be adjusted to produce maximal, moderate, or minimal incisor retraction, but like all closing mechanisms with a long range of action, it must be monitored carefully. (Redrawn from Siatkowski RE. *Am J Orthod Dentofac Orthop*. 1997;112:393–402, 484–495.)

preformed delta-shaped closing loops, it is important to adjust the loop so that the vertical legs are in contact before the loop is used (see Fig. 16.6A), in order to both be able to know how much it has been activated and be sure that the legs will come back into contact to create a rigid fail-safe wire that stops further movement.

It also is important that the design be as simple as possible because more complex configurations are less comfortable for patients, more difficult to fabricate clinically, and more prone to breakage or distortion. An elegant solution to the design of a closing loop that would provide optimum and nearly constant moment-to-force ratios at variable activations was offered by Siatkowski in his Opus loop (Fig. 16.8).[4] Engineering analysis, as the Opus loop demonstrates very nicely, shows that a relatively complex design is required to produce the best control of moment–force ratios. The possibilities of clinical problems from increased complexity always must be balanced against the potentially greater efficiency of the more complex design. The Opus loop has not been widely adopted because of concerns about its complexity and sturdiness. Clinical experience suggests that the average adolescent orthodontic patient can—and probably will—destroy almost any orthodontic device that is not remarkably resistant to being distorted.

A third design factor relates to whether a loop is activated by opening or closing. All else being equal, a loop is more effective when it is closed rather than opened during its activation. On the other hand, a loop designed to be opened can be made so that when it closes completely, the vertical legs come into contact, effectively preventing further movement and producing the desired fail-safe effect. A loop activated by closing, in contrast, must have its vertical legs overlap. This creates a transverse step, and the archwire does not develop the same rigidity when it is deactivated. The design with opening of the loop to activate it is preferred because its fail-safe property is more desirable than the better spring quality of closing the loop.

Now, let's apply what we have learned to the correction of the bimaxillary protrusion and Class II and III camouflage.

Correction of Bimaxillary Protrusion

Bimaxillary protrusion requires retraction of the protruding incisors. With only a few exceptions, it is treated by extraction of first premolars in both dental arches and controlled repositioning of the anterior segment of the arches into the extraction site. The objective is optimal improvement in dentofacial appearance and lip function. Clinical management differs depending on how much incisor retraction is planned. Orthodontists traditionally have spoken about this in terms of how much anchorage would be needed to produce the desired amount of retraction, and for the most part we will use the anchorage terminology here, although sometimes it is more direct to focus on just the desired tooth movement.

Let's begin with the usual situation, moderate posterior anchorage to retract the incisors slightly more than the posterior teeth would move forward and allow some tipping to upright the incisors as they are retracted. Then we can discuss how moderate anchorage could be upgraded to maximum anchorage, which would be needed for maximum retraction of the protruding incisors and/or active torque to move the incisor roots further than the crowns. Finally, we will close the discussion with minimum posterior anchorage, for which the goal would be less incisor retraction and more forward movement of the posterior segments.

Moderate Anchorage Situations

Most patients with bimaxillary protrusion fall into the moderate anchorage category, meaning that after alignment of the incisors to correct crowding has been completed, it is desired to close the remainder of the premolar extraction space with a 50:50 or 60:40 ratio of anterior retraction to posterior protraction.

Space Closure With 22-Slot Edgewise

In general, space closure in moderate anchorage situations often is done in two steps to better control posterior anchorage: first retracting the canines, sliding them along an 18 × 25 or 19 × 25 steel archwire with a NiTi spring or elastic that delivers about 200 g of force, and second, retracting the four incisors (Fig. 16.9). For the canine retraction, a posterior stop on the archwire, usually in front of the first molar tube, is needed. This stop has the effect of incorporating all the teeth except the canine into the anchorage unit. A-NiTi coil springs are preferred because they produce an almost ideal light constant force and there is no danger that the teeth will tip excessively.

In the lower arch the second stage can be continued, sliding along an 18 × 25 wire or a closing loop, often a T-loop in 18 × 25 steel; in the upper arch a closing loop is preferred when greater torque of the incisors is needed, as it often is (see Fig. 16.2). This two-stage closure will produce an approximately 60:40 closure of the extraction spaces, varying somewhat depending on whether second molars are included in posterior anchorage and the incisor torque requirement. En masse sliding leads to 50:50 closure at best, even with bi-dimensional wires that are smaller posteriorly in an effort to avoid friction (because binding is still present).

Although the two-step procedure is predictable and has excellent fail-safe characteristics, which explains why it remains commonly used, it takes longer to close space in two steps than one. One-step closure with the 22-slot appliance has been available with a segmented arch technique based on incorporating the anterior teeth into a single segment, and both the right and left posterior teeth

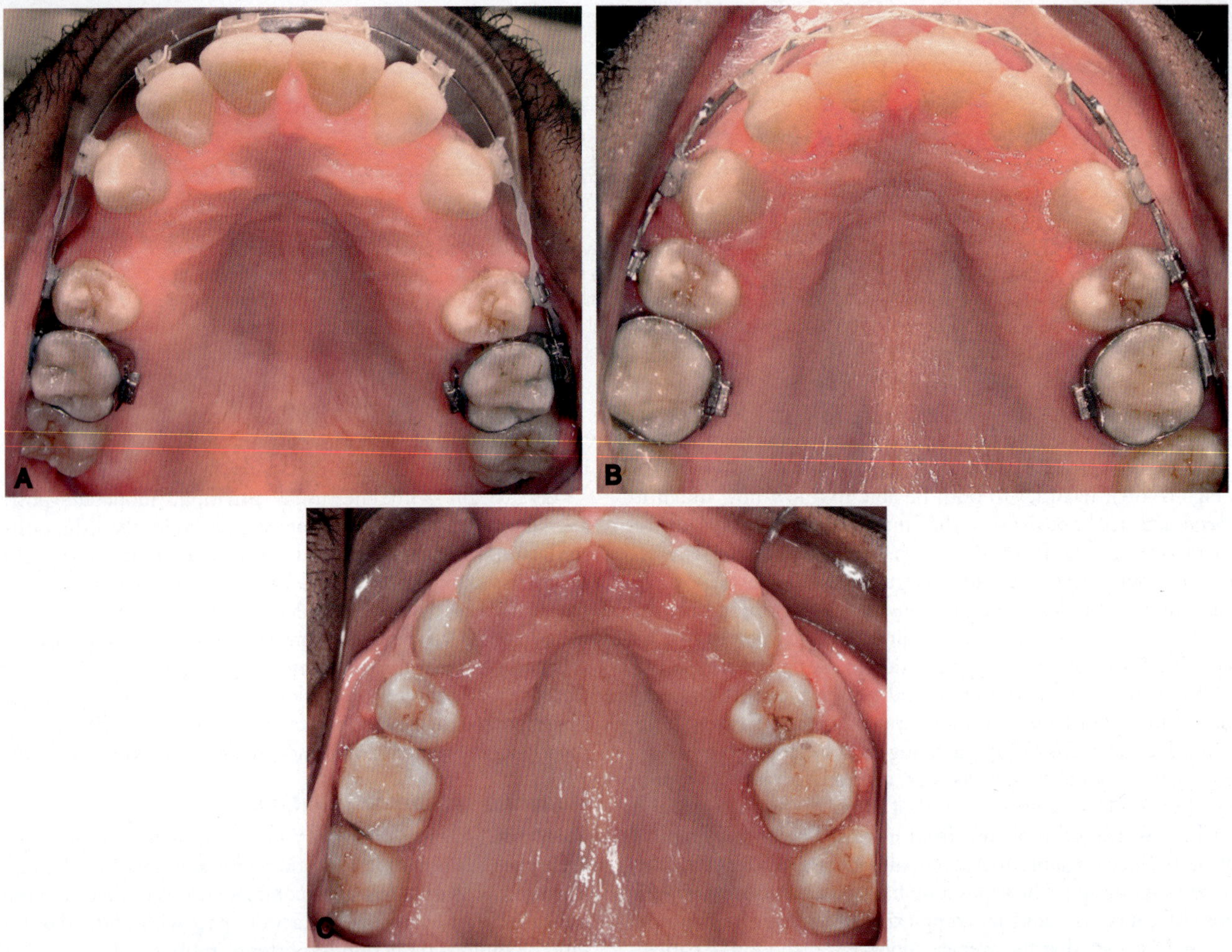

• **Fig. 16.9** Two-step space closure after extraction of maxillary first premolars. (A) Beginning closure with elastic chain being used to slide the canines distally along the archwire. (B) Canines retracted and closing loops in the archwire distal to the lateral incisors being used to retract the anterior segment. (C) Treatment complete with premolar spaces closed and torque of incisors properly controlled.

also into a single segment, with the two sides connected by a stabilizing lingual arch. A retraction spring (Fig. 16.10) is used to connect these stable bases, and the activation of the spring is varied to produce the desired pattern of space closure. These springs are very effective, and with careful initial activation, an impressive range of movement can be produced before reactivation is necessary.[5] The greatest disadvantage of this technique is not its increased complexity but that it does not exhibit fail-safe properties. Without a rigid connection between the anterior and posterior segments, there is nothing to maintain arch form and proper vertical relationships if a retraction spring is distorted or activated incorrectly.

Now that preformed closing loops are available in 19 × 25 TMA, one-step closure with a fail-safe design also can be done with 22-slot brackets as it often is with the 18-slot appliance (see later). This is faster than the older two-stage closure. It is not as fast as the segmented arch technique, but it is safer and less complex.

Space Closure With 18-Slot Edgewise

In contrast to the 22-slot edgewise appliance, the 18-slot appliance fits well with the design principles for closing loops discussed earlier. An excellent closing loop for 18-slot edgewise is a delta-shaped loop in 16 × 22 steel wire that is activated by opening (see Fig. 16.5). The wire slides through the brackets and tubes only when it is being activated. After that, as the closing loop returns to its original configuration, the teeth move with the archwire, not along it, so there is no resistance to sliding. It allows accurate activation, provides the appropriate root-paralleling moment via gable bends, and fails safely when the loop closes completely.

There are two ways to hold the archwire in its activated position. The simplest is by bending the end of the archwire gingivally

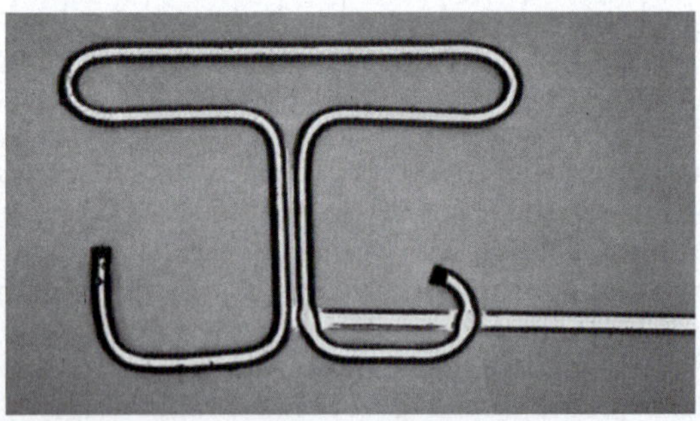

• **Fig. 16.10** Composite retraction spring designed by Burstone for use with the segmented arch technique, consisting of 18-mil beta-titanium (beta-Ti) wire (the loop) welded to 17 × 25 beta-Ti. This spring can be used for either en masse retraction of incisors or canine retraction.

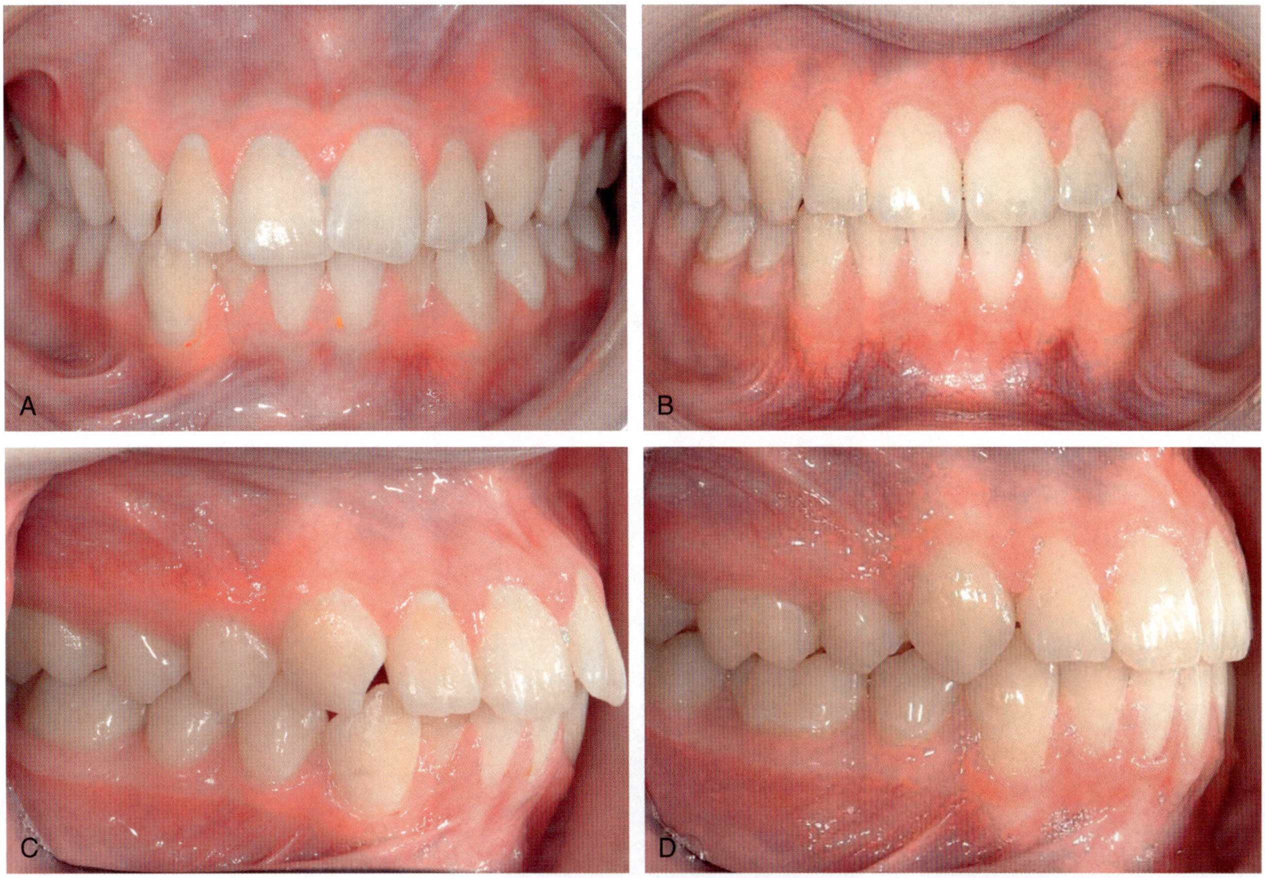

• **Fig. 16.11** Treatment of bimaxillary protrusion with four-premolar extraction. (A and C) Before treatment with mild crowding and incisor protrusion. (B and D) After treatment with crowding resolved and proper retraction of incisors to create improved dental esthetics. (Courtesy Dr. T. Shaughnessy.)

behind the last molar tube. The alternative is to place an attachment—usually a soldered tieback (see Fig. 16.7) on the posterior part of the archwire so that a ligature can be used to tie the wire in its activated position. With the 16 × 22 loop, it is usually necessary to remove the archwire and reactivate the gable bends after 3 to 4 mm of space closure, but a quick reactivation is all that is needed at most appointments during space closure. If it is anticipated that a closing loop archwire will not have to be removed for adjustment (i.e., the distance to be closed is 4 mm or less), bending the posterior end of the wire is satisfactory. It can be quite difficult to remove an archwire that has been activated by bending over the end, however, and it saves time in the long run to use tiebacks for closing loop archwires that will have to be removed and readjusted.

A reasonably typical correction of moderate bimaxillary protrusion is shown in Figs. 16.11 and 16.12. The improved facial appearance is apparent. As we have noted, Edward Angle was wrong in saying that facial appearance is always best with arch expansion and that extraction is never needed—and that is equally incorrect when it is said now. For a patient with bimaxillary protrusion, it is important at the treatment planning stage to establish the optimum position of the incisors—that is, how much incisor retraction is needed—and then structure the orthodontic mechanics to produce the desired outcome.

Maximum Incisor Retraction (Maximum Anchorage)

The same basic approach is needed with any appliance when maximum anchorage is needed: increased reinforcement of posterior anchorage and decreased strain on that anchorage. A sequence of steps to do that, along with space closure as outlined earlier, would be as follows.

Reinforcement With Stabilizing Lingual Arches

Stabilizing lingual arches must be rigid and should be made from 36-mil or 32 × 32 steel wire. These can be soldered to the molar bands, but it is convenient to be able to remove them, and Burstone's designs (see Chapter 10) are preferred. The resulting increase in posterior anchorage, although modest, will change the ratio of anterior retraction to posterior protraction to approximately 2 : 1.

It is important for a lower stabilizing lingual arch to lie behind and below the lower incisors so that it does not interfere with their retraction. If 36-mil round wire is used, the lower lingual arch is more conveniently inserted from the distal than from the mesial of the molar tube. The maxillary stabilizing lingual arch is a straight transpalatal design. Because maximum rigidity is desired for anchorage reinforcement, an expansion loop in the palatal section of this wire is not recommended unless a specific indication exists for including it.

Lingual arches for anchorage control should be removed after space closure is complete. Their presence during the finishing stage of treatment, after extraction spaces have been closed, is not helpful and may interfere with final settling of the occlusion.

Reinforcement With Headgear and Interarch Elastics

Extraoral force against the maxillary posterior segments is an obvious and direct method for anchorage reinforcement. It is possible to place extraoral force directly against the mandibular posterior segments, but it is more practical to use Class III elastics to transfer

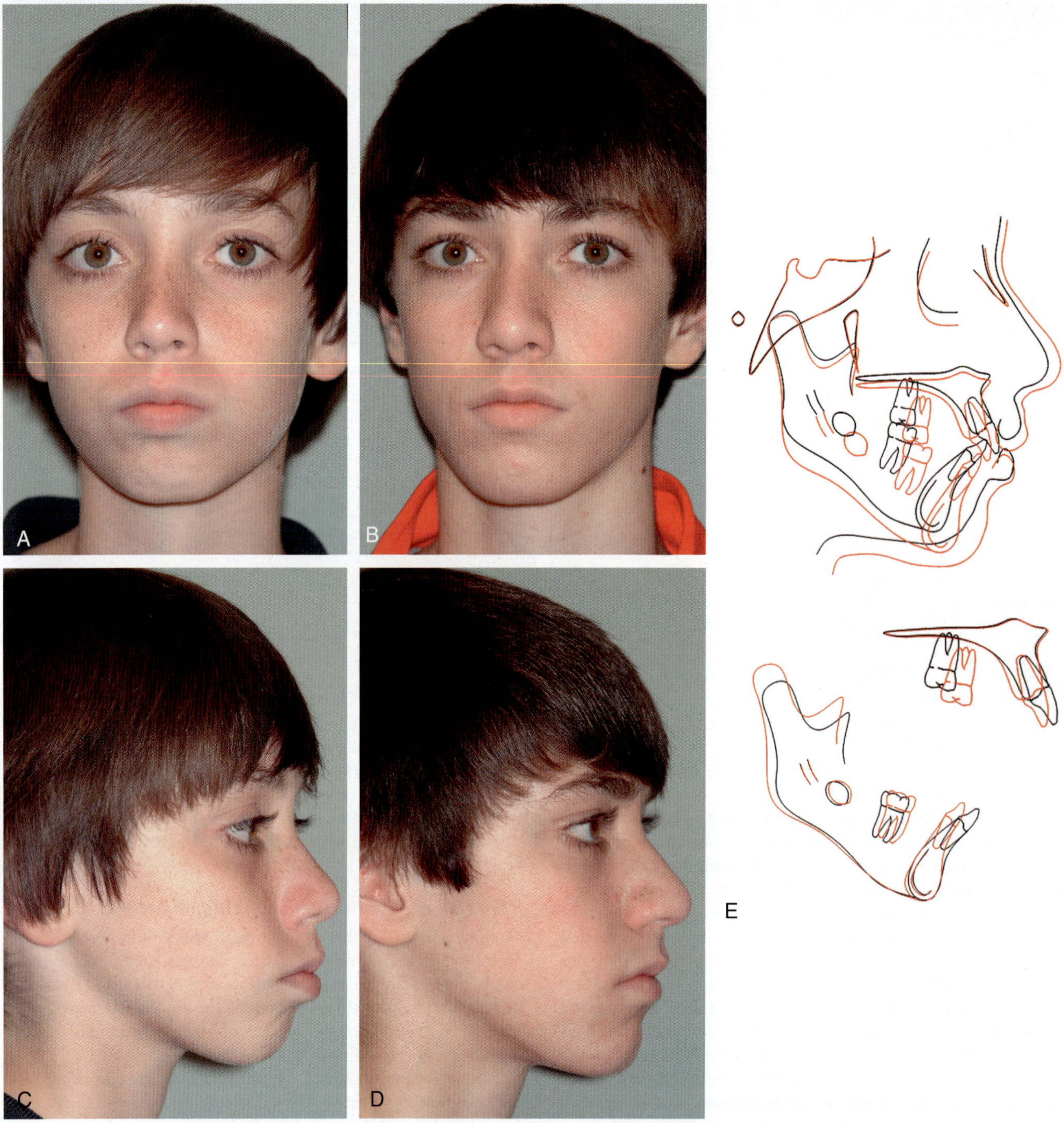

• **Fig. 16.12** Facial images and cephalometric tracings of the bimaxillary protrusion, premolar extraction case shown in Fig. 16.11. (A and C) before treatment. Note lip protrusion and the muscle strain needed for lip closure. (B and D) After treatment the lip posture is relaxed, facial convexity is reduced, and overall facial balance is improved. (E) Cephalometric superimpositions showing mandibular growth to improve chin projection as well as uprighting of upper and lower incisors. Proper anchorage management by the orthodontist during premolar space closure resulted in the desired combination of molar forward movement and incisor retraction to achieve the desired final tooth position. (Courtesy Dr. T. Shaughnessy.)

the extraoral force from the upper to the lower arch. Depending on how well the patient cooperates, additional improvement of retraction, perhaps to a 3 : 1 or 4 : 1 ratio, can be achieved.

Two-Step Frictionless Retraction

Individualized retraction of the canines with auxiliary springs before a second stage of incisor retraction with closing loops is an attractive method for reducing the strain on posterior anchorage and is a readily available with a modern appliance. For use of the retraction spring, an auxiliary tube on the first molars is needed. An auxiliary tube on the canine is unnecessary because the retraction spring can fit directly into the canine bracket. The PG spring designed by Gjessing is an efficient current design (Fig. 16.13)[6] but is somewhat complex to fabricate and activate.

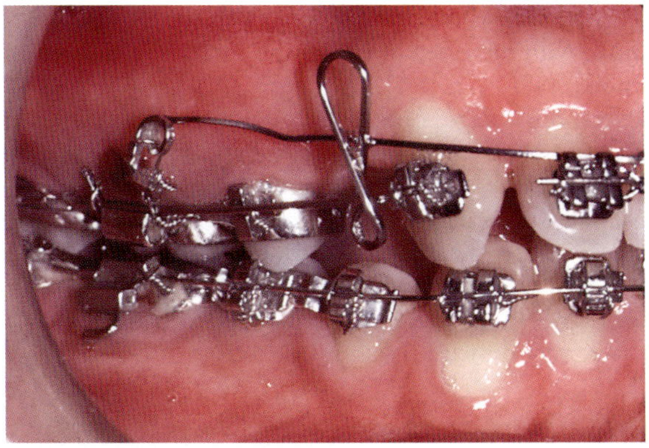

• **Fig. 16.13** For canine retraction, the Gjessing retraction spring offers excellent control of forces and moments and probably is the most effective current design of a spring for this purpose. In this patient, canine retraction is being done simultaneously with intrusion of the incisor segment.

After the canine retraction, closing loops, either in a continuous archwire or with a segmented arch approach, are then used for the second stage of retraction of the incisors.

Frictionless canine retraction with springs of this type presents two problems. The first is that it is difficult to control the position of the canine in all three planes of space as it is retracted. If the canine is pulled distally from an attachment on its buccal surface, the point of attachment is not only some distance occlusal but also buccal to the center of resistance. This means that without appropriate counterbalancing moments, the tooth will tip distally and rotate mesiobuccally. Both a root-paralleling moment and an antirotation moment must be obtained by placing two different gable bends in the same spring. Control of the vertical position of the canine, particularly after the gable bends in two planes of space have been placed, can be a significant problem.

Second, much more than with en masse retraction using segmented mechanics, segmental retraction of canines is not failsafe. The canine is free to move in three-dimensional space, and there are no stops to prevent excessive movement in the wrong direction if a spring is improperly adjusted or becomes distorted. Loss of vertical control is particularly likely. A missed appointment and a distorted spring can lead to the development of a considerable problem, and patients must be monitored carefully.

Retraction With Skeletal Anchorage

Skeletal anchorage for retraction of protruding incisors is the only way to close extraction spaces totally by retracting the anterior arch segment. The options are bone screws in the palate stabilizing a transpalatal arch to provide indirect anchorage to the posterior arch segment (see Fig. 10.49), or bone screws in the dental alveolus between the second premolar and first molar (see Fig. 10.48). Directly attaching a spring to the alveolar screw generates an upward and backward direction of pull; stabilizing the posterior teeth with palatal screws gives a direction of force parallel to the occlusal plane.

Until recently, it was thought that skeletal anchorage was equally effective with individual bone screws in the alveolar process or linked bone screws in the palate, but this is no longer correct. There are two lines of evidence leading to that conclusion. First, two randomized clinical trials of methods for anchorage control in maxillary incisor retraction concluded that, surprisingly, alveolar bone screws were no more effective in maintaining the posterior anchorage than a Nance-type lingual arch with an acrylic pad behind the maxillary incisors (see Fig. 11.55E).[7,8] It was not so much that the Nance appliance was effective as that it and the alveolar bone screws were equally ineffective. In contrast, palatal anchorage has now been shown to be quite effective in preventing mesial movement of the posterior teeth during retraction of incisors into premolar extraction sites,[9] especially when bilateral screws are placed in the anterior palate.[10] For maximum retraction of maxillary incisors, therefore, indirect anchorage from screws in the anterior palate (see Fig. 20.43) is now preferred.

The major advantage of skeletal anchorage in retraction of the anterior segment is that it offers vertical as well as anteroposterior control of the teeth.[11] To create the desired display of the incisors, they may need to be intruded as well as moved lingually, and although this is possible without bone screws or miniplates (see Fig. 9.48), it is complex and potentially difficult to manage.

There are three options for skeletal anchorage for maximum retraction of mandibular incisors: bone screws in the alveolar process, bone screws in the front of the ramus, or anchors placed vertically into the buccal projection of the mandibular body below the molars (see Fig. 10.51). Although there has not been a study to document that an anchor in the mandibular body is more effective than a mandibular alveolar bone screw, it seems likely that for incisor retraction, screws in mandibular alveolar bone would perform similarly to those in the maxilla and that an attachment in the mandibular body would be equivalent to palatal anchorage for maxillary retraction. Placing such an anchor is easier and less invasive than placing a long screw into the ramus.

The major disadvantage of skeletal anchorage for maximum incisor retraction in either arch is that it makes over-retraction of the incisor segments possible. The treatment objective is to improve the patient's dentofacial appearance and decrease social problems related to it. Retracting the anterior teeth too much makes the patient look worse, not better, as lip support is decreased and the nasolabial fold is accentuated. This is more of a problem in Class II or Class III camouflage than correction of bimaxillary protrusion, and is discussed further later.

Other applications of skeletal anchorage, including distal movement of the entire dental arch to reduce incisor protrusion, are presented in some detail in Chapter 20.

Minimum Incisor Retraction

Why would there be a need to close extraction spaces if retracting protruding incisors was not a goal of treatment? That could be the case if there were unanticipated residual spaces after alignment of crowded teeth, when space closure was needed after extraction of hopelessly carious teeth, or when some teeth (most likely mandibular second premolars) were congenitally missing (Fig. 16.14). As with any problem requiring anchorage control, the approaches to reducing the amount of incisor retraction when closing extraction spaces involve reinforcement of anchorage (the anterior teeth in this situation) and reduction of strain on that anchorage. An obvious strategy, implemented at the treatment planning stage, is to incorporate as many teeth in the anterior anchor unit as possible. All other factors being equal, the amount of incisor retraction will be less the further posteriorly in the arch an extraction space is located.

A second possibility for reinforcing incisor anchorage is to place active lingual root torque in the incisor section of the archwires, maintaining a more mesial position of the incisor crowns at the expense of somewhat greater retraction of the root apices (see Fig. 16.3). As the figure shows, what is a disadvantage when incisors are being retracted becomes an advantage when, for all practical purposes, the incisors are the anchorage.

A third possibility for maximizing forward movement of posterior teeth is to break down the posterior anchorage, moving the posterior teeth forward one tooth at a time. To close a second premolar extraction site (or the space where a second premolar was congenitally missing), it may be desired to stabilize the eight anterior teeth and to bring the first molars forward independently, creating a space between them and the second molars before bringing the second molars anteriorly. This strategy can readily be combined with increased torque of the anterior teeth to minimize retraction.

Skeletal anchorage, created by placing bone screws in either arch in the canine region, is the easiest and most effective way to close an extraction space by bringing posterior teeth forward (see Fig. 16.14). This is particularly advantageous when more forward movement is needed on one side than the other (Fig. 16.15). In both minimum and maximum retraction, temporary anchorage devices (TADs) now make it much easier to handle what previously were very difficult situations.

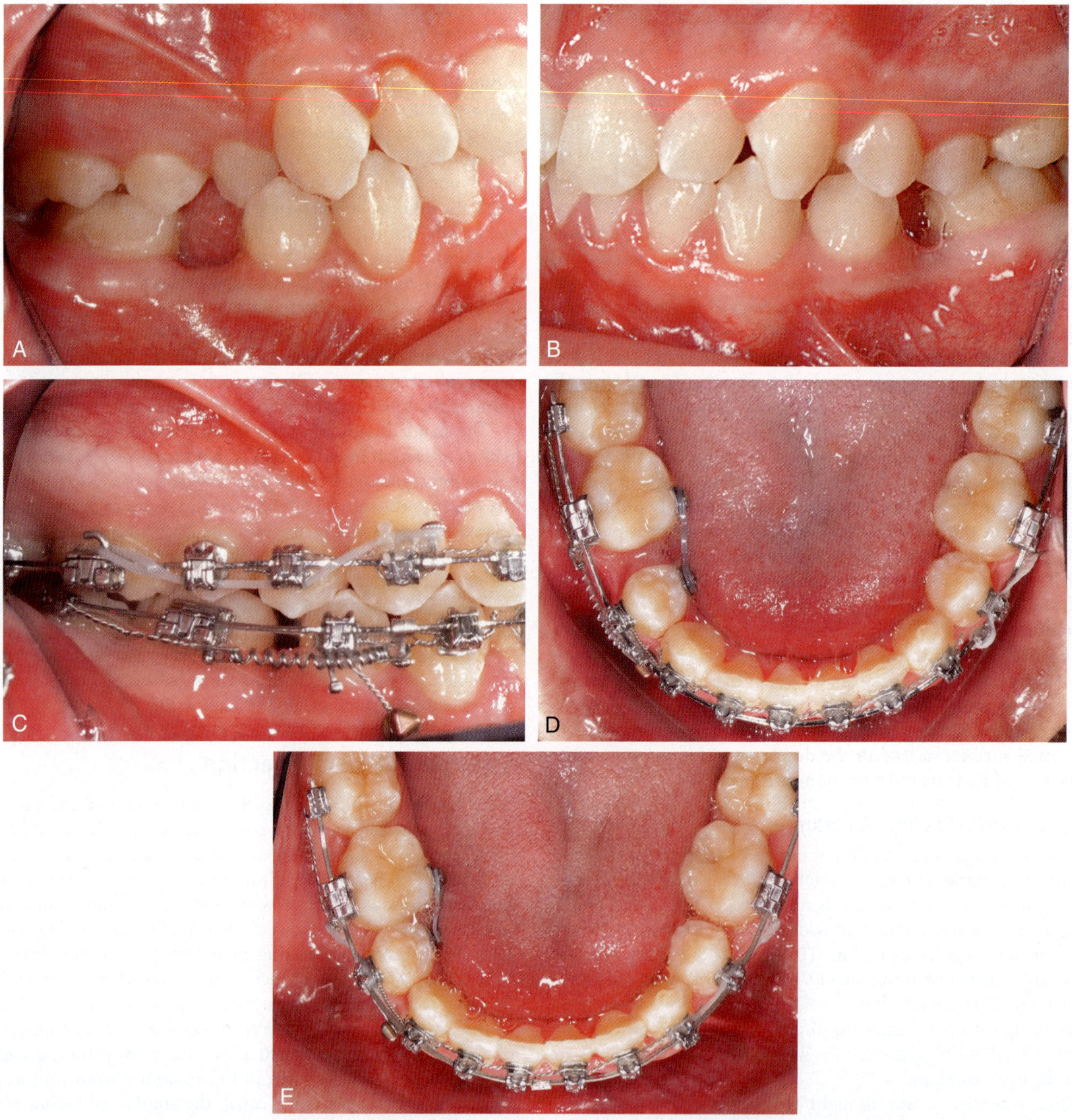

• **Fig. 16.14** (A and B) For this patient, a goal of treatment was closure of the space where mandibular second premolars were missing by bringing the mandibular molars forward, with more movement needed on the right side. (C) A bone screw was placed in the dentoalveolar process between the right canine and first premolar, and those teeth were stabilized by tying them to the archwire (indirect anchorage), and then the spaces were closed with sliding mechanics (D and E). (Courtesy Dr. N. Scheffler.)

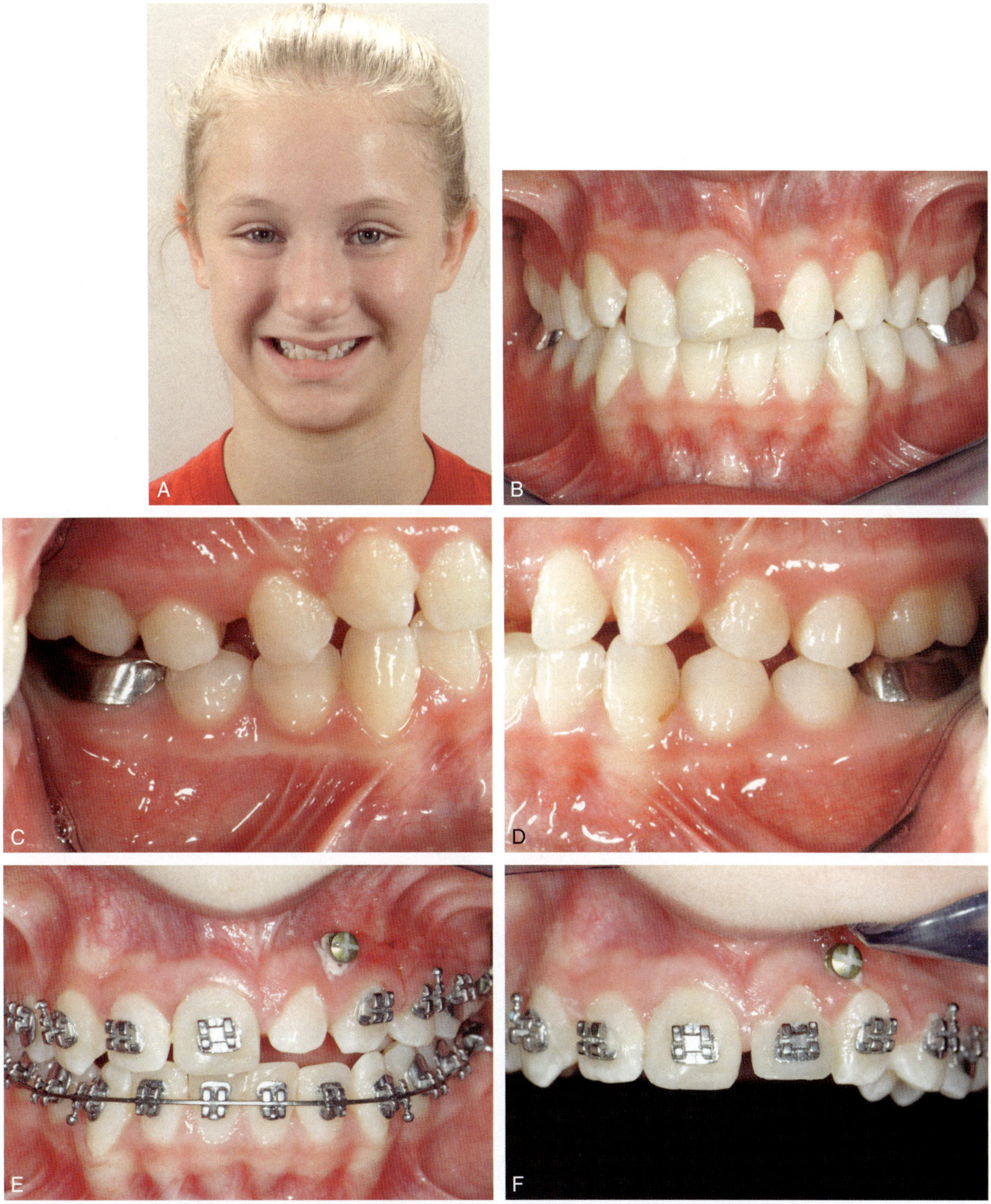

• **Fig. 16.15** (A) This girl lost her maxillary left central incisor as a result of trauma at age 8, and by the time she was seen by the orthodontist at age 11, the left lateral incisor had moved mesially into the central incisor space. (B–D) Intraoral views at age 11. The treatment plan was to use the lateral incisor as a replacement for the central incisor, intruding it to allow leveling of the gingival margin with the right central, then build it up so that it would be the correct size during the finishing orthodontics, and ultimately use a laminate veneer as part of the final restoration. The canine would be recontoured to make it an acceptable lateral incisor. (E) A bone screw was placed between the lateral incisor and canine as anchorage to bring the left posterior teeth anteriorly. (F) When the lateral was in the central spot and a Class II molar relationship had been obtained on the left side, a temporary buildup was done to bring the lateral incisor close to the width desired at the end of treatment, the canine was recontoured to serve as a lateral incisor (see Fig. 7.14), and brackets were placed to reposition these teeth.

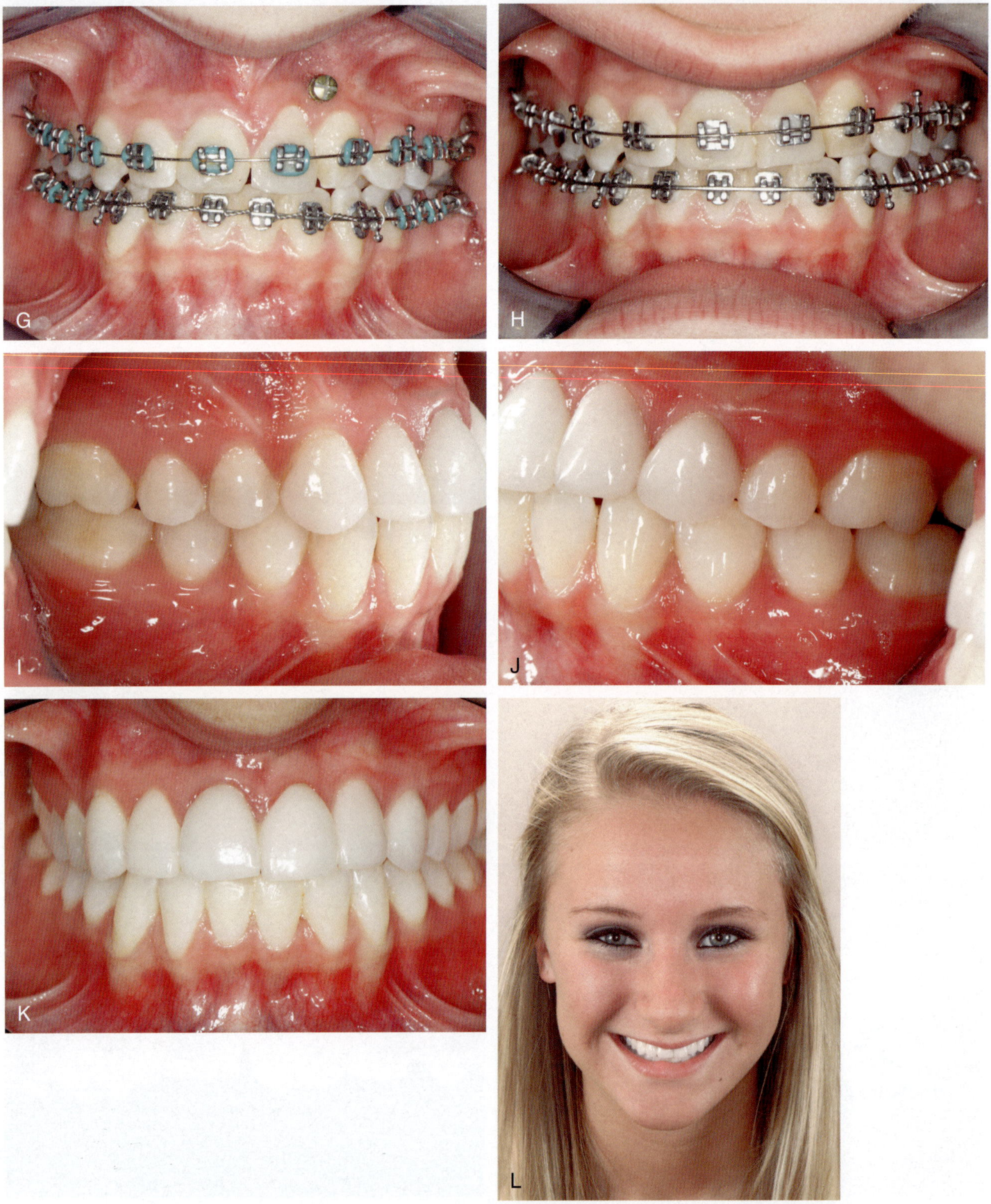

• Fig. 16.15, cont'd (G) Progress in alignment, with the bone screw still in place. At that point, a goal of treatment was to bring the gingival margins to approximately the correct levels for a central and lateral incisor, which required elongating the lateral and then shortening the crown, and then a diode laser was used to refine the gingival contours. (H) Toward the end of treatment, after the gingival recontouring. (I–K), Intraoral views at age 13, after completion of orthodontics and placement of a veneer on the left lateral, and (L) the facial view at that time. She was very pleased with the outcome, but a better smile arc could have been obtained by making the veneer on the lateral slightly longer and slightly elongating the right central (see section on micro-esthetics in Chapter 7).

Class II Correction in Adolescents

There are two major possibilities for correction of Class II malocclusion in adolescents: (1) differential growth of the jaws, guided by extraoral force or a functional appliance or (2) differential anteroposterior movement of the upper and lower teeth, with or without differential closure of extraction spaces. These approaches are not mutually exclusive, but even when growth modification is successful, it typically provides only a partial correction of a full-cusp Class II or Class III malocclusion. Some tooth movement almost always is needed to complete the correction of the molar relationship.

Differential Growth in Adolescent Class II Treatment

The use of extraoral force or functional appliances to influence jaw growth has been discussed in some detail in Chapter 14. The point was made there that Class II growth modification is most effective during the adolescent growth spurt, and that for most patients a preliminary period of preadolescent treatment with headgear or a removable functional appliance is not more effective and is less efficient than just waiting for the growth spurt.

Does that mean that beginning Class II treatment should always wait until the early permanent dentition? Often, but not always. The different timing of skeletal growth in males and females must be kept in mind when this approach is used. During adolescence, the mandible tends to grow forward more than the maxilla, providing an opportunity to improve a skeletal Class II jaw relationship. Girls mature considerably earlier than boys and are often beyond the peak of the adolescent growth spurt before the full permanent dentition is available and comprehensive orthodontic treatment can begin. Boys, who mature more slowly and have a more prolonged period of adolescent growth, are much more likely to have a clinically useful amount of anteroposterior growth during the early permanent dentition period.

When either extraoral force (headgear) or a functional appliance is used to modify growth in patients with Class II problems, a favorable response includes both restraint of maxillary growth and differential forward mandibular growth. For patients who are already in the adolescent growth spurt in the mixed dentition, there is nothing wrong with a first phase of removable functional appliance treatment and then a fixed appliance to obtain detailed occlusal results. A removable functional appliance, however, is unlikely to provide a satisfactory result in the early permanent dentition because it will have to be modified or discontinued when fixed appliance treatment begins. Also, when the permanent canines and premolars have erupted, it is advantageous to go ahead with alignment and transverse and vertical positioning of the dentition while growth modification is also occurring. Headgear is much more compatible with the fixed appliances needed for comprehensive treatment, and most varieties of fixed functional appliances are also compatible with the concurrent use of fixed appliances.

Many clinicians would like to believe that Class II elastics (or fixed springs that have the same effect) can influence growth as well as move teeth. If so, of course, all you would need would be Class II elastics. Unfortunately, that approach rarely succeeds. In an adolescent in the early permanent dentition period, a rigidly coupled fixed functional appliance such as the Herbst appliance effectively corrects Class II molar relationships (with varying combinations of differential growth and forward displacement of mandibular teeth). For cooperative patients whose lower incisors are already at their forward limit from an esthetic or stability point of view, headgear can be quite effective and does not introduce a Class II elastics effect (lower incisors forward).

Headgear for Adolescent Growth Modification

An ideal patient for headgear in the early permanent dentition period is a 12- to 14-year-old boy with a Class II problem whose skeletal maturity is somewhat behind his stage of dental development and who has good growth potential (Fig. 16.16). Boys at age 13, it must be remembered, are on the average at the same stage of maturation as girls at 11, and significant anteroposterior skeletal growth is almost always continuing. On the other hand, girls at age 13 are, on the average, at the same developmental stage as boys at 15, and by that time clinically useful changes in jaw relationship from growth guidance are unlikely. For a patient of either gender who is beyond the mixed dentition period but still in the adolescent growth spurt, there is no reason to wait for alignment and leveling to be completed before beginning treatment with a headgear or a fixed functional appliance, especially given that every passing day decreases the probability of a favorable growth response.

Although the main purpose of headgear is growth modification, some tooth movement in all three planes of space inevitably accompanies it because the extraoral force is delivered to the teeth. With headgear for Class II correction, when there is good vertical growth and the maxillary molars are allowed to elongate, the maxillary teeth erupt downward and backward, and spaces may open up in the maxillary arch. Even though the extraoral force is applied against the first molar, space does not always develop between the first molar and second premolar. Instead, the second premolar and, to a lesser degree, the first premolars often follow the molars. The result is often a space distal to the canines, along with a partial reduction of overjet as the jaw relationship improves (Fig. 16.17).

When this result occurs, the preferred approach is to consolidate space within the maxillary arch at a single location, using elastomeric chains to bring the canines and incisors into an anterior segment and the molar and premolars into a posterior segment. When the molar relationship has been corrected, the residual overjet is then reduced by retracting the incisors in this nonextraction patient in exactly the same way as in a patient who had a first premolar extraction space (see the following discussion). Extraoral force should be continued until an intact maxillary arch has been achieved. Discontinuing it when only the molar relationship has been corrected is unwise, both because the maximum skeletal effect probably has not been obtained at that point and because the retraction of the incisor teeth requires posterior anchorage, which can be reinforced by the headgear.

Fixed Functional Appliances for Adolescent Growth Modification

As we noted in Chapter 14, the Herbst appliance became the most popular functional appliance in the late 20th century because of its demonstrated effectiveness in correcting Class II malocclusion. With experience, it became clear that it was most effective during adolescent growth in patients who were already in the early permanent dentition period, so that a fixed appliance could be used to control mandibular incisor protrusion and other possible side effects.

In the early permanent dentition, space opening within the maxillary arch rarely occurs when a Herbst appliance or some of

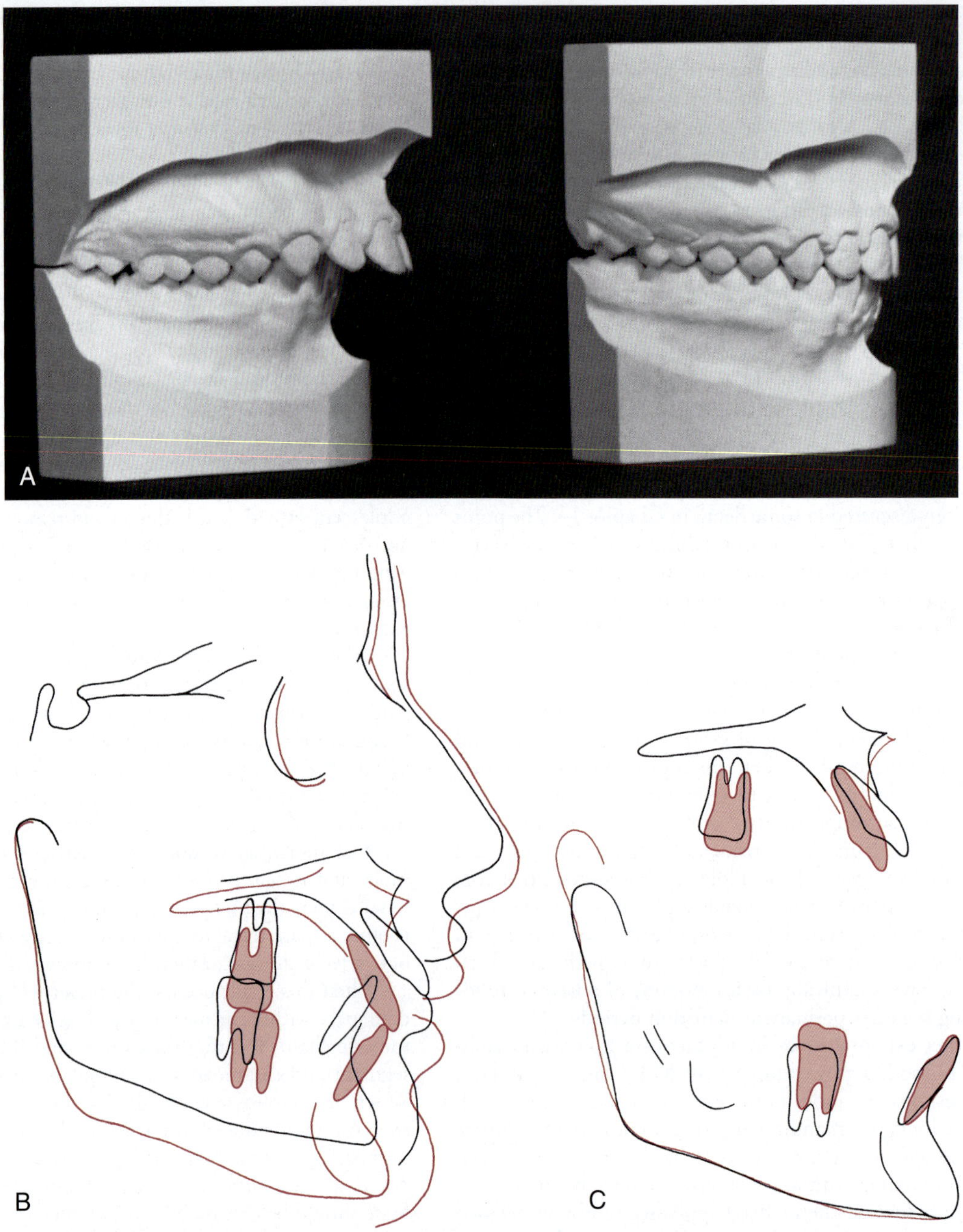

• **Fig. 16.16** Class II correction in a 13-year-old boy by using extraoral force to the maxilla. (A) Dental casts before and after treatment. (B and C) Cephalometric superimposition showing treatment changes. Note the large amount of vertical growth, which allowed the maxilla and maxillary dentition to be displaced distally as they moved vertically while the mandible grew downward and forward. As the maxillary and mandibular superimpositions show, overbite was corrected by relative intrusion (i.e., the lower incisors were held at the same vertical level while the molars erupted). There was relatively more eruption of the mandibular than the maxillary molar, reflecting the upward and backward direction of headgear force, and only a small amount of distal movement of the upper molars.

its modern variants (see Fig. 10.7) are used. Bonding the teeth that are available (canines and incisors in both arches, maxillary but usually not mandibular premolars) allows alignment and stabilization of the lower incisors while molar correction is occurring and facilitates the transition to a regular fixed appliance, which usually occurs after 9 to 12 months of Herbst treatment. The Herbst appliance is compatible with both labial and lingual fixed appliances.[12]

Class II Camouflage

In patients who have reasonable jaw relationships, correcting the excessive overbite that is the hallmark of a Class II problem largely by tooth movement is quite possible, with or without correcting the molar relationship. This is acceptable treatment, of course, only if the patient's facial appearance as well as dental alignment and occlusion are satisfactory—thus the earlier statement about

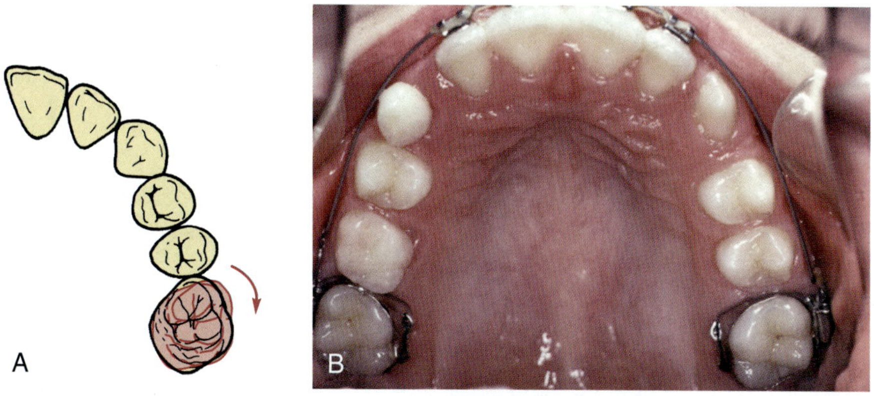

• Fig. 16.17 (A) In patients with Class II malocclusion, the upper molars usually are rotated mesially, and part of the apparent backward movement of the first molar is a distal rotation of the buccal cusps as the tooth rotates around its lingual root. The inner bow of a headgear facebow should be adjusted to produce this type of rotation. (B) Space tends to open within the maxillary arch when extraoral force to the upper first molars is used and the patient grows well, as in this patient after 12 months of headgear treatment during the adolescent growth spurt. Note that as the molars moved distally, the gingival fiber attachments produced distal movement of the premolars, opening space between these teeth and the canines. When a complete fixed appliance is placed at this stage, one of the first steps is consolidation of the space distal to the canines.

reasonable jaw relationships. Moderate skeletal Class II jaw relationships that are still present after orthodontic treatment often are no longer noticeable enough to be a problem, and therefore the patients with less severe skeletal Class II problems can be treated with tooth movement to camouflage the jaw discrepancy. The patients with more severe problems will need surgical mandibular advancement—and as noted in Chapter 7, it is the patient's decision as to whether surgery would be needed, not the doctor's.

There are three major ways to correct Class II malocclusion with tooth movement: distal movement of upper molars, differential anteroposterior tooth movement using extraction spaces, and nonextraction treatment that consists primarily of forward movement of the lower arch. We will consider them in that order.

Distal Movement of Upper Molars

The concept of "distal driving" the maxillary posterior teeth has a long orthodontic history. After early cephalometric studies in the 1940s showed that little or no distal movement of upper molars was produced by the Class II elastic treatment of that era, headgear was reintroduced as a means of moving the upper molars back. Skeletal anchorage (miniplates at the base of the zygoma or linked screws in the palate, but not alveolar bone screws) now is the most effective way to accomplish distal movement.

Although the modern methods discussed later have improved the situation, Class II correction by distal movement of upper molars has definite limits that are important to understand and respect. With headgear, it is now clear that significant distal positioning of the upper posterior teeth relative to the maxilla occurs primarily in patients who have vertical growth and elongation of the maxillary teeth so that the molars and premolars are tipped distally as they erupt. Without this vertical growth, it is difficult to produce more than 2 to 3 mm of distal movement of the upper molars, unless the upper second molars are extracted (see later). With skeletal anchorage above the roots of the teeth, 4 to 6 mm of distal movement is quite possible, but moving molars back requires space behind them, and second molar extraction may be required for major distalization. If second molars are to be distalized, early removal of third molars is advised; otherwise they may become significantly impacted and difficult to extract.

In patients with mild-to-moderate skeletal Class II malocclusion, the upper molars are likely to have rotated mesially around the lingual root, and merely correcting the rotation changes the occlusal relationship in a Class I direction (see Fig. 10.30). This can be done with a transpalatal lingual arch, an auxiliary labial arch, or the inner bow of a facebow. Sometimes upper molars are so mesially rotated that it is difficult or impossible to insert a facebow until the rotation has been partially corrected with a more flexible appliance (such as a heavy labial arch, typically 36-mil steel, inserted into the headgear tubes and tied over an initial alignment archwire). Correction of rotated maxillary first molars is the first step in Class II treatment of almost every type.

Anchorage Systems for Distal Movement

Mesial movement of teeth is easier than distal movement, simply because there is much more resistance to distal movement. Successful distal movement of molars therefore requires more anchorage than can be supplied by just the other teeth.

Headgear and Class II Elastics

The problem with headgear for tooth movement always has been that force of moderate intensity with long duration is needed, but headgear tends to supply relatively high force with only medium duration even in cooperative patients. Unless second molars are extracted (see later), significant distal movement of first molars (>2 mm) with headgear occurs only when the molar is extruded simultaneously, which is acceptable in a patient with substantial growth in height of the ramus, but otherwise leads to unfavorable downward and backward rotation of the mandible. High-pull headgear is not very effective in distalizing molars.

In theory, force from Class II elastics also can be used to push the upper molars distally, by using a sliding jig to concentrate the force on the molars. This was a mainstay of the original Tweed

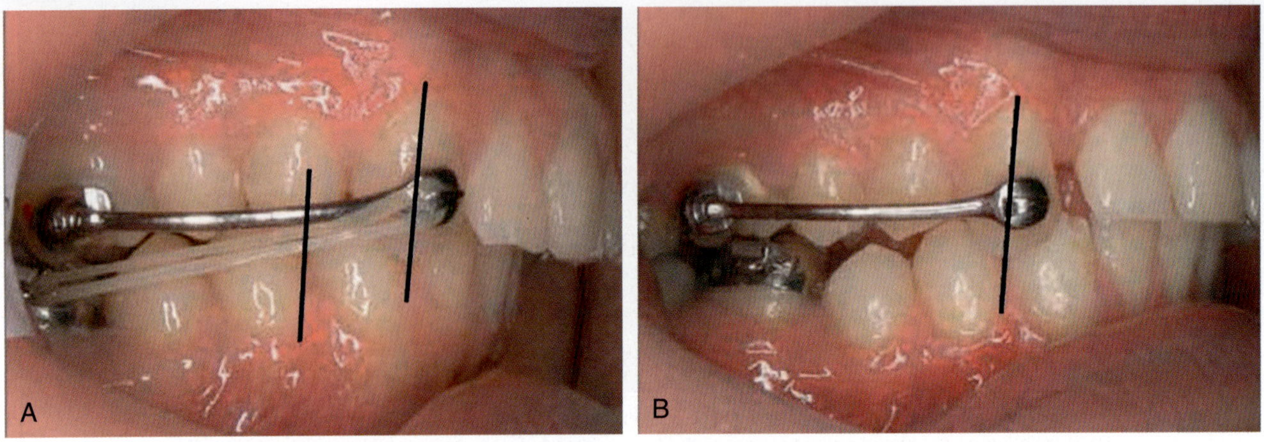

• **Fig. 16.18** Carriere Motion appliance used to apply Class II elastic force to upper molars in a Class II situation. (A) The elastic places a posterior force on the upper canine, then force is transferred to the upper molar. (B) Molar correction to Class I malocclusion is achieved, but the side effects of the Class II elastic wear are apparent. Extrusion of lower molar and loss of lower anchorage are visible, as is extrusion of the upper canine from the vertical force of the Class II elastic. Some of the lower molar extrusion and tipping can be reduced by using an overlay lower clear tray appliance.

technique, but as with Class II elastics in general, there is the risk of considerably more mesial movement of the lower teeth than distal movement of the upper teeth. The modern variant of the sliding jig is the Carriere Motion appliance shown in Fig. 16.18. As with the other techniques using Class II elastics, the lower molars extrude as the lower teeth move forward and the upper anterior teeth will extrude. In general, the major use of Class II elastics to a sliding jig, or any similar device, would be to accentuate rotation of the upper molar as a component of correcting the molar relationship, with no bodily distal movement expected.

Skeletal Anchorage

Palatal Anchorage. The idea that the relative stability of the anterior palate was a good possibility for obtaining additional anchorage goes back to the mid-20th century, far preceding TADs in the palate. Although removable appliances contact the palate, they are not effective in moving molars back, probably because they do not fit well enough. The Nance lingual arch, with a pad against the palatal rugae behind the central incisors, has long been considered an adjunct to preventing forward movement of maxillary molars. A fixed appliance that stabilizes the premolars and includes a plastic pad contacting the rugae—the pendulum appliance (Fig. 16.19) is the best example—was thought to be effective and was briefly popular in the late 20th century. Fortunately, most patients tolerate bulky palatal appliances such as this one with minimal problems, but contacting the palatal tissue has the potential to cause significant tissue irritation, to the point that sometimes the appliance has to be removed.

A greater problem is that however the molars were moved distally, they must be held there while the other teeth are then retracted to correct the overjet. It is one thing to move molars back, and something else to maintain them in that position. Follow-up studies with the pendulum appliance showed that space obtained by pushing the molars back with it was largely lost during later space closure, to the point that overjet reduction often was disappointing.[13]

Miniplate Anchorage. An alternative for retraction of the entire maxillary arch is miniplates on each side at the base of the zygomatic arch (Fig. 16.20). This works well as direct anchorage to move the entire arch posteriorly as a single unit if the anterior teeth are well aligned, or as a combined direct and indirect approach. This consists of direct anchorage to move the molars distally to create enough space for anterior alignment and retraction, and then indirect anchorage to stabilize the posterior segment while the incisors are moved back.[14] Both approaches work well, but invasive surgery is required to place and again to remove the miniplates.

It also is possible to use alveolar bone screws for anchorage to distalize molars and then stabilize them while the anterior teeth are retracted. This is no longer recommended because the bone screws must be repositioned during tooth movement and there is a risk of anchorage failure with single screws.

Palatal Bone Screw Anchorage. The bone of the anterior palate is the best location in the mouth for bone screws because of the thickness and density of the bone, and indirect skeletal anchorage from this area is the most effective way to move molars distally and hold them there while the other teeth are retracted into this area. This is so much more effective than pressure against palatal soft tissues that the older techniques for palatal anchorage can be considered obsolete.

If all that is needed is distal movement of the maxillary arch, indirect anchorage from two small screws on either side of the midpalatal suture is adequate to first move the molars distally and then hold them there while the premolars and anterior teeth are retracted. Hourfar and colleagues have published a series of cases that demonstrate how a palatal appliance supported by two bone screws can both expand the arch transversely and distalize upper molars.[15]

In a study based on 3D analysis of tooth position and orientation, Duran et al. noted that with direct force from a jackscrew in the midline of the palate against the maxillary first molars, effects in all three planes of space were observed.[16] As part of the mean 5 ± 2 mm distal movement of the first molars, on average they were intruded 0.5 mm, moved about 0.7 mm toward the midline, and rotated mesiobuccally 5 ± 3 degrees. Distal tipping, with a mean of 10 degrees, was a component of the distal movement. The method was precise, the wide variability in the responses was typical of outcome studies, and the midline jackscrew for tooth movement was not the best way to do that because of the heavy intermittent force—but this can be considered confirmation of previous findings that transverse expansion is needed when molars are moved distally, and that intrusion would be expected if the anchor is in the depth of the palate.

To demonstrate that distal movement of upper molars with bone screw anchors is possible even in adults, Kook et al. studied a group of young adults.[17] They found that the upper molars were moved back 3.3 ± 2 mm with a mild degree of distal tipping. The upper incisors were also retracted in this group about 3 mm and the occlusal plane was tipped because of intrusion of the molars and extrusion of the incisors.

Skeletal anchorage or not, two objects cannot occupy the same space at the same time, and there is only so much room at the rear of the maxillary arch. This means that in adolescents, extraction of the second molars may be necessary, and if second molars are distalized, early extraction of the third molars is indicated so that they do not end up impacted. In patients who have well-formed maxillary third molars, extraction of the second molars is a better idea than it might sound initially, because maxillary third molars usually erupt into the second molar extraction space nicely,

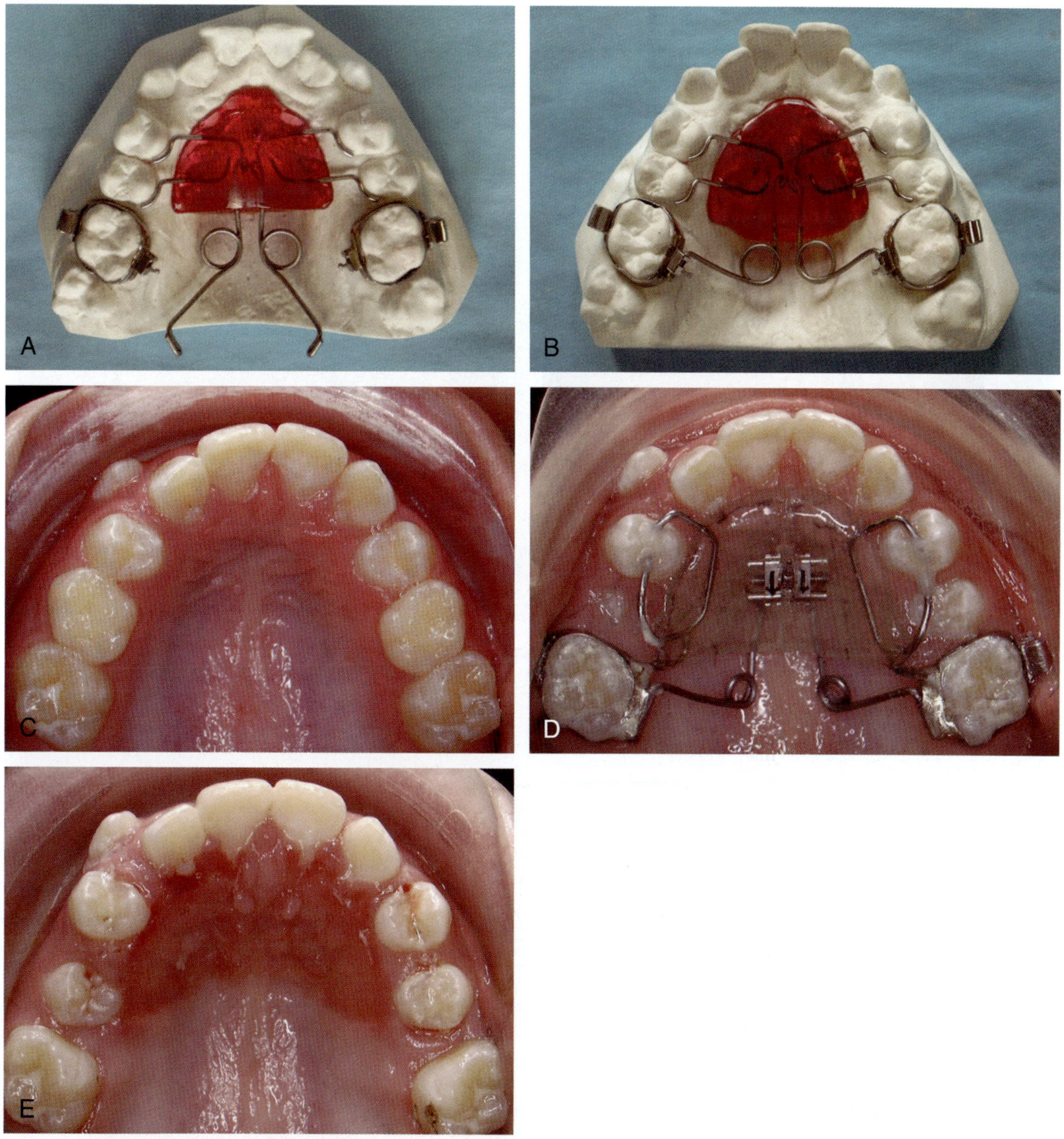

• **Fig. 16.19** Pendulum appliance for molar distalization. (A and B) Appliance on cast before and after activation of the springs. These are formed from beta-titanium (beta-Ti) wire and should deliver 200–250 g of force (steel wire is too stiff; it produces too much force). (C) Occlusal view of a patient with the maxillary canines nearly blocked out of the arch (in an individual who can afford some increase in maxillary incisor prominence). (D) Pendulum appliance with both a jackscrew for transverse expansion and molar distalizing springs (this modification is called the *T-Rex appliance*). (E) Removal of the appliance. Note the increase in space in the arch and the irritation of the palatal tissue beneath the appliance. Both are typical responses.

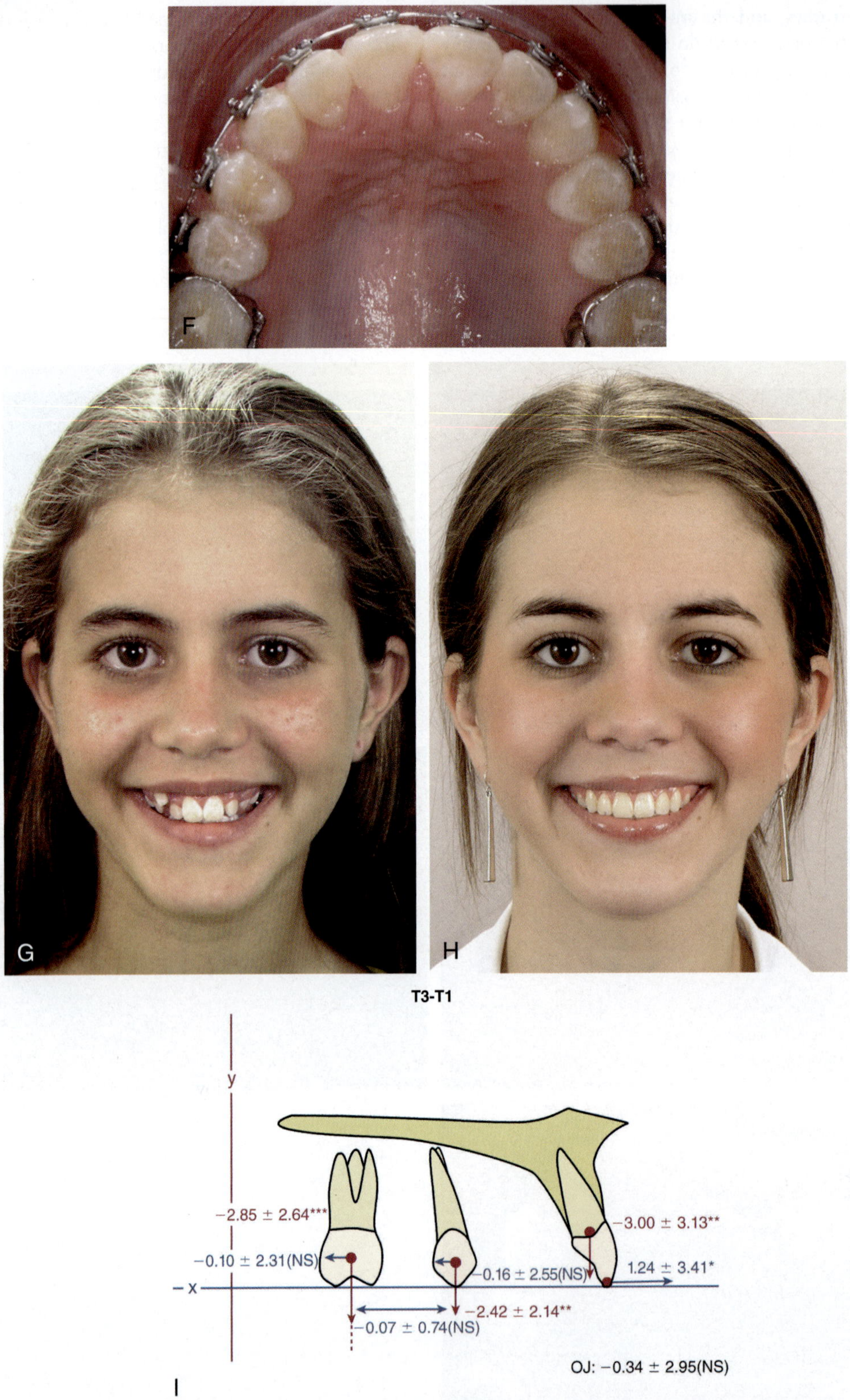

• **Fig. 16.19** (F) Alignment of the upper arch completed. (G and H) Initial and posttreatment smiles. (I) Mean changes in tooth position relative to the maxilla in a sample of 35 Class II patients treated with a first phase of pendulum appliance molar distalization followed by comprehensive fixed appliance treatment, with a mean treatment duration of 3.1 ± 0.6 years. Note the small average net distalization of the molars relative to the maxilla. In the final analysis, successful correction of the Class II malocclusion was due more to jaw growth, transverse expansion of the dental arches, and forward movement of the lower incisors than to distalization of upper molars. (Courtesy Professor A. Darendeliler.)

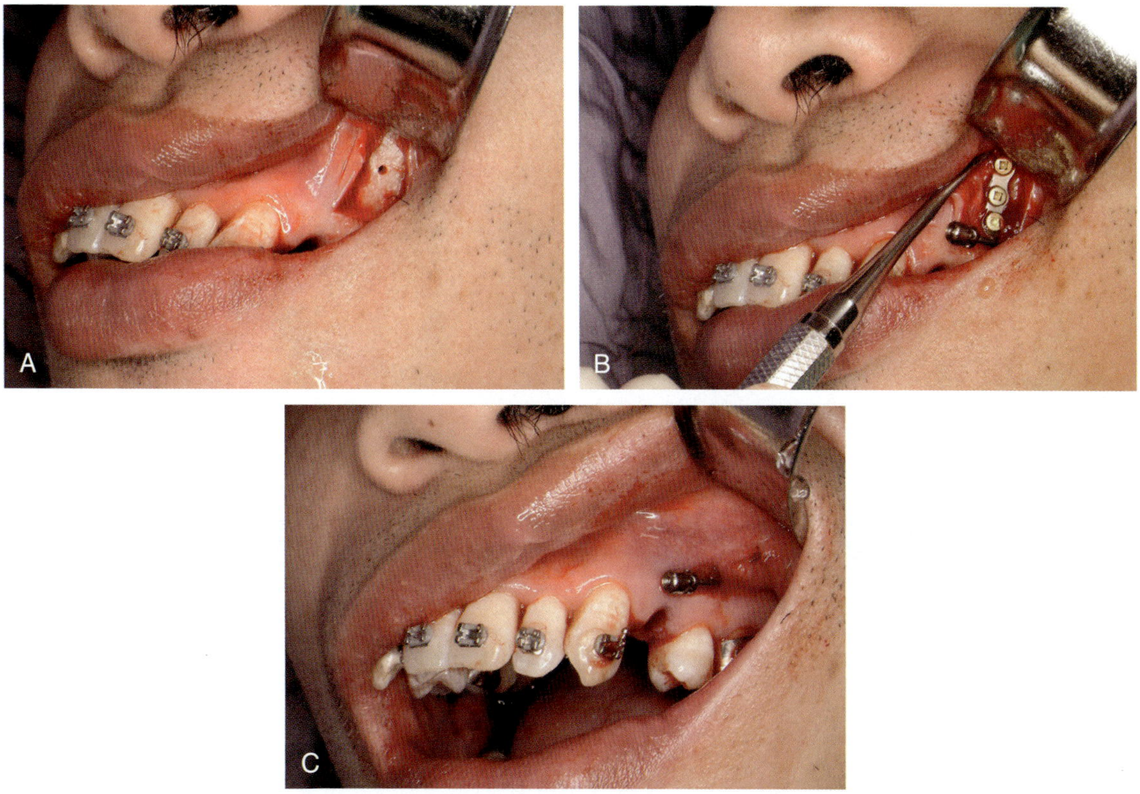

• **Fig. 16.20** Placement of a bone anchor at the base of the zygoma for maximum retraction of protruding maxillary incisors. (A) Exposure of the zygomatic buttress area; initial hole for screw drilled. (B) Anchor in place, secured by three bone screws. (C) Soft tissue covering the anchor, with only the tube for attachment of a retraction spring exposed in the mouth.

bringing bone with them (Fig. 16.21). The same 75% to 80% chance that maxillary third molars would be satisfactory replacements for the second molars presumably would apply with use of skeletal anchorage, as it did with headgear for distalization.[18]

Occasionally, unilateral molar distalization is indicated, typically when a unilateral Class II malocclusion is present and there is a dental midline discrepancy. Extraction of one-second molar facilitates this treatment, and the third molar usually replaces the missing second molar quite satisfactorily. Unilateral cervical headgear can be used for this treatment plan, but skeletal anchorage is preferred now because it is quicker and easier on the patient.

It is difficult to distalize the upper teeth too much with headgear or palatal anchorage. Skeletal anchorage is so effective that overretraction of the upper incisors is possible, which of course becomes unsuccessful camouflage. This makes it even more important to establish the desired final position of the incisors in planning treatment and then control tooth movement to reach this goal. In one sense, skeletal anchorage makes it possible to do what only surgery could do previously: move the maxillary dentition back too much.

Differential Anteroposterior Tooth Movement Using Extraction Spaces

There are two reasons for extracting teeth in orthodontics, as discussed in detail in Chapter 7: (1) to provide space to align crowded incisors without creating excessive protrusion and (2) to allow camouflage of moderate Class II or Class III jaw relationships when correction by growth modification is not possible. A patient with both Class II (or III) problems and crowding is a difficult problem because the same space cannot be used for both purposes. The more extraction space is required for alignment, the less is available for differential movement in camouflage, and vice versa.

An important part of treatment planning is deciding which teeth to extract and how the extraction spaces are to be closed (i.e., by retraction of incisor teeth, mesial movement of posterior teeth, or some combination). These decisions determine the orthodontic mechanics.

Class II Camouflage by Extraction of Upper First Premolars

In the late 20th century, it was claimed by some dentists that extraction of upper first premolars would lead to later temporomandibular dysfunction (TMD) problems. The theory, to the extent that the proponents of this claim had one, was that retracting the upper incisors would inevitably lead to incisor interferences, and this would cause TMD. The claim was never supported by any evidence, and research data have refuted it.[19] It is important to limit first premolar extraction for camouflage of Class II malocclusion to the appropriate patients and not to retract the incisors too much, but if done properly, it can be an excellent treatment method.

With this approach, the objective is to maintain the existing Class II molar relationship, closing the first premolar extraction space largely by retracting the protruding incisor teeth (Fig. 16.22). Anchorage must be reinforced, but one method, Class II elastics

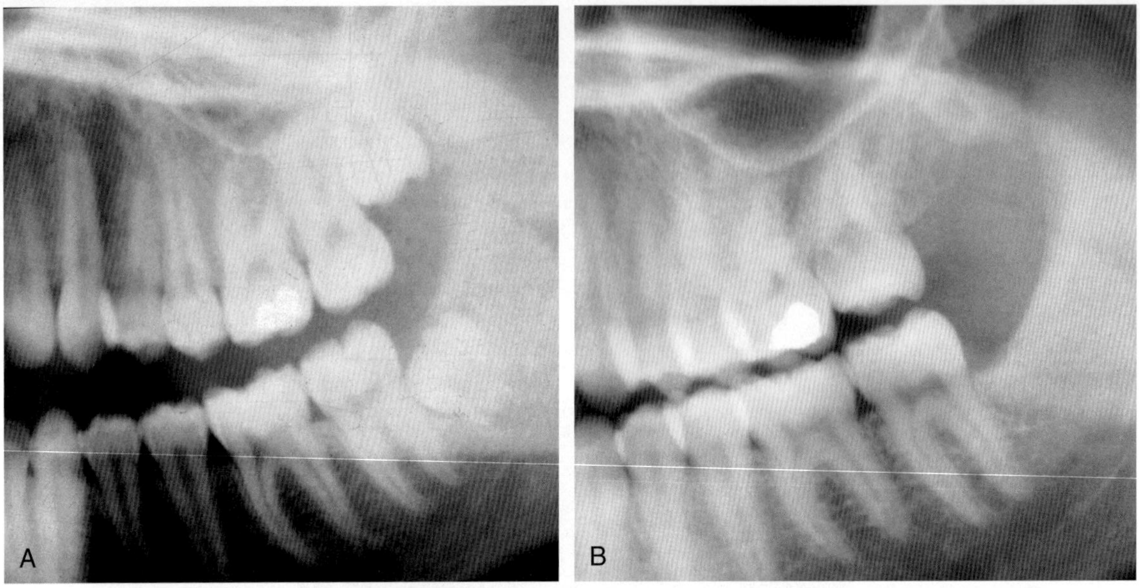

• **Fig. 16.21** (A) In this patient the treatment plan was extraction of the maxillary left second molar so that the first molar and premolars on that side could be moved distally to correct a yaw of the maxillary arch. (B) After treatment, with the third molar already erupting into the second molar extraction site. Eventually the remaining three third molars would be scheduled for extraction. A well-formed maxillary third molar can be a satisfactory replacement for an extracted second molar and usually erupts in a way that facilitates the replacement.

from the lower arch, is specifically contraindicated unless the lower incisors need to be moved forward (which rarely is the case). The remaining possibilities are extraoral force to the first molars, a stabilizing lingual arch, retraction of the maxillary anterior segment with extraoral force directly against these teeth, or skeletal anchorage.

Excellent reinforcement of posterior anchorage can be obtained with extraoral force only if it is applied consistently and for long durations. The more constant the headgear wear, the less a stabilizing lingual arch will be needed, but headgear for anchorage in Class II camouflage is rarely used now because poor patient compliance is likely. A stabilizing lingual arch augments the posterior anchorage full-time and is likely to be more effective.

It seems intuitively obvious that a lingual arch with a button against the palatal tissue should be more effective than a straight transpalatal lingual arch, but when first molars are being stabilized in a premolar extraction case, this is not necessarily true. As we noted earlier, anchorage from palatal soft tissue can be troublesome; more important, the effect of the stabilizing lingual arch is primarily to prevent the molars from rotating mesiolingually around their palatal root and secondarily to prevent them from tipping mesially. A straight transpalatal lingual arch is as effective as one with a palatal button in preventing rotation (Fig. 16.23), and for most patients, the marginally better stabilization with a palatal button is not worth the cost in tissue irritation. Note that this is true when a lingual arch is used to stabilize molars, but not true when the lingual arch is used to stabilize premolars, as in the molar distalization technique discussed earlier. When pushed mesially, premolars tip more than they rotate, and a palatal button on a lingual arch is at least a minimal step toward stabilizing them.

In addition to headgear and/or lingual arch stabilization, all the strategies described in Chapter 10 for reducing strain on anchorage (i.e., minimizing binding and friction, retracting canines individually, skeletal anchorage) are appropriate with upper first premolar extraction and can be brought into use.

Retracting protruding maxillary anterior teeth with headgear attached to the archwire (often called J-*hook headgear*) totally avoids strain on the posterior teeth and once was attractive from that point of view. This technique has two major disadvantages: (1) as with any headgear that provides too few hours and too much force, the force system is unfavorable for tooth movement and (2) there is significant binding and friction, not only where teeth slide along the archwire but also within the headgear mechanism itself because the headgear wires that attach to the teeth tend to bind against their protective sleeves.

This makes it difficult to control the amount of force, and more net force on one side than the other may lead to an asymmetric response. In fact, with J-hook headgear it is unusual if space does not close faster on one side than the other. Only if the headgear is worn nearly full-time (including school hours) will efficient tooth movement be obtained. For these reasons, headgear for direct retraction of the incisor segment is no longer recommended.

Skeletal anchorage in these premolar extraction cases is a straightforward way to reinforce anchorage, and retraction of the six anterior teeth can usually be managed satisfactorily with a single bone screw between the second premolar and first molar (see Fig. 10.47). In adolescents, use of TADs is necessary only if maximum retraction of the anterior segment without any elongation of the incisors is desired, a situation more likely to be encountered in adults.

Extraction of Maxillary and Mandibular Premolars

Correction of Class II buccal segment relationships with extraction of all four-first premolars implies that the mandibular posterior segments will be moved anteriorly nearly the width of the extraction space. At the same time, the protruding maxillary

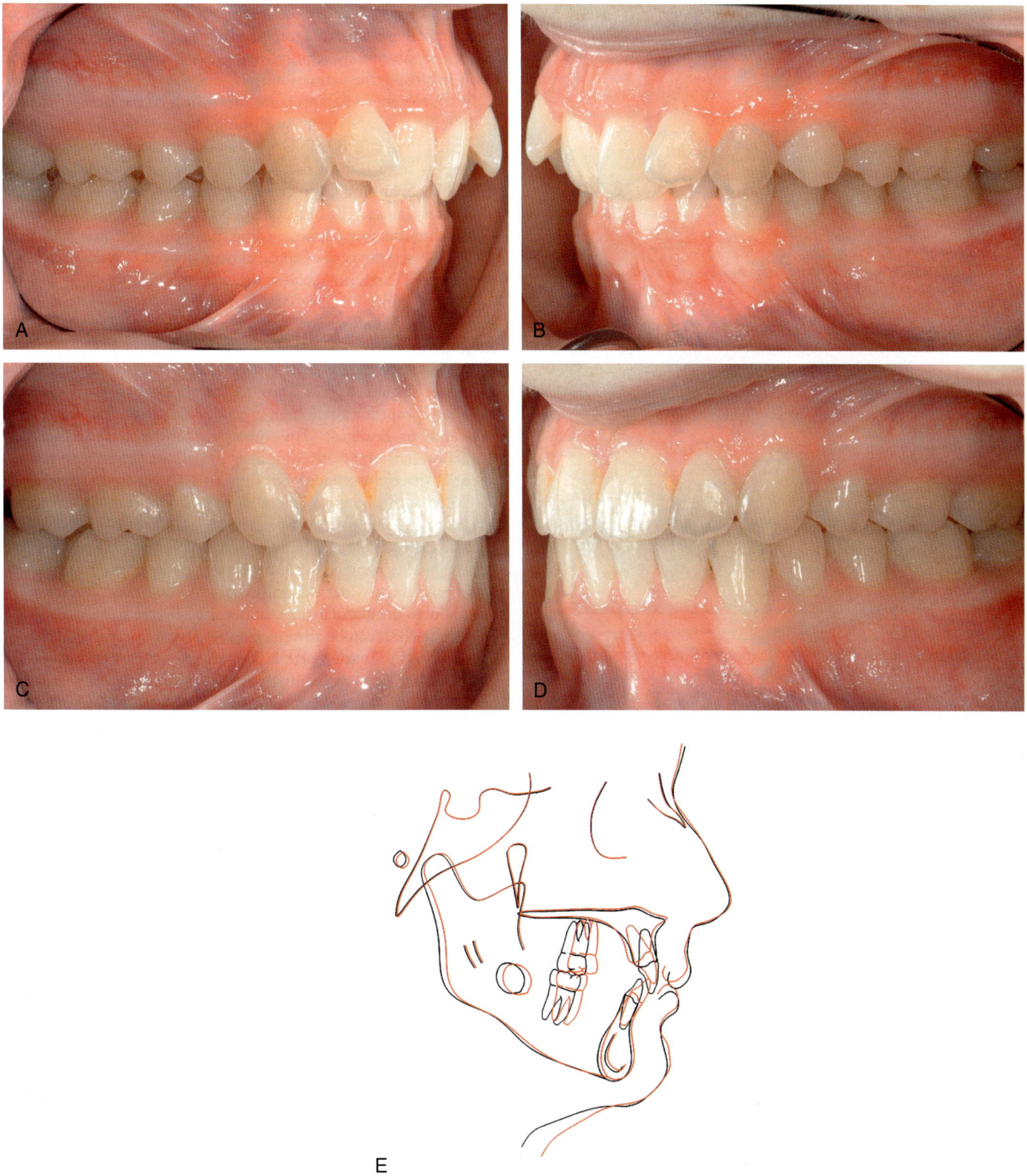

• **Fig. 16.22** An example of the camouflage of a Class II malocclusion by extraction of maxillary premolars. (A and B) Before treatment the molars and canines are Class II and the maxillary central incisors are retroclined in a division 2 pattern. (C and D) After treatment the molars remain Class II but the canines are in an ideal Class I position and the inclination of the incisor has been corrected to allow ideal overbite and overjet. (E) Cephalometric superimposition showing the dental and skeletal changes during treatment.

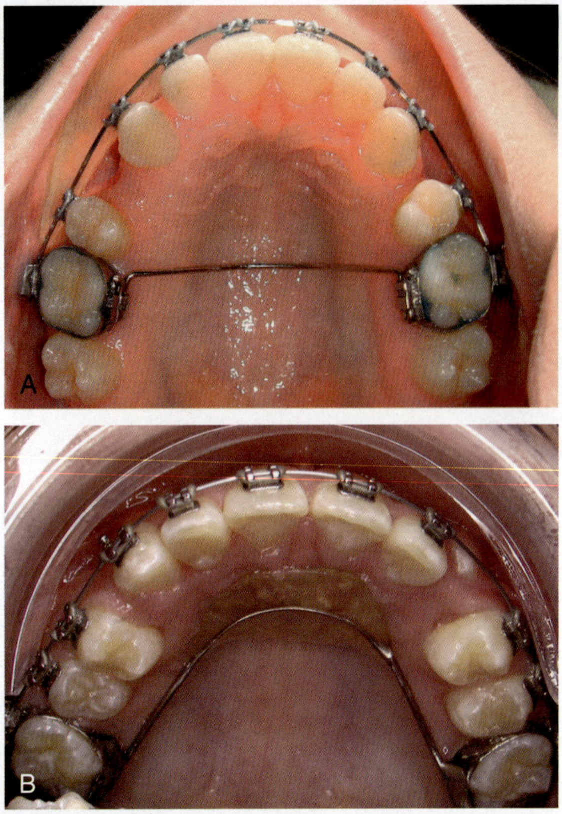

• **Fig. 16.23** (A) A transpalatal lingual arch without an adjustment loop is designed to reinforce anchorage by preventing molar rotation. (B) The Nance lingual arch projects forward into an acrylic pad against the palatal rugae, the most stable part of the palate—but there may be a soft tissue reaction to pressure in that area.

anterior teeth will be retracted with minimal forward movement of the maxillary buccal segments. This, in turn, implies (although it does not absolutely require) that Class II elastics will be used to assist in closing the extraction sites.

With the edgewise appliance, the width of the brackets makes it difficult to close space by tipping the crowns as in the Begg approach, but it is possible to structure anchorage so that space closure by retraction of the maxillary anterior teeth and protraction of the mandibular posterior segments occurs without the use of Class II elastics. The best control is achieved with the segmented arch technique, using space-closing springs in each arch fabricated specifically for the type of space closure desired (see the discussion of closure of extraction spaces earlier in this chapter).

A more common approach with the edgewise appliance is to extract maxillary first and mandibular second premolars, thus altering the anchorage value of the two segments (Fig. 16.24). With this approach, routine space-closing mechanics will move the lower molars forward more than the upper, particularly if maxillary posterior anchorage is reinforced with a stabilizing lingual arch or headgear. This upper first-lower second premolar extraction pattern greatly simplifies the mechanics needed for differential space closure with continuous-arch edgewise technique.

Occasionally, however, mesial movement of the lower first molar into a second premolar extraction space is difficult to produce. This is particularly likely when the second premolar was congenitally missing and a retained second primary molar is to be extracted, because with the wider extraction space to be closed, bone resorption reduces the alveolar ridge dimensions before space closure can be completed. It can be advantageous to remove only the distal root of the second primary molar, leaving the mesial part of the primary tooth in place (with a calcium hydroxide pulpotomy and temporary restoration) until the permanent tooth has been brought forward

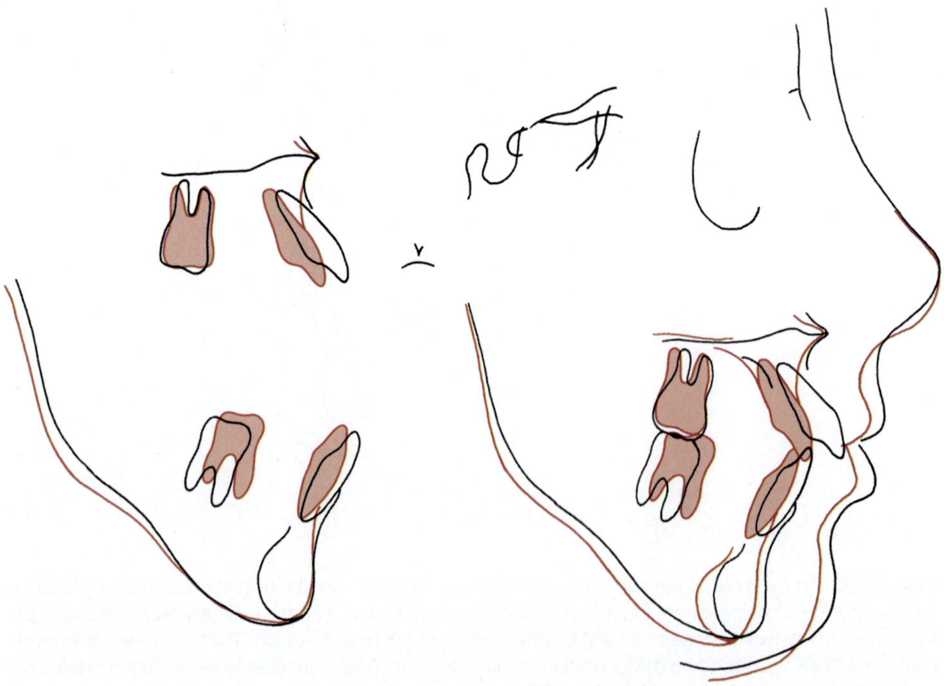

• **Fig. 16.24** Cephalometric superimposition showing the result of treatment with extraction of upper first and lower second premolars. Even with second premolar extraction, some retraction of the mandibular incisors may occur, but most of the space closure will be by mesial movement of the lower molar. This adult patient experienced no growth, and a slight downward and backward rotation of the mandible occurred.

for that half of the total distance. Then the remaining half of the primary tooth is extracted, and space closure completed.[20]

Nonextraction Correction With Interarch Elastics

Without extraction spaces, Class II elastics produce molar correction largely by mesial movement of the mandibular arch, with only a small amount of distal positioning of the maxillary arch, and can produce far too much protrusion of lower incisors (Fig. 16.25). When some forward movement of the mandibular dentition is desired, the amount of force varies with the amount of tipping that is allowed. With a well-fitting rectangular wire in the lower arch, approximately 250 g per side is needed to displace one arch relative to the other. With a lighter round wire in the lower arch, half that amount of force should be used. Incorporating the lower second molars into the appliance and attaching the elastics to a mesial hook on this tooth increase the anchorage and give a more horizontal direction of pull than hooking the elastic to the first molar.

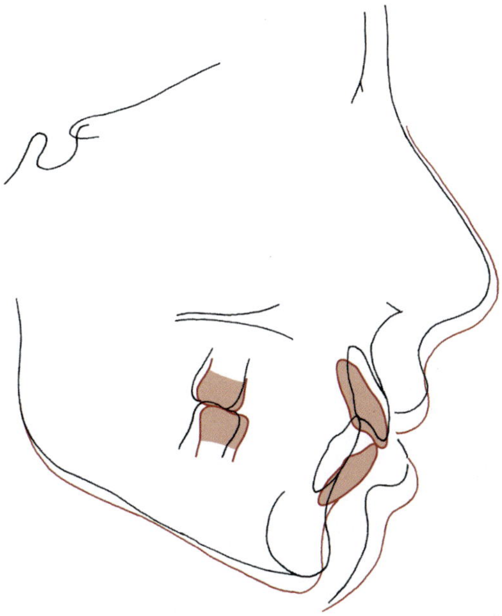

• Fig. 16.25 Cephalometric superimposition showing the response to Class II elastics in a girl in whom this was the major method for correcting a Class II malocclusion. Note that with rectangular archwires, some torque of the upper incisors was obtained. Both the downward-backward rotation of the mandible (perhaps less in this patient than often occurs) and the considerably greater forward displacement of the lower teeth than retraction of the upper teeth are typical. This amount of lower incisor protrusion is undesirable because of both the lip protrusion and lack of stability without permanent retention.

It is important to keep in mind that with or without extraction, Class II elastics produce not only anteroposterior and transverse effects but also a vertical force (Fig. 16.26). This force elongates the mandibular molars and the maxillary incisors, rotating the occlusal plane up posteriorly and down anteriorly. If the molars extrude more than the ramus grows vertically, the mandible itself will be rotated downward (see Fig. 16.25). Class II elastics are therefore contraindicated in nongrowing patients who cannot tolerate some downward and backward rotation of the mandible. The rotation of the occlusal plane, in and of itself, facilitates the desired correction of the posterior occlusion, but even if elongation of the lower molars can be tolerated because of good growth, the corresponding extrusion of the maxillary incisors can be unsightly.

Class II elastics, in short, may produce occlusal relationships that look good on dental casts but are less satisfactory when skeletal relationships and facial esthetics are considered. Because of this, applying heavy Class II force for 9 to 12 months as the major method for correcting a Class II malocclusion rarely produces an acceptable result. Using Class II elastics for 3 or 4 months at the completion of treatment of a patient with Class II malocclusion to obtain good posterior interdigitation, however, is often acceptable.

Class III Camouflage

Class III camouflage would be based on a combination of retraction of lower incisors and forward movement of maxillary incisors and, of course, would be successful only if the malocclusion was corrected without harming the facial appearance. In theory, Class III elastics could do this, but they also have a significant extrusive component, tending to elongate the upper molars and the lower incisors (see Fig. 16.26). In a short-face patient with a large mandible, rotating the mandible downward and backward, within limits, can help treatment of a Class III problem.

As we have noted previously, retracting the lower incisors is likely to make the chin look more, not less, prominent. For this reason, the reverse of the most popular approach to Class II

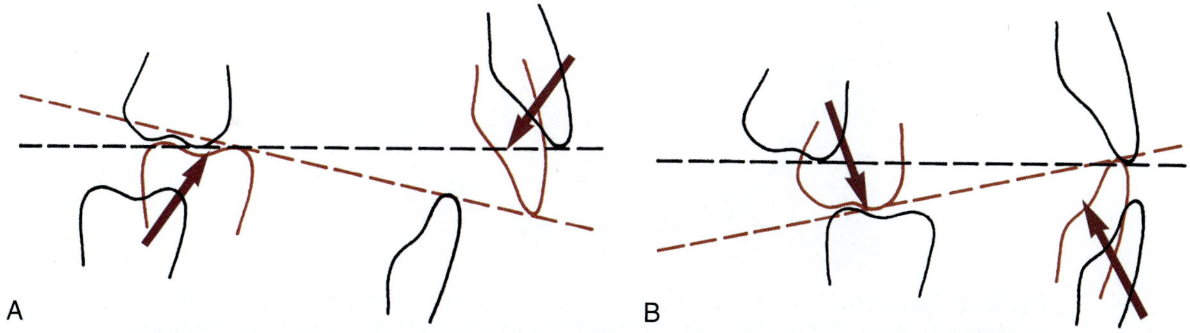

• Fig. 16.26 Rotation of the occlusal plane with Class II (A) and Class III (B) elastics. The rotation of the occlusal plane helps correct the molar relationship, but it can be deleterious in some patients because elongation of the molars may cause undesirable rotation of the mandible or undesirable tooth–lip relationships.

camouflage, extraction of mandibular first and maxillary second premolars with use of Class III elastics, rarely is a good plan for patients of European descent. They do not usually have mandibular dental protrusion and often cannot tolerate the increased anterior face height that Class III elastics tend to create. It may be a satisfactory plan in Asian patients, who often do have protrusion of lower incisors relative to the mandible and are more likely to tolerate downwards and backward rotation of the mandible.

A better approach to camouflage in patients of European descent with a moderately severe Class III problem is extraction of one lower incisor, which prevents major retraction of the lower teeth, while the maxillary incisors are moved facially with some tipping allowed. The combination of upright mandibular incisors and proclined maxillary incisors often leads to good dental occlusion rather than the expected tooth-size problem (Fig. 16.27), but a set-up, digital or plaster, should always be done when one lower incisor extraction is considered to verify the probable occlusal outcome. Another approach to camouflage a moderate Class III problem is removal of mandibular premolars while carefully controlling lower incisor retraction. Figs. 16.28 and 16.29

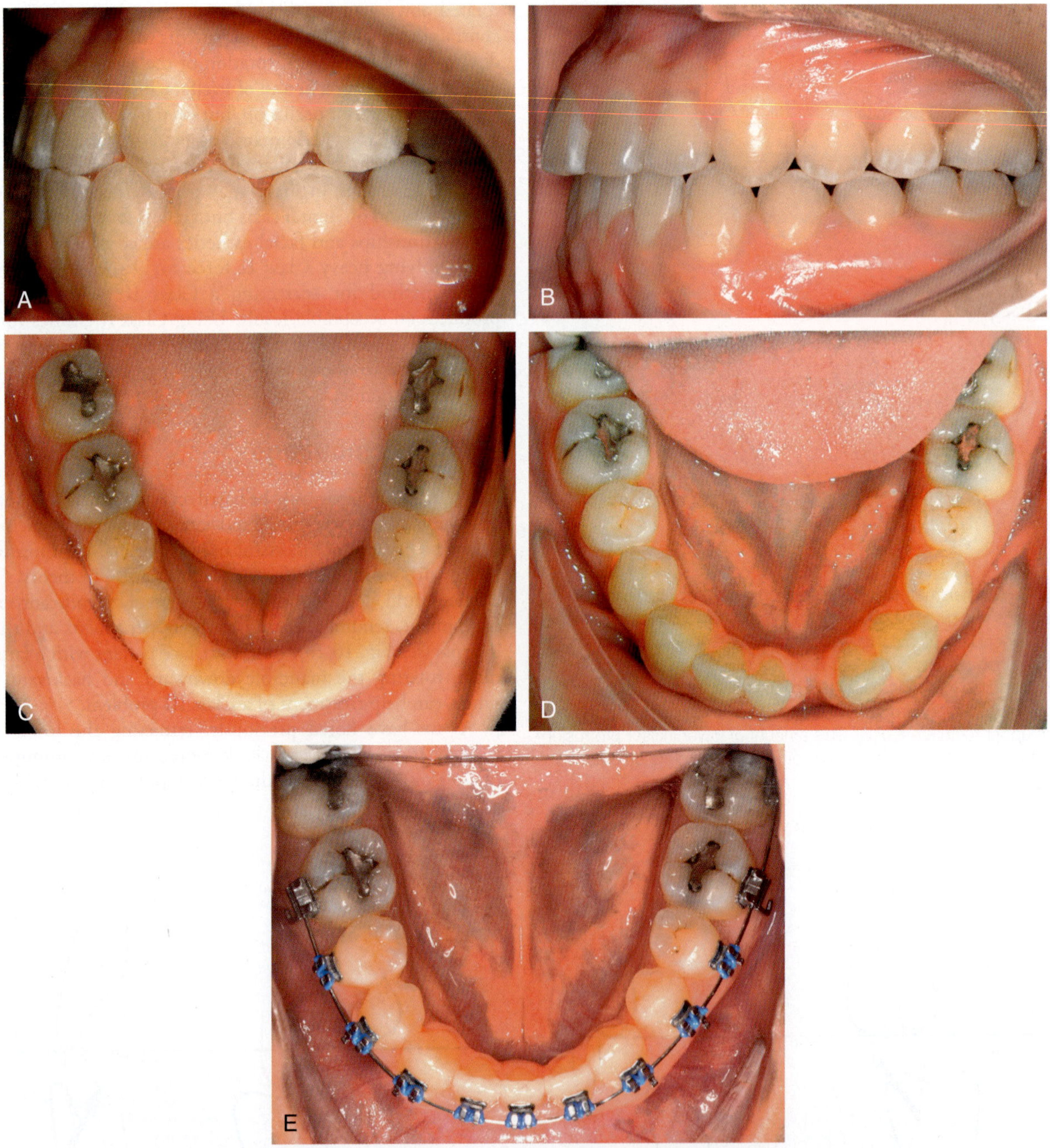

• **Fig. 16.27** Camouflage of a Class III malocclusion using the extraction of a single mandibular incisor. (A) Late mandibular growth after comprehensive treatment resulted in an end-to-end incisor relationship and a Class III tendency. (B) After extraction of the lower left central incisor and space closure to improve the incisor relationship. (C) Lower arch before incisor extraction. (D) Lower arch with incisor removed. (E) Fixed appliances used to close incisor extraction space and slightly retract mandibular incisors.

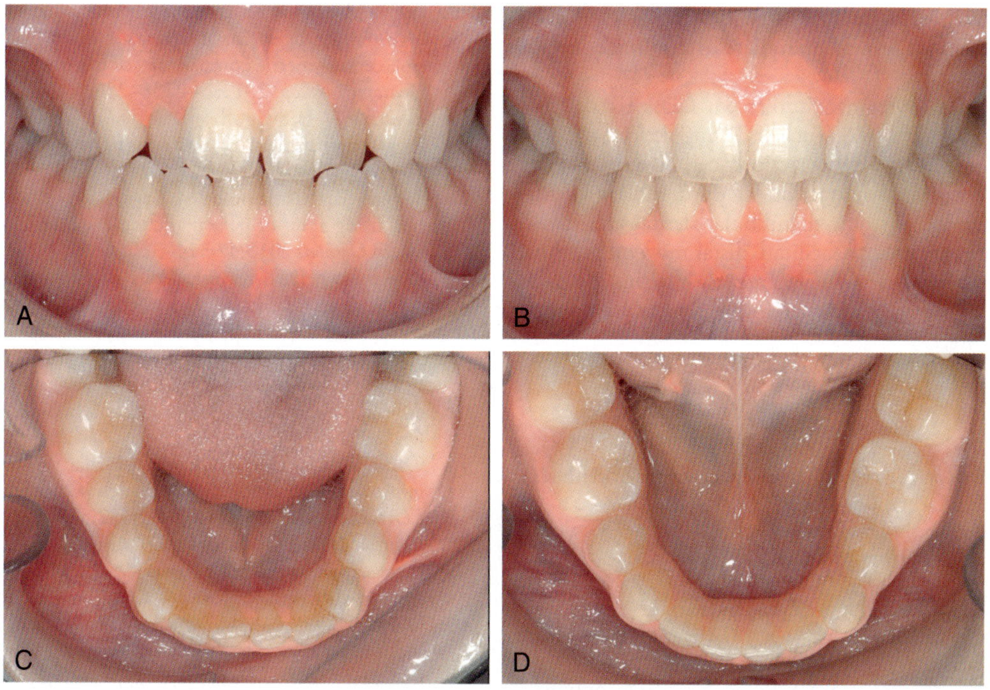

• **Fig. 16.28** Treatment of a mild Class III malocclusion with extraction of four second premolars. (A and C) Before treatment with anterior crossbite and mild crowding. (B and D) After premolar extraction and fixed appliance treatment. (Courtesy Dr. T. Shaughnessy.)

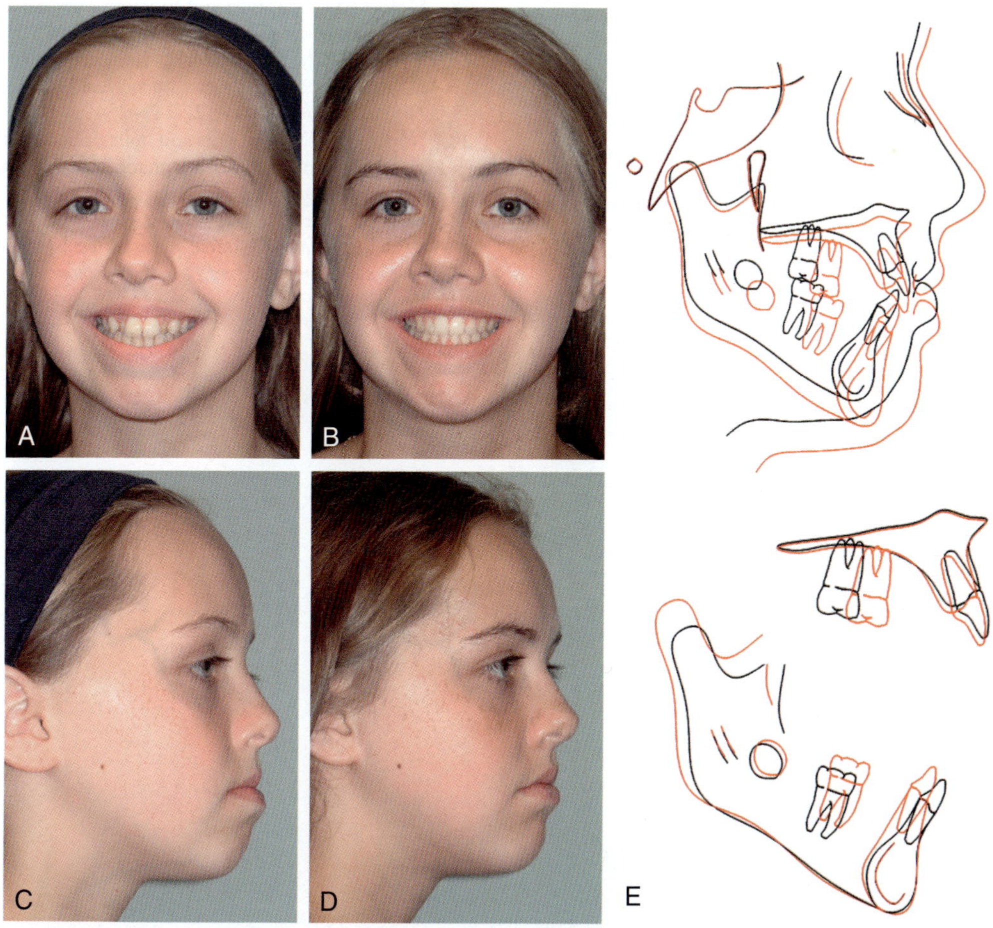

• **Fig. 16.29** Facial images and cephalometric tracings of the mild Class III case shown in Fig. 16.28. (A and C) Before treatment with lower lip eversion resulting in profile imbalance. (B and D) After second premolar extraction and fixed appliance treatment demonstrating improved facial profile and lip balance. (E) Cephalometric tracing showing dental and soft tissue changes as a result of treatment. Note the minimal upper incisor retraction possible with extraction of second premolars and proper management of anchorage. (Courtesy Dr. T. Shaughnessy.)

show an example of this treatment approach using extraction of maxillary and mandibular second premolars to minimize incisor change.

For Asian (or rarely, other) late adolescent Class III patients with major protrusion of the lower incisors, using skeletal anchorage to move the whole lower arch posteriorly can be quite helpful in correcting the problem.[21] Extraction of third molars is usually needed in order to move the mandibular dental arch back. If second molars are extracted to facilitate distal movement, third molars may erupt as satisfactory replacements, but this is not as likely as in the maxillary arch and therefore is not recommended as a routine procedure.

References

1. Booth FA. *Optimum Forces With Orthodontic Loops* [MS thesis]. University of Texas Dental Branch; 1971.
2. Techalertpaisarn P, Versluis A. Effect of apical portion of T-, sloped L-, and reversed L-closing loops on their force systems. *Angle Orthod.* 2017;87:104–110.
3. Ronay F, Kleinert W, Melsen B, et al. Force system developed by V bends in an elastic orthodontic wire. *Am J Orthod Dentofac Orthop.* 1989;96:295–301.
4. Siatkowski RE. Continuous archwire closing loop design, optimization and verification. Parts I and II. *Am J Orthod Dentofac Orthop.* 1997;112(393–402):484–495.
5. Nanda R, Uribe FA. *Atlas of Complex Mechanics.* Elsevier; 2017.
6. Eden JD, Waters N. An investigation into the characteristics of the PG canine retraction spring. *Am J Orthod Dentofac Orthop.* 1994;105:49–60.
7. Lagravere MO, Carey J, Heo G, et al. Transverse, vertical, and anteroposterior changes from bone-anchored maxillary expansion vs traditional rapid maxillary expansion: a randomized clinical trial. *Am J Orthod Dentofac Orthop.* 2010;137:304e1–304e12. discussion 304–305.
8. Sandler J, Murray A, Thiruvenkatachari B, et al. Effectiveness of 3 methods of anchorage reinforcement for maximum anchorage in adolescents: a 3-arm multicenter randomized clinical trial. *Am J Orthod Dentofac Orthop.* 2014;146:10–20.
9. Lee J, Miyazawa K, Tabuchi M, et al. Midpalatal miniscrews and high-pull headgear for anteroposterior and vertical anchorage control: cephalometric comparisons of treatment changes. *Am J Orthod Dentofac Orthop.* 2013;144:238–250.
10. Hourfar J, Ludwig B, Bister D, et al. The most distal palatal ruga for placement of orthodontic mini-implants. *Eur J Orthod.* 2015;37:373–378.
11. Wilmes B, Nienkemper M, Ludwig B, et al. Upper-molar intrusion using anterior palatal anchorage and the Mousetrap appliance. *J Clin Orthod.* 2013;47:314–320.
12. Wiechmann D, Schwestka-Polly R, Pancherz H, et al. Control of mandibular incisors with the combined Herbst and completely customized lingual appliance—a pilot study. *Head Face Med posted.* 2010;6:3.
13. Byloff FK, Darendeliler MA. Distal molar movement using the pendulum appliance. Part I. Clinical and radiological evaluation. *Angle Orthod.* 1997;67:249–260.
14. Cornelis MA, De Clerck HJ. Maxillary molar distalization with miniplates assessed on digital models: a prospective clinical trial. *Am J Orthod Dentofac Orthop.* 2007;132:373–377.
15. Hourfar J, Ruff CJ, Wilmes B, Ludwig B, Kanavakis G. Rapid maxillary expansion and upper-molar distalization with a miniscrew-supported hybrid appliance. *J Clin Orthod.* 2016;50(8):476–484.
16. Duran GS, Görgülü S, Dindaroğlu F. Three-dimensional analysis of tooth movements after palatal miniscrew-supported molar distalization. *Am J Orthod Dentofac Orthop.* 2015;150:188–197.
17. Kook YA, Bayome M, Trang VT, et al. Treatment effects of a modified palatal anchorage plate for distalization evaluated with cone-beam computed tomography. *Am J Orthod Dentofac Orthop.* 2014;146:47–54.
18. Moffitt AH. Eruption and function of maxillary third molars after extraction of second molars. *Angle Orthod.* 1998;68:147–152.
19. Rinchuse DJ, Rinchuse DJ, Kandasamy S. Evidence-based versus experience-based views on occlusion and TMD. *Am J Orthod Dentofac Orthop.* 2005;127:249–254.
20. Northway WM. The nuts and bolts of hemisection treatment: managing congenitally missing mandibular second premolars. *Am J Orthod Dentofac Orthop.* 2005;127:606–610.
21. Kook YA, Park JH, Bayome M, et al. Distalization of the mandibular dentition with a ramal plate for skeletal Class III malocclusion correction. *Am J Orthod Dentofac Orthop.* 2016;150:364–377.

17

Comprehensive Treatment: Finishing

BRENT E. LARSON AND WILLIAM R. PROFFIT

CHAPTER OUTLINE

After the teeth are well aligned, extraction spaces are closed with tooth roots reasonably parallel, deep bite or open bite has been corrected, and the teeth in the buccal segments are in a normal Class I relationship, the final stage of treatment is to get the details correct.

In the Begg technique, major root movements of both anterior and posterior teeth still remained to be done at the finishing stage, to obtain root paralleling at extraction sites and proper torque and axial inclination of tipped incisors, and this was accomplished with auxiliary springs. In the modern modified Begg technique, using Tip-Edge brackets, auxiliary springs are augmented with rectangular archwires in stage 3 (Fig. 17.1).

With contemporary edgewise techniques, much less treatment remains to be accomplished at the finishing stage, but minor versions of these same root movements are likely to be required. In addition, in most cases some adjustment of individual tooth positions is required in order to get marginal ridges level, obtain precise in-out positions of teeth within the arches, and generally overcome any discrepancies produced by errors in either bracket placement or appliance prescription. In some cases, it is necessary to alter the vertical relationship of incisors as a finishing procedure, either correcting moderately excessive overbite or closing a mild anterior open bite. The focus is not just on dental alignment and occlusion—the appearance of the teeth also must be kept in mind.

Although many variations are inevitable to meet the demands of specific cases, it is possible to outline a logical sequence of archwires for continuous arch edgewise technique, and this has been attempted in Box 17.1. The sequence is based on two concepts: (1) that the most efficient archwires should be used, so as to minimize clinical adjustments and chair time, and (2) that it is necessary to fill (or nearly fill) the bracket slot in the finishing stage with appropriately flexible wires to take full advantage of the modern appliance. That means that at this stage the wires should be 17 × 25 in 18-slot brackets and 21 × 25 in 22-slot brackets; the desired degree of bending or torsional stiffness is varied by using different archwire materials. Appropriate use of the recommended finishing archwires and variations to deal with specific situations in finishing are reviewed in some detail later.

Adjustment of Individual Tooth Positions

At the finishing stage of treatment, it is likely that up-down and in-out relationships of some teeth will need minor change, and the root position of some teeth may require adjustment (whether teeth were extracted or not). If the appliance prescription and bracket positioning were perfect, such adjustments would be unnecessary. Given the variations in both individual tooth anatomy and bracket placement that are encountered frequently, in many cases some adjustment of tooth positions is needed at this point.

When it becomes apparent that a bracket is poorly positioned, usually it is time-efficient to rebond the bracket rather than place compensating bends in archwires. This is particularly true when the inclination of the tooth is incorrect so that angulated step bends in wires would be required. After the bracket is rebonded, however, a flexible wire must be placed to bring the tooth to the correct position. Rectangular steel finishing wires are too stiff in bending

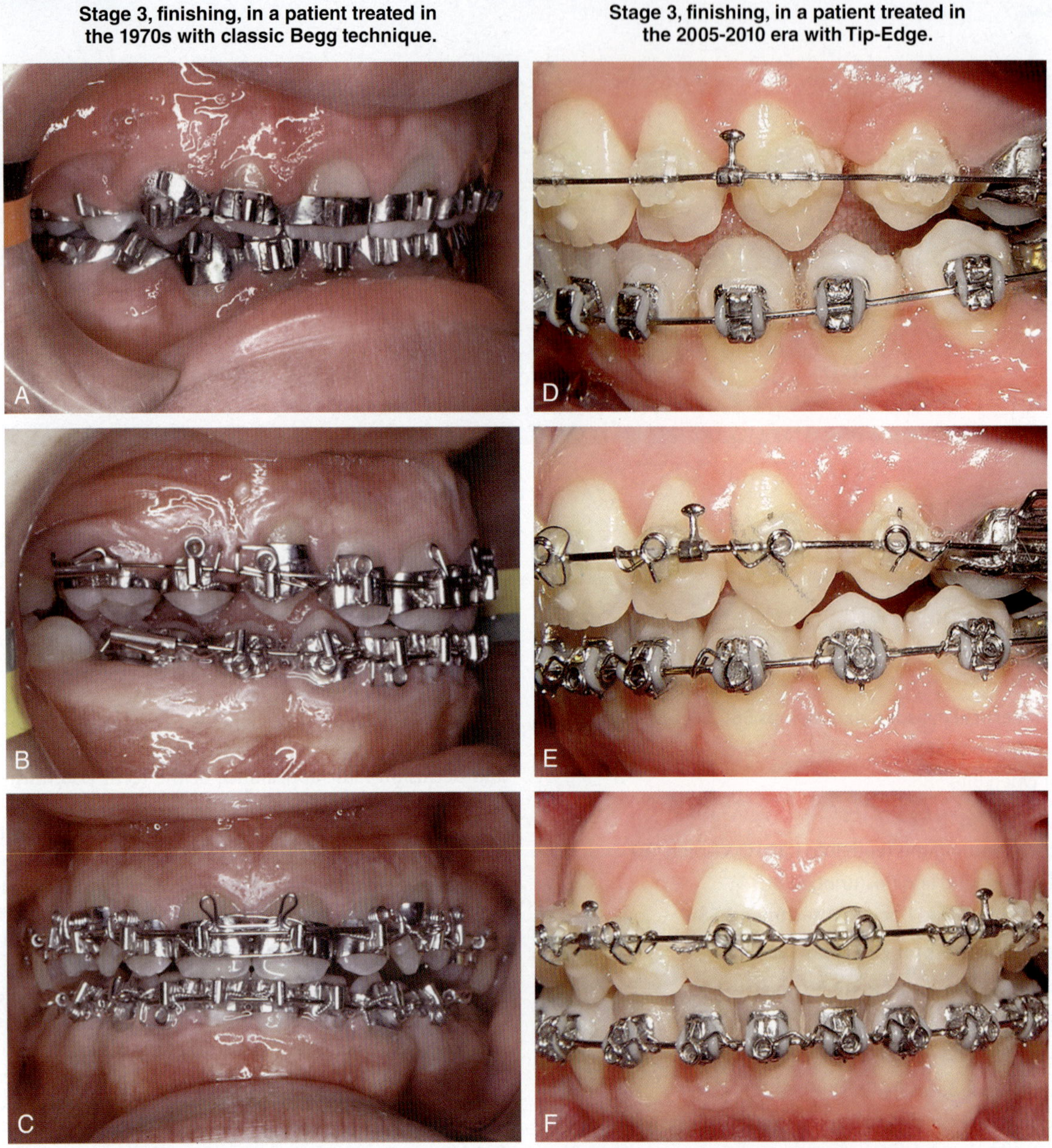

• **Fig. 17.1** Stage 3, Finishing, Comparing a Patient Treated With the Classic Begg Technique in the 1970s with One Treated in the 2005–10 Era With Tip-Edge, a Successor to Classic Begg. (A) The Begg appliance in a patient who has undergone premolar extraction and space closure and is ready for the finishing stage of treatment. Note the ribbon arch bracket turned upside down from the way Edward Angle positioned it. Archwires are pinned into place. (B) Uprighting springs and a torquing arch in place. The uprighting springs (used here on lateral incisors, canines, and second premolars) fit into the vertical tube portion of the bracket and are hooked underneath the base archwire to create root-positioning moments. An auxiliary torquing arch is threaded over the archwire and places a lingual force against the tooth above the bracket slot. (C) Anterior view of the torquing arch and uprighting springs. Stage 3, Finishing, in a Patient Treated in the 2005–10 Era With Tip-Edge. (D) The finishing stage of treatment with Tip-Edge, a modern extension of the Begg appliance, after tipping the teeth to close space and retract protruding incisors in this patient with Class II problems who had upper premolar extractions. (E) Auxiliary uprighting "SideWinder" springs (seen here on the maxillary lateral incisor, canine, and second premolar) are used for root positioning, with a different type of spring for the incisors where torque is desired, and a rectangular archwire serves as a template and prevents overcorrection. Note the improvement in both inclination of incisors and root paralleling at the extraction sites. (F) Frontal view. Note that the auxiliary spring for torque to incisors now is quite different from the Begg torquing arch or its equivalent for use as an edgewise auxiliary (see Fig. 17.6).

• BOX 17.1 Sequence of Archwires, Continuous Arch Edgewise Technique

18-Slot Appliance

Nonextraction

14 or 16 superelastic NiTi (A-NiTi)
16 steel (accentuated/reverse curve)
17 × 25 M-NiTi (only if roots displaced)
17 × 25 beta-Ti
17 × 25 steel

Extraction

14 or 16 superelastic NiTi
16 steel (accentuated/reverse curve)
16 × 22 steel closing loops
17 × 25 beta-Ti (if roots displaced, usually needed)
17 × 25 steel

22-Slot Appliances

Nonextraction

16 A-NiTi
16 steel (accentuated/reverse curve)
18 steel (accentuated/reverse curve)
21 × 25 M-NiTi
21 × 25 beta-Ti

Extraction

16 A-NiTi
16 steel (accentuated/reverse curve)
18 steel (accentuated/reverse curve)
19 × 25 steel, A-NiTi coil springs
or 18 × 22 steel T-loop or 19 × 25 beta-Ti delta loop
21 × 25 M-NiTi (if roots displaced, usually needed)
21 × 25 beta-Ti

For a typical adolescent patient with malocclusion of moderate severity. (Wire sizes in mil.)

A-NiTi, Austenitic (superelastic) NiTi; *beta-Ti*, beta-titanium (TMA); *M-NiTi*, martensitic (elastic, not superelastic) NiTi; *NiTi*, nickel-titanium.

for tooth positioning for both the 18- and the 22-slot appliances. In the 18-slot appliance, 17 × 25 beta-titanium (beta-Ti) usually is satisfactory. In the 22-slot appliance, 21 × 25 martensitic nickel-titanium (M-NiTi) often is the best choice; 21 × 25 beta-Ti is too stiff in bending, and smaller TMA wires fit too loosely in the bracket. Minor in-out and up-down adjustments, typically to obtain perfect canine interdigitation and level out marginal ridge heights, can be performed simply and easily by placing mild step bends in the finishing archwires.

If the choice is step bends, they must be placed in a flexible full-dimension wire, the next-to-last wire in the typical sequence shown in Box 17.1. Obviously, any step bends placed in the next-to-last wire (17 × 25 beta-Ti or 21 × 25 M-NiTi) must be repeated in the final wire that is used for torque (17 × 25 steel or 21 × 25 beta-Ti). Note that NiTi archwires (both M-NiTi and austenitic nickel-titanium [A-NiTi]) are *not* recommended for torquing. They simply do not have the torsional properties to be effective (see Chapter 9).

Although the position of a V-bend relative to the adjacent brackets is critical in determining its effect, the position of a step bend is not a critical variable. It makes little difference whether a step bend is in the center of the interbracket span or offset to either side.

Midline Discrepancies

A relatively common problem at the finishing stage of treatment is a discrepancy in the midlines of the dental arches. This can result from either a preexisting midline discrepancy that was not completely resolved at an earlier stage of treatment or asymmetric closure of spaces within the arch. Minor midline discrepancies at the finishing stage are no great problem, but it is quite difficult to correct large discrepancies after extraction spaces have been closed and occlusal relationships have been nearly established.

As with any discrepancy at the finishing stage, it is important to establish as clearly as possible exactly where the discrepancy arises. Although coincident dental midlines are a component of functional occlusion—all other things being equal, a midline discrepancy will be reflected in how the posterior teeth fit together—it is undesirable esthetically to displace the maxillary midline, bringing it around to meet a displaced mandibular midline. If a dental midline discrepancy results from a skeletal asymmetry, it may be impossible to correct it orthodontically, and treatment decisions will have to be made in the light of camouflage versus surgical correction (see discussion in Chapter 7).

Fortunately, midline discrepancies in the finishing stage usually are not this severe and are caused only by lateral displacements of maxillary or mandibular teeth that are likely to be accompanied by a mild Class II or Class III relationship on one side. In this circumstance, the midline can often be corrected by using asymmetric Class II (or Class III) elastic force. As a general rule, it is more effective to use Class II or Class III elastics bilaterally with heavier force on one side than to place a unilateral elastic. However, if one side is totally corrected while the other is not, patients usually tolerate a unilateral elastic reasonably well. It is also possible to combine a Class II or Class III elastic on one side with a diagonal elastic anteriorly to bring the midlines together (Fig. 17.2). This approach should be reserved for small discrepancies because asymmetric elastic use has asymmetric vertical side effects capable of producing an unesthetic anterior occlusal plane cant. Prolonged use of Class II or Class III elastics during the finishing stage of treatment should be avoided. Coordinated steps in the archwires also can be used to shift the teeth of one arch more than the other.[1]

An important consideration in dealing with midline discrepancies is the possibility of a mandibular shift contributing to the discrepancy. This can arise easily if a slight discrepancy in the transverse position of posterior teeth is present. For instance, a slightly narrow maxillary right posterior segment can lead to a shift of the mandible to the left on final closure, creating the midline discrepancy. The correction in this instance, obviously, must include some force system to alter the transverse arch relationships (usually careful coordination of the maxillary and mandibular archwires, perhaps reinforced by a posterior cross-elastic). Occasionally, the entire maxillary arch is slightly displaced transversely relative to the mandibular arch so that with the teeth in occlusion, relationships are excellent, but there is a lateral shift to reach that position. Correction again would involve posterior cross-elastics but in a parallel pattern (i.e., from maxillary lingual to mandibular buccal on one side and the reverse on the other side.

Tooth-Size Discrepancies

Correction of tooth-size discrepancy or compensation for it must be part of the initial treatment plan, but many of the steps to deal with these problems are taken in the finishing stage of treatment.[2] Interproximal enamel reduction (IPR) is the usual strategy

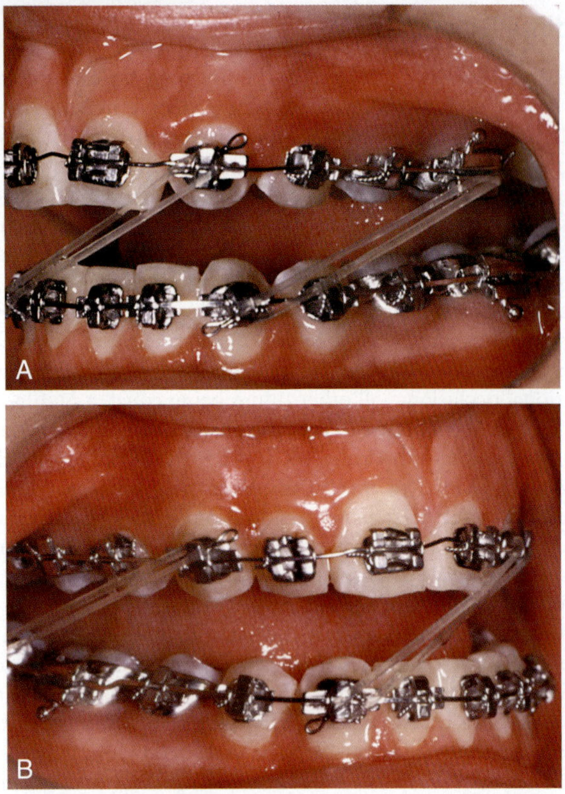

• **Fig. 17.2** (A and B) Midline correction can be approached with any combination of asymmetric posterior and anterior diagonal elastics. In this patient, a combination of Class II, Class III, and anterior diagonal elastics is being used (a "parallel elastics" arrangement), with a rectangular archwire in the lower arch and a round wire in the upper arch, in an attempt to shift the maxillary arch to the right.

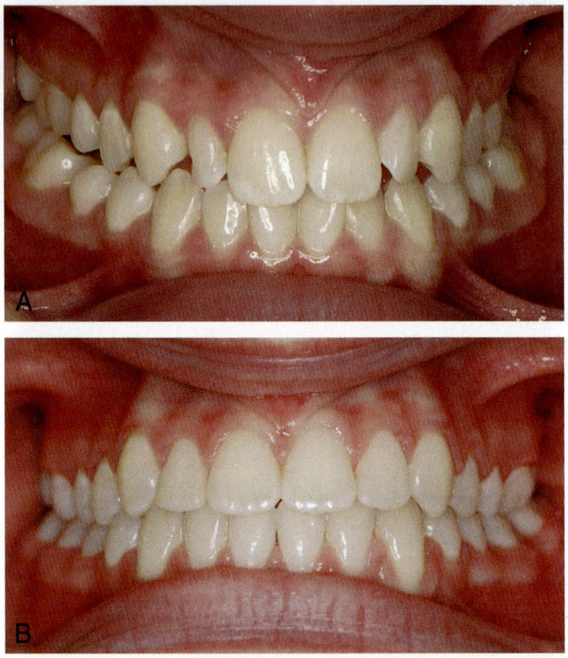

• **Fig. 17.3** Small maxillary lateral incisors create tooth-size discrepancy problems that may become apparent only late in treatment. (A) Small maxillary lateral incisors, one of which is distorted, before treatment. (B) After treatment in which space was created mesial and distal to the laterals so that laminates could be placed to bring the teeth to normal size and appearance.

to compensate for discrepancies caused by excess tooth size. When the problem is tooth-size deficiency, it is necessary to leave space between some teeth, which may or may not ultimately be closed by restorations. As a general guideline, a 2-mm tooth-size discrepancy noted from Bolton analysis is the threshold for clinical significance[3] (i.e., it is predicted such a large discrepancy will necessitate steps to deal with it during treatment), but at the finishing stage, you get to see how accurate the prediction really was.

One of the advantages of a bonded appliance is that interproximal enamel can be removed at any time. When IPR is part of the original treatment plan, most of the enamel reduction should be done initially, but final reduction can be deferred until the finishing stage. This procedure allows direct observation of the occlusal relationships before the final tooth-size adjustments are made. A topical fluoride treatment always is recommended immediately after IPR is done.

Tooth-size problems are often caused by small maxillary lateral incisors. Leaving a small space distal to the lateral incisor can be esthetically and functionally acceptable, but a composite resin buildup is usually the best plan for small incisors (Fig. 17.3). Precise finishing is easier if the buildup is done during the finishing stage of the orthodontic treatment. This can be accomplished simply by removing the bracket from the small tooth or teeth for a few hours while the restoration is done, then replacing the bracket and archwires (but bonding to a laminate veneer may damage the surface, so a buildup to establish tooth size is okay, but a veneer should be delayed). It is important to verify that the root position is close to ideal before restoration, because change in root position after buildup can alter esthetics by changing contact points and embrasure relationships. If the restoration is delayed until the orthodontic treatment is completed, it should be done as soon as possible after the patient is in retention. This requires an initial retainer to hold the space, and a new retainer immediately after the restoration is completed. The main reason for waiting until after the orthodontic appliance has been removed would be to allow any gingival inflammation to resolve.

More generalized small deficiencies can be masked by altering incisor position in any of several ways. To a limited extent, torque of the upper incisors can be used to compensate: leaving the incisors slightly more upright makes them take up less room relative to the lower arch and can be used to mask large upper incisors, whereas slightly excessive torque can partially compensate for small upper incisors. These adjustments require third-order bends in the finishing archwires, done manually or as a new archwire from altering the wire prescription in SureSmile and similar systems for robotic wire-bending. It is also possible to compensate by slightly tipping teeth or by finishing the orthodontic treatment with mildly excessive overbite or overjet, depending on the individual circumstances.[4]

Root Paralleling

In the original Begg technique (see Fig. 17.1A–C), the moments necessary for root positioning were generated by adding auxiliary springs into the vertical slot of the Begg (ribbon arch) bracket. In the modified Begg technique using the Tip-Edge appliance, root paralleling is accomplished with uprighting springs, very much as it was with traditional Begg treatment (see Fig. 17.1D–F). Rectangular wire is used primarily for torque (faciolingual root movement), not the mesiodistal root movement needed for root paralleling after teeth were allowed to tip during space closure.

During space closure with the edgewise appliance, it is almost always a goal of treatment to produce bodily tooth movement, preventing the crowns from tipping toward each other. If proper moment-to-force ratios have been used, little if any root paralleling will be necessary as a finishing procedure. On the other hand, it is likely that at least a small amount of tipping will occur in some patients and therefore some degree of root paralleling at extraction sites will often be necessary. If brackets were not oriented correctly at the time of placement, root separation or paralleling may be needed in nonextraction cases (this is most likely on maxillary lateral incisors and premolars). It is wise to obtain a panoramic radiograph when major tooth movement has been completed, to check for both root-positioning errors and root resorption that might dictate ending treatment early or taking a break from the final active treatment for 3 to 4 months to allow cementum to heal.

The same approach used for root positioning in Begg technique can be employed with the edgewise appliance if it includes a vertical slot behind the edgewise bracket that allows an uprighting spring to be inserted and hooked beneath a base archwire. When only steel archwires were available, this approach often was used, but in contemporary edgewise practice, it has been almost totally abandoned in favor of angulated bracket slots that produce proper root paralleling when a flexible full-dimension rectangular wire is placed.

With the 18-slot appliance, the typical finishing archwire is either 17 × 22 or 17 × 25 steel. These wires are flexible enough to engage narrow brackets even if mild tipping has occurred, and the archwire will generate the necessary root paralleling moments. If a greater degree of tipping has occurred, a more flexible full-dimension rectangular archwire is needed. To correct more severe tipping, a 17 × 25 beta-Ti (TMA) or even a 17 × 25 nickel-titanium (M-NiTi, not superelastic A-NiTi) wire might be needed initially, with a steel archwire used for final expression of torque.

With wider 22-slot brackets on the canines and premolars and with the use of sliding rather than loop mechanics to close extraction sites, there is usually even less need for root paralleling as a finishing procedure. But with 22-slot brackets, if teeth have tipped even slightly into an extraction space or if other root positioning is needed, steel archwires (19 × 25 steel, for instance) are much too stiff. A 21 × 25 beta-Ti wire is the best choice for a finishing archwire under most circumstances, and if significant root positioning is needed, 21 × 25 M-NiTi should be used first.

Although superelastic NiTi (A-NiTi) wires perform much better than elastic NiTi (M-NiTi) wires in alignment, this is not true of their performance as rectangular finishing wires. The great advantage of A-NiTi is its very flat load-deflection curve, which gives it a large range. In the finishing stage, however, appropriate stiffness at relatively small deflections, rather than range, is the primary consideration. A-NiTi wires usually deliver less force than their M-NiTi counterparts (this will depend on how the manufacturer manipulated the wire as it was produced [see Chapter 9]), and if rectangular NiTi wires are used in the finishing stage, M-NiTi almost always is the better choice. Why? Because it provides adequate force for root movement and less range, both of which are needed for precise tooth positioning. Occasionally, a severely tipped tooth will be encountered (almost always because of a bracket positioning error), and a greater range of action is needed. This may indicate use of a rectangular A-NiTi wire initially, then M-NiTi. An alternative, usually practical only if the edgewise brackets have a vertical slot or tube, is a Burstone auxiliary root-uprighting spring (Fig. 17.4).

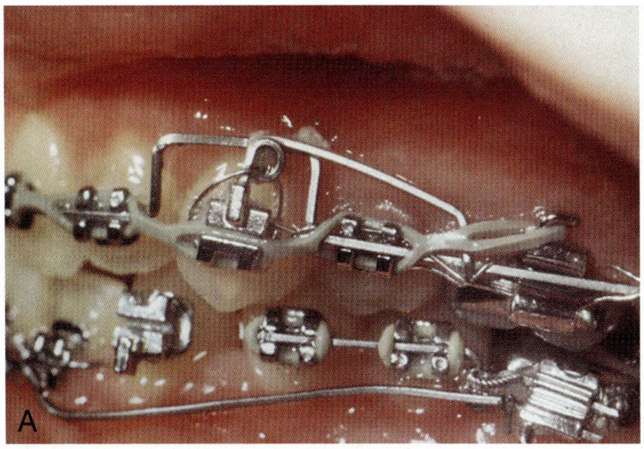

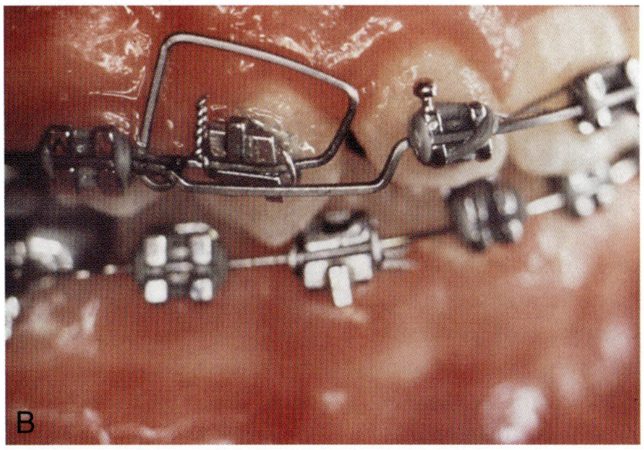

• **Fig. 17.4** (A) An uprighting spring to the maxillary canine, placed in a vertical tube incorporated into the canine bracket, in segmented arch technique. Note that the base archwire bypasses the canine. (B) An auxiliary root-positioning spring welded to the base archwire and tied into the edgewise bracket slot of a maxillary canine, with the base archwire bypassing the canine. Both approaches remain useful for correction of severe root-paralleling problems, but with the introduction of contemporary straight-wire appliances, use of auxiliary uprighting springs in edgewise technique has largely been replaced by resilient nickel-titanium (NiTi) or beta-titanium (beta-Ti) continuous archwires in preangulated brackets. (Courtesy Dr. C. Burstone.)

A root-paralleling moment is a crown-separating moment in edgewise technique just as it is in any other technique. Either the teeth must be tied together or the entire archwire must be tied back against the molars (Fig. 17.5) to prevent spaces from opening. Not only extraction sites but also maxillary incisors must be protected against this complication. When a full-dimension rectangular wire is placed in the maxillary arch, spaces are likely to open between the incisors in nonextraction as well as extraction cases. Tying the maxillary incisors together, which can be done conveniently with a segment of elastomeric chain from the mesial bracket of one upper lateral incisor across to the mesial bracket of the other, is necessary during finishing.

Torque

Lingual Root Torque of Incisors

If protruding incisors tipped lingually more than desired while they were being retracted, lingual root torque as a finishing procedure may be required. In the Begg technique, the incisors were deliberately tipped back during the second stage of treatment, and lingual root torque was a routine part of the third stage of treatment. As with root paralleling, this was accomplished with an auxiliary appliance that fit over the main or base archwire. The

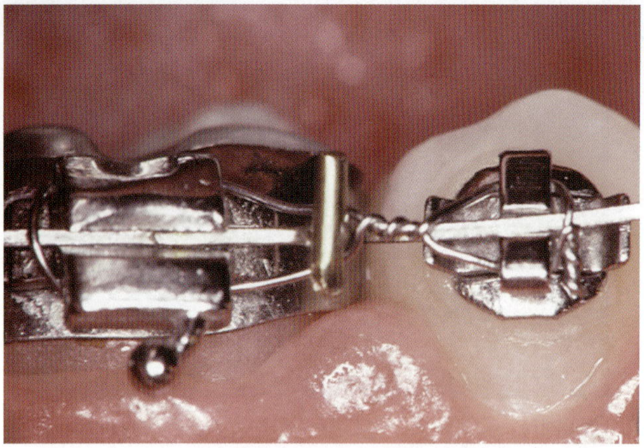

• **Fig. 17.5** A rectangular archwire that incorporates active root-paralleling moments or torque must be tied back against the molar teeth to prevent space from opening within the arch. If the ligature used to tie back the archwire is cabled forward and also used to tie the second premolar, the tieback is less likely to come loose.

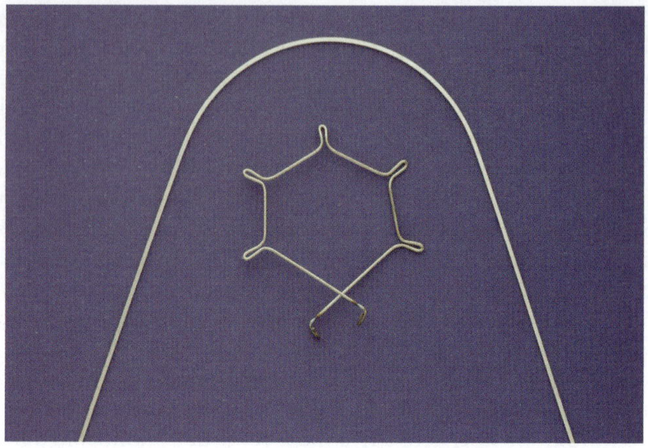

• **Fig. 17.6** Torquing auxiliary archwires exert their effect when the auxiliary, originally bent in a tight circle as shown, is forced to assume the form of a base archwire over which it will be placed. This tends to distort the base archwire, which should therefore be relatively stiff—at least 18-mil steel.

torquing auxiliary is a "piggyback arch" that contacts the labial surface of the incisors near the gingival margin, creating the necessary couple with a moment arm of 4 to 5 mm (see Fig. 17.1C).

These piggyback torquing arches can be used in edgewise technique in the same way (see Fig. 15.30D). Although they come in several designs, the basic principle is the same: the auxiliary arch, bent into a tight circle initially, exerts a force against the roots of the teeth as it is partially straightened out to normal arch form (Fig. 17.6).

A torquing force to move the roots lingually is also, of course, a force to move the crowns labially (see Fig. 16.3). In a typical patient with a Class II malocclusion, anchorage is required to maintain overjet correction while upper incisor roots are torqued lingually. For that reason, Class II elastics are likely to be necessary when active lingual root torque is needed during the final stage of Class II treatment.

With a modern edgewise appliance, only moderate additional incisor torque should be necessary during the finishing stage. With the 18-slot appliance, a 17 × 25 steel archwire has excellent properties in torsion, and torque with this archwire is entirely feasible. Built-in torque in the bracket slot means that it is unnecessary to place torquing bends in the archwire, making the accomplishment of torque as a finishing procedure relatively straightforward.

With the 22-slot appliance, full-dimension steel rectangular wires are far too stiff for effective torquing (see Fig. 9.11). If incisors have been allowed to tip too much lingually, correcting this merely by placing a rectangular steel archwire in a torque-prescription bracket is not effective because the wire creates too much torsional force and has a very limited range. Before brackets with built-in torque and titanium archwires were available, torquing auxiliaries were commonly used with the 22-slot appliance. One of the great virtues of torque-slot brackets is that tipping of incisors, for the most part, can be prevented during retraction and space closure. In addition, full-dimension M-NiTi or beta-Ti archwires can be used to torque incisors with 22-slot brackets (provided the brackets have torque built in), further reducing any need for auxiliary arches. For these reasons, torquing auxiliaries for 22-slot edgewise have almost disappeared from contemporary use, except when upright incisors are to be corrected by tipping the crowns facially. The auxiliaries are probably the best way to do this.

One torquing auxiliary, however, deserves special mention: the Burstone torquing arch (Fig. 17.7). It can be particularly helpful

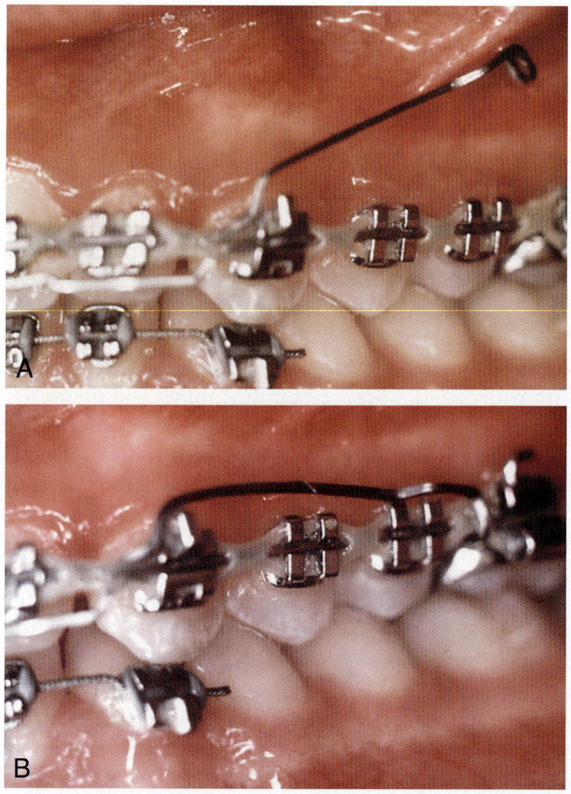

• **Fig. 17.7** The Burstone torquing auxiliary (also see Fig. 9.44) is particularly useful in Class II division 2 cases in which maxillary central incisors need a large amount of torque. The torquing auxiliary is full-dimension steel wire (21 × 25 or 17 × 25, in 22- or 18-slot brackets, respectively) that fits in the brackets only on the incisors. It can be used only on the centrals or on the centrals and laterals, as shown here. The base arch (preferably also full-dimension rectangular wire) extends forward from the molars through the canine or lateral incisor brackets, then steps down and rests against the labial surface of the teeth to be torqued. When the torquing auxiliary is passive (A), its long posterior arms are up in the buccal vestibule. It is activated (B) by pulling the arms down and hooking them beneath the base archwire mesial to the first molar. The segment of the base arch that rests against the labial surface of the central incisors is tied back to the molar buccal tubes (see Fig. 17.5), which prevents the crowns from going forward, and the result is efficient lingual root torque.

in patients with Class II division 2 malocclusion whose maxillary central incisors are severely tipped lingually and require a long distance of torquing movement, while the lateral incisors need little if any torque. Because of the long lever arm, this is the most effective auxiliary. It is equally effective with the 18- or 22-slot appliance. If all four incisors need considerable torque, use of a wire spanning from the molar auxiliary tube to the incisors, with a V-bend so that the incisor segment receives the greater moment, is a highly efficient approach.[5]

Three factors determine the amount of torque that will be expressed by any rectangular archwire in a rectangular slot: the torsional stiffness of the wire, the inclination of the bracket slot relative to the archwire, and the tightness of the fit between the archwire and the bracket. The variations in torque prescriptions in contemporary edgewise brackets are discussed in Chapter 10. These variations largely reflect different determinations of the average contour of the labial and buccal surfaces of the teeth, but some differences are also related to the expected fit of archwires.

With the 18-slot appliance, it is assumed that the rectangular archwires used for finishing will fit tightly in the bracket slot (i.e., that the finishing archwires will have a minimum dimension of 17 mil). With the 22-slot appliance, on the other hand, some prescriptions have extra built-in torque to compensate for rectangular finishing archwires that will have more clearance. Torque will not be expressed to the same extent with a 19 × 25 wire in a 22-slot bracket as with a 17 × 25 wire in an 18-slot bracket. The difference amounts to several degrees of difference in incisor inclination. The "effective torque" of various wire-bracket combinations is shown in Table 17.1. Obviously, when the torque prescription for a bracket is established, it is important to know what finishing wires are intended.

TABLE 17.1 Effective Torque

		BRACKET TORQUE ANGLE (DEGREES)		
		10	20	30
Wire Size	Play (Degrees)	Effective Torque		
18-Slot Bracket				
16 × 16	10.9	0.0	11.1	19.1
16 × 22	9.3	0.7	12.7	20.7
17 × 25	4.1	5.9	17.9	25.9
18 × 18	1.5	8.5	20.5	28.5
18 × 25	1.0	9.0	21.0	29.0
22-Slot Bracket				
16 × 22	21.9	0	0.1	8.1
17 × 25	15.5	0	6.5	13.5
19 × 25	9.6	0.4	12.4	20.4
21 × 25	4.1	5.9	17.9	25.9
21.5 × 28	1.8	8.2	20.2	28.2

Based on nominal wire and/or slot sizes; actual play is likely to be greater.
From Semetz F. Qualität und Normung orthodontischer Produkte aus der Sicht des Herstellers. *Kieferorthop Mitteil.* 1993;7:13–26.

For full expression of the torque built into brackets in the 22-slot appliance, the best finishing wire is usually 21 × 25 beta-Ti. This wire's torsional stiffness is less than that of 17 × 25 steel (see Fig. 9.11), but the shorter interbracket distances with 22-slot twin brackets bring its performance in torsion close to that of the smaller steel wire. Braided rectangular steel wires are available in a variety of stiffnesses, and the stiffest of these in 21 × 25 dimension can also be useful in 22-slot finishing. A solid 21 × 25 steel wire cannot be recommended because of its stiffness and the resulting extremely high forces and short range of action. If a solid steel wire of this size is used (the major reason would be surgical stabilization), it should be preceded by 21 × 25 beta-Ti.

Some clinicians are reluctant to use full-dimension archwires in 22-slot brackets, but it should be kept in mind that full torque expression will never be achieved with undersized wires without extreme bracket prescriptions or placement of major twist bends in the wires, and even then it is difficult to obtain adequate torque routinely.

Buccal Root Torque of Premolars and Molars

It should be kept in mind that buccal root torque of maxillary premolars can be an important esthetic consideration in positioning these teeth. It is surprisingly common that at the end of fixed appliance treatment, maxillary canines and premolars are tipped facially because the prescription in many modern brackets provides negative torque (lingual crown torque) for these teeth (see Table 10.2). Zachrisson has pointed out that this negatively affects smile esthetics, especially in patients with narrow and tapered arch forms, by making the canines less prominent and causing the first premolars to almost disappear on smile. To obtain a broader and more pleasing smile, the solution is not to further expand across the premolars, but to use buccal crown torque so that the crowns are uprighted (Figs. 17.8 and 17.9).[6] This gives the appearance of a broader smile without the risk of relapse that accompanies arch expansion. Long-term data indicate that the inclinations of these teeth remain the way they were at the end of treatment, so changing the torque is stable.[7]

Research into what patients see as important in dental esthetics did not confirm this subtle effect as important in affecting patient perceptions of the appearance of the teeth. Although some lay people noticed it, the majority simply had no idea what they were looking at. Orthodontists are much more likely to appreciate the esthetic effect of this uprighting, which may also provide better interdigitation of first premolar lingual cusps.

Correction of Vertical Incisor Relationships

If the first two stages of treatment have been accomplished perfectly, no change in the vertical relationship of incisors will be needed during the finishing stage of treatment. Minor adjustments are often needed, however, and major ones are occasionally required. At this stage, anterior open bite is more likely to be a problem than residual excessive overbite, but either may be encountered.

Excessive Overbite

Before attempting to correct excess overbite at the finishing stage of treatment, it is important to carefully assess why the problem exists and particularly to evaluate two things: (1) the vertical relationship between the maxillary lip and maxillary incisors and (2) anterior face height. If the display of the maxillary incisors on

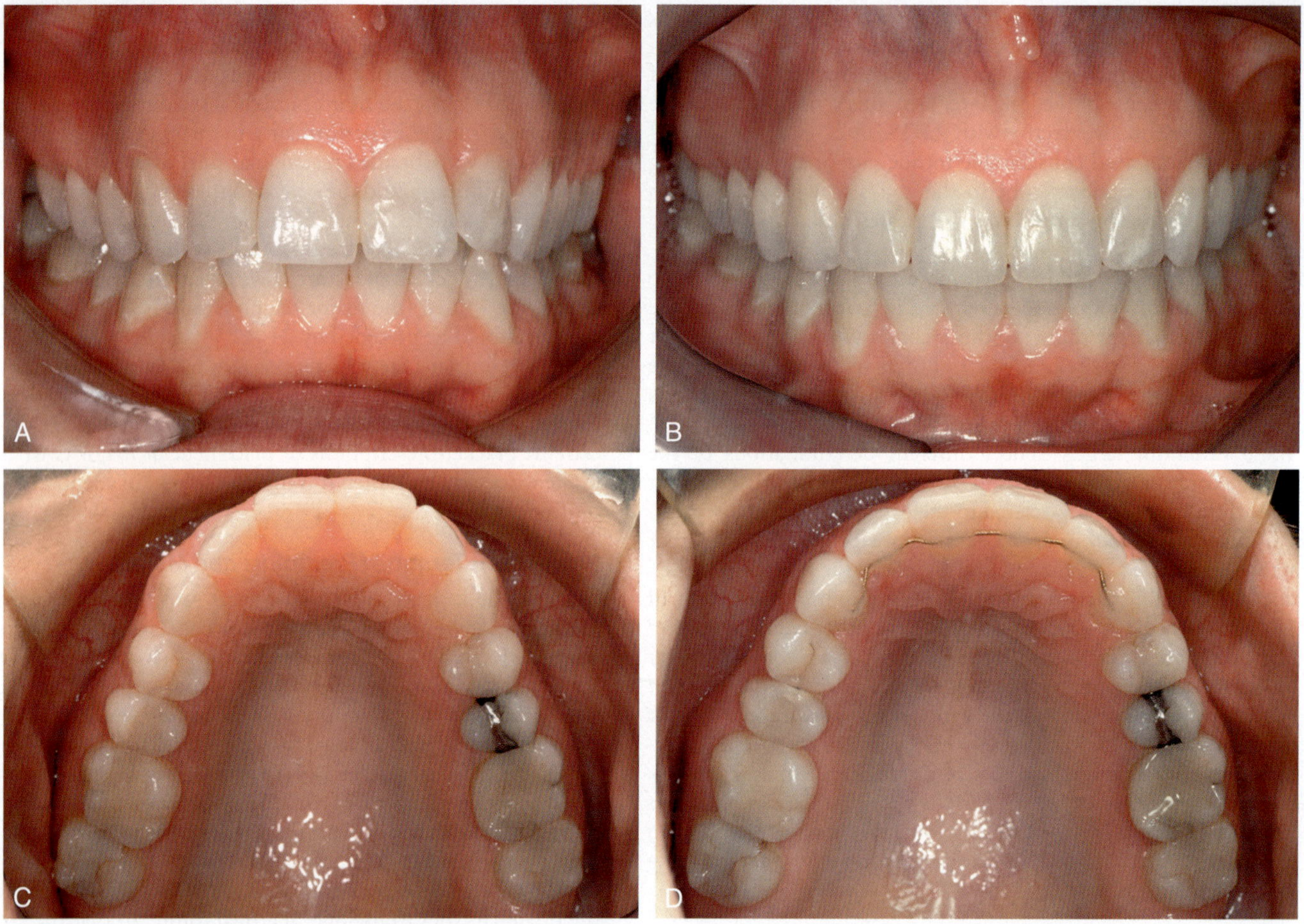

• **Fig. 17.8** For this patient the maxillary arch looks narrow because the canine and premolars are tipped lingually, but significant expansion across the canines and premolars is not necessary. Instead, torque to the canines and especially to the premolars so that these teeth are uprighted faciolingually without major expansion improves the appearance of the dentition, and the torque changes are stable in a way that expansion is not. (A and B) Before treatment. (C and D) After treatment that included torque to upright the canines and premolars. (Courtesy Dr. B. Zachrisson.)

smile is appropriate, it is important to maintain this and make any overbite correction by repositioning the lower incisors. If display is excessive, intrusion of the upper incisors would be indicated. If face height is short, elongating the posterior teeth slightly (almost always, the lower posterior teeth) would be acceptable; if face height is long, intrusion of incisors would be needed.

If intrusion is indicated and a rectangular finishing archwire is already in place, the simplest approach is to cut this archwire distal to the lateral incisors and install an auxiliary intrusion arch that is tied to this segment in the appropriate place. Remember that when a maxillary auxiliary intrusion arch is used, a stabilizing transpalatal lingual arch may be needed to maintain control of transverse relationships and prevent excessive distal tipping of the maxillary molars (see Fig. 15.23). The greater the desired vertical change in incisor position, the more important it will be to have a stabilizing lingual arch in place and vice versa. Small corrections during finishing usually do not require placement of a lingual arch.

Alternatively, if slight elongation of the posterior teeth is indicated, step bends in a flexible archwire would be satisfactory. The intermediate archwire before the final torquing archwire is the one for implementation of these step bends (17 × 25 TMA with the 18-slot appliance, 21 × 25 M-NiTi with the 22-slot appliance). An auxiliary depressing arch for overbite correction can be effective, but only if the base archwire is a relatively small round wire (see Chapter 15), so this is not the preferred approach for a modest amount of final overbite correction.

Anterior Open Bite

As with deep bite, it is important to analyze the source of the difficulty if an anterior open bite persists at the finishing stage of treatment, and as with deep bite, the relationship of the upper incisors to the lip and anterior face height is critical in determining what to do. If the open bite results from excessive eruption of posterior teeth, whether from a poor growth pattern or excessive use of interarch elastics (Fig. 17.10), correcting it at the finishing stage can be extremely difficult. The most effective approach to intrusion of posterior teeth is skeletal anchorage. Placing miniplates or palatal anchors at the finishing stage to accomplish this implies that the earlier stages of treatment were not completed satisfactorily, but this might be necessary in some patients with a severe long face pattern of growth.

If no severe problems with the pattern of facial growth exist, however, a mild open bite at the finishing stage of treatment often is due to an excessively level lower arch. This condition is managed best by elongating the lower but not the upper incisors, thereby creating a slight curve of Spee in the lower arch. Because of the stiffness of the rectangular archwires used for finishing, even with

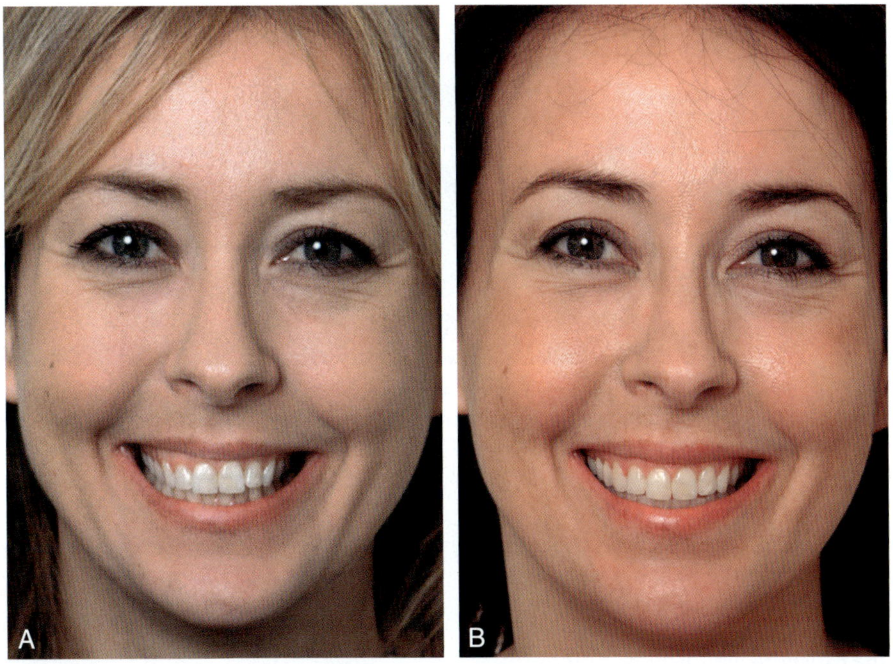

• **Fig. 17.9** (A and B) Same patient as Fig. 17.8. Note the improvement in smile esthetics and "width of the smile" produced by torque to the canines and premolars. This can be obtained most readily by changing the bracket prescription to decrease or eliminate the negative torque in most current prescription brackets for maxillary canines and premolars (see Table 10.3). (Courtesy Dr. B. Zachrisson.)

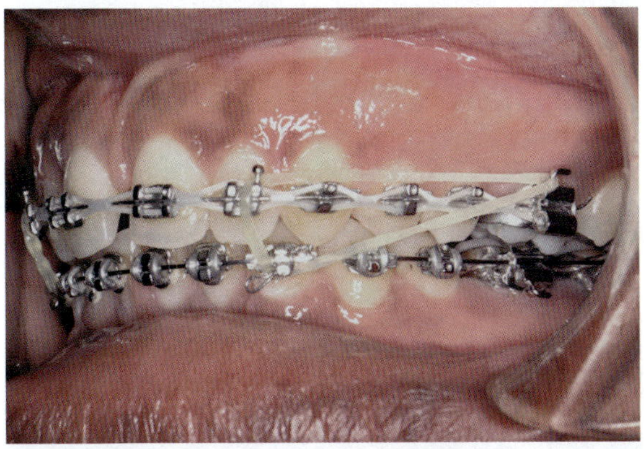

• **Fig. 17.10** Class III elastics tend to extrude upper molars, and their use can lead rapidly to the development of anterior open bite. Use of a triangular Class III elastic, as shown here, helps to control the open bite tendency. Class II elastics can do the same thing by extruding lower molars, and the bite opening can be reduced by a similar triangulation. Use of Class III or Class II elastics, of course, presupposes that some elongation of the molars is acceptable.

an 18-slot edgewise appliance, it is futile to use vertical elastics to deepen the bite without altering the form of the archwires. Steps in an appropriately flexible lower archwire, while maintaining a stiffer upper wire, can be effective when supplemented with light vertical elastics (Fig. 17.11). Obviously, if display of the upper incisors is inadequate, elongation of those teeth to close the bite would be indicated, and the same approach with the flexible or stabilizing archwires reversed would be indicated. Elongating the lower incisors to close a moderate anterior open bite is a quite stable procedure. Elongating the upper incisors is less stable and compromises facial esthetics if it makes them too prominent. This should be kept in mind when vertical repositioning of incisors is planned.

Final "Settling" of Teeth

At the conclusion of treatment with the edgewise appliance, it is not uncommon for a full-dimension rectangular archwire, no matter how carefully made, to hold some teeth slightly out of occlusion. The more precisely a stiff finishing archwire fits the brackets and the more bends that have been used to compensate for bracket positioning, the more likely it is that some teeth will be almost but not quite in occlusion. This phenomenon was recognized by the pioneers with the edgewise appliance, who coined the term "arch-bound" to describe it. They found that with precisely fitting wires, it was almost impossible to get every tooth into solid occlusion, although one could come close. From the early days of edgewise treatment to the present, therefore, a final step of bringing the teeth into occlusion, appropriately called "settling" the teeth, has been needed.

Methods for Settling the Teeth Into Ideal Occlusion

There are three ways to settle the occlusion:

- Replacing the rectangular archwires at the very end of treatment with light round arches that provide some freedom for movement of the teeth (16 mil in the 18-slot appliance, 16 or 18 mil in the 22-slot appliance) and using light vertical elastics to bring the teeth together
- Using laced posterior vertical elastics after removing the posterior segments of the archwires
- Using a tooth positioner or a limited series of aligners after the bands and brackets have been removed

Replacing full-dimension rectangular wires with light round wires at the very end of treatment was the original method for settling, recommended by Tweed and perhaps by other edgewise pioneers earlier. As we noted earlier, it is simply not correct that

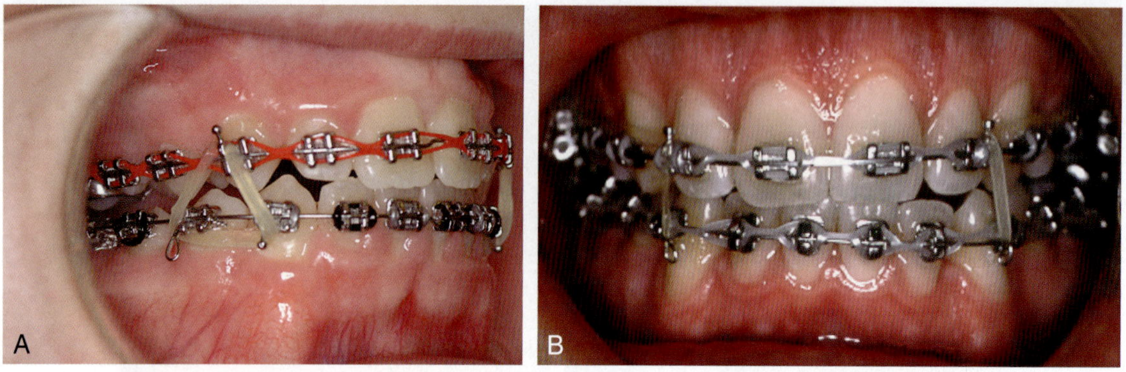

• **Fig. 17.11** Vertical elastics, (A) bilaterally in the triangular hook-up shown here in conjunction with an anterior box elastic or (B) as an anterior box elastic alone, can be used to help close a mild anterior open bite at the end of treatment, but this is effective only if the archwires are contoured to allow the tooth movement. Elastics cannot overpower a stiff archwire that is maintaining the open bite.

when edgewise brackets are used, the final archwires should be full-dimension rectangular ones. That idea went out with Angle—or should have. These light final arches must include any first- or second-order bends used in the rectangular finishing arches. It is usually unnecessary for the patient to wear light posterior vertical elastics during this settling, but they can be used if needed. These light arches will quickly settle the teeth into final occlusion and should remain in place for only a few weeks at most.

The difficulty with undersized round wires at the end of treatment is that some freedom of movement for settling posterior teeth is achieved, but precise control of anterior teeth is lost. It was not until the 1980s that orthodontists realized the advantage of removing only the posterior part of the rectangular finishing wire, leaving the anterior segment (typically canine-to-canine) in place, and using laced elastics to bring the posterior teeth into tight occlusion (Fig. 17.12).[8] This sacrifices a large degree of control of the posterior teeth and therefore should not be used in patients who had major rotations or posterior crossbite. For the majority of patients who had well-aligned posterior teeth from the beginning, however, this is a remarkably simple and effective way to settle the teeth into their final occlusion. It is the last step in active treatment for most patients at present. Light, not heavy, force is needed.

A typical arrangement is to use light ¾-inch elastics, with a Class II or Class III direction, depending on whether slightly more correction is desired. An alternative is to use a pair of 5/16- or ⅜-inch interarch elastics on both sides in a vertical triangle. These elastics should not remain in place for more than 2 weeks, and 1 week usually is enough to accomplish the desired settling. At that point the fixed appliances should be removed and the retainers placed.

Because it occurs after the orthodontic appliance has been removed, the use of a tooth positioner or aligners for final settling is discussed after the section on removing bands and bonded brackets.

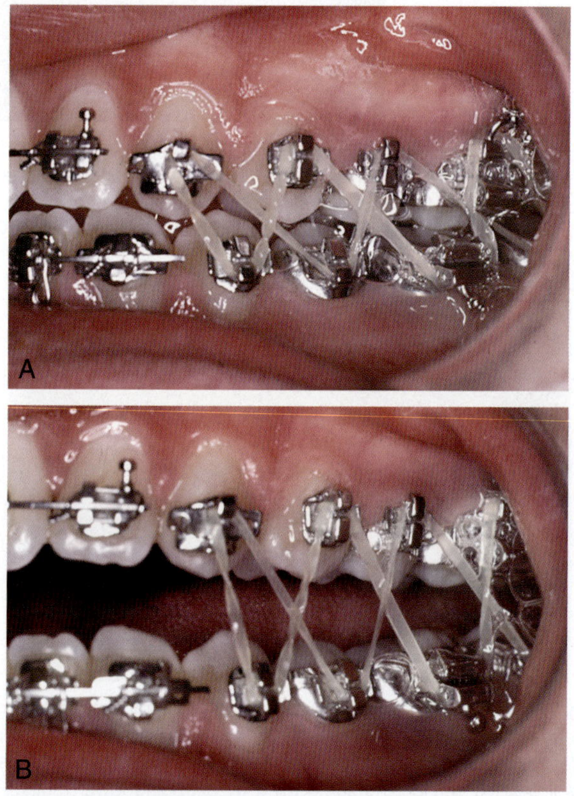

• **Fig. 17.12** (A and B) Laced elastics for settling the posterior teeth into final occlusion at the end of treatment, after the posterior wire segments have been removed. The elastics can be used either with light round archwires or (usually preferred) with rectangular segments in the anterior brackets and no wire at all posteriorly. With this method, the last step in treatment is cutting the rectangular finishing archwires distal to the lateral incisors or canines and removing the posterior segments, followed by 1 to 2 weeks of settling with the light elastics before debonding and debanding.

Control of Rebound and Posturing

After Class II or Class III correction, the teeth tend to rebound back toward their initial position despite the presence of rectangular archwires. Because of this, it is important to slightly overcorrect the occlusal relationships. In a typical patient with Class II anterior deep bite, the teeth should be taken to an end-to-end incisor relationship, with both overjet and overbite totally eliminated, before discontinuing Class II elastics or another type of Class II corrector. This provides some latitude for the teeth to rebound before final settling is accomplished.

Sometimes when Class II elastic force or its equivalent is used, patients begin to posture the mandible forward so that the occlusion looks more corrected than it really is; if the appliances are removed at that point, the patient is likely to slip back toward a

Class II molar relationship and increased overjet. This should not be confused with rebound, which is due only to tooth movement. Rebound is a 1- to 2-mm phenomenon; posturing can lead to 4 to 5 mm of relapse, and obviously it is important to detect it and continue treatment to a true correction.

These considerations lead to the guidelines for finishing treatment when interarch elastics have been used:

- When an appropriate degree of overcorrection has been achieved, the force used with the elastics should be decreased or the wear interval reduced (8–12 h/day) while the elastics are continued for another appointment interval.
- At that point, interarch elastics should be discontinued, 4 to 8 weeks before the orthodontic appliances are to be removed, so that changes due to rebound or posturing can be observed. It is better to tell the patient that he or she is getting a vacation from the elastics and that some further elastic wear may be necessary if changes are observed, rather than saying that elastics are no longer needed. If changes do occur, that makes it easier for patients to accept that the vacation is over and another period of elastics is needed.
- If the occlusion is stable, as a final step in treatment the teeth should be brought into a solid occlusal relationship without heavy archwires present by using one of the methods described earlier.

Removal of Bands and Bonded Attachments

Removal of bands is accomplished by breaking the cement attachment and then lifting the band off the tooth, which sounds simpler than it is in some instances. For upper molar and premolar teeth, a band-removing instrument is placed so that first the lingual then the buccal surfaces are elevated (Fig. 17.13). A welded lingual bar is needed on these bands to provide a point of attachment for the pliers if lingual hooks or cleats are not a part of the appliance. For the lower posterior teeth, the sequence of force is just the reverse: the band remover is applied first on the buccal then on the lingual surface.

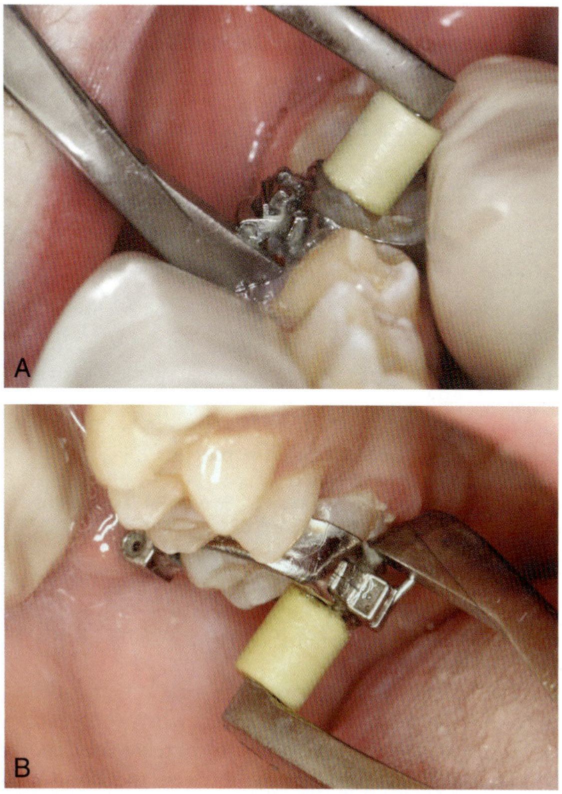

• **Fig. 17.13** Removal of molar bands with band-removing pliers. (A) Lower posterior bands are removed primarily with pressure from the buccal surface. (B) Upper posterior bands are removed with pressure primarily against the lingual surface, which is easier when a lingual tube (as shown here), cleat, or other attachment was welded to the band initially.

Bonded brackets must be removed, insofar as possible, without damaging the enamel surface. This is done by creating a fracture within the resin bonding material or between the bracket and the resin, and then removing the residual resin from the enamel surface. With metal brackets, applying special pliers to the base of the bracket so that the bracket bends (Fig. 17.14) is the safest method. This has the disadvantage of destroying the bracket so that it cannot be reused, but protecting the enamel is usually is a more important consideration.

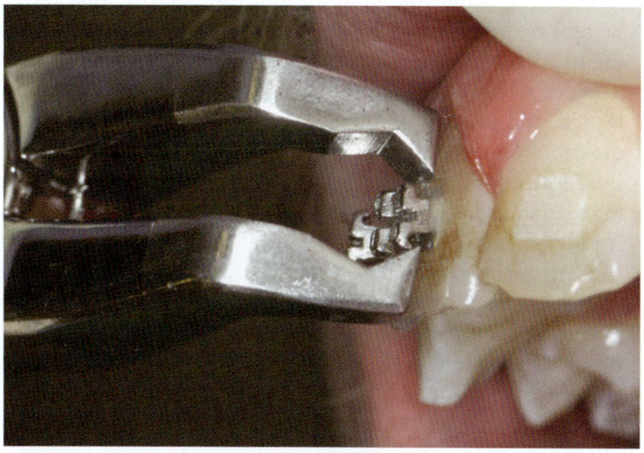

• **Fig. 17.14** Removal of bonded metal brackets. Special pliers can be used to flex the bracket and fracture the bonding resin, which usually results in much of the resin being left on the tooth surface.

Enamel damage from debonding metal brackets has been considered rare, but soon after ceramic brackets were introduced, there were reports of enamel fractures and removal of chunks of enamel when they were debonded (see Chapter 10 for a more detailed discussion). A recent study evaluated how frequently enamel fragments were found on the bracket base of mechanically debonded maxillary anterior teeth (canine-to-canine).[9] Data from this study are summarized in Table 17.2.

The differences between the groups for enamel damage and bracket fracture are statistically significant and clearly show that damage at debonding is more likely with ceramic than metal brackets. The damage rate with ceramic brackets was significantly less for ceramic brackets bonded with a resin-modified glass-ionomer cement (which is discussed in some detail in Chapter 10). The size of the enamel fragments varied with both types of brackets. Only a few patients (4%) had what would be considered major damage.

These data confirm previous reports that it also is easy to fracture a ceramic bracket while attempting to remove it, and if that happens, large pieces of the bracket must be ground away with a diamond stone in a handpiece. This is time consuming and must be done carefully to avoid enamel damage, so it can be considered an undesirable complication. These problems arise because ceramic brackets have little or no ability to deform—they are either intact or broken. Shearing stresses are applied to the bracket to remove it, and the necessary force can become alarmingly large.

TABLE 17.2 Enamel Presence on Debonded Brackets

	METAL BRACKETS	CERAMIC BRACKETS		
	Two-Step Etch-and-Bond $n = 150$	Two-Step Etch-and-Bond $n = 144$	Self-Etching Primer $n = 126$	RMGIC[a] $n = 66$
% Presence of enamel	13.3	30.2	38.2	19.7
% Bracket fracture	0	26.2	6.2	12.1

[a]Modified glass-ionomer cement (see discussion in Chapter 10).
RMGIC, Resin-modified glass-ionomer cement.
Summarized from Cochrane NJ, Lo TWG, Adams GG, Schneider PM. Quantitative analysis of enamel on debonded orthodontic brackets. *Am J Orthod Dentofac Orthop.* 2017;152(3):312–319.

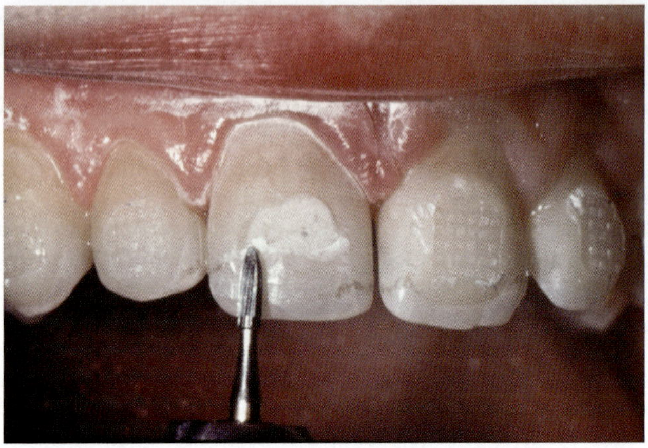

• **Fig. 17.15** On debonding, the bond failure usually occurs between the base of the bracket and the resin, leaving excess resin on the tooth. Removing excess bonding resin is best accomplished with a smooth 12-fluted carbide bur, followed by pumicing. The carbide bur is used with a gentle wiping motion to remove the resin.

There are three approaches to these problems in debonding ceramic brackets:

- Modify the interface between the bracket and the bonding resin to increase the chance that when force is applied, the failure will occur between the bracket and the bonding material. Chemical bonds between the bonding resin and the bracket can be too good, and most manufacturers now have weakened them or abandoned chemical bonding altogether. As the aforementioned data show, this has not eliminated fracture as a problem—all the ceramic brackets in the study were designed for mechanical, not chemical, bonding.
- Use heat to soften the bonding resin so that the bracket can be removed with lower force. Electrothermal and laser instruments to heat ceramic brackets for removal now are available. There is no doubt that less force is needed when the bracket is heated, and research findings indicate that there is little patient discomfort and minimal risk of pulpal damage.[10] Nevertheless, the ideal solution would be to perfect the third approach, so that ceramic brackets can be debonded without heating as readily as metal ones.
- Modify the bracket so that it breaks predictably when debonding force is applied. One advantage of a metal slot in a ceramic bracket is that then the bracket can be engineered to fracture in the slot area, which makes it much easier to remove.

Because each manufacturer of ceramic brackets has engineered the bracket for a specific removal technique, it is important to follow the manufacturer's recommendations to avoid enamel or bracket fracture. Several ceramic brackets have specific removal pliers designed to make removal easy and predictable for the clinician.

Cement left on the teeth after band removal can be removed easily by scaling, but residual bonding resin is more difficult to remove and removing fragments of a bonded ceramic bracket is even more difficult. For removing bonding resin, the best results are obtained with a 12-fluted carbide finishing bur at moderate speeds in a dental handpiece (Fig. 17.15).[11] This bur cuts resin readily but has little effect on enamel. Topical fluoride should be applied when the cleanup procedure has been completed, however, because some of the fluoride-rich outer enamel layer may be lost with even the most careful approach.

A practical solution to retained residual ceramic bracket material is to carefully remove the bulk of the material with a diamond bur, being certain to not contact the tooth. Then remove the bonding resin with a finishing bur. This is a reasonably rapid method and conserves the finishing burs that are rapidly destroyed by the ceramic bracket material.

Positioners and Aligners for Finishing

An alternative to segmental elastics or light round archwires for final settling is the use of a removable appliance to guide the teeth into their final position. Historically, a full-arch tooth positioner, an elastic device into which a patient bites repetitively to generate small amounts of tooth movement was the available option. Positioners were used regularly to assist in finishing after Begg and edgewise treatment in the pre-straight-wire era but now have almost disappeared from routine use, perhaps more completely than they really should have. More recently, the option of a limited series of aligners has become practical. These aligners are often made in the office using techniques described in Chapter 10 and shown in Fig. 10.12.

A tooth positioner is most effective if it is placed immediately following removal of the fixed orthodontic appliance. Normally, it is fabricated by removing the archwires 4 to 6 weeks before the planned removal of the appliance, taking impressions of the teeth and a registration of occlusal relationships, and then resetting the teeth in the laboratory, incorporating the minor changes in position of each tooth necessary to produce appropriate settling (Fig. 17.16). All erupted teeth need to be included in the positioner to prevent supereruption. As part of the laboratory procedure, bands and brackets are trimmed away, and any band space is closed.

The positioner is then fabricated by forming an elastic material (formerly rubber, then usually polyurethane, possibly now a flexible thermoformed material) around the repositioned and articulated casts, producing a device with the inherent elasticity to move the teeth slightly to their final position as the patient bites into it.

A limited series of clear aligners can also be used to guide the teeth into the desired ideal position immediately after the removal of bands and brackets (Fig. 17.17). Like the tooth positioner, this technique takes advantage of the widened PDL spaces that occur during active tooth movement to rapidly guide teeth into

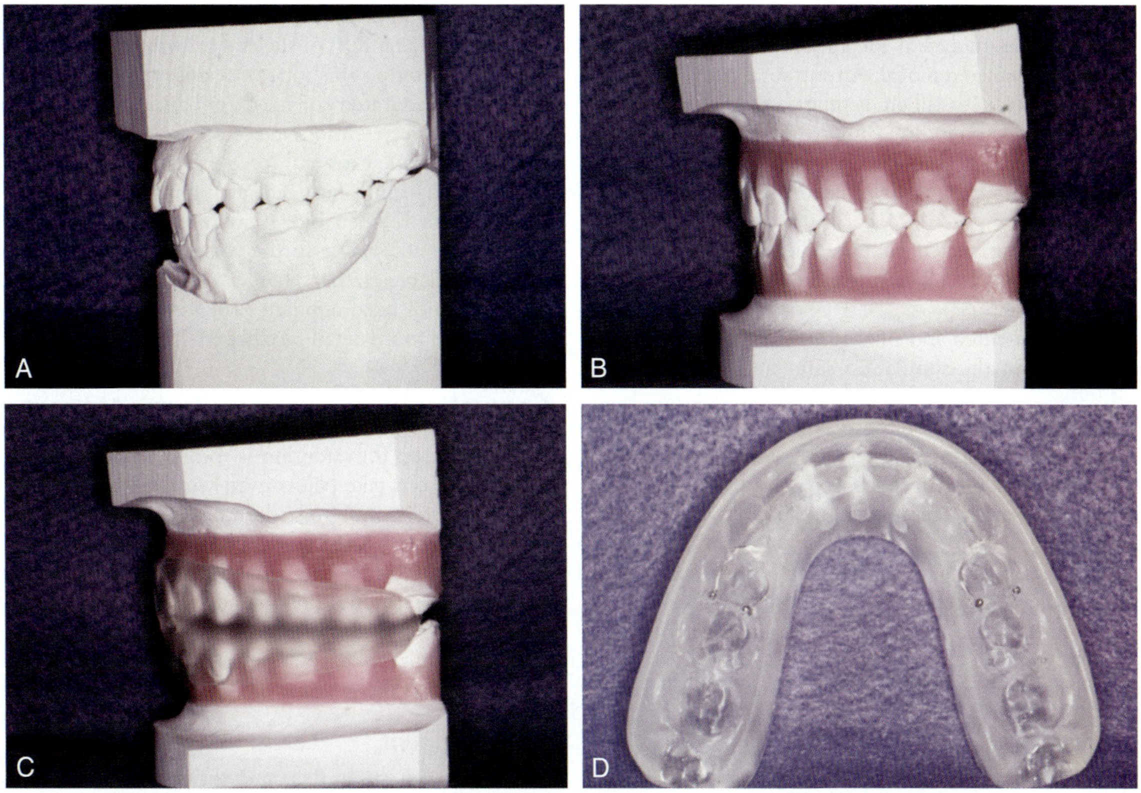

• **Fig. 17.16** Use of a positioner for finishing. (A) Dental casts after appliance removal. (B) The positioner set-up. Often the positioner impression is taken 1 month before debanding, with bands and brackets carved off the teeth in the laboratory, so the positioner can be delivered immediately after the appliance is removed. (C) Transparent positioner on set-up. (D) Maxillary occlusal view of the positioner. Note the clasps in the premolar region that help to prevent space from opening. Their use is particularly important when a positioner is used in a maxillary premolar extraction case.

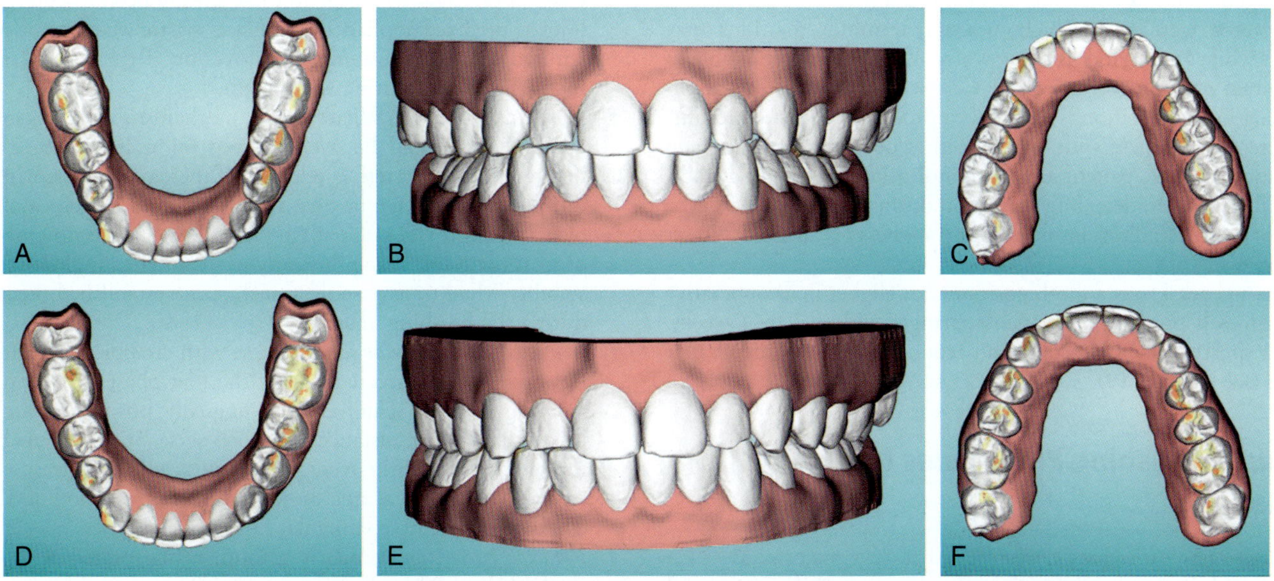

• **Fig. 17.17** Finishing aligners used following fixed appliance treatment to complete tooth positioning not done during the time in braces. Screen captures images of a patient whose braces were removed early because of poor oral hygiene and developing white spots. (A–C) The initial complete buccal crossbite still partially present when braces are removed leaving the upper arch wider than the lower and occlusal contacts only on the cusps (orange contacts on images). (D–F) The situation improved after the wear of eight stages of in-office aligners fabricated to improved the occlusal situation—note the improved occlusal contacts now on marginal ridges and in fossae.

position. The typical approach is to remove the archwires and any bands or brackets on the molars at the appointment prior to the planned complete appliance removal. An intraoral scan, with the incisor and premolar brackets still on, is then completed and archwires are then replaced—extending only to the premolars—and the patient is reappointed for the final appliance removal.

The limited series of aligners is fabricated using the following steps:

- Digital models are constructed from the intraoral scan and software tools are used to virtually remove the remaining brackets on premolars and incisors.
- The models are segmented and small adjustments to the tooth position are made in the simulation software to idealize the final result.
- Depending on the amount of tooth adjustment, a series of stages (usually 2–5) are created to reach the ideal position and 3D models are printed of each stage.
- Standard thermoforming techniques are used to create the aligners.

When the patient returns for their final appliance removal, the bands and brackets are removed and the aligners are delivered.

The use of a tooth positioner or aligners to produce the final settling has two advantages: (1) it allows the fixed appliance to be removed somewhat earlier than otherwise would have been the case (particularly important in situations of poor oral hygiene) and (2) it serves not only to reposition the teeth but to allow a reduction of gingival inflammation prior to final retainer construction. The use of positioners or aligners for finishing also have some disadvantages. First, they require a considerable amount of laboratory fabrication time and therefore are an additional expense—but that can be minimized with in-office aligner fabrication. Second, settling with a positioner tends to increase overbite more than the equivalent settling with light elastics. This is a disadvantage in the majority of orthodontic patients who had a deep overbite initially but can be advantageous if the initial problem was an anterior open bite. Also, a positioner does not maintain the position of de-rotated teeth well, which means that minor rotations may recur while a positioner is being worn. An aligner is better able to maintain rotation corrections. Finally, with any removable appliance, good cooperation is essential to produce the desired results. Severe malalignment with rotated teeth, a deep bite tendency, and an uncooperative patient are contraindications for use of a traditional positioner; deep bite correction during treatment would be less of a contraindication for finishing aligners because of its lesser thickness.

As a general rule, a tooth positioner or aligner in a cooperative patient will produce the possible changes within 2 to 4 weeks. Final (posttreatment) records and retainers can be made at that time (see Chapter 19).

Special Finishing Procedures to Avoid Relapse

Relapse after orthodontic treatment has two major causes: (1) continued growth by the patient in an unfavorable pattern and (2) tissue rebound after the release of orthodontic force.

Control of Unfavorable Growth

Changes resulting from continued growth in a Class II, Class III, deep bite, or open bite pattern contribute to a return of the original malocclusion and in that sense constitute relapse. These changes are due to the pattern of skeletal growth, not just to tooth movement. Controlling this type of relapse requires a continuation of active treatment after the fixed appliances have been removed.

This "active retention" takes one of two forms. One possibility is to continue extraoral force in conjunction with orthodontic retainers (high-pull headgear at night, for instance, in a patient with a Class II open bite growth pattern). The other, which is much more acceptable to the patient, is use of a modified functional appliance rather than a conventional retainer after the completion of fixed appliance therapy. This important subject is discussed in more detail in Chapter 19.

Control of Rebound After Tooth Movement

A major reason for retention is to hold the teeth until soft tissue remodeling can take place. Even with the best remodeling, however, some rebound from the application of orthodontic forces occurs, and indeed the tendency for rebound after interarch elastics are discontinued has already been discussed. There are two ways to deal with this phenomenon: (1) overtreatment, so that any rebound will only bring the teeth back to their proper position and (2) adjunctive periodontal surgery to reduce rebound from elastic fibers in the gingiva.

Overtreatment

Because it can be anticipated that teeth will rebound slightly toward their previous position after orthodontic correction, it is logical to position them at the end of treatment in a slightly overtreated position. Only a small degree of overtreatment is compatible with precise finishing of orthodontic cases as described previously, but it is nevertheless possible to apply this principle during the finishing phase of treatment. Consider four specific situations:

- *Correction of Class II or Class III malocclusion.* Overtreatment of 1 to 2 mm to accommodate for the expected rebound after Class II or Class III correction has already been discussed. As long as the fixed appliance is in place, elastic wear can be reinstituted to obtain a complete correction if there is excessive rebound (or if posturing is detected).
- *Crossbite correction.* Whatever the mechanism used to correct crossbite, it should be overcorrected by at least 1 to 2 mm before the force system is released. If the crossbite is corrected during the first stage of treatment, as should be the case, the overcorrection will gradually be lost during succeeding phases of treatment, but doing this early in treatment should improve stability when transverse relationships are established precisely during the finishing phase.
- *Crowded and irregular teeth.* Just as with crossbites, irregularities can be overcorrected during the first phase of treatment, carrying a tooth that has been lingually positioned slightly too far labial, for instance, and vice versa. It is wise to hold the teeth in a slightly overcorrected position for at least a few months. As a general rule, however, it is not wise to build this overcorrection into rectangular finishing archwires.
- *Rotation correction.* Similarly, a tooth being rotated into position in the arch benefits from being over-rotated. Maintaining an over-rotated position can be done by adjusting the wings of single brackets, or by maintaining a rotation wedge in place with twin brackets. Rotated teeth should be maintained in an overcorrected position as long as possible, but even then, these teeth are often candidates for the periodontal procedures described next.

Adjunctive Periodontal Surgery: Sectioning Elastic Gingival Fibers

A major cause of rebound after orthodontic treatment is the network of elastic supracrestal gingival fibers. As teeth are moved to a new position, these fibers are stretched, and they remodel very slowly. If the pull of these elastic fibers could be eliminated, a major cause of relapse of previously irregular and rotated teeth should be eliminated. In fact, if the supracrestal fibers are sectioned and allowed to heal while the teeth are held in the proper position, relapse caused by gingival elasticity is greatly reduced.

Surgery to section the supracrestal elastic fibers is a simple procedure that does not require referral to a periodontist unless possible gingival recession is an esthetic concern. It can be carried out by either of two approaches.

The first method, originally developed by Edwards,[12] is called *circumferential supracrestal fibrotomy* (CSF). After infiltration with a local anesthetic, the procedure consists of inserting the sharp point of a fine blade into the gingival sulcus down to the crest of alveolar bone. Cuts are made interproximally on each side of a rotated tooth and along the labial and lingual gingival margins unless, as is often the case, the labial or lingual gingiva is quite thin, in which case this part of the circumferential cut is omitted. No periodontal pack is necessary, and there is only minor discomfort after the procedure. It now is possible to make these cuts with a laser rather than a knife, and a study in Iran indicated that the laser-assisted CSF was as effective as the original procedure and produced less pain and bleeding. Those researchers reported that irradiation with a gallium-aluminum-arsenide laser at four points around incisors also gave equivalent results.[13]

An alternative method is to make an incision in the center of each gingival papilla, sparing the margin but separating the papilla from just below the margin to 1 to 2 mm below the height of the bone buccally and lingually (Fig. 17.18). This is said to reduce the possibility that the height of the gingival attachment will be reduced after the surgery, and it is particularly indicated for esthetically sensitive areas (e.g., the maxillary incisor region). Nevertheless, there is little if any risk of gingival recession with the original or laser-assisted CSF procedures unless cuts are made across thin labial or lingual tissues. From the point of view of improved stability after orthodontic treatment, the surgical procedures appear to be equivalent.

Neither CSF nor the papilla-dividing procedure should be done until malalignment of teeth has been corrected and the teeth have been held in their new position for several months. This means that either the surgery should be done a few weeks before removal of the orthodontic appliance or, if it is performed at the same time the appliance is removed, a retainer must be inserted almost immediately. It is easier to do the CSF procedure after the orthodontic appliances have been removed, although it can be carried out with appliances in place. An advantage of the papilla-dividing procedure may be that it is easier to perform with the orthodontic appliance still in place. The problem with placing a retainer immediately after the surgery is that it contacts soft tissue in a sore area, but full-time retention is needed until the soft tissues heal, and this is accomplished best by still having the fixed appliance in place.

Experience has demonstrated that sectioning the gingival fibers is an effective method to control rotational relapse but does not control the tendency for crowded incisors to again become irregular. The primary indication for gingival surgery therefore is a tooth or teeth that were severely rotated. This surgery is not indicated for patients with crowding without rotations.

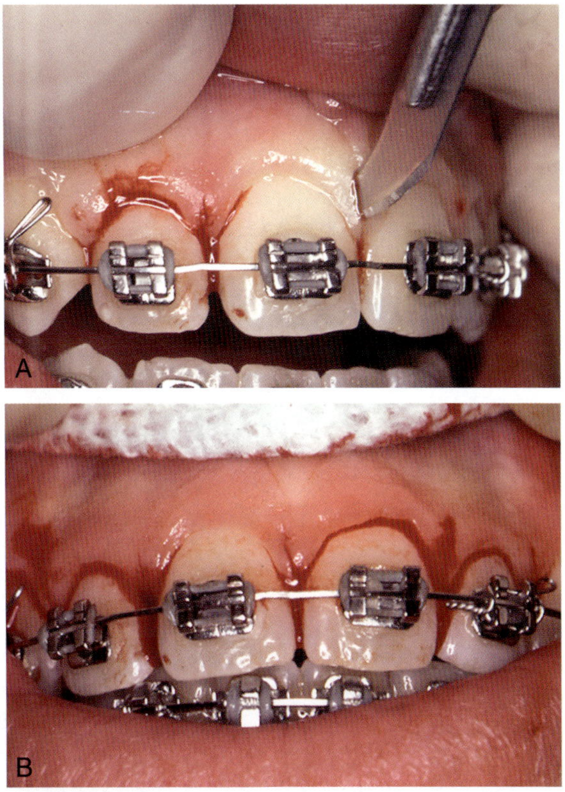

• **Fig. 17.18** The "papilla split" procedure is an alternative to the "around the tooth" circumferential supracrestal fibrotomy approach for sectioning gingival circumferential fibers to improve posttreatment stability. It is particularly indicated for esthetically sensitive areas such as the maxillary anterior region. Vertical cuts are made in the gingival papillae without separating the gingival margin at the papilla tip. (A) The blade inserted to make the vertical cut. (B) View at completion of the papilla splits before sutures are placed. Another advantage of this procedure is that it is easier to perform with an orthodontic appliance and archwire in place.

Micro-Esthetic Procedures in Finishing

Micro-esthetic considerations in the display and shape of the teeth have been discussed previously in Chapter 6. As a general rule, the soft tissue considerations should be dealt with first, and enameloplasty should be deferred until initial alignment has been achieved and rotations have been corrected.

Recontouring the Gingiva to Improve Tooth Proportions and Display

Height-width ratios of teeth are greatly affected by the extent to which gingiva covers the upper part of the crown, and this issue should be addressed before recontouring of the teeth is done. Note that for the patient shown in Fig. 17.19, the height-width ratio of the maxillary incisors was well below the normal proportion because the upper portion of the crowns was covered by gingiva. Careful probing established that removal of the gingiva to the level of the

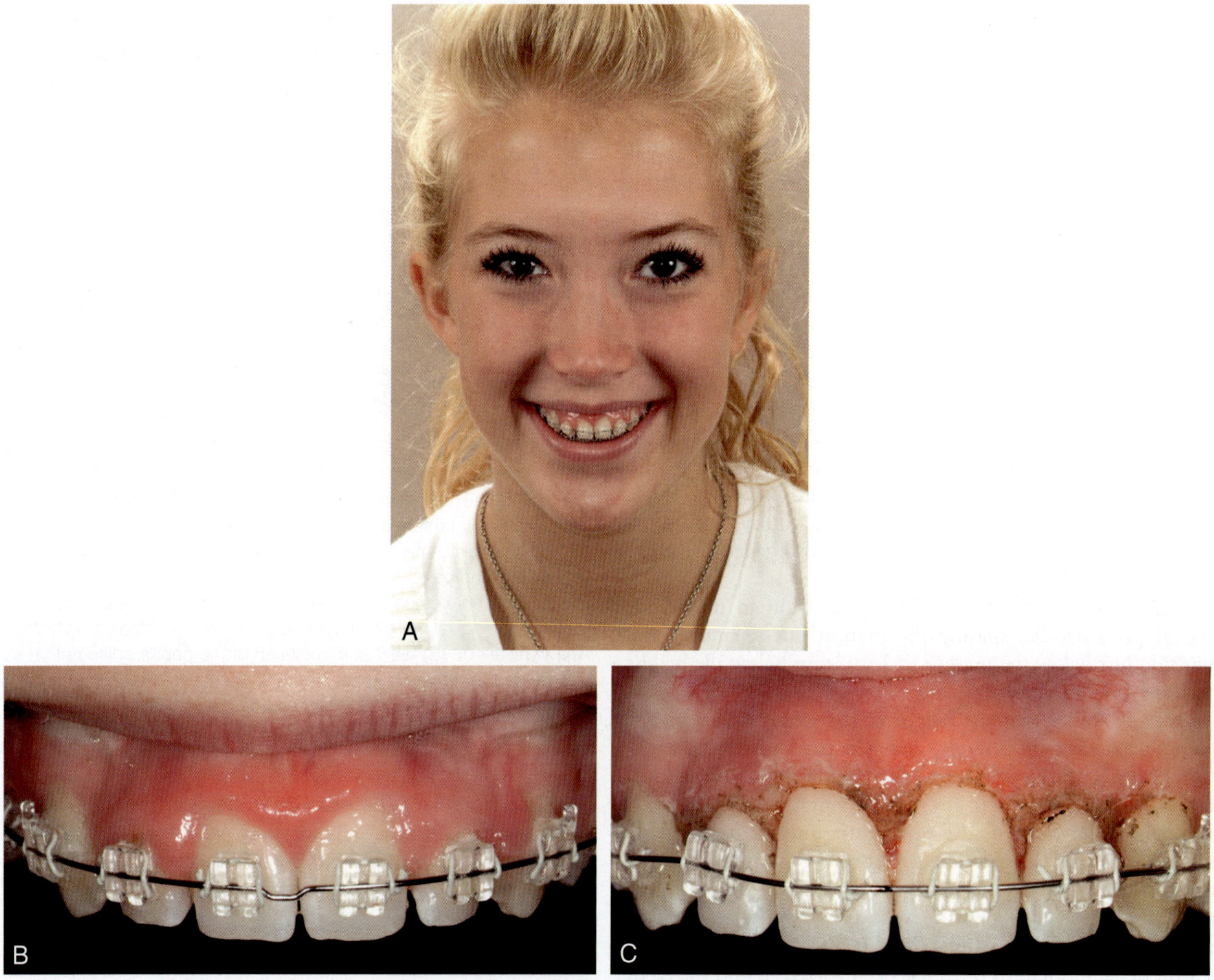

• **Fig. 17.19** (A) For this patient near the end of orthodontic treatment, the inadequate display of the maxillary incisors was primarily due to short clinical crowns because of gingival overgrowth. (B) In this view of the close-up smile, note that the zenith of both central incisor crowns, especially the right central, is too far distal, and that the contour of the gingiva over both lateral incisors is excessive. Probing established that removal of excessive tissue to the level of the cementoenamel junction was possible. (C) The appearance of the teeth and gingiva immediately after laser recontouring of the gingiva.

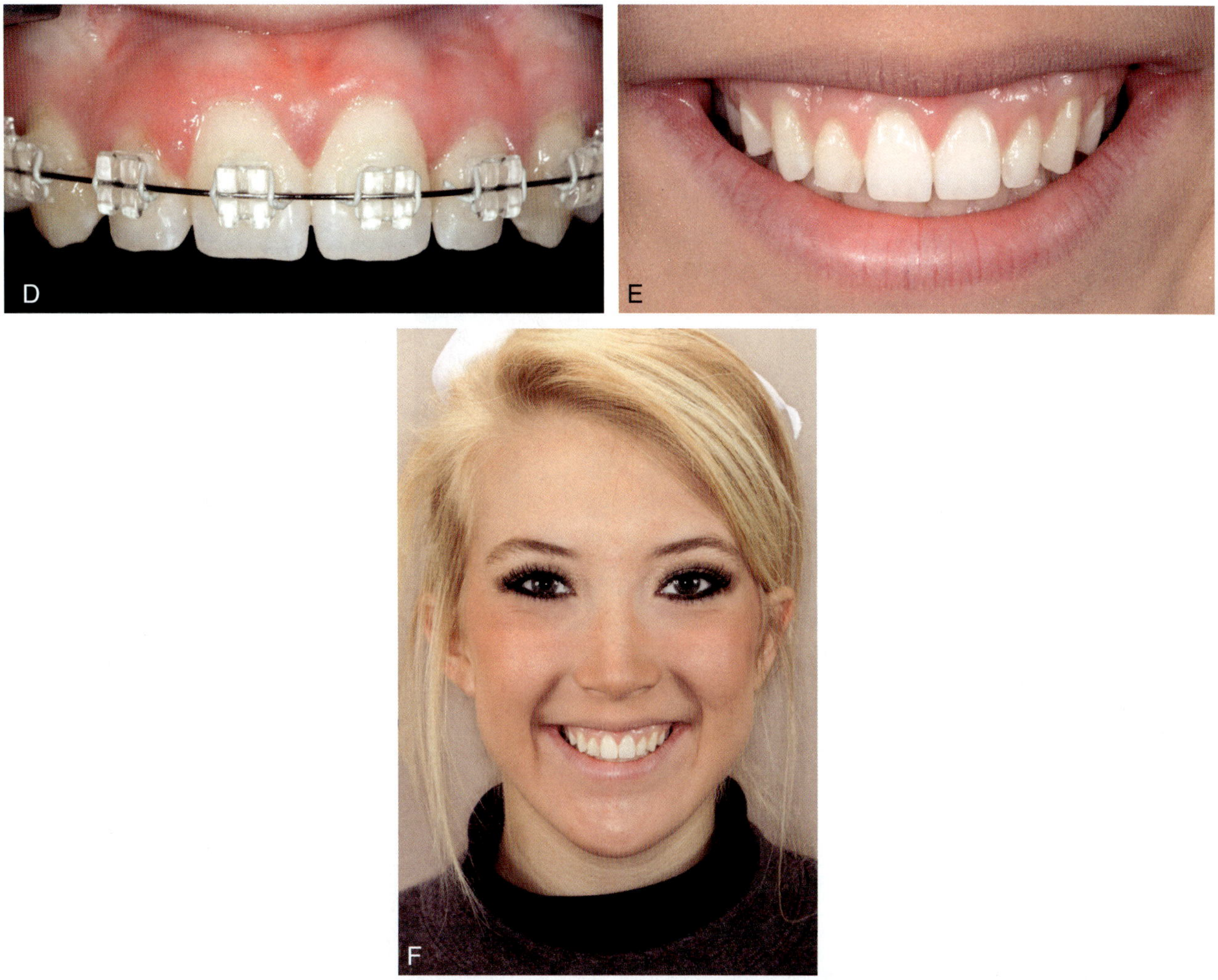

• **Fig. 17.19, cont'd** (D) Two weeks later. (E) Three months later, close-up, and (F) full-face smile at end of treatment.

cementoenamel junction was possible, and a diode laser (940 nm, EZlase, Biolase Technology) was used to do this. The effect was an improvement in both tooth proportionality and incisor display.

Reshaping the Teeth for Enhanced Esthetics

For many years, dentists have defined tooth shape and morphology in terms of (1) ideal ratios of tooth dimensions, which are affected by the extent to which the gingival tissues cover or expose the crown as discussed earlier and (2) definitions of tooth shape and contour. Much of modern esthetic dentistry is based on these dimensions and definitions.[14] Identification and treatment of micro-esthetic characteristics can greatly enhance orthodontic outcomes,[15] and therefore this process is an important part of both diagnosis and treatment.

Soft tissue recontouring often is done as a first step in treatment. This allows ideal vertical placement of brackets at the beginning of treatment so that gingival margins and placement of incisal edges can be optimized and provides time for healing so that the apparent proportions of the teeth will not be affected by soft tissue changes. Enamel recontouring should not be done until after the initial phase of orthodontic alignment because if a tooth rotation is corrected, the perception of its width is changed while the height is not, giving a misleading height-width ratio. After alignment, reshaping of the teeth can be carried out as desired but should be completed before the end of the finishing stage of treatment.[16]

Consider the patient shown in Fig. 17.20, whose chief concern was protruding teeth. She had been treated as an adolescent to reasonably good occlusion and dental alignment but now wanted enhancement of her appearance on smile.

Micro-esthetic considerations on clinical evaluation were:

- Vertical height differences for both the maxillary teeth and gingival margins.
- Different height-width ratios for the central incisors.
- Central incisors disproportionately larger than lateral incisors.

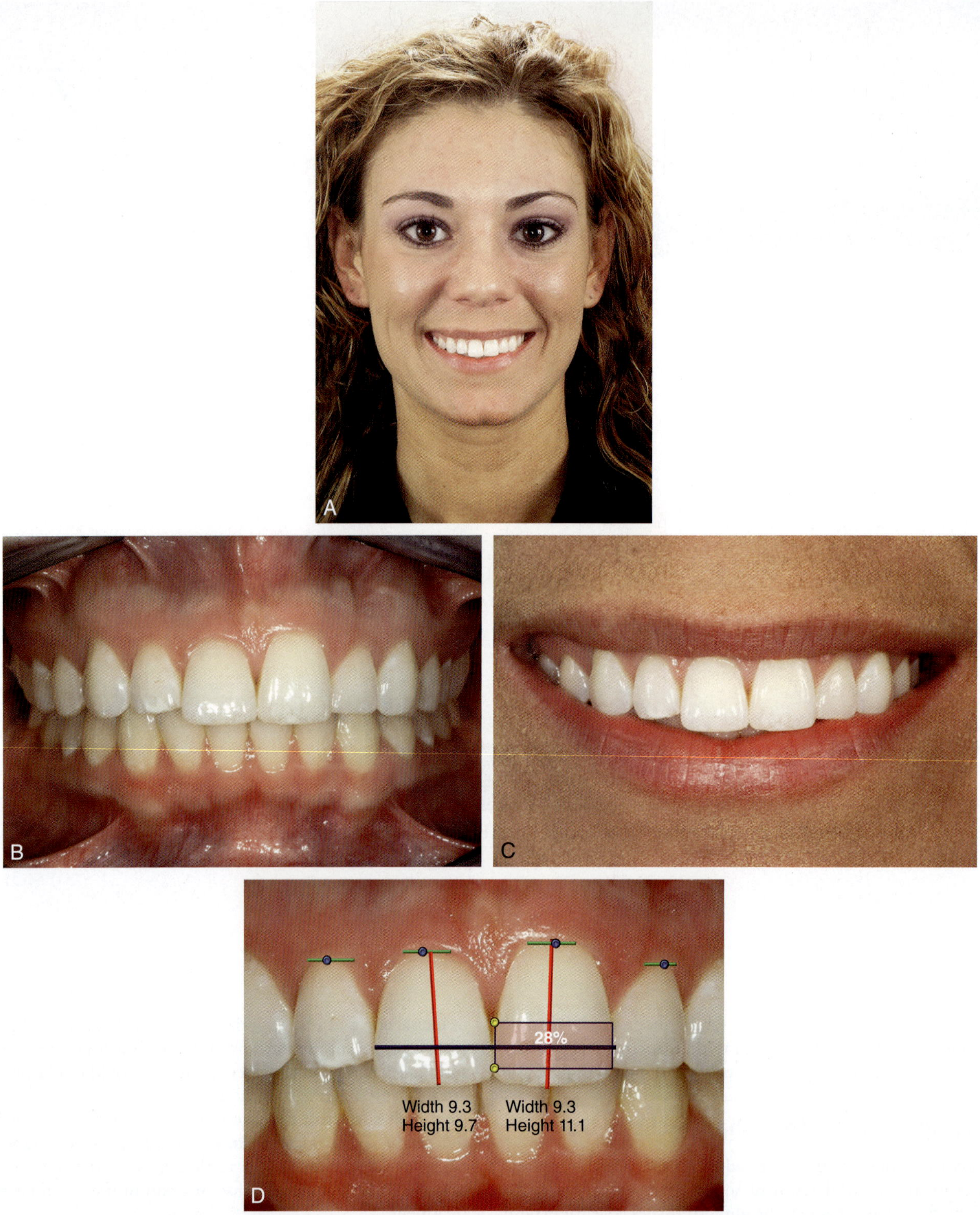

• **Fig. 17.20** (A) This patient had a chief complaint of protruding teeth. She had been treated as a child to a good occlusion and acceptable smile esthetics. (B and C) She had reasonably well-aligned teeth with good overbite/overjet and smile arc but (1) disparate incisal edges and gingival margins; (2) a 1 : 1 height-width ratio for the right central incisor, with a more appropriate 8 : 10 ratio for the left central; and (3) an excessive gingival embrasure between the centrals, which is often referred to as a "black triangle." (D) Assessment of micro-esthetic characteristics showed that the gingival zeniths (denoted by the blue dots) were well placed, being slightly distal to the long axes of the centrals and coincident to the long axes of the lateral incisors. The excessive gingival embrasure and black triangle were the result of the short connector of only 28% (shown by the box over the left central). The ideal connector length should comprise 50% of the central incisor height.

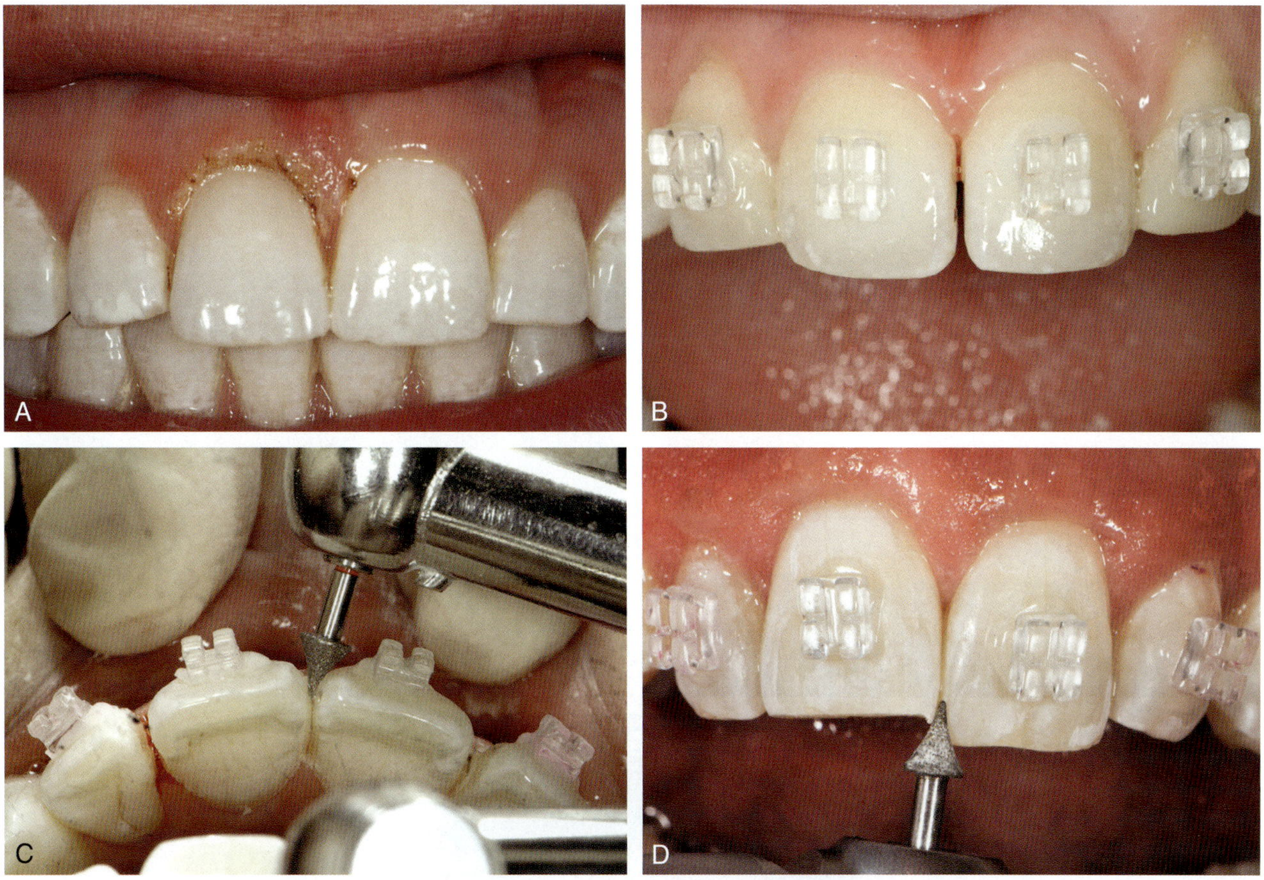

• **Fig. 17.21** For the patient shown in Fig. 17.20, the height of the right central was shorter than normal, and after periodontal probing demonstrated that adequate tissue could be removed without compromising the gingival attachment, a laser-assisted gingivectomy was carried out. (A) Immediately after the laser procedure. A gingival dressing was not needed because of the coagulation created by the laser. (B) After initial alignment of the teeth, a fine carbide bur was used to lengthen the connector between the centrals and brackets. (C) The interproximal reshaping resulted in line angles that required finishing with a cone-shaped diamond bur. (D) Once the space was closed, the mesial corners of the teeth were shaped to refine the incisal embrasures, and the height of the right central crown and the bracket positions were adjusted so that when the incisal edges were level, the gingival margins would also be level.

- Short connector length between the central incisors. The ideal connector length for these teeth is 50% of the height of the central incisors, and in this case the connector length was only 28%.
- An excessive gingival embrasure between the central incisors, resulting in a "black triangle."

The micro-esthetic treatment plan and order of treatment (Fig. 17.21) were as follows:

- Correct the height-width ratios for the central incisors. The ratio for the left central incisor was acceptably close to ideal; the right central incisor needed to be lengthened if possible. The gingival probing depth for the right central was 3 mm; reducing the sulcus depth with a laser-assisted gingivectomy would improve the crown height by 1 to 2 mm.
- Address the width proportions. Because the lateral incisors had normal width while the central incisors were unusually wide, narrowing the central incisors by removing interproximal enamel to improve the height-width ratio was the next step. Doing this only on the mesial surfaces would decrease or eliminate the black triangle between the centrals and increase the connector length. This would result in line angles that would require rounding of the embrasures as the final step in enameloplasty.
- Close the space created by reshaping the centrals, and as the final step in enameloplasty, reshape the incisal embrasures to finish the connector and embrasure form.
- After completion of treatment and removal of the orthodontic appliances, polish the enamel surfaces.

The patient's smile after treatment (Fig. 17.22) demonstrates the value of attention to the finishing details so that the characteristics of esthetic teeth are attained.

For a patient with malformed or damaged teeth, the orthodontist needs to interact with a restorative dentist, often both during and at the conclusion of active orthodontic treatment (Fig. 17.23). Temporary restorations so that all teeth are approximately the correct size make orthodontic finishing much easier. Modern restorative procedures, especially the use of laminate veneers, can make a significant difference in the quality of the final result. The orthodontic-restorative interaction is discussed in more detail in Chapter 20.

These micro-esthetic finishing procedures are a simple way to enhance the orthodontic result in a way that patients readily perceive and appreciate.

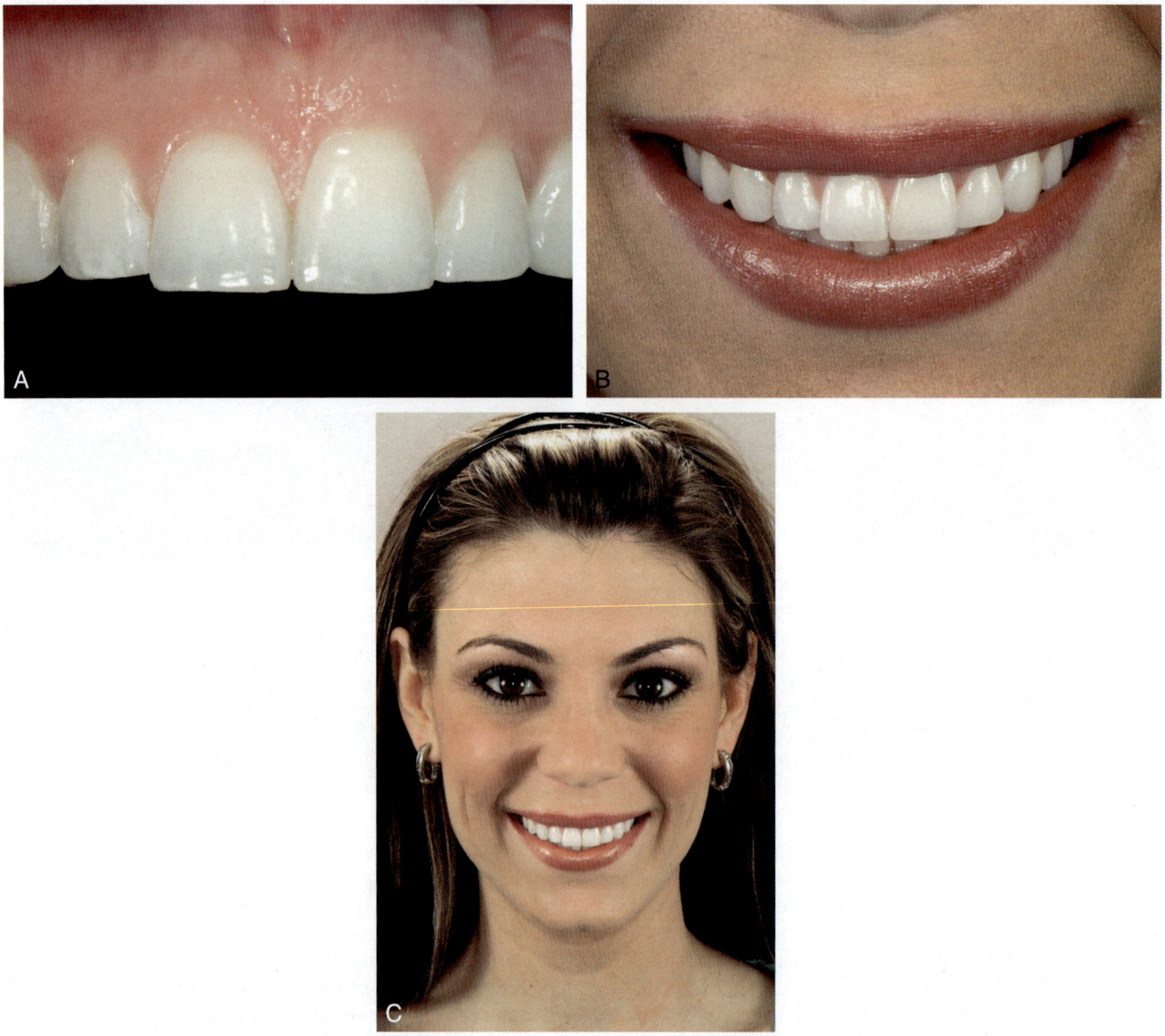

• **Fig. 17.22** Same patient as Figs. 17.20 and 17.21. (A) The desired contact placement, embrasures, and connector length were successfully attained. (B) The final close-up smile and (C) the final full-face smile. The comparison between Figs. 17.20A and 17.22C demonstrates the effect of improving tooth display and contours.

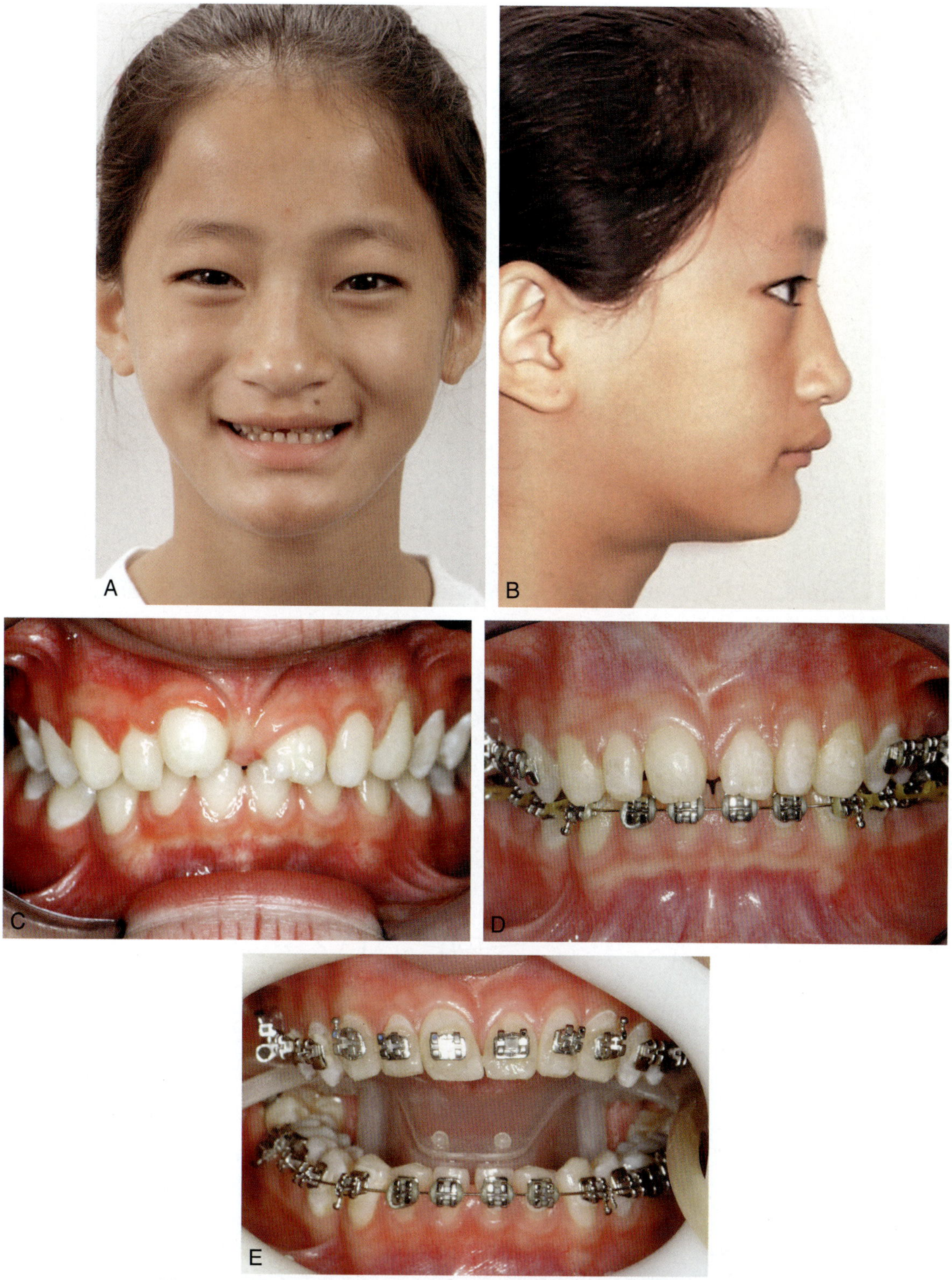

• **Fig. 17.23** (A) Pretreatment smile, (B) profile view, and (C) intraoral view of an 11-year-old girl with malformed maxillary central incisors. Note the short face height, everted upper lip, and short crown heights. Treatment was deferred until age 12½, when she had become quite concerned about the "no teeth" appearance of her smile and was judged to be beginning her adolescent growth spurt. It then was directed toward extrusion of posterior teeth to gain greater face height by using both cervical headgear and vertical elastics. (D) At age 14, after 18 months of treatment, the maxillary brackets were removed so temporary laminates could be placed to improve the proportions of the incisors and increase incisor display. (E) Then brackets were replaced at a more gingival level and treatment was continued.

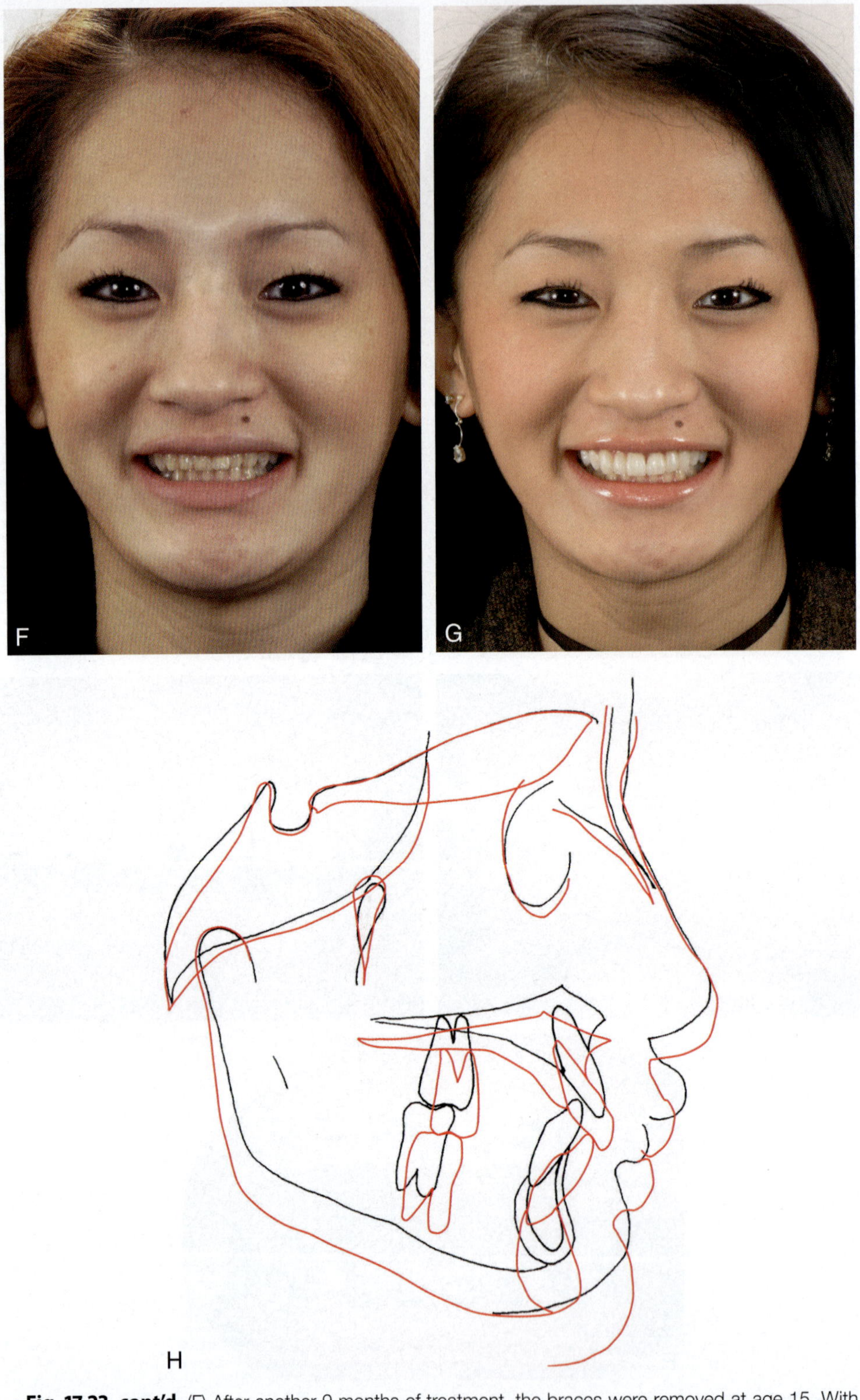

• Fig. 17.23, cont'd (F) After another 9 months of treatment, the braces were removed at age 15. With the temporary laminates still in place, the smile arc was flatter than ideal. (G) At age 18 permanent laminates were placed on the incisor teeth, with a further improvement in the appearance of the smile. (H) Cephalometric superimposition from age 12½ *(black)* to age 15 *(red)*, showing the increase in face height and eruption of posterior and anterior teeth that occurred during orthodontic treatment. The increase in face height and balance created by the orthodontic treatment made it possible to provide excellent restorations for the malformed teeth, and the restorations were a critical element in achieving the overall result.

References

1. Gianelly AA. Asymmetric space closure. *Am J Orthod Dentofacial Orthop*. 1986;90:335–341.
2. Grauer D, Heymann GC, Swift Jr. EJ. Clinical management of tooth size discrepancies. *J Esthet Restor Dent*. 2012;24:155–159.
3. Othman S, Harradine N. Tooth size discrepancies in an orthodontic population. *Angle Orthod*. 2007;77:668–674.
4. Fields HW. Orthodontic-restorative treatment for relative mandibular anterior excess tooth size problems. *Am J Orthod*. 1981;79:176–183.
5. Isaacson RJ, Rebellato J. Two-couple orthodontic appliance systems: torquing arches. *Semin Orthod*. 1995;1:31–36.
6. Zachrisson BU. Buccal uprighting of canines and premolars for improved smile esthetics and stability. *World J Orthod*. 2006;7:406–412.
7. Zachrisson BU. Maxillary expansion: long-term stability and smile esthetics. *Am J Orthod Dentofac Orthop*. 2002;121:432–433. (abstracted from *World J Orthod*. 2001;2:266–272).
8. Steffen JM, Haltom FT. The five-cent tooth positioner. *J Clin Orthod*. 1987;21:528–529.
9. Cochrane NJ, Lo TWG, Adams GG, Schneider PM. Quantitative analysis of enamel on debonded orthodontic brackets. *Am J Orthod Dentofac Orthop*. 2017;152:312–319.
10. Feldon PJ, Murray PE, Burch JG, et al. Diode laser debonding of ceramic brackets. *Am J Orthod Dentofac Orthop*. 2010;138:458–462.
11. Eliades T, Gioka C, Eliades G, et al. Enamel surface roughness following debonding using two resin grinding methods. *Eur J Orthod*. 2004;26:333–338.
12. Edwards JG. A long-term prospective evaluation of the circumferential supracrestal fiberotomy in alleviating orthodontic relapse. *Am J Orthod Dentofac Orthop*. 1988;93:380–387.
13. Jahanbin A, Ramazanzadeh B, Ahrari F, et al. Effectiveness of Er:YAG laser-aided fiberotomy and low-level laser therapy in alleviating relapse of rotated incisors. *Am J Orthod Dentofac Orthop*. 2014;146:565–572.
14. Spear FM, Kokich VG, Mathews DP. Interdisciplinary management of anterior dental esthetics. *J Am Dent Assoc*. 2006;137:160–169.
15. Raj V. Esthetic paradigms in the interdisciplinary management of maxillary anterior dentition—a review. *J Esthet Restor Dent*. 2013;25:295–304.
16. Sarver DM. Enameloplasty and esthetic finishing in orthodontics—Identification and treatment of microesthetic features in orthodontics. Part 1. *J Esthet Restor Dent*. 2011;23:296–302. part 2, 23:303–313, 2011.

18 Clear Aligners in Adolescents

MATTHEW E. LARSON, BRENT E. LARSON, AND REGINA BLEVINS

CHAPTER OUTLINE

Development of Aligner Treatment

Advancements in clear aligner fabrication and biomechanics have expanded orthodontic treatment options in the last few decades. Although some analog techniques existed to fabricate "aligners" for many years, mass production of aligners was not feasible until digital software and 3D printing became more cost-effective. Therefore virtually no orthodontic patients were treated with clear aligners until Align Technology received FDA clearance for the Invisalign system in 1998. Since that time, many advances have been made to achieve better treatment results more efficiently with aligners, dramatically changing the orthodontic landscape. Recent orthodontic industry estimates now indicate that more than 30% of orthodontic cases treated in the United States are treated with aligners.[1]

Described simply, aligners are digitally designed custom plastic trays that slowly transition tooth position from the current malocclusion to the final desired alignment, seen in select staging of a digital setup in Fig. 18.1. Currently, this is mainly displacement driven—gradually moving the tooth position from the original position to the desired final with a set amount of displacement each tray. Ideally, since teeth respond to force, this planning process should evolve to a more force-driven solution, as some systems have started to utilize. Initial planning is typically done by designing an ideal final outcome, but it is unlikely that all treatment goals are able to be met by the initial round of aligners.

Each stage in the digital setup is printed as a 3D model and used to fabricate a clear aligner. That aligner is worn for a set period of time to ideally move all teeth into that planned position. Currently, the most common wear schedule is changing to a new aligner once every week (7 days), but other wear schedules like 10- and 14-day wear are seen as well, especially where significant posterior movements are planned.[2] With more remote monitoring software now available, sometimes this wear schedule is more fluid—transitions to new aligners are made once the desired movements are seen.

In general, tracking of the aligners is monitored by the doctor at set periods during treatment to catch any deviations from the initial plan, but in many cases alterations to the plan involve a refinement scan to work up a supplemental plan. This contrasts with appointments using fixed appliances, where alterations can be done with wire selection, repositions, elastic changes, and IPR at any visit.

In complex cases with many challenging movements, orthodontists now often prioritize certain goals in the initial attachment design and staging, such as extraction space closure, openbite correction, or the most challenging rotations. Additional, less challenging movements are then prioritized in the next stages of aligners with optimized attachment design for those movements. In some respects, this mimics a fixed appliance treatment with progress records and subsequent bracket repositioning appointments.

Aligner Versus Fixed Appliance Treatment

At its core, the diagnosis and goals of orthodontic treatment remain unchanged with aligner treatment. Orthodontists still rely on the same biology of tooth movement, utilization and limitation of expected growth, and alveolar boundary conditions. However, the biomechanics of applying these forces to the teeth do change even though the biological response of the periodontal ligament stays the same. This change is due to the force from aligners being delivered by plastics with a much smaller elastic range than metal archwires and the fact that these plastics suffer from time-dependent changes to force (i.e. creep—see Chapter 9).

Benefits and Limitations of Aligners

Undoubtedly, the largest benefits of clear aligner therapy are esthetics, ease of oral hygiene, and lack of food restrictions. These are the benefits that drove innovative developments in aligner therapy in its infancy when most tooth movement could be done much more efficiently with traditional brackets and wires. These benefits and others are listed in Table 18.1 and are described later.

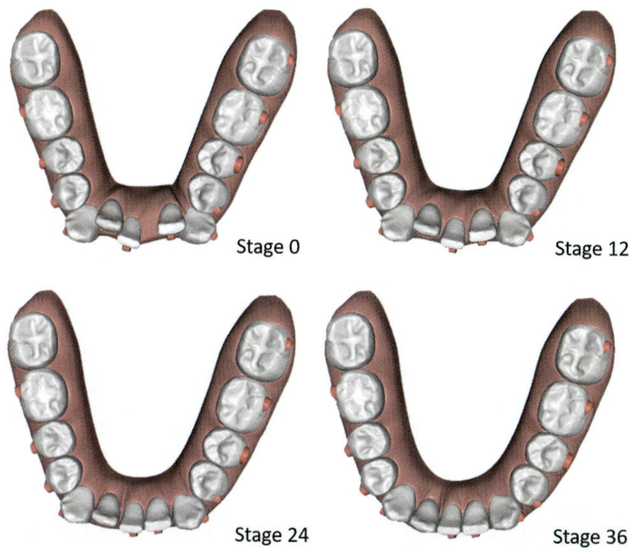

• **Fig. 18.1** Example of several stages in the digital staging of the planned movements in the mandibular arch with aligners. Each aligner has a small range of action, so the series of trays sequentially move the teeth from the initial position to the planned final position. Note that these movements should ideally be planned to allow proper force application and spacing during treatment—it may not be equal movements in each stage to the final position.

TABLE 18.1 Benefits of Aligners Versus Traditional Braces

Benefits of Traditional Braces	Benefits of Aligners
• Consistent force application • Easier adjustments to treatment plan mid-treatment • Easier to add adjunctive appliances (RPE, FORSUS, elastics, etc.) • Easier mechanics for deep bites, extrusion, and severe rotations	• Esthetics • Ease of cleaning • No food restrictions • Handle unique tooth anatomy easily • Treatment will be digitally planned • Good mechanics for intrusion, vertical control, and limited movements

In terms of esthetics, aligners have the potential to be nearly invisible depending on the specific plastic material used and its processing. However, if models are printing with a large layer size, a "stair-step" effect can be seen in the aligners (Fig. 18.2). Also, many movements are more consistently achieved with attachments placed on the teeth (described in more detail throughout this chapter), which has the potential to change the esthetics in the anterior area. Prior to starting treatment, patients should be informed of any potential need for anterior attachments and their potential esthetic impact.

Another benefit discussed with clear aligners is oral hygiene. Cleaning is undoubtedly more straightforward with aligners, as the aligners can be removed for routine brushing and flossing. This has been shown in a systematic review to lead to a significant reduction in plaque index in a mid-term follow-up and probing depths in a long-term follow-up.[3] In this same review, many periodontal indexes did not have a significant difference between aligners and braces, though, with a need for more high-level evidence being recommended. However, this potential improvement in oral hygiene does not mean there is no increased risk of decalcification with aligners. Drinking acidic or sugary liquids with aligners in place, or replacing aligners prior to cleaning will promote decalcification under the aligners. In this case, saliva will not be able to provide buffering to the same degree as normal naturally due to the aligner interfering with the contact of the saliva with the teeth. The pattern of decalcification in these cases is very different than with braces, as seen in Fig. 8.30, with more widespread involvement and inclusion of the cusp tips and incisal edges.

Clear aligners allow for no food restrictions as long as the trays are removed when eating. One challenge faced during fixed appliance therapy is reinforcing a diet that does not cause appliance

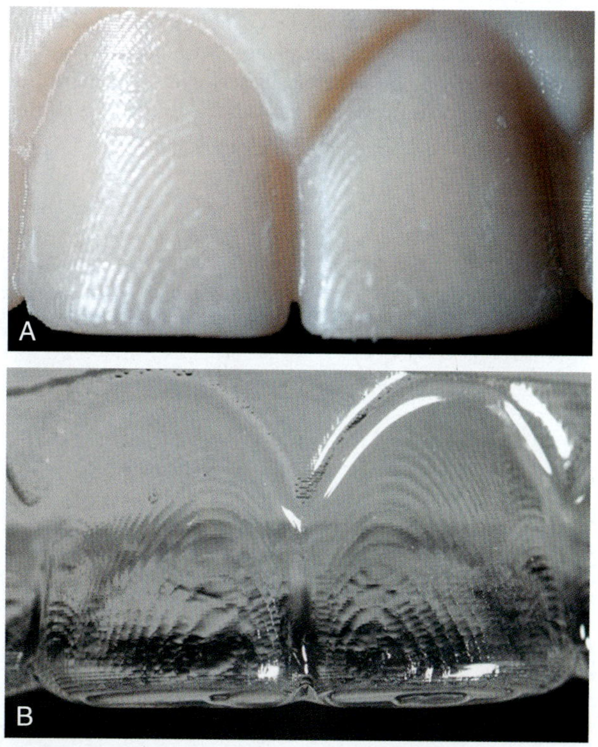

• **Fig. 18.2** Example of the "stair-step" effect possible with the fabrication of aligners with a larger layer thickness. (A) Close-up of the 3D printed model showing the stair-step ridges from the layered printing process. (B) Image of the aligner showing the same teeth with the stair-step ridges now transferred to the aligner by the thermoforming process.

breakage and the associated setback in treatment time. This means avoiding hard and chewy foods, including nuts, corn on the cob, apples, uncooked carrots, hard candy, and chewy candy. For some patients, this can be a significant lifestyle change and if the changes are not made, significant breakage will occur. These restrictions are not needed with aligners, avoiding this concern.

When wearing clear aligners, there will be two layers of plastic between the teeth that prop the bite open slightly and prevent wear on opposing teeth. There is discussion that this thickness of plastic may also promote intrusive force on the posterior, therefore making it easier to intrude posterior teeth and manage openbite cases. While this concept is not supported by evidence at this time, it is clear that the digital planning process at the least helps maintain the vertical position of posterior teeth, avoiding inadvertent extrusion that easily occurs with fixed appliances in high-angle cases.

An additional benefit of custom appliances, like aligners, is the ability to handle unusual geometry more consistently. Tooth anatomy as shown in Fig. 18.3 illustrates geometries that can be challenging for typical bracket placement but can be easily integrated into an aligner digital treatment plan.

Keep in mind that a few of these advantages refer more to the digital, custom nature of clear aligners. It is important to note that some of the same benefits can be found with digital, custom braces as discussed in Chapter 10. Other benefits of aligners: esthetics, ease of cleaning, and the ability to eat any food are unique to the appliance itself.

Treatment Goals and Virtual Setup

Orthodontic treatment planning should start from a prioritized problem list, then defined treatment objectives, and finally appliance selection to meet those objectives (see Chapters 6 and 7). Some orthodontic problems can be efficiently treated with aligners, some can be treated less predictably with aligners, and some cases are not good candidates for aligners without a hybrid technique (where some limited fixed appliances are used). A summary of different case types that fall under these categories is listed in Table 18.2.

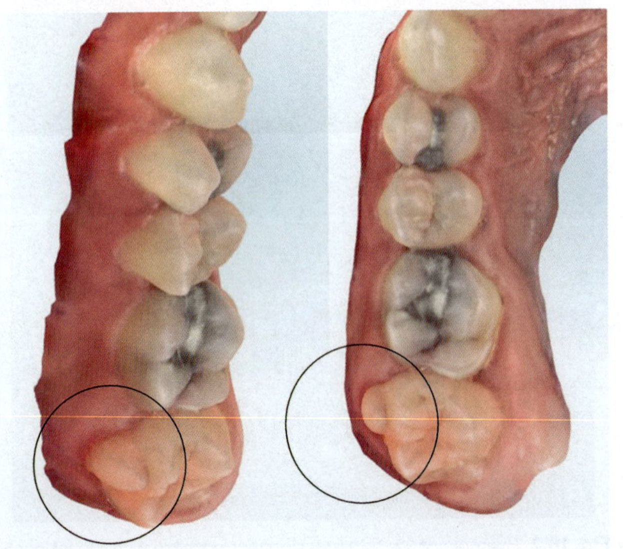

• **Fig. 18.3** Two images of an anomalous upper right second molar with an extra cusp on the facial surface (*circled*). Placing a bracket for fixed appliance treatment on this tooth would be nearly impossible but there is no problem using aligners on such a tooth.

One benefit of digital treatments like aligners is the final outcome and occlusion can be simulated at the start of treatment. This can be extremely beneficial in cases with tooth-size discrepancies (Bolton discrepancies), other unusual tooth anatomy, or where significant change to the archform or occlusion is required. It is interesting to note that the Bolton ratios were developed as a tool to help predict the optimum tooth-size ratio to achieve an ideal overjet because setting up physical models to see predicted occlusions was too labor intensive to do for all cases. With current technology, it is nearly as efficient to actually perform a full digital setup as it is to calculate a Bolton tooth-size ratio that may not be accurate for reasons such as the incisor torque compensations as a result of the relationship of the skeletal bases.

Examples of where the virtual treatment simulation can be useful are shown in Figs. 18.4 and 18.5. In the first case (Fig. 18.4), the barrel-shaped incisors and the potential need for composite buildups to change the tooth shape can be seen and discussed at the start of treatment. This visualization allows better informed consent prior to treatment rather than the patient or family being surprised that the spacing did not appear fully closed later in treatment. In the second case (Fig. 18.5), the final digital setup can be used to explain the treatment goals and why extraction of a lower incisor and interproximal reduction is recommended. It is critical to remember that this is a computer simulation guided by aligning landmarks on the teeth—it does NOT reflect biology, alveolar boundaries, or stable treatment goals. At the end of the day, it is a tool to be utilized by an educated clinician to help guide treatment planning.

In regard to treatment timing with adolescent aligner treatment, most considerations involving growth are identical to those that have been previously discussed with orthodontic treatment in general. A unique consideration with aligners is related to handling tooth eruption. Aligners are fabricated from an initial impression or intraoral scan, so tooth anatomy in the aligners is set at that point. There is the ability to incorporate eruption wells, or voids,—however, it is a generic space for passive eruption. If teeth are not present or further erupt during treatment, an updated scan

TABLE 18.2 Summary of Case Types and Their Predictability When Treating With Aligners

Problems Efficiently Treated With Aligners	Problems Less Predictably Treated—Possible but Not as Efficient	Problems Unreliably Treated Without Adjunctive Methods
Mild to moderate crowding	Severe crowding	Severe crowding—unable to engage tooth well with aligners
Mild to moderate spacing	Severe spacing	Spacing needing significant root movement
Mild vertical changes	Moderate vertical changes	Severe vertical changes
Mild A-P changes	Moderate A-P changes	Severe A-P changes
Single tooth crossbites	Mild-to-moderate dental transverse changes	Skeletal transverse changes (expansion)
		Tooth impactions

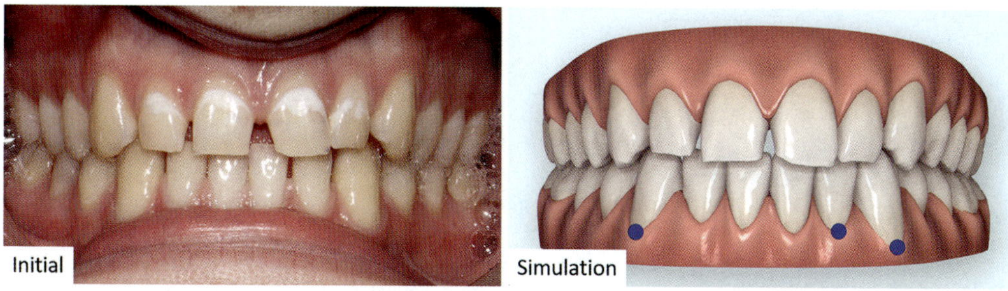

• **Fig. 18.4** Initial clinical photos of a patient with generalized anterior spacing and significantly tapered incisors. A simulated final position for the same patient that helps communicate to the family the amount of space closure possible with orthodontics and the remaining correction needing adjunctive restorative treatment.

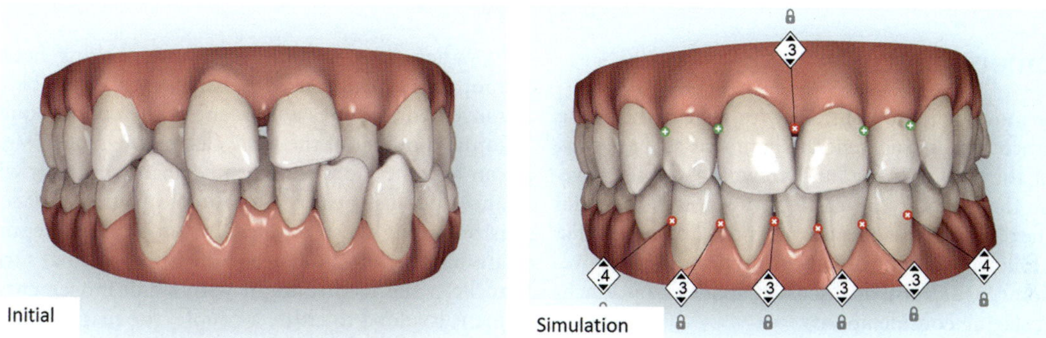

• **Fig. 18.5** Initial clinical photo of an adult patient with a significant tooth-size discrepancy and the simulated changes needed to achieve positive overjet. In this situation, both a lower incisor extraction and lower interproximal reduction (IPR) are needed to create positive overjet if no posterior bite correction is done.

is required for better adaptation. On one hand, this can be relatively easy with intraoral scanning and prolonged treatment has less decalcification risk than fixed appliances. On the other hand, it does mean fully "engaging" erupting teeth is generally slower with aligners. If patient desires and treatment goals are amenable to delaying treatment until full eruption of teeth, that is generally the most efficient for treatment.

Management Differences With Aligners

Although the diagnosis and treatment goals for aligner patients are similar to patients with fixed appliances, managing the orthodontic treatment process with clear aligners has significant differences. From the start, a complete digital setup is done to an idealized final position. Aligners are made from this digital plan unless a significant variation occurs and an updated refinement scan and plan are needed. Minor variation in aligner-tooth tracking can ideally be recognized early and corrected by better compliance with wear, additional time in the current tray before advancing, or checking interproximal contacts for binding.

Since aligners are removable, there are fewer issues that arise that can cause unexpected emergency, or comfort, appointments. Occasionally, attachments or buttons for elastics may need to be rebonded, but those issues are not as critical as broken wires or loose brackets that can cause pain or unwanted tooth movement. Although it can be more challenging to achieve significant root movement with aligners, this can be a slight benefit from a management perspective at times because it also is less likely to see unwanted root movement.

Since the treatment plan is set at the start and there are minimal risks of undesired tooth movement with aligners, it is possible to go longer intervals between treatment visits when using aligners. Most practices see aligner patients every 8 to 16 weeks. Additionally, remote monitoring tools using artificial intelligence (AI) can be utilized with clear aligners to help catch tracking issues sooner, which makes fewer in-office visits a viable option. However, these tools are still relatively new and undergoing constant revisions, and studies have found these AI tools to be inconsistent.[4]

If significant tracking issues occur, an updated digital scan (or impression) is needed to reset the staging for the aligners. This essentially repeats and refines the treatment planning process. The response to the initial aligners can be used to adjust the attachment design, speed of movements, and any overcorrection built into the plan.

One of the barriers many clinicians see to aligner treatment in adolescent is the additional cost. Outsourcing aligner fabrication can be expensive. This expense can be offset by the reduced number of visits and therefore reduced doctor and staff time.

Another large challenge for aligner treatment is managing compliance. Although many adolescents are compliant with aligner wear during treatment, it is a time of many life changes. Any interruptions in aligner wear can suddenly cause fit issues and lead to significant delay in treatment progress. Additionally, if compliance is poor, it can necessitate transitioning to braces—one study found this occurred in one out of six patients between the two offices studied,[5] but this will vary based on final goals and costs associated with transitioning to braces. This leads to further costs and inefficiencies for treatment. Overall, aligner treatment is an exciting and valuable addition to the tools orthodontists can use, but efficiently implementing in a practice takes thoughtful planning.

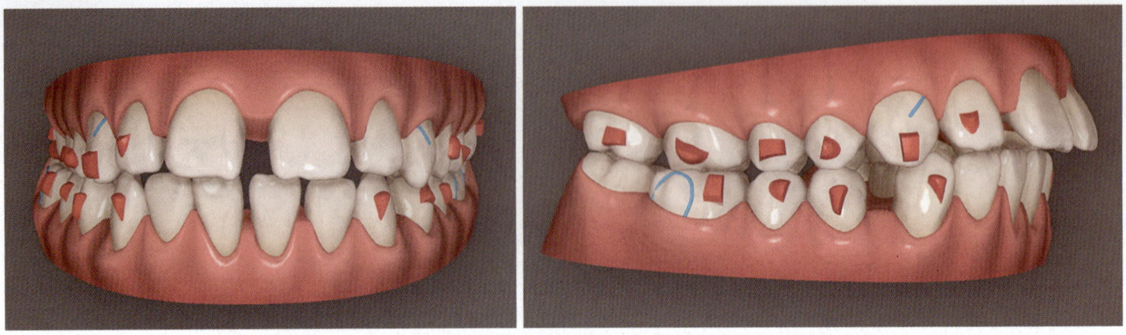

• **Fig. 18.6** Digital plan showing attachment design for space closure (and class II correction). Note that minimal anterior attachments are needed as the required movements are largely controlled tipping.

Tooth Alignment Concepts

The first type of movements to consider with aligner therapy is intra-arch movements including general alignment such as rotations, leveling of the arch, spacing, and crowding. These movements depend on the flexibility of plastic between each tooth (as opposed to the flexibility across the arch or inter-arch mechanics discussed in the following sections). For each type of tooth movement, general biomechanics will be discussed, followed by attachment design and staging considerations.

Simple Spacing

Although challenges can occur, aligners are generally a good option for treatment of simple spacing. Many cases with anterior spacing also have associated proclination, so the ideal movement would be to tip teeth more upright. This lends itself to treatment with aligners, as creating couples with aligners is more challenging than with fixed appliances. Therefore, tipping teeth is relatively easy while root movement is hard.

To maximize the control of tooth movement with aligners it is desirable to have aligner surface contact with the tooth. Although in theory only a point force is required to create tooth movement, better engagement helps prevent any side effects in other directions while moving towards the final planned position. This is an advantage in cases with spacing since it allows contact in the interproximal region until the space is closed.

Attachments

When tipping incisors lingually to close space, there is good surface area across the facial surface of the incisors to generate force to tip back teeth. When vertical control or root tip is needed along with programmed lingual tipping, then attachments might be warranted.

In cases with generalized spacing, geometric (relative) extrusion will occur when tipping incisors lingually. If it is undesirable for the bite to deepen from this relative extrusion, posterior attachments to seat the aligners and provide an intrusive force to the anterior teeth are needed. If extrusion of teeth is desired during space closure, such as with a mild anterior openbite, then anterior attachments are needed to keep anterior teeth seated into the aligner during space closure. Fig. 18.6 shows an example where slight geometric extrusion was needed, and minimal anterior attachments were required. Good correction of the spacing was obtained with well-planned staging and good patient compliance (Fig. 18.7).

When there is more significant spacing between teeth and root movement is needed, attachments may be desired. Bodily movement requires a moment of the couple equal and opposite to the moment of the force closing the space. With aligners, this can become more complicated than treatment with fixed appliances because at times it is unclear what surface of the aligner is providing these couples. In some cases, keeping visible space around the tooth to engage the interproximal surfaces is enough to keep the teeth upright with small movements. If an attachment is added to create a couple, the magnitude of the moment is determined by the force multiplied by the distance between them. Therefore, attachments should either be broad or divided into two separate attachments to provide an efficient couple (Fig. 18.8).

Staging and Planning

Staging movements during space closure follow the principles just discussed. To keep good interproximal engagement, general space closure should be achieved equally to keep good engagement of the aligner around the tooth, with all spaces closing towards the end of treatment. If a specific contact is closed at the start of treatment near larger spaces, it may be advantageous to open that contact until the large spaces are fully closed to improve control. (This is an important part of staging in extraction cases that will be discussed in more detail later [Fig. 18.9].)

One other interesting challenge with clear aligners is ensuring that spaces are completely closed. Since the greatest potential error with intraoral scanning is in the representation of tooth shape in the interproximal areas, it is predicting interproximal contact that is affected. Complete space closure is relatively straightforward with braces, as elastic chain or closing loops provide a continuous force that closes spacing until the contacts are touching. The slight inaccuracies in scanning, production errors with aligners, as well as complications due to displacement driven movements with a relatively low-stiffness material all combine to make completely closing spaces with aligners a challenge that may require additional planning.

One method to improve the predictability of fully closing contacts is overcorrection aligners. These aligners provide a "virtual" elastic chain to the teeth by over-closing the contacts. The default in Invisalign is to only tighten the anterior contacts, but overclosing all contacts or just specific contacts can also be planned. The benefit of this type of technique is that the aligners can be pre-planned without a separate appointment. However, they do not accurately predict where spacing may remain. If overcorrection aligners are worn while contacts are already fully closed, they

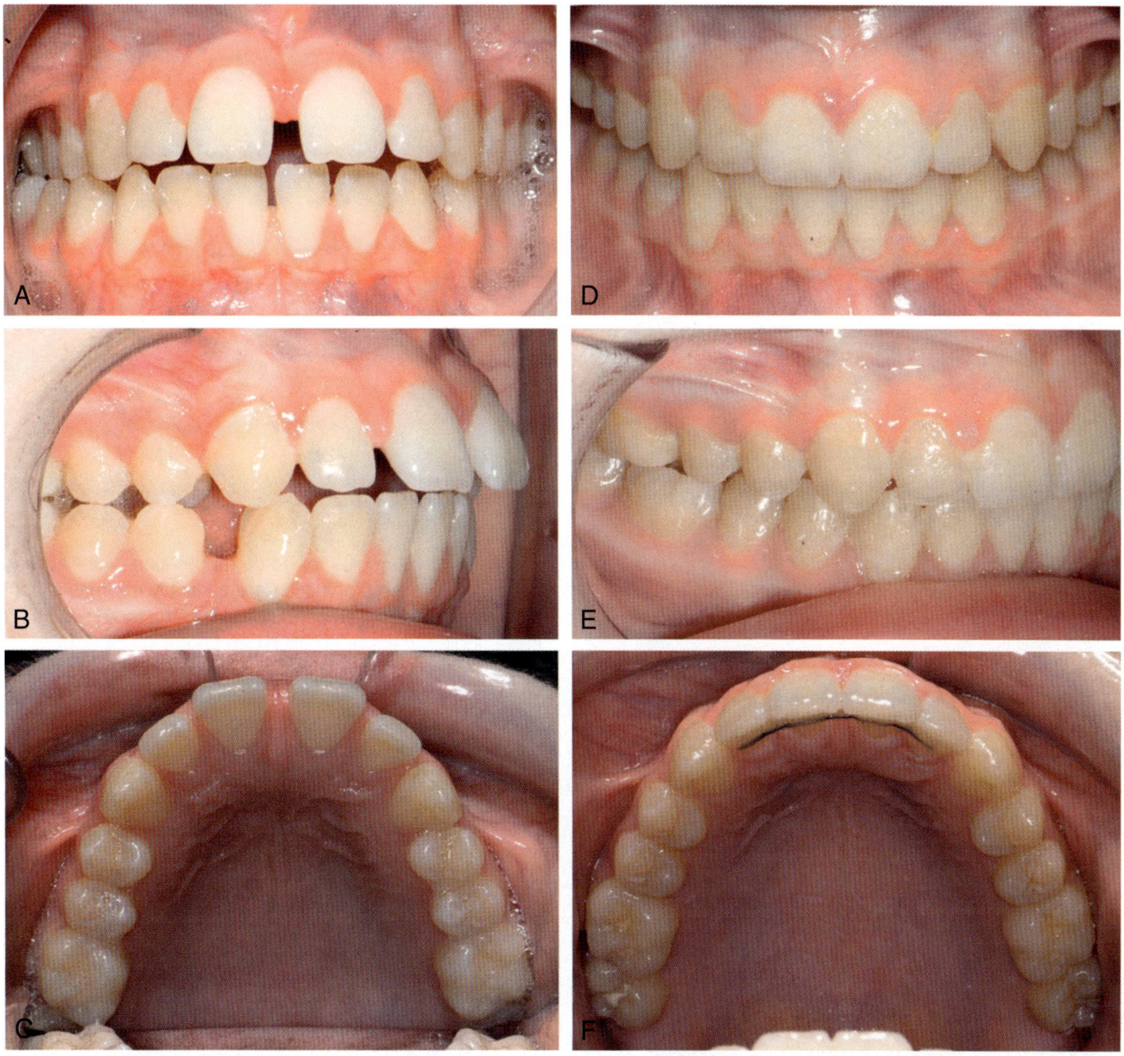

• **Fig. 18.7** Initial (A–C) and final clinical photos (D–F) for the case shown in Fig. 18.6. Space closure was efficiently achieved with minimal anterior attachments. Additionally, the posterior crossbite, class II posterior occlusion, and mild anterior openbite were also corrected.

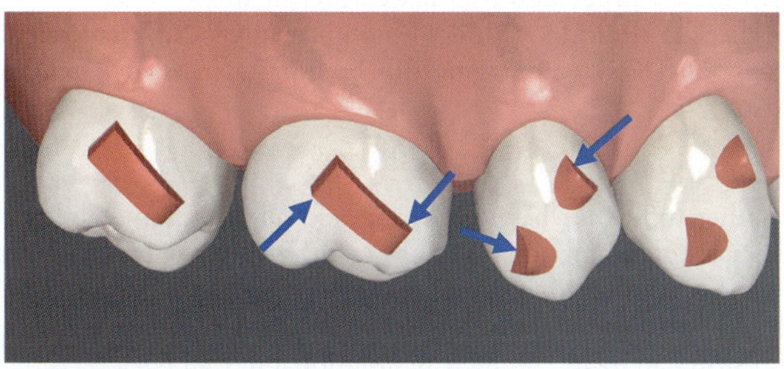

• **Fig. 18.8** Examples of attachment to provide a couple on posterior teeth to help with root control. Either a broad attachment (shown on molars) or two smaller paired attachments (shown on premolars) can provide this force. The *arrows* demonstrate the forces delivered to the attachments by the aligner to generate the couple.

can inadvertently cause unseating, slipped contacts, or unwanted intrusion.

Another common method to help close spaces is to precisely measure the remaining spacing with a leaf gauge (Fig. 18.10) and ensure those contacts are fully closed in the refinement plan. If deemed necessary, those specific contacts can be planned for "virtual" IPR that will not actually be performed clinically but will help ensure contacts are closed.

Mild Crowding

Treatment of mild crowding can be done very consistently with aligners but can initially be challenging as there are some differences in biomechanics compared to fixed appliances.

First, correction of tooth rotations requires space for correction. Although this appears simple in theory, clinicians need to be more cognizant of this during aligner treatment. Braces will naturally create space as the deviations in the wire with rotated teeth will tend to push teeth apart slightly during alignment. Also, although the arch dimensions with fixed appliances are guided by the archwire, the incisors will procline and posterior teeth can expand as needed for crowding resolution during alignment. This can occasionally be a negative with poor planning as teeth can procline to the extreme of causing dehiscence. However, in most cases, simple crowding with fixed appliances can be addressed tooth to tooth by engaging an initial NiTi archwire.

This is in contrast to aligner design, where each aligner controls the incisor position and arch width. Space needs to be deliberately

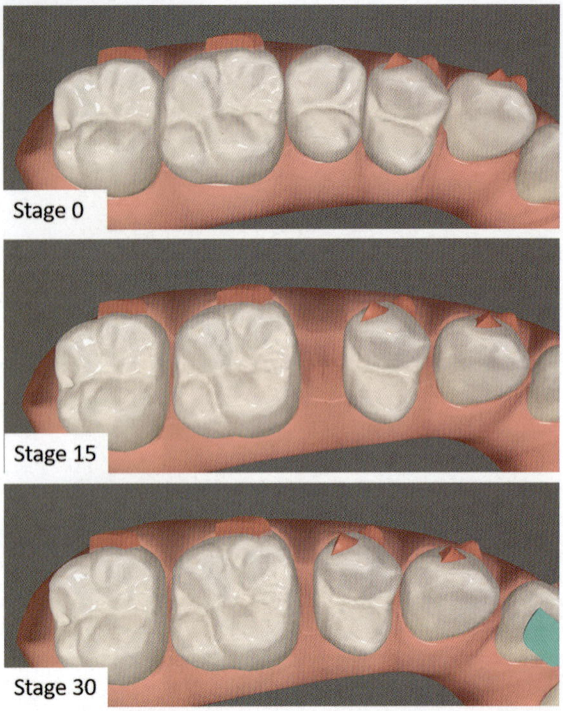

• **Fig. 18.9** Three select stages from an aligner sequence demonstrating the concept of opening interproximal contacts slightly during space closure to produce maximal engagement of the aligner around the tooth. This helps maintain tooth control and the open contacts can be closed tightly in the final stages.

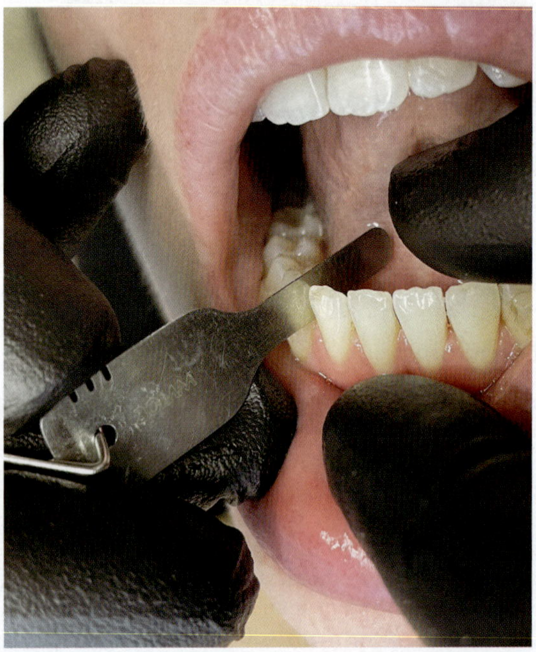

• **Fig. 18.10** Demonstration of a leaf gauge used to precisely measure the space between teeth. The leaf gauge set provides a series of gauges of varying thickness, usually from 0.1 to 0.5 mm, to measure interproximal space. Precisely knowing the space between teeth helps insure the accuracy of a digital setup and can also measure the amount of IPR completed in order to match the amount prescribed in the digital plan.

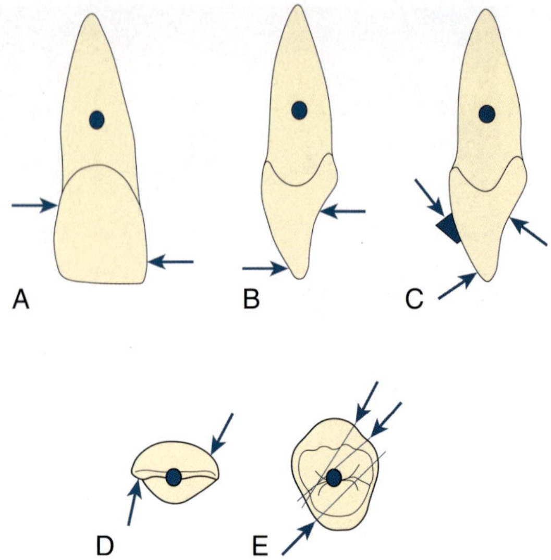

• **Fig. 18.11** Examples of force application with aligners. Note that because the effects of friction are generally minimal, all force application by the plastic is applied perpendicular to the tooth surface. (A) For mesial-distal tipping, force application can frequently be applied reasonably well to the crown of the tooth assuming that space is present for the aligner to engage the proximal surface. (B) This is often shown as an example of how torque is generated with aligners, but these force vectors are not perpendicular to the surface, therefore not realistic. (C) This is the accurate direction of the vectors shown in B. Since these forces are intrusive, note that a seating attachment is typically required to avoid unwanted side effects. (D) Rotation can be applied to incisors relatively easily without attachments. (E) More rounded premolar teeth have significant issues with rotations as all applied forces, without attachments tend to pass very close to the center of resistance making rotation inefficient.

created and verified that it is above the known error in the system. Teeth that appear to barely pass by each other during a digital setup and staging will often be found to bind in the mouth. Ensuring that no binding occurs can be improved by programming visible spaces around teeth during derotation or ensuring "zero collision tolerance" where the software makes sure no overlap occurs. Even with these considerations in place, interproximal contacts should be checked clinically with floss at regular intervals. Interproximal reduction (IPR) or restaging can be done as needed if binding exists.

Attachments

Another difference between braces and aligners is the ability to generate rotation moments on the teeth. With a fixed twin bracket on a tooth, a rotational moment can easily be created by engaging an archwire. Additionally, forces from elastic chains or progressing to a stiffer archwire can increase rotational movements.

Aligners have difficulty applying rotational moments to most teeth with the exception of incisors. This is because, with the exception of some minor forces with friction, aligners apply forces perpendicular to the tooth surface or attachment (Fig. 18.11). For incisors, this can still create effective rotational moments. For canines or premolars, there are only small rotational moments as the distance between the line of action of the perpendicular force and the center of resistance is limited. This can be improved by attachment design but overcorrection of rotations may still be needed in the virtual plan. Maxillary lateral incisors will tend to intrude during derotation so additionally seating attachments are desirable on those teeth.

Complex Crowding

As rotations and overall crowding become more significant, dealing with the limitations of aligners is more challenging. By following the basic principles of good attachment design and space creation, challenging cases can be treated efficiently with aligners. Fig. 18.12 shows an adolescent with crowding treated with clear aligners. Attachment design and the prescribed IPR are shown in Fig. 18.13.

In some severe cases, adjunctive appliances that improve rotation forces may be needed. One method of improving rotational moments is bonding buttons and using elastics or power chain to create additional rotational force (Fig. 18.14). This helps provide a direct rotational moment application and the aligners help prevent unwanted side effects in other planes of space that may occur with the elastic chain alone. More complex methods of adjunctive treatment can also be done, but those are described in the "Hybrid Treatment" section.

It is important to note that with all these intra-arch movements, the amount of correction seen intraorally will be different than the displacements shown on the digital plan. This is likely due to multiple reasons, including stress relaxation within the plastic, compliance issues, or just due to the fact that an ideal displacement does not necessarily produce an ideal force system to move the tooth to that location. Current research estimates that 50% of planned movements are realized [6] and that refinements are often needed for ideal correction. Keep in mind that this does not mean aligners are not a useful tool, but they do require some amount of over-engineering and revision not unlike fixed appliances needing bracket repositioning or bends in the archwire.

Management of A–P, Vertical, and Transverse Correction

The other types of movement to consider with aligners are the overall alignment of the arches in three planes of space. This includes A–P movements that require inter-arch mechanics, vertical changes that require more planning across the overall arch with aligners, and transverse changes that also may require planning across the arch and inter-arch mechanics.

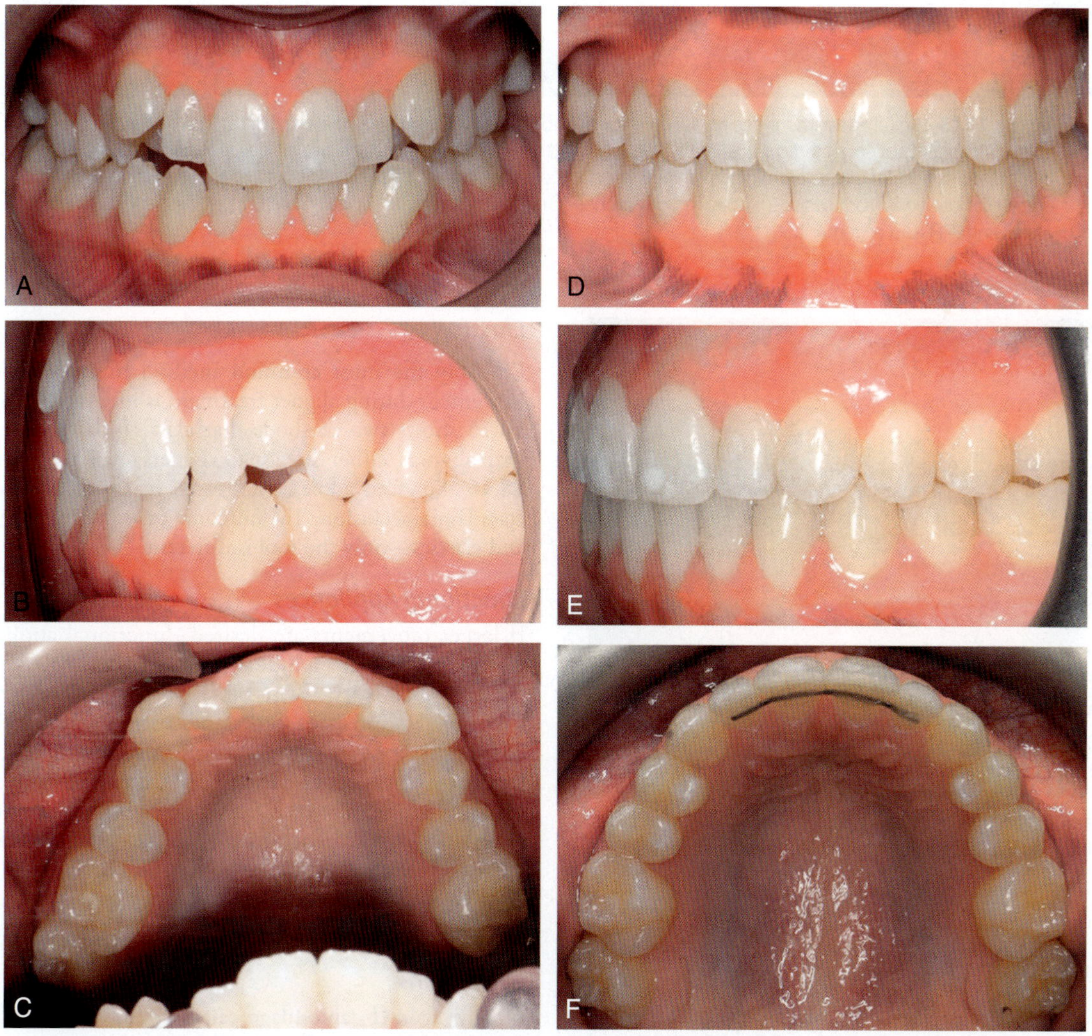

• **Fig. 18.12** Pretreatment and posttreatment clinical photographs of an adolescent with significant crowding and irregularity treated successfully with aligners. (A–C) The pretreatment presentation with a class I posterior relationship. (D–F) The same views after aligner treatment demonstrating resolution of the crowding and maintenance of the posterior occlusal relationship.

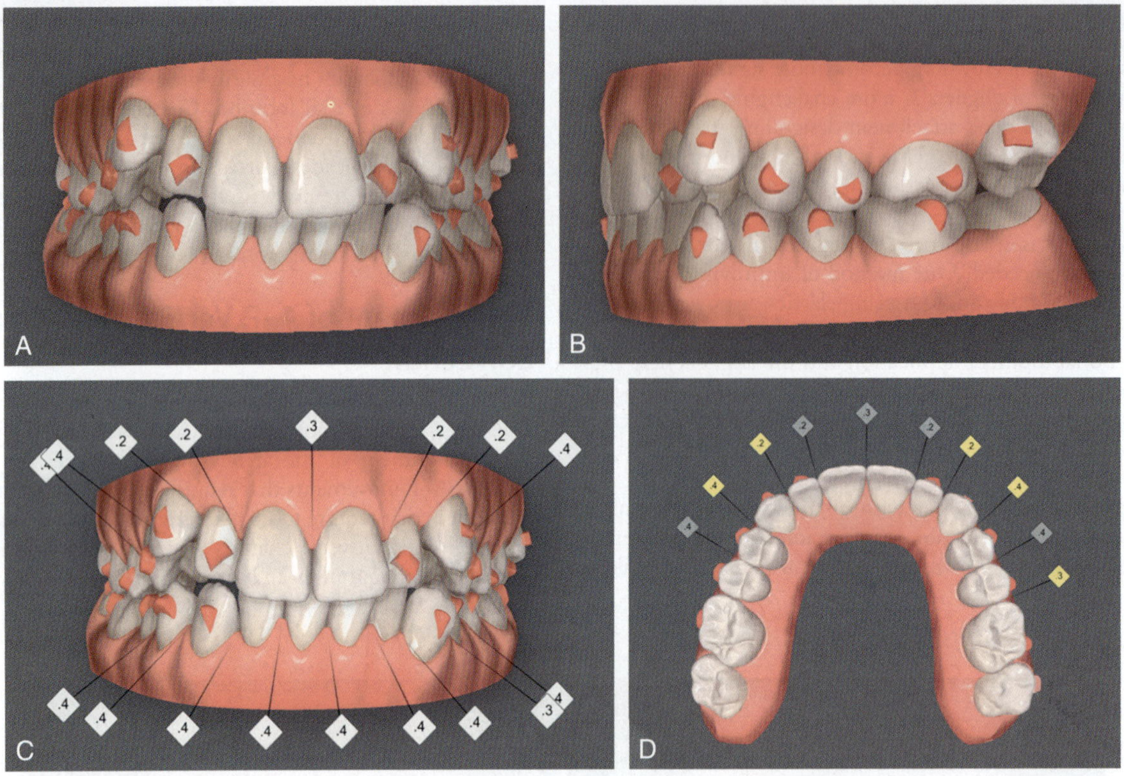

• **Fig. 18.13** Digital attachment design and IPR for the adolescent patient shown in Fig 10.12. The more complex planned tooth movements require attachments on most posterior teeth and the upper lateral incisors (A and B). To create space for alignment while maintaining an acceptable incisor position, IPR was required in most interproximal locations from molar to molar in both arches (C). (D) The expected upper arch form and incisor position following IPR and alignment.

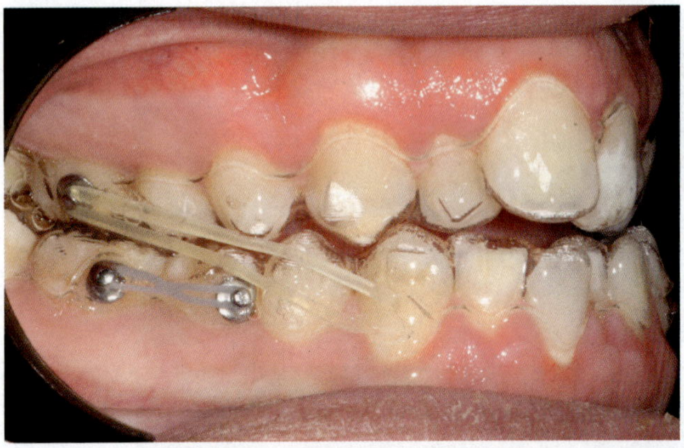

• **Fig. 18.14** Correction of a significant rotation of the lower right second premolar aided by the addition of bonded buttons on the premolar and the molar connected by an elastic chain to provide an additional rotational force. Note that this can be done as aligners are being worn for general tooth alignment and class III elastics are used for A–P correction.

Class II correction

In many respects, the general treatment options for class II correction are the same as discussed in Chapter 16, including dento-alveolar movement, encouraging differential growth, and orthodontic camouflage. However, how to apply forces to achieve these goals differs with aligners.

Elastics

Probably the most common method to achieve dento-alveolar movement during aligner treatment is inter-arch elastic wear. Fig. 18.15 shows two methods that class II elastics can be attached with aligners, either directly to aligners or to buttons on teeth. Fig. 18.16 shows an adolescent treated using aligners to correct her class II malocclusion. The outcome mirrors treatment with braces and elastics—only the tool is different.

Functional Appliances

If larger movements are desired, functional appliances can be utilized. This can include a Herbst or MARA appliance prior to aligner delivery, Twin Block wear followed by aligners, or functional appliances built into the aligner design like the Invisalign MA system. Please note that although all of these functional appliances can appear to produce skeletal changes, systematic research finds that much of the movement is dento-alveolar.[7–9] Treatment of an adolescent class II patient with a MARA and aligners is shown at several stages in Figs. 18.17 and 18.18 show the incisor changes that resulted in overjet correction.

Extractions

Finally, class II camouflage can be done with removal of upper premolars. Due to difficulties closing extraction spaces, these cases may be better suited to fixed appliances as shown in Fig. 16.22. However, with good mechanics and case selection, acceptable results can be achieved.

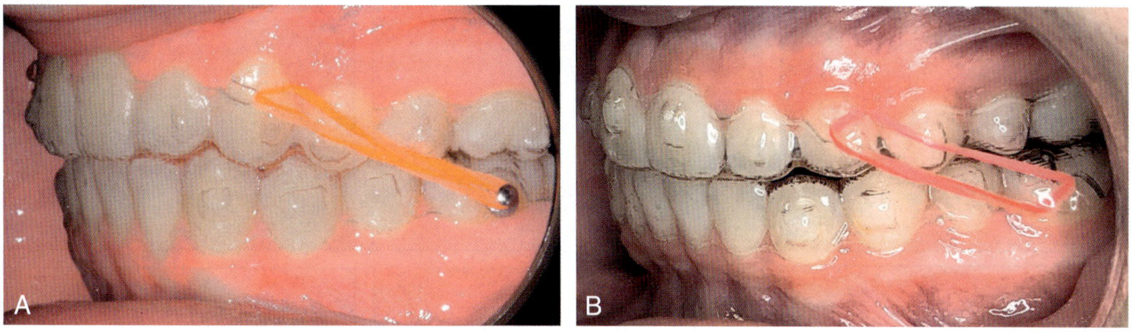

• **Fig. 18.15** Two methods of using class II elastics with aligners. (A) Elastic connected to a hook in the aligner in the maxilla and to a bonded button on the mandibular molar. A cutout for the molar is included in the design stage to allow full seating of the lower aligner without contacting the button. (B) Elastic is connected to hooks in the aligner plastic in both upper and lower aligners. The hooks are included in the design stage when class II elastics are planned.

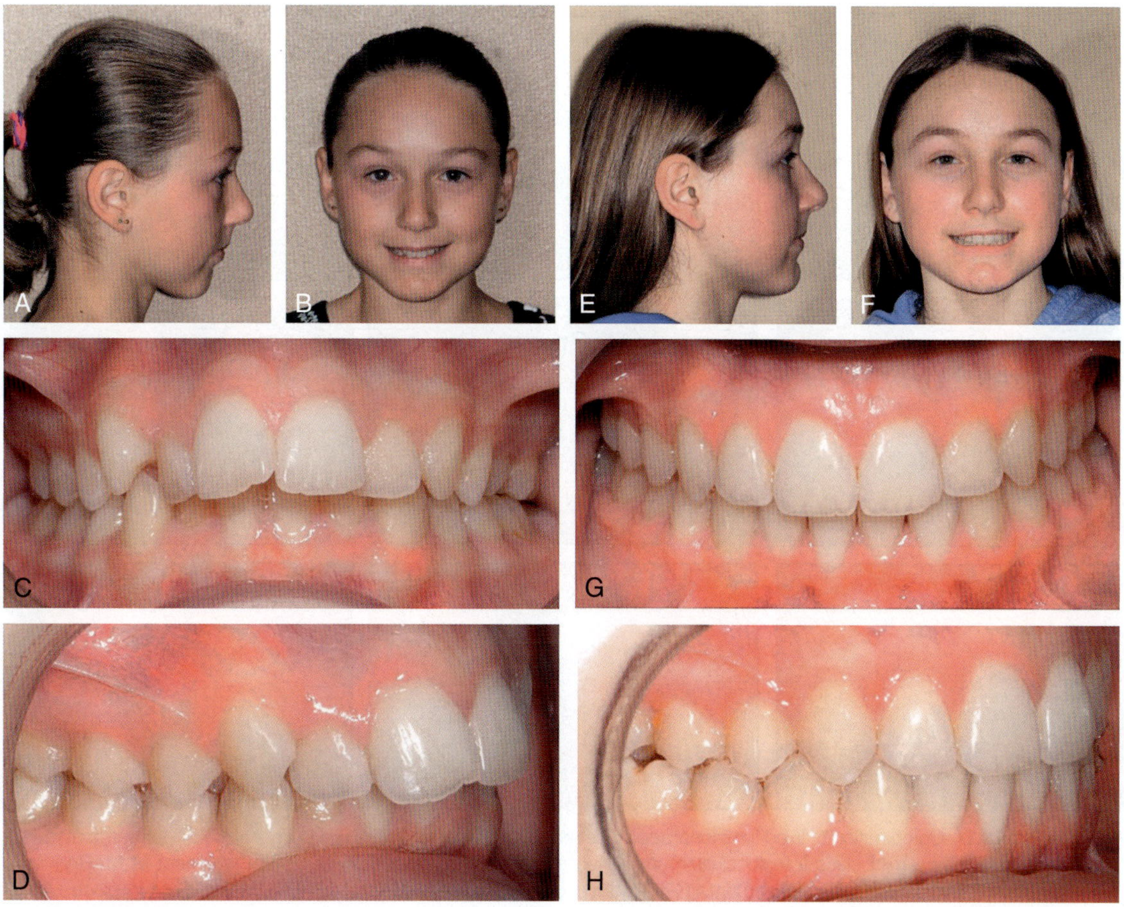

• **Fig. 18.16** Class II malocclusion in an adolescent treated with aligners andclass II elastics. (A–D) Initial presentation with convex profile, midline discrepancy, and class II molar and canine relationship on the right side. (E–H) Posttreatment clinical photos showing straightening of the profile with growth, coincident midlines, and correction of the right side molar and canine relationship.

It is important to mention that, in general, class II mechanics will tend to tip back maxillary incisors and therefore maintaining proper incisor torque is important to achieve the desired final incisor position with complete correction to class I. This is critical to consider when treating with clear aligners, as significantly less root movement will occur compared to the planned outcome.[10] Torque will need to be overcorrected in order to maintain torque control during treatment.

Class III Correction

Mechanics for class III correction are very similar to those utilized in class II correction just with reversed force vectors

Elastic correction setups with either cuts in the aligners or buttons on the teeth can be utilized. One scenario where this can be useful is treatment of late class III growth where negative overjet develops sometime after comprehensive treatment. Aligners with

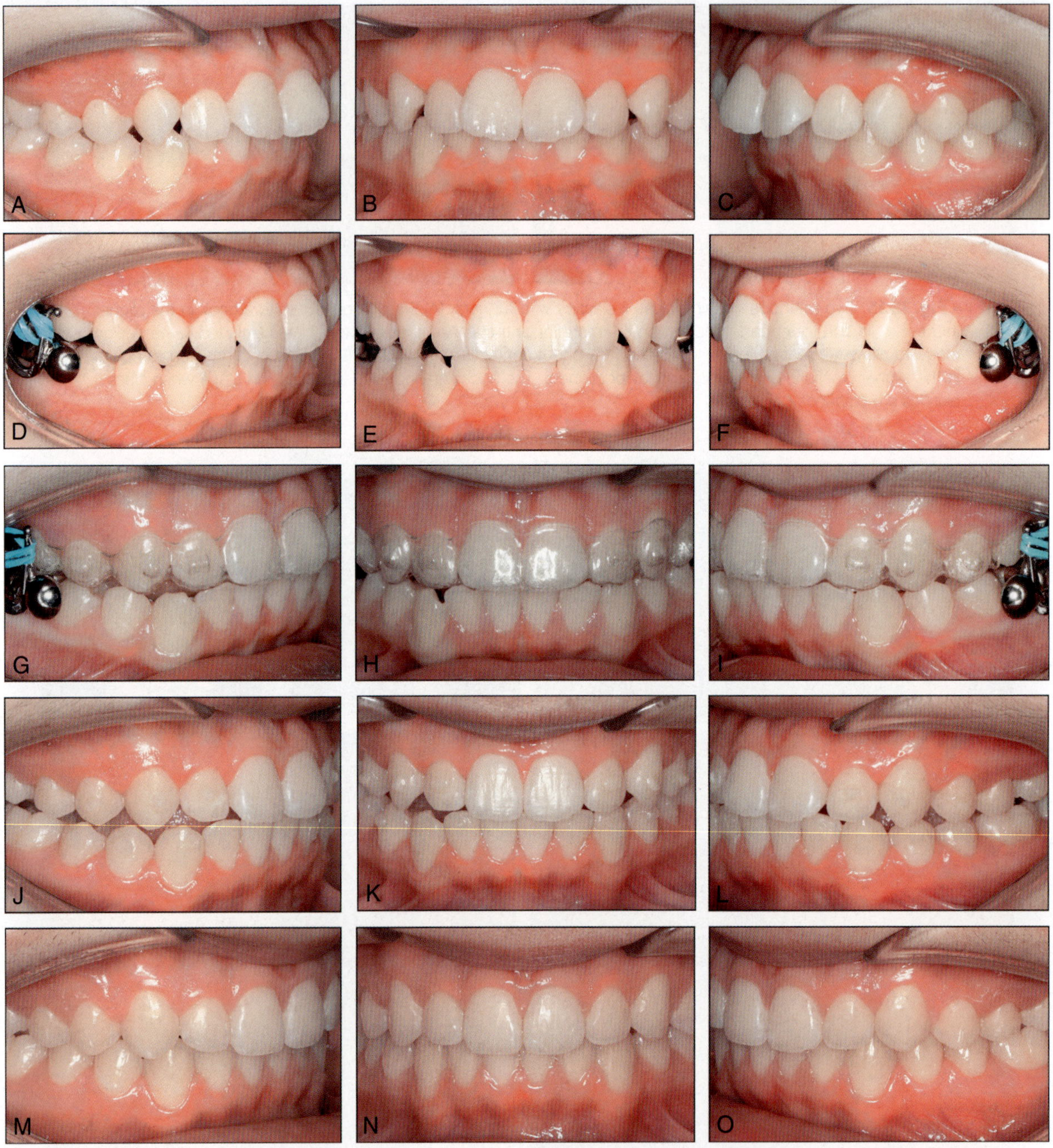

• **Fig. 18.17** Combination of fixed functional appliance and aligner treatment in an adolescent. (A–C) Pretreatment photos showing mild class II malocclusion, increased overjet and mild irregularity. (D–F) Placement of MARA appliance for mandibular advancement. (G–I) Addition of upper aligner while MARA appliance is still in place. (J–L) Removal of MARA after overcorrection of the class II relationship, ready for refinement aligners. (M–O) Posttreatment result with ideal alignment and occlusion. (Courtesy Dr. Neil Kravitz.)

relatively minimal movement and class III elastics can be utilized to predictably regain positive overjet if only limited movement is needed (Fig. 18.19). More complex class III treatment may be possible with excellent patient cooperation and favorable growth response but is less predictable. Fig. 18.20 shows a developing class III malocclusion that was treated with aligners and elastics to an acceptable occlusal and facial result. The change was a combination of tooth movement and rotation of the mandible down and back to help mask the class III skeletal relationship.

Interproximal reduction (IPR) is another commonly utilized method to help improve overjet in cases with a class III tendency. This is best suited to cases with a mandibular tooth-size excess with molars close to class I. Additional IPR can be done to camouflage mild class III cases where the molars are not in class I occlusion, but keep in mind, each 1 mm of retraction requires roughly 2 mm of IPR. For example, if the molars are a quarter-cusp class III (or roughly 2 mm), then 4 mm of IPR (2 mm each side) would be required to create positive overjet. Clearly, this will quickly

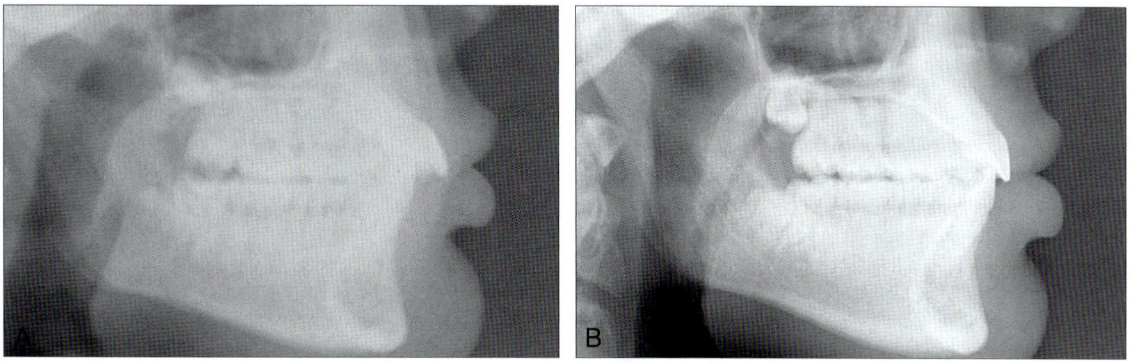

• **Fig. 18.18** Pretreatment (A) and posttreatment (B) cephalometric views of the patient in Fig. 10.17 showing much improved incisor position and improvement of the mento-labial fold following correction of the class II malocclusion with a MARA and aligners. (Courtesy Dr. Neil Kravitz.)

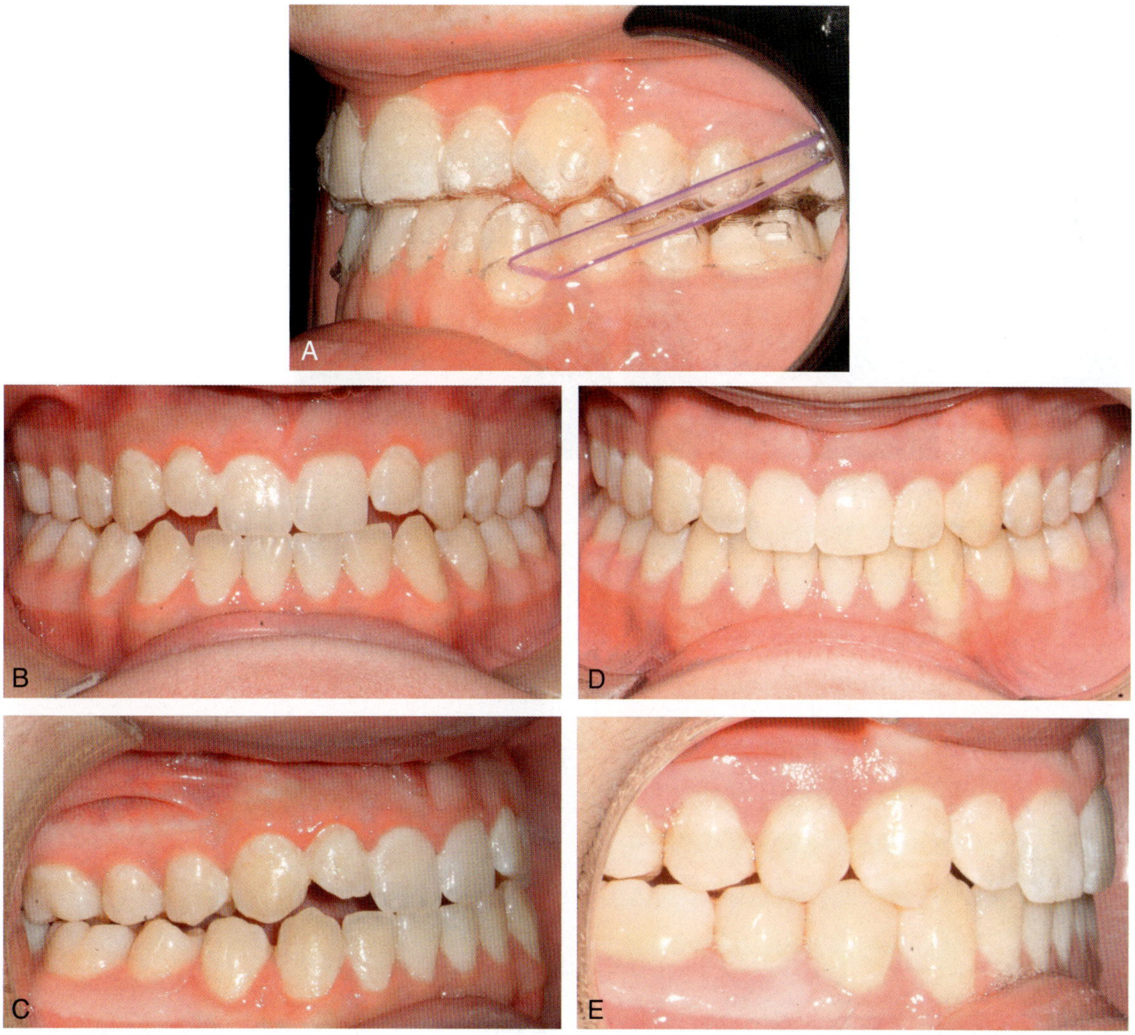

• **Fig. 18.19** Treatment of mild class III with aligners and elastics. (A) Class III elastics worn from a bonded button on the upper molar to a hook in the lower aligner. (B and C) Mild class III malocclusion with end-to-end incisor contact following late adolescent growth. (D and E) Same patient following aligner and elastic treatment showing a much improved incisor relationship.

go beyond reasonable amounts of IPR in more severe cases but remains a useful tool in mild cases.

If the class III malocclusion is more severe, camouflage with lower tooth removal or full correction with orthognathic surgery may be viable treatment options. Orthodontic camouflage with lower premolar removal has the same challenges as with any premolar space closure with aligners. Removal of a lower incisor can be a reasonable treatment option depending on the occlusion and this smaller space can be more predictably closed with good aligner mechanics. Mechanics for more complex space closure and setups for orthognathic surgery are covered in more depth in Chapter 21.

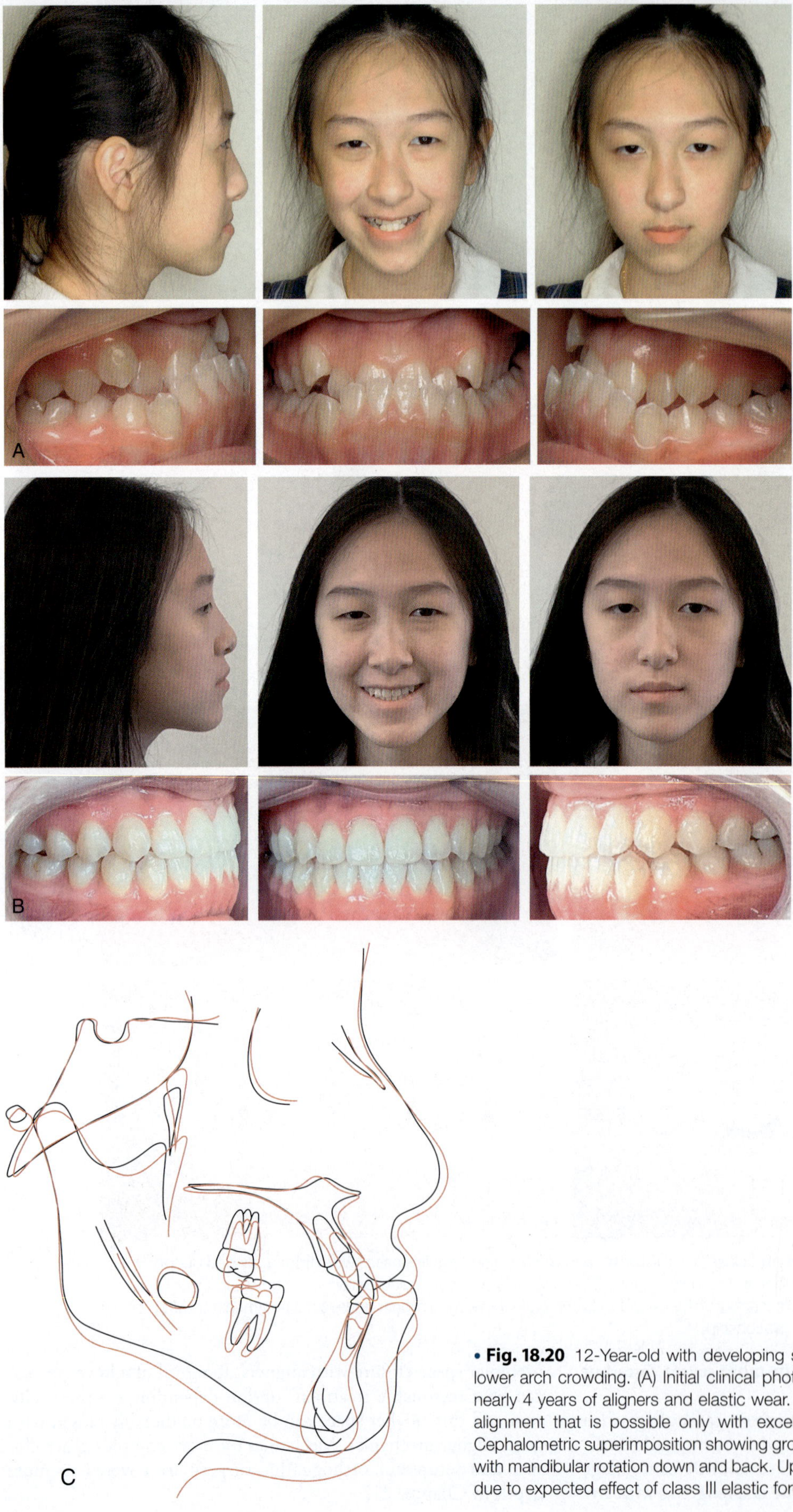

• **Fig. 18.20** 12-Year-old with developing severe class III malocclusion with upper and lower arch crowding. (A) Initial clinical photographs. (B) Final clinical photographs after nearly 4 years of aligners and elastic wear. Note improved facial balance, smile arc and alignment that is possible only with excellent cooperation and favorable growth. (C) Cephalometric superimposition showing growth directed vertically as a result of treatment with mandibular rotation down and back. Upper incisors and molars were moved forward due to expected effect of class III elastic force.

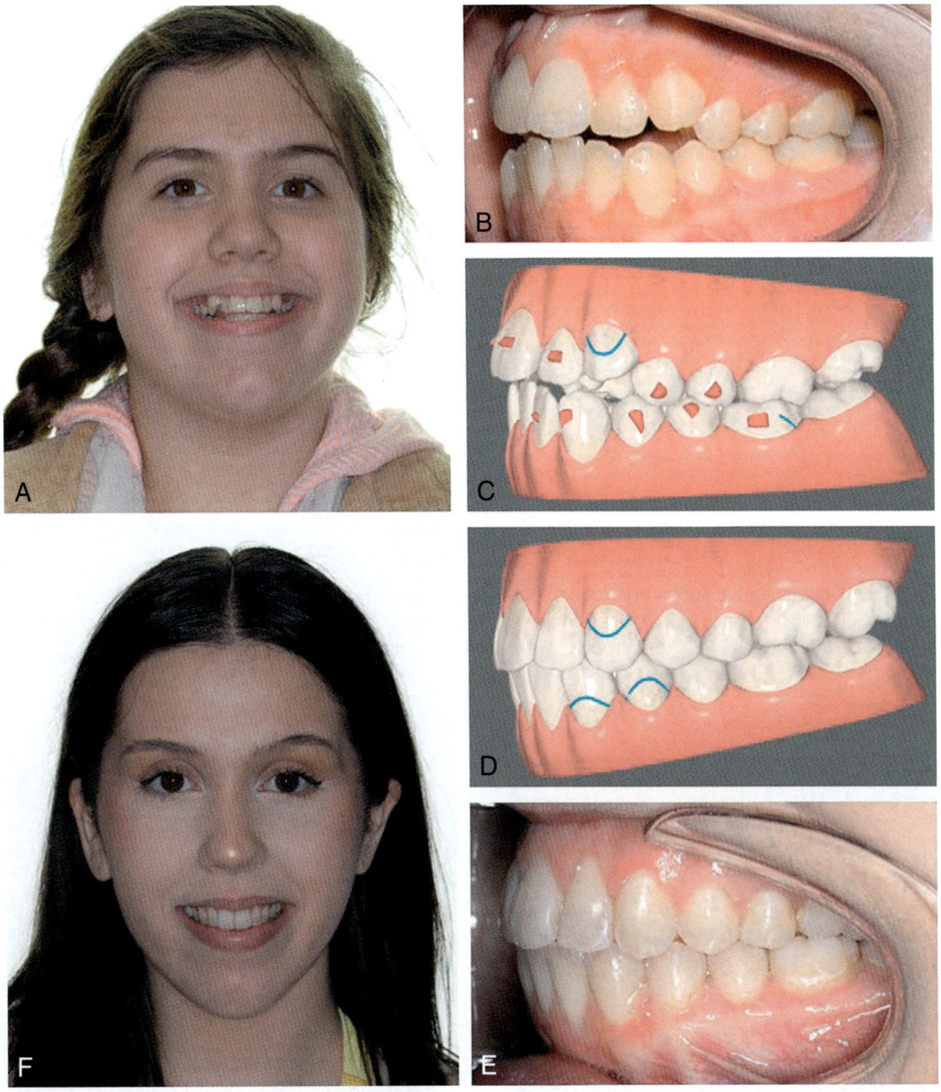

• **Fig. 18.21** 12-year-old with an anterior openbite treated with aligners. (A) Initial frontal photo showing openbite, irregular alignment and a flat smile arc. (B) Initial intraoral photo demonstrating the extent of the openbite. (C) Digital attachment design including upper anterior incisor attachments to aid in extrusion. Also note the cutout for bonded button placement on the upper left canine. (D) Final alignment and occlusion design in final refinement. (E) Final intraoral photograph mirroring the planned tooth position in D. (F) Final facial result showing improved alignment and consonant smile arc.

Openbite Correction

Anterior openbite correction remains a challenging area in orthodontics, but aligner treatment can be very useful in mild to moderate open bites. This is because the thickness of the plastic in the posterior may support posterior intrusion and can allow anterior extrusion. Importantly, since the aligners are digitally designed, there are fewer inadvertent vertical side effects causing posterior tooth extrusion which tend to further open the bite.

Several protocols have been suggested for closing open bites, but all rely on anterior extrusion, posterior intrusion, or some combination of the two. A case example of attachment design and the digital setup for an adolescent malocclusion is shown in Fig. 18.21. This nearly 12-year-old displayed an anterior openbite, flat smile arc, and a mild increase in lower face height. Note that direct extrusion along the long axis leaves very little surface area for engagement. With more significant extrusion, it is typically desirable to first move teeth labially to create space, then simultaneously retract and extrude them. This increases the surface area for engagement during extrusion. All methods of posterior intrusion or anterior extrusion will not fully express clinically, with potentially two-thirds of the programmed bite closure being realized,[11] so overcorrection should be built into the plan. The clinical treatment resulted in positive overbite, a more consonant smile arc, but didn't improve the overall lower face height. A cephalometric superimposition of the patient shown in Fig. 18.21 can be seen in Fig. 18.22. The openbite was corrected largely by upper incisor extrusion, controlling molar eruption during growth and avoiding further opening of the mandibular plane.

Deep Bite Correction

In contrast to anterior openbite correction, deep bite correction can be a challenging movement with aligners as it is more difficult

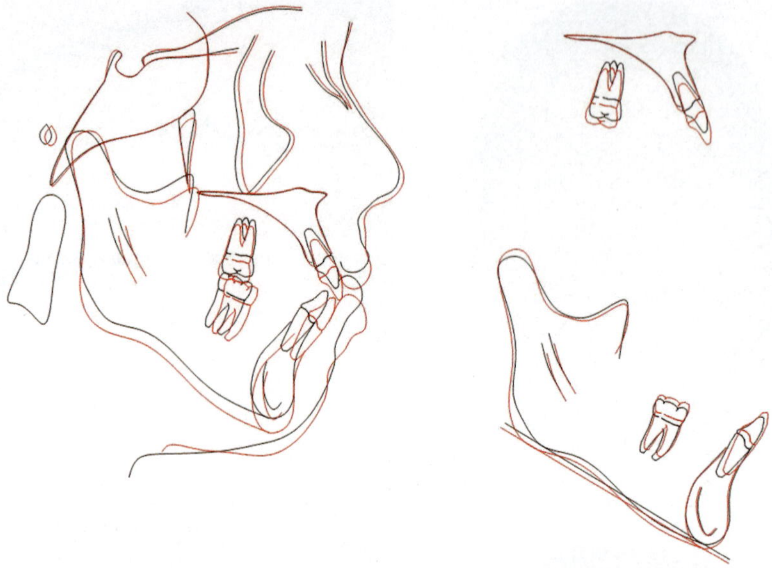

• **Fig. 18.22** Cephalometric superimposition of openbite patient in Fig. 10.21. Upper incisor extrusion exceeded molar eruption and the mandibular plane remained stable allowing openbite correction while maintaining facial balance. Note that molars were not intruded, but eruption matched vertical ramus growth to avoid lengthening the face.

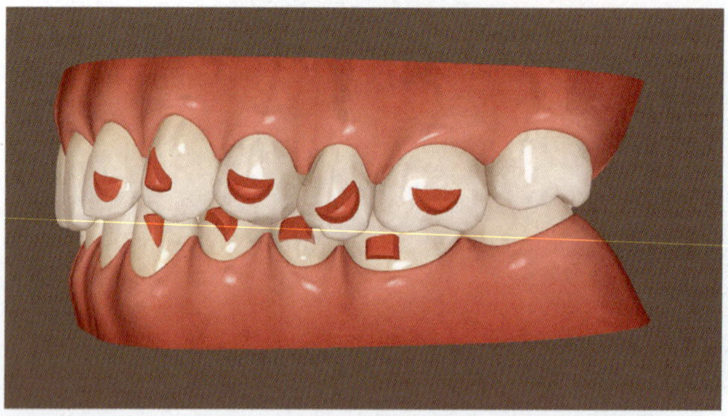

• **Fig. 18.23** Example of attachment design for treatment of anterior deep bite. Adequate posterior attachments are required to provide retention of aligner and delivery of the arch leveling force. This example includes a combination of traditional rectangular attachments and optimized deep bite attachments—the important point is there must be good posterior retention.

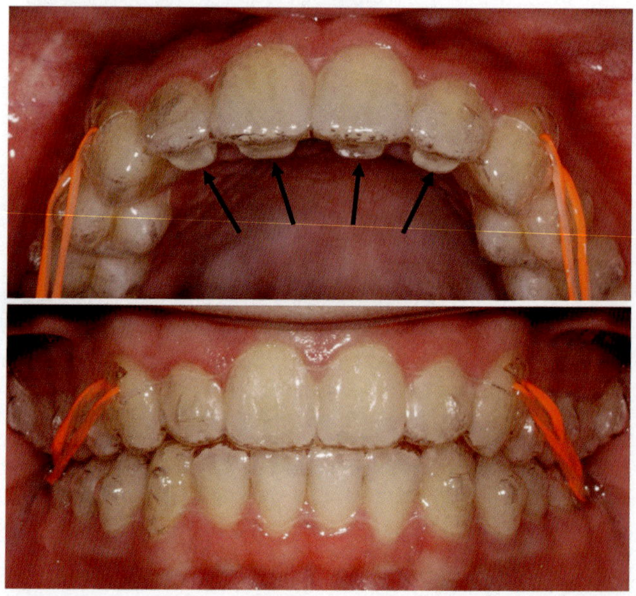

• **Fig. 18.24** Bite ramps added for more efficient correction of deep bite malocclusions. The arrows point to bite ramps on the lingual of the four upper incisors. These prevent the posterior teeth from touching and allow more efficient extrusion of premolars to level the arches.

to generate forces to intrude anterior teeth or allow posterior extrusion when occluding on two layers of plastic. Unfortunately, it is also a very common movement required during aligner treatment, especially in cases with posttreatment relapse of lower crowding or upper spacing.

Providing intrusive forces on anterior teeth will create reciprocal extrusive forces on posterior teeth. Without posterior attachments, aligners will unseat in the back eliminating any significant force application to correct the deep bite. Attachment design in these cases focuses on strong posterior aligner retention (Fig. 18.23), but even with large attachments, the force levels to level the occlusal planes tend to be lower than what fixed appliances can generate.

To allow more predictable posterior extrusion and improve intrusive forces on the anterior teeth, bite ramps can be placed behind the maxillary anterior teeth to remove posterior occlusal bite forces that prevent lower premolar extrusion. These bite ramps can be placed on select teeth where further correction is needed, such as the upper incisors shown in Fig. 18.24.

Finally, deep bite correction depends on the force activation over the entire length of the arch, which is why when using fixed appliances it is helpful to incorporate second molars and move to stiff archwires. Using aligners with relatively low stiffness, small

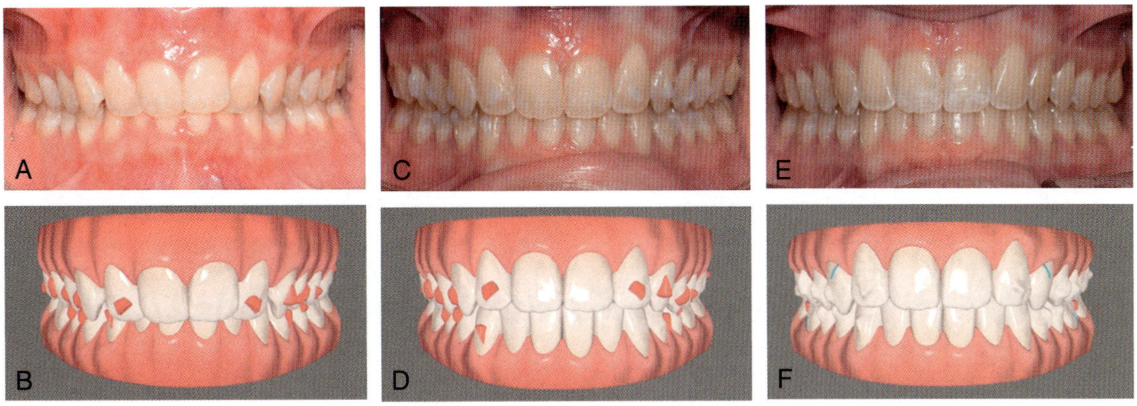

• **Fig. 18.25** Clinical example of the predictable under-expression of deep bite correction planned in the digital aligner design. (A) Original deep bite malocclusion. (B) Attachment design for aligner treatment. (C and D) Planned and actual deep bite correction for first set of aligners. (E and F) Planned final refinement result and actual clinical result at the completion of treatment.

displacements will not create much force. In multiple studies, only 33% of the predicted deep bite correction was found to express clinically.[12,13] Therefore deep bite correction needs to be significantly overcorrected in the virtual setup even when using the mechanics just mentioned. Fig. 18.25 shows the amount of overbite correction programmed into the aligners versus the actual clinical result in a representative case.

Transverse Correction

The final plane of space to consider with aligners is the transverse dimension. Changes to arch width can be made with fixed expanders, aligners alone with mindful attachment design, or with inter-arch elastics.

For adolescent patients where sutural expansion is possible, orthopedic expansion with a fixed rapid palatal expander (RPE) provides the most consistent width correction in cases with a skeletal discrepancy. Expansion can be carried out with a typical expansion protocol (see Chapter 13) prior to aligners. Once expansion is complete, stabilization with a bonded TPA for minimal aligner interference is possible, or the expander can be left in place for stabilization and those teeth supporting the expander can simply be avoided in the initial aligners. Miniscrew-assisted rapid palatal expanders (MARPEs) can also be used in older adolescence and can be maintained during aligner wear if they are purely bone-borne (Fig. 18.26).

If the desired transverse correction is dental or if the plan is to compensate dentally for a mild skeletal discrepancy, correction with the aligners alone can be attempted. This becomes more challenging with larger movements and with more involved teeth. If there are teeth not in crossbite both mesial and distal to a tooth in crossbite, that correction will be easier. With any method, overcorrection of the transverse movement is required. Supporting this recommendation for overcorrection is a study from the University of Minnesota that compared digital aligner setups with actual clinical outcomes and concluded that transverse changes in the maxilla are often not fully achieved.[14]

Cross elastics can be used to support transverse correction, but care needs to be taken to minimize extrusive side effects. These extrusive effects are generally better controlled with aligners because of the temporary posterior intrusive forces seen as a result of wearing two layers of plastic between the teeth.

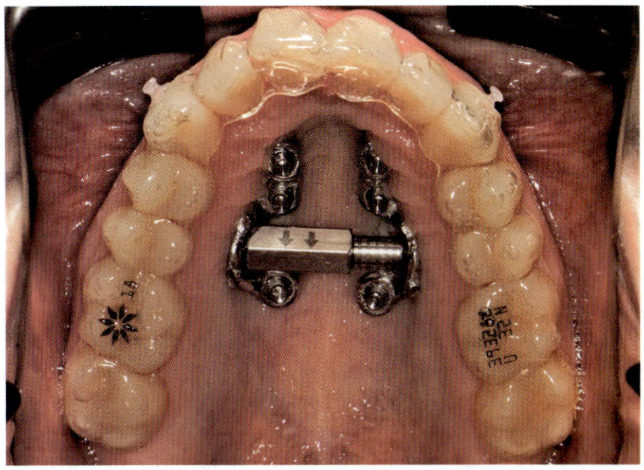

• **Fig. 18.26** Aligner worn with a miniscrew-assisted rapid palatal expander to allow alignment while stabilization of maxillary expansion is taking place.

Hybrid Treatment

Just as braces alone cannot correct every malocclusion, aligners also need additional techniques to improve treatment results in certain cases. This can include inter-arch elastics for bite correction, intra-arch elastics for displaced teeth, buttons and elastic chains for severe rotations, partial fixed appliances, or even full braces for a shorter duration than typical comprehensive treatment. Simple hybrid techniques utilizing elastics, fixed functional appliances, and expanders were covered in their relevant sections already. Some more complex hybrid options are discussed below.

Management of Impacted or Ectopic Teeth

Impactions and severely ectopic teeth are an area where aligners alone are unable to provide the desired force to the teeth. A clear aligner alone cannot provide force underneath the gingival tissue and connecting traction force directly to a removable appliance is challenging. A few different hybrid techniques are available which allow these cases to be treated largely with aligners.

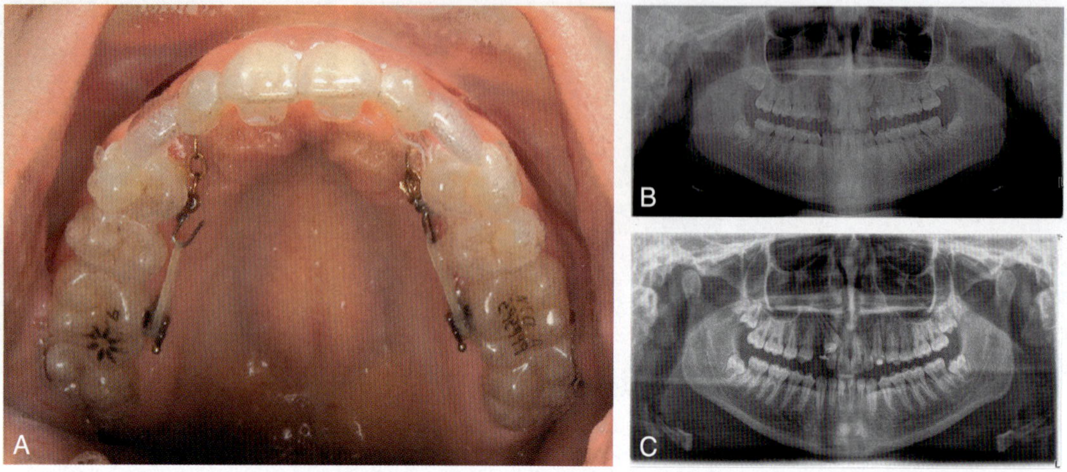

• **Fig. 18.27** Bilateral impacted maxillary canines treated with aligners. (A) Elastics placed from molar hooks to hooks connected to the impacted canines providing a distally directed force. (B and C) Initial and progress panoramic images showing the improvement in canine position as a result of the treatment approach shown in (A).

The first method is elastics added by the patient that are worn from a hook connected to the impacted tooth to the aligner (Fig. 18.27). This will rely on good compliance with elastic wear and it requires an adequate span for elastic activation that can be difficult to obtain in some situations.

The second method is limited fixed attachments, using a transpalatal arch, a temporary anchorage device (TAD), or limited brackets (Fig. 18.28).[15] This may be an option if a patient does not wish to have any significant degree of fixed appliance treatment but does require a more consistent force system for predictable movement of the impacted tooth. It is important to note that these methods should be limited to situations where fixed appliances are refused or unable to be utilized. Currently, the treatment of choice for impacted teeth remains fixed appliances.

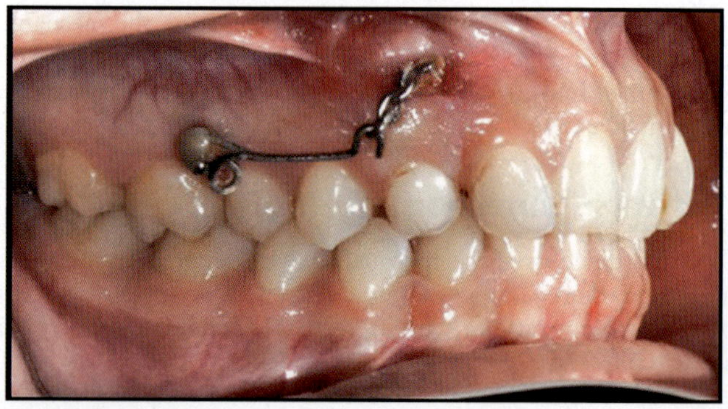

• **Fig. 18.28** Temporary anchorage device (TAD) used to provide traction force to impacted maxillary canine. Lack of attachments on the teeth allow aligners to be worn during the time that traction force is delivered to the canine. (Reprinted with permission from Capuozzo R, De Felice ME, Caruso S, Gatto R, Caruso S. Upper canine extrusion using temporary anchorage devices and clear aligners. *J Clin Orthod*. 2023;57(1):63–72.)

Management of Complex Space Closure or Root Uprighting

There are a number of patients where the majority of orthodontic problems can be managed with aligners but select problems in the case would require fixed appliances. In these situations, hybrid treatment can be a reasonable option. An example of this could be complex space closure, especially in situations of severe tipping or where TADs may be needed for anchorage. Many of these issues are more commonly seen in adults and are discussed in more depth in Chapter 21.

A frequently seen issue in adolescent cases that may require partial fixed appliances is an impacted lower second molar. Cases with severe tipping typically require hybrid treatment because creating an uprighting force with an aligner requires force application on the mesial surface that is not accessible. A large attachment can help with this force application, but limited fixed appliances are typically more efficient.

Likewise, in cases with needing TADs to support significant space closure, hybrid treatment with limited fixed appliances is often a more efficient treatment option. This is often the situation when closing larger spaces such as protraction of the second and third molars to compensate for the loss of an upper first molar as seen in Fig. 18.29.

Finishing Treatment Started With Fixed Appliances

During orthodontic treatment with fixed appliances, challenges can occur that may lead to the braces being removed prior to all treatment goals being achieved (see Fig. 17.17). The most common concern is oral hygiene, where white spot lesions begin forming around the brackets. There are also occasions where fixed appliances are requested to be removed for a special event like senior school pictures, prom, or simple burn out after an extended treatment time. In these cases, it is advantageous to have an option to meet the remaining treatment goals if possible. Please note that this aligner finishing relies on good compliance with aligner wear, which may be challenging in some scenarios just mentioned.

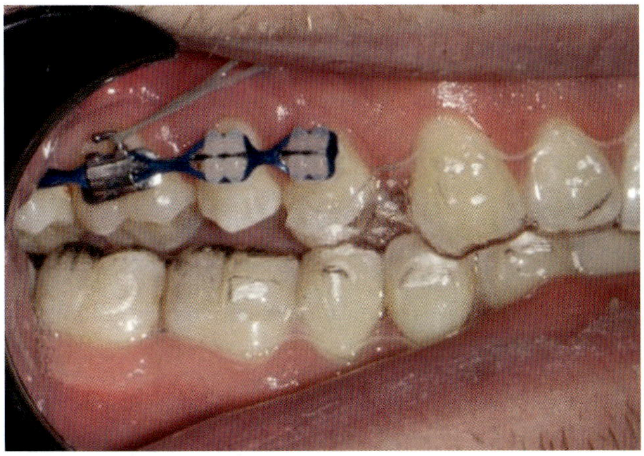

• **Fig. 18.29** Hybrid treatment designed to protract an upper second and third molar to eliminate the need for restorative replacement of the missing first molar. Limited fixed appliances are used to control root position while the teeth are protracted by the force of an elastic chain to a TAD (not visible under the lip). Aligners are in place during this time to align other parts of the upper and lower arches. Once the posterior teeth are fully protracted, a new intraoral scan is taken to plan the final aligners to complete the tooth movement.

Strategies for Success

Providing effective and efficient treatment with clear aligners relies on having good initial treatment goals, a good digital plan and treatment staging, and then proper monitoring of treatment progress. Strategies for designing successful aligner treatment are discussed below.

Digital Setups and Staging

Hopefully at this point it is clear that successful orthodontic treatment starts with proper diagnosis and treatment goals. Digital setups are wonderful tools, but they do not have the biological limits that provide constraints within the mouth. In a treatment simulation, any amount of crowding can be corrected without extraction, any openbite closed non-surgically, and any amount of expansion obtained. It is the knowledge of the clinician coupled with the tools in the software that can create realistic treatment goals.

Knowing that programmed movements will not fully express means that some amount of overcorrection is needed in the digital setup. A brief list of common movements and anticipated overcorrections is shown in Table 18.3.

In addition to overcorrection of some movements initially, care should be taken in refinement setup to assess how well certain movements progressed in the initial trays. Every patient is unique and different amounts of programmed movement may be needed.

In terms of staging movements, some key principles are important:

1. Teeth need space to move: Ensure contacts are open for rotations or extrusion. Binding will prevent movements, so clinically checking contacts at each visit helps identify problem areas.
2. Surface area and aligner retention are key: Ensure large attachments are used where needed. Keeping slightly open contacts and rescanning if there are changes in tissue level ensures the best aligner retention.

TABLE 18.3 List of Tooth Movements and Recommended Overcorrections for Digital Aligner Setups

Movement	Initial Overcorrection Recommended
Rotations	3–5 degrees, either initially or in refinement
Spacing	Virtual closing chain in the final stages or plan to address in refinement
Open bites	Heavy anterior contacts and light posterior contacts
Deep bites	1–2 mm openbite in anterior and heavy premolar contacts mimicking a reverse curve wire
Transverse correction	3 mm overcorrection per side (roughly bringing maxillary lingual cusps nearly to the mandibular buccal cusps)
Anterior torque	10 degrees past ideal (overcorrection)

3. Move smoothly to the final position using all aligners: Although some round-tripping of movements may be needed to open contacts or other reasons, typically movements should move smoothly to the final digital plan. Depending on the digital technician or staging algorithms, sometimes the most displaced tooth doesn't start moving until halfway through treatment, or all movements progress at maximum speed until complete. Both can reduce the chances of ideal tracking.
4. In complex cases, prioritize certain movements in the initial set of aligners: Then, when planning other smaller movements in refinement aligners, different attachments better designed for those movements can be utilized. For some situations, prioritizing certain movements with each digital setup and attachment design can increase predictability.

Attachment Design

Attachment design for individual movements is discussed where relevant for those types of movements. However, some overall design principles are important to consider as well.

Some aligner companies—mainly Invisalign at this stage—have "optimized" attachments that not only involve a bonded attachment to the tooth but are linked to modifications within the aligner fabrication to help assist certain movements. For example, an optimized rotation attachment may create additional activation in the direction of the rotation and clearance on the opposite side for the tooth to move. At this time, those attachments need to be removed in refinement and re-added as needed to keep those additional activations. Put another way, any attachment left on during refinement is simply noted as the new geometry of that tooth—that may be sufficient for many uses (for example, large posterior attachments for retention during deep bite correction) but some attachments may be removed and reworked in refinement to create the best force system for the remaining movements.

It is also important to think about the value of each attachment—many movements are possible without attachments. Sometimes, there is a tendency to overuse attachments so nearly every tooth has one. Also, remember that aligners do not place force solely on the attachment. In fact, most treatment would progress poorly if that was the case. Aligners can provide forces over multiple surfaces of the tooth surface, so occasionally the main purpose of the attachment is to just improve the seating of the tooth in the aligner so the force can be applied as designed.

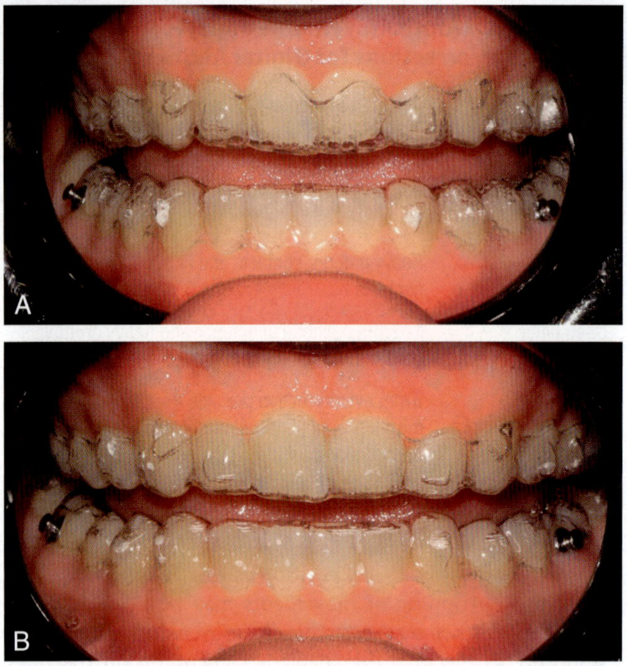

• **Fig. 18.30** Comparison of a poor-fitting aligner (A) and the same patient with a new, well-fitting aligner (B). Note in image A the air gap at the incisal edge of the upper incisors and the cusps of the lower premolars. The presence of these visible gaps generally means the teeth are not tracking properly and that a new intraoral scan and new aligner trays are needed to regain control of the tooth movement.

Case Monitoring and Compliance

In general, since fewer issues typically occur outside the office that can have adverse effects on the teeth, in-office visits are scheduled less frequently with aligners than fixed appliance cases. Patients are provided 6 to 12 aligners (or sometimes even more) to wear for 1 week each. When teeth track well with the planned movement, this works very well. However, when teeth do not track well, time is lost until it is recognized. Therefore, patient education on what to watch for or some form of virtual monitoring where patients send photos for office assessment is important. Fig. 18.30 shows an example of good and poor-fitting aligners.

In cases where there are minor issues with a tooth tracking, checking the contacts and performing light IPR may be enough to recapture the tooth with increased time in that aligner stage. Additionally, there are pliers that can deform the aligners to provide additional pressure to move teeth, as shown in Fig. 18.31. These can used to dimple the plastic to increase retention, help recapture a non-tracking tooth, or assist in finishing at the end of treatment.

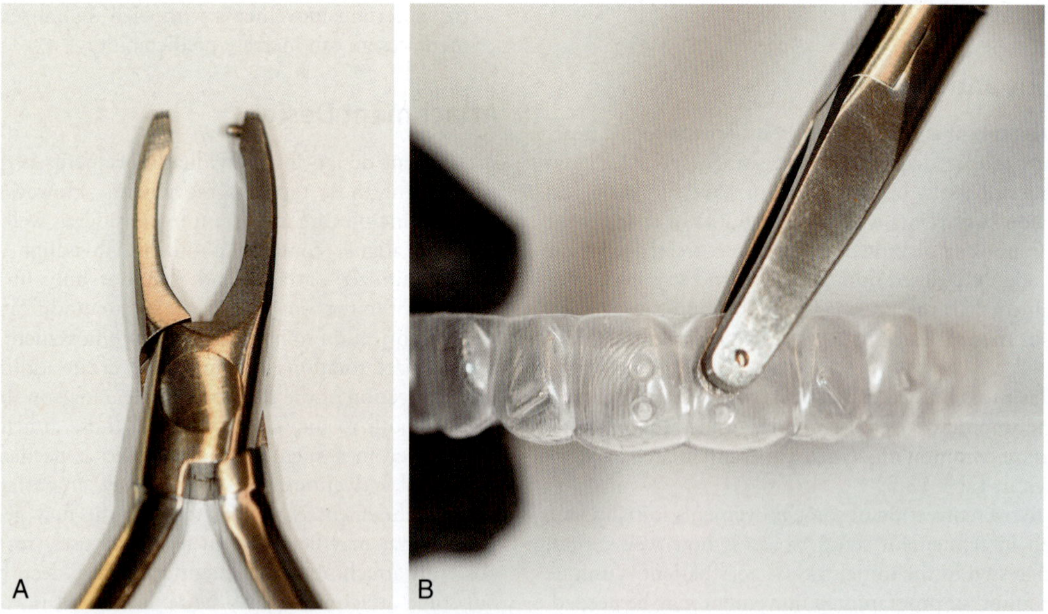

• **Fig. 18.31** Specially designed pliers can be used to intentionally deform, or dimple, the plastic of aligners to provide additional pressure for tooth movement or aligner retention. (A) shows a close-up of the plier, and (B) shows the plier being used to dimple the central incisor areas of an aligner to provide better rotation.

References

1. Levin RP. *2022 Orthodontic Practice Performance Survey*. Orthodonticproductsonline.com; 2023. orthodonticproductsonline.com/practice-management/business-development/2022-orthodontic-practice-performance-survey.
2. Al-Nadawi M, Kravitz ND, Hansa I, Makki L, Ferguson DJ, Vaid NR. Effect of clear aligner wear protocol on the efficacy of tooth movement. *Angle Orthod*. 2021;91(2):157–163. https://doi.org/10.2319/071520-630.1.
3. Crego-Ruiz M, Jorba-García A. Assessment of the periodontal health status and gingival recession during orthodontic treatment with clear aligners and fixed appliances: A systematic review and meta-analysis. *Med Oral Patol Oral Cir Bucal*. 2023;28(4):e330–e340. https://doi.org/10.4317/medoral.25760. Published 2023 Jul 1.
4. Ferlito T, Hsiou D, Hargett K, et al. Assessment of artificial intelligence-based remote monitoring of clear aligner therapy: a prospective study. *Am J Orthod Dentofacial Orthop*. 2023;164(2):194–200. https://doi.org/10.1016/j.ajodo.2022.11.020.
5. Kravitz ND, Dalloul B, Zaid YA, Shah C, Vaid NR. What percentage of patients switch from Invisalign to braces? A retrospective study evaluating the conversion rate, number of refinement scans, and length of treatment. *Am J Orthod Dentofacial Orthop*. 2023;163(4):526–530.
6. Haouili N, Kravitz ND, Vaid NR, Ferguson DJ, Makki L. Has Invisalign improved? A prospective follow-up study on the efficacy of tooth movement with Invisalign. *Am J Orthod Dentofacial Orthop*. 2020;158(3):420–425.
7. Glaser BJ, Tai SK, Blevins R, Daher S. Prospective multicenter investigation of Invisalign treatment with the mandibular-advancement feature: an interim report. *J Clin Orthod*. 2022;56(8):458–463.
8. O'Brien K, Wright J, Conboy F, et al. Effectiveness of early orthodontic treatment with the Twin-block appliance: a multicenter, randomized, controlled trial, Part 1: Dental and skeletal effects. *Am J Orthod*. 2003;124:234–343.
9. Cacciatore G, Ugolini A, Sforza C, Gbinigie O, Plüddemann A. Long-term effects of functional appliances in treated versus untreated patients with Class II malocclusion: a systematic review and meta-analysis. *PLoS One*. 2019;14:e0221624.
10. Hong YY, Zhou MQ, Cai CY, et al. Efficacy of upper-incisor torque control with clear aligners: a retrospective study using cone-beam computed tomography. *Clin Oral Investig*. 2023;27(7):3863–3873. https://doi.org/10.1007/s00784-023-05006-1.
11. Blundell HL, Weir T, Byrne G. Predictability of anterior open bite treatment with Invisalign. *Am J Orthod Dentofacial Orthop*. 2023;S0889-5406(23)00301-3. doi:10.1016/j.ajodo.2023.04.017
12. Burashed H, Sebai RE. Quantifying the efficacy of overbite reduction in patients treated with clear aligners using optimized versus conventional attachments. *J World Fed Orthod*. 2023;12(3):105–111. https://doi.org/10.1016/j.ejwf.2023.03.003.
13. Shahabuddin N, Kang J, Jeon HH. Predictability of the deep overbite correction using clear aligners. *Am J Orthod Dentofacial Orthop*. 2023;163(6):793–801. https://doi.org/10.1016/j.ajodo.2022.07.019.
14. Grünheid T, Loh C, Larson BE. How accurate is Invisalign in nonextraction cases? Are predicted tooth positions achieved? *Angle Orthod*. 2017;87(6):809–815.
15. Capuozzo R, De Felice ME, Caruso S, Gatto R, Caruso S. Upper canine extrusion using temporary anchorage devices and clear aligners. *J Clin Orthod*. 2023;57(1):63–72.

19
Retention

BRENT E. LARSON AND WILLIAM R. PROFFIT

CHAPTER OUTLINE

At sporting events, no matter how good things look for one team late in the game, the saying is "It's not over until it's over." In orthodontics, although the patient may feel that treatment is complete when the appliances are removed, or the last aligner is finished, an important stage lies ahead. Orthodontic control of tooth position and occlusal relationships must be withdrawn gradually, not abruptly, if excellent long-term results are to be achieved. The plan of retention is critical and should be included in each patient's original treatment plan.

Why Is Retention Necessary?

A number of factors can be cited as influencing long-term results, including gender, posttreatment growth, type of malocclusion, magnitude of the pretreatment irregularity, and quality of the orthodontic treatment.[1,2] Most orthodontic treatment results are potentially unstable, and therefore retention is necessary for three major reasons that are summarized in Fig. 19.1:

- The gingival and periodontal tissues are affected by orthodontic tooth movement and require time for reorganization when the appliances are removed.
- The teeth may be in an inherently unstable position after the treatment, so soft tissue pressures constantly produce a relapse tendency.
- Changes produced by continued growth may alter the orthodontic treatment result.

Even if the teeth are in a position that should be stable and there is no further growth, retention is still vitally important until gingival and periodontal reorganization is completed. If the teeth are placed in an unstable position, as often is the case following significant arch expansion, gradual withdrawal of orthodontic appliances is of no value. The only possibilities are accepting relapse or using permanent retention. Finally, whatever the situation, retention cannot be abandoned until growth is essentially completed.

Reorganization of the Periodontal and Gingival Tissues

Widening of the periodontal ligament (PDL) space and disruption of the collagen fiber bundles that support each tooth are normal responses to orthodontic treatment (see Chapter 8). In fact, these changes are necessary to allow orthodontic tooth movement to occur. Even if tooth movement stops before the orthodontic appliance is removed, restoration of the normal periodontal architecture will not occur as long as a tooth is strongly splinted to its neighbors, as when it is attached to a rigid orthodontic archwire. For that reason, holding the teeth with passive archwires cannot be considered the beginning of retention. Bone bending as each tooth is displaced slightly relative to its neighbor as the patient chews is necessary for recovery from the splinting effect of a fixed orthodontic appliance. Once the teeth can respond individually to the forces of mastication, reorganization of the PDL occurs over a 3- to 4-month period, and the slight mobility present at appliance removal disappears.

This PDL reorganization is important for stability because of the periodontal contribution to the equilibrium that normally controls tooth position. To briefly review our current understanding of the pressure equilibrium (see Chapter 5 for a detailed discussion), the teeth normally withstand occlusal forces because of the shock-absorbing properties of the periodontal system. More important for orthodontics, small but prolonged imbalances in tongue-lip-cheek pressures or pressures from gingival fibers that would otherwise produce tooth movement are resisted by "active

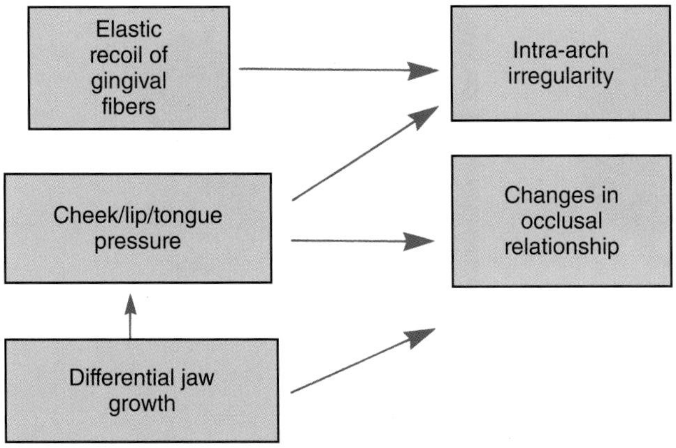

• **Fig. 19.1** The major causes of relapse after orthodontic treatment are elastic recoil of gingival fibers, which can cause intra-arch irregularity; cheek/lip/tongue pressures, which can affect both tooth alignment and occlusal relationships; and differential jaw growth, which can change occlusal relationships. Gingival fibers and soft tissue pressures are especially potent in the first few months after treatment ends, before PDL reorganization has been completed. Unfavorable growth is the major contributor to long-term changes in occlusal relationships.

stabilization" due to PDL metabolism. It appears that this stabilization is caused by the same force-generating mechanism that produces eruption. The disruption of the PDL produced by orthodontic tooth movement probably has little effect on stabilization against occlusal forces, but it reduces or eliminates active stabilization. This means that immediately after orthodontic appliances are removed, teeth will be unstable in the face of occlusal and soft tissue pressures that can be resisted later. That is why every patient needs retainers for at least a few months.

The gingival fiber networks are also disturbed by orthodontic tooth movement and must remodel to accommodate the new tooth positions. Both collagenous and elastic fibers are present in the gingiva, and Reitan showed many years ago that the reorganization of both occurs more slowly than in the PDL.[3] Within 4 to 6 months, the collagenous fiber networks within the gingiva have normally completed their reorganization, but the elastic supracrestal fibers remodel extremely slowly and can still displace a tooth more than a year after removal of an orthodontic appliance. In patients with severe rotations, sectioning the supracrestal fibers around teeth that initially were severely rotated, at or just before the time of appliance removal, is a recommended procedure because it reduces relapse (see Fig. 17.18 and the discussion of fiberotomy). It is clear that any adjunctive procedures such as fiberotomy or low-level laser treatment could potentially help with stability but cannot reduce the need for mechanical retention.[4]

This timetable for soft tissue recovery from orthodontic treatment outlines the principles of retention against intra-arch instability. These are:

- The direction of potential relapse can be identified by comparing the position of the teeth at the conclusion of treatment with their original positions. Teeth will tend to move back in the direction from which they came, primarily because of elastic recoil of gingival fibers but also because of unbalanced tongue-lip forces.
- Teeth require daily (at least 12 h/day) retention after comprehensive orthodontic treatment for the first 3 to 4 months after a fixed orthodontic appliance is removed. Because data from removable Hawley retainers with sensors show that median wear time is about 8 hours per day and rarely exceeds 12 hours but that retainers are reasonably effective if worn at this level,[5] orthodontists have learned to ask for wear every day and for more hours than they really expect.
- To promote reorganization of the PDL, the teeth should be free to flex individually during mastication, as the alveolar bone bends in response to heavy occlusal loads during mastication (see Chapter 8). This requirement can be met by a removable appliance worn regularly except during meals or by a fixed retainer that is not too rigid.
- Because of the slow response of the gingival fibers, retention should be continued for at least 12 months if the teeth were quite irregular initially but can be reduced to part-time after 3 to 4 months. After approximately 12 months, it may be possible to discontinue retention in nongrowing patients, but gradual discontinuation of the appliances can test this process and the stability.
- More precisely, in the absence of growth, the teeth should be stable by 1 to 2 years after treatment if they ever will be. Some patients who are not growing will require permanent retention because of lip, cheek, and tongue pressures that are too great for active stabilization to balance.
- Patients who will continue to grow, however, usually need retention until growth has slowed to the low levels that characterize adult life.

Occlusal Changes Related to Growth

A continuation of growth is particularly troublesome in patients whose initial malocclusion resulted largely or in part from the pattern of skeletal growth. Skeletal problems in all three planes of space tend to recur if growth continues (Fig. 19.2) because most patients continue in their original growth pattern as long as they are growing. Transverse growth is completed first, which means that long-term transverse changes are less of a problem clinically than changes from late anteroposterior and vertical growth.

Comprehensive orthodontic treatment is usually carried out in the early permanent dentition, and the duration is typically between 12 and 30 months. This means that active orthodontic treatment is likely to conclude at age 14 to 15, whereas anteroposterior and particularly vertical growth often do not subside even to the adult level until several years later. In late adolescence, continued growth in the pattern that caused a class II, class III, deep bite, or open bite problem in the first place is a major cause of recurrence after orthodontic treatment and requires careful management during retention.

Long-term studies of adults have shown that very slow growth typically continues throughout adult life, and the same pattern that led to malocclusion in the first place can contribute to a deterioration in occlusal relationships many years after orthodontic treatment is completed.[6]

Retention When a Class II Growth Pattern Exists

Recurrence of a class II relationship must result from some combination of tooth movement (forward in the upper arch, backward in the lower arch, or both) and differential growth of the maxilla relative to the mandible (Fig. 19.3). As might be expected, tooth movement caused by local periodontal and gingival factors can be an important short-term problem, whereas differential jaw growth is a more important long-term problem because it directly alters jaw position and this contributes to repositioning of teeth.

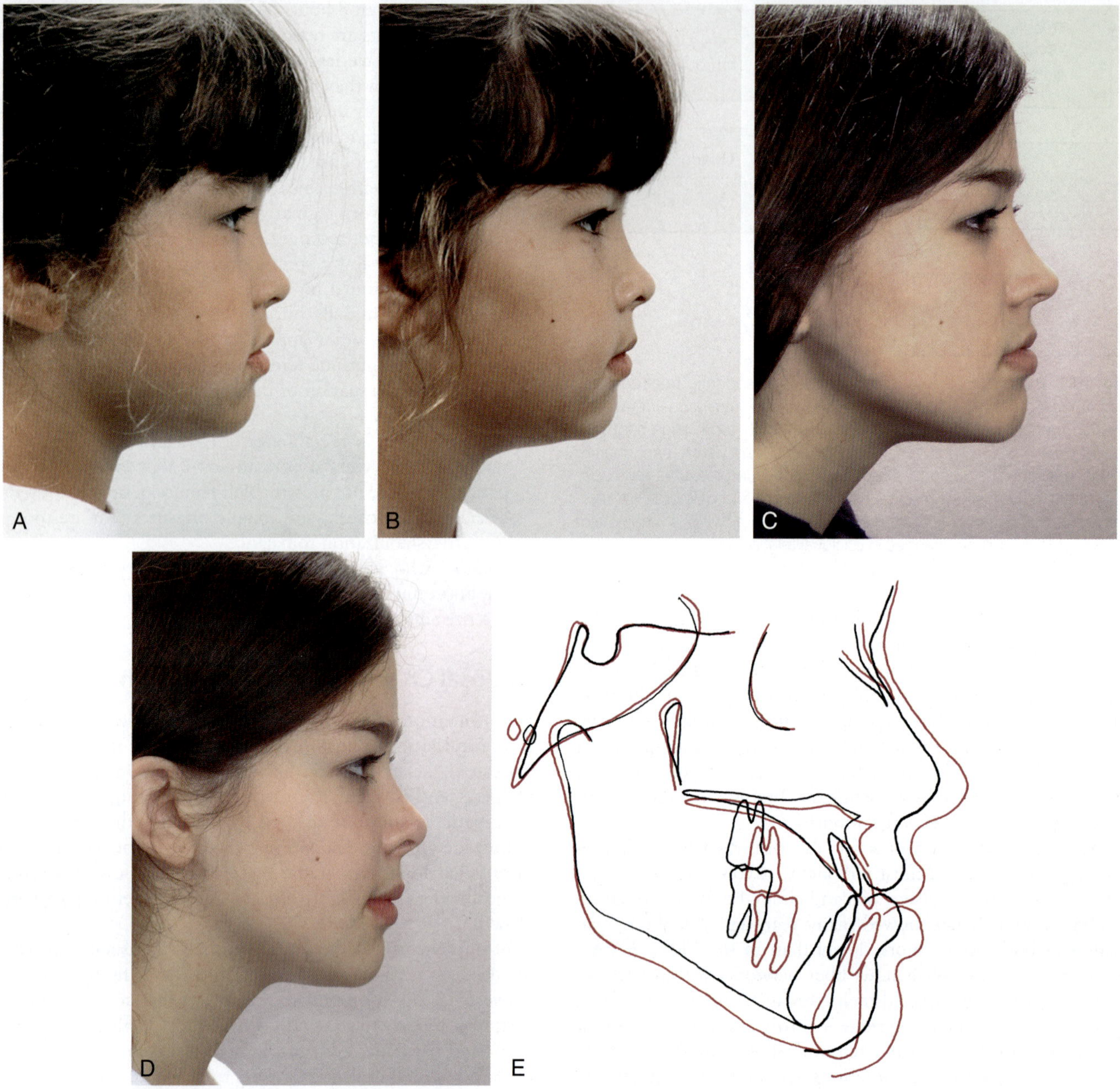

• **Fig. 19.2** Growth after early treatment of a class III problem is likely to cause the problem to recur, as in this girl. (A) Profile at age 7, before treatment. (B) Age 8, after treatment with reverse-pull headgear (facemask). (C) Five years later, after the adolescent growth spurt. (D) After orthognathic surgery, at age 17—which was not done until she showed no further mandibular growth during the previous year. (E) Cephalometric superimposition showing the pattern of growth from the end of the facemask treatment *(black)* through adolescence to just before surgery *(red)*.

Overcorrection of the occlusal relationships as a finishing procedure is important in controlling tooth movement that would lead to class II relapse. Even with good retention, 1 to 2 mm of anteroposterior change caused by adjustments in tooth position is likely to occur after treatment, particularly if class II elastics were employed. This change occurs relatively quickly after active treatment stops.

In class II treatment it is important not to move the lower incisors too far forward, but this can happen easily with class II elastics. In this situation, lip pressure will tend to upright the protruding incisors, leading relatively quickly to crowding and return of both overbite and overjet. Often this occurs only a few months after full-time retainer wear is discontinued. As a general guideline, if more than 2 mm of forward repositioning of the lower incisors occurred during treatment, permanent retention is very likely to be required.

The slower long-term recurrence that occurs in some patients results primarily from differential jaw growth. In patients with class II problems, this can be controlled in either of two ways. The first, if headgear was used in treatment, is to continue its use on a reduced basis (at night, for instance) in conjunction with a retainer to hold the teeth in alignment. This requires leaving the first molar bands on when everything is removed at the end of active treatment. It is quite satisfactory in well-motivated patients

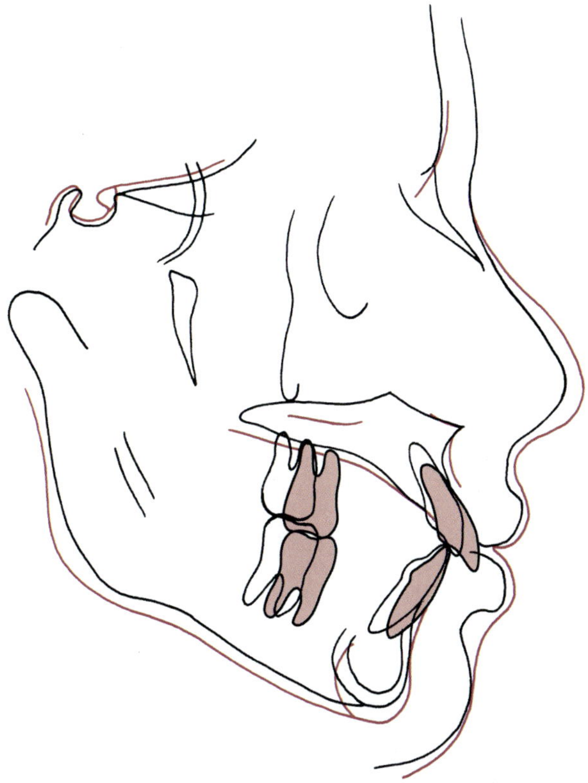

• **Fig. 19.3** Cephalometric superimposition demonstrating growth-related relapse in a patient treated to correct a class II malocclusion. *Black*, Immediate posttreatment, age 13; *red*, recall, age 17. After treatment, both jaws grew downward and forward, but mandibular growth did not match maxillary growth, and the maxillary dentition moved forward relative to the maxilla. As in class III patients, early class II treatment has little or no effect on the underlying growth pattern.

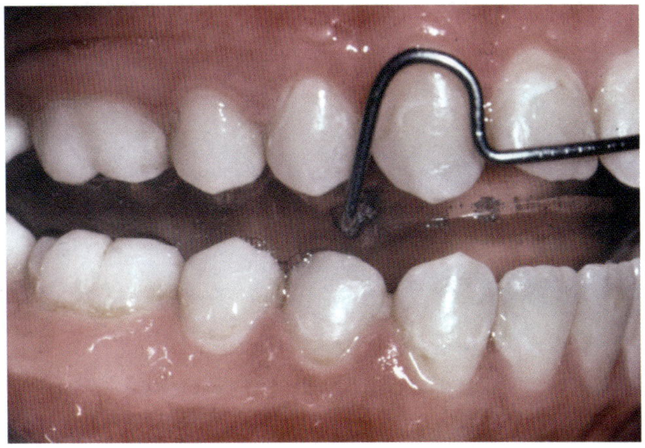

• **Fig. 19.4** In patients in whom further growth in the original class II pattern is expected after active treatment is completed, a functional appliance worn at night can be used to maintain occlusal relationships. In a typical class II deep bite patient, acrylic over the lower posterior teeth is trimmed away so that these teeth can erupt slightly while other teeth are tightly controlled.

who have been wearing headgear and are willing to continue it during retention and is compatible with traditional retainers that are worn full-time initially—but compliance with headgear use becomes a problem with all but the most cooperative patients.

The other method is to use a functional appliance of the activator or Bionator type to hold both tooth position and the occlusal relationship (Fig. 19.4). To the patient, this intraoral device is just another variety of retainer, and compliance is less of a problem. If the patient does not have excessive overjet, as should be the case at the end of active treatment, the construction bite for the functional appliance is taken without any mandibular advancement; the idea is to prevent a class II malocclusion from recurring, not to actively treat one that already exists.

A potential difficulty is that the functional appliance will be worn only part-time, typically just at night, and daytime retainers of conventional design also will be needed to control tooth position during the first few months. Use of a functional appliance as an extra retainer from the beginning makes sense for a patient with a severe growth problem. For patients with less severe problems, in whom continued growth may or may not cause relapse, it may be more rational to use only conventional maxillary and mandibular retainers initially and replace them with a functional appliance to be worn at night if relapse is beginning to occur after a few months.

This type of retention is often needed for 24 months or more after the daytime retainer has been discontinued in patients who had a skeletal problem initially. The guideline is this: the more severe the initial class II problem and the younger the patient at the end of active treatment, the more likely that either headgear or a functional appliance will be needed during retention to maintain the class II correction. It is better and much easier to prevent relapse from differential growth than to try to correct it later.

Retention When a Class III Growth Pattern Exists

Retention after correction of a class III malocclusion early in the permanent dentition period can be frustrating, because recurrence from continuing mandibular growth is very likely and extremely difficult to control (see Fig. 19.3). Applying a restraining force to the mandible, as from a chin cup, is not nearly as effective in a patient with class III malocclusion as a modified functional appliance in a patient with class II issues. If face height is normal or excessive after orthodontic treatment and recurrence occurs from mandibular growth, surgical correction after the growth has expressed itself may be the only answer. In mild class III problems, a positioner may be enough to maintain the occlusal relationships during posttreatment growth.

Retention After Deep Bite Correction

Correcting excess overbite is an almost routine part of orthodontic treatment, and therefore most patients require control of the vertical overlap of incisors during retention to prevent relapse from uncontrolled incisor eruption. Posttreatment growth in a short face pattern, of course, makes recurrence of excessive overbite more likely. Controlling this is accomplished most readily by using a removable upper retainer made so that the lower incisors will encounter the baseplate of the retainer if they begin to slip vertically behind the upper incisors (Fig. 19.5). The procedure, in other words, is to build a potential biteplate into the retainer, which the lower incisors will contact if the bite begins to deepen. The retainer does not separate the posterior teeth.

Because vertical growth continues into the late teens, a maxillary removable retainer with a bite plane often is needed for several years after fixed appliance orthodontics is completed. Bite depth can be maintained by wearing the retainer only at night, after stability in other regards has been achieved.

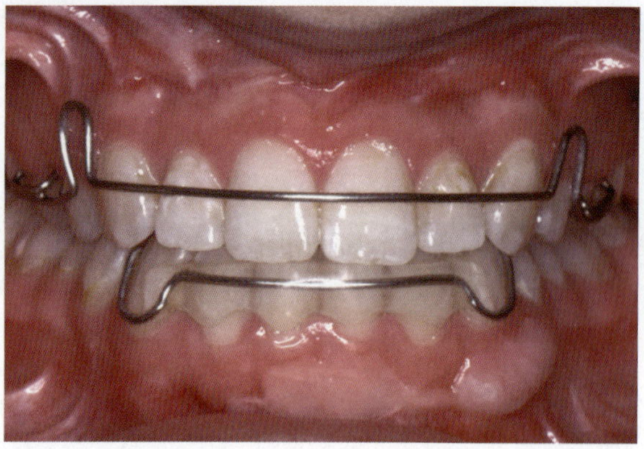

• **Fig. 19.5** Control of the vertical position of teeth in retention is as important as controlling alignment in patients who had a deep bite or open bite initially. For this patient who was treated for a deep bite, the lower incisors contact the palatal acrylic of the upper Hawley retainer, while the upper incisors contact the facial surface of the lower Moore retainer. This prevents incisor eruption that would lead to return of excessive overbite.

Retention After Anterior Open Bite Correction

Relapse into anterior open bite can occur by any combination of depression of the incisors and elongation of the molars. Active habits (of which thumb-sucking is the best example) can produce intrusive forces on the incisors, while at the same time leading to an altered posture of the jaw that allows posterior teeth to erupt. If thumb-sucking continues after orthodontic treatment, relapse is all but guaranteed. Tongue habits, particularly tongue-thrust swallowing, are often blamed for relapse into open bite, but the evidence to support this contention is not convincing (see discussion in Chapter 5). In patients who do not place some object between the front teeth, return of open bite is almost always the result of elongation of the posterior teeth, particularly the upper molars, without any evidence of intrusion of incisors (Fig. 19.6). Controlling eruption of the upper molars therefore is the key to retention in patients with an open bite.

The preferred method to do that is a palate-covering removable appliance (modified Hawley retainer, discussed later) with bite blocks between the posterior teeth to create several millimeters of jaw separation (Fig. 19.7). This stretches the patient's soft tissues to provide a force opposing eruption. As we have noted previously, bite blocks are ineffective in intruding posterior teeth, but they are capable of impeding eruption. High-pull headgear to the upper molars, in conjunction with a standard removable retainer to maintain tooth position, also can be effective, but the intraoral appliance is better tolerated and controls eruption of lower as well as upper posterior teeth. Excessive vertical growth and eruption of the posterior teeth often continue until late in the teens or early twenties, so retention also must continue well beyond the typical completion of active treatment.

The recent increase in reports of successful treatment of mild open bite malocclusion with clear aligners has led to suggestions that vacuum-formed retainers with thickened plastic over the posterior occlusal surfaces may be useful for retention of these patients. The theory is that this would provide enough of a bite block effect to prevent posttreatment eruption of the posterior teeth and that patient compliance would be better, but no good data exist. As we have noted in Chapter 10, individual cases of open bite correction with aligners often show more incisor extrusion than posterior intrusion, and a recent study from the

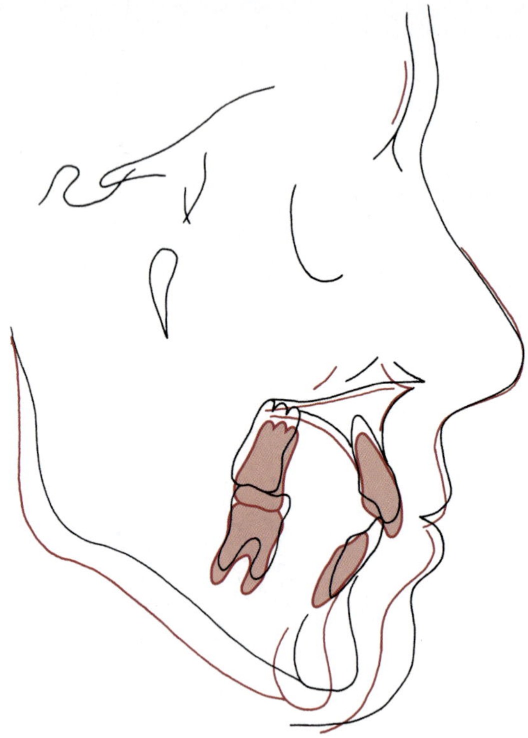

• **Fig. 19.6** Four years after removal of the orthodontic appliances and a reasonable correction of the malocclusion, this 18-year-old with a long face growth pattern has an anterior open bite, 5 mm of overjet with an end-on molar relationship, and severe crowding of the mandibular incisors. Relapse of this type is associated with little or no mandibular growth and a downward and backward mandibular rotation as the maxilla grows downward and upper posterior teeth erupt. The incisor crowding is due to uprighting and lingual repositioning of the incisors as the mandibular rotation thrusts them into the lower lip.

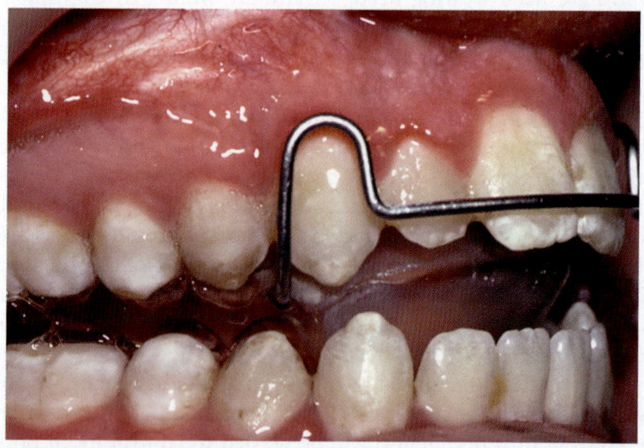

• **Fig. 19.7** Controlling the eruption of posterior teeth during late vertical growth is the key to preventing open bite relapse. There are two major approaches to accomplishing this: a maxillary retainer with bite blocks (or a functional appliance) to impede eruption, as shown here in a patient soon after his severe open bite was corrected, or high-pull headgear. In a patient with the long-face growth pattern, one or the other must be continued as a nighttime retainer through the late teens. Although high-pull headgear can be quite effective in a cooperative patient, a removable appliance with bite blocks is a better choice for most patients for two reasons: it controls eruption of both the upper and lower molars, and usually it is better accepted because it is easier to wear.

University of Washington indicated that this is the more likely outcome.[7] It is possible that open bite retention with vacuum-formed retainers also would work mostly by encouraging eruption of anterior teeth. More trials are needed to clarify their usefulness in retaining open bite cases.

Retention of Lower Incisor Alignment

Not only can continued skeletal growth affect occlusal relationships, it also has the potential to alter the position of teeth. If the mandible grows forward or rotates downward, the effect is to carry the lower incisors into the lip, which creates a force tipping them distally. For this reason, continued mandibular growth in normal or class III patients is strongly associated with crowding of the lower incisors. Incisor crowding also accompanies the downward and backward rotation of the mandible seen in skeletal open bite problems (see Fig. 19.3). A retainer in the lower incisor region is needed to prevent crowding from developing until growth has declined to adult levels.

It often has been suggested that orthodontic retention should be continued, at least on a part-time basis, until the third molars have either erupted into normal occlusion or been removed. The implication of this guideline, that pressure from the developing third molars causes late incisor crowding, is almost surely incorrect (see Chapter 5). On the other hand, because eruption of third molars or their extraction usually does not take place until the late teen years, the guideline is not a bad one in its emphasis on prolonged retention in patients who are continuing to grow.

Most adults, including those who underwent orthodontic treatment and once had perfectly aligned teeth, end up with some crowding of lower incisors at 5-year or longer recall. It seems likely that late mandibular growth is the major contributor to this crowding tendency. Steinness et al. noted that the amount of lower incisor crowding in untreated individuals was three times greater than in those who had a fixed lingual retainer,[8] documenting the need for maintaining these teeth against the lingual tipping that accompanies late forward growth of the mandible. However, several studies have shown that which individuals will have posttreatment crowding cannot be predicted from the characteristics of the original malocclusion or variables associated with treatment. It makes sense therefore to routinely retain lower incisor alignment until mandibular growth has declined to adult levels (i.e., until the late teens in girls and into the early 20s in boys). A recent Cochrane review indicated that there is currently not enough evidence to recommend one retention approach over another for maintaining alignment, so it is best practice to make the decision based on each individual patient and their wishes.[9]

Timing of Retention: Summary

Retention is needed for all patients who underwent treatment with fixed orthodontic appliances, or aligners, to correct intra-arch irregularities. It should be:

- Daily (essentially full-time) for the first 3 to 4 months, except that removable retainers not only can but should be removed while eating, and fixed retainers should be flexible enough to allow displacement of individual teeth during mastication (unless periodontal bone loss or other special circumstances require permanent splinting)
- Continued on a part-time basis for at least 12 months to allow time for remodeling of gingival tissues.
- If significant growth remains, continue part-time until completion of growth.

For practical purposes, this means that nearly all patients treated in the early permanent dentition will require retention of incisor alignment at least until their late teens, and in those with skeletal disproportions initially, part-time use of a functional appliance or extraoral force probably will be needed.

Removable Retainers

Hawley Retainers

Well into the 21st century, the most common removable retainer for the maxillary arch was the Hawley retainer, designed in the 1920s as an active tooth-moving device to close spaces between maxillary incisors and before then serving as a retainer. It incorporates clasps on molar teeth and a characteristic outer bow with adjustment loops, usually spanning from canine to canine (Fig. 19.8). Because it covers the palate, it automatically provides a potential bite plane to control overbite.

The ability of this retainer to provide some tooth movement was an important asset with fully banded fixed appliances because when bands are removed, small spaces between the teeth will be present. With bonded attachments, there is no longer any need to close spaces with a retainer, but it is important that the retainer allow the posterior teeth to settle into occlusion after appliance removal, and slightly trimming the acrylic lingual to the posterior teeth so that an eruption path exists is an important clinical adjustment of the Hawley retainer. The outer bow provides excellent control of the incisors even if it is not adjusted to retract them, especially if the anterior section has acrylic added to fit more tightly, or perhaps even better, if the anterior segment is formed from a clear polymer (see Fig. 19.8D). This modification also improves the esthetics of the retainer.

When first premolars have been extracted, one function of a retainer is to keep the extraction space closed, which the standard design of the Hawley retainer may not do. Even worse, the standard Hawley labial bow extends across a first premolar extraction space, tending to wedge it open. A common modification of the Hawley retainer for use in extraction cases is a bow soldered to the buccal section of Adams clasps on the first molars so that the action of the bow helps hold the extraction site closed.

Alternative designs for extraction cases are to wrap the labial bow around the entire arch, using circumferential clasps on second molars for retention, or to bring the labial wire from the baseplate between the lateral incisor and canine and bend or solder a wire extension distally to control the canines. The latter alternative does not provide an active force to keep an extraction space closed but avoids having the wire cross through the extraction site and gives positive control of canines that were initially positioned labially. The loop of the traditional Hawley design does not provide this.

The clasp locations for a Hawley retainer must be selected carefully because clasp wires crossing the occlusal table can disrupt rather than retain the tooth relationships established during treatment. Circumferential clasps on the terminal molar may be preferred over the more effective Adams clasp if the occlusion is tight.

Remember that an important design element for the Hawley retainer is to bring the acrylic behind the upper incisors high enough to control bite depth. For any patient who once had an excessive overbite, light contact of the lower incisors against the baseplate of the retainer is desired.

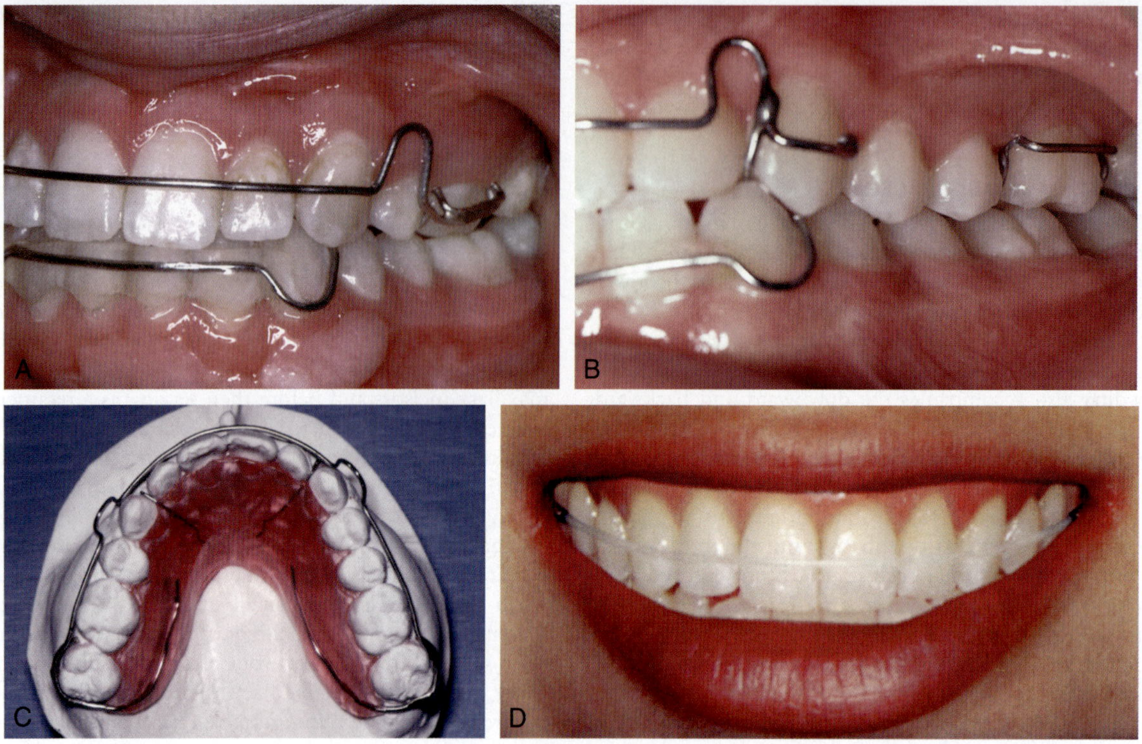

• **Fig. 19.8** A canine-to-canine anterior bow and clasps on molars are the characteristic features of the Hawley retainer design. (A) A Hawley retainer for a patient with maxillary premolar extractions, with the anterior bow soldered to Adams clasps on the first molars so that the extraction site is held closed. (B) The adjustment loop of the Hawley anterior bow often keeps the wire from having full contact with the canines. If good control of the canines is needed, as in this patient whose canines were facially positioned before treatment, a wire that extends across the canines can be soldered to an anterior bow that crosses distal to the lateral incisor. (C) In a patient whose second molars have erupted, a wraparound outer bow soldered to C-clasps on the second molars provides a way to avoid interference as the retainer wire crosses the occlusion, but a bow with such a long span will be quite flexible. (D) A removable maxillary retainer with a clear outer bow, which fits more tightly than a metal wire and is better esthetically but cannot be adjusted to modify tooth positions without starting over with a new retainer.

Spring (Clip) Retainers

A second major type of removable orthodontic retainer is the spring or spring-clip retainer, which consists of a plastic bar (usually wire-reinforced) along the labial and lingual surfaces of the teeth. Retainers of this type are particularly indicated when the goal is to prevent spaces from reopening. In the mandibular arch, canine-to-canine clip-on retainers are used frequently, occasionally extending to include the first premolars (Fig. 19.9). Maxillary anterior spring retainers can be useful in adults with long clinical crowns, but usually would not be tolerated in younger patients because of occlusal interferences.

In a mandibular extraction case, usually it is a good idea to extend a canine-to-canine wraparound distally on the lingual aspect only to the central groove of the first molar (Fig. 19.10). This is called a *Moore retainer*. It provides control of the second premolar and the extraction site but must be made carefully to avoid lingual undercuts in the premolar and molar region. The extension of the retainer beyond the canines also makes it less likely that the retainer will be inadvertently swallowed if it becomes loose.

Clear (Vacuum-Formed) Retainers

A retainer made with a clear heat-softened plastic that is pressure formed down tightly over the teeth with a vacuum-forming device, or positive-pressure machine, is another form of retainer that wraps around the dentition (Fig. 19.11). Although, in today's world, these retainers are often fabricated with positive-pressure machines like the Biostar (Great Lakes Dental Technologies, Tonawanda, NY) they were historically made with suction, or vacuum, and are therefore still often referred to as vacuum-formed retainers, or VFRs. Because the material is transparent and thin, a vacuum-formed retainer is all but invisible, and most patients prefer them. At present this is the most widely used retainer for the maxillary arch, and patients using a clear retainer report greater satisfaction with their treatment than those with other types of retainers.[10] In terms of effectiveness of maintaining incisor alignment, there is no difference between these retainers and a bonded wire retainer.[11] This implies excellent compliance, and it does seem that patients are more likely to wear a clear retainer regularly.

As with anything else, there are limitations to vacuum-formed retainers:

- The thickness of the material over the occlusal surface of the teeth can become a problem, especially if both the upper and lower arches are retained in this way, because separation of the posterior teeth in occlusion may develop. Posterior occlusion is better at 6 months with a Hawley retainer than a vacuum-formed one for just the maxillary arch, but there is no difference at longer-term recall.[12] The combination of a vacuum-formed upper and a fixed lower retainer is better than maxillary and mandibular vacuum-formed retainers.

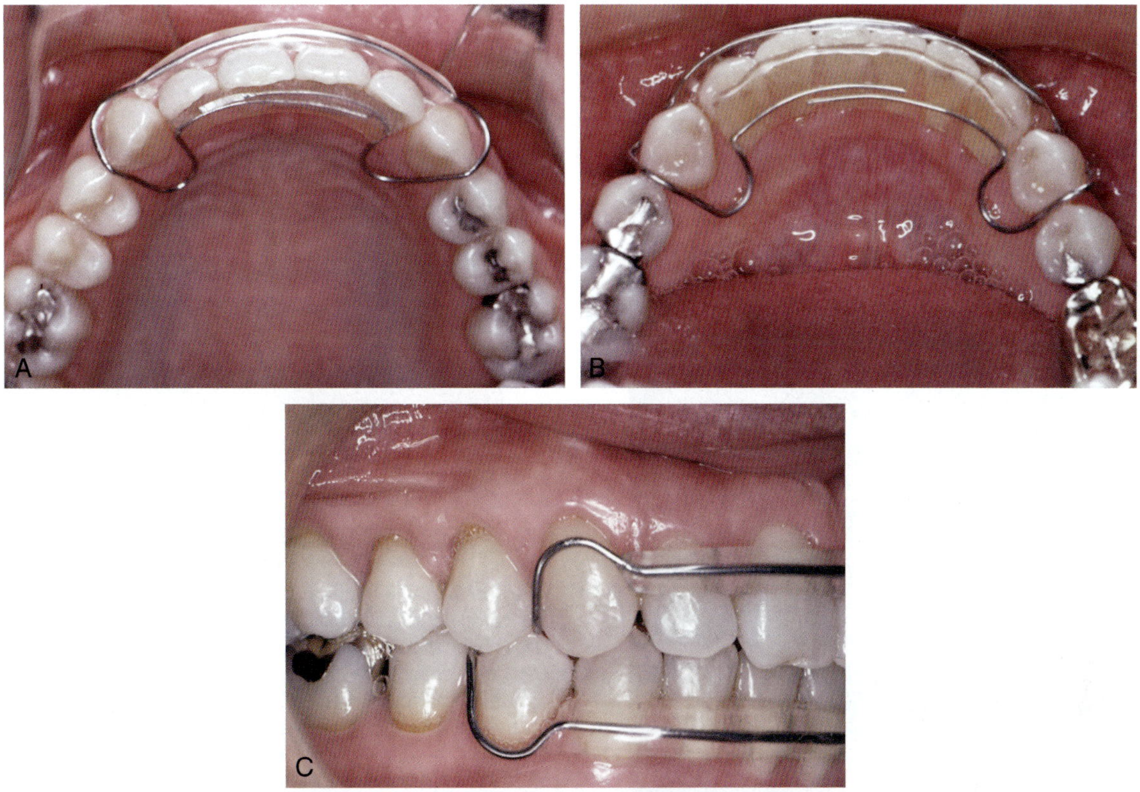

• **Fig. 19.9** (A) A removable maxillary spring retainer that controls alignment of the incisors is rarely used because the Hawley retainer does that while controlling maxillary posterior teeth as well while offering vertical control of the lower incisors. Its primary indication is for patients who had major spacing of the upper incisors initially. In contrast, the clip-on design, shown in Fig. 19.10, is preferred as a removable lower retainer over the Hawley design because undercuts lingual to the lower molars make it difficult to place a lower retainer that extends posteriorly. (B) If desired, a maxillary (or mandibular) 3-3 spring retainer can be extended to one or both first premolars. This is indicated primarily when the canine(s) had been displaced facially before treatment. (C) Anterior spring retainers 3-3 in the maxilla and 4-4 in the mandible in a patient who had maxillary and mandibular anterior spacing before treatment.

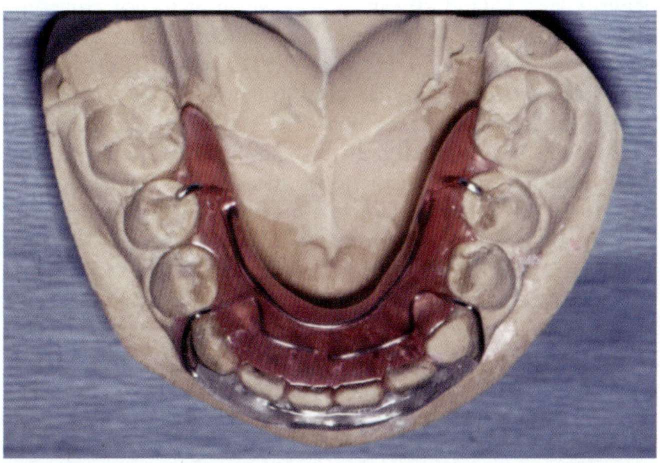

• **Fig. 19.10** For a mandibular retainer, the wire Hawley bow is less effective than a wire-reinforced acrylic bar that tightly contacts the lower incisors. This Moore design has almost completely replaced the Hawley design for lower removable retainers that extend to the posterior teeth. Note that the retainer contacts the upper lingual surface of the first molars but does not extend into the lingual undercuts.

- The retainer maintains alignment but does not control deepening of the bite as well as a palate-covering Hawley retainer.
- The vacuum-formed retainers have less transverse rigidity and therefore may not be as effective at maintaining palatal expansion as a Hawley retainer.
- After 6 to 9 months, a vacuum-formed retainer tends to crack and discolor to the point that it has to be replaced. This is highly variable and some newer plastic materials are promising better long-term survival.

It is widely accepted now that use of the final aligner as a retainer in a clear aligner case (see Chapters 18 and 21) is not as effective as the use of other retainer types, because a more flexible, and less durable, material is used for active aligners. A more rigid material designed specifically for use as a retainer is preferred.

Positioners as Retainers

A tooth positioner also can be used as a removable retainer, either fabricated for this purpose alone, or more commonly, continued as a retainer after initially serving as a finishing device. As discussed in Chapter 17, positioners are now used primarily as finishing devices for patients with an open bite. A positioner does have one major advantage over a standard removable or

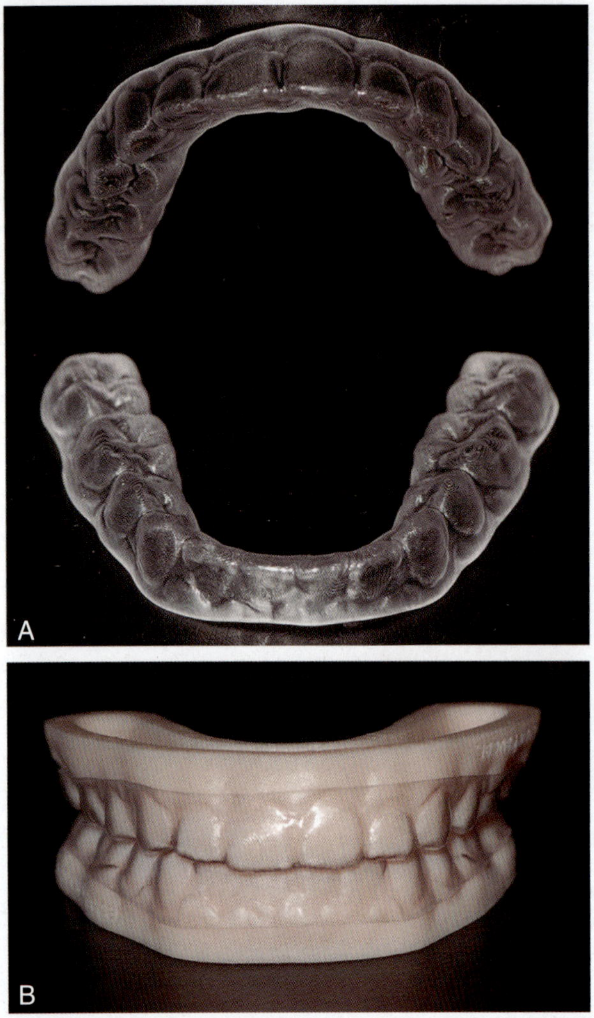

• **Fig. 19.11** Vacuum-formed retainers (A) Upper and lower thermoformed retainers fabricated for maintaining tooth position following active orthodontic treatment. (B) The same retainers shown on the 3D printed models used to fabricate the retainers. This retainer type is often preferred by patients because it is nearly invisible when worn and generally does not affect speech articulation.

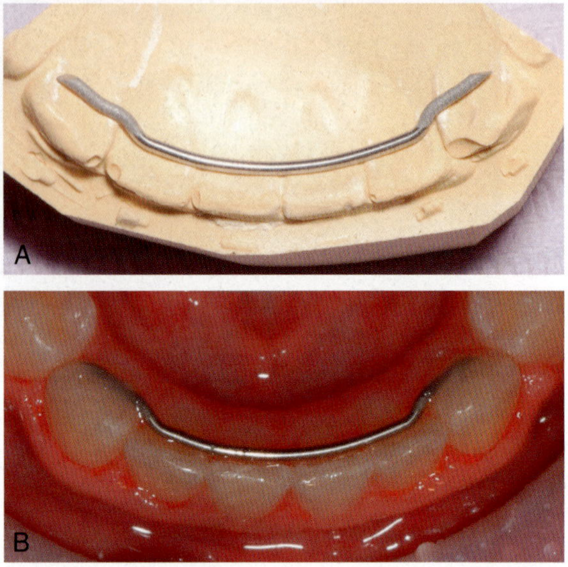

• **Fig. 19.12** (A) A bonded canine-to-canine retainer in the lower arch is fabricated on a lower cast, often with a carrier to hold it in position while it is being bonded. The ends of the wire are microetched to provide the needed retention when embedded in the composite pads. (B) A bonded canine-to-canine retainer, with composite retention pads, in place. The composite should be flowed smoothly over the wire to provide a continuous, smooth contour with the tooth to avoid plaque accumulation and breakage from chewing forces.

wraparound retainer, though; it maintains the occlusal relationships as well as intra-arch tooth positions. With preformed positioners now available (Ortho-Tain, Winnetka, IL), this can be a consideration for patients with an unfavorable growth pattern. A recent review indicated that positioners of this type were as effective as the combination of a maxillary vacuum-formed retainer and a bonded lingual incisor retainer with or without interproximal stripping.[13]

Fixed Retainers

Fixed (bonded) orthodontic retainers are normally used where intra-arch instability is anticipated and prolonged retention is planned.[14] There are three major indications:

- Maintenance of lower incisor position during late growth
- Diastema maintenance
- Maintenance of posterior tooth position in adults

Let's consider them in that order.

Maintenance of Lower Incisor Position During Late Growth

Lower incisor crowding that develops in the late teen years is largely due to late growth of the mandible in the normal growth pattern. Especially if the lower incisors have previously been irregular, even a small amount of differential mandibular growth between ages 16 and 20 can cause a return of incisor crowding. This is relapse because it is caused by tooth movement, but it also is a form of recurrence in that it is related to forward growth of the mandible relative to the other facial structures.

An excellent retainer to hold these teeth in alignment is a fixed lingual bar, attached only to the canines and resting against the flat lingual surface of the lower incisors above the cingulum (Fig. 19.12). This prevents the incisors from moving lingually and is also reasonably effective in maintaining correction of rotations in the incisor segment.

Fixed canine-to-canine retainers must be made from a wire heavy enough to resist distortion over the rather long span between these teeth. Usually 28- or 30-mil steel is used for this purpose. With this design, a bonded retainer can remain in place for many years. Although there has been concern about a long-term effect on periodontal health because of the difficulty of flossing with a retainer in place, long-term recall of patients who had worn a bonded lower retainer for more than 20 years showed no negative effect on periodontal health.[15] In fact, those who were still wearing the retainer many years later tended to be in better health than those who had lost their retainer or had it removed. A similar finding was made in a recent national survey of periodontal health in South Korea: those with previous orthodontic treatment had better periodontal health in the long term.[16]

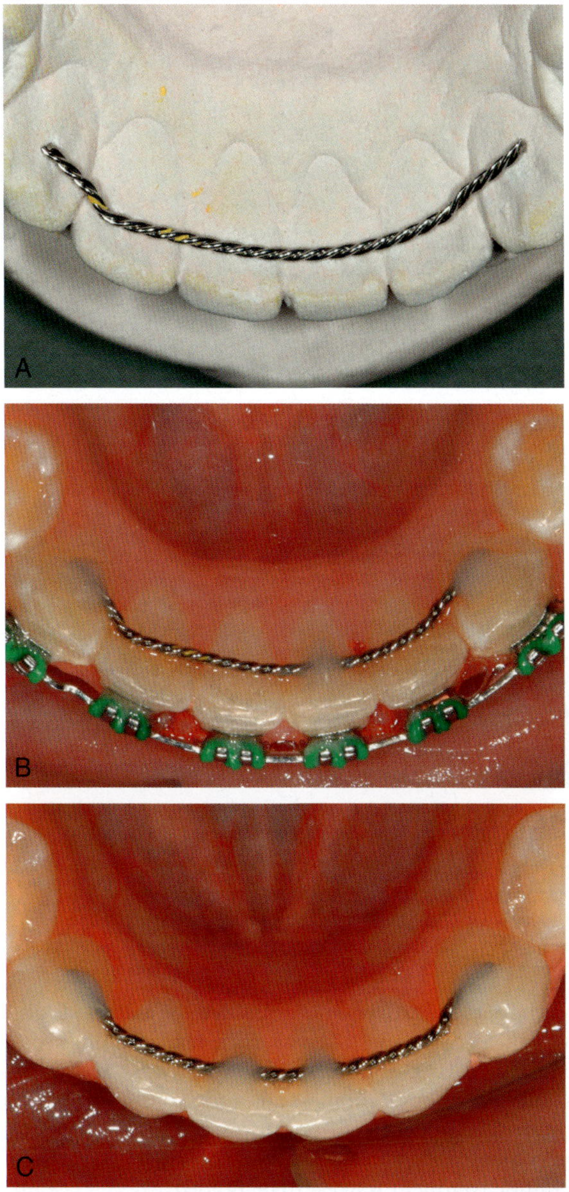

• **Fig. 19.13** It is desirable to place a bonded lingual retainer in the lower arch immediately after removing the active appliance, and often the best way to do that is to bond the retainer just before removing the archwire and brackets. (A) Adapting a piece of passive 0.032 twist wire on an impression of the lingual surface of the lower teeth, adjusting it to fit above the cingulae of the incisors and canines. (B) The retainer being bonded to the canines and one lower incisor before archwire and bracket removal. (C) The completed retainer. This design, with bonding of the canines and central but not lateral incisors, is an effort to combine some movement of the incisors during function with a larger wire for better stability. No data yet exist to compare it with other fixed lingual retainers. (Courtesy Dr. T. Shaughnessy.)

It is also possible to bond a fixed lingual retainer to all or some of the incisor teeth. The major indication for this variation is a tooth or teeth that have been severely rotated. Whatever the type of retainer, however, it is desirable not to hold the teeth rigidly during retention. For this reason, if the span of the retainer wire is reduced by bonding an intermediate tooth or teeth, a more flexible wire should be used. A good choice for a fixed retainer with adjacent teeth bonded (Fig. 19.13) is a braided steel archwire of 17.5-mil diameter. A springy wire of this type must be completely passive when bonded in place.

For long-term stability, enough movement of the mandibular incisors to promote maturation of the supporting bone is important, and the canine-to-canine fixed retainer allows this without restraint. But it does not resist rotation as well as a smaller flexible wire bonded to all incisors. On the other hand, with all the teeth bonded, bond failure and long-term problems are a greater risk.

Maintenance of Diastema Closure

A second indication for a fixed retainer is a situation in which teeth must be permanently or semi-permanently bonded together to maintain the closure of a space between them. This is always the case when a diastema between maxillary central incisors has been closed. Even if a frenectomy has been carried out (see Fig. 15.22), there is a tendency for a small space to open between the upper central incisors. A removable retainer is not a good choice for prolonged retention of a central diastema. In troublesome cases, the diastema is closed when the retainer is in place but opens up quickly when it is removed. This "jiggling" tooth movement that accompanies the back-and-forth closure is potentially damaging to the periodontium and should be avoided.

The best retainer for this purpose is a bonded section of flexible wire, as shown in Fig. 19.14. The wire should be contoured so that it lies near the cingulum to keep it out of occlusal contact. The object of the retainer is to hold the teeth together while allowing them some ability to move independently during function, hence the importance of a flexible wire.

If generalized spacing existed between maxillary or mandibular incisors, a bonded section of flexible wire attached to more teeth can be used to keep the teeth together, extending lateral-to-lateral in the same way as a retainer to maintain alignment (Fig. 19.15). Extending the bonded wire to the canines or premolars can be done but it greatly increases the chance of bonding failure and is indicated only rarely.

Inadvertent Tooth Movement With Fixed Lingual Retainers

Recent experience has shown an unexpected hazard with fixed lingual retainers: the wires, even those carefully fabricated to be passive, can produce unexpected long-term changes. Fortunately, this happens rarely. Unfortunately, the extent of change when it does occur can be far beyond trivial (Fig. 19.16).[17] Until recently, most orthodontists were unaware that this occurred; those who had seen it thought it was just bad luck with one or two of their patients. Now it is clear that patients with fixed retainers in place need regular observation, by a family dentist if not the orthodontist, because remarkable changes can develop slowly over time before the patient notices the changes and decides to see someone about it.

Loss of lower incisor alignment from inadvertent tooth movement is more likely when wires break (Fig. 19.16A). This is most likely with smaller dimension wires bonded to all the anterior teeth. When a wire breaks, it is likely to become distorted at the same time, and that can lead to activation of the wire even if it was originally placed in a passive state. Lower canine-to-canine wires must be larger and are unlikely to break. Perhaps more important, if the bond to one canine is lost, the retainer is likely to break loose from the other one, and if not, the patient will almost surely notice the loose wire.

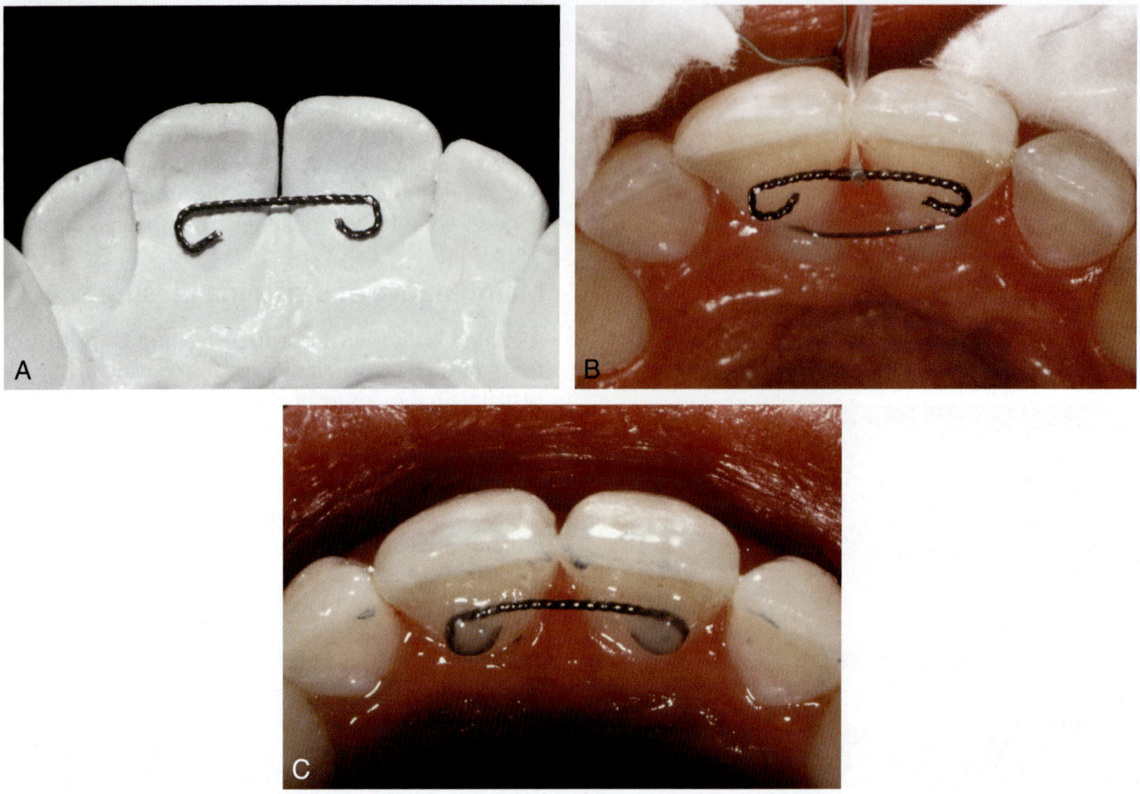

• **Fig. 19.14** Bonded lingual retainer for maintenance of a maxillary central diastema. (A) Use of 17.5-mil twist wire contoured to fit passively on the dental cast. (B) A wire ligature is passed around the necks of the teeth to hold them tightly together while the retainer is bonded. The wire retainer is held in place with dental floss passed around the contact, and (C) composite resin is flowed onto the cingulum of the teeth, over the wire ends. Note that the retainer wire is positioned gingivally to avoid contact with the lower incisors. A Hawley retainer or vacuum-formed retainer can be worn to stabilize other teeth in the presence of a bonded segment of this type.

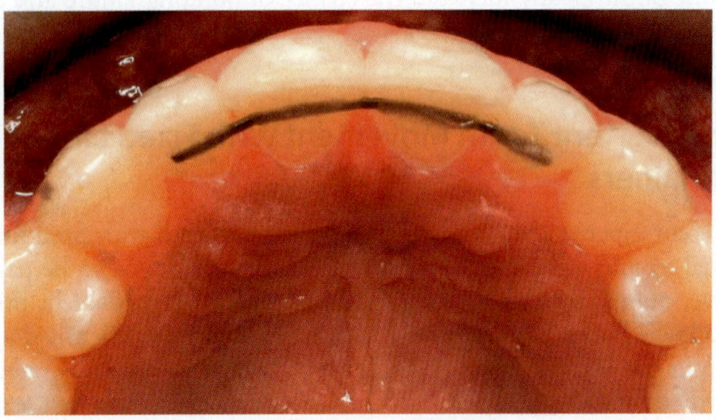

• **Fig. 19.15** A section of wire, usually bonded just to the four maxillary incisors, also can be used to maintain alignment of maxillary incisors that were severely displaced. A wire segment such as this also can be used to prevent deepening of the bite as lower incisors erupt. In this case a 0.027″ × 0.011″ ribbon archwire was used to minimize occlusal interference (Courtesy Retanium, Reliance Orthodontic Products, Itasca, IL).

It is quite possible, however, for problems to arise even when the retainer remains bonded (Fig. 19.16B and C). With spiral wires, tooth movement due to a wire that was slightly distorted as it was being bonded could be the problem, and downward deflection of the wire could occur if the bonds to the incisors failed but the canines remained bonded. As the figures show, displacement of the tooth roots by inadvertent torque forces is as likely as displacement of the crowns, and this may cause fenestration of the labial or lingual alveolar cortical bone. Retreatment is needed in such cases, and can be quite complex and time-consuming in order to correct both alignment and root displacement. For patients with severe root displacement, coordinated periodontal surgery and orthodontic treatment is likely to be needed.

Inadvertent tooth movement also can become a problem with a bonded diastema retainer, such as the one shown in Fig. 19.16D. If the bonded retainer wire is placed in an active state, or it becomes active through occlusal trauma, the roots of the central incisors will slowly move in opposite directions. This is much more likely when a spiral, or twisted, wire is used as the retainer and for that reason this wire type should be avoided when possible.

This experience makes it plain that long-term professional supervision of fixed lingual retainers is needed. Patients with fixed retainers should be seen in the initial retention period by the orthodontist, perhaps for the first 2 years when bond failure rates are greatest. After 2 years, it would seem most practical for the patient's dentist to inspect the fixed retainer at regular dental examinations.

Maintenance of Spaces in the Dental Arch

A fixed retainer is also the best choice to maintain a space where an implant (or bridge pontic) eventually will be placed. There often is a delay in placing the restoration that will serve, among other functions, as a permanent orthodontic retainer. If further

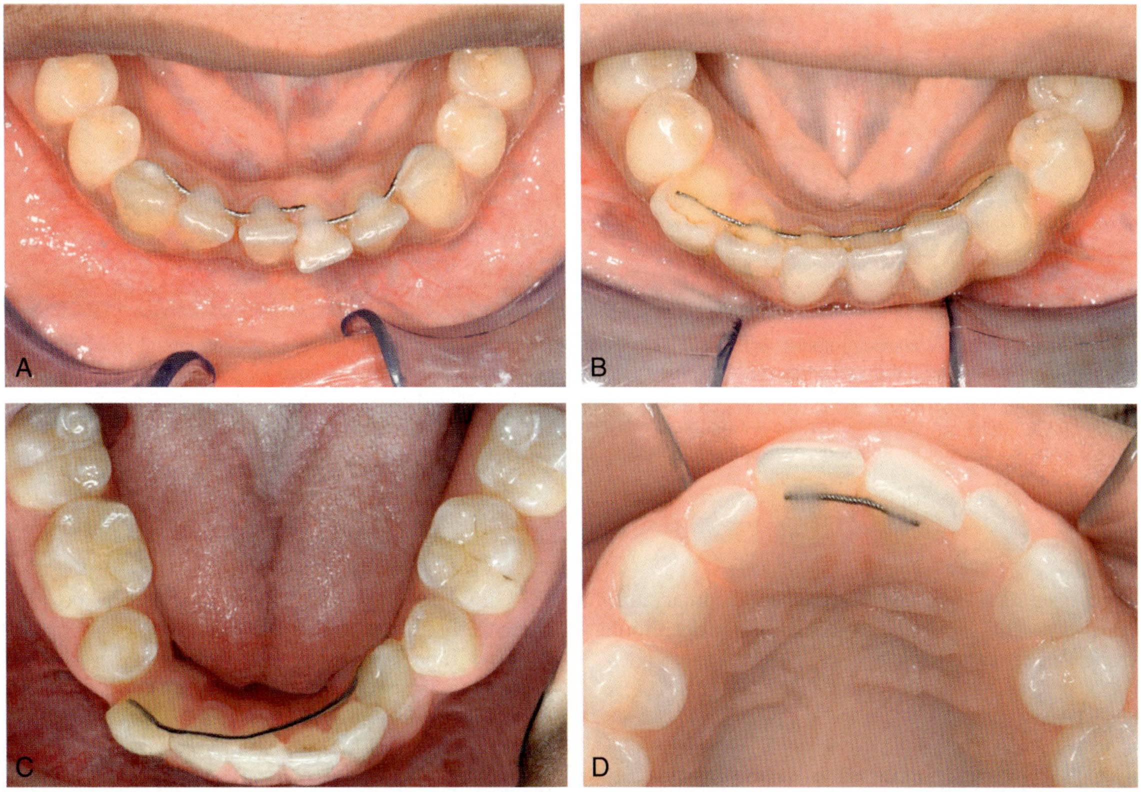

• **Fig. 19.16** Inadvertent tooth movement from fixed lingual retainers (A) For this patient, after breakage of the wire in the midline, the left incisors were tipped facially and the canine was torqued lingually. The other segment showed less effect, but root movement of the right canine also occurred. (B) This individual had the lingual retainer wire completely intact. It became active from biting forces or other trauma, and resulted in gradual facial tipping of the right canine and torque of the right lateral incisor and central incisor in opposite directions. (C) This twist wire retainer was still secured at both canines but had debonded from the incisors. Note the skewing of the arch form and the severe torque in opposite directions on the canines. (D) Bonded retainers to maintain closure of a maxillary central incisor also can produce inadvertent tooth movement. Eight years after placement of a bonded retainer, central incisors showing active torque expressed from what should have been a passive wire. (Courtesy Dr. T. Shaughnessy.)

periodontal therapy or bone grafting is needed after the teeth have been positioned, several months or even a year can pass, and a fixed retainer is much better than a removable one.

The preferred retainer for maintaining space for posterior restorations is a heavy intracoronal wire bonded to the adjacent teeth (Fig. 19.17). Obviously, the longer the span, the heavier the wire should be. Placing the wire gingivally, out of occlusion, decreases the chance that it will be displaced or distorted by occlusal forces.

Anterior spaces need a replacement tooth, which can be attached to a removable retainer (Fig. 19.18). This approach guarantees nearly full-time wear and is satisfactory for short periods. After a few months, especially if an implant or permanent bridge will be delayed for a long time while adolescent vertical growth is completed, it is better to place a fixed retainer in the form of a temporary bonded bridge.

The major objection to any fixed retainer is that it makes interproximal hygiene procedures more difficult, especially in the lower anterior area. In this sense, there is both bad and good news: there is greater plaque buildup when a multistrand wire is bonded to all the lower anterior teeth than when a heavier round wire is bonded only to the canines, but a wire bonded to all the teeth is more effective in maintaining alignment.[18] It is possible to floss between

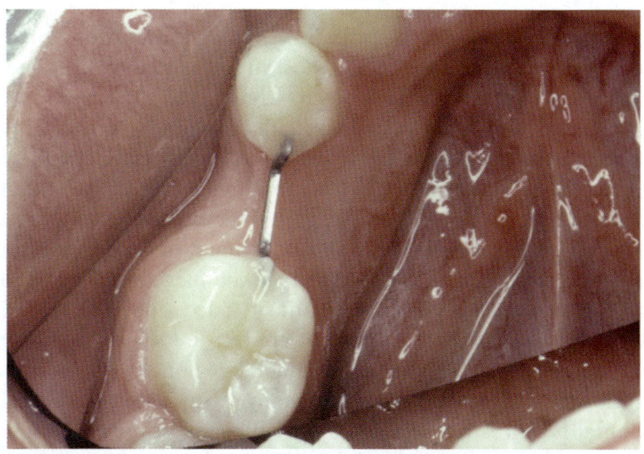

• **Fig. 19.17** A fixed retainer to maintain space for eventual replacement of a missing second premolar. A shallow preparation has been made in the enamel of the marginal ridges adjacent to the extraction site, and a section of 21 × 25 wire, stepped down away from the occlusion, is bonded as a retainer.

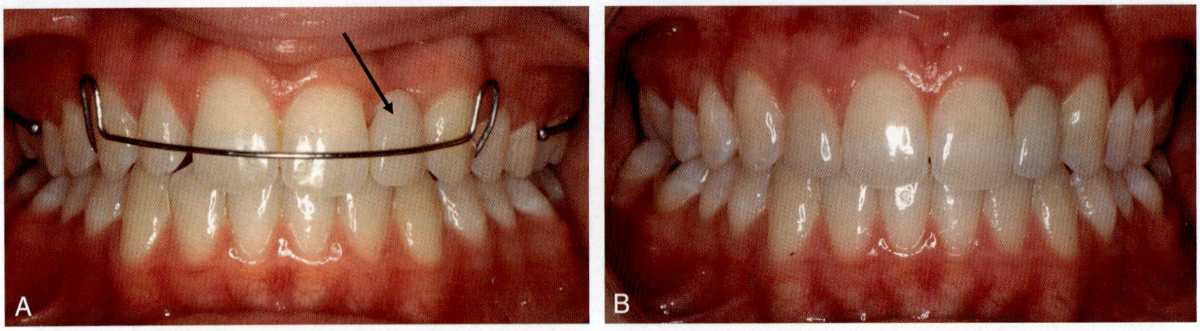

• **Fig. 19.18** (A) Hawley retainer with pontic added to maintain space for the missing upper left lateral incisor (*arrow*) following orthodontic treatment provides esthetic retention during the time needed for growth completion prior to implant placement. Note that the upper right lateral is small and also in need of restoration. (B) Same patient after left lateral incisor implant restoration and veneer restoration on right lateral incisor. The retainer in A was successful in keeping the appropriate space during the transition period until final restorations were possible.

teeth that have a fixed retainer across the interdental contact areas by using a floss-threading device, and the orthodontist should teach and strongly encourage this.

Active Retainers

"Active retainer" is a contradiction in terms because a device cannot be actively moving teeth and serving as a retainer at the same time. It does happen, however, that relapse or growth changes after orthodontic treatment lead to a need for some tooth movement during retention. This usually is accomplished with a removable appliance that continues as a retainer after it has repositioned the teeth; hence the name. A typical Hawley retainer, if used initially to close a small amount of band space, can be considered an active retainer, but the term usually is reserved for two specific situations: realignment of irregular incisors with spring retainers or aligners and management of class II or class III relapse tendencies with modified functional appliances.

Realignment of Irregular Incisors

Re-crowding of lower incisors is the major indication for an active retainer to correct incisor position. The shape of the incisor crowns can contribute to re-crowding,[19] but the cause of the problem in these cases usually is late mandibular growth that tipped the incisors lingually. If late crowding has developed, it is often necessary to reduce the interproximal width of lower incisors before realigning them, so that the crowns are not forced labially into an obviously unstable position. Not only does interproximal reduction of contacts reduce the mesiodistal width of the incisors, decreasing the amount of space required for their alignment, but it also flattens the contact areas. This increases the inherent stability of the arch in this region. If IPR is done cautiously and judiciously, data indicate that long-term periodontal health is not affected by the increase in root proximity that would be an inevitable side effect.[20]

Interproximal enamel can be removed with either abrasive strips, thin disks in a handpiece, or thin flame-shaped diamond stones. Obviously, enamel reduction should not be overdone, but if necessary, the width of each lower incisor can be reduced up to 0.5 mm without going through the interproximal enamel. If an additional 2 mm of space can be gained, reducing each incisor 0.25 mm per side (Fig. 19.19), it is usually possible to realign these teeth after moderate relapse.

After interproximal reduction to achieve appropriate space, there now are two ways to complete the realignment: an active canine-to-canine spring retainer, or a short series of aligners produced in-office with a three-dimensional (3D) printer. The steps in making such an active retainer are (1) reduce the interproximal width of the incisors and apply topical fluoride to the newly exposed enamel surfaces; (2) prepare a laboratory model on which the teeth can be reset into alignment; and (3) fabricate an alignment device to fit the model (Fig. 19.20). The 3D printer technology to achieve alignment would be the same as with other applications of in-office aligners and is discussed in Chapters 18 and 21.

If there is more than a modest degree of relapse, however, a fixed appliance for retreatment must be considered. With bonded brackets on the lower arch from premolar to premolar, space can be opened and superelastic nickel-titanium (NiTi) wires can be used to bring the incisors back into alignment quite efficiently (Fig. 19.21). It is wise to include some interproximal reduction when this is done, at least enough to flatten the contact areas. Permanent retention obviously will be required after the realignment, so a bonded lingual retainer should be placed before the brackets are removed.

Correction of Occlusal Discrepancies: Modified Functional Appliances as Active Retainers

It is possible to describe an activator as consisting of maxillary and mandibular retainers joined by an interocclusal bite block. Although even the simplest activator is more complex than that (see Chapter 13), the description does illustrate the potential of a modified functional appliance to simultaneously maintain the position of teeth within the arches while altering, at least minimally, the occlusal relationships.

A typical use for an activator or Bionator as an active retainer would be in a male adolescent who had slipped back 2 to 3 mm toward a class II relationship after early correction. It would look exactly like the functional appliance retainer (see Fig. 19.4), except that the bite was taken to advance the mandible the 2 to 3 mm needed to correct the occlusion. If the patient still is experiencing

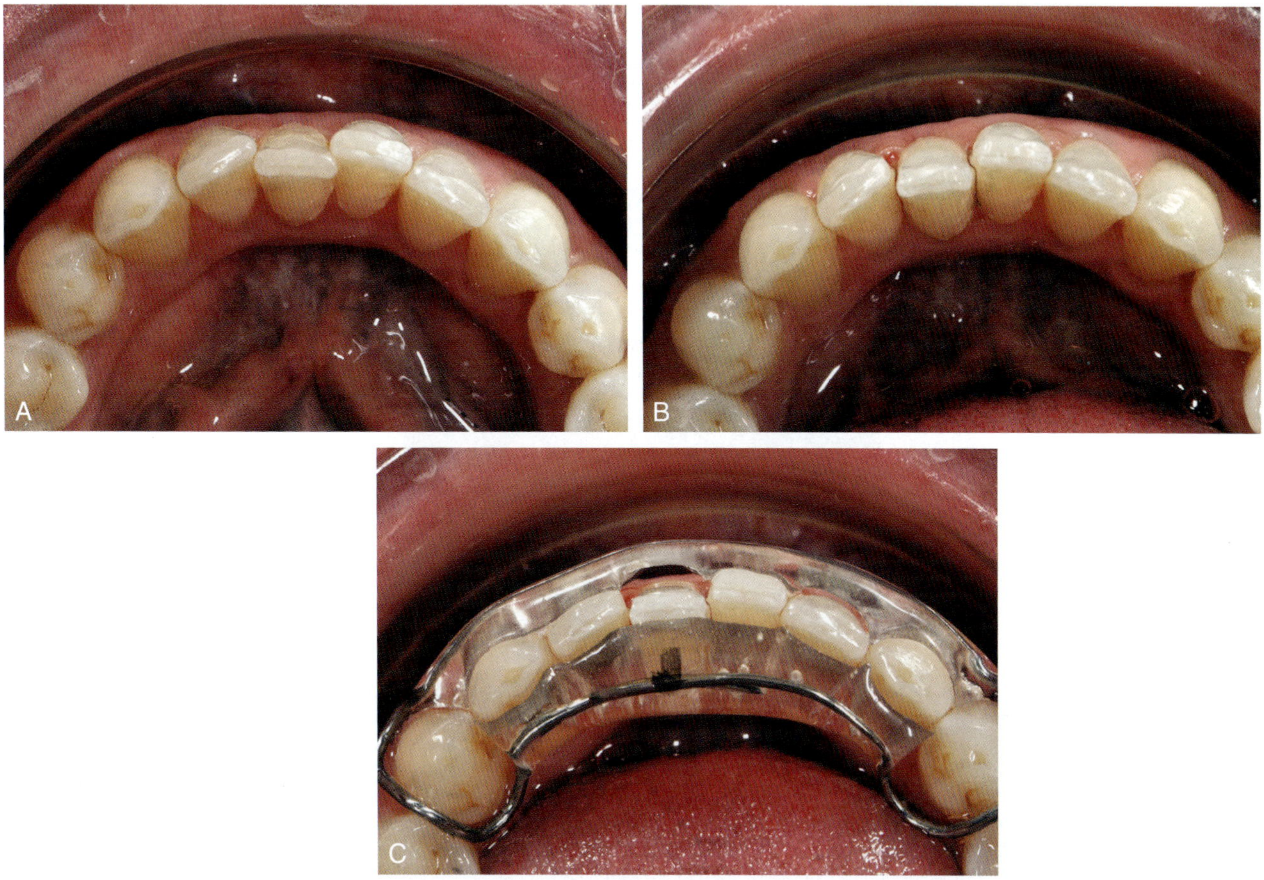

• **Fig. 19.19** Removal of interproximal enamel to facilitate alignment of crowded lower incisors. (A and B) Before and after use of a carbide-coated strip to remove enamel. The surfaces are polished after the stripping is completed. Topical fluoride should be applied immediately after stripping procedures because the fluoride-rich outer layer of enamel has been removed. (C) A canine-to-canine clip-on active retainer for this patient immediately after placement. It was made as described in Fig. 19.20 and must be worn full-time until the teeth are back in alignment.

some vertical growth (almost all boys younger than age 18 fall into this category), it may be possible to recover the proper occlusal position of the teeth. Differential anteroposterior growth is not necessary to correct a small occlusal discrepancy—tooth movement is adequate—but some vertical growth is required to prevent downward and backward rotation of the mandible. For all practical purposes, this means that a functional appliance as an active retainer can be used in teenagers but is of no value in adults. Stimulating skeletal growth with a device of this type simply does not happen in adults, at least to a clinically useful extent.

The use of a functional appliance as an active retainer differs from its use as a pure retainer. With use as a retainer, the objective is to control growth, and tooth movement is largely an undesirable side effect. In contrast, an active retainer is expected primarily to move teeth—no significant skeletal change is anticipated. An activator or Bionator as an active retainer is indicated only if not more than 3 mm of occlusal correction is sought. Over this distance, correction can be achieved by restraining the eruption of maxillary teeth posteriorly and directing the erupting mandibular teeth anteriorly.

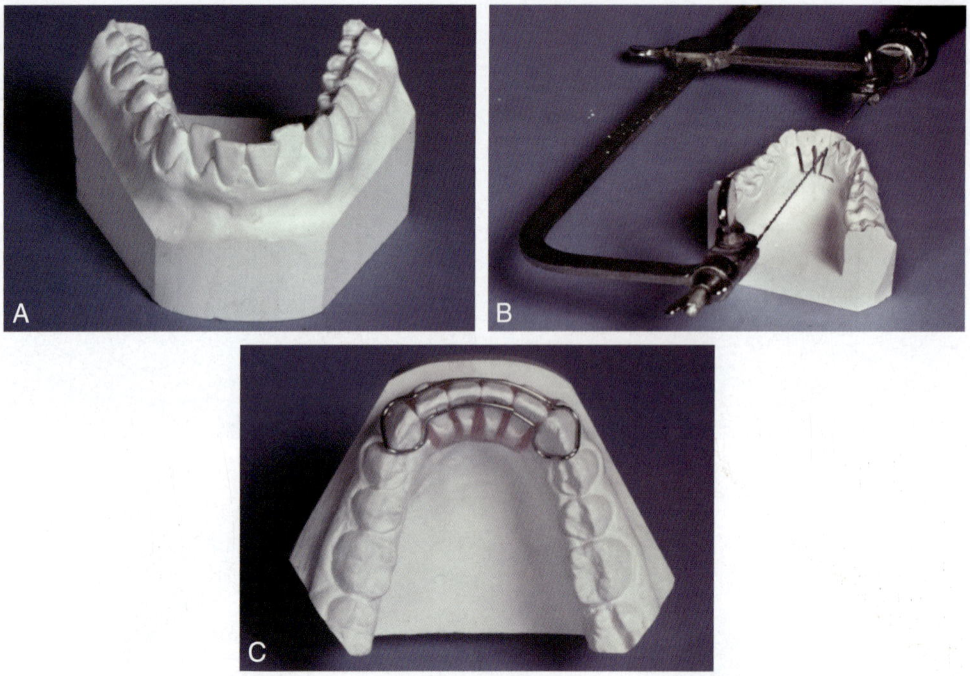

• **Fig. 19.20** Steps in the fabrication of a canine-to-canine clip-on spring appliance to realign lower incisors. (A) Re-crowded incisors in a patient who decided not to wear their removable retainer. After appropriate interproximal reduction, an impression is made for a laboratory cast. (B) A saw-cut is made beneath the teeth through the alveolar process to the distal of the lateral incisors, and cuts are made up to but not through the contact points. (C) The incisor teeth are broken off the cast and broken apart at the contact points, creating individual plaster teethh; then the teeth are reset in wax in proper alignment. 28-mil steel wire is contoured around the labial and lingual surface of the teeth as shown, with the wire overlapping behind the central incisors. A covering of acrylic is added over the labial part of the wire, completing the aligner, which then looks exactly like a canine-to-canine spring retainer. If the appliance is used as an aligner, however, full-time wear is essential until the teeth are back in position.

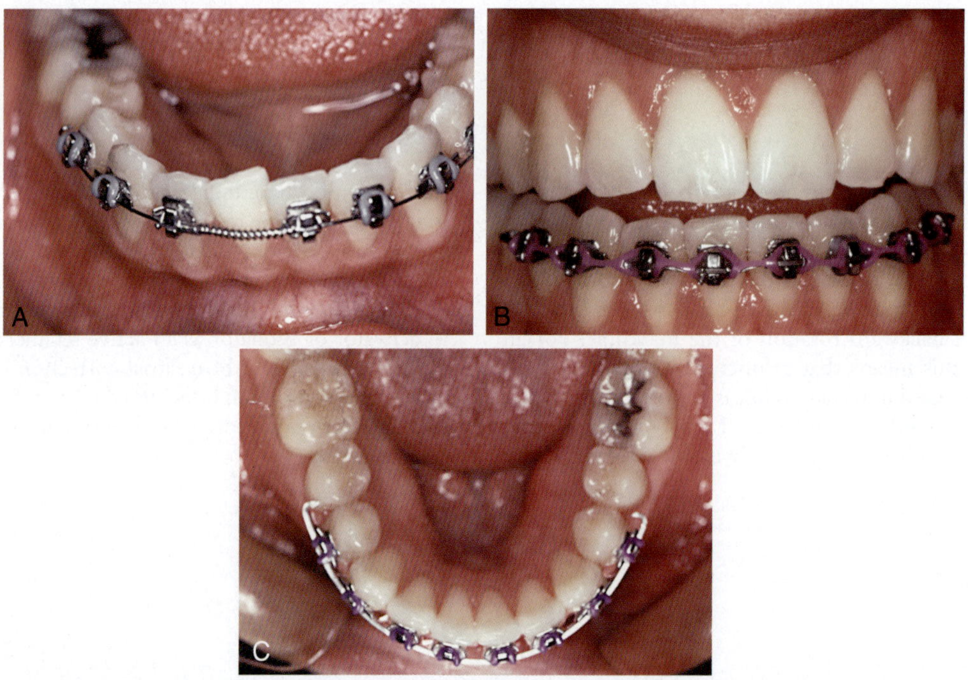

• **Fig. 19.21** For this patient who was concerned about crowding of lower incisors several years after orthodontic treatment, excessive interproximal reduction would have been required to gain realignment with a clip-on spring appliance. In that circumstance, a partial fixed appliance with bonded brackets only on the segment to be realigned is the most practical approach. (A) Bonded appliance from first premolar to first premolar, with a coil spring on 16-mil round steel wire to open space for the rotated and crowded right central incisor. (B and C) Alignment of the incisors on rectangular nickel-titanium (NiTi) wire after space was opened, which was completed 4 months after treatment began. At this point a fixed lingual retainer can be bonded before the brackets and archwire are removed.

References

1. Ormiston JP, Huang GJ, Little RM, et al. Retrospective analysis of long-term stable and unstable orthodontic treatment outcomes. *Am J Orthod Dentofacial Orthop*. 2005;128:568–574.
2. Joondeph DR, Huang G, Lirrle R. Stability, retention, and relapse. In: Graber TM, Vararsdall RL, Vig KWL, Huang G, eds. *Orthodontics: Current Principle and Techniques*. 6th ed. Mosby; 2017.
3. Reitan K. Tissue rearrangement during the retention of orthodontically rotated teeth. *Angle Orthod*. 1959;29:105–113.
4. Al-Moghrabi D, Algharbi M, Arqub SA, Alkadhimi A, Fleming PS. The effectiveness of adjuncts or alternatives to the use of orthodontic retainers in preserving posttreatment outcomes: a systematic review. *Am J Orthod Dentofacial Orthop*. 2023 Jan;163(1):9–21. e3.
5. Schott TC, Schlipf C, Glasl B, et al. Quantification of patient compliance with Hawley retainers and removable functional appliances during the retention phase. *Am J Orthod Dentofacial Orthop*. 2013;144:533–540.
6. Behrents RG. *A Treatise on the Continuum of Growth in the Aging Craniofacial Skeleton*. University of Michigan Center for Human Growth and Development; 1984.
7. Khosravi R, Cohanim B, Hujoel P, et al. Management of overbite with the Invisalign appliance. *Am J Orthod Dentofacial Orthop*. 2017;151:691–699.
8. Steinnes J, Johnsen G, Kerosuo H. Stability of orthodontic treatment outcome in relation to retention status. *Am J Orthod Dentofacial Orthop*. 2017;151:1027–1033.
9. Littlewood SJ, Millett DT, Doubleday B, Bearn DR, Worthington HV. Retention procedures for stabilizing tooth position after treatment with orthodontic braces. *Cochrane Database Syst Rev*. 2016;2016(1): Update in: *Cochrane Database Syst Rev*. 2023;5.
10. Mollov ND, Lindauer SJ, Best AM, et al. Patient attitudes toward retention and perceptions of treatment success. *Angle Orthod*. 2010;80:468–473.
11. Tynelius GE, Bondemark L, Lilja-Karlander E. Evaluation of orthodontic treatment after 1 year of retention—a randomized controlled trial. *Eur J Orthod*. 2010;32:542–547.
12. Mai W, He J, Meng H, Jiang Y, et al. Comparison of vacuum-formed and Hawley retainers: a systematic review. *Am J Orthod Dentofacial Orthop*. 2014;145:720–727.
13. Tynelius EG, Petrén S, et al. Five-year postretention outcomes of three retention methods—a randomized controlled trial. *Eur J Orthod*. 2015;37:345–353.
14. Zachrisson BU. Long-term experience with bonded retainers: update and clinical advice. *J Clin Orthod*. 2007;41:728–737.
15. Booth FA, Edelman JM, Proffit WR. Twenty-year follow-up of patients with permanently bonded mandibular canine-to-canine retainers. *Am J Orthod Dentofacial Orthop*. 2008;133:70–76.
16. Sim HY, Kim HS, Jung DU, et al. Association between orthodontic treatment and periodontal diseases: results from a national survey. *Angle Orthod*. 2017;87:651–657.
17. Shaughnessy TG, Proffit WR, Samara SA. Inadvertent tooth movement with fixed lingual retainers. *Am J Orthod Dentofac Orthop*. 2016;149:277–286.
18. Al-Nimri K, Al Habashneh R, Obeidat M. Gingival health and relapse tendency: a prospective study of two types of lower fixed retainers. *Aust Orthod J*. 2009;25:142–146.
19. Shah AA, Elcock C, Brook AH. Incisor crown shape and crowding. *Am J Orthod Dentofacial Orthop*. 2003;123:562–567.
20. Zachrisson BU, Nyøygaard L, Mobarak K. Dental health assessed more than 10 years after interproximal enamel reduction of mandibular anterior teeth. *Am J Orthod Dentofacial Orthop*. 2007;131:162–169.

SECTION 7

Treatment for Adults

Adult orthodontics has been the fastest growing type of orthodontic treatment in recent years, going from a relative rarity before the 1980s to a commonplace procedure today. In the United States, adults (those older than 18 at the start of treatment) now comprise more than one-fourth of all patients receiving comprehensive orthodontic treatment. A similar trend is occurring worldwide in orthodontic practices, trailing the US percentage in less-developed countries but steadily increasing everywhere. Adult orthodontics, at this point, is a major component of orthodontic practice.

This does not mean that treatment procedures can be the same as for adolescents or children. Perhaps the biggest difference is that for adults, other types of dental treatment are almost always required, which makes interdisciplinary interaction and cooperation a necessity from the beginning. The prevalence of periodontal problems increases with age, and even young adults seeking orthodontic treatment may require some level of periodontal care. As adult patients become older, orthodontic treatment must be done in the context of a mature dentition with worn teeth and restorative implications, not a new one as with adolescents. The absence of growth in adults (or more accurately, the very small increments of continuing growth) means that growth modification is not a treatment option—everything must be accomplished with tooth movement, restorative dentistry, or orthognathic surgery. So, skeletal anchorage and camouflage can play larger roles. In a sense, planning orthodontic treatment for adults can be easier because there are no uncertainties related to the amount and direction of growth, but comprehensive treatment for adults requires a high level of technical skill, knowledge of other disciplines, and an advanced understanding of biomechanics.

Several other considerations are particularly important in the treatment of adults:

1. Treatment planning must involve all the dentists who will play a role in the treatment. It cannot be done by the orthodontist in isolation. With a group of practitioners, an important question is "Who is the conductor of this orchestra?" This, of course, depends on the details of treatment, but when replacement of teeth or extensive restorations are necessary, the planning almost has to start with what the prosthodontist or restorative dentist wants, and the extent to which those desires can be met.
2. Given that many specialties are usually involved in diagnosis, treatment decisions, and treatment delivery, it makes even more sense to start the treatment with the final result in mind. This can be accomplished with a diagnostic setup or digital treatment simulation that can be used as a diagnostic and communication tool among the treatment team and between them and the patient, and coordination of this with the facial goals of treatment.
3. Ideal dental occlusion and facial appearance are not necessarily an appropriate treatment goal, even for adults who will have comprehensive treatment and specialty care, but the facial paradigm should be influential in priority and goal setting. There is a difference between realistic treatment that is focused on the patient's problems and ideal treatment aimed at perfection. This must be evaluated for various treatment procedures in the context of time, cost and risk versus benefit to the patient, so discussion of treatment options and genuinely informed consent are very important.
4. Adults react to being orthodontic patients differently than children and adolescents in two ways: almost always they are intensely interested in their treatment and want to understand what is happening and why, so they require more clinical time in explanations; and either they experience more pain than younger patients or are less tolerant of it, so medication for pain control may be more important.

5. Disease control is essential before orthodontics can begin. As we have noted earlier in this book, this means bringing both dental and periodontal disease under control, which may add endodontics and oral surgery to the types of treatment. Clearly, advanced age brings into play other health conditions and medications not faced in adolescents that may impact the tooth movement mechanisms.

In the chapters that follow, Chapter 20 focuses on orthodontic treatment in interaction with other dental specialists except maxillofacial surgeons, and Chapter 22 adds orthognathic surgery to the considerations in planning and implementing coordinated treatment. Although the focus is on orthodontics in both chapters, a discussion of treatment procedures by other dental specialists is included in the discussion of interdisciplinary treatment, as it must be. In Chapter 22, the surgical options and the surgeon-orthodontist interaction in the 3-D planning and management of orthodontic and surgical treatment receive particular attention. Chapters 20 and 22 include discussions of obstructive sleep apnea as an adjunctive orthodontic treatment and its relationship to orthognathic surgical planning, respectively. A new addition to this edition of the book is Chapter 21 which focuses on the use of clear aligner treatment in the adult population. Like the new Chapter 18 on aligner treatment for adolescents, Chapter 21 emphasizes how the unique challenges of adult treatment can effectively be managed with aligners by using the foundation concepts of biomechanics and understanding the biology of tooth movement.

20

Special Considerations in Treatment for Adults

DAVID M. SARVER, WILLIAM R. PROFFIT, HENRY W. FIELDS, BENJAMIN T. PLISKA, AND TORU DEGUCHI

CHAPTER OUTLINE

Adjunctive Versus Comprehensive Treatment

In general, orthodontists consider adults as those whose growth is essentially completed. The mean cutoff age for females is 18 (which means for some slow maturers it would be later), but for males it is 20 or 21, simply because males are often still growing up to that age. Patients who seek orthodontic treatment beyond those ages fall into two quite different groups: (1) younger adults (typically younger than 35, often in their 20s) who desired but did not receive comprehensive orthodontic treatment as youths and now seek it as they become financially independent and (2) an older group, typically in their 40s or 50s, who have other dental problems and need orthodontics as part of a larger treatment plan.

For the first group, the goal is to improve their quality of life. They usually seek the maximum improvement that is possible. They may or may not need extensive treatment by other dental specialists but frequently need interdisciplinary consultation. The second group's goal is quite different. They usually seek to maintain what they have, not necessarily to achieve as ideal an orthodontic result as possible. For them, orthodontic treatment is needed to meet specific goals that would make control of dental disease and restoration of missing teeth easier and more effective, so the orthodontics is an adjunctive procedure to the larger periodontal and restorative goals.

Adjunctive orthodontic treatment, particularly the simpler procedures, often can be carried out within the context of general dental practice. In adults, growth has been essentially completed and is no longer a variable requiring major consideration in managing treatment, and the types and magnitude of tooth movement required for most adjunctive procedures are straightforward. Adjunctive treatment does not require familiarity with the principles of comprehensive orthodontic treatment, but it does presume an understanding of orthodontic diagnosis and treatment planning.

In contrast, the discussion of comprehensive treatment for adults in the latter part of this chapter builds on the principles discussed in Chapters 15–17 and focuses on the aspects of comprehensive treatment for adults that are different from treatment for adolescents. Comprehensive orthodontics for adults tends to be difficult and technically demanding. The absence of growth means that growth modification to treat jaw discrepancies is not possible. The only possibilities are tooth movement for camouflage or orthognathic surgery, but applications of skeletal anchorage are now broadening the scope of orthodontics to include some patients who would have required surgery even a few years ago. Applications of skeletal anchorage are discussed and illustrated in detail in this chapter; a discussion of skeletal anchorage versus surgery follows in Chapter 22.

Adjunctive orthodontic treatment for adults is, by definition, tooth movement carried out to facilitate other dental procedures necessary to control disease, restore function, and/or enhance appearance. Usually, it involves only a part of the dentition, and the primary goal usually is to make it easier or more effective to replace missing or damaged teeth. Making it easier for the patient to control periodontal problems is a frequent secondary goal and sometimes the primary goal. The treatment duration tends to be a few months, rarely more than a year, and long-term retention often is supplied by the restorations. Whether one or several practitioners are involved, adjunctive orthodontics must be coordinated carefully with the periodontal and restorative treatment.

In contrast, the goal of comprehensive orthodontics for adults is the same as for adolescents: to produce the best combination of dental and facial appearance, dental occlusion, and stability of the result to maximize benefit to the patient. Comprehensive orthodontics requires either a complete fixed orthodontic appliance or a high level of skill in managing clear aligner therapy. Intrusion of some teeth is likely to be needed, orthognathic surgery may be considered to improve jaw relationships, and the duration of treatment exceeds 1 year. Adults receiving comprehensive treatment are the main candidates for esthetically enhanced appliances; the prime examples are ceramic facial brackets, clear aligners, and lingual appliances. The complexity of the treatment procedures means that an orthodontic specialist is likely to be significantly more efficient in delivering the care.

Principles of Adjunctive Treatment

Treatment Goals

Whatever the occlusal status originally, the goals of adjunctive treatment should be to:

- Improve periodontal health by eliminating plaque-harboring areas and improving the alveolar ridge contour adjacent to the teeth.
- Establish favorable crown-to-root ratios and position the teeth so that occlusal forces are transmitted along the long axes of the teeth.
- Facilitate restorative treatment by positioning the teeth so that:
  - More ideal and conservative techniques (including implants) can be used.
  - Optimal esthetics can be obtained with bonding, veneers, or full-coverage porcelain restorations.

Typically, adjunctive orthodontic treatment will involve any or all of several procedures:

1. Repositioning teeth after extractions or bone loss so that implants can be placed, or more ideal fixed or removable partial dentures can be fabricated.
2. Aligning anterior teeth to allow more esthetic restorations or successful splinting while maintaining good interproximal bone contour and embrasure form.
3. Correcting crossbite if this compromises jaw function (not all crossbites do)
4. Forcing eruption of badly broken-down teeth either to:
   - Expose sound root structure on which to place crowns, or
   - Level bone margins and regenerate alveolar bone.

An old rule says that to make clear what something is, it helps to point out what it isn't but might be mistaken for. So, some important corollaries:

- Orthodontic treatment for temporomandibular dysfunction (TMD) should not be considered adjunctive treatment.
- Although intrusion of teeth can be an important part of comprehensive treatment for adults, it probably should be managed by an orthodontist even as an adjunctive procedure because of the technical difficulties involved and the possibility of periodontal complications. As a general guideline in treatment of adults with periodontal involvement and bone loss, lower incisor teeth that are excessively extruded are best treated by reduction of crown height, which has the added advantage of improving the ultimate crown-to-root ratio of the teeth. For other teeth, tooth-lip relationships must be kept in mind when crown-height reduction is considered.
- Crowding of more than 3 to 4 mm should not be attempted by stripping enamel from the contact surfaces of the anterior teeth. It may be advantageous to strip posterior teeth to provide space for alignment of the incisors, but this requires a complete orthodontic appliance and cannot be considered adjunctive treatment.

Diagnostic and Treatment Planning Considerations

Planning for adjunctive treatment requires two steps: (1) collecting an adequate diagnostic database and (2) developing a comprehensive but clearly stated list of the patient's problems, taking care not to focus unduly on any one aspect of a complex situation. The importance of this planning stage in adjunctive orthodontic treatment cannot be overemphasized because the solution to the patient's specific problems may involve the synthesis of many branches of dentistry. In adjunctive treatment, the restorative dentist usually is the principal architect of the treatment plan, and the use of orthodontics (whether an orthodontist is or is not part of the treatment team) is to facilitate better restorative treatment.

Nevertheless, the steps outlined in Chapter 6 should be followed when the problem list is being developed. The interview and clinical examination are the same whatever the type of orthodontic treatment. Diagnostic records for adjunctive orthodontic patients, however, differ in several important ways from those for adolescents and children.

For this adult and dentally compromised population, the records should usually include individual intraoral radiographs to supplement the panoramic radiograph that often suffices for younger and healthier patients (Fig. 20.1). When active dental disease is present, the panoramic radiograph does not give sufficient detail. The revised guidelines from the U.S. Food and Drug Administration in 2014 (see Table 6.8) should be followed in determining exactly what radiographs are required in evaluating the patient's oral health status. The American Board of Orthodontics now requires evidence of pretreatment periodontal condition for all adult patients.[1]

For adjunctive orthodontics with a partial fixed appliance, pretreatment cephalometric radiographs usually are not required, but it is important to anticipate the impact of various tooth movements on facial esthetics. In some instances, the computer prediction methods used in comprehensive treatment (see Chapter 7) can be quite useful in planning adjunctive treatment. Articulator-mounted casts or digital simulated articulated casts are likely to be needed because they facilitate the planning of associated restorative procedures.

Once all the problems have been identified and categorized, the key treatment planning question is: can the occlusion be restored within the existing tooth positions, or must some teeth be moved to achieve a satisfactory, stable, healthy, and esthetic result? The goal of providing a physiologic occlusion and facilitating other dental treatment has little to do with Angle's concept of an ideal occlusion. At this point, it is important to consider the difference between realistic and idealistic treatment planning. In older patients, searching for an "ideal" result could involve more treatment than would really benefit the patient.

Obviously, the time needed for any orthodontic treatment depends on the severity of the problem and the amount of tooth movement desired, but with efficient use of orthodontic appliances, it should be possible to reach the objectives of adjunctive treatment within 6 months. As a practical matter, this means that

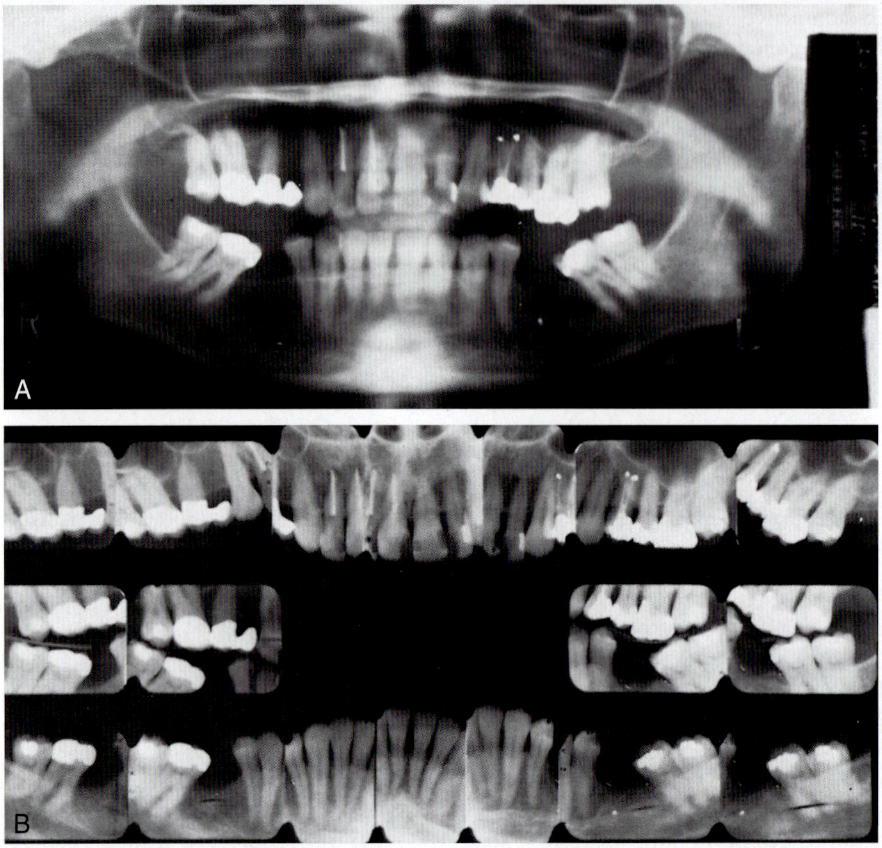

• **Fig. 20.1** (A and B) For the periodontally compromised adults who are the usual candidates for adjunctive orthodontics, periapical radiographs of the areas that will be treated, as well as a panoramic radiograph, usually are needed. Periodontal disease now is the major indication for periapical radiographs. For this patient who is a candidate for adjunctive orthodontic treatment, adequate detail of root morphology, dental disease, and periodontal breakdown is obtained only from carefully taken periapical radiographs.

like comprehensive orthodontics, most adjunctive orthodontics cannot be managed well with traditional removable appliances. It requires either fixed appliances or a sequence of clear aligners to get the job done in a reasonable time frame. In addition, it is becoming increasingly apparent that skeletal anchorage makes adjunctive tooth movement more effective and efficient. For adjunctive treatment, this is almost always in the form of alveolar bone screws.

Biomechanical Considerations

Characteristics of the Orthodontic Appliance

When a partial fixed appliance is to be used for adjunctive treatment, with the possible exception of alignment of anterior teeth, an edgewise appliance with biomechanical characteristics like those of twin brackets is preferred. The rectangular bracket slot permits control of buccolingual axial inclinations, the relatively wide bracket helps control undesirable rotations and tipping. If a larger slot size is used, it allows the use of stabilizing wires that are somewhat stiffer than ordinarily might be used in comprehensive treatment.

Recently, further developments in clear aligner therapy (see Chapter 10) have resulted in an effective removable appliance that can be well suited to alignment of anterior teeth. Removable appliances of the traditional plastic-and-wire type are rarely satisfactory for adjunctive (or comprehensive) treatment. They are often uncomfortable and are likely to be worn for too few hours per day to be effective. With clear aligners, both discomfort and interference with speech and mastication are minimized, and patient cooperation improves. The better appearance of a clear aligner is also a factor in choosing it to align anterior teeth.

Despite this esthetic advantage, there are biomechanical limitations. Control of root position is difficult with clear aligners, and bonded attachments to teeth and modifications of the aligners are needed to produce several important types of tooth movement (see Table 18.2). If these limitations are not important, clear aligners can be considered for adjunctive orthodontics. If they are, most adults who are candidates for adjunctive treatment will accept a visible fixed appliance.

Modern edgewise brackets of the straight-wire type are designed for a specific location on an individual tooth. Placing the bracket in its ideal position on each tooth implies that every tooth will be repositioned if necessary to achieve ideal occlusion (Fig. 20.2A). Because adjunctive treatment is concerned with only limited tooth movements, it is usually neither necessary nor desirable to alter the position of every tooth in the arch. For this reason, in a partial fixed appliance for adjunctive treatment, the brackets are placed in an ideal position only on teeth to be moved, and the remaining teeth to be incorporated in the anchor system are bracketed so that the archwire slots are closely aligned (Fig. 20.2B). This allows the anchorage segments of the wire to be engaged passively in the brackets with little bending. Passive engagement of wires produces minimal disturbance of teeth that

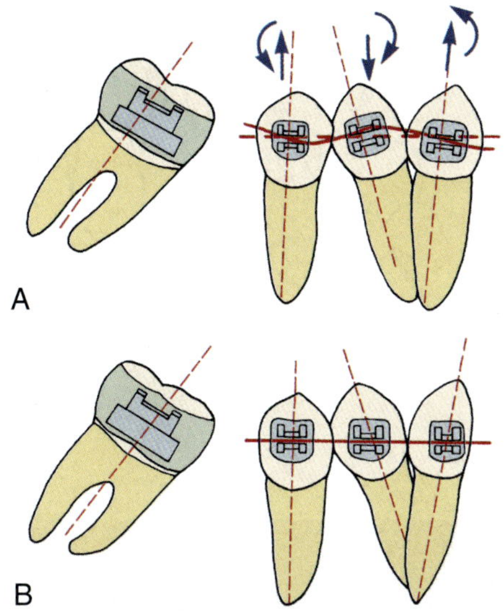

• **Fig. 20.2** (A) Brackets placed in the "ideal" position on moderately irregular anchor teeth for molar uprighting. For adjunctive orthodontic treatment, movement of the anchor teeth usually is undesirable, but a straight length of wire will move them if the brackets are positioned in this way. (B) Brackets placed in the position of maximum convenience, lined up so that a straight length of wire can be placed without moving the anchor teeth. This makes things easier if no movement of the anchor teeth is desired. For adjunctive orthodontic procedures such as molar uprighting, we recommend the use of fully adjusted "straight-wire" 22-slot brackets and working archwires that are somewhat smaller than the bracket slot to reduce unwanted faciolingual movement of anchor teeth even though the brackets are lined up in the other planes of space.

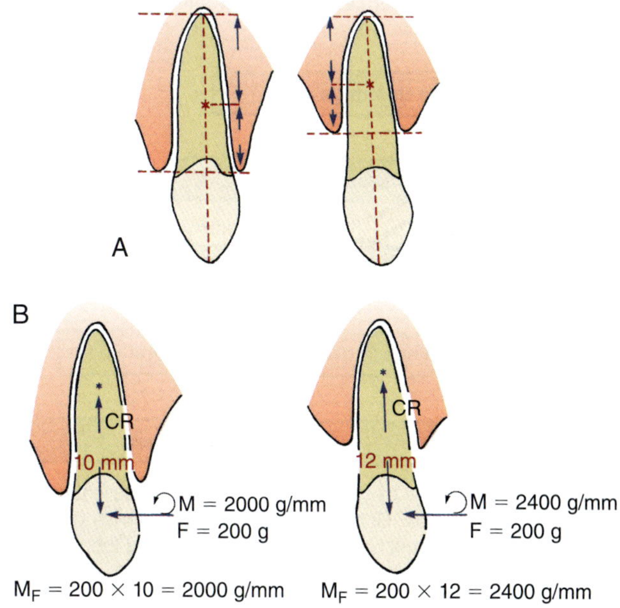

• **Fig. 20.3** (A) The center of resistance of a single-rooted tooth lies approximately 6/10 of the distance between the apex of the tooth and the crest of the alveolar bone. Loss of alveolar bone height, as for the tooth on the right, moves the center of resistance closer to the root apex. (B) The magnitude of the tipping moment produced by a force is equal to the force times the distance from the point of force application to the center of resistance. If the center of resistance moves apically, the tipping moment produced by the force (M_F) increases, and a larger countervailing moment produced by a couple applied to the tooth (M_C) would be necessary to produce bodily movement. This is almost impossible to obtain with traditional removable appliances and very difficult with clear aligners, even when bonded attachments are added. For all practical purposes, a fixed appliance is required if root movement is the goal in patients who have experienced loss of alveolar bone height. *CR*, Center of resistance; *F*, force; *M*, moment of force.

are in a physiologically satisfactory position. This important point is illustrated in more detail in the sections on specific treatment procedures that follow.

Effects of Reduced Periodontal Support

Because patients who need adjunctive orthodontic treatment have often lost alveolar bone to periodontal disease before it was brought under control, the amount of bone support of each tooth is an important consideration. When bone is lost, the periodontal ligament (PDL) area decreases, and the same force against the crown produces greater pressure in the PDL of a periodontally compromised tooth than a normally supported one. The absolute magnitude of force used to move teeth must be reduced when periodontal support has been lost. In addition, the greater the loss of attachment, the smaller the area of supported root and the further apical the center of resistance will become (Fig. 20.3). This affects the moments created by forces applied to the crown and the moments needed to control root movement. In general terms, tooth movement is quite possible despite bone loss, but lighter forces and relatively larger moments are needed.

Timing and Sequence of Treatment

In the development of any orthodontic treatment plan, the first step is control of any active dental disease (Fig. 20.4). Before any tooth movement, active caries and pulpal pathology must be eliminated by using extractions, restorative procedures, and pulpal or apical treatment as necessary. Endodontically treated teeth respond normally to orthodontic force, if all residual chronic inflammation has been eliminated.[2] Before orthodontics, teeth requiring restorations should be restored with well-placed amalgams or composite resins. Restorations requiring detailed occlusal anatomy should not be placed until any adjunctive orthodontic treatment has been completed because the occlusion inevitably will be changed. This could necessitate remaking crowns, bridges, or removable partial dentures.

Periodontal disease also must be controlled before any orthodontics begins because orthodontic tooth movement superimposed on poorly controlled periodontal health can lead to rapid and irreversible breakdown of the periodontal support apparatus.[3] Scaling, curettage (by open flap procedures, if necessary), and gingival grafts should be undertaken as appropriate. Surgical pocket elimination and osseous surgical procedures should be delayed until completion of the orthodontic phase of treatment because significant soft tissue and bony recontouring occurs during orthodontic tooth movement. Clinical studies have shown that orthodontic treatment of adults with both normal and compromised periodontal tissues can be completed without loss of attachment, if there is good periodontal therapy both initially and during tooth movement.[4]

During this preparatory phase, the patient's enthusiasm for treatment and ability to maintain good overall oral hygiene should be carefully monitored. Adjunctive orthodontics has the potential to do more harm than good in patients who cannot or will not

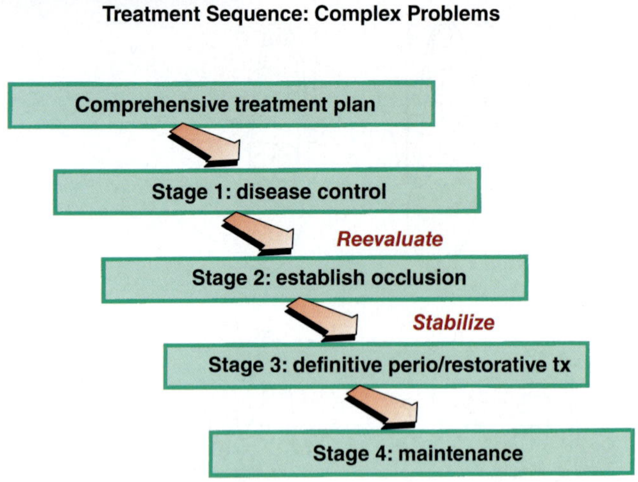

• **Fig. 20.4** The sequence of steps in the treatment of patients requiring adjunctive orthodontics. Orthodontics is used to establish occlusion but only after disease control has been accomplished, and the occlusion should be stabilized before definitive restorative treatment is carried out.

maintain good oral hygiene. If disease can be controlled, however, adjunctive orthodontics can significantly improve the final restorative and periodontal procedures.

Adjunctive Treatment Procedures

Uprighting Posterior Teeth

Treatment Planning Considerations

When a first permanent molar is lost during childhood or adolescence and not replaced, the second molar drifts mesially and the premolars often tip distally and rotate as space opens between them. As the teeth move, the adjacent gingival tissue becomes folded and distorted, forming a plaque-harboring pseudopocket that may be virtually impossible for the patient to clean (Fig. 20.5). Repositioning the teeth eliminates this potentially pathologic condition and has the added advantage of simplifying the ultimate restorative procedures.

When molar uprighting is planned, several interrelated questions must be answered:

- If the third molar is present, should both the second and third molars be uprighted? For many patients, distal positioning of the third molar would move it into a position in which good hygiene could not be maintained or it would not be in functional occlusion. In these circumstances, it is more appropriate to extract the third molar and simply upright the remaining second molar tooth. If both molars are to be uprighted, the biomechanical requirements change, and the technique must be modified as described later.
- How should the tipped teeth be uprighted? By distal crown movement (tipping), which would increase the space available for an implant or bridge pontic, or by mesial root movement, which would reduce or even close the edentulous space? For most patients, treatment by distal tipping of the second molar and a bridge or implant to replace the first molar is preferred (Fig. 20.6). If extensive ridge resorption has already occurred, particularly in the buccolingual dimension, closing the space by mesial movement of a wide molar root into the narrow alveolar ridge will proceed very slowly. If uprighting with space closure is to be done successfully, skeletal anchorage in the form of

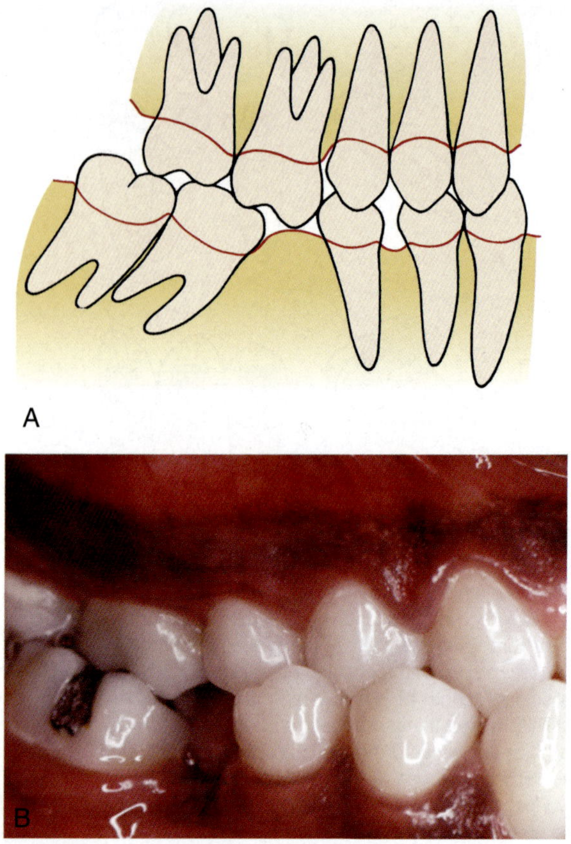

• **Fig. 20.5** (A) Loss of a lower molar can lead to tipping and drifting of adjacent teeth, poor interproximal contacts, poor gingival contour, reduced interradicular bone, and supra-eruption of unopposed teeth. Because the bone contour follows the cementoenamel junction, pseudopockets form adjacent to the tipped teeth. (B) Note the loss of alveolar bone in the area where a mandibular first molar was extracted many years previously. Mesial drift and tipping of the second molar has closed half the space. The patient's posterior crossbite, however, is unrelated to early loss of the molar.

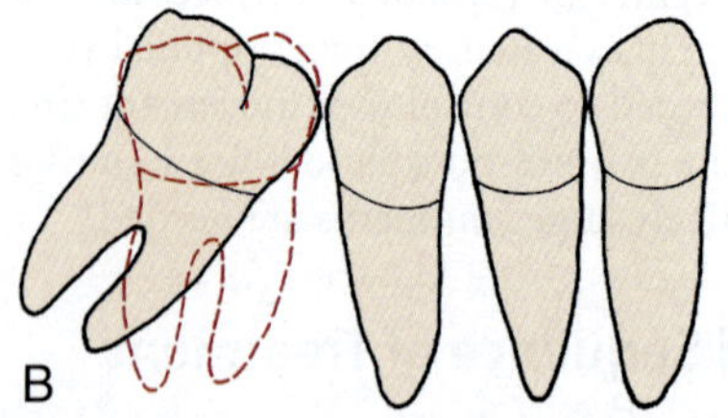

• **Fig. 20.6** (A) Uprighting a tipped molar by distal crown movement leads to increased space for a bridge pontic or implant, whereas uprighting the molar by mesial root movement (B) reduces space and might eliminate the need for a prosthesis, but this tooth movement can be very difficult and time-consuming to accomplish, especially if the alveolar bone has resorbed in the area where a first molar was extracted many years previously (see Fig. 20.39).

a temporary skeletal anchorage often is needed, and the treatment time can be as much as 3 years.

- Is extrusion of a tipped molar permissible? Uprighting a mesially tipped tooth by tipping it distally, which leaves the root apex in its pretreatment position, also extrudes it. This has the merit of reducing the depth of the pseudopocket found on the mesial surface, and because the attached gingiva follows the cementoenamel junction while the mucogingival junction remains stable, it also increases the width of the keratinized tissue in that area. In addition, if the height of the clinical crown is systematically reduced as uprighting proceeds, the ultimate crown-root length ratio will be improved (Fig. 20.7). Unless slight extrusion or crown-height reduction is acceptable, which is usually the case, the patient should be considered to have problems that require comprehensive treatment and treated accordingly.
- Should the premolars be repositioned as part of the treatment? This will depend on the position of these teeth and the restorative plan, but in many cases the answer is *yes*. It is particularly desirable to close spaces between premolars when uprighting molars because this will improve both the periodontal prognosis and long-term stability. In some instances, uprighting the molar and then moving the premolar back against it will provide a better site mesial to the premolar for an implant.

In molar uprighting, the treatment time will vary with the type and extent of the tooth movement. Uprighting one, second molar by distal crown tipping proceeds much more rapidly than mesial root movement. Failure to eliminate occlusal interferences will prolong treatment. The simplest cases should be completed in 8 to 10 weeks, but uprighting two molars in the same quadrant could easily take 6 months, and the complexity of doing this puts it at the outer limit of adjunctive treatment with a partial fixed appliance.

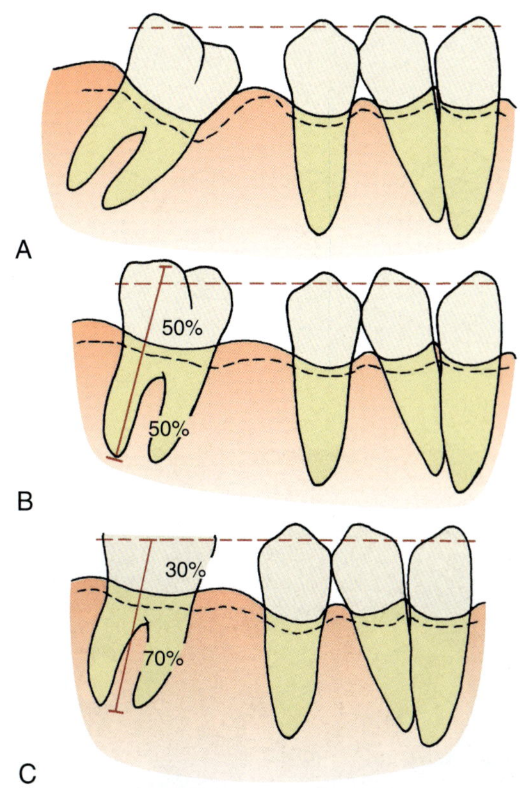

• Fig. 20.7 (A to C) Uprighting a tipped molar increases the crown height while it reduces the depth of the mesial pocket. Subsequent crown reduction decreases occlusal interference and also improves the ratio of crown height to supported root length of the molar, so reducing the height of the molar crown is a routine part of molar uprighting.

Appliances for Molar Uprighting

Distal Crown Tipping

A partial fixed appliance to upright tipped molars consists of bonded brackets on the premolars and canine in that quadrant and either a bonded rectangular tube on the molar or a molar band. A general guideline is that molar bands are best when the periodontal condition allows, which means for all practical purposes they would be used in younger and healthier patients. The greater the degree of periodontal breakdown around the molar to be uprighted, the more a bonded attachment should be considered.

Where the premolar and canine brackets should be placed depends on the intended tooth movement and occlusion. If these teeth are to be repositioned, the brackets should be placed in the ideal position at the center of the facial surface of each tooth. However, if the teeth are merely serving as anchor units and no repositioning is planned, then the brackets should be placed in the position of maximum convenience where minimum wire bending will be required to engage a passive archwire (see Fig. 20.2).

If the molar is only moderately tipped, treatment can often be accomplished with a flexible rectangular wire. In a 0.022 slot appliance, the best choice is 17 × 25 austenitic nickel-titanium (A-NiTi) that delivers approximately 100 g of force. With this material, a single wire may complete the necessary uprighting (Fig. 20.8). A braided rectangular steel wire also can be used but is more likely to require removal and reshaping. It is important to relieve the occlusion as the tooth tips upright. Failure to do this may cause excessive tooth mobility and increase treatment time.

If the molar is severely tipped, a continuous wire that uprights the molar will have side effects (which almost always are undesirable) on the position and inclination of the second premolar. For that reason it is better to carry out the bulk of the uprighting by using an auxiliary uprighting spring (Fig. 20.9). After preliminary alignment of the anchor teeth, if necessary, stiff rectangular wire (19 × 25 steel) maintains the relationship of the teeth in the anchor segment, and the auxiliary spring is placed in the molar auxiliary tube. It is formed from either 17 × 25 beta-titanium (beta-Ti) wire without a helical loop or 17 × 25 steel wire with a loop added to provide more springiness. The mesial arm of the helical spring should be adjusted to lie passively in the vestibule and on activation should hook over the archwire in the stabilizing segment. It is important to position the hook so that it is free to slide distally as the molar uprights. In addition, a slight lingual bend placed in the uprighting spring is needed to counteract the forces that tend to tip the anchor teeth buccally and the molar lingually (Fig. 20.9C).

Can distal tipping of a single molar on both sides be done at the same time? Yes, but then a bonded lingual stabilizing wire canine-to-canine should be placed to control the incisor position (Fig. 20.9D).

Mesial Root Movement

If mesial root movement is desired, an alternative treatment approach is indicated. Skeletal anchorage is required if the goal is to close the old extraction space (see Fig. 20.39). If a small amount of mesial movement to prevent opening too much space is the goal, a single T-loop sectional archwire of 17 × 25 stainless steel or 19 × 25 beta-Ti wire can be effective (Fig. 20.10).

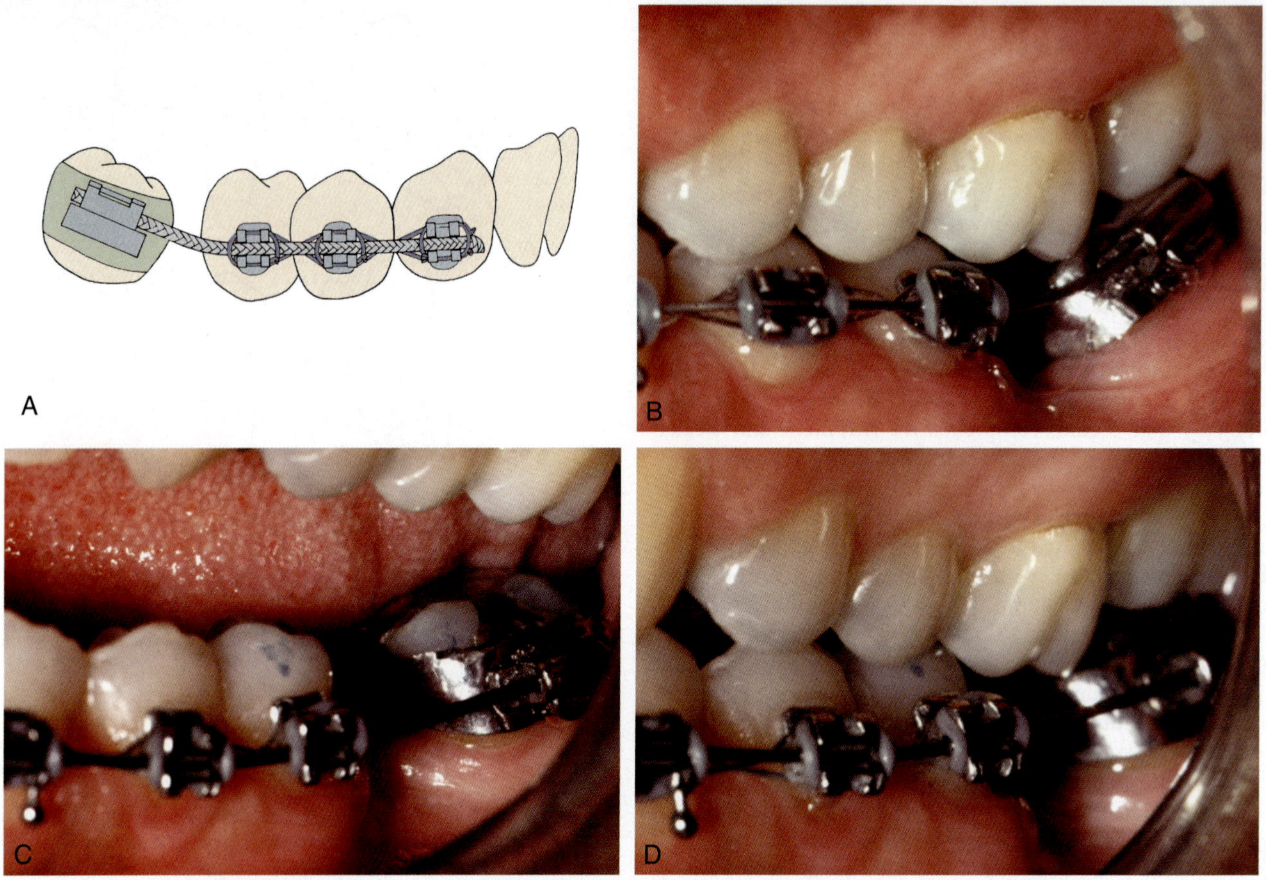

• **Fig. 20.8** Fixed appliance technique for uprighting one molar with a continuous flexible wire. (A) Initial bracket alignment is achieved by placing a light flexible wire such as 17 × 25 austenitic nickel-titanium (A-NiTi) from molar to canine. (B) Molar uprighting with a continuous martensitic nickel-titanium (M-NiTi) wire. (C) Progress 1 month later. (D) Uprighting essentially completed 2 months later.

After initial alignment of the anchor teeth with a light flexible wire, the T-loop wire is adapted to fit passively into the brackets on the anchor teeth and gabled at the T to exert an uprighting force on the molar. Insertion into the molar can be from the mesial or distal side. If the treatment plan calls for maintaining or closing rather than increasing the pontic space, the distal end of the archwire should be pulled distally through the molar tube, opening the T-loop by 1 to 2 mm, and then bent sharply gingivally to maintain this opening. This activation provides a mesial force on the molar that counteracts distal crown tipping while the tooth uprights (Fig. 20.10D). If opening the space is desired, the end of the wire is not bent over so the tooth can slide distally along it.

The T-loop appliance also is indicated if the molar to be uprighted is severely tipped but has no occlusal antagonist. In that circumstance, a T-loop minimizes the extrusion that accompanies uprighting, which can be excessive with the other methods when there is no antagonist.

Final Positioning of Molar and Premolars

Once molar uprighting is almost complete, often it is desirable to increase the available pontic space and close open contacts in the anterior segment. This is done best by using a relatively stiff base wire, with a compressed coil spring threaded over the wire to produce the required force system. With 22-slot brackets, the base wire should be 18-mil round or 17 × 25 steel. It should engage the anchor teeth and the uprighted molar more or less passively and extend through the molar tube, projecting about 1 mm beyond the distal end. An open coil steel spring (0.009-in. wire, 0.030-in. lumen) is cut so that it is 1 to 2 mm longer than the space, slipped over the base wire (Fig. 20.11), and compressed between the molar and distal premolar. This provides a force of approximately 150 gm to move the premolars mesially while continuing to tip the molar distally. The coil spring can be reactivated without removing it by compressing the spring and adding a split stop to maintain the compression (Fig. 20.11B).

Uprighting Two Molars in the Same Quadrant

Because the resistance offered when uprighting two molars is considerable, only small amounts of tooth movement should be attempted unless comprehensive orthodontic treatment with a complete fixed appliance is planned. The goal should be a modest amount of distal crown tipping of both teeth, which typically would leave space for a premolar-sized implant or pontic. In the lower arch, a bonded canine-to-canine lingual stabilizing wire (which is similar to a bonded retainer) is needed to control the position of the anterior teeth (see Fig. 20.9D). Trying to upright both the second and third molars bilaterally at the same time is not a good idea; significant movement of the anchor teeth is inevitable unless skeletal anchorage is used.

When both the second and the third molars are to be uprighted, the third molar should carry a single rectangular tube and the second molar a bracket. Because the second molar is usually more severely tipped than the third molar, increased flexibility of the wire mesial and distal to the second molar is required. The best

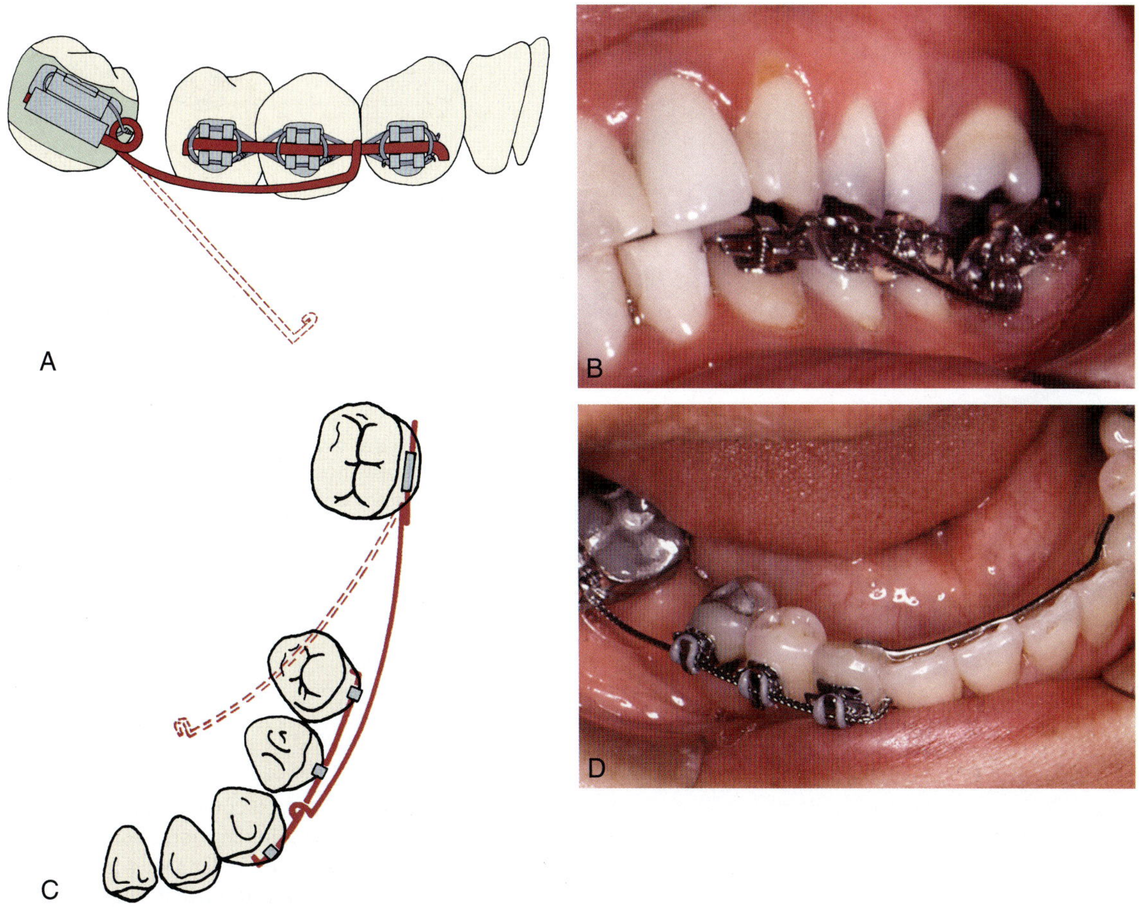

• **Fig. 20.9** Uprighting with an auxiliary spring. (A) If the relative alignment of the molar precludes extending the stabilizing segment into the molar bracket, then a rigid stabilizing wire, 19 × 25 stainless steel, is placed in the premolars and canine only (often with the brackets positioned so this wire is passive—see Fig. 20.2). The mesial arm of the uprighting spring lies in the vestibule before engagement, and the spring is activated by lifting the mesial arm and hooking it over a stabilizing wire in the canine and premolar brackets. (B) Auxiliary uprighting spring to molar just after initial placement. Note the helix bent into the steel wire that forms the spring to provide better spring qualities. (C) Because the force is applied to the facial surface of the teeth, an auxiliary uprighting spring tends not only to extrude the molar but also to roll it lingually, while intruding the premolars and flaring them buccally. To counteract this side effect, the uprighting spring should be curved buccolingually so that when it is placed into the molar tube, the hook would lie lingually to the archwire before activation *(dashed line)*. (D) Better control of anchorage, with either a continuous wire or an auxiliary spring, is obtained when a canine-to-canine stabilizing wire is bonded on the lingual surface of these teeth.

approach is to use a highly flexible wire initially—17 × 25 A-NiTi usually is a good choice—and then proceed to a TMA wire of the same size. Excessive mobility of the teeth can result from failure to reduce occlusal interferences.

Retention

After molar uprighting, the teeth are in an unstable position until the implant or prosthesis that will provide long-term retention is placed, and a retainer is needed. If an auxiliary uprighting spring was used, a wire shaped as shown in Fig. 20.12A works well. Especially if an implant is planned, there may be a considerable delay while a bone graft heals, and the implant becomes integrated. If retention is needed for more than a few weeks, the preferred approach is to remove the orthodontic appliance and place an intracoronal wire splint (19 × 25 or heavier steel wire) bonded into shallow preparations in the abutment teeth (Fig. 20.12B). This type of splint causes little gingival irritation and can be left in place for a considerable period, but it would have to be removed and rebonded to allow bone grafting and implant surgery.

Crossbite Correction

Posterior crossbites frequently are corrected using "through the bite" elastics from a conveniently placed tooth in the opposing arch, which moves both the upper and lower tooth (Fig. 20.13A). This tips the teeth into the correct occlusion but also tends to extrude them, which can change occlusal relationships throughout the mouth. These elastics should be used only for a short time.

Often it is desirable to move the maxillary teeth more than the mandibular. One way to do that is to have several teeth in the lower arch stabilized by a heavy archwire segment (Fig. 20.13B–D).

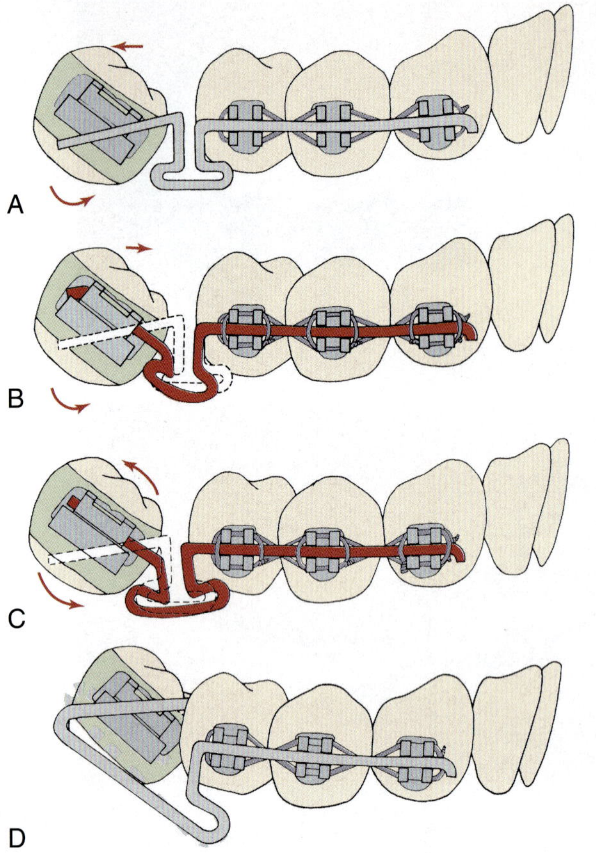

• **Fig. 20.10** (A) T-loop spring in 17 × 25 steel wire, showing the degree of angulation of the wire before it is inserted into the molar tube that is necessary to upright a single-tipped molar. (B) If a T-loop is activated by pulling the distal end of the wire through the molar tube and bending it, the tooth cannot move distally. This generates a moment that results in molar uprighting by mesial root movement with space closure. (C) A T-loop for uprighting by distal tipping. Note that the tooth can move back by sliding along the wire. (D) Modification of a T-loop that can be used to upright a severely tipped or rotated molar by distal tipping. The wire is inserted into the distal end of the tube on the molar. The additional wire in the loop provides a longer range of action, but the uprighting is still by distal crown tipping.

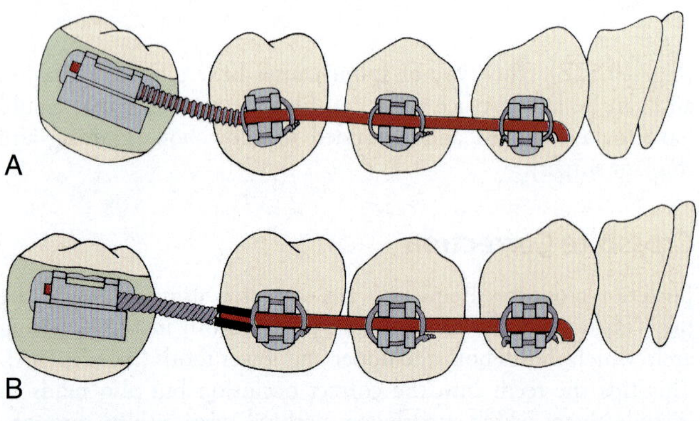

• **Fig. 20.11** (A) A compressed coil spring on a round wire (usually 18-mil steel) may be used to complete molar uprighting while closing remaining spaces in the premolar region. (B) The coil spring can be reactivated by compressing it against a split spacer crimped over the archwire just behind the premolar bracket.

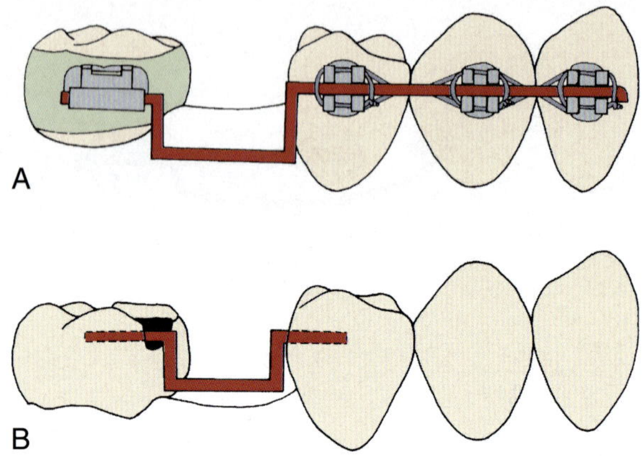

• **Fig. 20.12** A molar that has been uprighted is unstable and must be maintained in its new position until a fixed bridge or implant is placed to stabilize it. There are two ways to provide temporary stabilization: (A) a heavy rectangular (19 × 25) steel wire engaging the brackets passively and (B) an intracoronal splint (often called an A-*splint*) made with 19 × 25 or 21 × 25 steel wire that is bonded in shallow preparations in the proximal enamel with composite resin. This causes minimal tissue disturbance. The intracoronal splint is preferred, particularly if retention is to be continued for more than a few weeks.

Of course, the same approach could be used in reverse to produce more movement of a mandibular tooth. Sometime that is the case when a mesially tipped lower molar also is in buccal crossbite. An auxiliary uprighting spring can move it lingually as it uprights by two modifications in design: omitting the inward bending of the spring before it is activated (see Fig. 20.9C) and making the spring from round wire.

If an anterior crossbite is due only to a displaced tooth and correcting it requires only tipping (as in the case of a maxillary incisor that was tipped lingually into crossbite), then a removable appliance or clear aligner may be used to tip the tooth into a normal position. However, that also produces an apparent intrusion and a reduction in overbite (Fig. 20.14). This can present a problem during retention because a positive overbite serves to retain the crossbite correction.

If a deep overbite accompanies an anterior crossbite, correcting it will be much easier if a temporary bite plane that frees the occlusion is added. This bite plane should be carefully constructed to contact the occlusal surfaces of all teeth to prevent any super-eruption during treatment. As soon as the patient can bite behind the tooth that was in crossbite, the bite plate should be removed. Establishing a good overbite relationship is the key to maintaining crossbite correction.

Extrusion

There are several methods to extrude selected teeth so that endodontic therapy or restorative dentistry can be completed. Essentially, with light continuous forces, teeth can be extruded and both the bone and gingival tissue will follow. That is true if the teeth are extruded with bands, brackets and archwires or clear trays. The mechanics of clear tray extrusion are discussed in Chapter 18 and 21.

When using fixed appliances there are two approaches: controlled extrusion or light continuous forces.

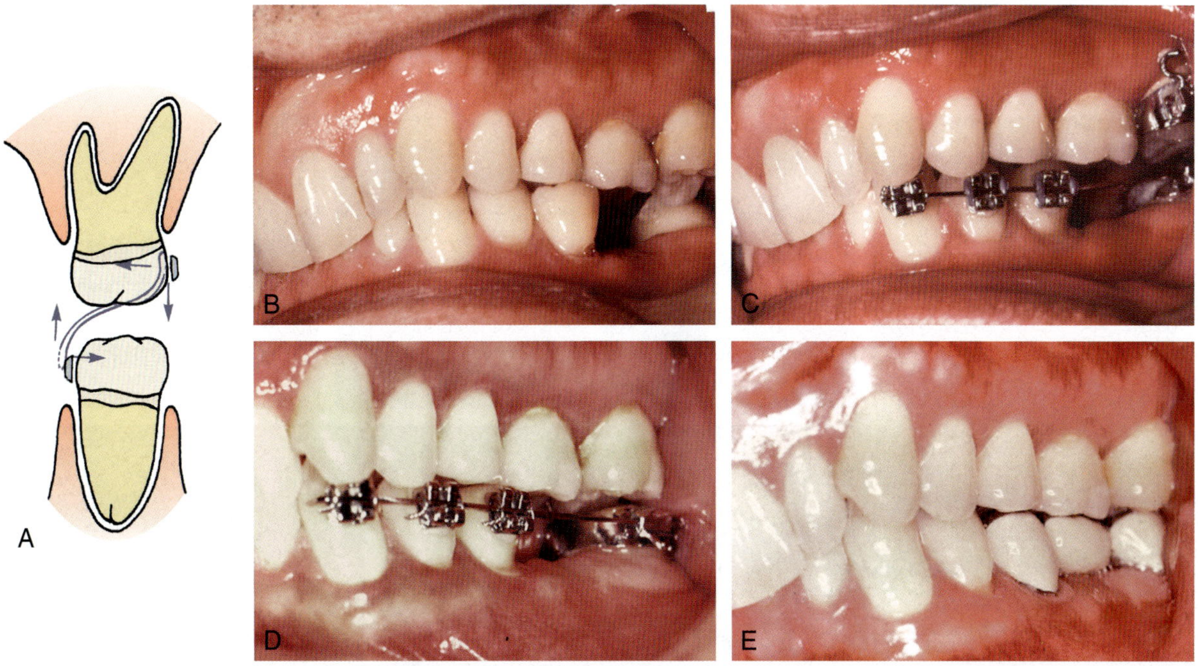

• **Fig. 20.13** (A) "Through the bite" or cross-elastics produce both horizontal and vertical forces and will extrude the teeth while moving them buccolingually. If these elastics are used to correct posterior crossbite in adults, care must be taken not to open the bite anteriorly too much. Cross-elastics are rarely indicated for an anterior crossbite. (B) Buccal crossbite of the second molars in a patient at age 50 who had lost the mandibular first molar years previously. The lower second molar had tipped mesially and lingually. (C) The standard orthodontic appliance for uprighting a lower molar was used, consisting of a band on the mandibular second molar, a bonded canine-to-canine mandibular lingual wire to augment anchorage, and bonded brackets on the facial aspect of the premolars and canine. In addition, a lingual cleat was placed on the lower band, and a band with a facial hook was placed on the maxillary second molar so that cross-elastics could be worn. (D) The molar uprighting was completed after the crossbite was corrected. (E) The completed bridge in place. This is classic adjunctive orthodontics. The anterior deep bite and incisor alignment were not problems for this patient and were not corrected.

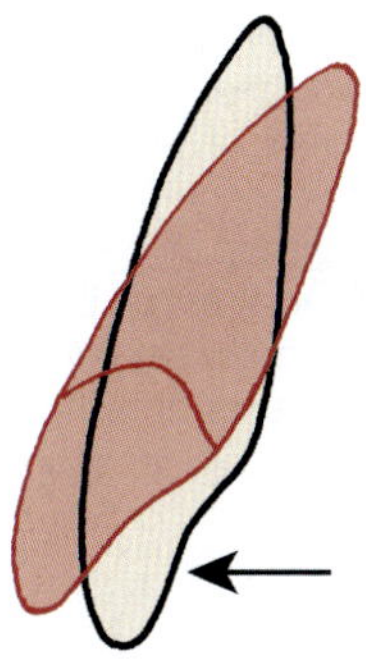

• **Fig. 20.14** A labially directed force against a maxillary incisor (from a removable or fixed appliance) will tip the tooth and cause an apparent intrusion of the crown, which reduces the overbite (or makes anterior open bite worse).

Controlled Extrusion

For teeth with defects in or adjacent to the cervical third of the root, controlled extrusion (sometimes called *forced eruption*) can be an alternative to light continuous forces combined with crown-lengthening surgery.[5] This procedure is designed to gain more clinical crown accompanied by limited if any surgery, but can be less predictable than ideal in this regard. The central idea is that heavy, nonphysiologic forces are used to rapidly extrude the tooth, (Fig. 20.15) so that the gingival margin does not follow and more of the tooth is exposed, with less need for surgical intervention.

Its potential advantages over extrusion with light continuous forces followed by crown-lengthening surgery are that extrusion of the tooth can allow isolation under a rubber dam for endodontic therapy when it would not be possible otherwise, and it allows crown margins to be placed on sound tooth structure while maintaining a uniform gingival contour that provides improved esthetics. In addition, the alveolar bone height is not compromised, the apparent crown length is increased, and the bony support of adjacent teeth is not compromised. But it usually is necessary to perform some, at least limited recontouring of the gingiva and often of the bone, to produce a contour even with the adjacent teeth and a proper biologic width (Fig. 20.15).

In general, control of apical infection should be completed before extrusion of the root begins. If so, preliminary endodontic treatment to relieve symptoms is done initially, and the tooth is maintained with a temporary root filling or other palliative treatment until it has been moved to a better position. For some patients, however, the orthodontic movement must be completed before definitive endodontic procedures because one purpose of extrusion may be to provide better access for endodontic and restorative procedures.

The distance the tooth should be extruded is determined by three things:

1. The location of the defect (e.g., fracture line, root perforation, or resorption site)

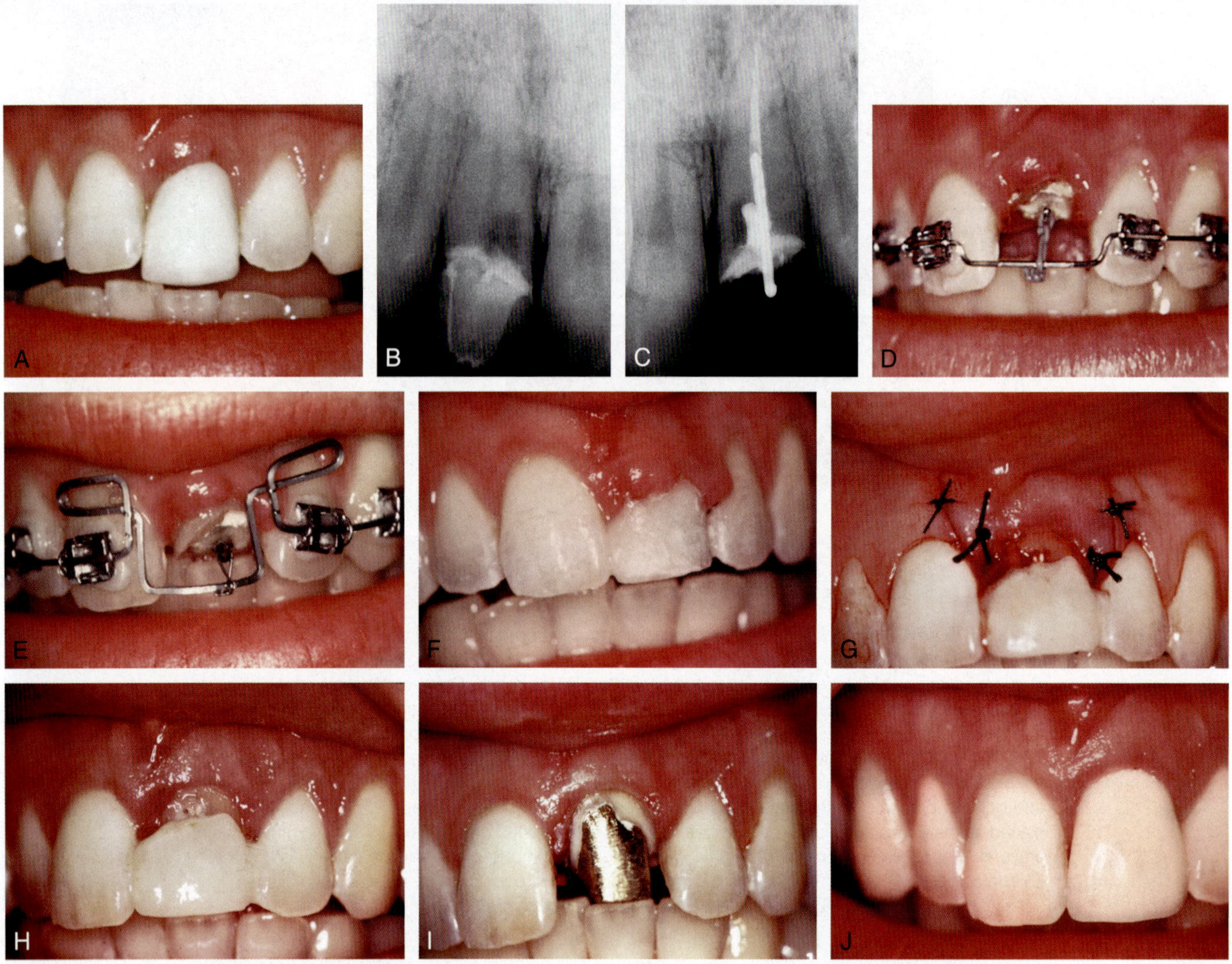

• **Fig. 20.15** Forced eruption can move a tooth that is unrestorable because of subgingival pathology into a position that allows treatment. (A) This central incisor had a crown placed after having been chipped previously, but now showed gingival inflammation and elongation. (B) A periapical radiograph revealed internal root resorption below the crown margin. (C) The treatment plan was endodontic treatment to arrest the internal resorption, then elongation of the root so that a new crown margin could be placed on sound root structure. (D) Initially, an elastomeric tie was used from an archwire segment to an attachment on the post that was cemented in the root canal. (E) Then loops in a flexible rectangular wire (17 × 25 beta-titanium [beta-Ti]) were used for quicker and more efficient tooth movement. (F) Four millimeters of elongation occurred in as many weeks, and a temporary restoration was placed. (G and H) An apically repositioned flap was used to create the correct gingival contour. (I and J) Then a coping and final ceramic crown were prepared. Extraction of the tooth was avoided, and a highly esthetic restoration was possible.

2. Space to place the margin of the restoration so that it is not at the base of the gingival sulcus (typically, 1 mm is needed)
3. An allowance for the biologic width of the gingival attachment (about 2 mm)

Thus, if a fracture is at the height of the alveolar crest, the tooth should be extruded about 3 mm; if it is 2 mm below the crest, 5 mm of extrusion would ideally be needed. The size of the pulp chamber or canal at the level of the margin of the future restoration also is a consideration—the wall of the tooth at that location must not be too thin. The crown-to-root ratio at the end of treatment should be 1: 1 or better. A tooth with a poorer ratio can be maintained only by splinting it to adjacent teeth.

Isolated one- or two-wall vertical pockets pose a particular esthetic problem if they occur in the anterior region of the mouth. Surgical correction may be contraindicated simply on esthetic grounds. Forced eruption of such teeth, with concomitant crown reduction, can improve the periodontal condition while maintaining excellent esthetics.

In general, extrusion can be as rapid as 1 mm per week without damage to the PDL, so 3 to 6 weeks is sufficient for almost any patient. Too much force, and too rapid a rate of movement, runs the risk of tissue damage, tooth devitalization, and ankylosis.

With any technique for controlled extrusion, the patient must be seen every 1 to 2 weeks to remove any occlusal contacts that would impede eruption (for instance, shorten the height of a temporary crown), control inflammation, and monitor progress. After active tooth movement has been completed, a period of at least 3 weeks but not more than 6 weeks of stabilization is needed to allow reorganization of the PDL. If a periodontal surgical procedure is needed to recontour the alveolar bone and/or reposition the gingiva, it can be done a month after completion of extrusion. As with molar uprighting, it is better to complete the definitive prosthetic treatment without extensive delay.

Conventional Orthodontic Extrusion

Because extrusion is the tooth movement that occurs most readily and intrusion is the movement that occurs least readily, ample anchorage is usually available from adjacent teeth. The appliance needs to be quite rigid over the anchor teeth, and flexible where it attaches to the tooth that is being extruded. A continuous flexible archwire (Fig. 20.16A) produces the desired extrusion but must be managed carefully because it also tends to tip the adjacent teeth toward the tooth being extruded, reducing the space for subsequent restorations and disturbing the interproximal contacts within the arch. A flexible cantilever spring to extrude a tooth (Fig. 20.16B), or a rigid stabilizing wire and an auxiliary elastomeric module or spring for extrusion (Fig. 20.16C) provide better control.

Currently, the preferred method is to use a heavy base wire and a light (usually NiTi) overlay wire to accomplish both stable adjacent tooth anchorage and light tooth moving forces. Because the predictability of the posttreatment gingival height and contour are poor and gingival surgery is nearly always needed regardless of the extrusion method chosen, this approach is relatively simple (Fig 12.9).

The basic principle for any approach to extrusion is there must be an anchor unit and some form of flexibility to provide the tooth moving force. There are some less elegant solutions than the overlay wire method that might appeal to those less likely to bend wire or use more complex biomechanics.

Two methods are suggested for extrusion in uncomplicated cases. The first employs a stabilizing wire, 19 × 25 or 21 × 25 stainless steel, bonded directly to the facial surface of the adjacent teeth (Fig. 20.17). A post and core with temporary crown and pin are placed on the tooth to be extruded, and an elastomeric module is used to extrude the tooth. This appliance is simple and provides excellent control of anchor teeth, but better control can be obtained when orthodontic brackets are used.

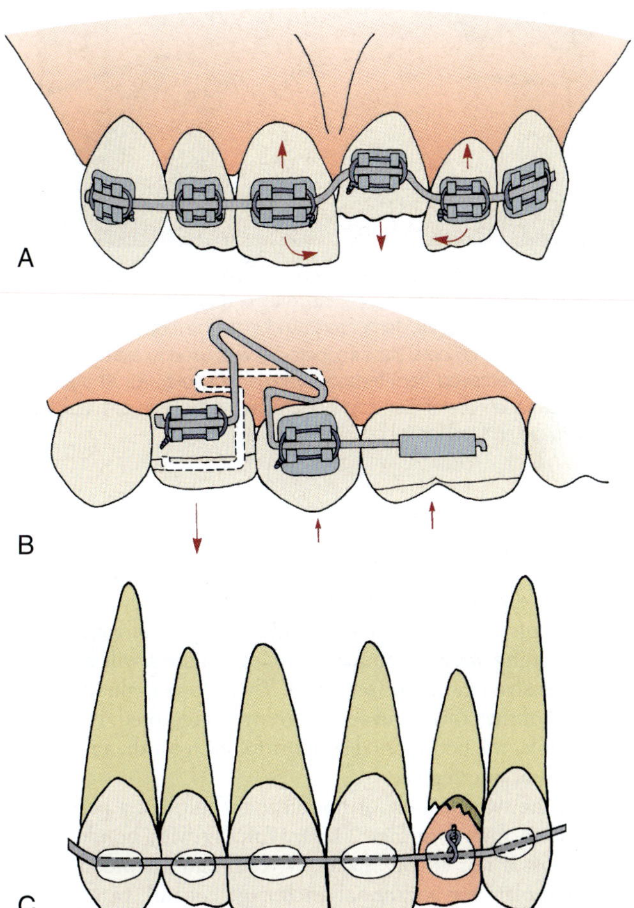

• **Fig. 20.16** (A) Although a continuous orthodontic wire activated as shown will produce the desired extrusive force, it will also cause the teeth on either side to tip toward each other, reducing the space available for the extruding tooth. (B) A segmental T-loop in a rectangular wire (17 × 25 steel in 18-slot brackets, 19 × 25 beta-titanium [beta-Ti] in 22-slot appliance) will extrude a tooth while controlling mesiodistal tipping of the anchor teeth. (C) Extrusion also can be done without conventional orthodontic attachments by bonding a 19 × 25 steel-stabilizing wire directly to the facial surface of adjacent teeth. An elastomeric module is stretched between the stabilizing wire and a pin placed directly into the crown of the tooth to be extruded. If a temporary crown is used for better esthetics while the extrusion is being done, it must be progressively cut away to make the tooth movement possible. (Courtesy Dr. L. Osterle.)

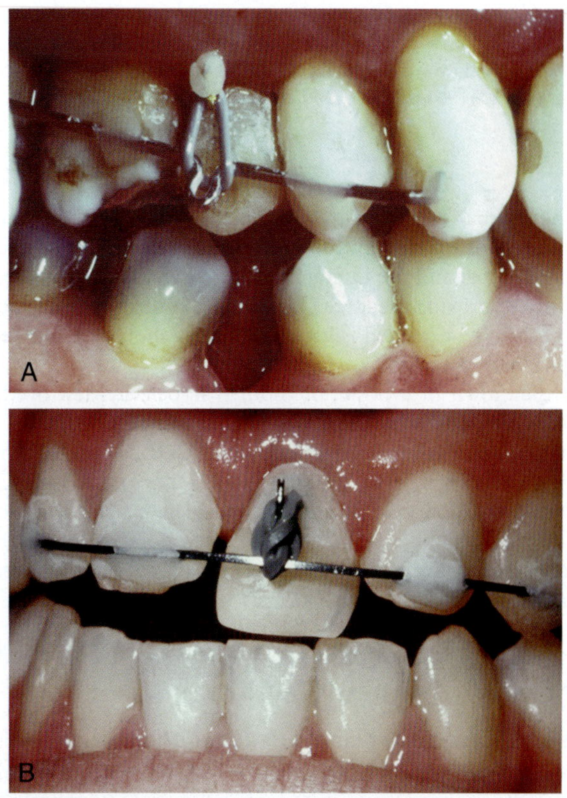

• **Fig. 20.17** (A) For extrusion of this fractured premolar so that a satisfactory permanent restoration could be made, an elastomeric module was stretched between the stabilizing wire and a pin placed directly into the crown of the premolar. (B) The same technique can be used to extrude an incisor. The temporary restoration placed on the tooth while it is being extruded needs to be reduced at frequent intervals. (Courtesy Dr. L. Osterle.)

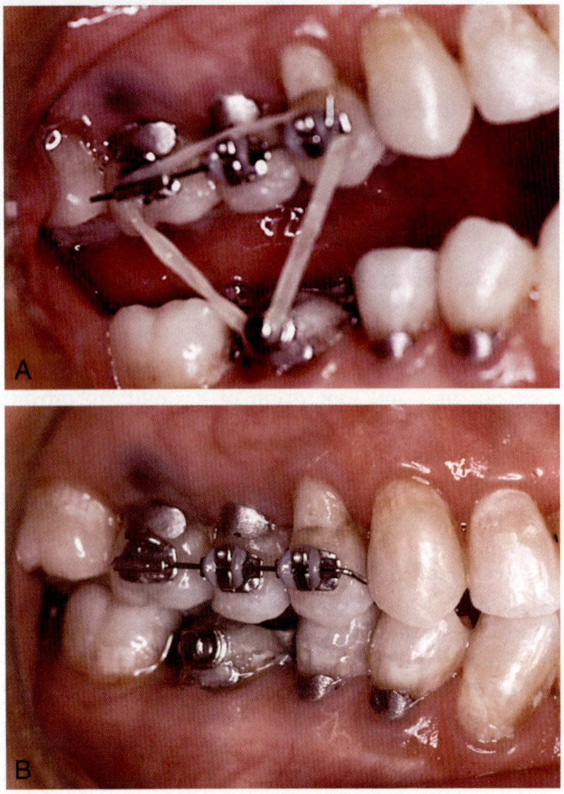

• **Fig. 20.18** For this patient in her 60 s, the facial surface of a lower first molar fractured to below the gingival margin. (A) The maxillary premolars and first molar were bonded and stabilized, and an elastic to a button bonded on the lower molar was used to elongate it to the point that (B) the fracture line was exposed and a satisfactory crown preparation was possible.

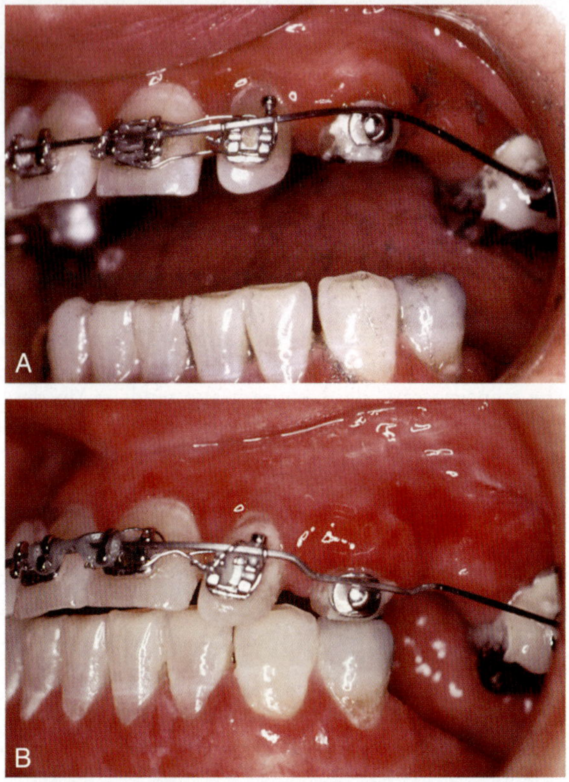

• **Fig. 20.19** A bridge attached to the maxillary left canine failed because of caries beneath the crown on the canine. After endodontic treatment, a button was bonded to an amalgam temporary buildup on the root, and (A) a continuous archwire (17 × 25 beta-titanium [beta-Ti]) was used to extrude the tooth; amalgam was removed from temporary buildup weekly. (B) At the point at which a permanent restoration could be placed, all the amalgam buildup had been removed and the tooth had been elongated 5 mm.

The alternative is to bond brackets to the anchor teeth, bond an attachment (often a button rather than a bracket) to the tooth to be extruded, and use interarch elastics (Fig. 20.18) or a flexible archwire to provide the force (Fig. 20.19). If the buccal surface of the tooth to be extruded is intact, a bracket should be bonded as far gingivally as possible.

If the crown of a posterior tooth is hopelessly destroyed, an orthodontic band with a bracket usually can be placed over the remaining root surface. An orthodontic band has the benefit of helping isolation procedures during emergency endodontic treatment. Once endodontic treatment is completed, a pin in the tooth can be used for the attachment, and a temporary crown can be placed if needed for esthetics. Adjacent teeth are bonded to serve as the anchor unit.

Alignment of Anterior Teeth

Diastema Closure and Space Redistribution

The major indication for adjunctive orthodontic treatment to correct malaligned anterior teeth is preparation for buildups, veneers, or implants to improve the appearance of the maxillary incisor teeth. The most frequent problem is a maxillary central diastema, which is often further complicated by irregular spacing related to small or missing lateral incisors (Fig. 20.20).

A "diagnostic setup" is very helpful in planning the correction of such problems. For this procedure, the study casts are duplicated and the malaligned teeth are carefully cut from the model, repositioned, and then waxed back onto the cast in a new position. If digital casts are available, a contemporary alternative is to do this on a computer screen, and this is part of routine treatment planning when a sequence of clear aligners will be used in comprehensive treatment (see later). This allows evaluation of the feasibility of the crown and root movements required, the anchorage available, the periodontal support for each tooth, and the possible occlusal interferences.

There are two possible orthodontic techniques: a partial fixed appliance as shown in Fig. 20.20, typically with bonded brackets on most if not all the maxillary teeth and a bonded tube on the first molars for additional anchorage control, or a sequence of clear aligners. With a fixed appliance, initial alignment is carried out by using a light wire such as 16-mil A-NiTi or 17.5-mil braided steel. This wire is replaced after the teeth are aligned with a 16- or 18-mil round steel wire, along which the teeth are repositioned with elastomeric modules or coil springs. There is always a tendency for the space to reopen after any degree of diastema closure. Bonding a flexible wire on the lingual surface of the incisors as a permanent retainer is recommended.

An alternative is the use of a sequence of clear aligners. These can be produced in two ways: (1) for modest amounts of tooth movement, aligners can be made in the office with relatively inexpensive computer software and three-dimensional (3D) printing (see Fig. 10.12) and (2) for more extensive tooth movement, a set

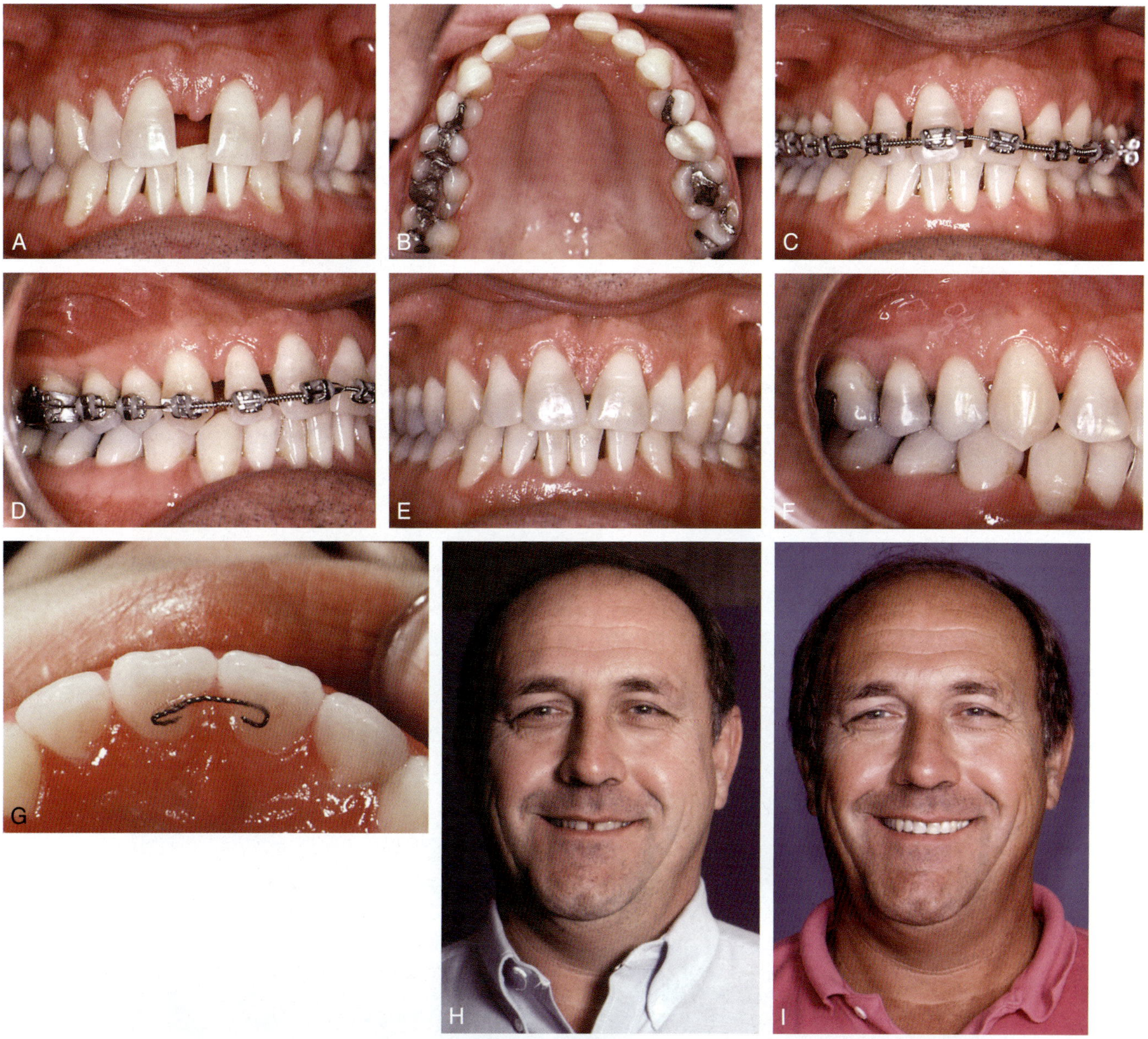

• **Fig. 20.20** If spacing of maxillary incisors is related to small teeth and a tooth-size discrepancy, composite buildups are an excellent solution, but satisfactory esthetics may require redistribution of the space before the restorations are placed, as in this patient who was concerned about his large central diastema. (A and B) Before treatment, age 48. (C and D) Redistribution of the space by using a fixed appliance with coil springs on a 16-mil steel archwire immediately before removal of the orthodontic appliance and placement of the restorations (to be done the same day). A 17.5-mil multistrand steel wire was used for initial alignment before the coil springs were placed. (E and F) Completed restorations (composite buildups). (G) Note the fixed retainer of bonded 21.5-mil multistrand wire on the lingual surface of the central incisors to prevent partial reopening of the midline space. Surgical revision of the frenum was not performed, partially in deference to the patient's age. (H) Appearance on smile before and (I) after treatment.

of 15 to 50 aligners can be fabricated on stereolithographic models created from computer models of the projected tooth movement. In adjunctive treatment, the first method is potentially quite useful. Tray production is described in Chapter 10, while clear tray treatment for adults is described in Chapter 21.

Crowded, Rotated, and Displaced Incisors

As a rule, spacing is the problem when maxillary incisors need realignment to facilitate other treatment. Crowding is usually the problem when alignment of the lower incisors is considered to provide access for restorations, achieve better occlusion, or enable the patient to maintain the teeth. In some cases, alignment of the incisors in both arches must be considered. The key question is whether the crowding should be resolved by expanding the arch, removing some interproximal enamel from each tooth to provide space,[6] or removing one lower incisor.

Expansion of a crowded incisor segment can be done with clear aligners, but if only the lower arch is to be treated, the esthetics of the appliance is not a consideration, and a partial fixed appliance is more efficient and cost-effective (Fig. 20.21). A segment of

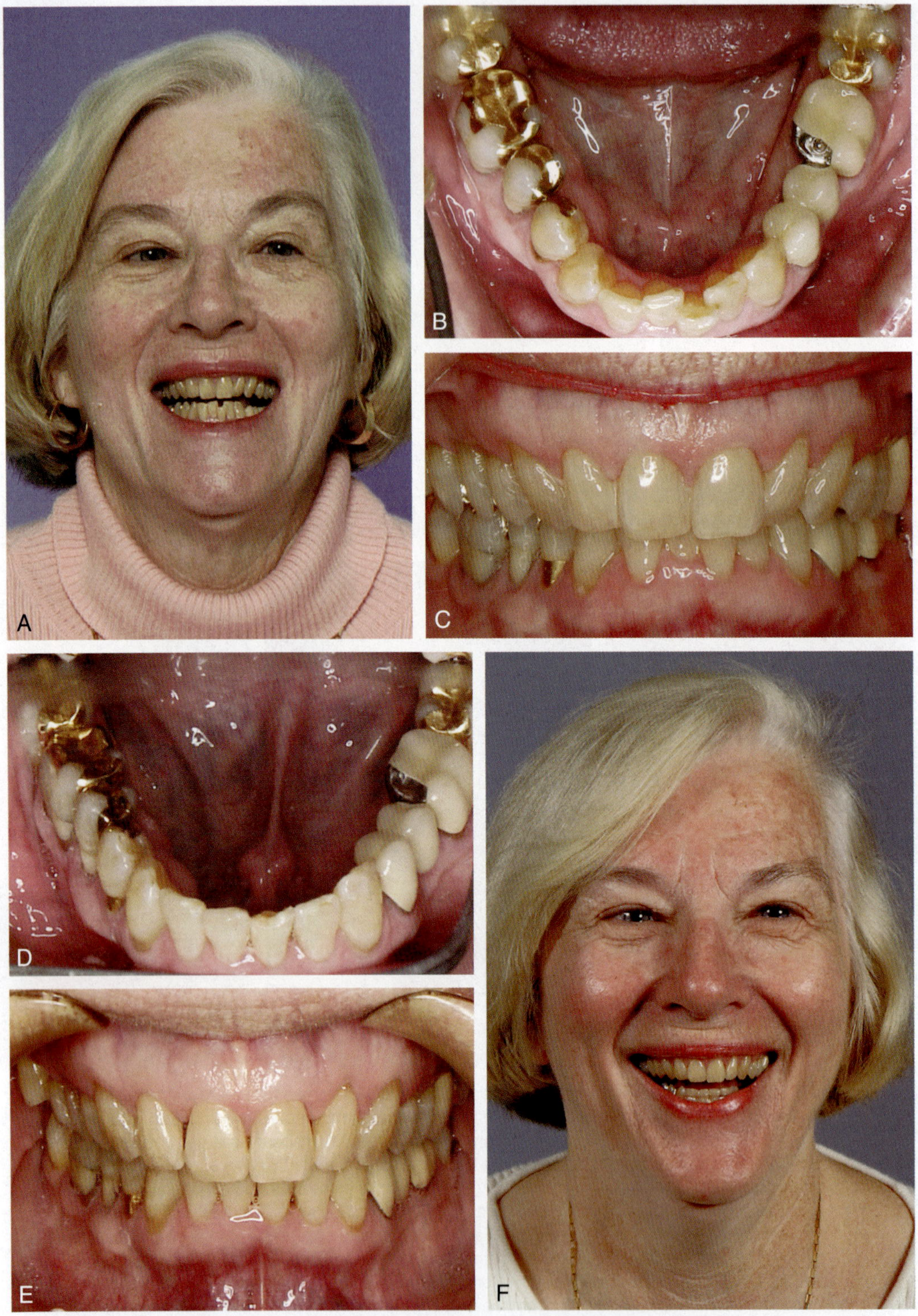

• **Fig. 20.21** In an adult with a damaged lower incisor (in this case, the left central incisor with a crown fracture) and incisor crowding, there were two treatment possibilities: extract the damaged tooth and use the space to align the remaining teeth or align the teeth with arch expansion and restore the damaged one. The decision had an esthetic component because the lower incisors are visible on smile in older individuals. In this patient, aligning the lower incisors without extraction would also require aligning the upper incisors, but this expansion would increase lip support and improve the overall facial appearance as well as the dental appearance. (A) Smile before treatment, after loss of one corner of the lower right central incisor. (B) Mandibular occlusal view. (C) Frontal view. Note the moderately deep bite and lack of overjet. The restorative dentist sought orthodontic consultation, thinking that extraction of the damaged tooth might be the best plan. The patient wanted the best esthetic result and accepted a period of treatment with a fixed appliance on both arches, after which the incisor would be restored. The orthodontic alignment required 5 months. (D) Mandibular occlusal view after alignment. (E) Frontal view. (F) Smile after restoration was completed.

A-NiTi wire, with stops to make it slightly advanced, usually is the best way to bring the teeth into alignment (see Fig. 15.3).

Stripping the contact points of the teeth to remove enamel can provide space for alignment of mildly irregular lower incisors, and either a fixed appliance or a clear aligner sequence can provide the tooth movement. This should be undertaken with caution, however, because it may have an undesirable effect on overjet, overbite, posterior intercuspation, and esthetics.[7] In severe crowding, removing one lower incisor and using the space to align the other three incisors can produce a satisfactory result and can be managed with clear aligner therapy if bonded attachments are part of the treatment plan (Fig. 20.22). The treatment time and difficulty, whatever the type of appliance, put this at or across the border of comprehensive treatment. Neither stripping nor incisor extraction should be undertaken without a diagnostic setup to verify feasibility.

Remember that stretched gingival fibers are a potent force for relapse after rotations have been corrected, and that good long-term stability may require a fiberotomy (see Chapter 17). Whether clear aligners or a fixed appliance was used, retention is necessary until restorative or other treatment is completed. This can be the final aligner in a sequence (although this may be too flexible to be a good retainer), a molded thermoplastic retainer after a fixed appliance is removed, a canine-to-canine clip retainer, or a bonded fixed retainer (see Chapter 19).

Obstructive Sleep Apnea-Related Orthodontic Procedures

Effectiveness of Oral Appliance Treatment

While worn during sleep these oral appliances work to protrude the mandible and associated soft tissues which increases the caliber of the airway, especially in the transverse dimension, thus reducing airway collapsibility. It is important to note, however, that despite the significant change in mandibular position and apparent increase in airway volume, only 29%–71% of patients will have their OSA resolve completely with appliance use[8], and roughly one-third of patients will see no therapeutic effect at all. It is now standard protocol that after the appliance is fitted and optimally titrated, a follow-up assessment is made by the referring physician, with polysomnography used to verify treatment efficacy.

Due to the significant amount of OSA patients ineffectively treated with mandibular advancing appliances, they have been considered an inferior treatment option to CPAP for managing OSA. However, while CPAP is more effective than mandibular advancing appliances at lowering the number of apneas during sleep, this may be offset by improved patient tolerance and adherence with oral appliance therapy. This concept of mean disease alleviation, where oral appliances are generally less effective, but used more, whereas CPAP is very effective but used much less often, is thought to be why more recent data has pointed to equivalent outcomes for cardiovascular and quality of life measures of disease even in cases of severe OSA.

Dental Side Effects of Obstructive Sleep Apnea Treatment

It should come as no surprise that mandibular advancing appliances used to manage obstructive sleep apnea, much like functional appliances to treat class II malocclusions, can cause significant tooth movement. The short term and temporary side effects of these appliances can include tooth or muscle soreness, dry mouth or alternatively excess salivation, and intraoral soft tissue irritation. Over the long term—and it is important to remember that for many patients prescribed mandibular advancing oral appliances, this can mean for the rest of their lives—the weight of holding the mandible and associated soft tissues forward is transmitted by the appliance to the dentition resulting in tooth movement. Studies examining occlusal changes after a period of 10 or more years have reported reductions in overjet and overbite of 2 to 3 mm with a wide amount of individual variation (Figs. 20.23 and 20.24). The formation of anterior crossbites is common, and the reductions in overjet appear to be progressive with each year of appliance use.[9] Interestingly, there is little skeletal movement or change in mandibular position observed over similar time periods, though significant proclination of the mandibular incisors and uprighting of the maxillary incisors can be expected.[10]

Perhaps less well recognized are the dental changes resulting from prolonged CPAP use (Fig. 20.25). Most commonly seen in patients who use a nasal mask type interface for their CPAP therapy, dental spacing due to proclination of the anterior teeth has been reported.[11] It is thought that as air is forced through the nose and down the pharynx, the tongue can be pushed forward against the teeth leading to their movement over time. As such it would be reasonable for patients who are prescribed this type of CPAP to be also provided with orthodontic retainers to prevent this unwanted side effect.

An open discussion about the likely occlusal side effects is an important part of the informed consent process prior to starting oral appliance treatment. For many patients, any inconvenience associated with altered occlusion is far outweighed by the quality-of-life improvements that accompany the better sleep and treatment of the significant comorbidities and health risks caused by OSA. However, over time the occlusal changes can reach a point where they are unacceptable to the patient leading them to seek orthodontic correction of what can be at times a severe malocclusion. Two critical issues need to be addressed before orthodontic treatment can be initiated. First, orthodontic treatment with either fixed appliances or removable aligners will typically preclude the patient from wearing their medically prescribed mandibular advancing oral appliance. Stopping treatment of OSA should only be done under the direction of a physician and alternative therapy such as CPAP will be needed to manage these patients. Secondly, upon completion of orthodontic correction of the malocclusion it would be illogical to have the patient return to using their oral appliance again, only to reform the malocclusion in a few years' time. Often patients will switch to CPAP or attempt surgical corrections to their disease.

Comprehensive Treatment in Adults

Psychologic Considerations

A major motivation for orthodontic treatment of younger patients is the parents' desire to do the best they can for their children. The typical child or adolescent accepts orthodontics in about the same rather passive way that he or she accepts going to school, summer camp, and the inevitable junior high school dance: as just another in the series of events that one must endure while growing up. Occasionally, of course, an adolescent actively resists orthodontic treatment, and the result can be unfortunate for all concerned if the treatment becomes the focus of an adolescent rebellion. In most instances, however, children tend not to become emotionally involved in their treatment.

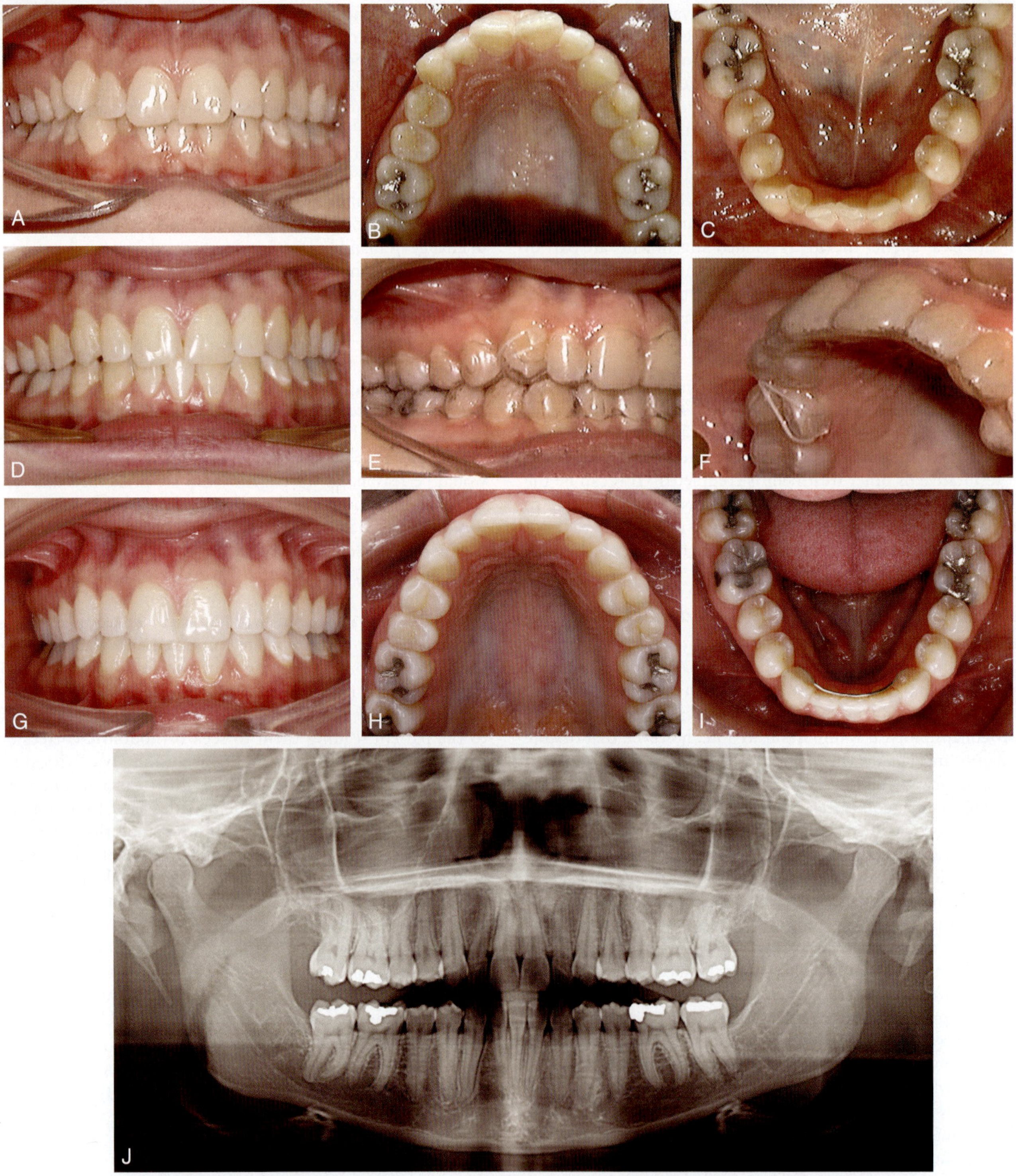

• **Fig. 20.22** This 24-year-old patient had a congenitally missing mandibular right lateral incisor and a retained but failing primary incisor and was selected for Invisalign treatment. (A) Frontal view. (B) Maxillary occlusal. Note the rotation of the maxillary right canine. (C) Mandibular occlusal. The plan was extraction of the primary incisor and closure of the extraction site with a series of Invisalign aligners and bonded attachments to produce the necessary rotation and root movement. Before treatment began, air-rotor stripping of the maxillary anterior teeth was done to reduce the tooth-size discrepancy. (D) Note the hard-to-see bonded attachments on the maxillary right canine and incisors and on the mandibular right canine and central incisor. The original plan called for 13 upper and 15 lower aligners, plus three overcorrection aligners. (E and F) After eight aligners it was noted that the maxillary right canine was not tracking, and an elastic to additional bonded attachments was used along with the aligner to further rotate it. New records were taken, and four upper and five lower revision aligners, with three revision overcorrection aligners, were fabricated. (G to I) Completion of treatment. A bonded canine-to-canine mandibular retainer was used, and the final maxillary aligner was continued at night as the maxillary retainer. (J) Panoramic radiograph at the completion of treatment. Total treatment time was 19 months (which included 2 months waiting for revision aligners). (Courtesy Dr. W. Gierie.)

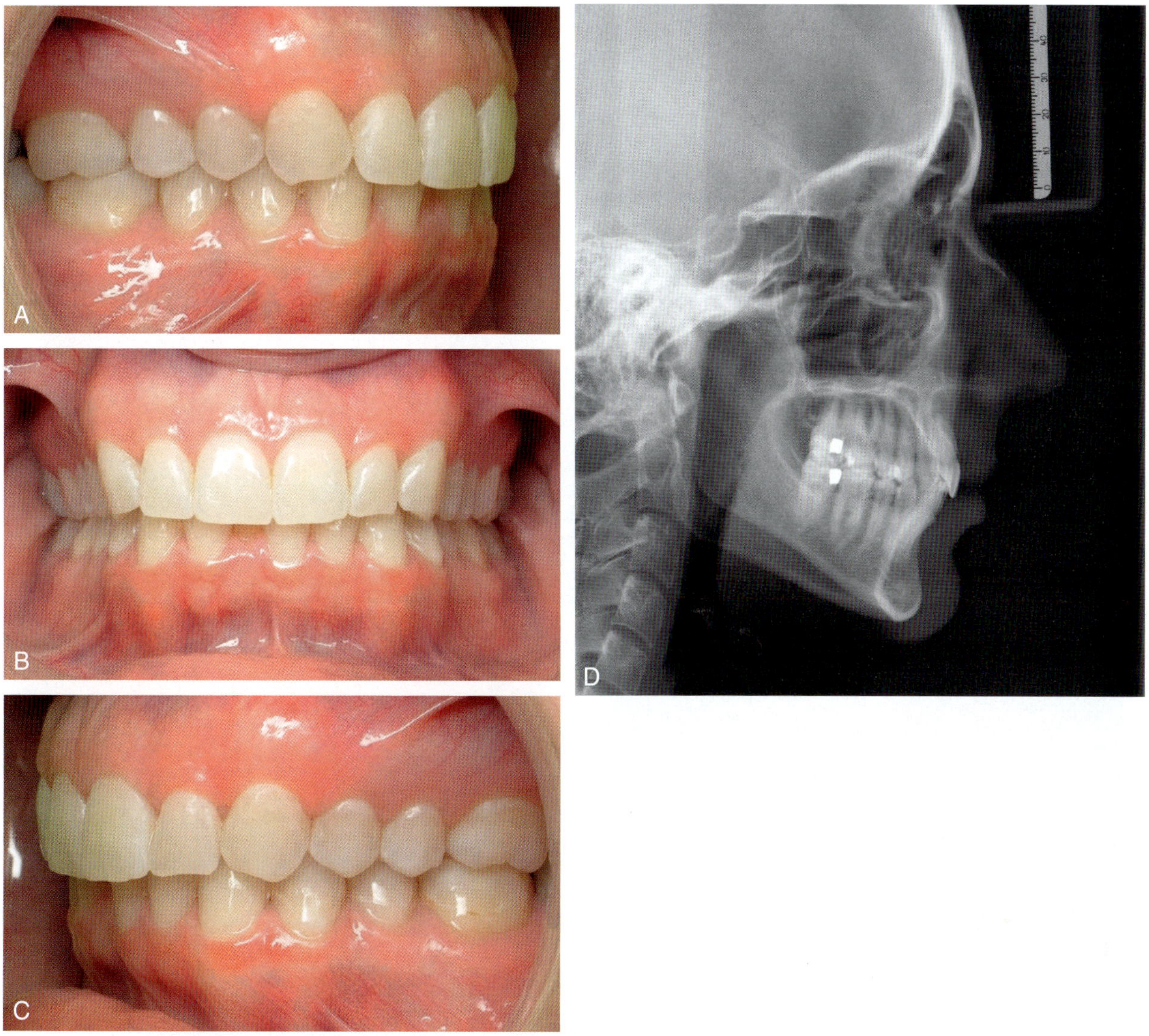

• **Fig. 20.23** Mandibular Advancing oral appliances can be an effective form of treatment for many adults with obstructive sleep apnea. While managing a serious disease with significant negative health effects, these appliances have a common side effect of tooth movement that can dramatically alter the occlusion in some patients. (A, B,C) Here you see the patient prior to initiating oral appliance therapy with a mandibular advancing appliance. They had a reasonable Class I occlusion and overbite and overjet. (D) The pretreatment cephalometric radiograph confirms the occlusion.

Adults in both the younger and older groups, in contrast, seek comprehensive orthodontic treatment because they themselves really want it. For the younger patients who are trying to improve their lot in life, exactly what they want is not always clearly expressed, and some young adults have a remarkably elaborate hidden set of motivations. It is important to explore why an individual wants treatment, and why now as opposed to some other time. This is the only way to avoid setting up a situation in which the patient's expectations for treatment cannot possibly be met. Sometimes, orthodontic treatment is sought as a final effort to improve personal appearance to deal with a series of complicated social problems. Orthodontic treatment obviously cannot be relied on to repair personal relationships, save jobs, or overcome a series of financial disasters. If the prospective patient has unrealistic expectations of that sort, it is much better to deal with them sooner than later.

Most adults in both the younger and older groups, fortunately, understand why they want orthodontics and are realistic about what they can obtain from it. One might expect those who seek treatment to be less secure and less well-adjusted than the average adult, but for the most part, they have a more positive self-image than average.[12] It apparently takes a good deal of ego strength to seek orthodontic treatment as an adult, and ego strength rather than weakness characterizes most potential adult patients. A patient who seeks treatment primarily because he or she wants it (internal motivation) is more likely to respond well psychologically than a patient whose motivation is the urging of others or

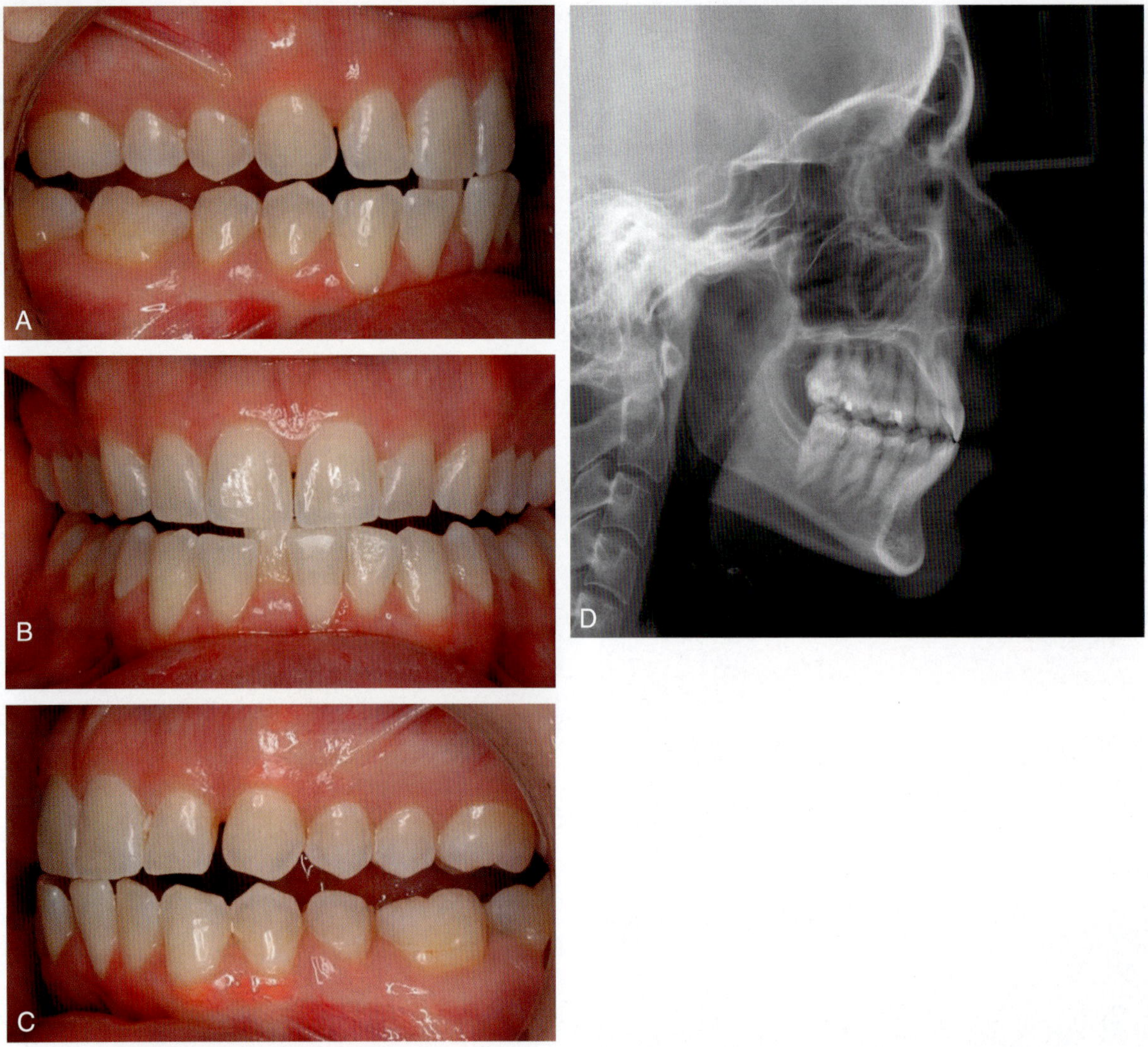

• **Fig. 20.24** (A–C) The patient's (from Fig. 20.23) obstructive sleep apnea was successfully managed with a Mandibular Advancing Appliance, but they also experienced the known side effects of mesial tipping and proclination of the lower dentition after 8 years of consistent nighttime wear. Note the posterior open bite and traumatic occlusion of the incisors. (D) The cephalometric radiograph confirms the malocclusion.

the expected impact of treatment on others (external motivation). Patients with an inadequate or pathologic personality (Fig. 20.26) are more likely to have a complex set of unrecognized expectations for treatment, the proverbial hidden agenda.

One way to identify the minority of individuals who may present problems because of their unrealistic expectations is to compare the patient's perception of his or her orthodontic condition with the doctor's evaluation. If the patient thinks that the appearance or function of the teeth is creating a severe problem, but an objective assessment simply does not corroborate that, orthodontic treatment should be approached with caution.

Even highly motivated adults are likely to have some concern about the appearance of orthodontic appliances. The demand for an invisible orthodontic appliance comes almost entirely from young adults or late adolescents who are concerned about the reaction of others to obvious orthodontic treatment. In an earlier era, this was a major reason for using removable appliances in adults, particularly the Crozat appliance in the United States (see Fig. 10.1).

All the possibilities for a better appearing appliance, however, can lead to potential compromises in orthodontic treatment. Ceramic brackets, although much better, inevitably make treatment more difficult because of the problems outlined in Chapter 10. Lingual appliances have been greatly improved since the turn of the 21st century and now make all types of tooth movement quite possible but still are technically difficult for the doctor to use efficiently and can be difficult for patients to tolerate. Clear aligners manage some types of tooth movement quite well but have difficulty with others (see Box 10.1). Small bonded attachments on teeth that require complex movements give the aligner a better purchase, partially overcoming this difficulty, but this makes the treatment much more complex.

Although there is nothing wrong with using the most esthetic appliance possible for an adult patient, the compromises associated with this approach should be thoroughly discussed in advance. It is unrealistic for a patient to expect that orthodontic treatment can be carried out without other people knowing about it. The whole issue of the visibility of the orthodontic appliances

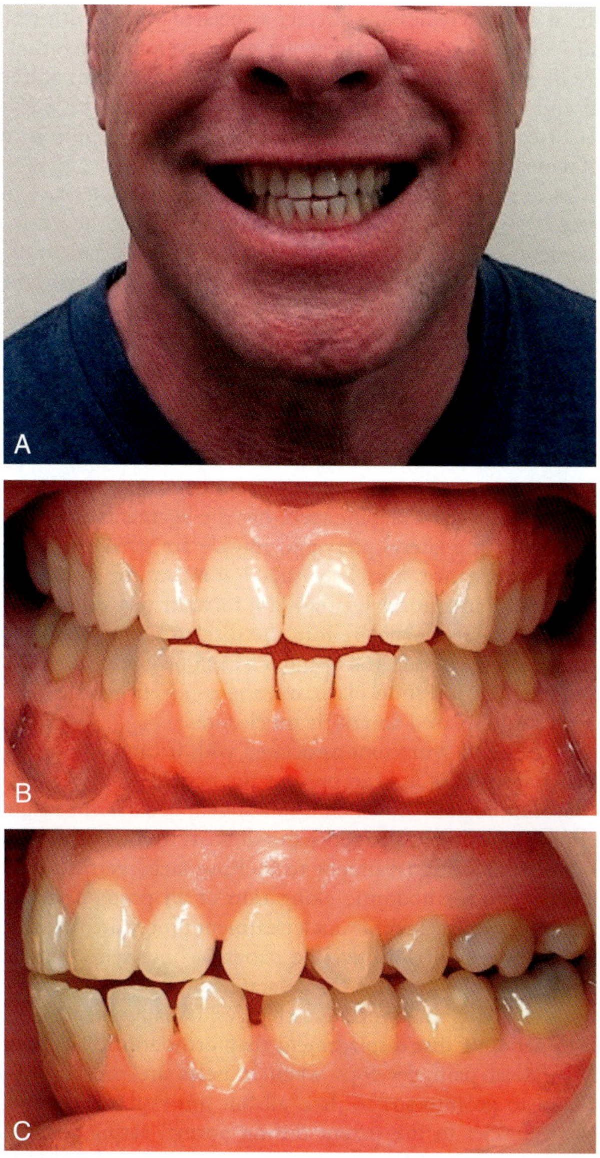

• **Fig. 20.25** In some patients, the pressure from CPAP therapy may cause the tongue to protrude forward while in use during sleep. (A–C) This can lead to increased proclination of the anterior teeth resulting in unwanted spacing and a reduction in overjet as seen here. Orthodontic retainers worn along with CPAP may prevent these changes from occurring.

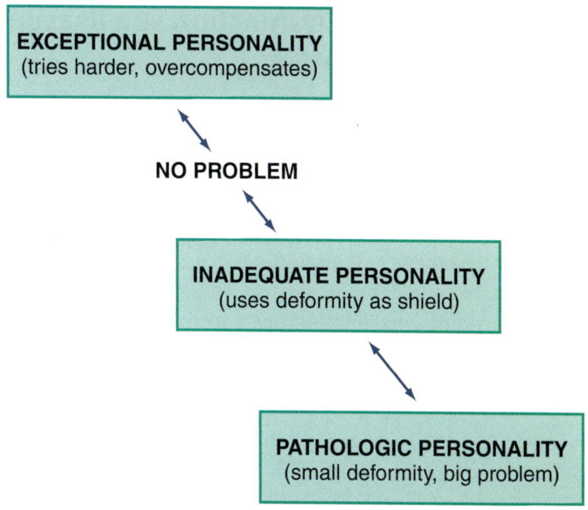

• **Fig. 20.26** Dentofacial deformity can affect an individual's life adjustment. Fortunately, most potential adult orthodontic patients fall into the "no problem" category psychologically. A few highly successful individuals (who nevertheless may seek treatment) can be thought of as almost overcompensating for their deformity with their exceptional personality, but they tend to be personable and very pleasant to work with. For some individuals, however, the orthodontic condition can become the focus for a wide-ranging set of social adjustment problems that orthodontics alone will not solve. These patients fall into the "inadequate personality" and "pathologic personality" categories; these patients are difficult and almost impossible, respectively, to help. An important aspect of orthodontic diagnosis for adults is understanding where a patient fits along this continuum.

is much less important, at least in the United States, than many patients fear. Orthodontic treatment for adults is certainly socially acceptable, and one does not become a victim of discrimination because of visible orthodontic appliances. In a sense, the patient's expectations become a self-fulfilling prophecy. If the patient faces others confidently, a visible orthodontic appliance causes no problems. Only if the patient acts ashamed or defensive is there likely to be any negative reaction from others.

The question of whether an orthodontic office should have a separate treatment area for adults, separated from the adolescents who still constitute the bulk of most orthodontic practices, is related to the same set of negative attitudes. Most comprehensive orthodontic treatment for adolescents is carried out in open treatment areas, not only because this is efficient but also because the learning effect from having patients observe what is happening to others is a positive influence in patient adaptation to treatment. Should adults be segregated into private rooms, rather than joining the group in the open treatment area? This is logical only if the adult is greatly concerned about privacy (which is truer of Europeans than Americans) or is vaguely ashamed of being an orthodontic patient.

Sometimes, for some adults, treatment in a private room may be preferable, but for most adults, learning from interacting with other patients helps them understand and tolerate the treatment procedures. There are positive advantages in having patients at various stages of treatment compare their experiences, and this is at least as beneficial to adults as to children, perhaps more so.

Although adults can be treated in the same area as adolescents, they cannot be handled in the same way. The typical adolescent's passive acceptance of what is being done is rarely found in adult patients, who want and expect a considerable degree of explanation of what is happening and why. An adult can be counted on to be interested in the treatment, but that does not automatically translate into compliance with instructions. Unless adults understand why they have been asked to do various things, they may choose not to do them, not in the passive way an adolescent might just shrug it off but from an active decision not to do it. In addition, adults, as a rule, are less tolerant of discomfort and more likely to complain about pain after adjustments and about difficulties in speech, eating, and tissue adaptation. Additional chair time to meet these demands should be anticipated.

These characteristics might make adults sound like less desirable orthodontic patients than adolescents, but this is not necessarily so. Working with individuals who are intensely interested in their own treatment and motivated to take care of their teeth can be a pleasant and stimulating alternative to the less-involved adolescents. If the expectations of both the doctor and the patient are realistic, comprehensive treatment for adults can be a rewarding experience for both.

Temporomandibular Dysfunction as a Reason for Orthodontic Treatment

TMD and temporomandibular (TM) pain rarely are encountered in children seeking orthodontic treatment, but TMD is a significant motivating factor for some adults who consider orthodontic treatment.[13] The relationship between dental occlusion and TMD is highly controversial, and it is important to view this objectively. Orthodontic treatment can sometimes help patients with TMD, but it cannot be relied on to correct these problems.[14] Patients need to understand what may happen to their symptoms during and after orthodontics.

Types of Problems

In diagnosis of TMD problems, patients are classified as being in one of four large groups: those with masticatory muscle disorders, TM joint disorders, chronic mandibular hypomobility, or growth disorders.[15] From the perspective of potential orthodontic treatment in adults, differentiating between the first two groups is particularly important (Fig. 20.27). Because muscle spasm and joint pathology can coexist, the distinction in many patients is difficult. Nevertheless, it is unlikely that orthodontics will relieve TMD symptoms in a patient who has internal joint problems or other nonmuscular sources of pain. Those who have myofascial pain or dysfunction, on the other hand, may benefit from improved dental occlusion. It is interesting that in males with severe malocclusion, occlusal characteristics are directly associated with health-related quality of life. Even though females with severe malocclusion are more likely to have TMD, this was not true for them, although pain and TMD do show a significant association. This suggests that correcting the malocclusion might be more helpful in male than female TMD patients.[16]

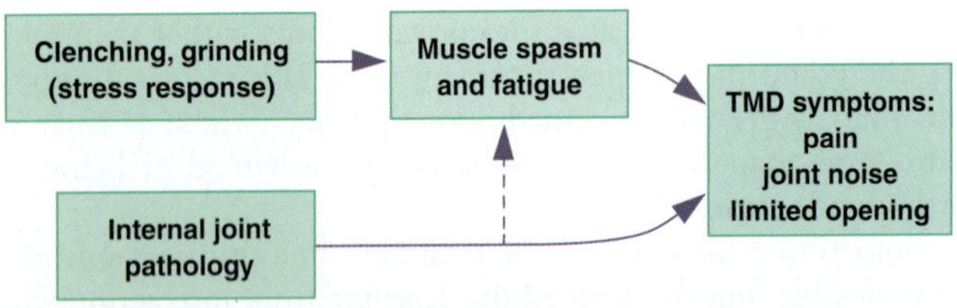

• **Fig. 20.27** Temporomandibular dysfunction *(TMD)* symptoms arise from two major causes: muscle spasm and fatigue, which almost always are related to excessive clenching and grinding in response to stress, and internal joint pathology. As a general guideline, patients with symptoms of muscle spasm and fatigue may be helped by orthodontic treatment, but simpler methods should be attempted first. Orthodontics alone is rarely useful for patients with internal joint pathology.

Almost all of us develop some symptoms of degenerative joint disease as we grow older, and it is not surprising that the jaw joints are sometimes involved (Fig. 20.28). Arthritic involvement of the TM joints is most likely to be the cause of TMD symptoms in patients who have arthritic changes in other joints of the body. A component of muscle spasm and muscle pain should be suspected in individuals whose only symptoms are in the TM joint area, even if radiographs show moderate arthritic degeneration of the joint.

Displacement of the disc (Fig. 20.29) is increasingly frequent as age increases and can arise from a number of causes. One possibility is trauma to the joint such that the ligaments that oppose the action of the lateral pterygoid muscle are stretched or torn. In this circumstance, muscle contraction moves the disk forward as the mandibular condyles translate forward on wide opening, but the ligaments do not restore the disk to its proper position when the jaw is closed. The result is a click on opening and closing, as the disk pops into place over the condylar head as the jaw opens but is displaced anteriorly on closure.

The click and symptoms associated with it can be corrected if an occlusal splint is used to prevent the patient from closing the jaw beyond the point at which displacement occurs. The resulting relief of pain influences patients and dentists to seek either restorative or orthodontic treatment to increase facial vertical dimension. However, orthodontic elongation of all posterior teeth to control disk displacement is not a treatment procedure that should be undertaken lightly. Often the patient whose symptoms have been controlled by a splint can tolerate its reduction or removal, without requiring major occlusal changes. Usually there are better ways of handling disc displacement than orthodontic treatment.

Myofascial pain develops when muscles are overly fatigued and tend to go into spasm. It is all but impossible to overwork the jaw muscles to this extent during normal eating and chewing. To produce myofascial pain, the patient must be clenching or grinding the teeth for many hours per day, presumably as a response to stress. Great variations are seen in the way different

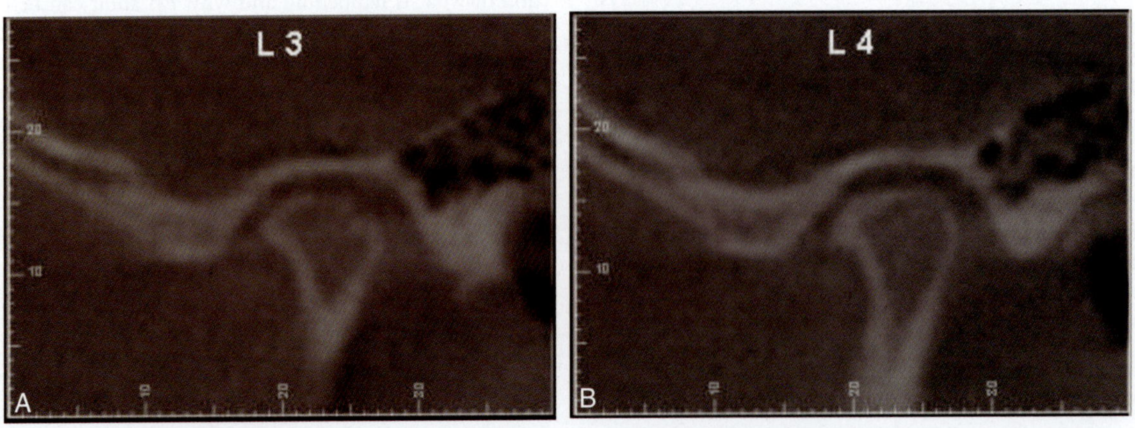

• **Fig. 20.28** Pathologic changes in the condylar head, as seen in cone beam computed tomography (CBCT) images from a large field-of-view scan. (A) Note the erosion of the distal surface of the condylar head and (B) the lipping of the anterior surface in the adjacent slice.

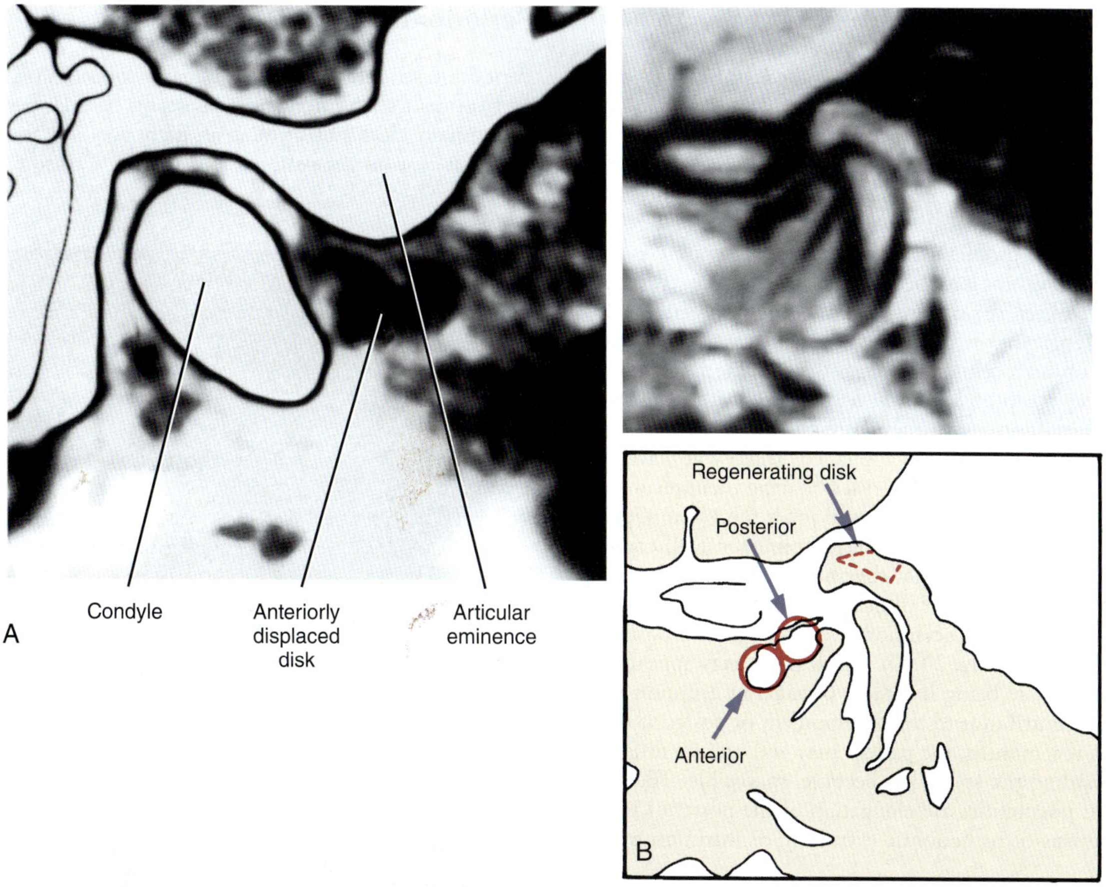

• **Fig. 20.29** Hard and soft tissue imaging of disk displacement in the temporomandibular joint. (A) Computed tomography view of a displaced mandibular disk, which can be visualized (as a darker area) in front of the condyle. (B) Magnetic resonance imaging (MRI) view of a displaced disk, with the anterior and posterior bands indicated on the adjacent sketch. There is evidence on this scan of a regenerating disk, as shown in the dashed area. MRI scans have largely replaced radiographic views for the diagnosis of disk displacement because the soft tissues can be seen more clearly and no ionizing radiation is required; cone beam computed tomography is preferred for visualization of bony changes.

individuals respond to stress, both in the organ system that feels the strain (many problems besides TMD are related to stress) and in the amount of stress that can be tolerated before symptoms appear (tense individuals develop stress-related symptoms before their relaxed colleagues do). For this reason, it is impossible to say that occlusal discrepancies of any given degree will lead to TMD symptoms, although recent multicenter research has at least clarified the possibilities.[17]

It is possible to demonstrate that some types of occlusal discrepancies predispose patients who clench or grind their teeth to the development of TMD symptoms. It must be kept in mind, however, that it takes two factors to produce myofascial pain: an occlusal discrepancy *and* a patient who clenches or grinds the teeth. Perhaps the most compelling argument against malocclusion as a primary cause of TMD is the observation that TMD is no more prevalent in patients with severe malocclusion than in the general population.[18] The dictum "let your teeth alone" would solve myofascial pain problems if it could be followed by the patient.

Treatment Indications

From this perspective, three broad approaches to myofascial pain symptoms can be considered: reducing the amount of stress; reducing the patients' reactions to stress; or improving the occlusion, thereby making it harder for patients to hurt themselves. Drastic alteration of the occlusion, by either restorative dental procedures or orthodontics, is logical only if the less invasive stress-control and stress-adaptation approaches have failed. In that circumstance, orthodontic treatment to alter the occlusion so that the patient can better tolerate parafunctional activity may be worth attempting. In some instances, this may involve orthognathic surgery to reposition the jaws.

The extent to which TMD symptoms in many adults disappear when comprehensive orthodontic treatment begins can be surprising and overly gratifying to those who do not understand the etiology of myofascial pain. Orthodontic intervention can appear almost magical in the way that TMD symptoms disappear long before the occlusal relationships have been corrected. The explanation is simple—orthodontic treatment makes the teeth sore, so grinding or clenching sensitive teeth as a means of handling stress does not produce the same subconscious gratification as previously. Then the parafunctional activity stops, and the symptoms vanish.

The changing occlusal relationships also contribute to breaking up the habit patterns that contributed to the muscle fatigue and pain. No matter what the type of orthodontic treatment, as long as treatment that produces strongly deflective contacts is avoided, symptoms are unlikely to be present while movement of a significant number of teeth is occurring. Prolonged use of Class II or Class III elastics may not be well tolerated in adults who have had TMD problems and should be avoided (for that matter, prolonged use of elastics should be avoided in most other adult patients as well).

The moment of truth for TMD patients who have had orthodontic treatment comes sometime after the orthodontic treatment is completed, when the clenching and grinding that originally caused the problem tend to recur. At that point, even if the occlusal relationships have been significantly improved, it may be impossible to keep the patient from moving into extreme jaw positions and engaging in parafunctional activity that produces pain. The use of interocclusal splints in this situation may be the only way to keep symptoms from recurring. In short, the miraculous cure that orthodontic treatment often provides for myofascial pain tends to disappear with the appliance. Those who have had symptoms in the past are always at risk of having them recur.

Occasionally, orthodontic treatment is made more complicated by previous splint therapy. If an occlusal splint for TMD symptoms covers the posterior but not the anterior teeth, the anterior teeth that have been taken out of occlusion begin to erupt again and may come back into occlusion even though the posterior teeth are still separated (Fig. 20.30). Clinically, it may appear that the posterior teeth are being intruded, but incisor eruption usually is a greater contributor to the development of posterior open bite. In only a few months, the patient may end up in a situation in which discarding the splint has become impossible. Then the only treatment possibilities are elongation of the posterior teeth, either with crowns or orthodontic extrusion, or intrusion of the anterior teeth.

Orthodontic intervention at this stage is difficult because TMD symptoms are likely to develop immediately if the splint is removed, and it is not possible to elongate the posterior teeth orthodontically without discarding or cutting down the splint. Placing orthodontic attachments on the posterior teeth and using light vertical elastics to the posterior segments is a method that can be used to bring the posterior teeth back into occlusion (Fig. 20.31) if the patient can tolerate this treatment. Some re-intrusion of the elongated anterior teeth is likely to occur, but a significant increase in face height is often maintained. This should be considered an unfortunate side effect, not something that might be beneficial.

Periodontal Considerations

Periodontal problems are rarely a major concern during orthodontic treatment of children and adolescents because periodontal disease usually does not arise at an early age and tissue resistance is higher in younger patients. For the same reasons, periodontal

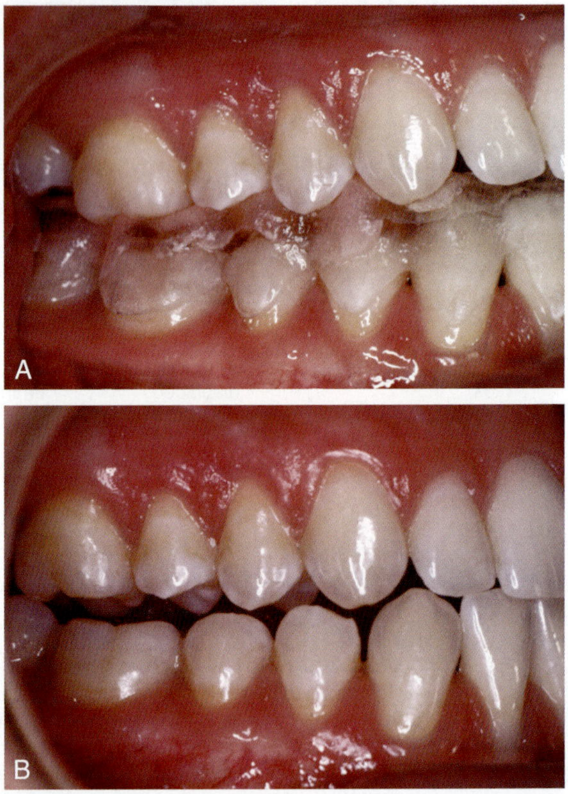

• **Fig. 20.30** (A) Occlusal relationships in a 24-year-old female who had worn a splint covering only her posterior teeth for the previous 18 months. (B) Note the posterior open bite when the splint was taken out. This was created by a combination of intrusion of the posterior teeth and further eruption of the anterior teeth. Orthodontic treatment to bring the posterior teeth back into occlusion required tranquilizers during treatment because she was uncomfortable without the splint until occlusion was reestablished.

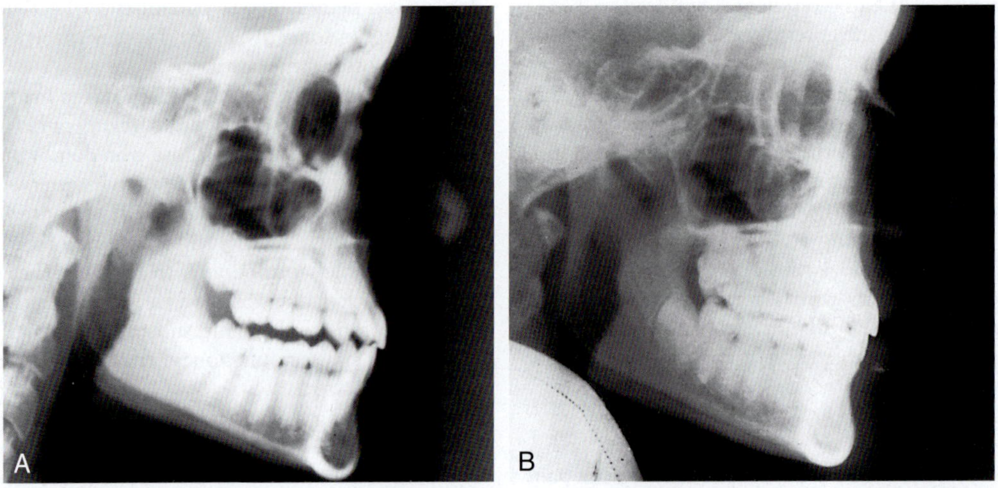

• **Fig. 20.31** Cephalometric radiographs for the patient shown in Fig. 20.30. Before (A) and after (B) orthodontic treatment to extrude the posterior teeth back into occlusion.

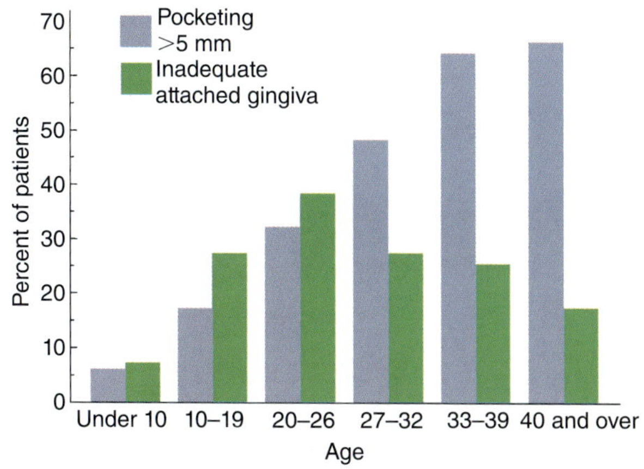

• **Fig. 20.32** The prevalence of periodontal pockets of 5 mm or more and prevalence of inadequate attached gingiva as a function of age in 1000 consecutive patients with severe orthodontic problems who were referred for possible surgical-orthodontic treatment. (Redrawn from Moriarty JD, Simpson DM. J *Dent Res*. 1984;63(Special Issue A):1249].)

considerations are increasingly important as patients become older, regardless of whether periodontal problems were a motivating factor for orthodontic treatment.

The prevalence of periodontal disease as a function of age in a large group of potential orthodontic patients with severe malocclusion is shown in Fig. 20.32. Note that up to the late 30 s, there is nearly a straight-line relationship between age and periodontal pocketing (defined here as the presence of pockets of 5 mm or more). In contrast, the prevalence of mucogingival problems peaks in the 20s. The odds are that any patient over the age of 35 has some periodontal problems that could affect orthodontic treatment, and mucogingival considerations are important in treatment of the younger adult group.

Periodontal disease is not a continuous and steadily progressive degenerative process. Instead, it is characterized by episodes of acute attack on some but usually not all areas of the mouth, followed by quiescent periods. It is obviously important to identify high-risk patients and high-risk sites. The best indicator that disease may be present is a history of disease. At present, persistent bleeding on gentle probing is the best indicator of active and presumably progressive disease, which is why it is important for the orthodontist to probe carefully during an orthodontic clinical examination. New diagnostic procedures to evaluate subgingival plaque and crevicular fluids for the presence of indicator bacteria, enzymes, or other chemical mediators now are clinically useful. These are likely to be used on potential orthodontic patients referred for further periodontal evaluation. There appear to be at least three risk groups in the population for progression of periodontal bone loss: those with rapid progression (about 10%), those with moderate progression (the great majority, about 80%), and those with no progression (about 10%).[19]

There is no contraindication to treating adults who have had periodontal disease and bone loss, as long as the disease has been brought under control (Fig. 20.33). Progression of untreated periodontal breakdown must be anticipated, however, and the patient's periodontal situation must receive major attention in planning and executing orthodontic treatment for adults.

Treatment of Patients With Minimal Periodontal Involvement

Any patient undergoing orthodontic treatment must take extra care to clean the teeth, but this is even more important in adult orthodontics. Bacterial plaque is the main etiologic factor in periodontal breakdown, and its effect is largely determined by the host response. Orthodontic appliances simultaneously make maintenance of oral hygiene more difficult and more important. In children and adolescents, even if gingivitis develops in response to the presence of orthodontic appliances, it almost never extends into periodontitis. This cannot be taken for granted in adults, no matter how good their initial periodontal condition.

The periodontal evaluation of a potential adult orthodontic patient must include not only the response to periodontal probing but also the level and condition of the attached gingiva. Labial movement of incisors in some patients can be followed by gingival recession and loss of attachment. The risk is greatest when irregular teeth are aligned by expanding the dental arch, which stresses and thins the gingiva, adding to the stress that might be created by gingival inflammation or toothbrush trauma. Once recession begins, it can progress rapidly, especially if there is little or no keratinized attached gingiva and the attachment is only alveolar mucosa.

It was once thought that the width of the gingival attachment was the major factor in whether recession occurred. The concept now is that two characteristics are important: the width of the attached gingiva (not all keratinized gingiva is attached) and the thickness of the gingival tissue. The width of the attached gingiva can be observed most readily by inserting a periodontal probe and observing the distance between the point at which the gingival attachment is encountered and the point at which the alveolar mucosa begins. Lingually tipped lower incisors in patients with a prominent chin have a high risk of recession, and thin gingival tissue probably is the reason.

For adult orthodontic patients, it is much better to prevent gingival recession than to try to correct it later. For this reason, a gingival graft (Fig. 20.34) must be considered in adults with minimal attached gingiva or thin tissue, particularly those for whom arch expansion will be used to align incisors and those who will have surgical mandibular advancement or genioplasty (see Chapter 22).

Moderate Periodontal Involvement

Before orthodontic treatment is attempted for patients who have preexisting periodontal problems, dental and periodontal disease must be brought under control. Preliminary therapy can include all aspects of periodontal treatment. It is important to remove all calculus and other irritants from periodontal pockets before any tooth movement is attempted, and it is often wise to use surgical flaps to expose these areas to ensure the best possible scaling. Is a bone graft slurry indicated to prevent bone dehiscence and gingival recession when significant arch expansion is planned for an adult? Data to indicate the point at which that might make a significant difference are lacking.

Treatment procedures to facilitate the patient's long-term maintenance, such as osseous recontouring or repositioned flaps to compensate for areas of gingival recession, are best deferred until the final occlusal relationships have been established. A period of observation following preliminary periodontal treatment to make sure that the patient's disease is adequately controlled and to allow healing after the periodontal therapy should precede comprehensive orthodontics.

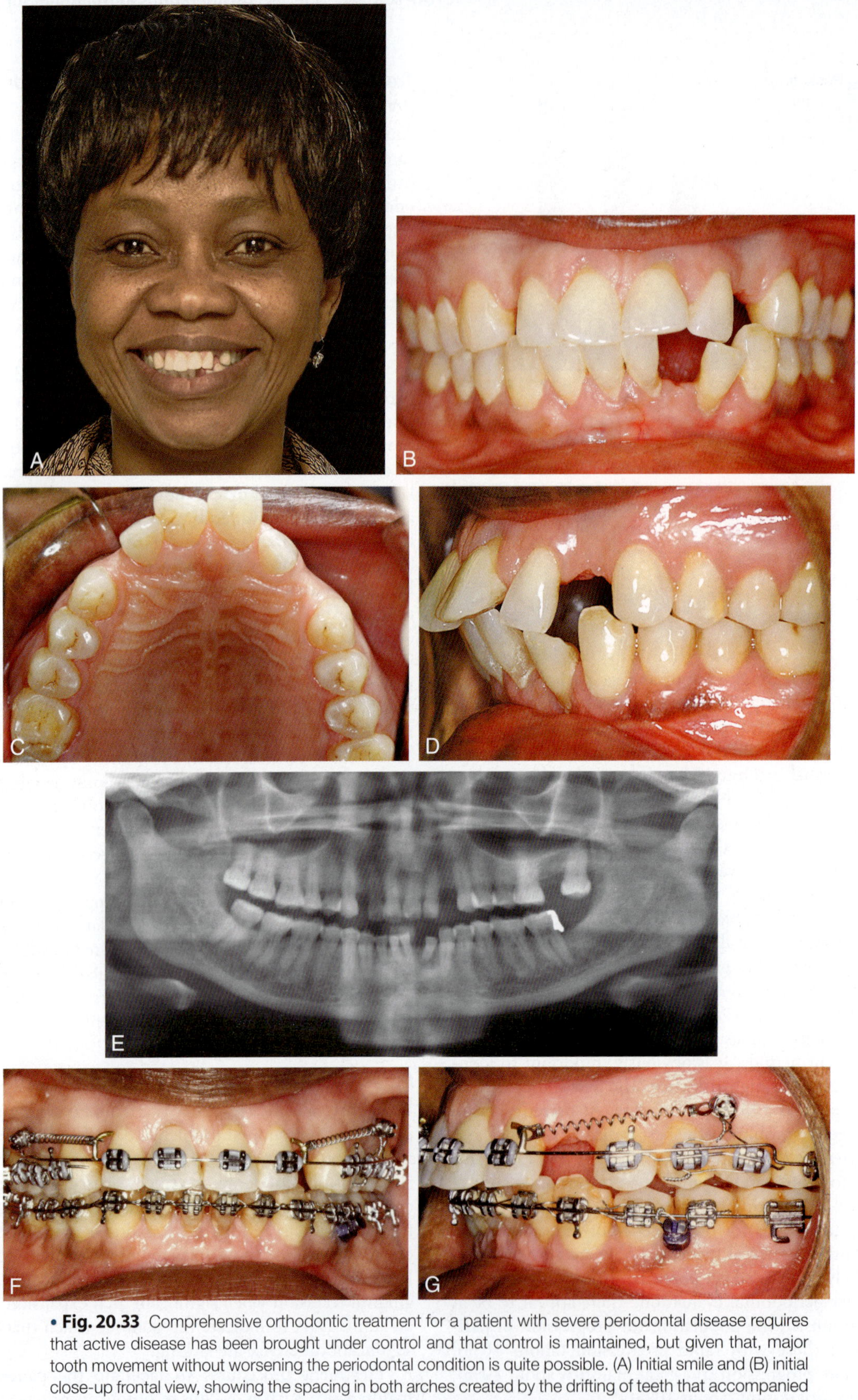

• **Fig. 20.33** Comprehensive orthodontic treatment for a patient with severe periodontal disease requires that active disease has been brought under control and that control is maintained, but given that, major tooth movement without worsening the periodontal condition is quite possible. (A) Initial smile and (B) initial close-up frontal view, showing the spacing in both arches created by the drifting of teeth that accompanied her severe periodontal problems. (C and D) Occlusal and lateral intraoral views before treatment. (E) Initial panoramic radiograph. She had moderately severe generalized periodontal disease with localized severe bone loss. After the periodontal disease was brought under control, she sought treatment to retract her protruding incisors and close the anterior spaces in both arches. The plan was to use skeletal anchorage (alveolar bone screws) in both arches to retract the incisors while maintaining normal overbite. Closure of the old maxillary left second molar extraction space was judged to be more than could be managed even with skeletal anchorage without compromising the symmetry of the anterior segment.

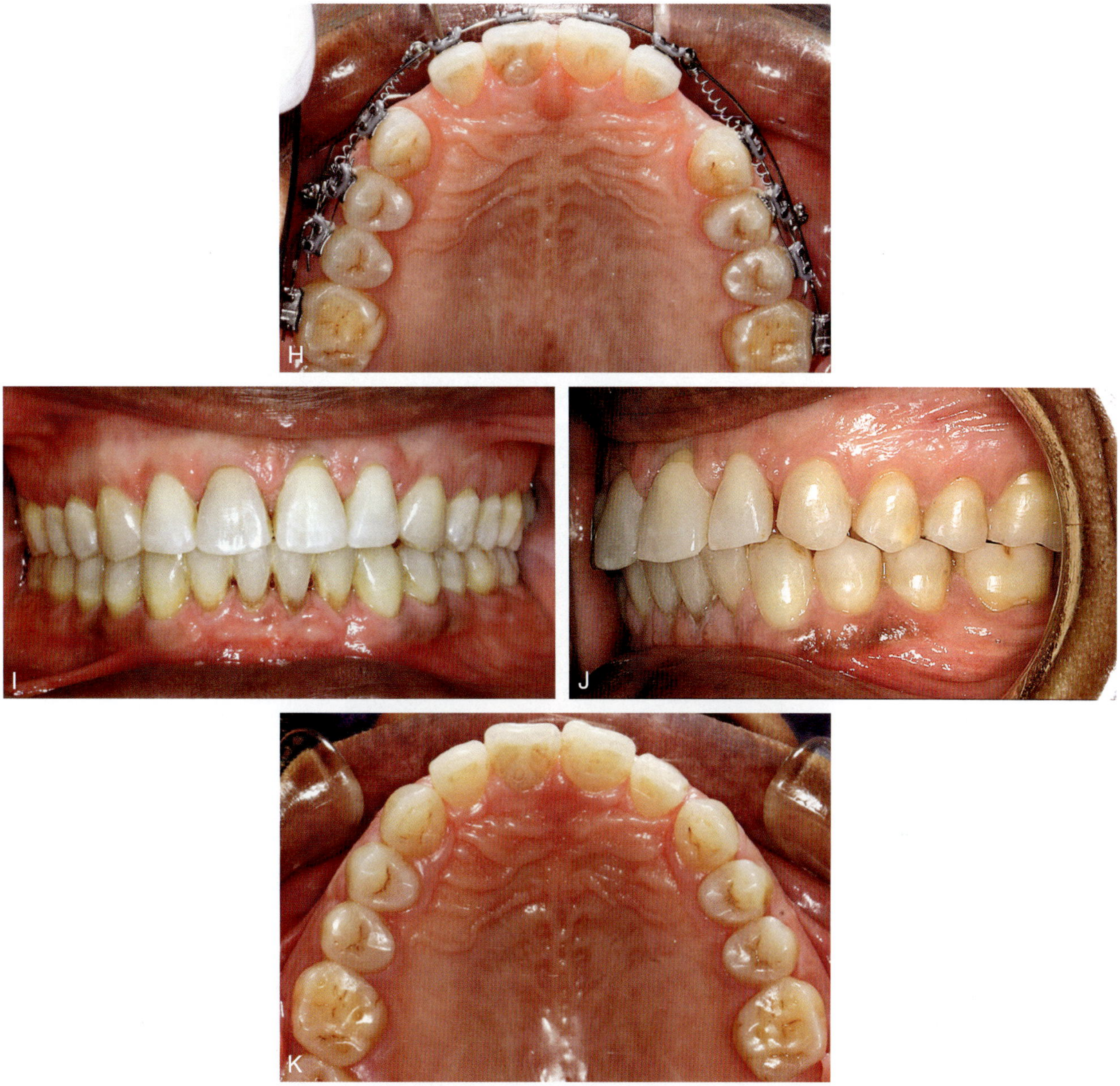

• Fig. 20.33, cont'd (F and G) Austenitic nickel-titanium (A-NiTi) coil springs and sliding mechanics were used for space closure in both arches, with screws placed between the first and second premolars in both arches. Note the combination of direct and indirect anchorage in the maxillary arch. (H) Occlusal view of temporary anchorage device (TAD)–supported space closure in the maxillary arch. (I–K) Age 58, after completion of orthodontic treatment that required 35 months. Note the improvement in dental alignment and occlusion, and the maintenance of her periodontal health.

Disease control also requires endodontic treatment of any pulpally involved teeth. There is no contraindication to the orthodontic movement of an endodontically treated tooth, so root canal therapy before orthodontics will cause no problems. Attempting to move a pulpally involved tooth, however, is likely to cause a flare-up of pulpitis and pain.

The general guideline for preliminary restorative treatment is that temporary restorations should be placed to control caries, with the definitive restorative dentistry delayed until after the orthodontic phase of treatment. Temporary restoration, however, should not be taken to mean the use of a short-lived material that will last only a few months. Composite resin is now the preferred temporary restorative material while orthodontics is being carried out. Cast restorations should be delayed until after the final occlusal relationships have been established.

Because the margins of bands can make periodontal maintenance more difficult, it is better to use a fully bonded orthodontic appliance for periodontally involved adults. Self-ligating brackets or steel ligatures are preferred for patients with periodontal

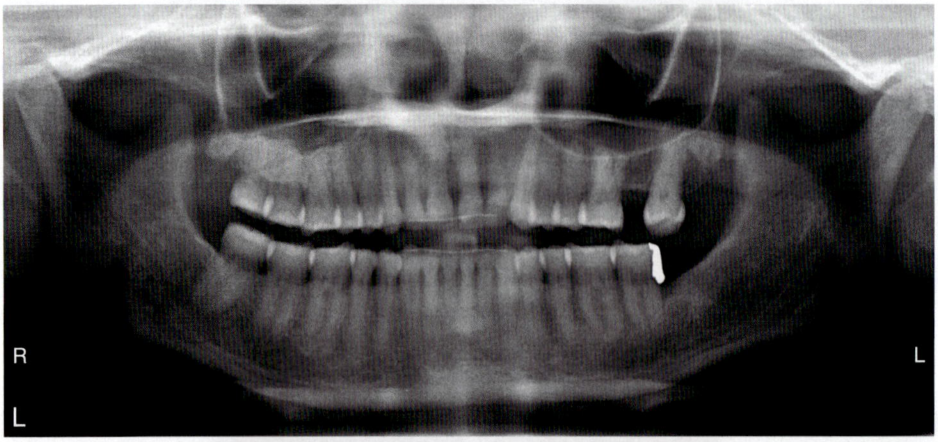

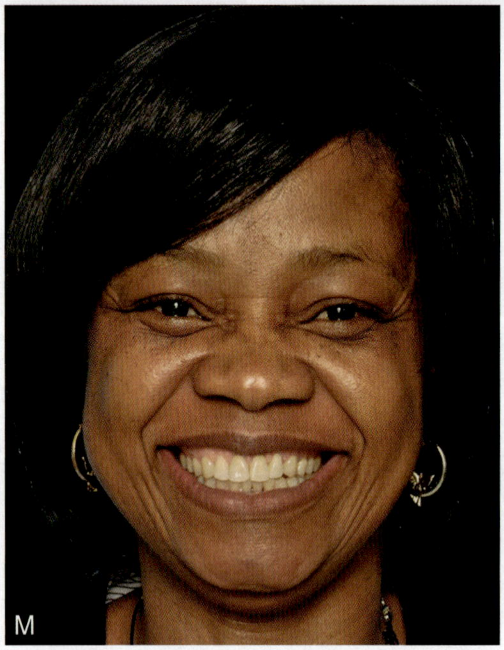

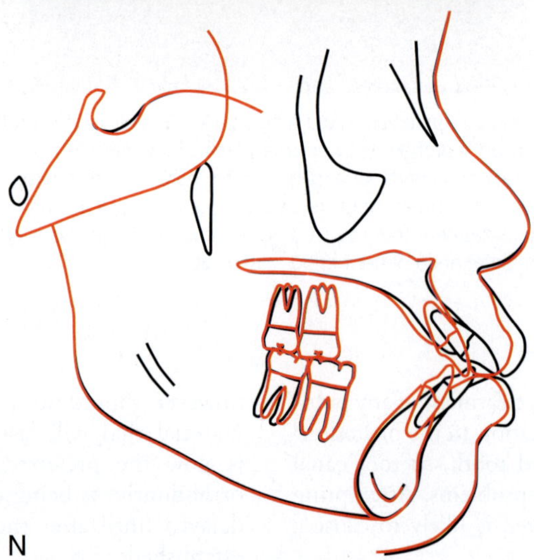

N

• **Fig. 20.33, cont'd** (L) Posttreatment panoramic radiograph. The overhang on the distal of the lower left first molar was removed during later restorative dentistry. (M) Posttreatment smile. (N) Cephalometric superimposition showing the major retraction of the incisors with no forward movement of the posterior teeth. (Courtesy Dr. D. Grauer.)

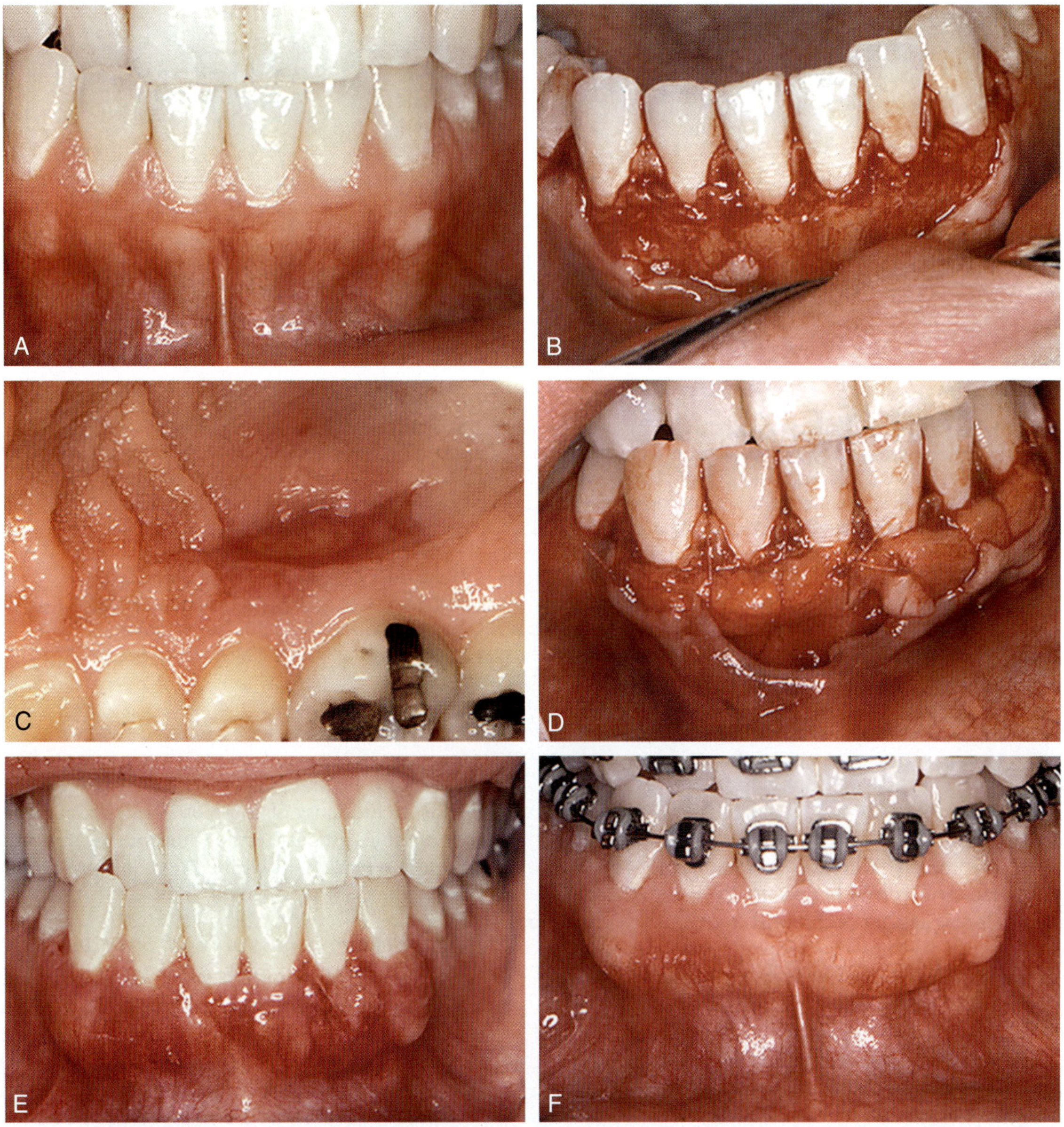

• **Fig. 20.34** In adults who will undergo comprehensive orthodontic treatment, gingival grafting to create adequate quantity and thickness of attached gingiva is important before orthodontic tooth movement is begun. (A) Lack of attached gingiva and thin gingival tissue in the mandibular anterior region in a patient whose lower incisors must be advanced to align them. Note the alveolar mucosa extending almost to the gingival margin on all anterior teeth. (B) Surgical preparation of a bed for grafting. (C) The palatal donor site for tissue for the gingival graft. (D) The graft sutured in place. (E) Healing 1 week later, showing incorporation of the grafts. (F) Initial alignment archwire in place 3 months later, with the gingival grafts creating both a thicker contour of the gingival tissue and a generous band of attachment. (Courtesy Dr. J. Moriarty.)

involvement, rather than elastomeric rings to retain orthodontic archwires, because patients with elastomeric rings have higher levels of microorganisms in gingival plaque.[20]

During comprehensive orthodontics, a patient with moderate periodontal problems must be on a maintenance schedule, with the frequency of cleaning and scaling depending on the severity of the periodontal disease. Periodontal maintenance therapy at 2- to 4-month intervals is the usual plan. Adjunctive chemical agents between appointments (including chlorhexidine if needed) also should be considered.

Severe Periodontal Involvement

The general approach to treatment for patients with severe periodontal involvement is the same as that outlined earlier, but the treatment itself must be modified in two ways: (1) periodontal maintenance should be scheduled at more frequent intervals, perhaps with the patient being seen as frequently for periodontal maintenance as for orthodontic appliance adjustments (i.e., every 4–6 weeks) and (2) orthodontic treatment goals and mechanics must be modified to keep orthodontic forces to an absolute minimum

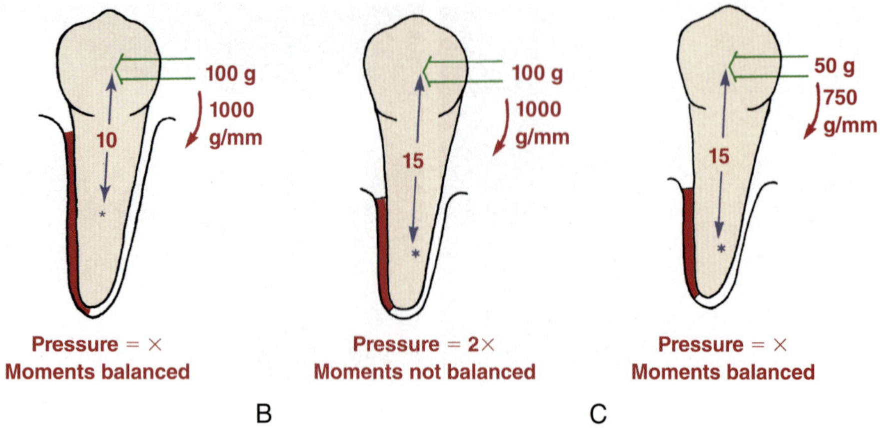

• **Fig. 20.35** Bone loss around a tooth that is to be moved affects both the force and the moment needed. (A) For optimum bodily movement of a premolar whose center of resistance is 10 mm apical to the bracket (i.e., normal height of alveolar bone support), a 100-gm force and a 1000 g-mm moment are needed. (B) The same force system would be inappropriate for an identical premolar whose bone support had been reduced by periodontal disease such that the periodontal ligament (PDL) area is half as large as it was originally, and the center of resistance is now 15 mm apical to the bracket. For such a tooth, the 100-g force would produce 1500 g-mm moment on a smaller PDL area with approximately twice the optimal pressure in the PDL, and the moment would not be large enough to prevent tipping. (C) The correct force system for the periodontally involved tooth would be a 50-g force and a 15 × 50 = 750 g-mm moment. Orthodontic movement of periodontally involved teeth can be done only with careful attention to forces (smaller than normal) and moments (relatively larger than normal).

because the reduced area of the PDL after significant bone loss means higher pressure in the PDL from any force (Fig. 20.35). Sometimes it is helpful to temporarily retain a tooth that is hopelessly involved periodontally, using it to help support an orthodontic appliance that will contribute to saving other teeth.

The crown-root ratio is a significant factor in the long-term prognosis for a tooth that has sustained periodontal bone loss. Shortening the crown has the virtue of improving the crown-root ratio. In adults with bone loss and an anterior deep bite, the orthodontist should not hesitate to remove part of the crown of elongated lower incisors as an alternative to intrusion, when this would both simplify orthodontic leveling of the arch and improve the periodontal prognosis. Reducing crown height of upper incisors must be approached cautiously because of the possible adverse effect on anterior tooth display, and often intrusion of abraded incisors so that the crown can be restored to normal height is a better approach.[21] It is interesting that even after severe periodontal problems have developed, orthodontic treatment can be carried out without further loss of alveolar bone *if* good control of the periodontal condition is maintained. Space closure in areas of major bone loss sometimes leads to an improvement in bone height if at least one wall of the periodontal pocket remains (Fig. 20.36). As part of informed consent, patients like this can be told that they can have comprehensive orthodontic treatment without undue risk of making their periodontal situation worse, but they should not be promised an improvement.

Prosthodontic-Implant Interactions

Adults seeking comprehensive orthodontic treatment often also have dental problems that require restorations. Such problems include loss of tooth structure from wear and abrasion or trauma, gingival esthetic problems, and missing teeth that require replacement with either conventional prosthodontics or implants.

Problems Related to Loss of Tooth Structure

The positioning of damaged, worn, or abraded teeth during comprehensive orthodontics must be done with the eventual restorative plan in mind. Early consultation with the restorative dentist obviously becomes important. There are four important considerations in deciding where the orthodontist should position teeth that are to be restored: the total amount of space that should be created, the mesiodistal positioning of the tooth within the space, the buccolingual positioning, and the vertical positioning. It is important to determine in advance whether the orthodontic goal is to level the incisal edges and marginal ridges, the gingival margins and contours, and/or the bone levels.

When tooth structure has been lost all the way beyond the normal contact point, the tooth becomes abnormally narrow, and restoration of the lost crown width, as well as height, is important. The orthodontic positioning must provide adequate space for the appropriate addition of the restorative material. The ideal position may or may not be in the center of the space mesiodistally; this would depend on whether the most esthetic restoration would be produced by symmetric addition on each side of the tooth or whether a larger buildup on one side would be better.

Similarly, the ideal buccolingual position of a worn or damaged maxillary tooth would be influenced by how the restoration was planned. If crowns are planned, the tooth should be in the center of the dental arch without tight contact with the opposing arch. But if a facial veneer is to be used for an incisor

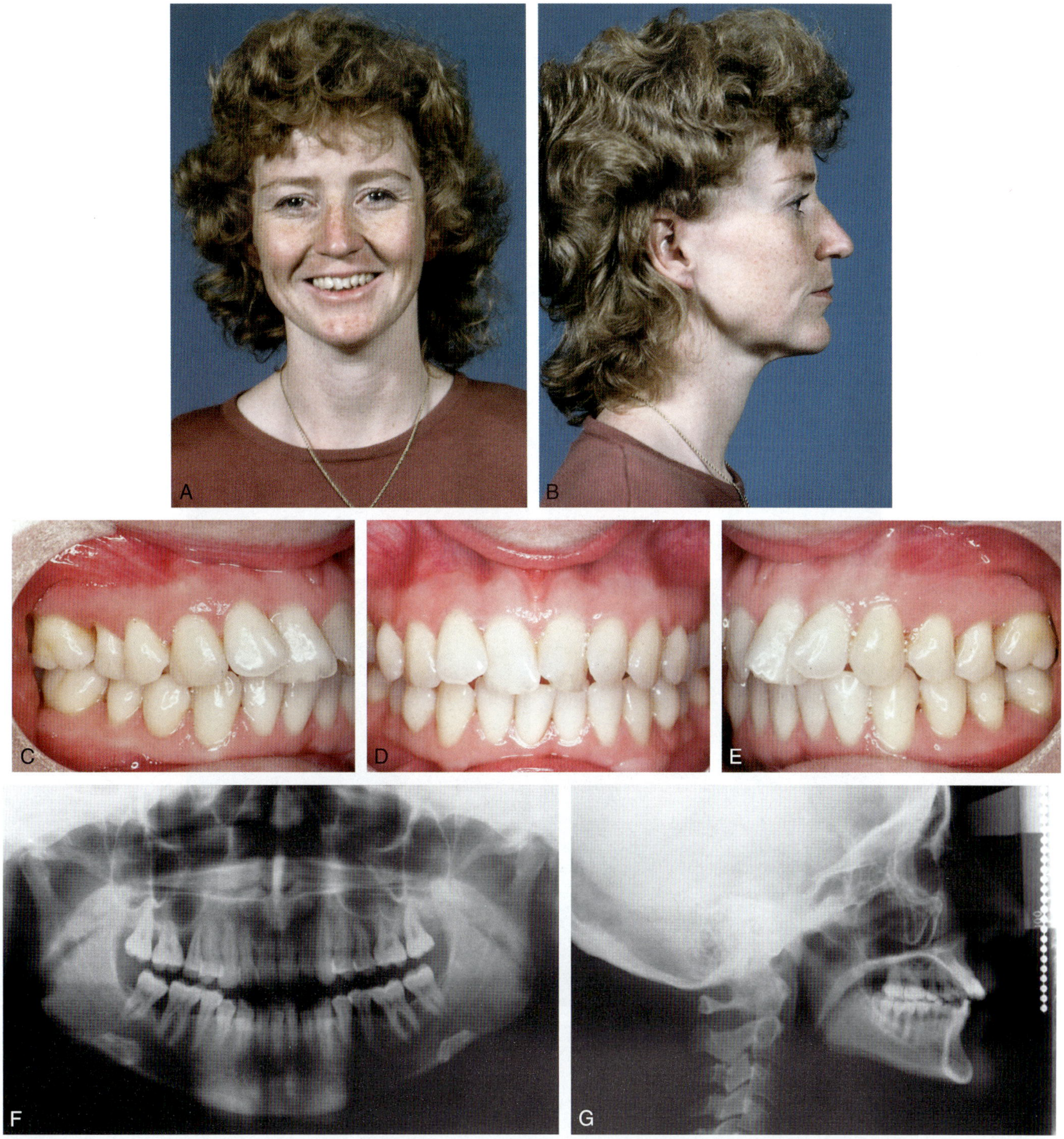

• **Fig. 20.36** (A–E) At age 27, this female sought orthodontic treatment because her periodontist thought that her periodontal disease could be controlled better if the alignment of her teeth were improved, and because she had never liked the appearance of her extremely crowded and irregular maxillary incisors. There was a full-cusp Class II molar relationship and minimal overbite. (F) The panoramic radiograph showed severe bone loss in multiple areas, but active disease was now under control. (G) The cephalometric radiograph showed a mild skeletal Class II jaw relationship, with moderate maxillary incisor protrusion. The treatment plan called for extraction of the maxillary left first premolar and the right second premolar (chosen because of the large periodontal defect distal to it, although this would make the orthodontic treatment more difficult). The extraction space, plus reduction of interproximal enamel to compensate for the tooth-size discrepancy created by the very large maxillary lateral incisors, would allow for alignment of the upper teeth without creating incisor protrusion.

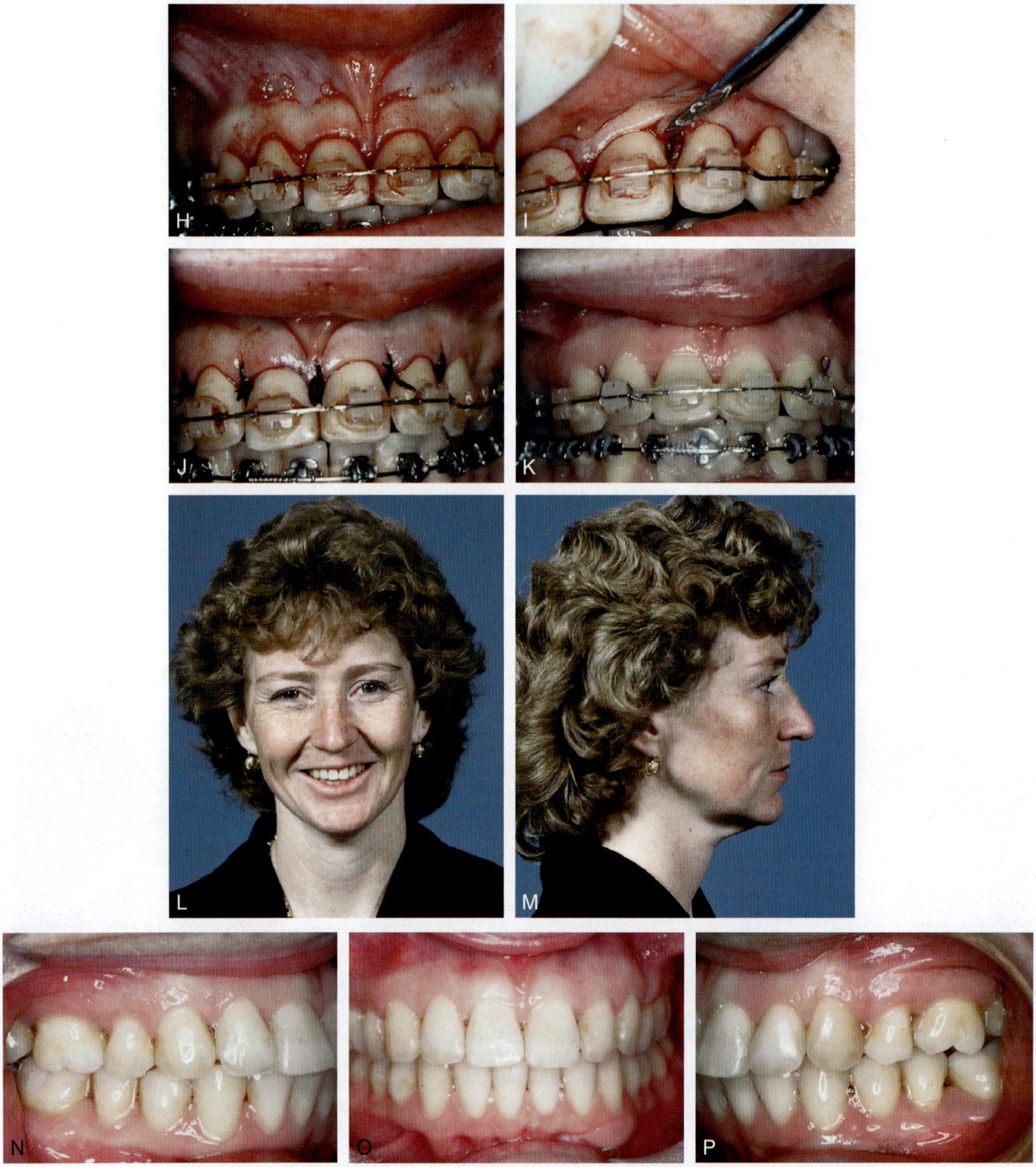

• **Fig. 20.36, cont'd** (H–J) Because of the severe rotations of the irregular maxillary incisors, after alignment was completed but with the orthodontic appliance still in place, repositioning of the maxillary frenum and sectioning of the elastic gingival fibers were carried out. (K) Three weeks later. (L–P) After 18 months of treatment, both the occlusion and the appearance of the teeth were greatly improved.

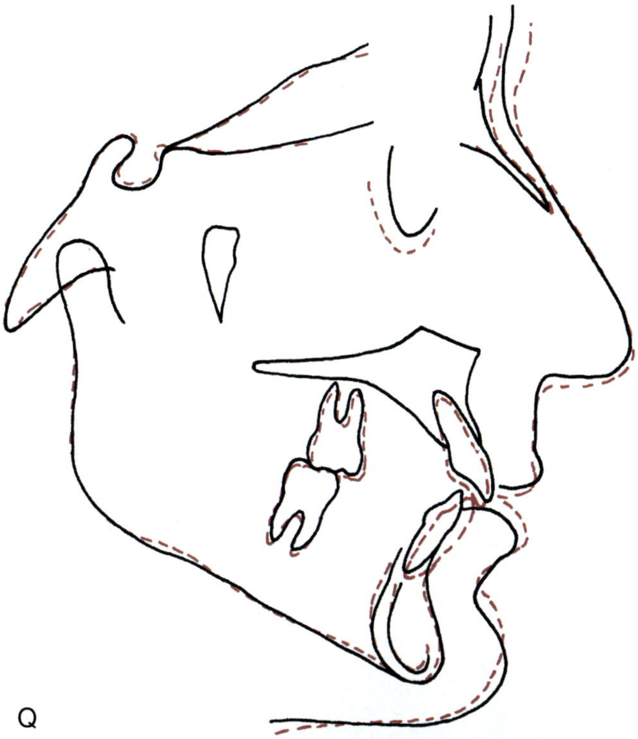

Q

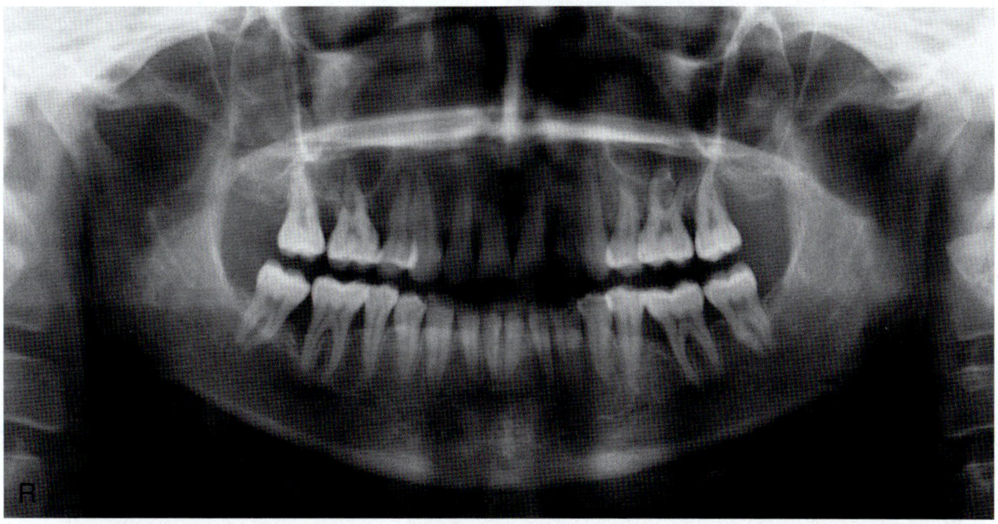

R

• **Fig. 20.36, cont'd** (Q) Cephalometric superimposition shows slight retraction of the maxillary incisors and mild proclination of the mandibular incisors, as was desired in this case. (R) Panoramic radiograph 1 year after the orthodontic treatment was completed. The periodontal condition remained under good control during and after the orthodontic treatment. Note the fill-in of alveolar bone in the area where the severely affected maxillary right second premolar was extracted. The periodontal defects remain in the lower arch but did not get worse during the extensive orthodontic treatment. (Periodontal surgery by Dr. R. Williams.)

or canine (Fig. 20.37), the orthodontist should place the tooth more lingually than otherwise would be the case, in contact with its antagonist in the lower arch, to accommodate the thickness of the veneer on the facial surface. Finally, better restorations can be done if the orthodontist provides slightly more space than is required, so there is room for the restorative dentist to finish and polish proximal surfaces. The slight excess space can then be closed with a retainer.

If only a small amount of tooth structure has been lost—for instance, if the incisal edge of one incisor has been fractured—it may be possible to smooth the fractured area and elongate the damaged tooth so that the incisal edges line up. The result, however,

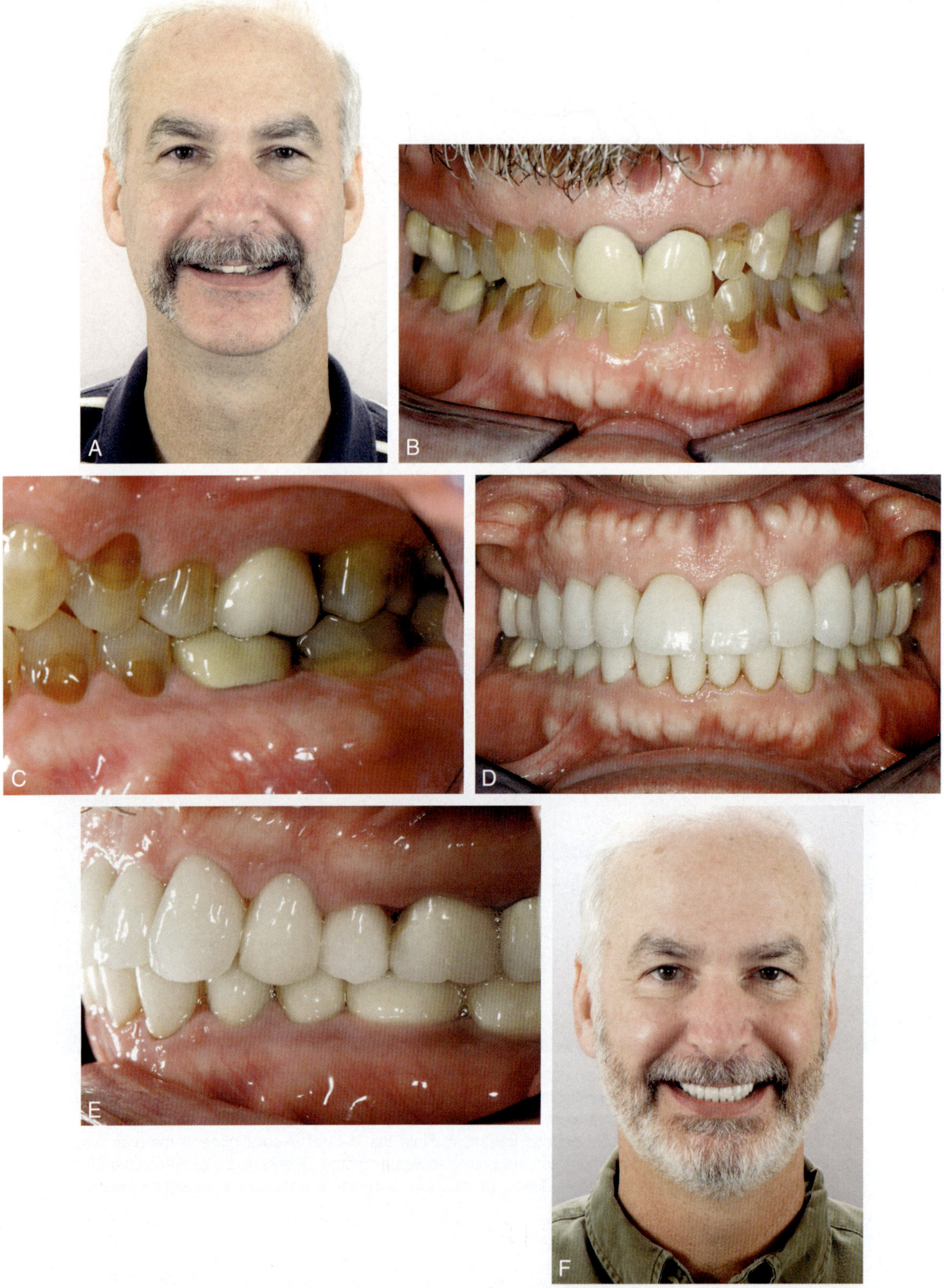

• **Fig. 20.37** (A) This 49-year-old male sought treatment to improve the appearance of his teeth, which were badly worn and stained. He was careful to minimize the display of his incisors on smile. (B) Crowns had been placed on the maxillary central incisors, but they were too short for their width. (C) The other teeth in both arches were badly worn and stained. The treatment plan was to align the teeth, opening some space to facilitate buildups and laminates. (D–F) Age 51, after treatment, with crowns and laminates for correction of the wear and staining that were placed after the end of active orthodontic treatment. The posttreatment smile, with as much display of lower as upper teeth, is appropriate for his age, although slightly longer restorations for the upper incisors would have been better. The patient chose to have the crowns and laminates made whiter than was consistent with his age, and obviously valued the contrast with his previous condition.

will be uneven gingival margins, which means that elongation of a fractured tooth must be done with caution and with consideration of the extent to which the gingival margins are exposed when the patient smiles. Before acceptably esthetic composite resin build-ups of anterior teeth were available, orthodontic elongation of fractured teeth was a more acceptable treatment approach than it is at present. Now, more than 1 to 2 mm of elongation rarely is a good plan unless the patient never exposes the gingiva.

Gingival Esthetic Problems

Gingival esthetic problems fall into two categories: those created by excessive and/or uneven display of gingiva and those created by gingival recession after periodontal bone loss.

The importance of maintaining a reasonably even gingival margin in the maxillary incisor area, especially when patients show the gingiva when they smile, is a factor in deciding on the best treatment when one lateral incisor is missing. Substituting a canine on one side will result in uneven gingival margins unless great care is taken to extrude the canine and reduce its crown height, even if the crown of the substituted canine is recontoured. If several teeth have been worn or fractured, extruding them can create an unesthetic "gummy smile" even if the gingival margins are kept at the same level across all the teeth. In that circumstance, it would be better to intrude the incisors to obtain a proper gingival exposure and then restore the lost crown height.

Dental esthetics are not just the teeth. A particularly distressing problem is created by gingival recession after periodontal bone loss in the maxillary incisor region, which creates "black triangles" between these teeth (see Fig. 6.44). The best approach to this problem is to remove some interproximal enamel so that the incisors can be brought closer together. This moves the contact points more gingivally, minimizing the open space between the teeth. The more bulbous the crowns were initially, the more successful this approach can be.

Missing Teeth: Space Closure Versus Prosthetic Replacement

Old Extraction Sites

In adults, closing an old extraction site is likely to be difficult. The problem arises because of resorption and remodeling of alveolar bone. After several years, resorption results in a decrease in the vertical height of the bone, but more important, remodeling produces a buccolingual narrowing of the alveolar process as well. When this has happened, closing the extraction space requires a reshaping of the cortical bone that comprises the buccal and lingual plates of the alveolar process. Cortical bone will respond to orthodontic force in most instances, but the response is significantly slower.

Closing an old mandibular first molar extraction site is very difficult, because mesial drift of the second and third molars and distal drift of premolars have partially closed it, and the molars have tipped mesially. In adjunctive treatment, as shown earlier (see Figs. 20.6 and 20.7), a mesially tipped second molar usually is uprighted by tipping it distally, and then an implant or bridge is placed. If comprehensive treatment is planned, should the space be closed by bringing the first molar mesially? This depends very much on the specific problems of an individual patient. Often, it is better judgment to open a partially closed old extraction site and replace the missing tooth. This decision should be considered carefully in consultation between the orthodontist and prosthodontist.

Panoramic radiographs of two patients with similar spacing in the lower arch after early loss of mandibular first molars—one who had distal tipping for bilateral uprighting of second and third molars, and the other who had bilateral space closure with mesial root movement—are shown in Figs. 20.38 and 20.39. Both had comprehensive treatment with the use of alveolar bone screws as anchorage. For the patient with space opening, the factor that determined treatment time was other aspects of the malocclusion; for the one with space closure, the long treatment time was primarily determined by the slow remodeling of cortical bone in the old extraction site.

Tooth Loss Due to Periodontal Disease

A space closure problem is also posed by the loss of a tooth to periodontal disease. Sometimes, closure of the space where a hopelessly involved tooth was extracted results in an improvement of the periodontal situation (see Fig. 20.36). Unless at least one bony wall remains, however, it is better to move teeth away from such an area in preparation for a prosthetic replacement, because normal bone formation cannot be expected as the tooth moves into the defect.

However, there is an exception. First molars and incisors are lost in some adolescents and young adults to aggressive juvenile periodontitis, which differentially attacks these teeth and is characterized by high levels of a specific microbe, *Aggregatibacter actinomycetemcomitans*. This problem is rare, but it is estimated to occur up to three times more frequently in African-American children, and in a sequence of cases detected in one county in Florida, all 60 children were black.[22] In the etiology of the disease, both immune and inflammatory responses to the bacteria in the gingival sulcus are important, and it appears that some bacteria may play a protective role. Once the disease process has been brought under control, which now typically involves antibiotic therapy, the causative agent largely disappears and the disease rarely recurs. Although bone around the first molars often is completely destroyed, neither the second molar nor the second premolar is significantly affected in most patients.

Orthodontic closure of the incisor spaces is rarely feasible because of loss of bone created by the disease, but in adolescent or young adult patients who lost first molars to aggressive local periodontitis, it often is possible to orthodontically close the extraction sites, bringing the second permanent molar forward into the area where the first molar was lost. Usually this does not require bone screws or implants for additional anchorage. The second molar brings its own investing bone with it, and the large bony defect disappears.

This favorable response is attributed to some combination of three factors: the relatively young patients, the fact that the original attack was almost entirely on the first molars, and the change in the bacterial flora. In an older patient who lost a first molar to periodontal disease, it is unlikely that the other teeth have been totally spared or that the bacterial flora have changed, and it would not be good judgment to attempt to close the space.

Comprehensive Orthodontics in Patients in Whom Implants Are Planned

In older patients with long-standing tooth loss, bone grafts often are necessary to widen the alveolar process where a future implant will be required. Usually, it is advantageous to go ahead with placement of grafts in areas that will receive implants while orthodontic treatment is being carried out in other areas of the mouth. The goal should be to have the patient ready for definitive

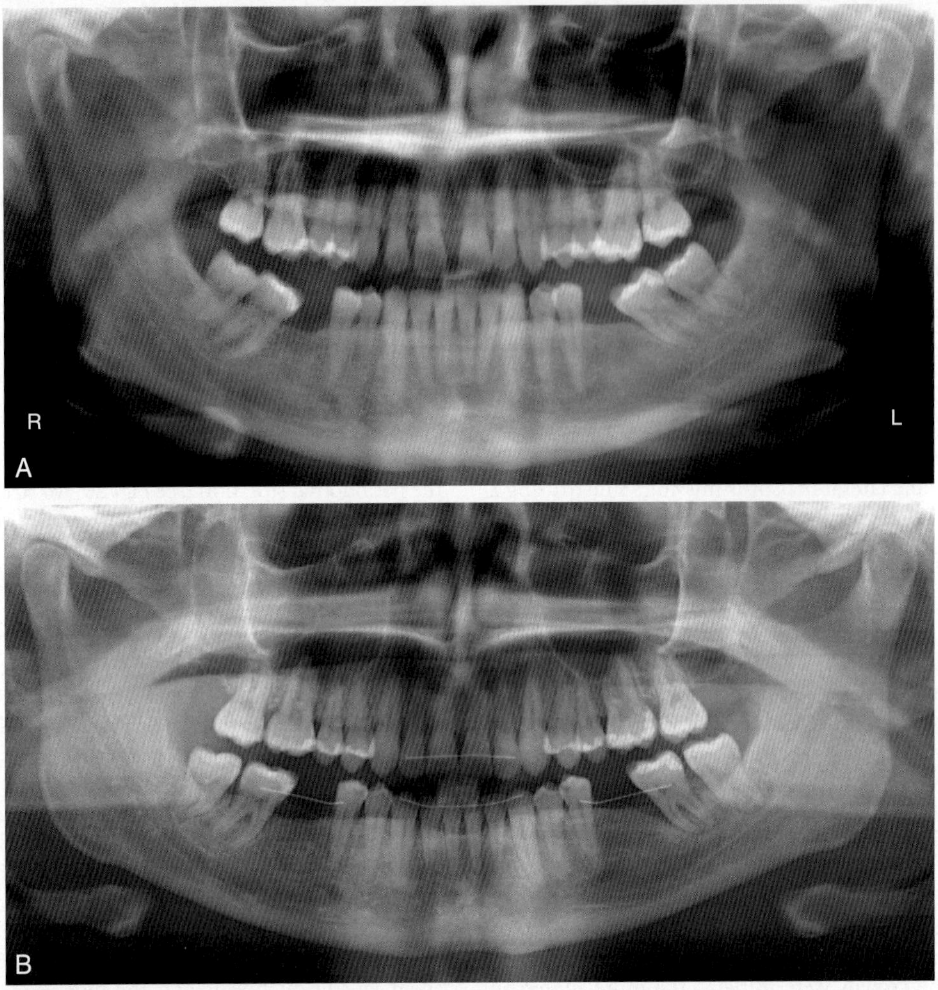

• **Fig. 20.38** (A) Panoramic radiograph of a 32-year-old patient who lost mandibular first molars years ago and now desired treatment to correct her malocclusion. She chose comprehensive fixed appliance treatment, including uprighting of both the second and third molars, opening space for replacement of the missing first molars with either implants or fixed bridges. Treatment time was 30 months. It would have taken about 6 months to upright only the first molars, but uprighting two molars on each side requires much more time, and it is difficult to maintain the occlusal relationships without a maxillary appliance. (B) Posttreatment radiograph. Uprighting the second molar does not create new bone but does tend to improve the periodontal condition; in this patient the persisting one-wall pocket on the mesial of the left second molar is much more treatable than it would have been without the uprighting. Note that fixed retainers are being used to maintain both incisor alignment and the position of the molars until restorations can be placed.

prosthodontic treatment as soon as possible after the orthodontic appliances are removed, rather than having a considerable delay while both grafts and implants are done.

After the grafts have matured to the point that implants can be inserted, it also may be possible to do the implant operation before all orthodontic treatment is finished. The implant surgical procedure itself rarely causes significant delay, and an osseointegration period during the orthodontic treatment is advantageous. A long delay caused by graft healing and maturation before implants can become a problem in orthodontic retention. Almost always, a fixed orthodontic retainer is the best choice to maintain a space for an implant. In the anterior area, patients often prefer a temporary resin-bonded bridge (Fig. 20.40), which must be removed for the implant operation and reinserted afterward unless immediate loading of the implant is feasible.

A damaged and ankylosed maxillary incisor or canine in a teenager poses a special problem when eventual replacement with an implant is planned. The ankylosed tooth interferes with orthodontic treatment to align the other teeth and can become quite unsightly, but alveolar atrophy will occur if the tooth is extracted before vertical growth is completed and the implant can be placed. In this situation, the alveolar bone can be "banked" by removing the crown of the offending tooth but retaining the endodontically treated root (Fig. 20.41), or simply decoronating the tooth without endodontic treatment. Either way, there is a better chance of successful implant placement later without a bone graft. Meanwhile, the orthodontic treatment can be completed with a pontic tied to an archwire, and then a more substantial resin-bonded bridge is worn until vertical growth is completed and it is safe to place the implant.

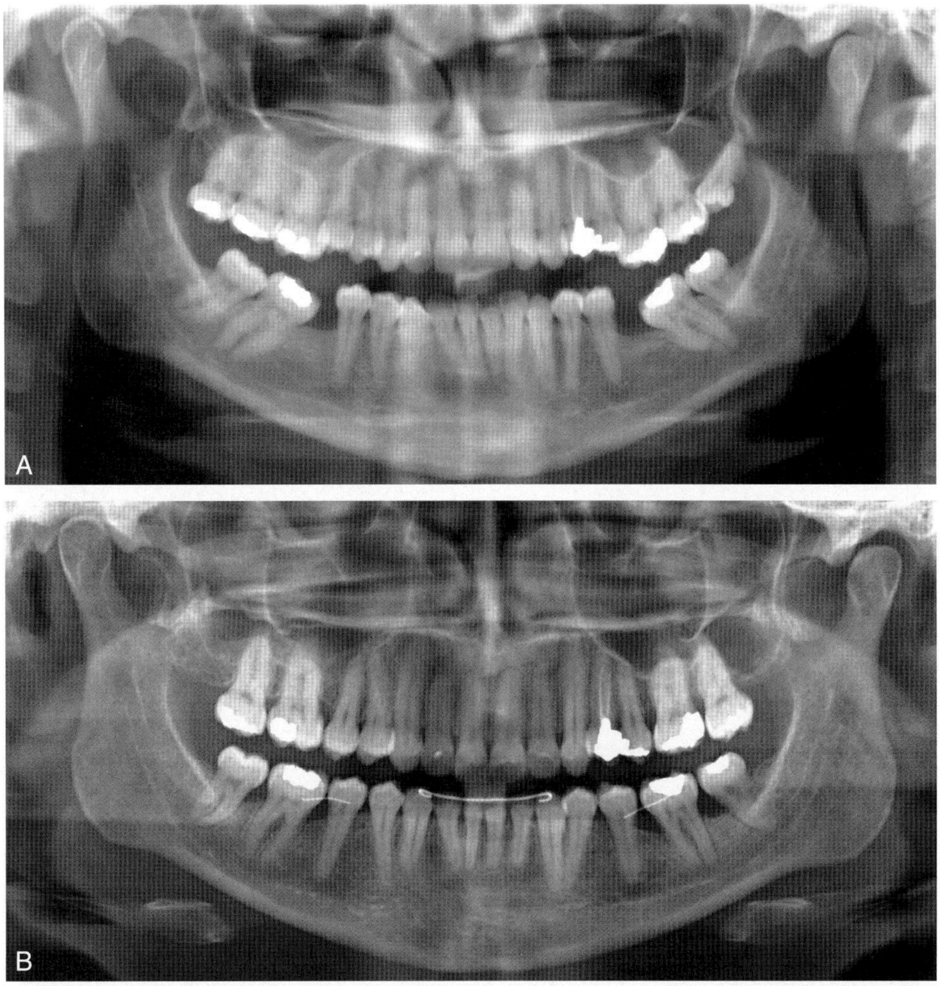

• **Fig. 20.39** (A) Panoramic radiograph of a 39-year-old patient who also lost mandibular first molars years ago. Comprehensive orthodontics was planned to align the anterior teeth in both arches, correct the supereruption of the maxillary first molars, and close the old extraction spaces. (B) After completion of treatment, which required 36 months primarily because tooth movement into old extraction spaces like this requires remodeling of cortical bone. Note that the periodontal situation on the mesial of the second molars remains less than ideal and that fixed retainers are being used to maintain closure of the extraction spaces, as well as incisor alignment.

However successful the treatment is up to that point, placing an implant too soon creates a major problem. The implant becomes the equivalent of an ankylosed tooth and will appear to intrude as vertical development continues and the other teeth erupt (Fig. 20.42). This creates a discrepancy of the gingival margins as well as the incisal edges, which is very difficult to manage even if the implant is removed and replaced with a new crown. With adult patients, this problem can occur later in life because slow vertical growth often continues into middle age.

Complex Treatment Procedures

Lingual Orthodontics

Progress in lingual orthodontics in the last few years has culminated in the development of techniques that overcome most of the previous difficulty in using this technology. The most advanced current lingual technique uses a custom-formed pad for each tooth to provide more secure bonding of the appliance, a low-profile bracket printed in a new proprietary alloy with bracket slots that are much more precise than those with edgewise brackets and made so that wires can be inserted from above, and computer-controlled wire-bending robots to generate the archwires. These changes in the appliance are described in Chapter 10 (see Fig. 10.38) and are further illustrated here.

In lingual orthodontics, the wire-bending robots are an important part of the system. They provide compensation for an unavoidable problem, the short distances between the teeth on the lingual aspect. For any wire, the shorter the span, the stiffer the material. The distances between the teeth along the archwire are so short that even with narrow brackets, it can be hard to align severely crowded lower incisors without reshaping the archwires, including the A-NiTi wire for initial alignment. Remotely forming the wires with a wire-bending robot makes this a much more

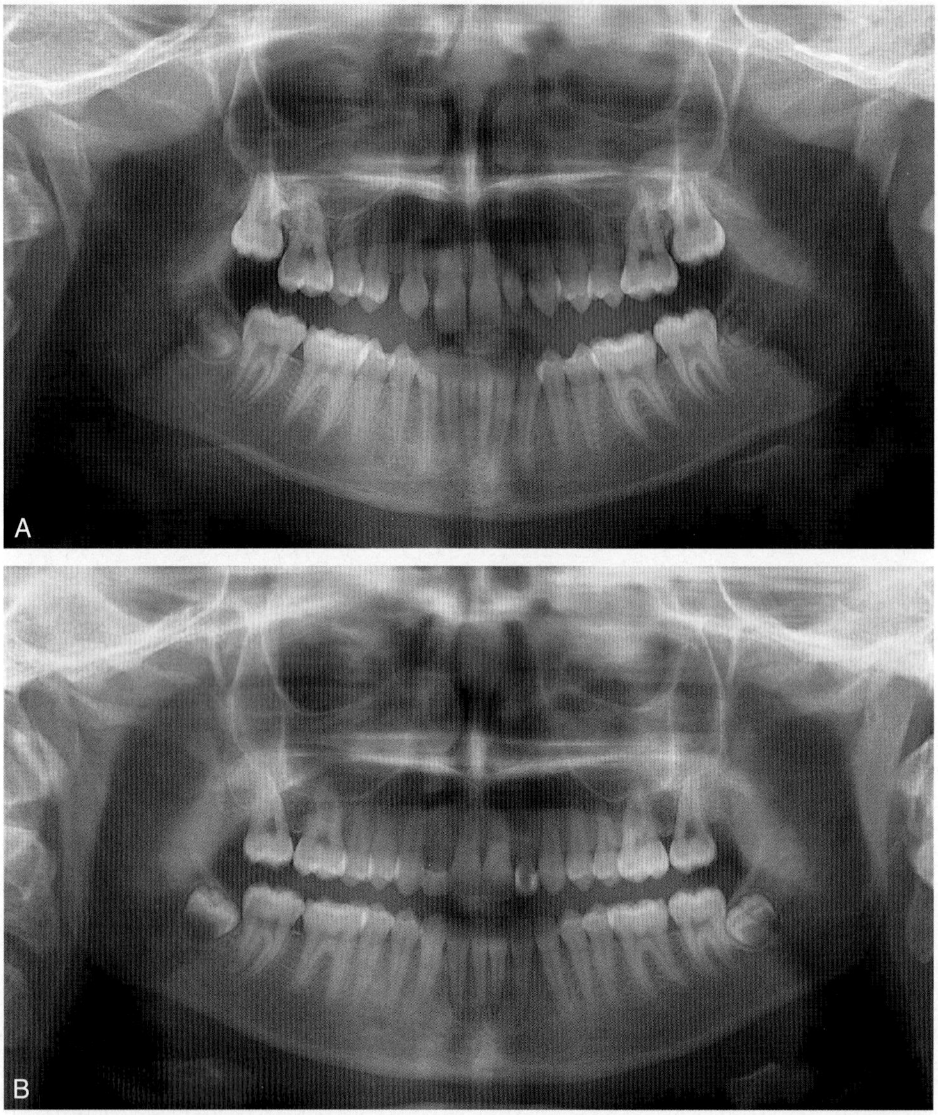

• **Fig. 20.40** For this girl, whose treatment is shown in Figs. 15.9 and 15.10, a bonded bridge to maintain space for an implant to replace the missing right lateral incisor was an important part of the treatment plan. (A) The panoramic radiograph just after the canine erupted shows it on the mesial side of the space, but moving it distally would help to correct the dental midline. (B) The posttreatment pan shows the buildups on the left lateral incisor and the bridge between the right canine and central incisor. Note that to obtain optimum esthetics, the crown of the lateral incisor has been oriented properly even though the dilacerated root then is tipped distally, which is appropriate in this situation. You also can see that there is adequate space for the implant. Perhaps the most important advantage of a bonded bridge is that it controls the position of the tooth roots during further eruption in late adolescence, in a way that a removable retainer with a pontic cannot. (Courtesy Dr. T. Shaughnessy.)

precise and less time-consuming procedure. One way to look at it is that although modern lingual orthodontic treatment is quite different from clear aligner therapy, it is based on computer technology to a similar extent.

With lingually bonded brackets and archwires, any type of tooth movement now can be produced quite efficiently, including root positioning at extraction sites and root torque. Steps in the lingual appliance treatment of a patient with a complex malocclusion are shown in Figs. 20.43 and 20.44.

An important question is the extent to which the treatment plan, represented by the setup of teeth from which the shape of archwires is derived, is achieved in the posttreatment alignment and occlusion of the teeth. For the lingual technique, this information was achieved by digital superimposition of the treatment outcome on the setup.[23] The data show (see Fig. 10.41) that there was a precise reproduction of the treatment goal in the tooth positions that were achieved, except that second molars were not positioned quite as accurately. Information of this type is not yet available for any of the other types of computer-oriented treatment methods. It has the potential to improve accuracy for all computer-aided design/computer-aided manufacturing (CAD/CAM) methods that now are being introduced into orthodontics and was used to improve the performance of the WIN system that followed Incognito.

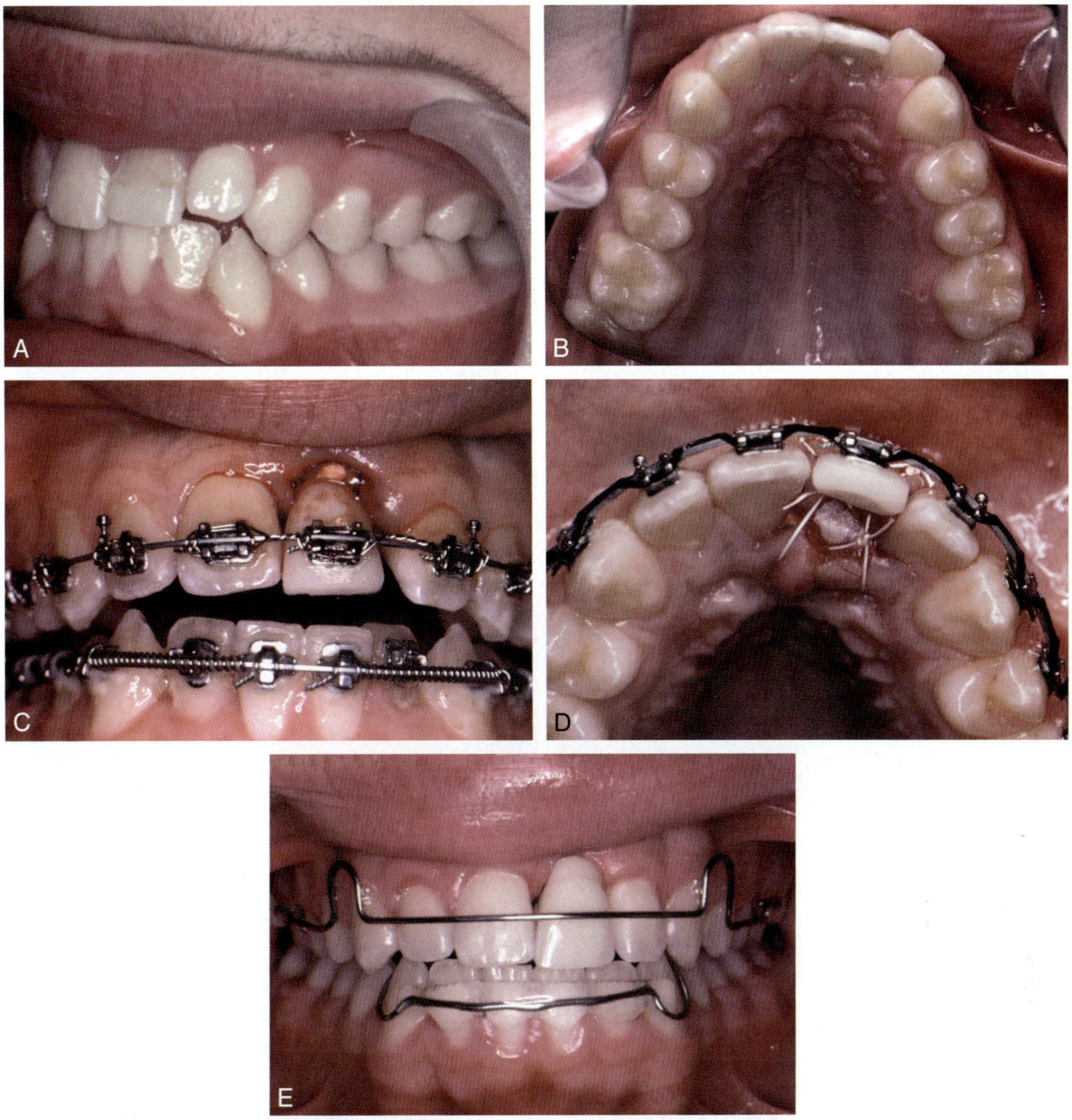

• **Fig. 20.41** This 14-year-old boy had a lingually displaced and ankylosed maxillary central incisor after a basketball injury. (A and B) Before treatment. It was not possible to correct the alignment of other teeth without removing the ankylosed tooth, which eventually would be replaced with an implant, but loss of alveolar bone in the area would result from early extraction. (C) The decision was to remove only the crown of the ankylosed tooth, retaining the root as a way of maintaining the alveolar bone. With an orthodontic appliance in place, a pontic was tied to the archwire when the crown was removed. The root was filled with calcium hydroxide, and gingival and palatal tissue (D) was sutured over it. (E) It then was possible to expand both arches and correct the malocclusion. At the end of active treatment, a pontic was placed on the orthodontic retainer as a temporary replacement. An implant was placed successfully at age 18.

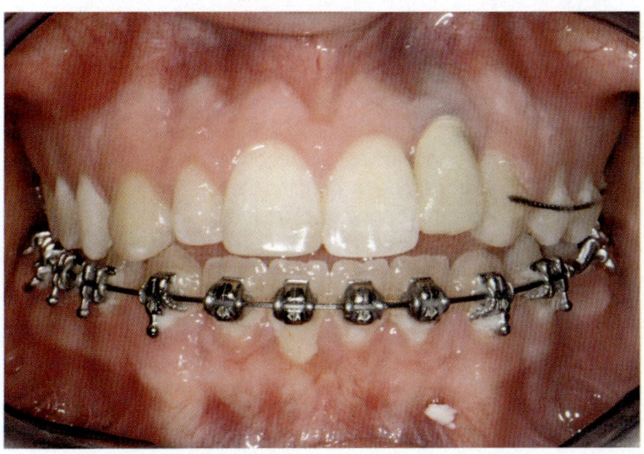

• **Fig. 20.42** For this patient, an implant to replace a missing maxillary lateral incisor was placed at age 15. At age 17, further vertical growth had led to unesthetic relative intrusion of the implant, with displacement of both the incisal edge and gingival margin. At this point, a longer crown on the implant is not a satisfactory solution. There is no good alternative to removing the implant, grafting the area, and placing a new implant.

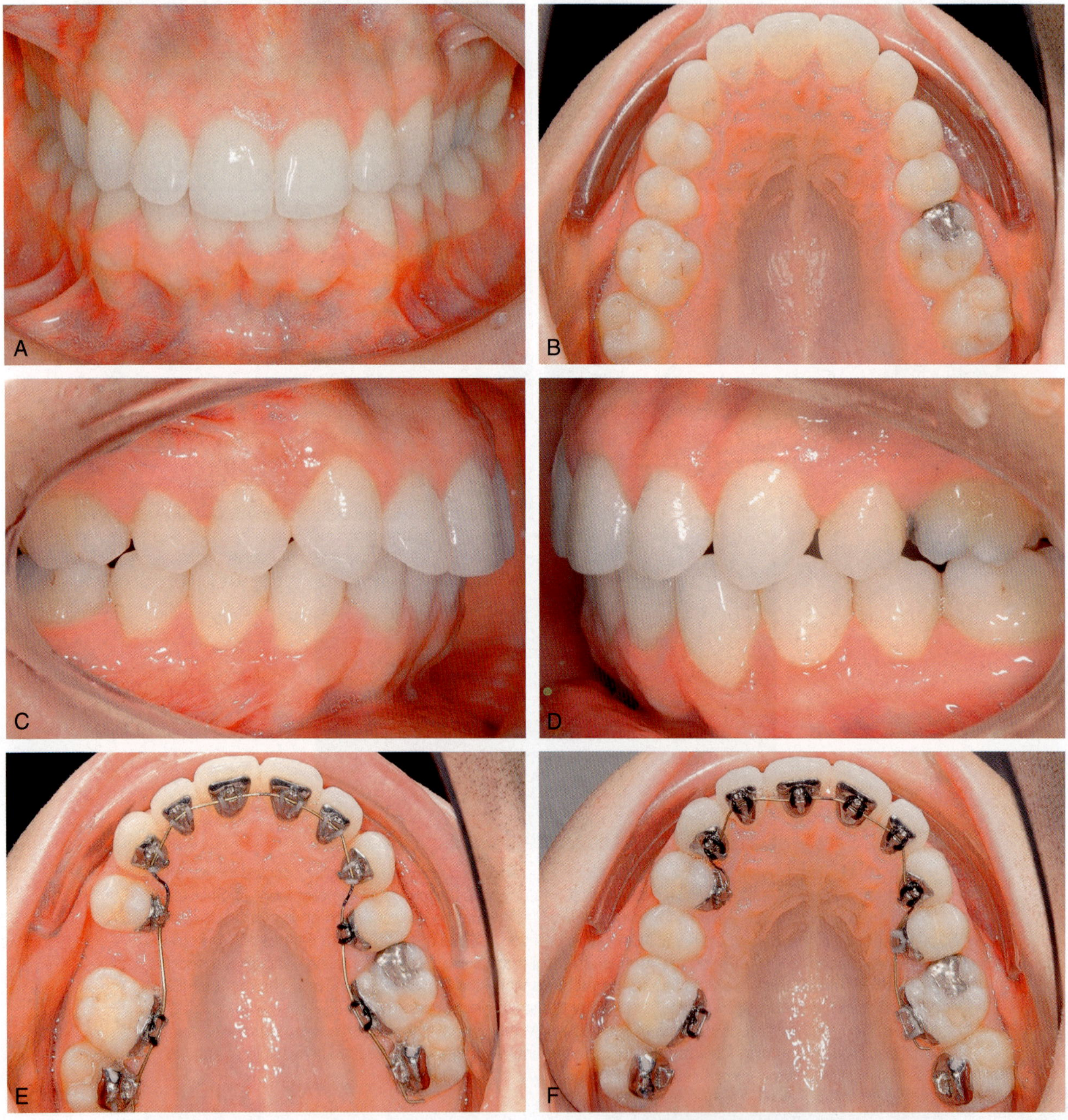

• **Fig. 20.43** The contemporary lingual appliance offers more precise archwire sizes and slots than current labial appliances, along with computer-formed archwires that allow better accomplishment of the planned occlusion—but the plan must be adjusted by the orthodontist to achieve placement of the dentition in the face. (A–D) Initial records for a patient with a midline discrepancy because of a missing maxillary left second premolar. The plan was to extract the other maxillary second premolar and close the space by bringing the maxillary arch around toward the midline. (E and F) The lingual brackets were indirectly bonded before the premolar extraction, and a light nickel-titanium (NiTi) archwire was used for initial alignment.

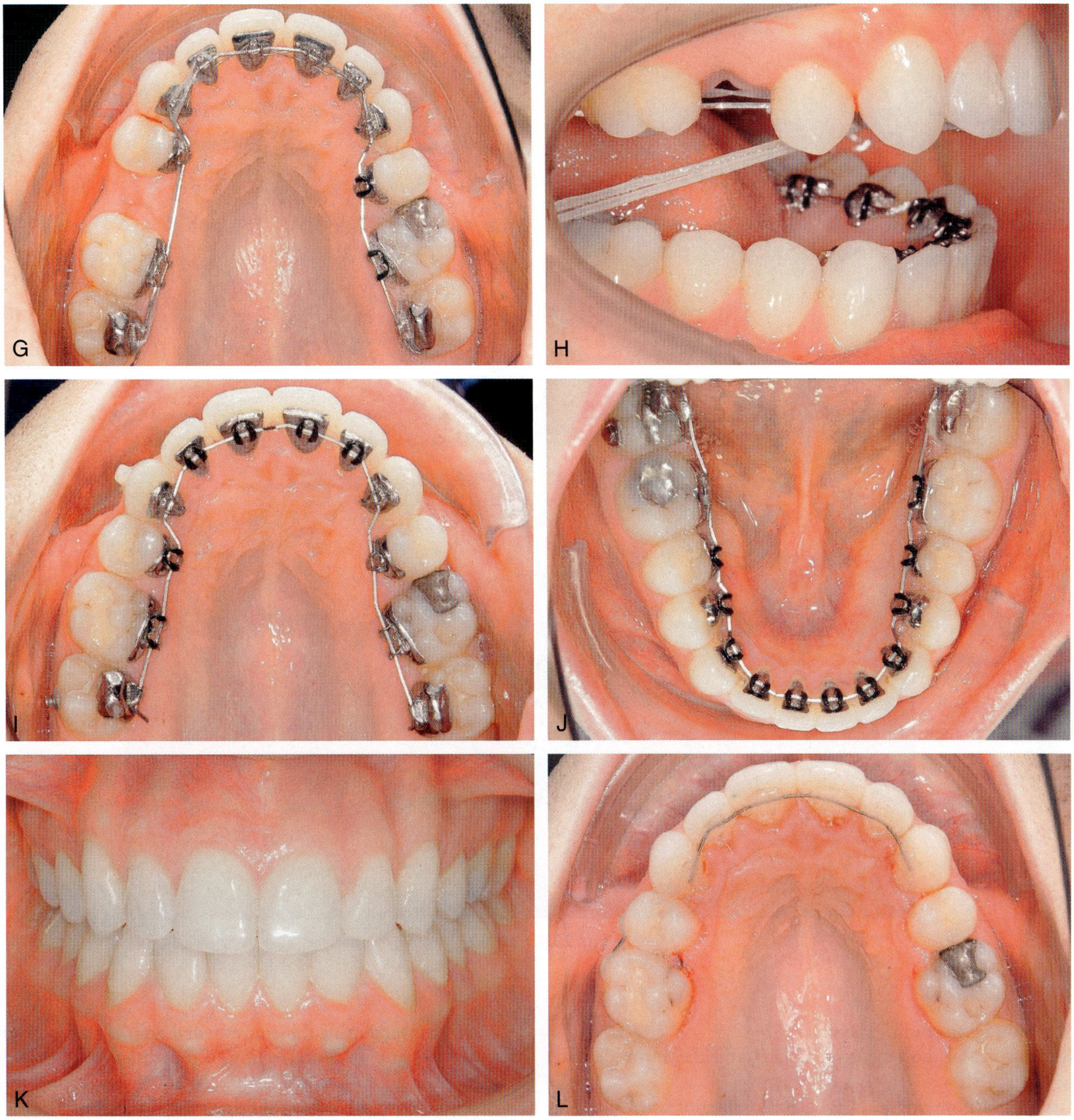

• **Fig. 20.43, cont'd** (G and H) Then the extraction space was closed by sliding on an undersized rectangular archwire, using a unilateral Class II elastic to swing the maxillary anterior teeth toward the midline. (I and J) Coordinated archwires toward the end of space closure. Note that a facial attachment for the Class II elastic was used after initial attachment of the elastic on the lingual aspect. (K–M) The completed correction of the malocclusion, and (N) the panoramic radiograph at the completion of treatment, before extraction of the impacted third molars. (Courtesy Dr. D. Wiechmann.)

Clear Aligner Therapy in Complex Cases

Treating complex cases with clear aligners is similar to treatment of less severe problems. Treatment still involves the use of a sequence of aligners that lead to a predicted endpoint, but there are three big differences: (1) the sequence of steps typically used by the computer system technicians typically needs to be modified, (2) the direction and amount of movement of teeth produced by the standard algorithms often are reduced, and (3) new records and a new set of revision aligners often are needed during the treatment process. These types of treatment for adults are addressed in Chapter 21.

Applications of Skeletal Anchorage

There are now four major applications for skeletal anchorage in treatment of adults:

1. Positioning individual teeth when no other satisfactory anchorage is available (usually because other teeth have been lost to dental or periodontal disease)

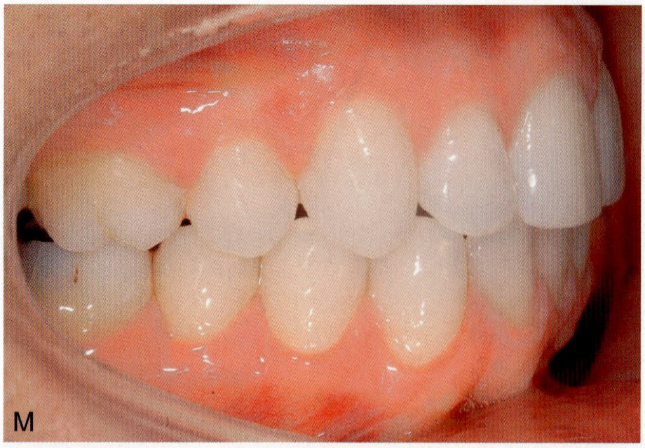

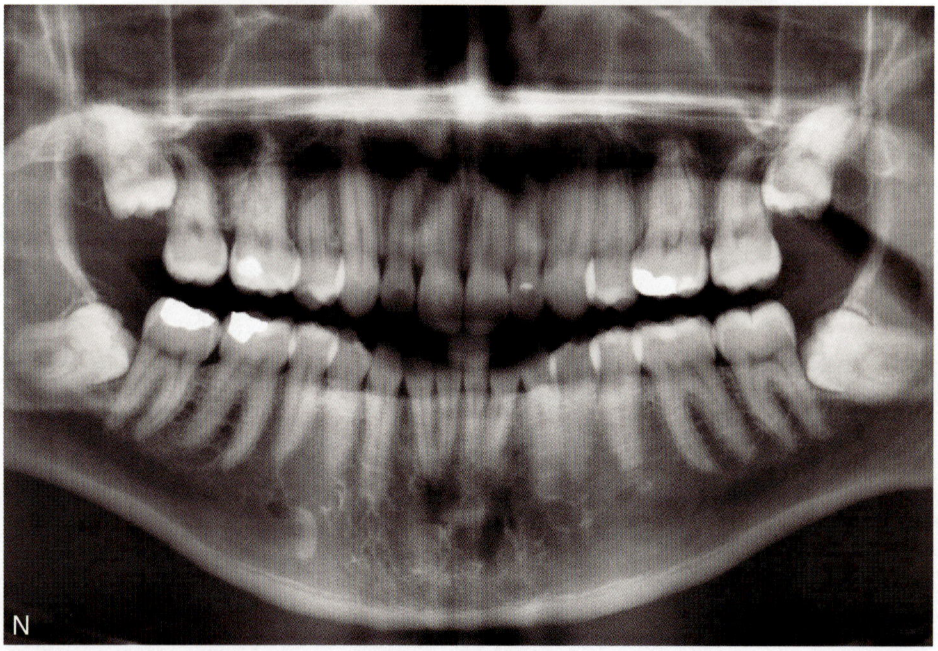

• **Fig. 20.43, cont'd**

2. Retraction of protruding incisors
3. Distal or mesial movement of molars (and the entire dental arch if needed)
4. Intrusion of posterior teeth to close an anterior open bite or anterior teeth to open a deep bite

Positioning of individual teeth and closing extraction spaces have been covered in Chapters 15 and 16; the more demanding applications in adults are discussed and illustrated here.

Retraction of Protruding Incisors

Retraction of maxillary anterior teeth into a premolar extraction site with bone screws in the palate as anchorage was one of the first applications of skeletal anchorage. An implant in the center of the palate can be used to stabilize a lingual arch that prevents movement of the molars to which it is attached (see Fig. 9.35), but stabilization away from the midline is better and both direct and indirect anchorage are available as desired (Fig. 20.45). Retraction of mandibular anterior teeth into an extraction site (which could be a molar as well as a premolar site) can be managed best with alveolar bone screws in the buccal shelf below the molars (see Fig. 10.51).

Distal movement of the entire dental arch is the most ambitious treatment plan for retraction of protrusion of incisors. This was impossible until skeletal anchorage became available but now can be done for both arches—if there is space behind the molars. Second molar extraction may be needed to provide that. For the maxillary arch, this is done most readily with miniplates below the zygomatic arch, but it also is possible with palatal anchorage. Distal movement of the mandibular arch can be accomplished with bone screws in the buccal shelf (Fig. 20.46) or in the mandibular ramus.

In Asian adults who had significant retraction of incisors to correct bimaxillary protrusion, bony spicules sometimes appear between the roots of the teeth (Fig. 20.47A). These have previously been labeled as bony exostoses, but new research at Yonsei University/University of North Carolina with 3D imaging has shown that this is not correct. Instead, as you can see in the 3D superimposition of CBCT images before and after treatment for the same patient (Fig. 20.47B), they are created by differential remodeling of alveolar bone as the teeth are moved posteriorly. The bone immediately adjacent to the tooth remodels the same distance as the tooth moved; in affected patients, bone between

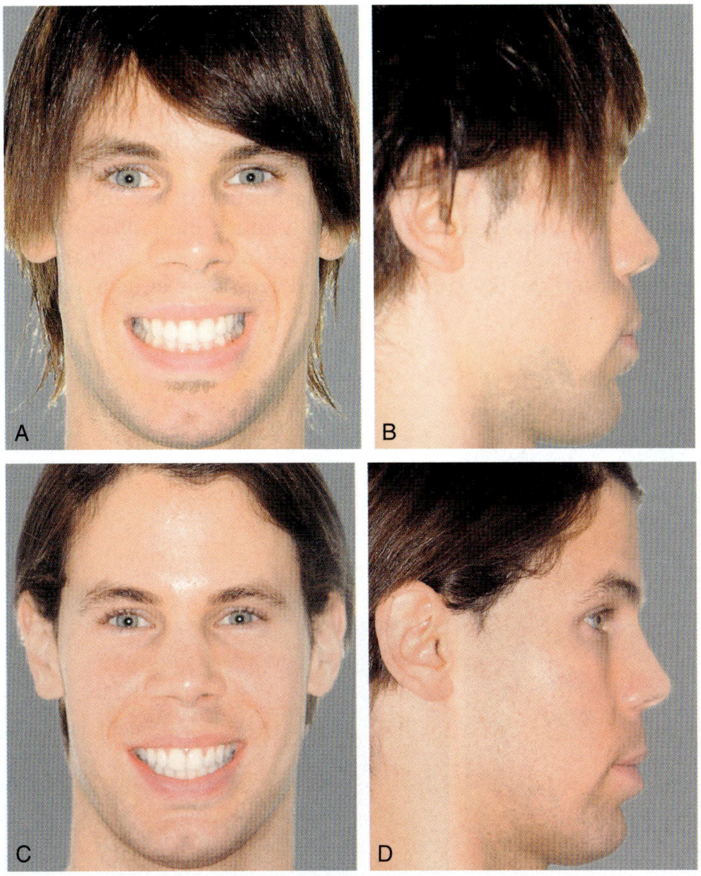

• **Fig. 20.44** For the patient in Fig. 20.43, facial images before (A and B) and after (C and D) treatment. Note the amount of correction of the maxillary dental midline to the skeletal midline. (Courtesy Dr. D. Wiechmann.)

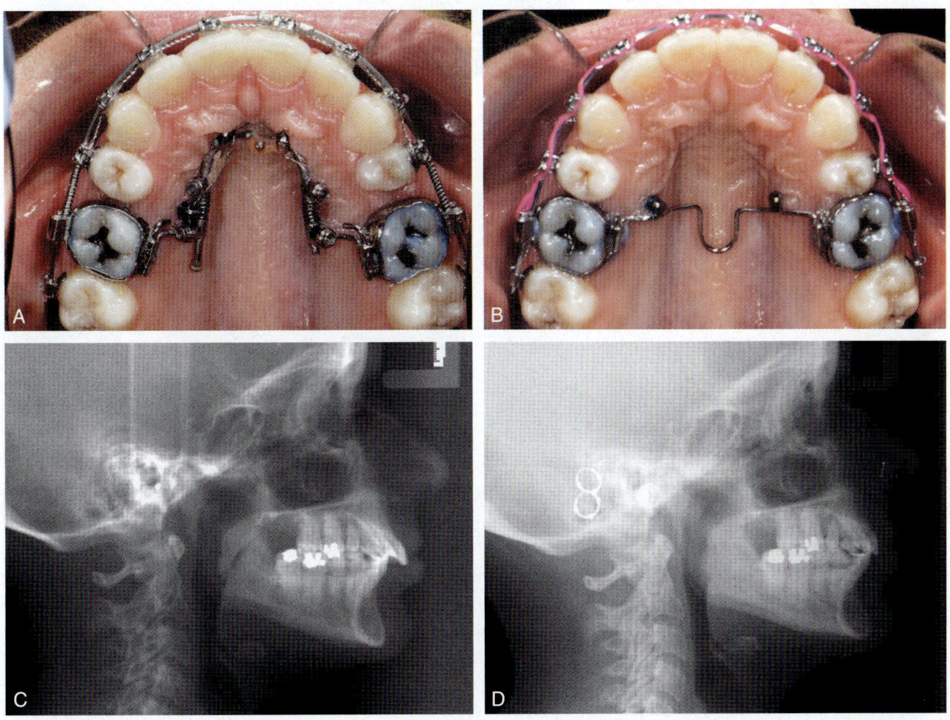

• **Fig. 20.45** (A) For this 28-year-old patient with protrusion of the maxillary arch and a partially corrected Class II malocclusion despite previous maxillary first premolar extraction, the treatment plan was palatal anchorage with bilateral bone screws for distalization of the entire maxillary arch. Initially, the molars were distalized to move them back to a Class II relationship rather than a super–Class II. (B) Then the palatal screws were used to stabilize the molars while the other teeth were retracted. (C) The pretreatment and (D) posttreatment cephalometric radiographs show the overjet reduction and attainment of the desired molar relationship. (Courtesy Dr. N. Scheffler.)

and over the teeth remodels less, and this creates irregular bony protrusions.

Why this occurs only in adults of Asian descent (or has not been noticed if it occurs in other populations) and why it occurs only in a minority of those who have incisor retraction, is not known at this point.

Retraction and Intrusion of Protruding Incisors. Protruding maxillary incisors usually are tipped facially and tipping them lingually is an obvious way to correct their axial inclination. This movement also brings the incisal edges downward, which is good if increasing incisor display and closing an anterior open bite are part of the treatment plan, but bad if maintaining or decreasing incisor display and correcting an anterior deep bite are needed. With segmented arch mechanics, maxillary incisors can be both retracted and intruded (see Fig. 9.48) if excellent anchorage is maintained with stabilizing lingual arches and headgear if necessary. This is technically much more difficult than just retraction of the incisors, which often can be managed with a stabilizing lingual arch and requires excellent patient cooperation. If retraction and

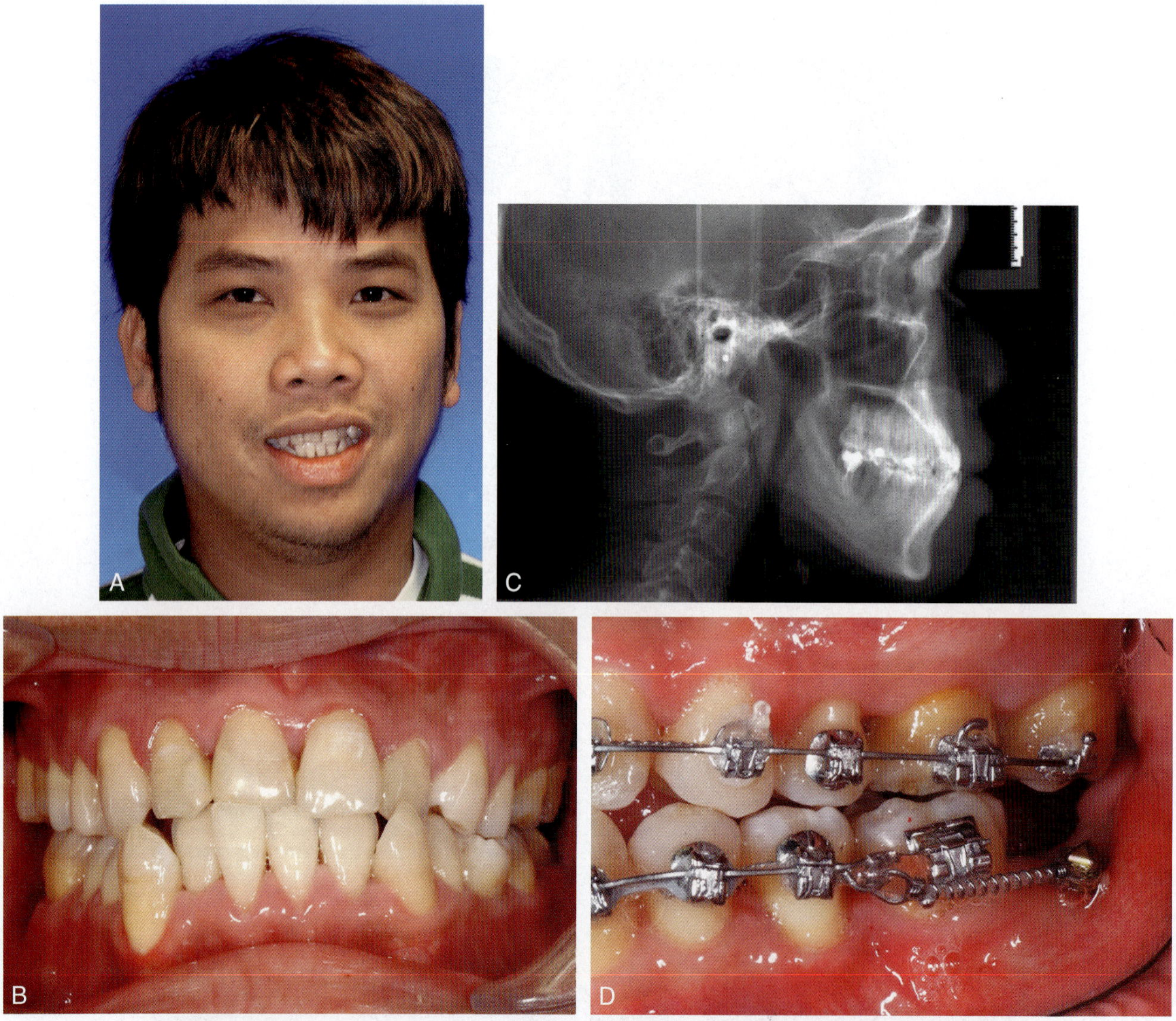

• **Fig. 20.46** For patients of European descent, it is rarely appropriate to correct a Class III tendency and anterior crossbite by retracting the lower incisors. Asians, however, often have a component of mandibular dental protrusion; if so, retracting the incisors or moving the entire mandibular arch distally can correct the crossbite without harm to the facial appearance. (A and B) Pretreatment smile and dental appearance, with crowding and moderate protrusion of the lower anterior teeth. (C) The pretreatment cephalometric radiograph showing the protrusion of the lower incisors. One mandibular second molar had been lost previously to caries, the other had been treated endodontically, and the third molars had been removed. The plan was extraction of the remaining mandibular second molar, with distalization of the entire arch to gain a better functional molar relationship, as well as correct the crossbite. (D) Bone screws were placed bilaterally in the buccal shelf of the alveolar process (which is preferred over a screw in the ramus when this area is available), and nickel-titanium (NiTi) springs were used to move the dental arch posteriorly.

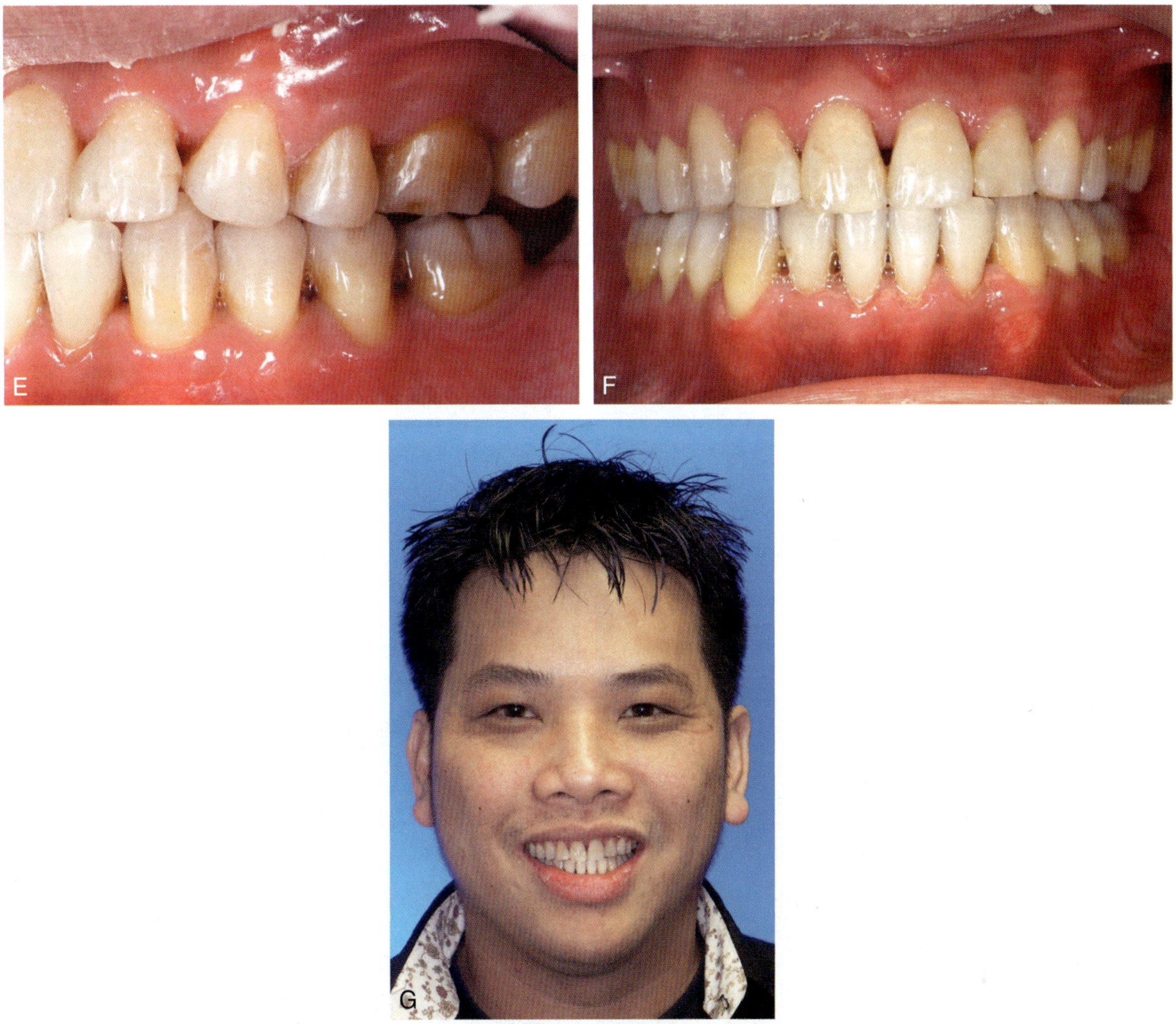

• **Fig. 20.46, cont'd** (E and F) The posttreatment dental appearance and (G) smile, with correction of the mandibular anterior crowding and crossbite. The smile was greatly improved, with little effect on apparent chin prominence. (Courtesy Dr. N. Scheffler.)

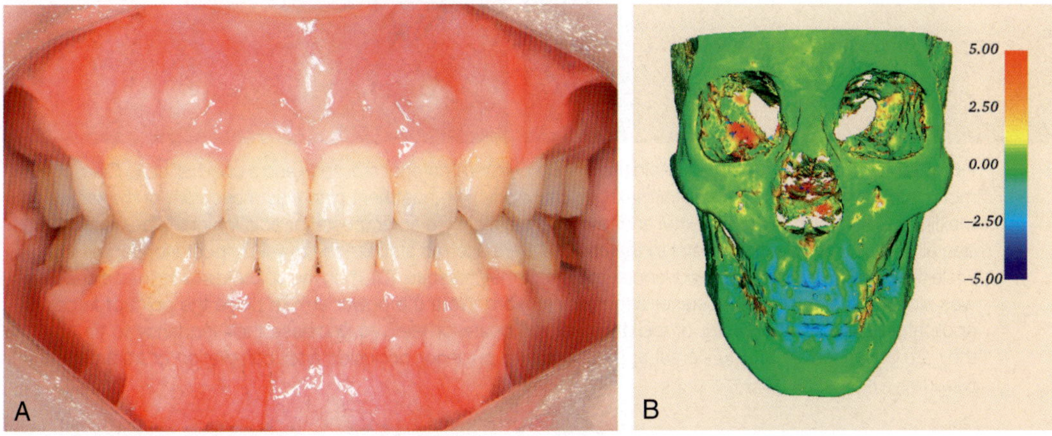

• **Fig. 20.47** (A) After orthodontic treatment to retract protruding incisors into first premolar extraction spaces, this adult developed bony protrusions between and over some of the teeth. These are not due to the formation of new bone on the surface of the alveolar process (exostosis), as previously thought. (B) Instead, as this color map superimposition of 3D images before and after treatment shows, the alveolar bone over the roots of the teeth remodels to follow the tooth movement, while less change occurs for some of the bone between or over the teeth. The green color indicates no change, the blue color shows backward movement, and the intensity of the color shows the amount of change. Note the dark blue around the roots of the anterior teeth, with light blue and green over the roots. The light orange color over the crowns of the posterior teeth indicates a small amount of transverse expansion of these teeth. (Courtesy Dr. J. C. Chung.)

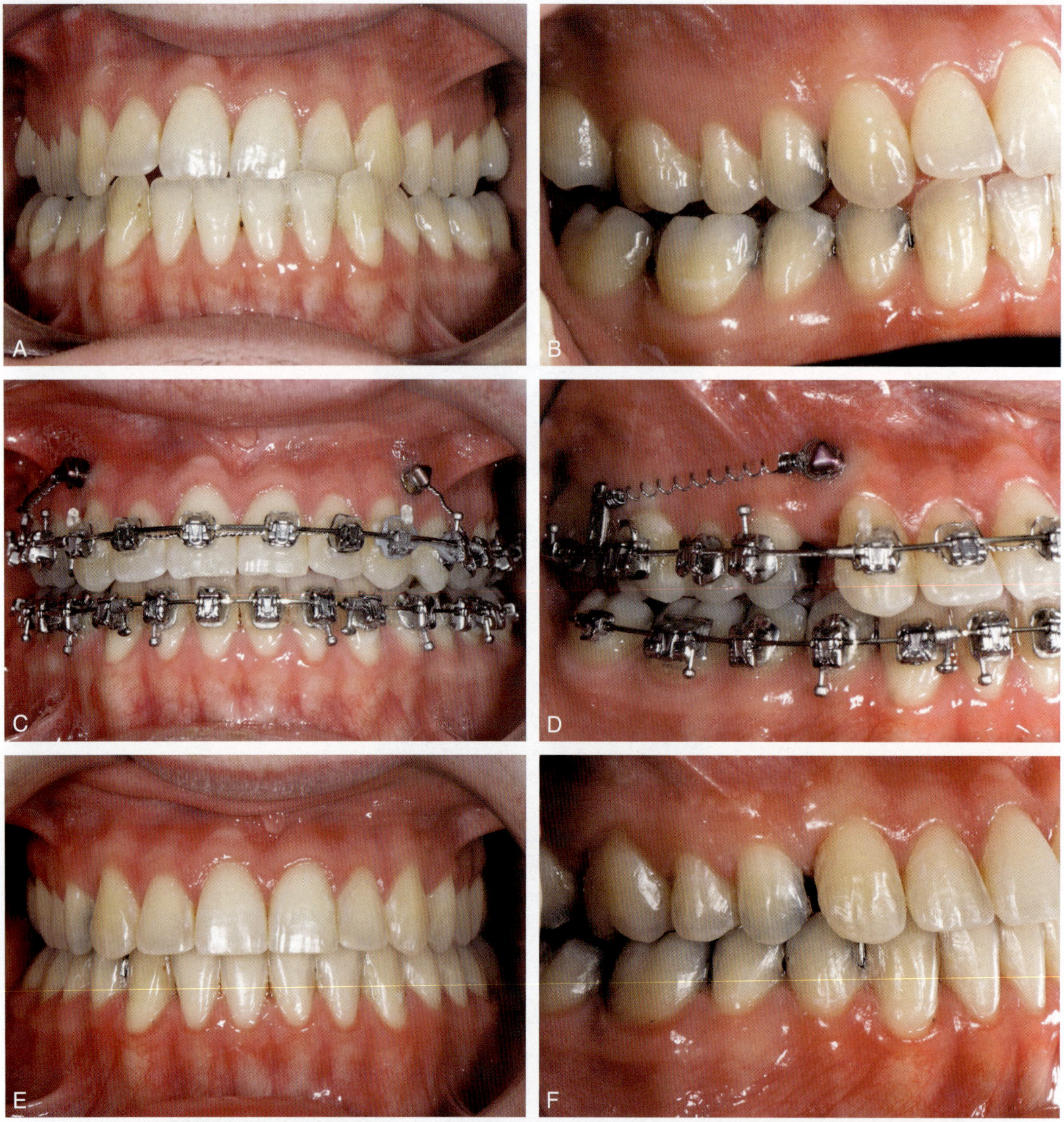

• **Fig. 20.48** (A and B) This 28-year-old male had a unilateral anterior crossbite and a one-half cusp Class III molar relationship, with mild skeletal maxillary deficiency. The treatment plan was movement of the entire maxillary arch forward, using skeletal anchorage to maintain the anteroposterior position of the mandibular dental arch. (C) Bone screws distal to the canines were used to stabilize the maxillary posterior segments while the maxillary incisors were advanced to correct the crossbite. (D) Then the space distal to the canines was closed by bringing the posterior segments forward. Note the power arm to place the point of force application closer to the center of resistance of the posterior teeth to decrease their tendency to tip as they are advanced. (E and F) Dental appearance and posterior occlusion after completion of treatment. (Courtesy Dr. N. Scheffler.)

intrusion are needed, skeletal anchorage now is recommended. With alveolar bone screws between the molar roots or miniplates at the base of the zygomatic arch, the direction of force, both upward and backward, is ideal for this purpose, and A-NiTi retraction springs provide a constant known force level.

Distal Movement of Molars or the Entire Dental Arch

Maxillary Distalization. Distal movement of the maxillary molars is one way to provide space in a crowded maxillary arch; distal movement of the entire maxillary dental arch would provide a way to correct a Class II malocclusion due to a forward position of the upper teeth on their skeletal base. For both types of movement, miniplates below the zygomatic arch or palatal bone screws provide a predictable outcome. Bone screws in the alveolar process interfere with root movement and are not recommended. Single bone screws in the infrazygomatic process away from the roots are a possibility but may not withstand the amount of force needed to move multiple teeth. The entire arch usually can be moved back 2 to 4 mm. More than that usually requires extraction of the second molars.

Mandibular Distalization. Moving the entire mandibular arch distally was simply impossible until skeletal anchorage became available. It can be done now by using a long bone screw into the mandibular buccal shelf or the ramus (usually less desirable)—but most American orthodontists still do not think of it in the two circumstances in which it can be helpful:

1. Class III malocclusion with a component of mandibular dental protrusion, which is almost never seen in Class III patients of European origin but does occur reasonably frequently in Asians, for whom this form of Class III camouflage can be quite acceptable (see Fig. 20.46).
2. Incisor protrusion created during treatment of severe crowding. This was avoided by extraction to prevent it until popularization of the idea that light forces and just the right self-ligating bracket somehow allowed nonextraction treatment without protrusion,[24] which of course it really didn't. In fact, lower incisor protrusion with Damon and similar self-ligating brackets is a common accompaniment to arch expansion. Use of skeletal anchorage during alignment to keep from advancing the incisors can produce a better relationship of the dental arch to basal bone.[25]

Molar Protraction. Space closure by bringing molars forward is accomplished most readily with indirect anchorage to stabilize the anterior dental segments, from bone screws in the palate for maxillary molar protraction and in the mandibular buccal shelf or ramus for the mandible (Figs. 20.48 and 20.49).

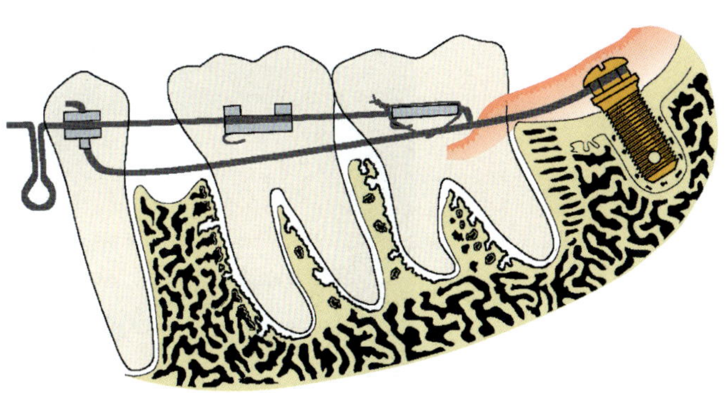

• **Fig. 20.49** Use of indirect anchorage from a bone screw in the mandibular ramus to move mandibular second and third molars forward to close an old mandibular first molar extraction site. The skeletal anchorage makes this movement possible when it otherwise would not be, but it is still quite slow because remodeling cortical bone in the collapsed alveolar area at the extraction site occurs very slowly. Treatment time typically is 2–3 years.

Intrusion

Intrusion of teeth in adults is a consideration in two situations: (1) overerupted maxillary incisors leading to excessive tooth and gingival display and/or anterior deep bite and (2) overerupted molars in anterior open bite with excessive face height. Occasionally intrusion of other teeth is indicated.

Intrusion of Incisors. In adolescents and young adults with excessive overbite, the choice between intrusion of incisors or extrusion of posterior teeth often can be resolved in favor of extrusion because vertical growth will compensate for it. In adults, the choice often must be intrusion, which is much more effective when skeletal anchorage in the form of miniplates or screws is available and when segmented rather than continuous archwires are used. The practical effect is to make both segmented arch treatment and skeletal anchorage more important in adults than in younger patients.

One potential problem with intrusion in adults with periodontal involvement is the prospect that a deepening of periodontal pockets might be produced by this treatment. Ideally, of course, intruding a tooth would lead to a reattachment of the periodontal fibers, but there is no basis for expecting this. What seems to happen instead is the formation of a tight epithelial cuff, so that the position of the gingiva relative to the crown improves clinically while periodontal probing depths do not increase. If good hygiene is maintained, clinical experience has shown that it is possible to maintain teeth that have been treated in this way and that root length and alveolar bone height are not greatly affected.[26]

The mechanotherapy needed to produce incisor intrusion in an adult is not different from the methods for younger patients described in some detail in Chapters 9 and 15. In adults, however, careful stabilization of dental arch segments during incisor intrusion is even more important, especially if the patient also has had periodontal bone loss. For those patients, skeletal anchorage via alveolar bone screws is particularly advantageous. Differential intrusion of maxillary incisors, with more intrusion on one side or intrusion on one side and extrusion on the other, also can be used to help correct a canted maxillary occlusal plane if the cant is not too severe (see the discussion of roll deformity in Chapter 6 and Fig. 15.28 to view an asymmetric intrusion arch).

Intrusion of Posterior Teeth to Close Anterior Open Bite. Most patients with anterior open bite have elongation of the maxillary and/or mandibular posterior teeth, so the mandible is rotated downward and backward. The maxillary incisor segment often is reasonably well positioned relative to the upper lip. Extrusion of the upper incisors to close the bite in a patient with this issue is neither esthetically acceptable nor stable. Intrusion of the maxillary posterior segments so that the mandible can rotate upward and forward is the ideal approach to treatment (Fig. 20.50). This was essentially impossible until segmental maxillary surgery was developed in the early 1970s so that the maxillary posterior segments could be moved upward. Skeletal anchorage to intrude the posterior teeth has the potential to create the same mandibular response (Fig. 20.51). This now makes orthodontic intrusion a possible alternative to surgery, at least for patients with the less severe long-face problems.

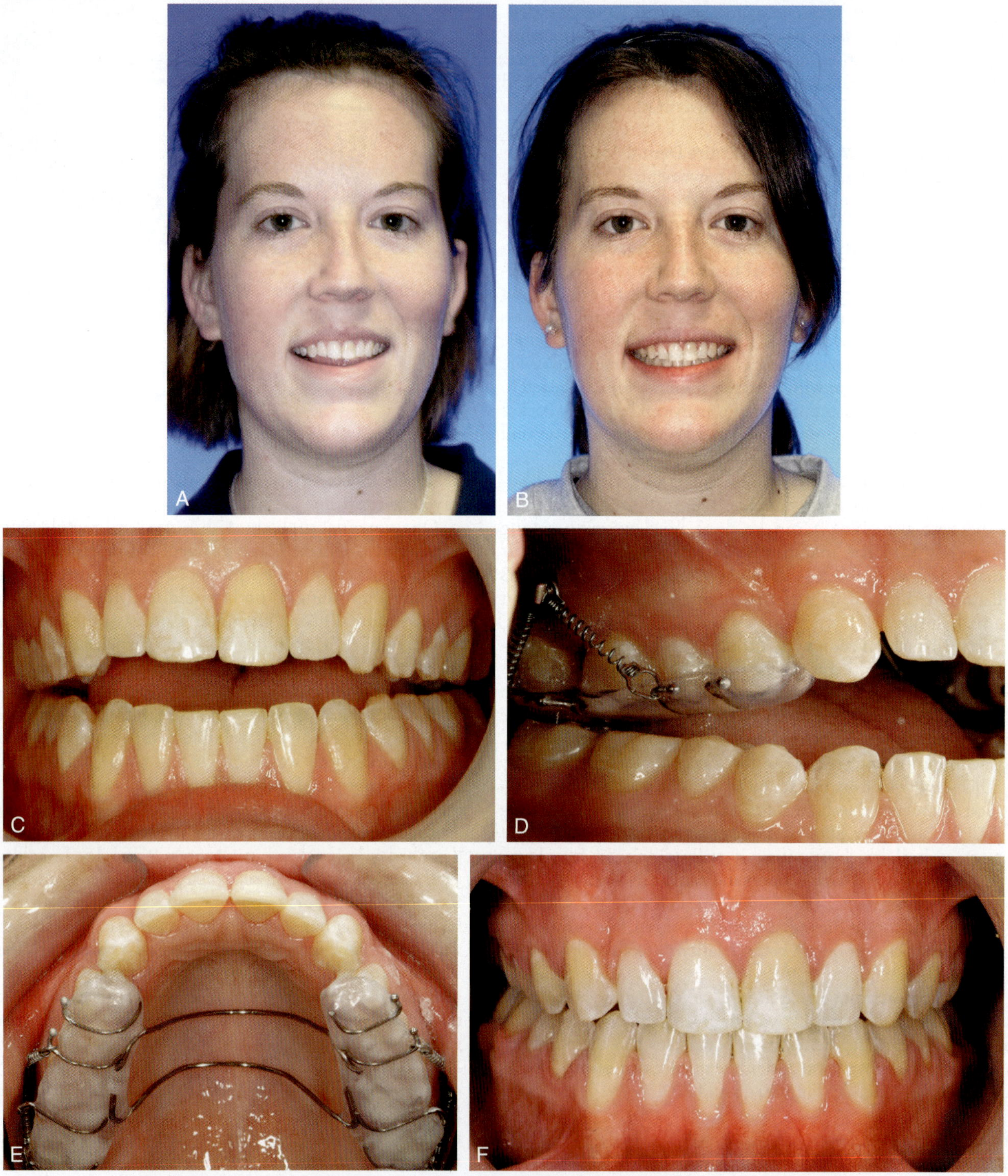

• **Fig. 20.50** Intrusion of maxillary posterior teeth can be effective treatment for an adult or late adolescent patient with a moderate long-face, open bite problem. (A) Age 26, before treatment for correction of anterior open bite and reduction of anterior face height. The chin was 2–3 mm off to the right, but this was not a problem. A chin deviation of less than 4 mm rarely is noticed—the patient was unaware of it. (B) Age 27, after treatment. Note the improved facial proportions as well as correction of the open bite. (C) Frontal intraoral view, showing the 6-mm anterior open bite and contact only on the distal aspect of the first molars and second molars. (D) Right lateral view with intrusion beginning. A long bone screw into the base of the zygoma is used for anchorage, with a modified Erverdi plate (AOB plate) used to control the teeth. (E) Palatal view of the AOB plate, showing the twin transpalatal arches connecting the splints, which must be off the palate initially so that they do not contact the soft tissues until intrusion is complete. (F) Open bite closed. The mild dental midline discrepancy, with mandibular dentition 2 mm off to the right, was not corrected because doing so would have pulled the maxillary midline off the midline of the face. (Courtesy Dr. N. Scheffler.)

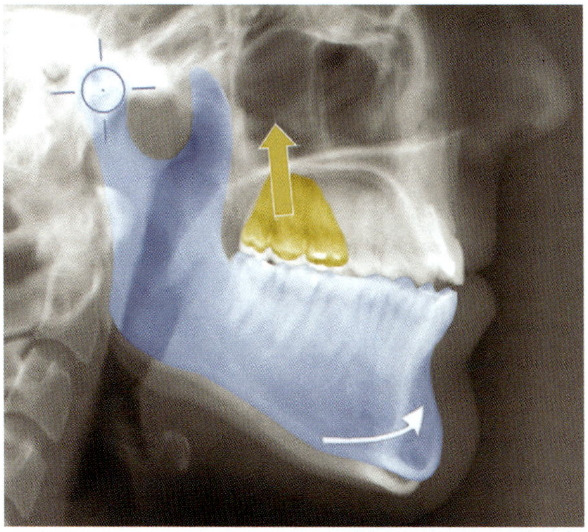

• **Fig. 20.51** Schematic drawing of mandibular rotation up and forward to correct anterior open bite by intrusion of maxillary posterior teeth. One of the assumptions with this technique is that the mandible will rotate to the correct anteroposterior position, and a major indication for orthognathic surgery for open bite patients is that the mandible would not rotate to the correct position without ramus osteotomy to shorten or lengthen it, or Le Fort I osteotomy to reposition the maxilla forward or back.

As the range of treatment with clear trays has broadened, correction of anterior open bite and deep bite has become possible, with the presumed mechanism for open bite being intrusion of posterior teeth. A recent review of experience at the University of Washington showed that a median gain of 1.5 mm in overbite was obtained in patients with open bite but that the effect was largely extrusion of incisors, not intrusion of molars.[27]

For intrusion of maxillary posterior teeth, miniplates at the base of the zygomatic arch (see Fig. 13.25) provide excellent anchorage. These plates are held with multiple screws and are covered by oral soft tissues. The fixture for attachment to the orthodontic appliance extends through the soft tissue, preferably at the junction between gingiva and mucosa. A major problem with miniplates is that they require more surgery than most orthodontists want to do, but at present many oral and maxillofacial surgeons have not been trained to do this procedure, and surgical help may not be available.

A long bone screw extending into the base of the zygomatic arch, which orthodontists with experience with alveolar bone screws can place, is a possible alternative. A screw of this type should be placed through attached gingiva if possible because bone screws placed in unattached tissue are at greater risk of infection and tissue overgrowth. Some preliminary separation of roots in the region in which the screw will be placed makes it easier to avoid root contact and is recommended (Fig. 20.52). The screw can be placed above and between the first and second molars (if some retraction of the maxillary arch might also be needed to assist with Class II correction) or above and between the first molar and second premolar (if the patient also has a mild Class III tendency and some mesial movement of the dental arch would help).

An ideal force system for intrusion is created by A-NiTi springs, which provide a relatively constant known force over a considerable range of activation. An upward force on the facial aspect of the posterior teeth is also a force to tip them facially, and control to prevent this is essential. Transpalatal lingual arches are one possibility, but controlling all the teeth in the segment being intruded is necessary. A bonded plate covering the occlusal surface of the teeth, fabricated so that it is off the palate enough to allow the intrusion, is the preferred method at present (see Fig. 20.50E).

As the mandible rotates upward and forward as the posterior teeth intrude, it may be advantageous to have a Class II or Class III component to the force so that the maxillary arch is moved a little forward or back as the intrusion occurs, to help in obtaining correct overjet at the end of treatment. This can be facilitated by adjusting the point of attachment of the spring to the plate (Fig. 20.53), as well as by locating the screw as described earlier.

Even with appropriate light force (not more than 200 g to a three-tooth posterior segment), intrusion does not occur as quickly as other types of tooth movement. Space closure and most other types of movement occur at the rate of about 1 mm per month. At best, posterior intrusion occurs at half that rate. Because 1 mm intrusion of maxillary posterior teeth should translate into about 2 mm of closure of anterior open bite, a 4-mm open bite often closes in as many months. At that point, the rest of a complete fixed appliance can be placed and the other necessary treatment can be completed while the intruded segment remains tied to the anchor screw or miniplate. After intrusion of the posterior segments, the same anchors used for that purpose easily can serve as anchorage for retraction or protraction of the maxillary arch.

Two publications in 2014 described this technique in more detail[28] and present the best data to date for outcomes with this technique.[29] The sample for the study is described in Box 20.1, and the outcomes are briefly summarized in Box 20.2. Based on jaw geometry, it was expected that there would be a 2-mm decrease in open bite (or increase in overbite) for every millimeter of posterior intrusion. All the patients were treated to at least 1 mm of overjet.

The outcomes are an excellent example of a clinical data set that is much easier to understand when the percentages of patients with clinically significant changes are shown, not just the means and standard variations for the whole sample. That usually is the case when there was large variability in the response to treatment and not a normal distribution around the mean, which occurs frequently in clinical outcome studies. For this study, changes in cephalometric measurements of more than 2 mm or 2 degrees were considered outside the range of measurement error and clinically significant, and changes greater than 4 mm or 4 degrees were considered highly clinically significant.

First, note the changes created by treatment as reported in the standard fashion of means and standard deviations (see Box 20.2).

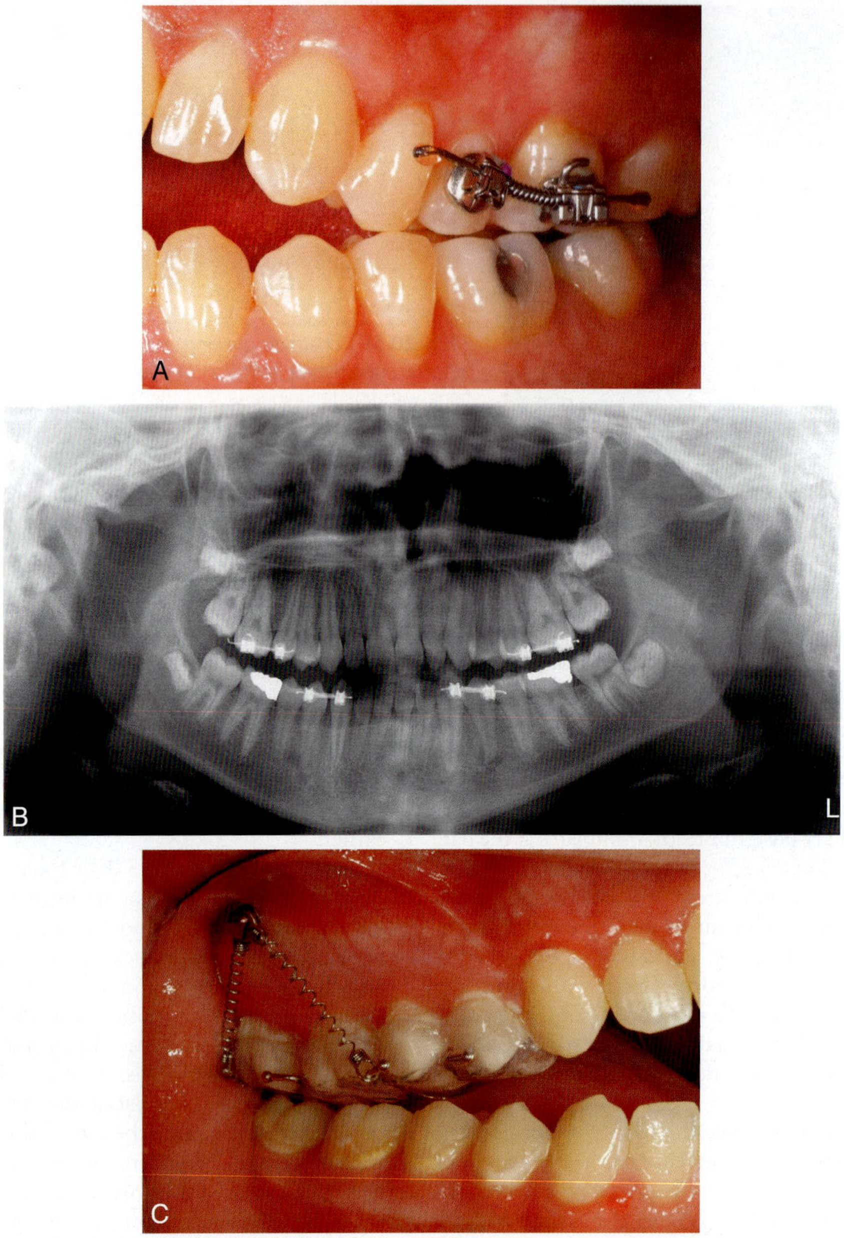

• **Fig. 20.52** (A) Before intrusion of the maxillary posterior segments to correct an anterior open bite, the roots of the second premolar and first molar are diverged to facilitate placing an alveolar bone screw between their roots. (B) A panoramic radiograph of a different patient being prepared for placement of bone screws for maxillary intrusion, showing the root divergence needed for placement of a long screw into the base of the zygomatic arch. (C) The bone screw being used as anchorage for intrusion, with use of a modified Erverdi appliance to prevent buccal tipping of the teeth in the intrusion segment. (Courtesy Dr. N. Scheffler.)

The mean amount of intrusion of the maxillary first molar, mean decrease in anterior face height, and mean increase in overbite all were significantly different from zero. But there were large standard deviations for all three changes, which indicates a large amount of variability in the results, and none of the patients had the expected amount of decrease in face height (2 mm for every 1 mm of posterior intrusion).

Now, look at Fig. 20.54, which shows the percentage of patients with clinically significant changes in anterior face height. Changes in anterior face height, of course, would reflect changes in the vertical position of the mandible as posterior teeth were intruded and the mandible rotated upward and forward to correct the anterior open bite. Changes at the later times during completion of treatment after intrusion was complete, and then at 1 and 2 years after treatment, would show how many patients experienced relapse or progressive change. This makes it apparent that the reported mean decrease in anterior face height of 1.7 mm is misleading. What really happened was that during active intrusion, 40% of the patients had 2.4 mm of decrease in face height and another 10% had more than 4 mm of decrease. One patient's face height increased rather than decreased.

Fig. 20.54 also shows the changes after overbite correction was completed and intrusion stopped. You can see that 20% of the patients had a clinically significant amount of relapse in face

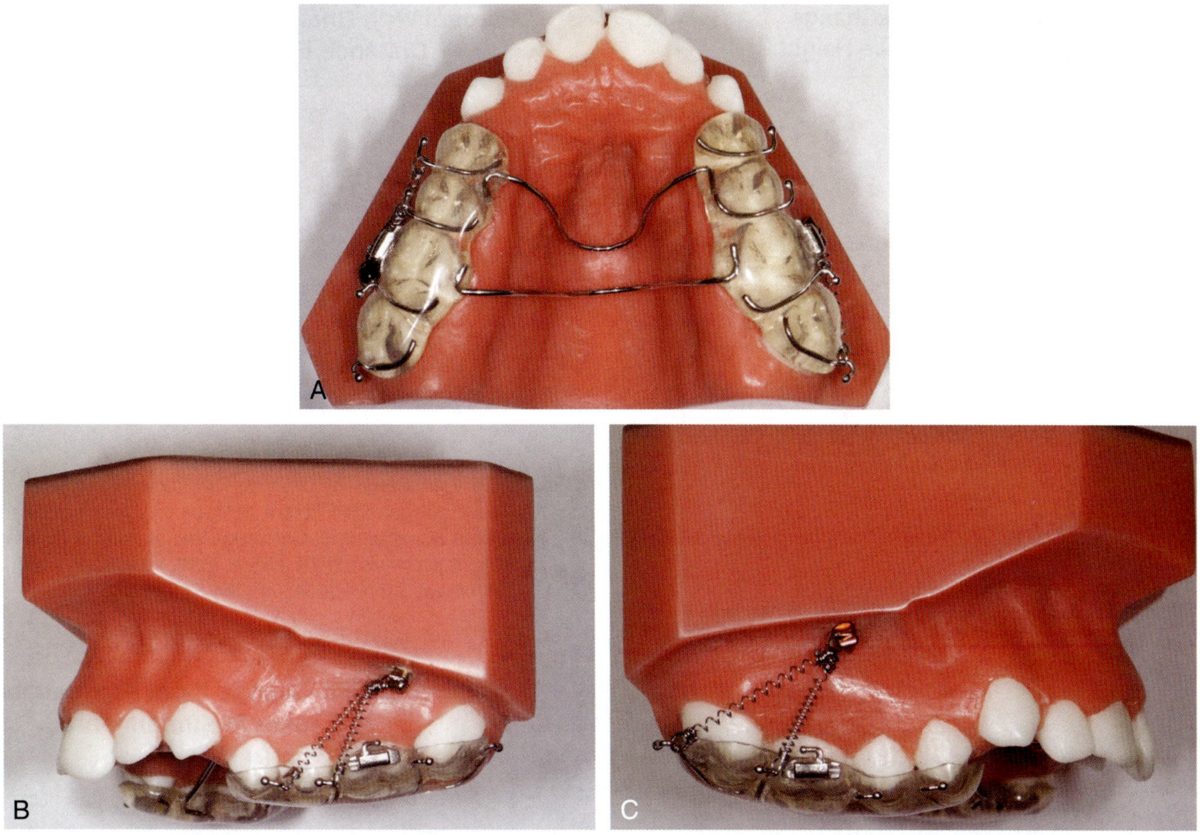

• **Fig. 20.53** (A) Occlusal splint for intrusion of maxillary posterior teeth. The lingual arches are off the palate, giving room for intrusion to occur without forcing them into the soft tissues. (B) Intrusion springs to the bone anchor with a Class II as well as vertical direction of force. (C) Intrusion springs with a Class III direction of pull. (Courtesy Dr. N. Scheffler.)

• BOX 20.1 Scheffler et al.: The Sample Consecutive Patients Treated Identically

- Maxillary intrusion splint
- Temporary anchorage device (TAD) at base of zygomatic buttress
- Nickel-titanium (NiTi) springs from TAD to splint, net intrusion force (about 100 g on each side)

Data Points (Cephalometric Radiographs)

- Pretreatment
- Completion of intrusion
- Completion of treatment
- One-year recall ($n = 27$)
- Two-year recall ($n = 25$)

• BOX 20.2 During Active Intrusion

Two millimeters of posterior maxillary intrusion should produce an approximately 4-mm decrease in anterior face height and an approximately 4-mm decrease in open bite, but often the results are less.

- Mean intrusion of maxillary first molar = 2.0 ± 1.6 mm
- Mean decrease in anterior face height = 1.7 ± 1.6 mm
- Mean increase in overbite = 1.8 ± 1.6 mm

Why Does This Happen?

- Because lower molars often erupt 0.6 ± 1.6 mm as the upper molars are intruded

height during the completion of treatment, and that some patients had changes in both directions after the end of treatment.

A clearer view of molar intrusion and relapse is shown in Fig. 20.55, which shows changes in the vertical position of the maxillary first molar to the palatal plane—that is, the actual amount of intrusion that was produced and then the amount of relapse. Note that two-thirds of the patients had more than 2 mm (clinically significant) of molar intrusion; then 10% had more than 2 mm of re-eruption during the last part of treatment, and by 2 years after treatment, 16% had experienced this amount of re-eruption. From the geometry of the mandible, you would expect about twice as much change in face height and overbite as the change in vertical molar position. Comparison with Fig. 20.54 makes it clear that the change anteriorly was not as much as the 1 : 2 ratio suggests.

You have already seen in Box 20.2 that eruption of lower molars was a major factor in achieving less mandibular rotation than was expected during active intrusion. Fig. 20.56 shows the number of patients with clinically significant lower molar eruption. Lower molar eruption during maxillary molar intrusion was the major reason for failure to obtain the expected change in anterior dimensions, and further eruption during the orthodontic treatment continued to be a factor in relapse—but almost no change beyond that was shown.

Fig. 20.57 shows the change for four critical dimensions from pretreatment to 1-year after treatment. This gives you the net changes over that time, essentially a look at the long-term outcomes. The percentages for increase in overbite are higher than

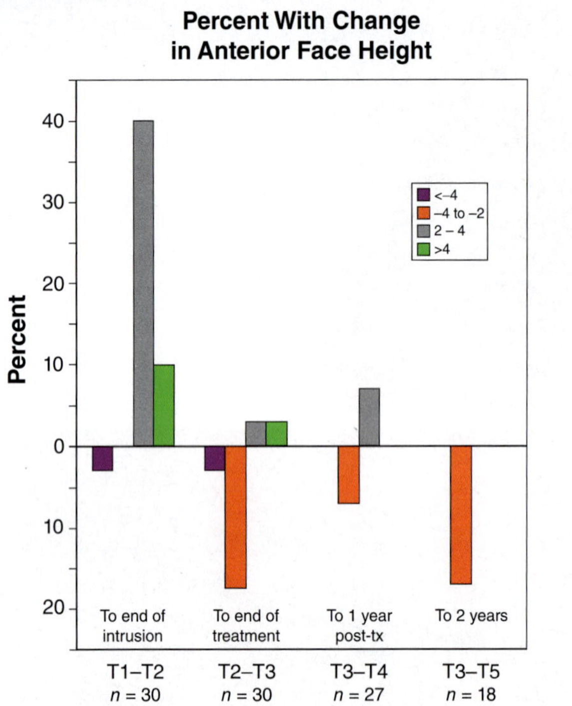

• **Fig. 20.54** Percentage of patients with clinically significant change in anterior face height with intrusion of posterior teeth. (Redrawn from Scheffler et al. Outcomes and stability in long face/open bite patients treated with TADs and a maxillary intrusion splint. *Am J Orthod Dentofacial Orthop*. 2014;146:594–602.)

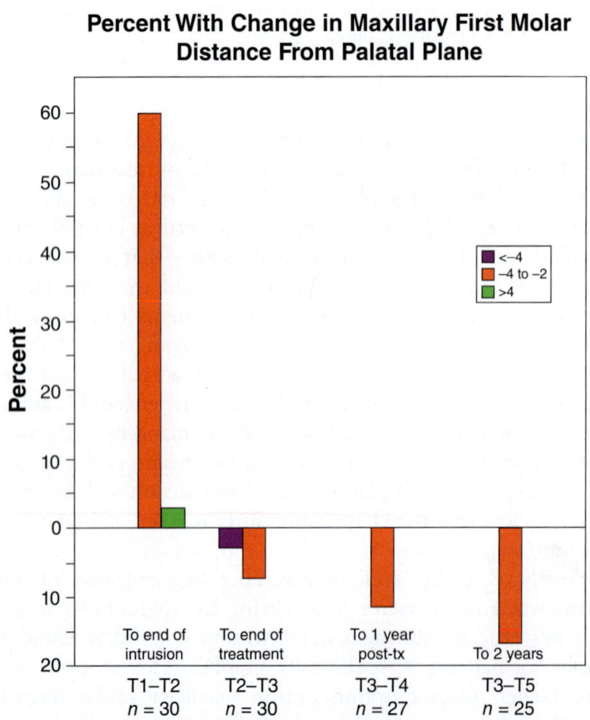

• **Fig. 20.55** Percentage of patients with change in the vertical position of the maxillary first molar relative to the palatal plane (true intrusion). Note that the number of patients with clinically significant decrease in face height (see Fig. 20.53) is less than would be expected from the geometric prediction of twice as much decrease in overjet and face height as intrusion of molars. (Redrawn from Scheffler et al. Outcomes and stability in long face/open bite patients treated with TADs and a maxillary intrusion splint. *Am J Orthod Dentofacial Orthop*. 2014;146:594–602.)

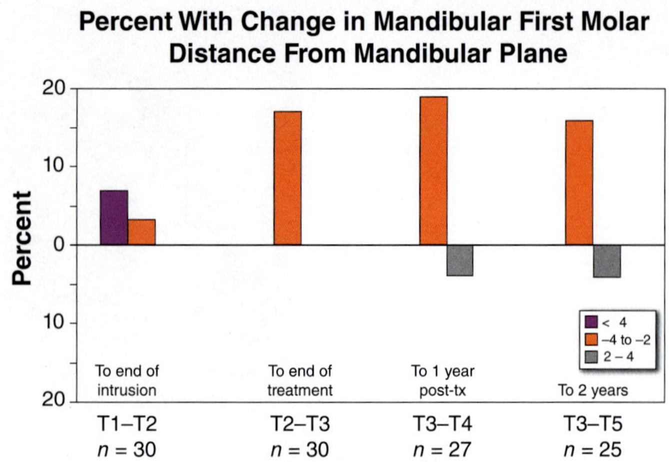

• **Fig. 20.56** Percentage of patients with clinically significant change in lower molar position from before intrusion to 2 years after treatment. (Redrawn from Scheffler et al. Outcomes and stability in long face/open bite patients treated with TADs and a maxillary intrusion splint. *Am J Orthod Dentofacial Orthop*. 2014;146:594–602.)

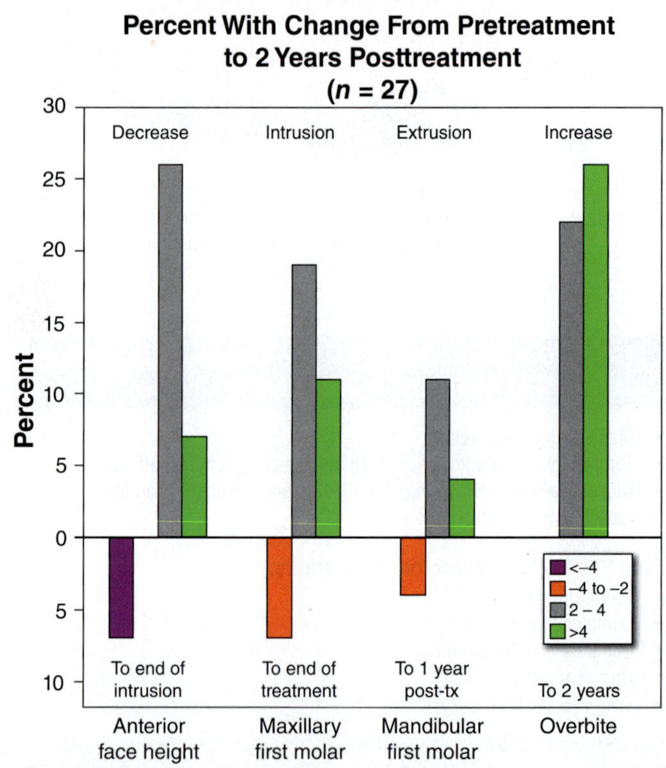

• **Fig. 20.57** Percentage of patients with changes in anterior face height, maxillary first molar vertical position, and mandibular first molar position from end of intrusion to 2 years after treatment. (Redrawn from Scheffler et al. Outcomes and stability in long face/open bite patients treated with TADs and a maxillary intrusion splint. *Am J Orthod Dentofacial Orthop*. 2014;146:594–602.)

for decrease in anterior face height. In fact, none of the patients had a return of open bite, although 20% went from positive overbite to zero overbite—that is, to an end-to-end incisor relationship. How did that happen? Because eruption of the incisors, which continued after the orthodontic treatment was completed, largely compensated for the further relapse in molar intrusion in a few patients, or for some downward movement of the maxilla (unexpected late growth) after treatment in the small number of patients in whom that occurred. It is interesting that late vertical growth also has been observed after surgical superior repositioning of the maxilla (see the comparison in Chapter 22 of this surgical procedure versus orthodontic intrusion).

Would the same outcomes occur if palatal rather than zygomatic buttress anchorage were used for posterior intrusion? No studies to answer that question have been presented, but there is no reason to think that how the teeth were intruded would change their response. After all, teeth have no way to know or care exactly how force against them was developed.

In summary:

- Maxillary molar intrusion can give satisfactory correction of moderately severe open bite (up to 6 mm in the long term from intrusion, more with extrusion of incisors).
- Control of lower molar eruption now is recognized as important in gaining the desired skeletal change and should be included routinely when maxillary molar intrusion is done (see Fig. 20.58).
- Clinical experience (unfortunately, not well documented beyond case reports) suggests that intrusion of both maxillary and mandibular posterior teeth can allow closure of more severe open bites
- Eruption of maxillary and/or mandibular incisors partially compensates for re-rotation of the mandible, so bite opening after open bite correction rarely occurs.
- It appears that Le Fort I surgery to superiorly reposition the maxilla is more likely to produce a significant shortening of anterior face height.

Are adults willing to accept as invasive a procedure as miniplates for maxillary posterior intrusion to correct severe anterior open bite? Especially when the only alternative is orthognathic surgery, most of them are. What was the treatment experience

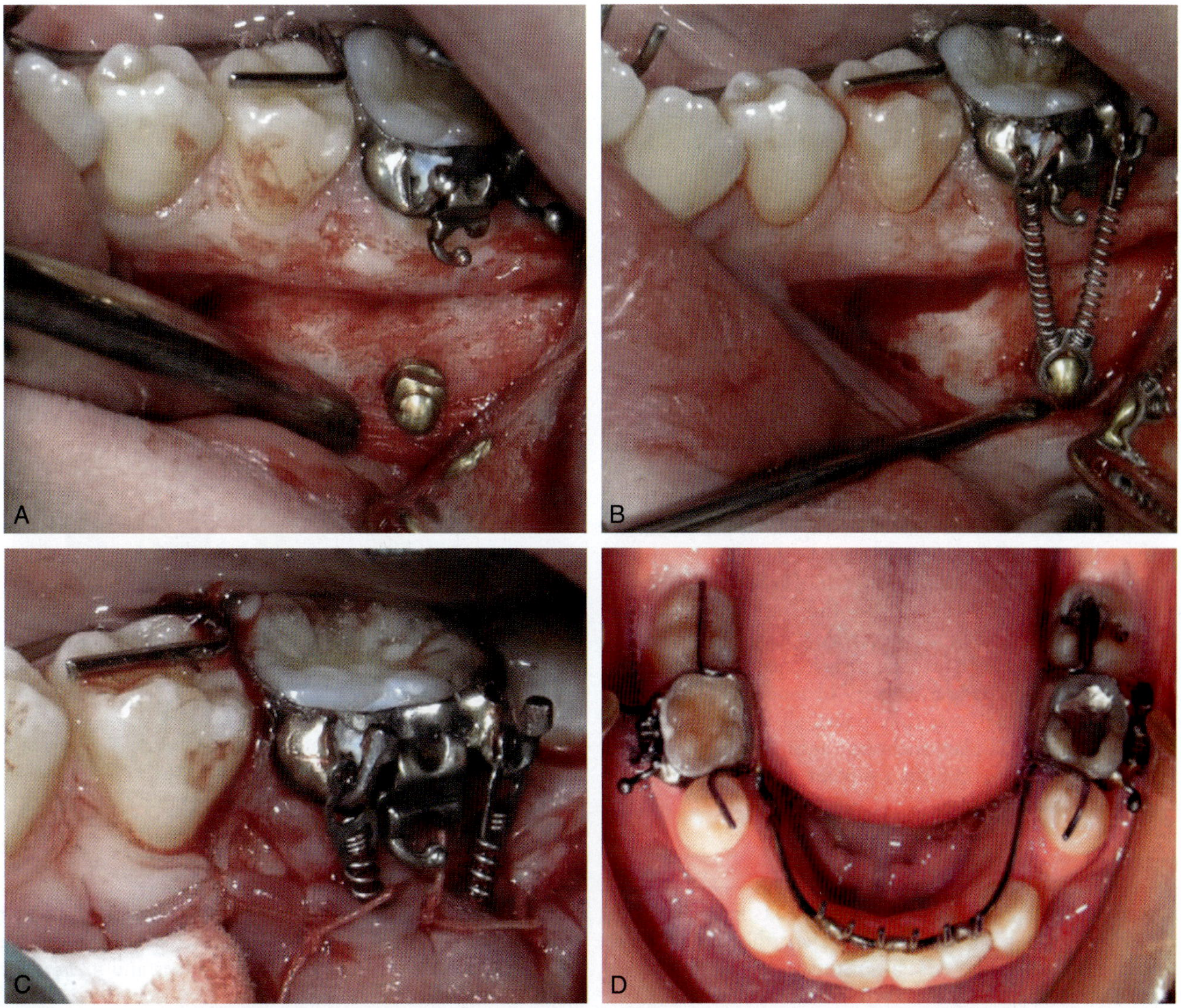

• **Fig. 20.58** Skeletal anchorage can be used to restrain eruption of lower molars or to intrude them, and if more than 6 mm closure of open bite is needed, intrusion of both upper and lower molars is needed. For mandibular posterior intrusion: (A) Alveolar bone screw placed between the molar and premolar roots; (B) nickel-titanium (NiTi) coil springs for intrusion; (C) gingival flap repositioned over the bone screw head; (D) occlusal view showing the wires to transfer force to the second molar and second premolar soldered to the molar bands. Note the adjustable lingual arch and spurs attached to the lingual arch to create tongue repositioning away from the open bite. (Courtesy Dr. J. Fisher.)

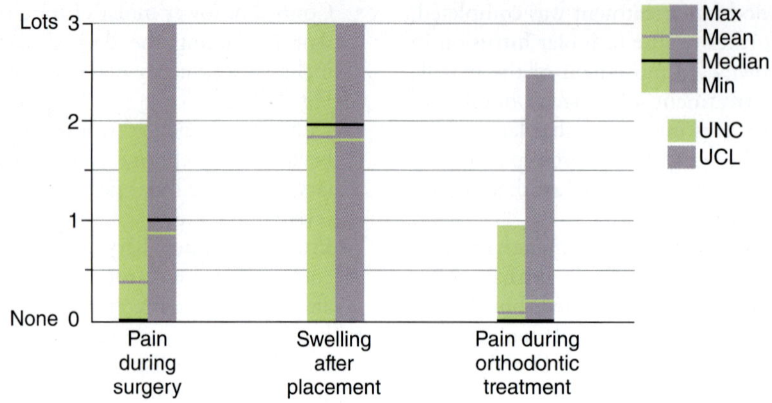

• **Fig. 20.59** Pain and swelling as reported by patients treated with miniplates as temporary skeletal anchors at University of North Carolina *(UNC)* and Université Catholique de Louvain *(UCL)*. (Redrawn from Cornelis MA, et al. Patients' and orthodontists' perceptions of miniplates used for temporary skeletal anchorage: a prospective study. *Am J Orthod Dentofacial Orthop*. 2008;133:18–24.)

like, and were they satisfied with the outcomes? The best data are for miniplates at the base of zygomatic arch, which show that problems with these multiscrew anchors are surprisingly small.[30] On a 1 to 4 scale, the mean score for pain associated with the operation was 1, minimal pain. Postsurgical swelling had a mean rating of 2, but a few patients gave it a score of 4, so it is important that patients not be surprised by the extent of swelling. There was essentially no pain or discomfort during the period of active intrusion (Fig. 20.59). After 1 year, 83% of the patients said that their experience with skeletal anchorage was better than they expected, and 73% said they did not mind having the miniplate anchor. The majority commented that they did not experience as much pain and discomfort as they thought they might.

The reaction of the doctors to miniplates was also favorable (Fig. 20.60). On a scale of 1 to 4 from very easy to very difficult, the surgeons who placed the skeletal anchorage rated the procedure as 1.7. The average time for a surgeon to place a single miniplate with two or three screws was 15 minutes. The orthodontists involved in these cases initially anticipated treatment of these patients to be somewhat or very difficult. However, with use of miniplates, the same cases were then considered to be very to moderately easy, and the orthodontists judged the complexity of use of skeletal anchorage to be very to moderately easy over all time points. At the 1-year time point, all the orthodontists said they would use miniplate anchorage again, and their average degree of satisfaction was 3.8 on a 4-point scale (3, moderately satisfied; 4, very satisfied).

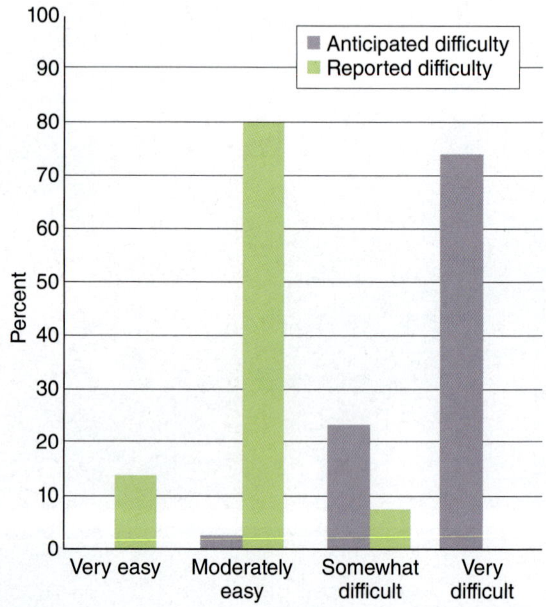

• **Fig. 20.60** Orthodontists' expectations at University of North Carolina (UNC) of difficulty of treating patients for whom miniplates as anchors were planned, and the actual difficulty these orthodontists reported. Although they had expected that almost all (98%) of the cases would be somewhat difficult or very difficult, they rated almost all the actual treatment as very easy (15%) or moderately easy (80%), and none as very difficult. (Redrawn from Cornelis MA, et al. Patients' and orthodontists' perceptions of miniplates used for temporary skeletal anchorage: a prospective study. *Am J Orthod Dentofacial Orthop*. 2008;133:18–24.)

Summary

Comprehensive orthodontic treatment for adults has gone from almost zero 55 years ago to nearly 30% of the orthodontic patient population at present. With skeletal anchorage, the range of treatment possibilities has greatly increased in recent years.

The effect on orthodontists of more treatment of adults has been greater involvement in the larger scope of dental treatment, simply because adults are much more likely to have problems that extend beyond their need for orthodontics. Most orthodontists now work more closely with dental colleagues in treatment of adults, rather than focusing almost totally on children and adolescents—and being more involved in other aspects of dentistry is stimulating and interesting, as well as important in achieving the best outcomes and greatest benefit for adult patients.

References

1. Grubb JE, Greco PM, English JD, et al. Radiographic and periodontal requirements of the American Board of Orthodontics: a modification in the case display requirements for adult and

periodontally involved adolescent and preadolescent patients. *Am J Orthod Dentofacial Orthop*. 2008;134:3–4.
2. Esteves T, Ramos AL, Pereira CM, et al. Orthodontic root resorption of endodontically treated teeth. *J Endod*. 2007;33:119–122.
3. Thilander B. Infrabony pockets and reduced alveolar bone height in relation to orthodontic therapy. *Semin Orthod*. 1996;2:55–61.
4. Ogihara S, Wang HL. Periodontal regeneration with or without limited orthodontics for the treatment of 2- or 3-wall infrabony defects. *J Periodontol*. 2010;81:1734–1742.
5. Ziskind D, Schmidt A, Hirschfeld Z. Forced eruption technique: rationale and technique. *J Prosthet Dent*. 1998;79:246–248.
6. Chudasama D, Sheridan JJ. Guidelines for contemporary air-rotor stripping. *J Clin Orthod*. 2007;41:315–320.
7. Grauer D, Heymann GC. Clinical management of tooth-size discrepancies. *J Esthet Restor Dent*. 2012;24:155–159.
8. Bamagoos AA, Sutherland K, Cistulli PA. Mandibular advancement splints. *Sleep Med Clin*. 2016;11:343–352. https://doi.org/10.1016/j.jsmc.2016.04.002. 2016.
9. Pliska BT, Nam H, Chen H, Lowe AA, Almeida FR. Obstructive sleep apnea and mandibular advancement splints: occlusal effects and progression of changes associated with a decade of treatment. *J Clin Sleep Med*. 2014;10:1285–1291. https://doi.org/10.5664/jcsm.4278. 2014.
10. Hamoda MM, Almeida FR, Pliska BT. Long-term side effects of sleep apnea treatment with oral appliances: nature, magnitude and predictors of long-term changes. *Sleep Med*. 2019;56:184–191. https://doi.org/10.1016/j.sleep.2018.12.012. Epub 2018 Dec 29. PMID: 30850300.
11. Pliska BT, Almeida FR. Tooth movement associated with CPAP therapy. *J Clin Sleep Med*. 2018;14(4):701–702. https://doi.org/10.5664/jcsm.7080. PMID: 29609723; PMCID: PMC5886451.
12. Phillips C, Broder HL, Bennett ME. Dentofacial disharmony: motivations for seeking treatment. *Int J Adult Orthod Orthognath Surg*. 1997;12:7–15.
13. Dahlström L, Carlsson GE. Temporomandibular disorders and oral health-related quality of life. A systematic review. *Acta Odontol Scand*. 2010;68:80–85.
14. Mohlin B, Axelsson S, Paulin G, et al. TMD in relation to malocclusion and orthodontic treatment. *Angle Orthod*. 2007;77:542–548.
15. Macfarlane TV, Kenealy P, Kingdon HA, et al. Twenty-year cohort study of health gain from orthodontic treatment: temporomandibular disorders. *Am J Orthod Dentofacial Orthop*. 2009;135: 692.e1–692.e8; discussion 692–693.
16. Rusanen J, Silvola AS, Tolvanen M, et al. Pathways between temporomandibular disorders, occlusal characteristics, facial pain, and oral health-related quality of life among patients with severe malocclusion. *Eur J Orthod*. 2012;34:512–517.
17. Slade GD, Ohrbach R, Greenspan JD, et al. Painful temporomandibular disorder: decade of discovery from OPPERA studies. *J Dent Res*. 2016;95:1084–1092.
18. Okeson JP. *Management of Temporomandibular Disorders and Occlusion*. 7th ed. Mosby-Elsevier; 2013.
19. Brown LJ, Brunelle JA, Kingman A. Periodontal status in the United States, 1988–91: prevalence, extent, and demographic variation. *J Dent Res*. 1996;75:672–683.
20. Türkkahraman H, Sayin MO, Bozkurt FY, et al. Archwire ligation techniques, microbial colonization, and periodontal status in orthodontically treated patients. *Angle Orthod*. 2005;75:231–236.
21. Bellamy LJ, Kokich VG, Weissman JA. Using orthodontic intrusion of abraded incisors to facilitate restoration: the technique's effects on alveolar bone level and root length. *J Am Dent Assoc*. 2008;139:725–733.
22. Shaddox LM, Huang H, Lin T, et al. Microbiological characterization in children with aggressive periodontitis. *J Dent Res*. 2012;91:927–933.
23. Grauer D, Proffit WR. Accuracy in tooth positioning with fully customized lingual orthodontic appliances. *Am J Orthod Dentofacial Orthop*. 2011;140:433–443.
24. Damon D. Treatment of the face with biocompatible orthodontics. In: Graber TM, Vanarsdall RL, Vig KWL, eds. *Orthodontic Principles and Techniques*. 4th ed. Elsevier/Mosby; 2005.
25. Lin J. *Creative Orthodontics Blending the Damon System and TADs to Manage Difficult Malocclusions*. Yong Chieh Co.; 2007.
26. Melsen B. Intrusion of incisors in adult patients with marginal bone loss. *Am J Orthod Dentofacial Orthop*. 1989;96:232–241.
27. Kosravi R, Cohanim B, Hujoel P, et al. Management of overbite with the Invisalign appliance. *Am J Orthod Dentofacial Orthop*. 2017;151:691–699.
28. Scheffler NR, Proffit WR. Skeletal anchorage technique for intrusion of maxillary posterior teeth in treatment of anterior open bite. *J Clin Orthod*. 2014;48:158–165.
29. Scheffler NR, Proffit WR, Phillips C. Outcomes and stability in long face / open bite patients treated with TADs and a maxillary intrusion splint. *Am J Orthod Dentofacial Orthop*. 2014;146:594–602.
30. Cornelis MA, Scheffler NR, Nyssen-Behets C, et al. Patients' and orthodontists' perceptions of miniplates used for temporary skeletal anchorage: a prospective study. *Am J Orthod Dentofacial Orthop*. 2008;133:18–24.

21

Clear Aligners in Adults

MATTHEW E. LARSON, BRENT E. LARSON, AND REGINA BLEVINS

CHAPTER OUTLINE

Aligners Versus Fixed Treatment in Adults

Many adults seeking orthodontic care are conscience of esthetics and prefer minimal disruptions to their normal lifestyle. Therefore it is not surprising that there is a large demand for clear aligner treatment in adults. Treatment can often be accomplished with good esthetics, although the attachments and aligners will be slightly visible—this can be a surprise for some patients expecting it to be completely "invisible." Additionally, aligner treatment offers more flexibility in appointment timing and length, including the potential for virtual visits at certain points. It is important to note that the initial diagnosis, attachment placement, interproximal adjustments, and attachment removal are all important steps in the aligner process that will require in-person visits.

Benefits and Limitations of Aligners

Overall benefits and limitations of aligner treatment in adults are very similar to those for adolescents discussed in Chapter 18 and detailed in Table 18.1. However, due to the fact that adult patients are non-growing and have had permanent teeth in the mouth for a longer period of time, some of these issues become more impactful.

First of all, as mentioned, adult patients are often conscious of esthetics and want the least disruption to their usual lifestyle. In most cases, this gives a preference towards aligner treatment versus traditional braces. However, depending on daily habits that may inhibit good aligner wear, like frequently sipping coffee throughout the morning or snacking throughout the day, braces are occasionally the more acceptable option. Also, some malocclusions can be treated more efficiently with one method or the other—for instance, minor alignment or spacing issues can typically be corrected easily with aligners, while braces may be better suited for correction of significant deep bites. A recent randomized controlled trial showed that for mild malocclusions, similar outcomes could be produced with aligners and braces, but the aligner treatment took several months longer, on average.[1]

Another difference in adult patients is the degree of exposed tooth structure—continued passive eruption typically leads to more tooth surface area being available to increase retention and improve aligner engagement. Also, it's more common to see heavily restored dentitions in adults. Porcelain and metal can be challenging surfaces to attach bonded brackets, so aligners can be preferable in those cases.

With aging, the velocity of tooth movement can also change. Iwasaki et al. found that for tooth translation, growing individuals had movement that was 1.5 times faster than non-growing subjects.[2] Therefore it can be hard to correctly plan the velocity of tooth movement during treatment. With braces, adjustments can be made to the wire activation at each appointment. However, with aligners, the provider may have to adjust the time of wear for each aligner (i.e. switch from changing every 7 to every 10 days) or the staging to make the incremental movements at a slower velocity (which involves fabrication of new trays). In adults, it can be challenging at times to know whether the lack of the teeth tracking with the aligners is due to poor compliance, poor aligner design or mechanics, or just slow biology.

Challenges in Adult Patients

Clear aligner treatment in adults can be challenging for the reasons listed with clear aligner biomechanics for adolescents in Chapter 18 along with the general challenges of adult treatment discussed in Chapter 20. Some key issues in this regard are lack of growth, presence of restorations, worn or missing teeth, increased need for multidisciplinary care, and patient compliance.

Since adult patients have largely completed their jaw growth and tooth eruption (recognizing that small changes continue throughout life), changes to occlusion can be more challenging. Specifically, since the skeletal base is not changing, anterior-posterior correction and vertical changes can be difficult, if not impossible, without surgery. These corrections must come only from tooth movement and not some combination of tooth movement and growth as is seen in adolescents. Additionally, vertical control becomes critical as there is no continued ramus growth to compensate for careless mechanics that may result in extrusion of posterior teeth.

In terms of tooth anatomy, it is common in adult patients to see effects of aging in their dentition. This can be related to localized tooth wear due to their specific malocclusion or to years of parafunction. Additionally, altered tooth anatomy can be related to restorations that were placed attempting to provide better alignment, or occlusal improvement, by changing crown shape while leaving the roots in a poor position. Also, it is more common to see periodontal disease, both in terms of bone loss and gingival recession, in adult patients. Sometimes this can be relatively minor, but without addressing the periodontal issues prior to treatment, it can worsen during the course of care. Finally, missing teeth are frequently encountered—in fact, idealizing space for implants is a common reason for adults seeking orthodontic treatment.

With the increased frequency of restorative and periodontal needs in adult patients, it is a high priority to have good communication with the patient's entire dental team before, during and after any aligner treatment. In the presence of periodontal disease, control of active disease and inflammation should be verified with the general dentist, or periodontist, prior to starting treatment. Final implant and buildup spacing should be coordinated early to ensure treatment is directly progressing to the endpoint that is agreed upon at the beginning. Thankfully, the digital planning tools essential to aligner treatment are amazing tools to simulate the final tooth size and position for collaborative planning purposes. Fig. 21.1 demonstrates the use of readily available tools to communicate a final restorative option to the restorative dentist in

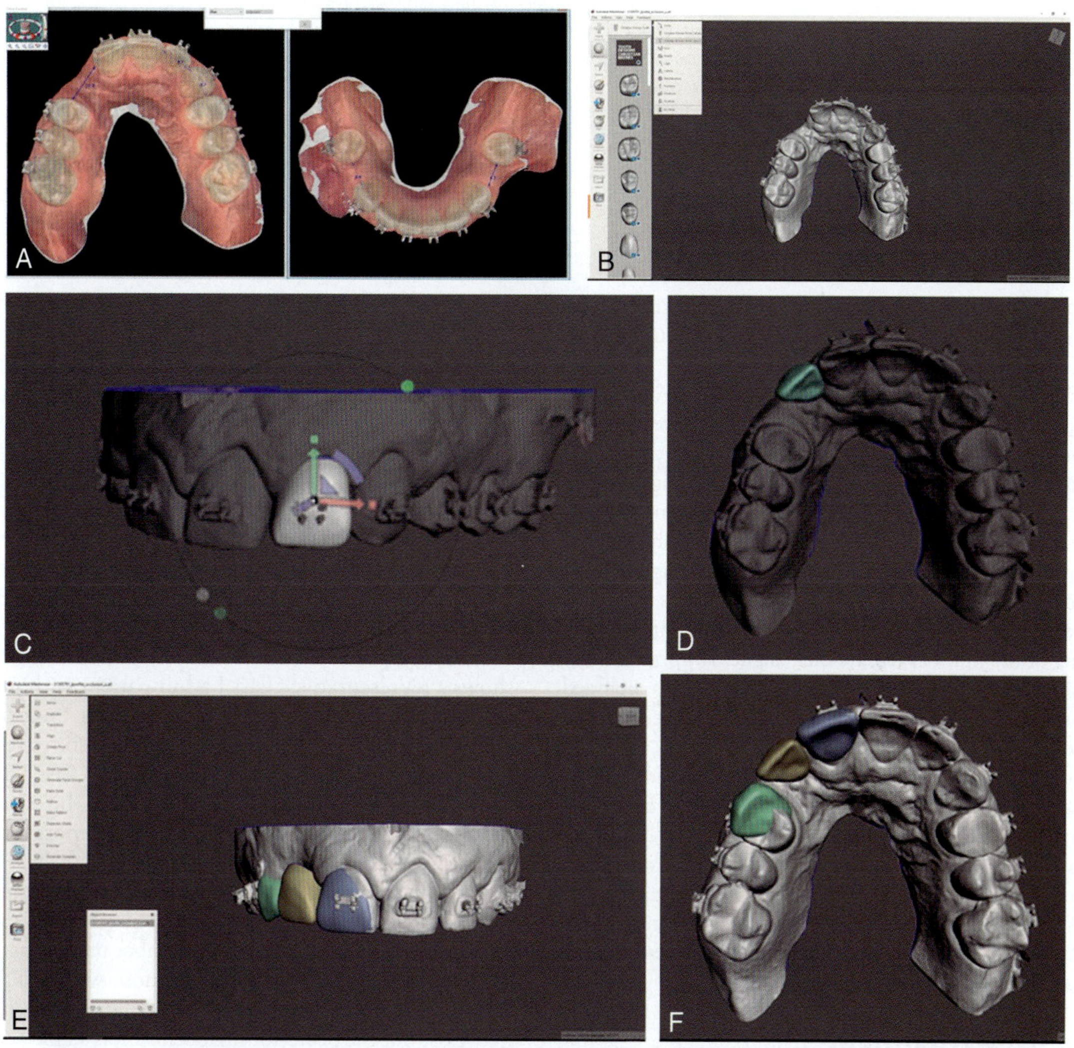

• **Fig. 21.1** Complex adult case with missing teeth needing orthodontic and restorative care. (A) Progress intraoral scan with brackets on. (B) Upper arch scan imported into Meshmixer (free 3D program for working with meshes) with tooth library installed. (C) Upper lateral incisor selected from the library and matched to the size of existing left lateral incisor. (D) Lateral incisor mirrored to the right side and placed into position. (E and F) Frontal and occlusal views of upper arch with lateral incisor replaced and similar techniques used to adjust the size of the central incisor and simulate the use of the premolar as the canine. These 3D simulations are very effective communication tools to insure all members of the dental team are visualizing an achievable outcome.

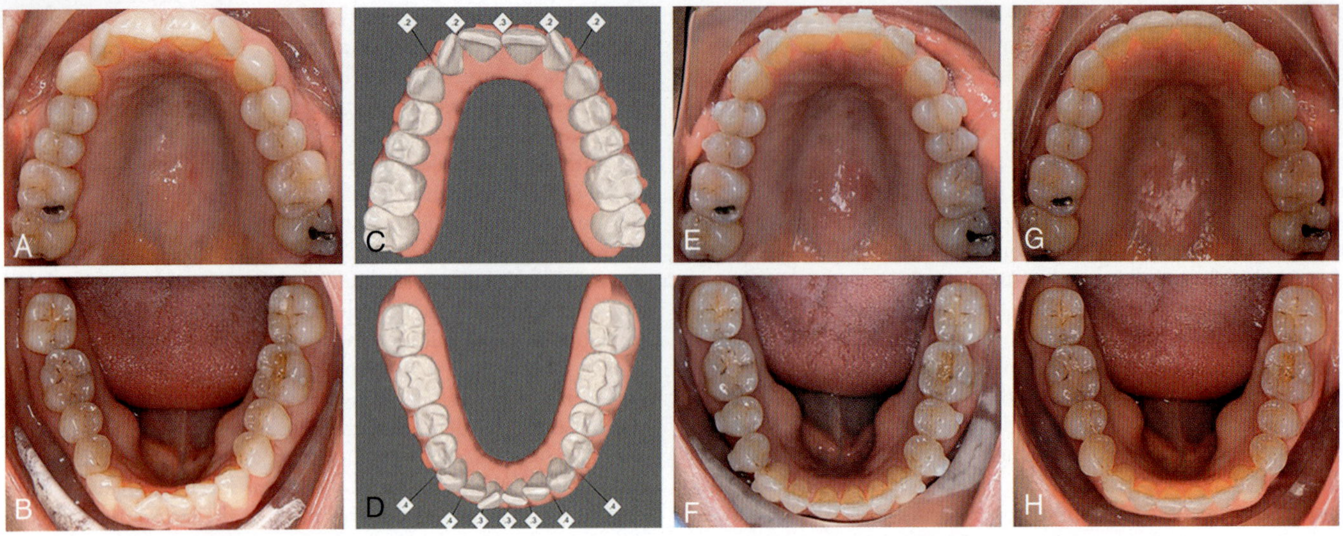

• **Fig. 21.2** Representative adult Class I malocclusion of mild difficulty treated successfully with aligners. (A and B) Initial presentation of upper and lower arches showing the intra-arch alignment needed. (C and D) Digital representation of the planned interproximal reduction to allow space for alignment while retaining acceptable incisor positioning. (E and F) Progress photos of the arches with attachments in place and with most alignment corrected. (G and H) Final photos showing the excellent alignment achieved as a result of thoughtful planning, appropriate tooth-size reduction and good aligner wear.

a complex adult with multiple missing teeth. This advanced level of 3D simulation allows the final occlusal plan to be adjusted with the input of the whole dental team.

One final challenge often seen in adults is compliance and burnout with aligner wear. The recommendation for aligner wear is typically to have the aligners in place for 20 to 22 hr/day. Some companies market "new technology" allowing reduced hours for aligner wear, but remember the full-time recommendation comes from biologic principles discussed in Chapter 8. Tooth movement typically does not start until at least 4 hours of force application, so there is significantly more daily movement that occurs in 20 versus 12 hours. Reduced hours of wear will require adjustments either to the amount of movement per aligner or the number of days each aligner is worn. A study using anonymous data from a self-report monitoring app analyzed data on a cohort of over 2500 adult patients and found that 36% had full compliance with full-time (22 hours) wear instructions, 38% had fair compliance and about 25% had poor compliance.[3] In addition to daily wear considerations, comprehensive aligner cases can take 12 to 36 months, while clinicians realize that many patients tolerate aligner wear well for about 12 months and then compliance tends to wane. The lesson is that for complex adult aligner cases that are expected to last more than 12 to 15 months, extra care should be taken to make sure the patient understands that long-term commitment is essential to treatment success.

Comprehensive Treatment

Although major changes to occlusion can be more difficult without growth, comprehensive orthodontic treatment that treats the occlusal discrepancy is still the goal in most adult cases. There are situations where compromises may need to be made in the occlusal correction or the alignment due to the patient's desire to avoid adjunctive fixed appliances, extractions, or orthognathic surgery. In these cases, informed consent is critical as the treatment may not lead to an ideal outcome due to the factors just discussed. In spite of these limitations, many comprehensive cases can be well treated with aligners, however, and the difficulty in correction of various malocclusion categories is described later.

Mild Difficulty

The most predictable aligner cases in adults consist of mainly intra-arch movements, with minimal inter-arch movements. In other words, crowding or spacing within each arch with minimal root movements will be the easiest patients to treat. Fig. 21.2 shows a representative Class I adult patient with moderate upper and lower crowding treated with aligners to correct the intra-arch alignment problems. Cases with crossbites (especially more than single-tooth crossbites), Class II or Class III occlusal relationships, deep bites or significant open bites, and situations requiring significant root movement are more challenging and are discussed below.

Even in cases with mild crowding, it is quite common in adults to use interproximal reduction as a method to create space for alignment. This can be due to a number of reasons. Bolton tooth-size discrepancies are easier to diagnose with a digital setup and easy to address in the digital plan. Mild A-P occlusal deviations may exist but the posterior malocclusion is stable and worth maintaining, so the treatment of choice is adjusting the overjet with appropriate IPR. Also, any issues with gingival recession, particularly with anterior tooth overlap, may also lead to black triangles (open gingival embrasures) between the teeth after alignment. This issue and the resolution that can be provided with aligners and IPR are shown in Fig. 21.3.

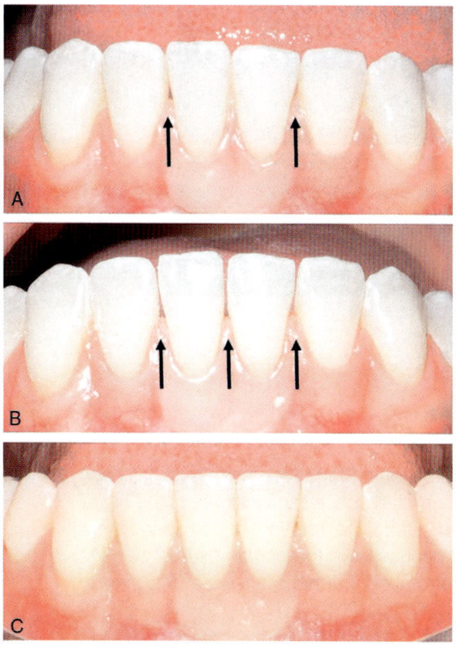

• **Fig. 21.3** Example of the use of interproximal reduction (IPR) and a limited number of aligners to eliminate open gingival embrasures (*black triangles*) that result when the gingival papilla does not fill the gingival embrasure. This is often an esthetic issue that is present in adults. (A) *Arrows* point to the open gingival embrasures present prior to treatment. (B) IPR completed producing spaces (*arrows*) and less tapered tooth morphology. (C) After wear of aligners to close the spaces and create a longer connector between teeth and therefore eliminating the open gingival embrasures.

Moderate Challenges

As a clinician's skill and experience with aligner use increases, more challenging cases can be treated, including more significant rotations, crossbites, A-P movements, and changes to overbite. However, a systematic review indicated that although aligners can produce similar outcomes to fixed appliance treatment, the predictability of many movements is still low and refinements will be needed in almost every case to compensate for this lack of predictability.[4,5] More significant crowding or spacing can be treated with similar principles to smaller movements, but it is even more critical to ensure adequate space is created between teeth to allow the desired movements and to verify that the teeth track in the aligner throughout treatment. This can be seen in the case shown in Fig. 21.4 and the select screenshots of the digital plan to correct the rotation shown in Fig. 21.5.

Changes to the A-P relationships of the dentition can also be made with aligners. It is important to note that for adults, this will be due to dental changes only, so planning should ensure teeth remain in a healthy position within alveolar bone. Methods of attaching elastics to achieve Class II/Class III bite correction are shown in Chapter 18. A case where the use of inter-arch elastics achieved successful occlusal correction is shown in Fig. 21.6. Note, this case also illustrates a few other important points in A-P bite correction in adults. First, derotation of upper molars is often critical in helping achieve proper molar correction in Class II malocclusions. The maxillary first molars typically rotate forward around the lingual root, so derotation around that lingual root will tend to distalize the buccal cusps tips and gain 1 to 2 mm of A-P correction. It is apparent that the restored dentition does not fit quite as well in the new class I position because the restorations were contoured to fit the original malocclusion, and also, the worn lower left central incisor is more obvious following overbite correction, so potential restorative work for this tooth after treatment should be discussed.

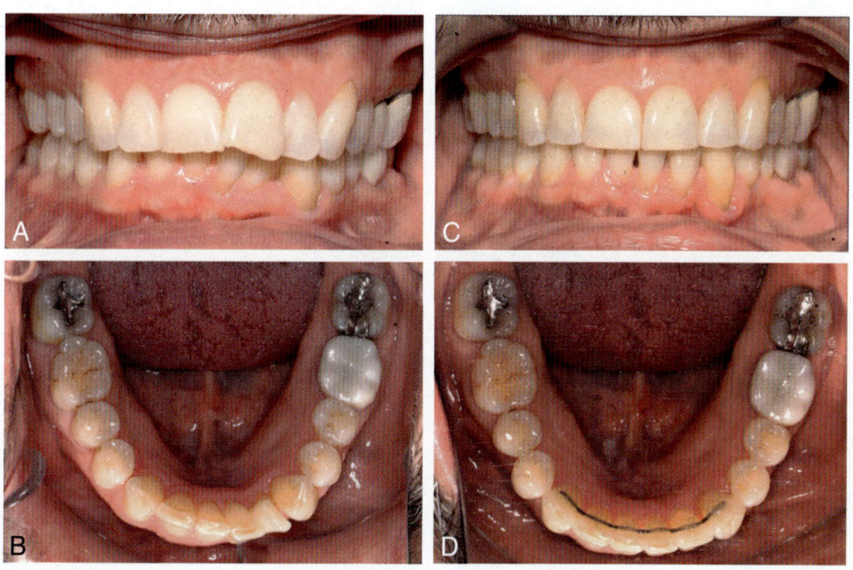

• **Fig. 21.4** Adult patient with a moderately challenging situation due to the significant rotation of the lower left lateral incisor. (A and B) Frontal and lower occlusal views of the initial presentation showing the nearly 90 degree rotation of the lateral incisor. (C and D) Same views after aligner treatment showing improved alignment in both arches, but particularly the full correction of the rotated lateral incisor. Note the use of a fixed retainer bonded to all six lower anterior teeth to prevent relapse of the incisor correction.

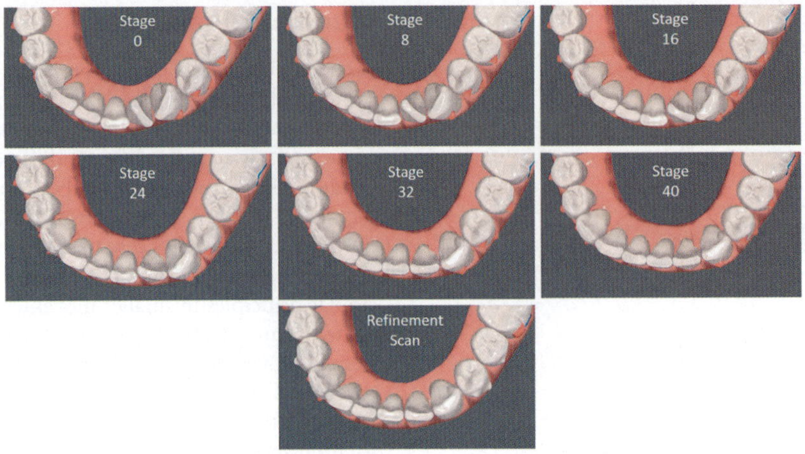

• **Fig. 21.5** Screenshots of the digital plan for the patient in Fig. 21.4. Note that at Stage 8 a small space has been created around the rotated incisor to allow rotation without collision. That small space is maintained in the digital plan through Stages 16, 24, and 32 as smooth rotation is planned. Once the rotation is complete, small space-closing movements occur by Stage 40. The Refinement Scan panel shows the actual result of the first series of aligners resulting in good, but not complete, correction of the rotation. Further trays were designed to complete the correction shown in Fig. 21.4.

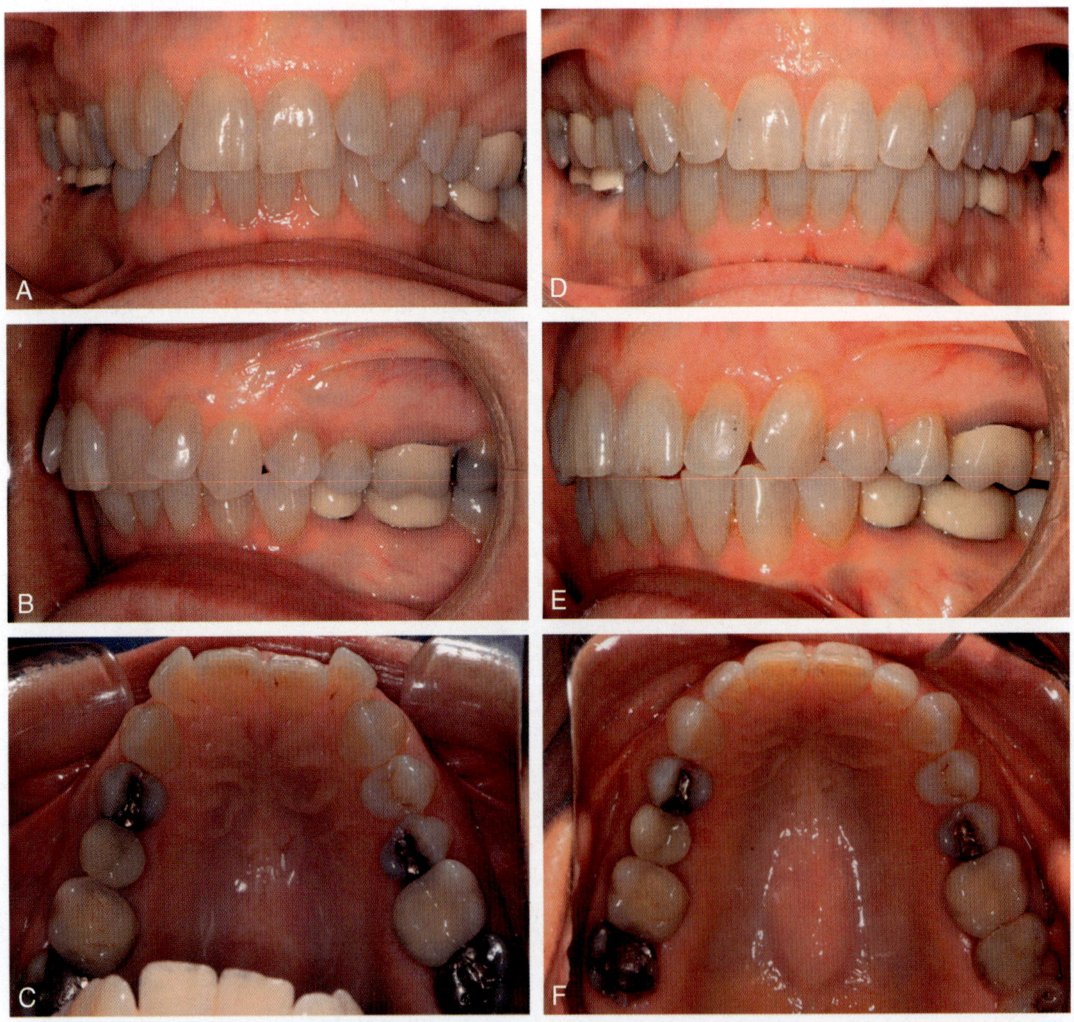

• **Fig. 21.6** Adult Class II malocclusion treated with aligners and class II elastics for A-P correction. (A–C) Pretreatment views of the malocclusion demonstrating a Class II molar and canine relationship along with significant incisor irregularities. (D–F) Same patient after aligner treatment with correction of the molar and canine relationship to Class I and much improved anterior tooth alignment. Note the need to derotate the upper molars for Class II correction and the challenge in dealing with restored teeth, whose shape was built to fit the previous malocclusion, making ideal tooth interdigitation difficult.

Complex Cases

Treating complex cases with Invisalign or other clear aligner alternatives can appear deceptively similar to treatment of less severe problems. Treatment still involves the use of a sequence of aligners that lead to a predicted endpoint, but there are four big differences: (1) the sequence of steps typically suggested by the computer algorithms and/or digital technicians typically needs significant modification, (2) the direction and amount of movement of teeth produced by the standard algorithms often are reduced, (3) it is more common to add adjunctive appliances (limited braces, TADs, etc.), and (4) progress records and a new set of revision aligners are needed, often more than once, during the treatment process.

What this means is a much greater involvement of the doctor during the planning and clinical management of these cases. Standard "ideal" setups created by a technician with standardized staging may produce reasonable results in mild to moderate cases, but in complex cases more significant overcorrection and intentional planning of the staging is required. As an example, in anterior open-bite closure, significant posterior open bites may need to be programmed in the digital plan to move the teeth to the desired finish (Fig. 21.7).

Additionally, when extractions are combined with aligners, like the case in Fig. 21.8, good anchorage is required either by using appropriate attachments or by creating space around the anchorage teeth during retraction (see Fig. 18.9). Also, attachment design and overall staging need to be well designed to maintain root control. Using these guidelines, properly selected extraction cases can be well treated with aligners when there is good patient compliance with prescribed aligner wear (Fig. 21.9).

Why would progress records and revision, or refinement, aligners more often be needed in complex situations? Experience has shown that as the amount of movement and treatment steps increase, it is better to set an initial goal that is intermediate to the final goal and then establish the sequence of aligners starting from that midpoint to complete the treatment. The golf analogy would be a chip and a short putt is likely to produce a better result than a really long putt. The similarity to fixed appliances would be to take progress records and reposition brackets to achieve the needed movement to reach the goals.

Hybrid Treatment

Hybrid treatment for adults utilizes similar methods as discussed for adolescent in Chapter 18, except the need for hybrid treatment increases due to the increased prevalence of tipped or missing teeth, occlusal changes, lack of growth, and other issues that make adult treatment more challenging.

With significant open bite, active splints attached to miniscrews as seen in Fig. 20.53 can be used prior to aligner treatment. This can change the clinical situation for the aligner treatment from a significant open-bite treatment to a mild open-bite case in need of only posterior setting and alignment.

Occasionally, a single arch is complex enough that treatment with fixed appliances and miniscrews may be required. In these cases, hybrid treatment can be possible, as shown in Fig. 21.10, where the unilateral open bite was closed using a hybrid technique.

Root Uprighting

In cases where teeth are missing, it is common to see teeth adjacent to the missing tooth tip into that space over time. A relatively common issue where adults benefit from adjunctive treatment is when additional space for the missing tooth needs to be created and idealized for implants, or the space potentially closed altogether if possible.

Root uprighting is possible with aligners alone, as in Fig. 21.11, when there is good surface area of tooth exposed and a large attachment, or attachments, can be placed to assist the movement. However, in many cases, there is not adequate exposed surface area, so placement of limited braces can be useful to create an efficient force system to upright that tooth either prior to aligner treatment or concurrently as shown in Fig. 18.29.

Deep Bite Correction

Finally, correction of deep bites can be achieved in adults with aligners.

Deep bite correction in adults is similar to what is described in Chapter 18 but is even more challenging due to the lack of vertical growth. This is illustrated in the patient shown in Fig. 21.12. Notice that anterior bite ramps (discussed in Chapter 18) can help with bite opening in deep bite cases, and retentive posterior attachments are critical. Also, this case would have been substantially more difficult if proclination of the incisors to correct the crowding was not a treatment goal. The cephalometric superimposition shows some true intrusion of incisors, but much of the deep bite correction happened due to incisor proclination. However, deep bite cases with generalized spacing are even more challenging, as the space closure will tend to upright the incisors and increase the overbite.

Mild to moderate deep bite cases can show a significant improvement using good mechanics with aligners alone. This will include anterior bite turbos, large posterior seating attachments, and proclination where possible.

In patients with a severe anterior overbite, discussing the potential for lower braces if minimal progress is observed or even committing to braces from the start can be wise. Unfortunately, severe overbite cases are often the once most important to fully correct in order to provide adequate space for planned restorative work. Additionally, if there is already significant lower tooth wear, there is no room to place lower braces both in terms of available tooth structure and the required occlusal clearance (Fig. 21.13). In this situation, treatment with aligners may be the best available option, even if not terribly efficient.

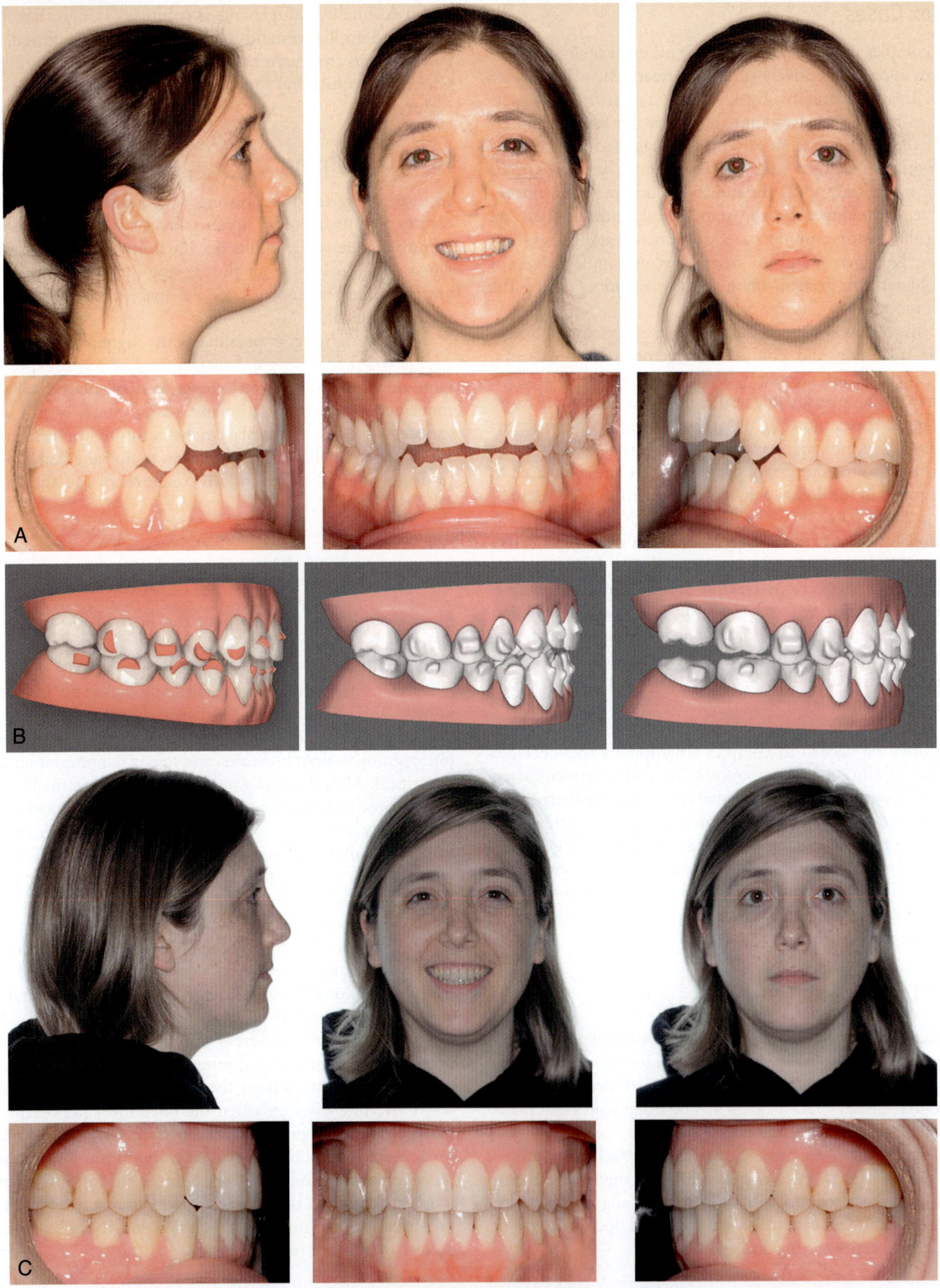

• **Fig. 21.7** Adult anterior open bite treated with aligners. (A) Pretreatment photographs showing significant anterior open bite and flat smile arc. (B) Select screen capture images showing the initial setup on the left with a slight posterior opening planned, the center image displays the actual result after the first series of trays, and the right image shows the exaggerated posterior opening required during refinement that allowed for complete correction. (C) Posttreatment photos demonstrating closure of the anterior open bite and improvement of the smile arc using the overcorrection principles demonstrated in B. Complex malocclusions such as this require significant provider monitoring and thoughtful adjustment to reach the desired outcome.

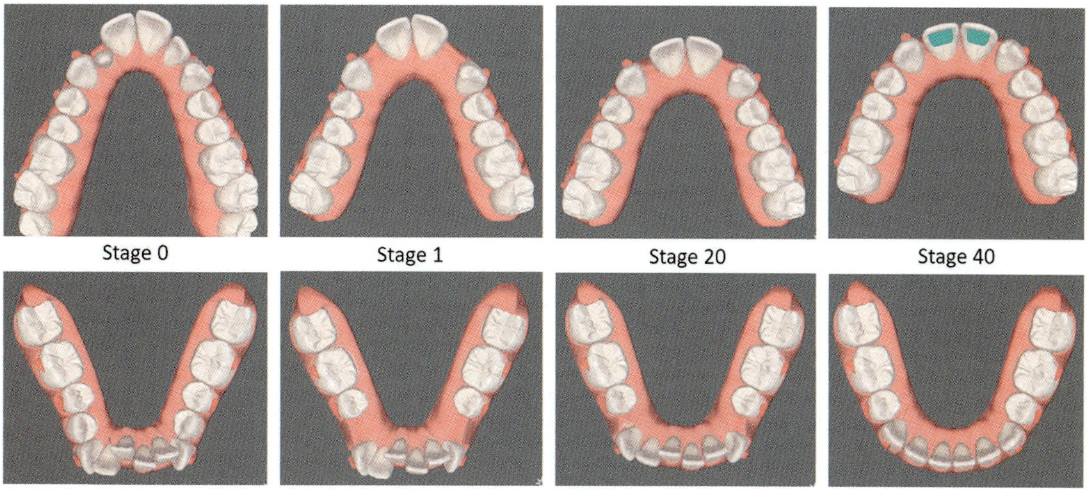

• **Fig. 21.8** Select screenshots of select stages of the digital plan for the adult extraction case shown in Fig. 21.9. This individual was treatment planned to have the upper lateral incisors and lower first premolars removed. Stage 0 shows the attachment design to provide anchorage for the planned tooth movements. Stage 1 shows the digital extraction of the teeth including the upper third molars. Stage 20 shows the sequential canine retraction in the lower arch and the archform changes beginning in the upper arch. Stage 40 shows the addition of bite ramps on the upper central incisors to control the overbite that tends to increase as the incisors are tipped lingually. Overall, this plan demonstrates the thoughtful selection of an extraction case that requires limited root movement and the sequential staging needed for successful plan implementation.

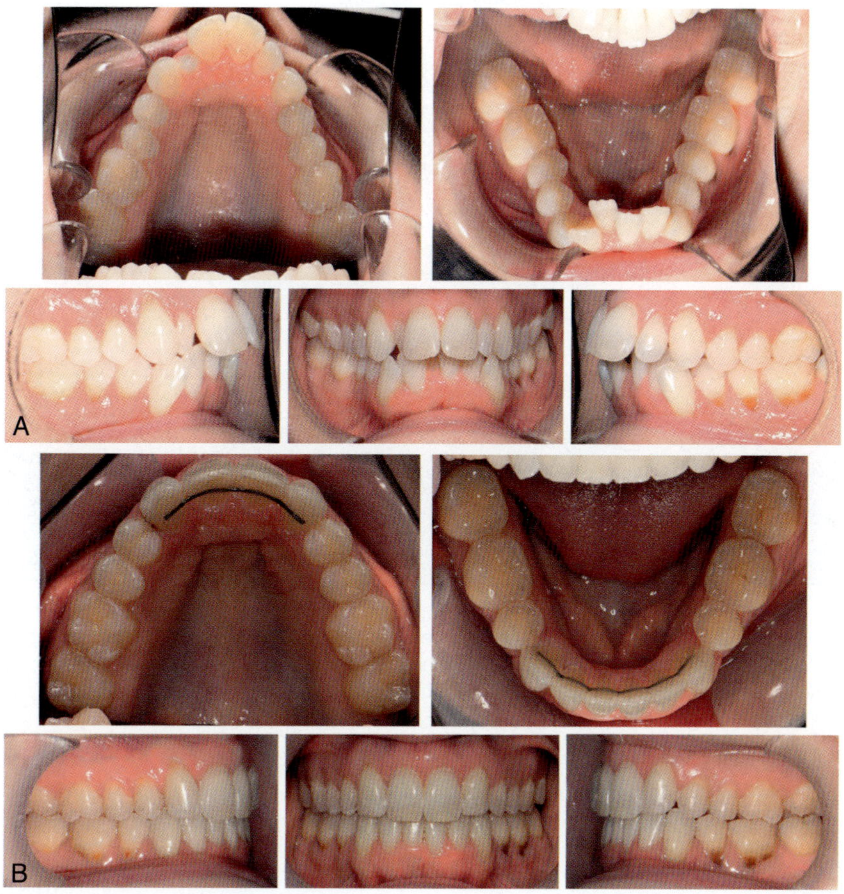

• **Fig. 21.9** Clinical treatment photographs of the patient whose digital plan appears in Fig. 21.8. (A) Intraoral pretreatment images of the adult planned for extractions and aligner treatment showing severe lower crowding, small upper lateral incisors, and generalized gingival recession. (B) Posttreatment images of the same patient after completion of aligner treatment using the digital plan presented in Fig. 21.8. The upper canines are substituted for the lateral incisors while the molar relationship remains class I. Bonded retainers are used in both arches—in the upper arch to maintain the space closure and in the lower arch to retain the alignment. The gingival recession remains largely unchanged because the tooth movement was planned to keep the roots within the existing alveolar housing.

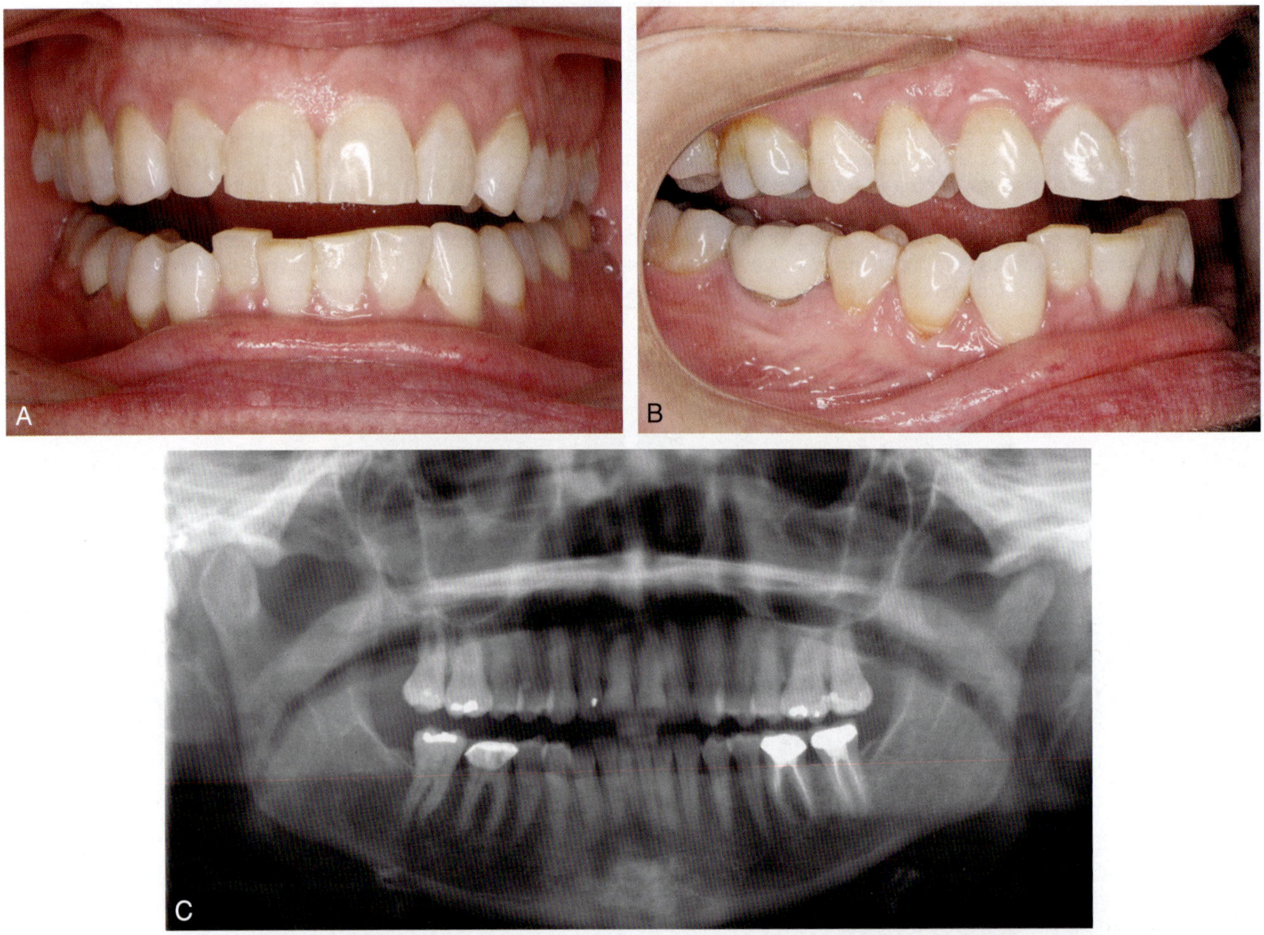

• **Fig. 21.10** Invisalign can be combined with fixed appliance treatment to achieve tooth movement that would be very difficult with Invisalign alone. (A and B) For this 47-year-old female, an unusual unilateral open bite had developed slowly over the previous 5 years, with little or no change during the last year. (C) The panoramic radiograph showed condylar asymmetry, with resorption of the left condyle that was tentatively attributed to osteoarthritis.

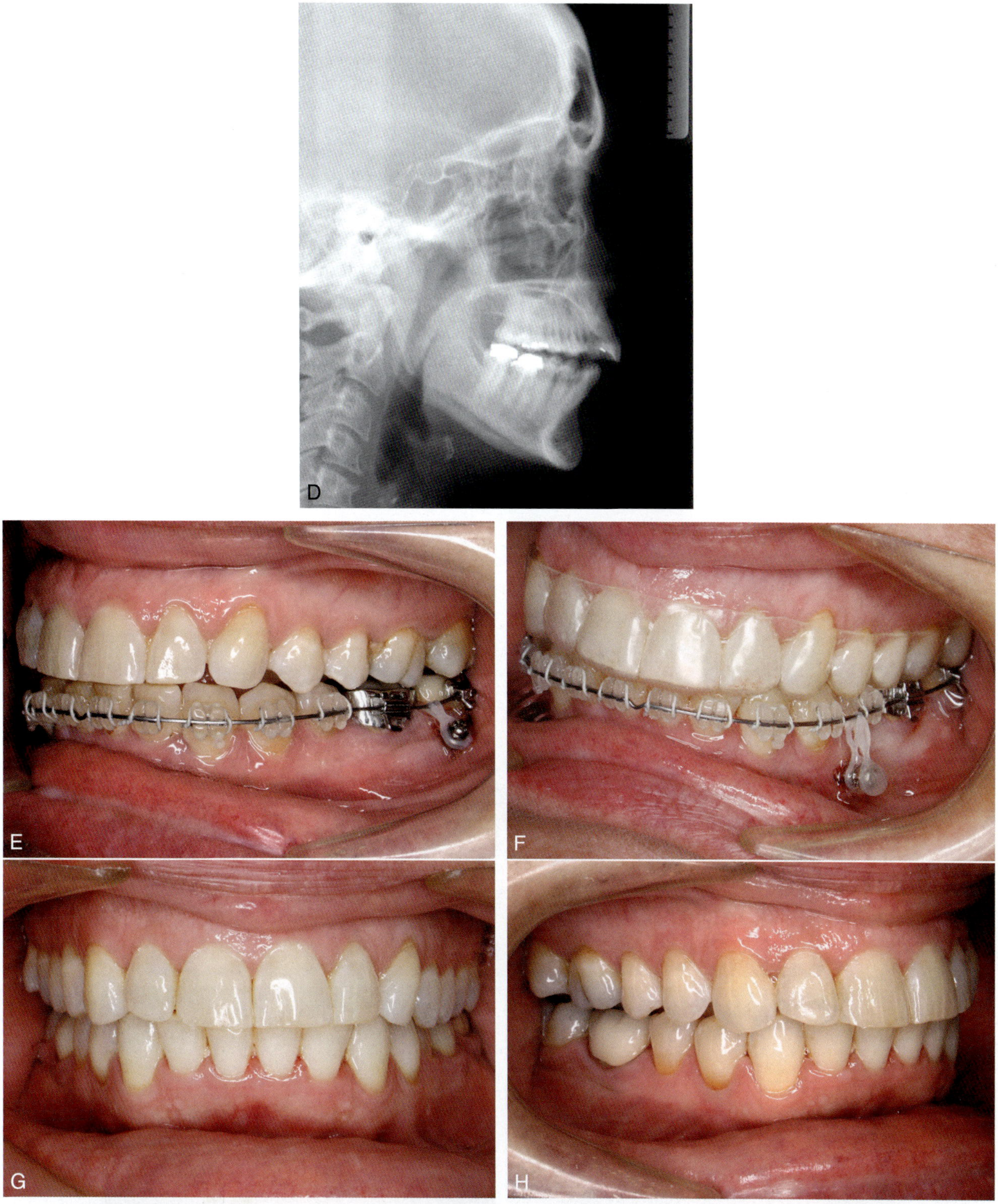

• **Fig. 21.10, cont'd** (D) The cephalometric radiograph showed a different vertical level of the mandibular posterior teeth on the two sides, and virtual intrusion of the mandibular posterior teeth on the left side indicated that this would allow the mandible to rotate upward and forward, closing the unilateral open bite and bringing her to nearly normal occlusion. The treatment plan was to use a fixed appliance in the lower arch with skeletal anchorage to close the posterior teeth on the left side and close the open bite, while aligning the upper arch with Invisalign and completing treatment with Invisalign in both arches. (E) Bone screw as anchorage for intrusion of the mandibular molars. (F) A second bone screw later for anchorage to intrude the premolars. While the intrusion was occurring, a series of aligners was used in the maxillary arch; note the final aligner being used as a retainer at this point in treatment. Once the bite was closed (which took 8 months), the expected relapse tendency was not observed during the next 6 months, and at that point a revision series of aligners was used over a period of another 4 months to complete the treatment. (G and H) Frontal and lateral posttreatment views. At 3 years' posttreatment *(not pictured)*, the mild posterior open bite on the right side had closed, and the anterior open bite correction was stable. (Courtesy Dr. W. Gierie.)

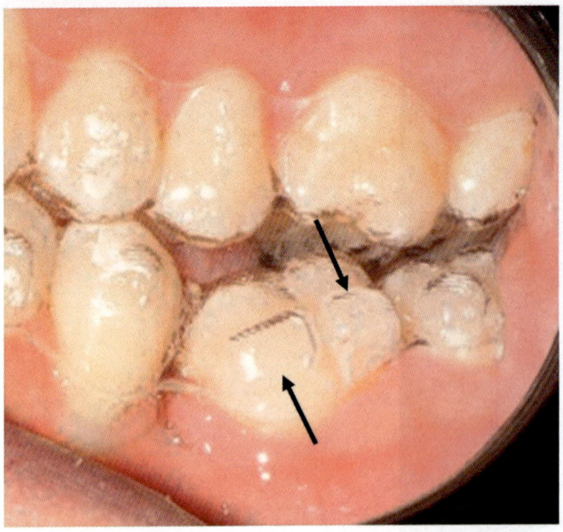

• **Fig. 21.11** An example of a tipped tooth that is able to be uprighted using aligners only. The exposed facial surface of the tipped molar is large enough to place two horizontal attachments in order to generate an uprighting couple on the tooth. The arrows demonstrate the two important places the aligner is engaging the attachments to provide the desired couple.

Limited Treatment

One unique advantage with aligners is that individual teeth can be moved without as many unwanted side effects to control. This is because it is more difficult in general to get root movement and therefore the undesired tooth movement. Also, movement can be limited to certain teeth, using the full dentition as anchorage to minimize side effects. This can be very advantageous in situations where limited, localized tooth movement is planned or needed such as in cases of orthodontic relapse where minor movements are needed to touch-up the alignment or to close small spaces that may have opened.

Crowding

A common occurrence following orthodontic treatment is minor relapse during retention. The small corrective movements that are needed to reverse these unwanted changes can be dealt with very efficiently with aligners. The big benefit is that you can predictably maintain the posterior occlusion while improving the position of the teeth needing correction. Occasionally, this can be done

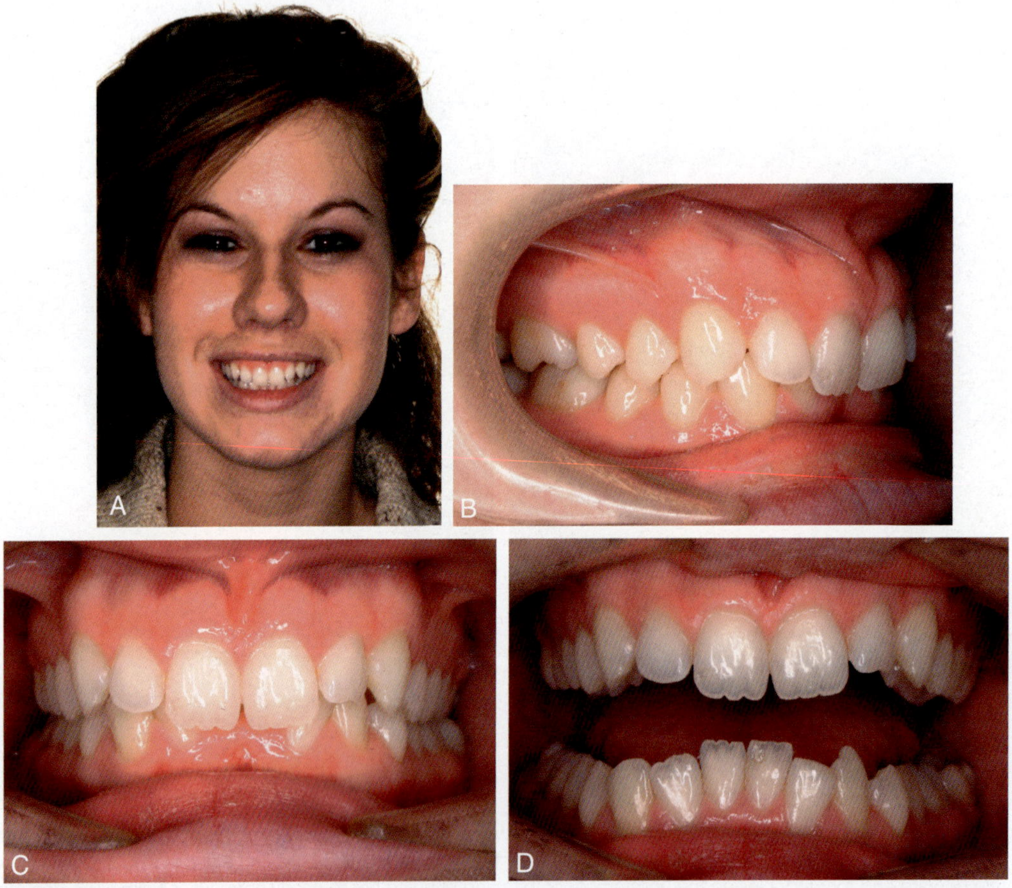

• **Fig. 21.12** Because Invisalign aligners provide light force, intrusion of teeth with aligners is quite possible. In a patient with a deep bite as shown here, an important question is the amount of intrusion of incisors versus extrusion of posterior teeth and increase in anterior face height. Bite ramps on the lingual aspect of maxillary incisors open the bite posteriorly and facilitate molar eruption; thickening of the aligner material over the posterior teeth would inhibit eruption. (A–D) Initial records for a young adult for whom intrusion of maxillary and mandibular central incisors was desired, along with a moderate increase in anterior face height. The plan was an initial stage of treatment with 23 aligners to an intermediate goal with forward movement and intrusion of the maxillary central incisors, followed by forward movement, alignment, and intrusion of the mandibular incisors, then new records and revision aligners to complete treatment.

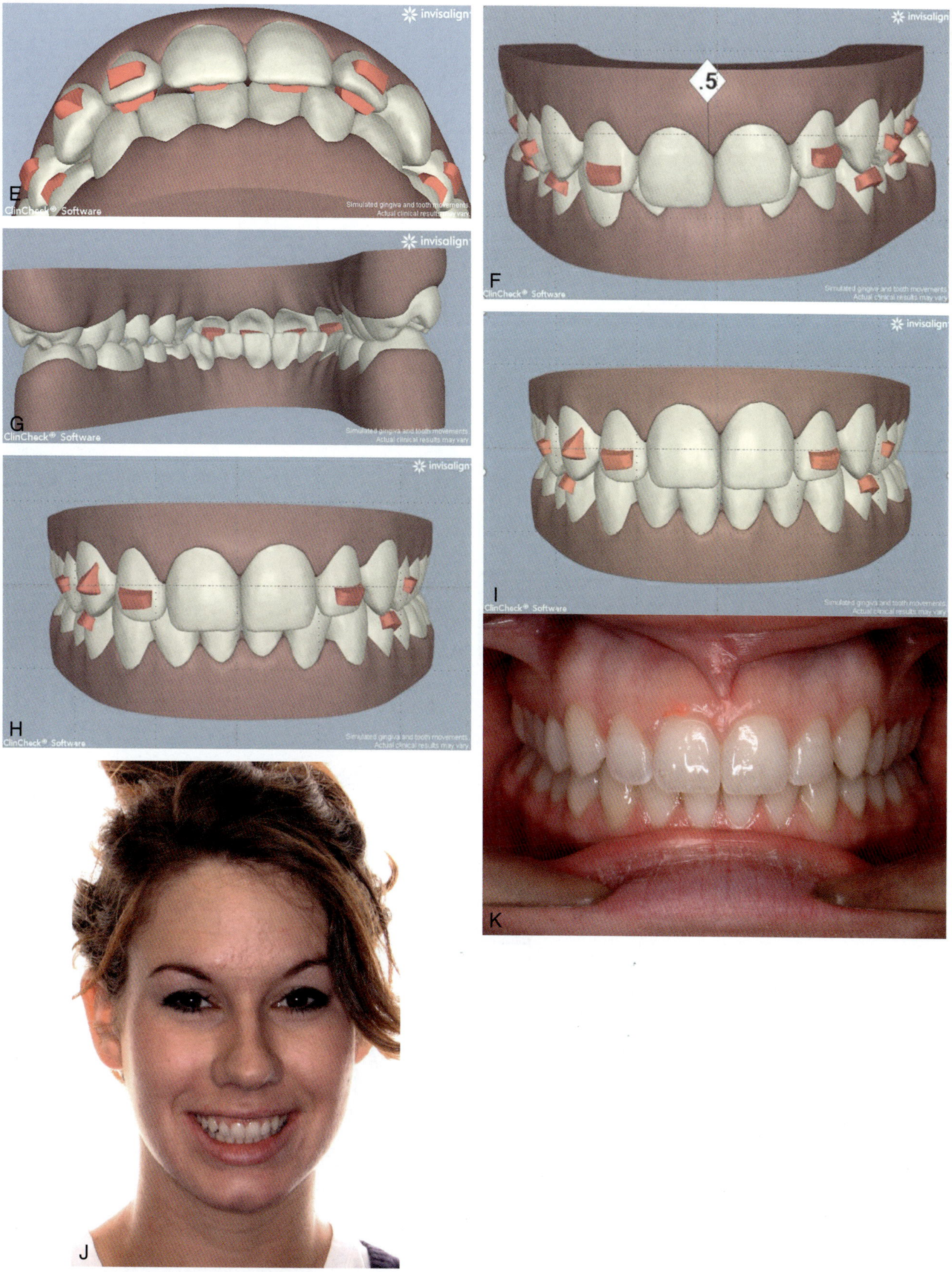

• **Fig. 21.12, cont'd** (E and F) ClinCheck stage 0, showing the bite ramps behind the upper incisors and attachments on the maxillary lateral incisors and canines to resist extrusion while the central incisors were intruded. Note the planned initial reshaping of the maxillary central incisors, repositioning their contact point downward. (G and H) ClinCheck stage 23, showing the expected overbite and alignment at that intermediate point, and (I) ClinCheck revision stage 10, at completion of treatment. (J and K) Smile and close-up of occlusion at end of treatment.

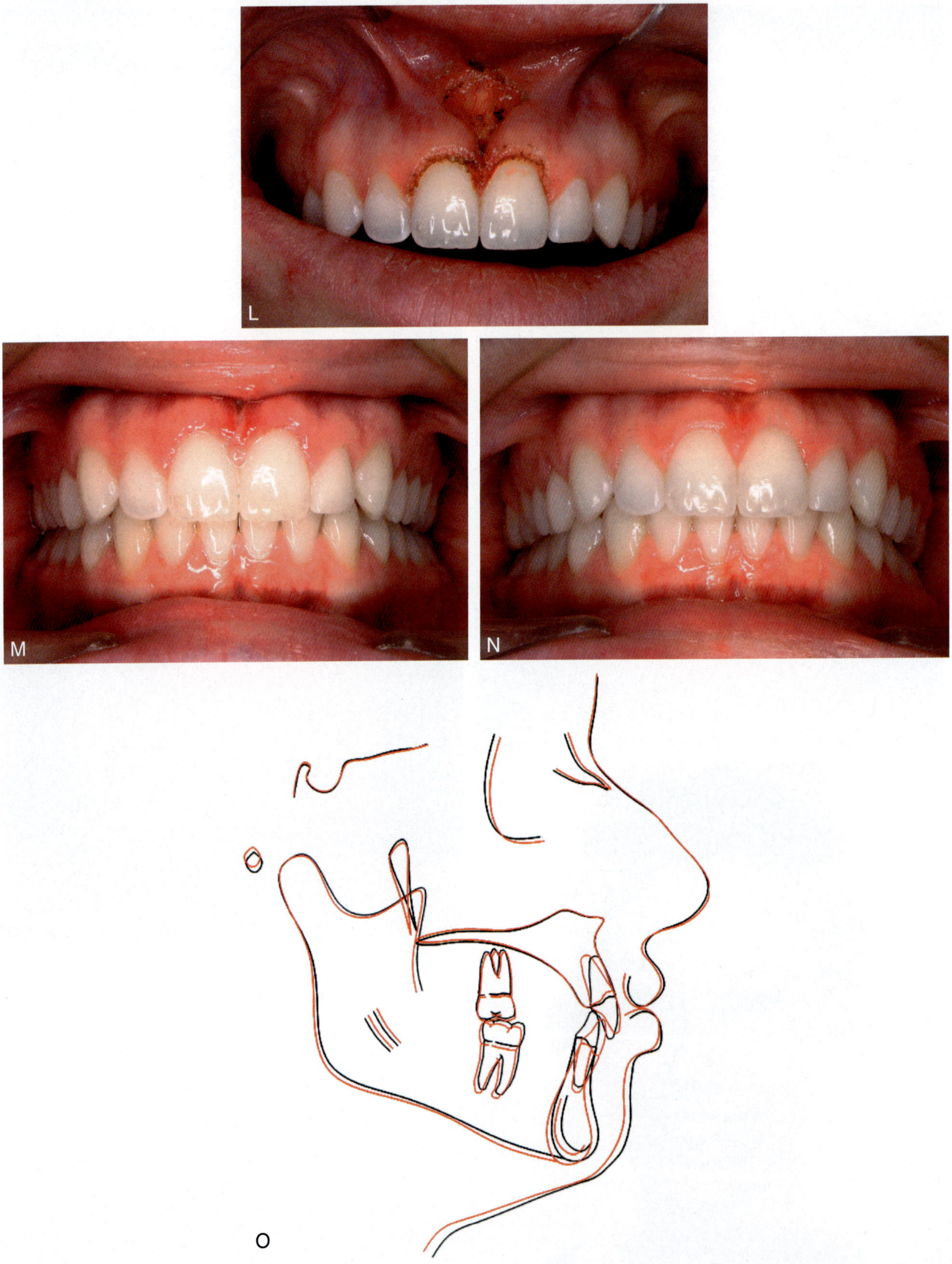

• Fig. 21.12, cont'd (L) The finishing stage of treatment was laser release of the tight maxillary central frenum and gingival recontouring of the central incisors to obtain the correct height-width proportion. (M) Healing at 1 week and (N) 2 weeks after the surgical procedure. (O) The superimposition tracing from beginning to end of treatment (23 months) shows that the desired amount of intrusion and mandibular rotation was achieved. A mandibular bonded 3-3 retainer and a maxillary clear retainer were placed. (Courtesy Dr. W. Gierie.)

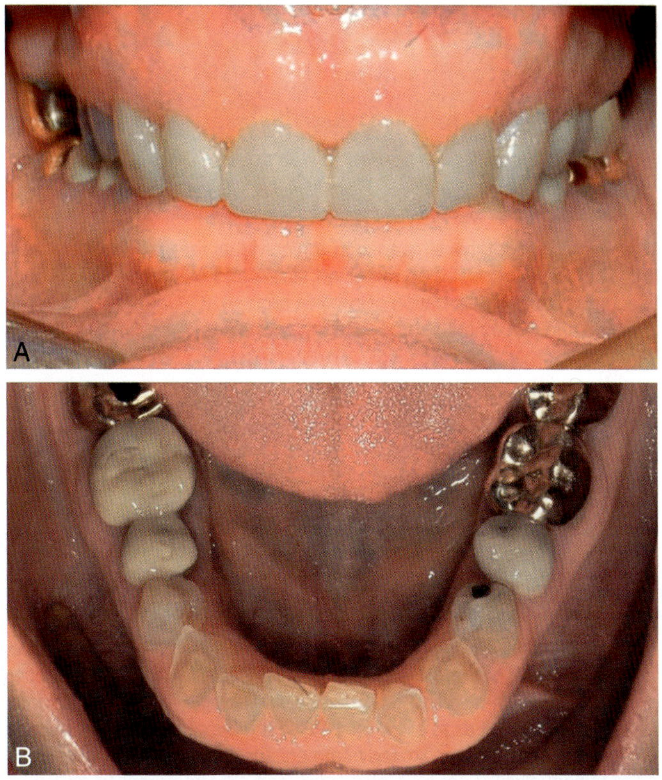

• **Fig. 21.13** Example of a deep bite adult malocclusion that may be an aligner case simply because the lower anterior teeth have been severely abraded. The increased overbite combined with the porcelain restorations on the upper anterior teeth have worn the dentition so significantly that the dentin is exposed and placement of fixed appliances is nearly impossible.

without attachments, but even if attachments are needed there are often significantly fewer than if bonded brackets are placed. An example of this is seen in Fig. 21.14, where a series of 10 aligners were worn for 2 weeks each. A minor refinement of 2 aligners was used after the initial 10 to optimize the result in 6 months.

Spacing

Another frequent patient concern seen in clinical practice is mild spacing, especially midline diastemas. Again, treatment can often be done with limited aligners with minimal or no attachments. However, care should be taken to check for Bolton tooth-size discrepancies and increased overbite, as both these issues will cause maxillary anterior spacing to reopen if not addressed during the limited treatment. Fig. 21.15 shows an example of an upper midline diastema where slight maxillary IPR was done to reduce the potential for black triangle formation and a greater amount of mandibular IPR was done to correct the tooth-size discrepancy. This situation also serves as an example of setting clear goals and expectations for adult treatment—this patient previously underwent comprehensive treatment and did not want to spend time or money working on midline correction. Although the midline discrepancy remains, the patient was very happy to achieve this result in 5 months of limited aligner treatment.

Minor Occlusal Changes

Finally, another area where limited treatment with aligners can provide a significant benefit to patients is with minor occlusal changes. These can happen for a number of reasons but can be improved with aligners in many cases.

One common issue is late mandibular growth or mandibular advancement appliances that posture the mandible forward at night to improve the airway—in these situations, the occlusion can change to an uncomfortable and traumatic edge-to-edge relationship causing wear. In these cases, such as shown in Fig. 21.16, limited aligners with Class III elastics can help restore positive overjet with good patient compliance.

Some additional occlusal changes that may be treated by limited aligners are supraeruption of posterior teeth from wear of a retainer or night guard without full occlusal coverage (only in very minor discrepancies), minor spaces before restorative work, mild class II relapse, or minor maxillary transverse changes leading to bite opening.

Other Challenges

Handling Missing Teeth

Missing teeth are another commonly encountered challenge with clear aligner treatment in adults. In the esthetic zone, few adults will accept having a visible space for months during treatment. A few common solutions are available for these situations:

- Painted aligners: Virtual pontic teeth are placed into the digital treatment plan leaving an empty tooth space in the aligners when they are manufactured. The teeth are ideally created slightly undersized so the full contour of the adjacent teeth can be engaged for more consistent tooth movement and control. The pontic paint of the correct shade is placed inside

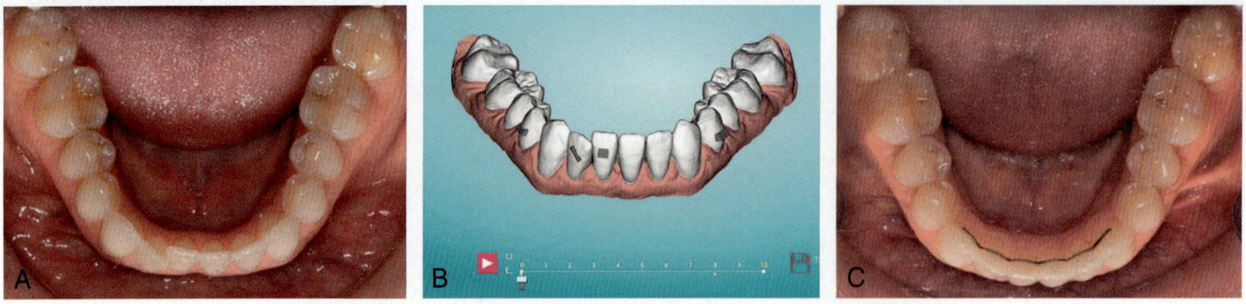

• **Fig. 21.14** (A) Mild lower incisor rotational relapse in an individual that previously underwent comprehensive orthodontic treatment. The posterior occlusion remained stable and only correction of the incisor rotation was desired. (B) Digital attachment plan for fabrication of in-office aligners. (C) Same individual with alignment restored using aligners for 6 months and placement of a bonded lower retainer to prevent the rotation from recurring.

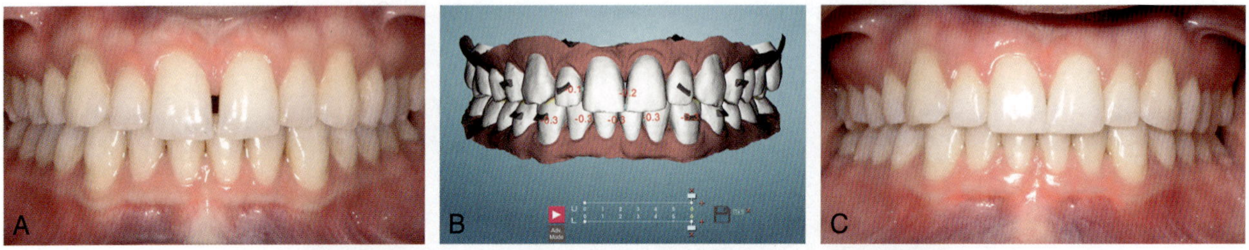

• **Fig. 21.15** (A) Upper midline diastema in an adult that occurred sometime after comprehensive orthodontic treatment. The overall alignment and occlusion remained stable but the spacing was a concern for the patient. (B) Screenshot of the original digital plan showing the attachments and IPR planned to address the existing mild lower anterior tooth-size excess as well as to allow mild IPR in the maxillary arch to prevent a black triangle from appearing after space closure. (C) Completed limited treatment showing diastema closure using aligners for about 5 months. Note that the patient elected not to pursue more complex treatment to address the midline discrepancy—an important decision to make prior to beginning the aligner treatment.

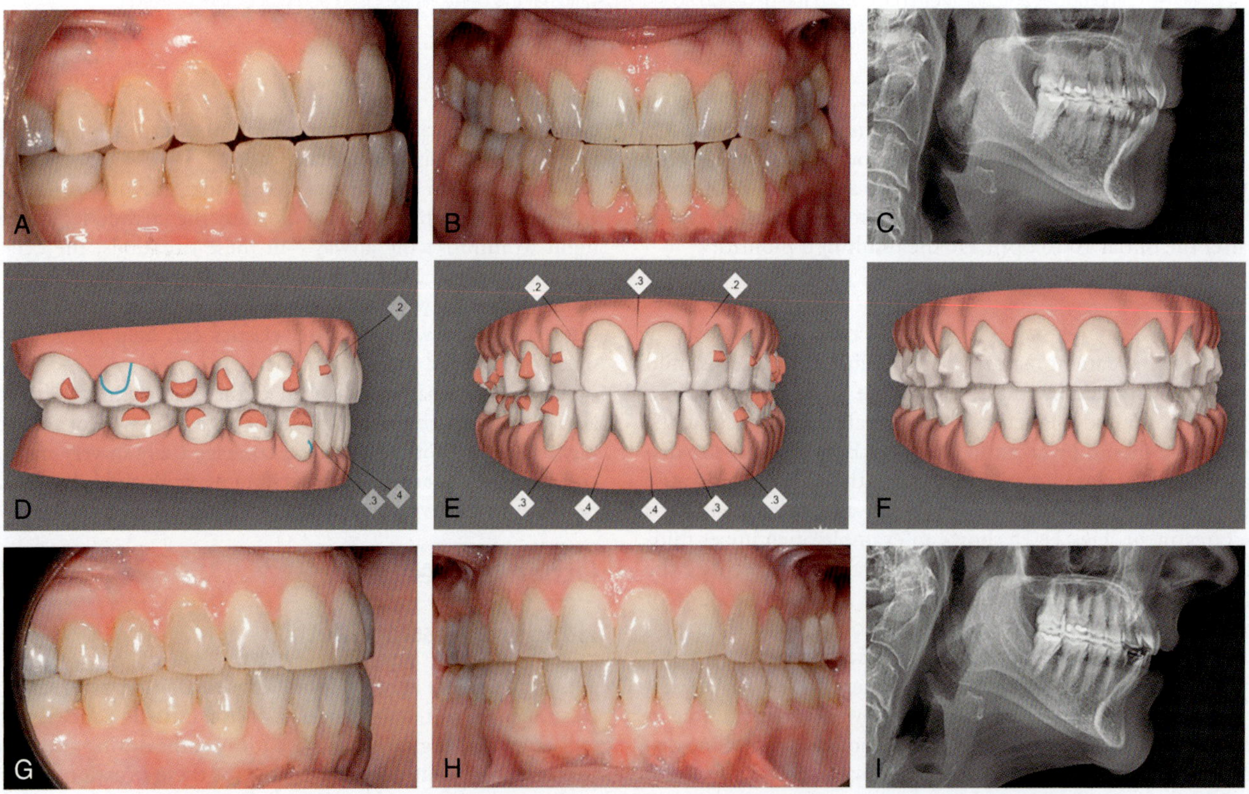

• **Fig. 21.16** Late mandibular growth can occasionally cause occlusal changes to occur in early adulthood even if the general alignment remains good. (A–C) A patient with continued growth on the right side following adolescent treatment resulting in a minor occlusal change, end-to-end incisor relationship and a midline deviation. (D and E) Digital plan for the first set of aligners—note attachments for aligner retention and cutouts for planned Class III elastic wear. (F) Refinement plan to further correct overjet and midlines. (G–I) Final result of the aligner treatment showing improvement in the overbite/overjet relationship and significant correction of the midline.

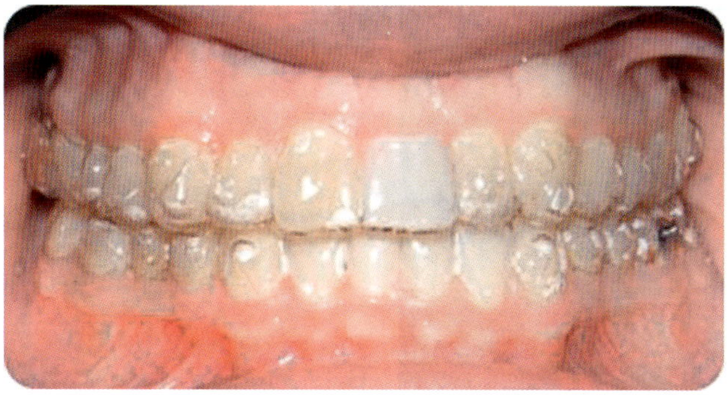

• **Fig. 21.17** The use of pontic paint to provide esthetic improvement for missing teeth during aligner treatment. The maxillary left central incisor is missing and a virtual pontic was created in the digital plan. The inside facial surface of the tooth space in the aligner is painted with the appropriate shade of pontic paint to make it appear as if a tooth is present.

the aligner on the facial surface of the missing tooth to make it appear as if there is a tooth in this location (Fig. 21.17). This is a common method but does require time to match the shade and additional employee time to paint each aligner in this manner.

- Removable pontic or pontic wax placed into each aligner: If the pontic shape remains consistent, a solid pontic can be placed in the aligner and moved from aligner to aligner by the patient as treatment progresses. If the pontic shape changes, a flexible tooth colored wax can be molded into each aligner. This allows the patient to change the pontic on their own, but because there is not a tight seal between the pontic and the aligner, discoloration can occur during wear.
- Placement of a cantilever bridge during treatment: Potentially the best method of handling a missing tooth is provisional replacement of the tooth. Typically, implant placement is not desired until after tooth movement when ideal spacing and occlusion has been created. However, if the adjacent tooth needs minimal tip or rotational changes, a cantilevered resin-bonded bridge, attached to the adjacent tooth, can provide a stable option during tooth movement.

Orthognathic Surgery

Detailed concepts and principles for combined orthodontic and orthognathic surgery treatment are presented in Chapter 22, but presurgical and postsurgical tooth movement to support orthognathic surgery can be accomplished with aligners just as with fixed appliances. The main variation is providing support for intermaxillary fixation or elastic wear during and immediately after surgery. With fixed appliances, this support is provided directly by the braces, wires, and surgical hooks attached to the patient's teeth. With aligners, in single-jaw cases, sufficient ligation may be obtained by bonding buttons to the posterior teeth and using elastic chain or steel ligature to hold the teeth into the surgical positioning splint while internal rigid fixation is placed. With more complex movements, TADs may be placed in each quadrant for more stable support.[6] It should be noted that some surgeons request that, even in aligner cases, fixed appliances be placed before surgery and that they be left in place for the immediate postsurgical healing period to allow for the most flexibility in dealing with any immediate postsurgical issues.

An additional difference is that aligner wear can be extremely challenging immediately after orthognathic surgery. Some surgeons prefer to discontinue aligner wear for a few weeks after surgery to allow natural settling of the occlusion. This may be possible if the presurgical setup is near ideal but continued wear of the surgical splint for several weeks may lead to more predictable surgical outcomes.

Fig. 21.18 shows two methods for providing support for the intermaxillary fixation needed during the orthognathic surgical procedure. First, a one-jaw mandibular advancement patient prepared for orthognathic surgery using aligners. The presurgical preparation was accomplished in 6 months and was aided by the fact that the patient was previously treated some years ago but did not proceed with the surgery at that point. Fixation during surgery was planned with buttons bonded to the posterior teeth. Second, more complex surgical movement require TADs placed in all quadrants to support fixation and postsurgical elastic wear.

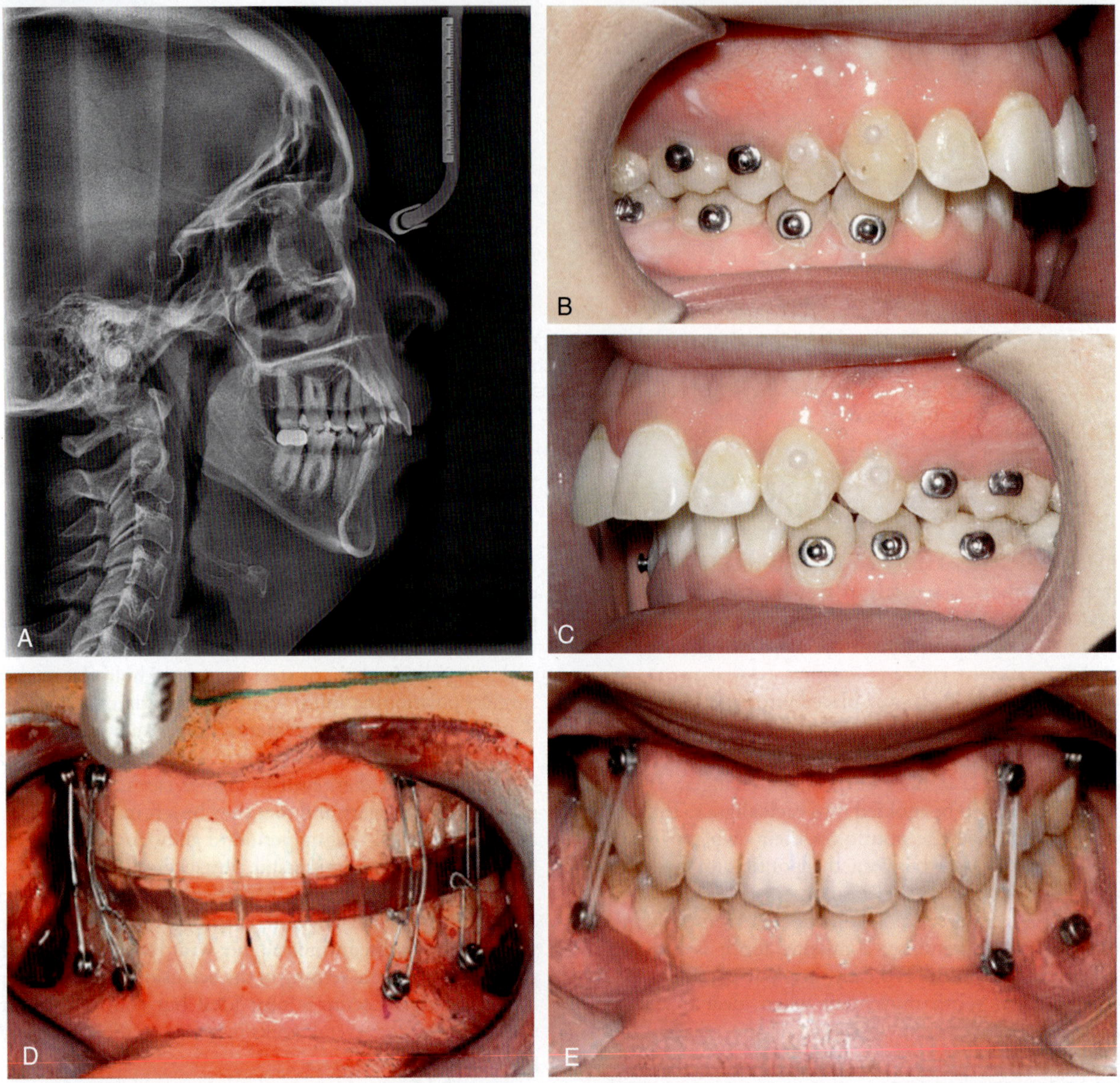

• **Fig. 21.18** Patient with a class II malocclusion due to mandibular deficiency prepared for orthognathic surgery with aligners. (A) Lateral cephalometric film demonstrating mandibular deficiency and the overjet created to allow for surgical advancement. (B and C) Bonded buttons added to the posterior teeth before surgery to provide attachment for the intermaxillary fixation needed while the fixation plates are attached and for guiding elastics after surgery. (D) In a different patient, TADs in all four quadrants used during surgery to fixate the maxillary and mandibular jaws into the occlusal splint to allow placement of rigid fixation plates. (E) TADs used in the postsurgical period to wear guiding elastics during the healing period. (From Parsaei Y, Uribe F, Steinbacher DM. Clear aligner therapy and orthognathic surgery. *J Clin Orthod*. 2022 Dec;56(12):692–707. PMID: 37158984.

References

1. Lin E, Julien K, Kesterke M, Buschang PH. Differences in finished case quality between Invisalign and traditional fixed appliances. *Angle Orthod*. 2022;92(2):173–179. https://doi.org/10.2319/032921-246.1.
2. Iwasaki LR, Liu Y, Liu H, Nickel JC. Speed of human tooth movement in growers and non-growers: selection of applied stress matters. *Orthod Craniofac Res*. 2017 Jun;20(Suppl 1):63–67.
3. Timm LH, Farrag G, Baxmann M, Schwendicke F. Factors influencing patient compliance during clear aligner therapy: a retrospective cohort study. *J Clin Med*. 2021 Jul 14;10(14):3103.
4. Robertson L, Kaur H, Fagundes NCF, Romanyk D, Major P, Flores Mir C. Effectiveness of clear aligner therapy for orthodontic treatment: a systematic review. *Orthod Craniofac Res*. 2020;23(2):133–142. https://doi.org/10.1111/ocr.12353.
5. Ke Y, Zhu Y, Zhu M. A comparison of treatment effectiveness between clear aligner and fixed appliance therapies. *BMC Oral Health*. 2019;19(1):24. https://doi.org/10.1186/s12903-018-0695-z. Published 2019 Jan 23.
6. Parsaei Y, Uribe F, Steinbacher DM. Clear aligner therapy and orthognathic surgery. *J Clin Orthod*. 2022;56(12):692–707.

22

Combined Surgical and Orthodontic Treatment

DAVID M. SARVER, WILLIAM R. PROFFIT, HENRY W. FIELDS, AND BENJAMIN T. PLISKA

CHAPTER OUTLINE

For patients whose orthodontic problems are so severe that neither growth modification nor camouflage offers a solution, surgery to realign the jaws or reposition dentoalveolar segments is the only possible treatment. Surgical treatment is not a substitute for orthodontics in these patients. Instead, it must be properly coordinated with orthodontics and other dental treatment to achieve good overall results. Dramatic progress in recent years has made it possible for combined treatment to correct many severe problems that simply were untreatable only a few years ago (Fig. 22.1).

Development of Orthognathic Surgery

Surgery for mandibular prognathism began early in the 20th century with occasional treatment that consisted of a body ostectomy, removing a molar or premolar tooth and an accompanying block of bone. Edward Angle, commenting on a patient who underwent treatment of this type over 100 years ago, described how the result could have been improved if orthodontic appliances and occlusal splints had been used. Although there was gradual progress in techniques for setting back a prominent mandible throughout the first half of the 20th century, the introduction of the sagittal split ramus osteotomy in 1957 marked the beginning of the modern era in orthognathic surgery.[1] This technique used an intraoral approach, which avoided the necessity of a potentially disfiguring skin incision. The sagittal split design also offered a biologically sound method for lengthening or shortening the lower jaw with the same bone cuts, thus allowing treatment of mandibular deficiency or excess (Fig. 22.2).

During the 1960s American surgeons began to use and modify techniques for maxillary surgery that had been developed in Europe, and a decade of rapid progress in maxillary surgery culminated in the development of the Le Fort I downfracture technique, which allowed repositioning of the maxilla in all three planes of space (Fig. 22.3).[2,3] By the 1980s it was possible to reposition either or both jaws, move the chin in all three planes of space, and reposition dentoalveolar segments surgically as desired. In the 1990s rigid internal fixation greatly improved patient comfort by making immobilization of the jaws unnecessary, and a better understanding of typical patterns of postsurgical changes made surgical outcomes more stable and predictable. With the introduction of facial distraction osteogenesis around the turn of the century and its rapid development since then, larger jaw movements and treatment at an earlier age became possible for patients with the most severe problems (usually related to syndromes).

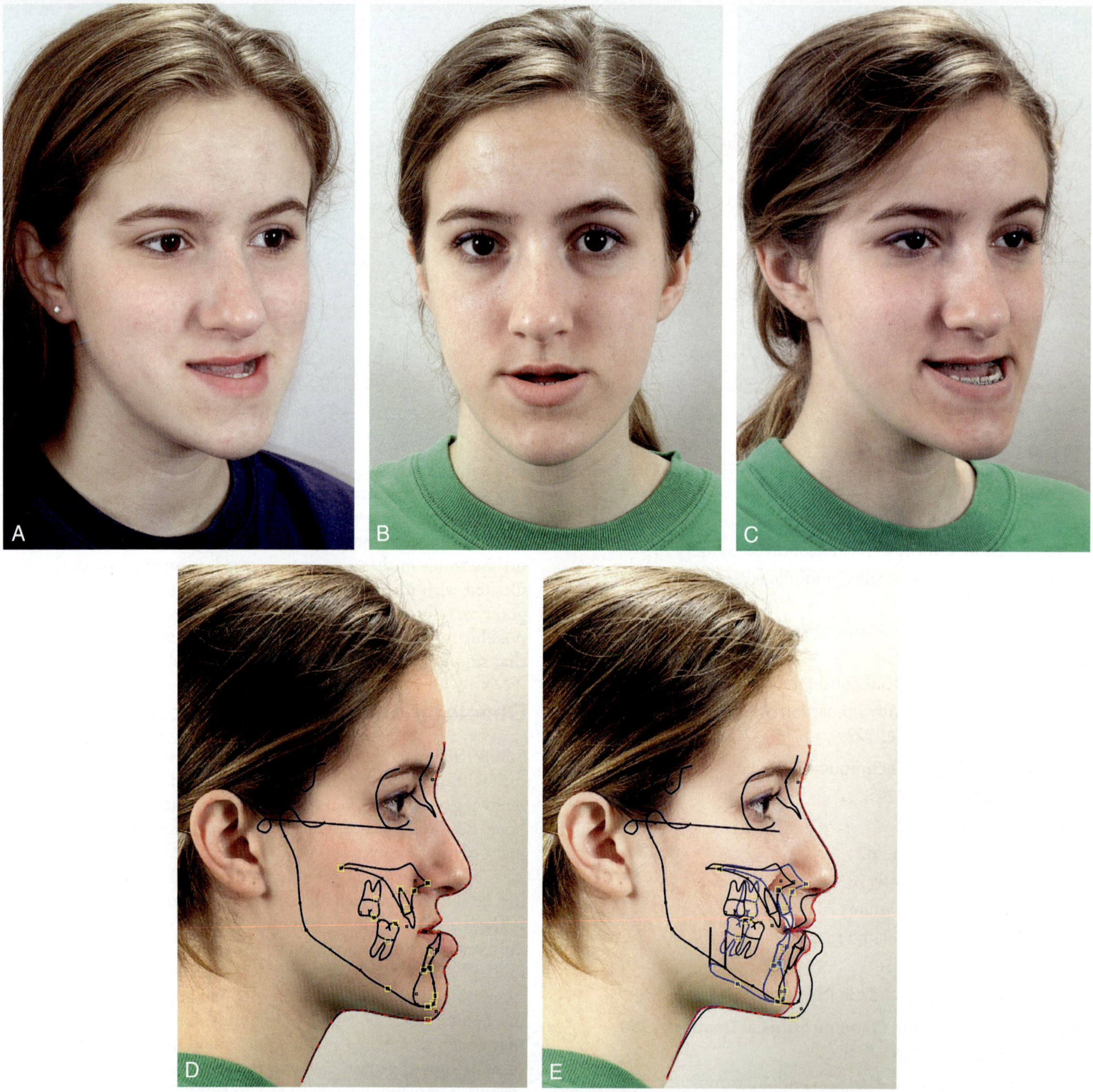

• **Fig. 22.1** (A) At age 14, when she was first seen for orthodontic consultation, this girl had significant anteroposterior and vertical maxillary deficiency (note the lack of maxillary incisor display on smile) and a large mandible. Although she had reached sexual maturity 3 years previously, the decision was to obtain a cephalometric radiograph and see her on 1-year recall to be sure that active mandibular growth had effectively ended before beginning orthodontic preparation for orthognathic surgery. Treatment was started at age 15, with the goal of removing dental compensation for the skeletal discrepancy. This required extraction of maxillary first premolars so that the proclined maxillary incisors could be retracted, with nonextraction treatment of the lower arch and some proclination of the lower incisors. Although she was in buccal crossbite, placing the dental casts in Class I occlusion showed that when the anteroposterior jaw discrepancy was corrected, transverse dental relationships would be approximately normal, so expansion of the maxillary arch was not necessary. (B and C) Age 17, after presurgical orthodontics, which temporarily made her facial appearance worse. It is important that patients understand in advance that this will occur. (D) The cephalometric tracing at that point was linked to the facial photograph so that predictions of various combinations of maxillary advancement and mandibular setback could be evaluated. (E) This prediction shows that anticipated effect of approximately equal advancement of the maxilla and setback of the mandible.

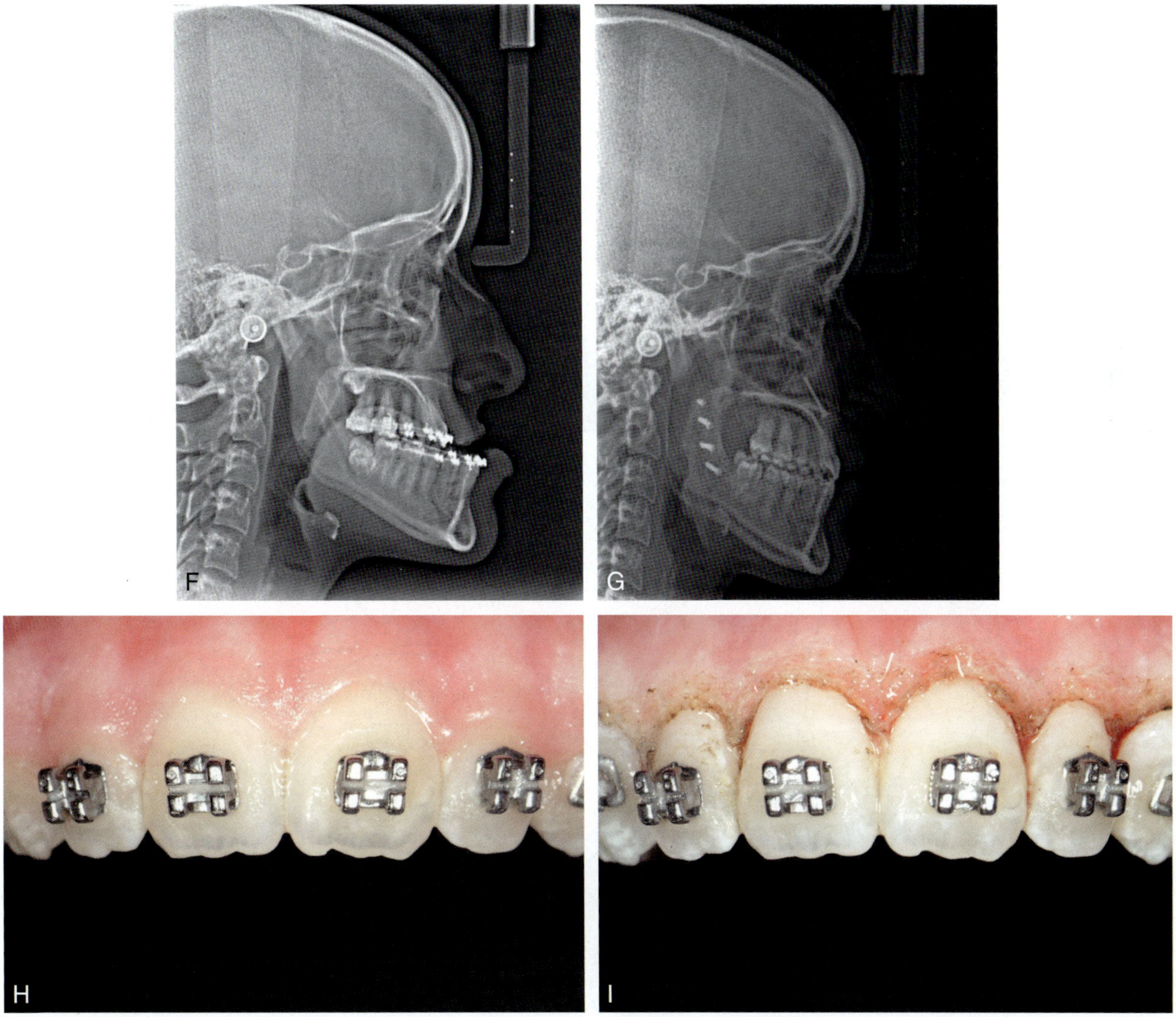

• **Fig. 22.1, cont'd** (F) The presurgical cephalometric radiograph. The surgical plan was 5 mm of maxillary advancement with some downward movement, 5 mm of mandibular setback, and rhinoplasty to correct the drooping nasal tip and decrease the width of the alar base. (G) Postsurgical cephalometric radiograph. (H) At the end of the postsurgical orthodontic treatment, the crowns of the central incisors were disproportionately wide for their height because of gingival overgrowth. (I) The gingival margins were recontoured with a diode laser.

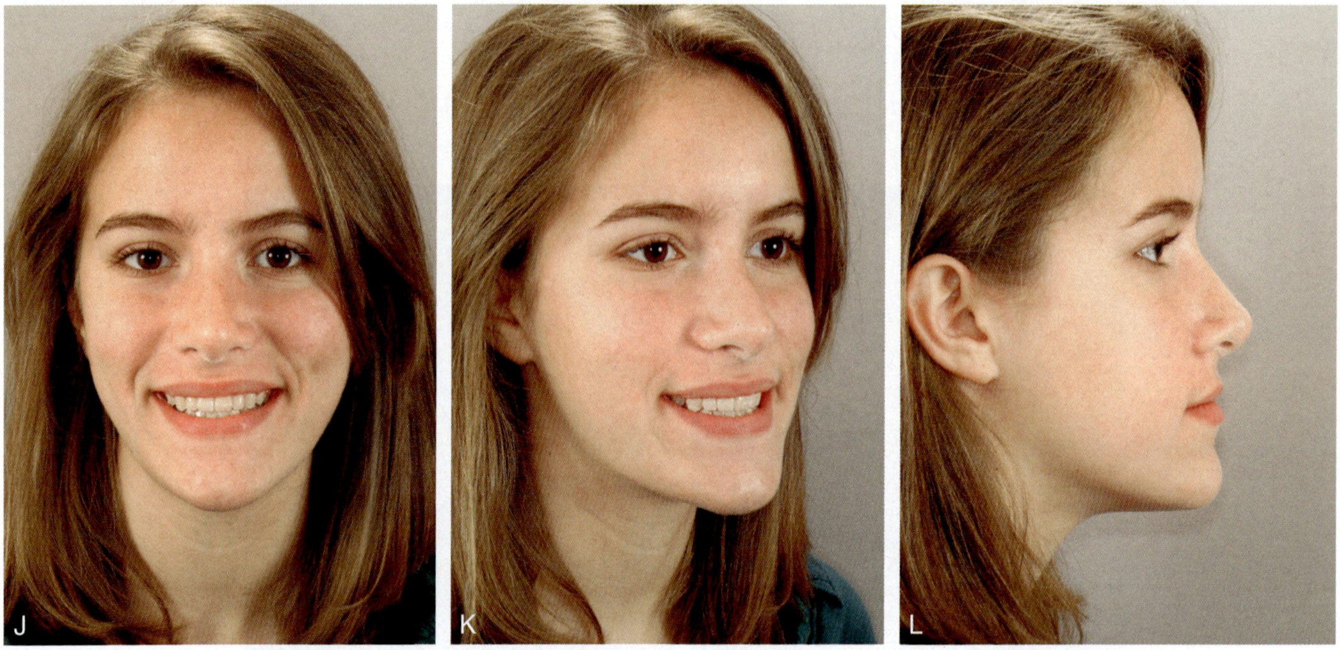

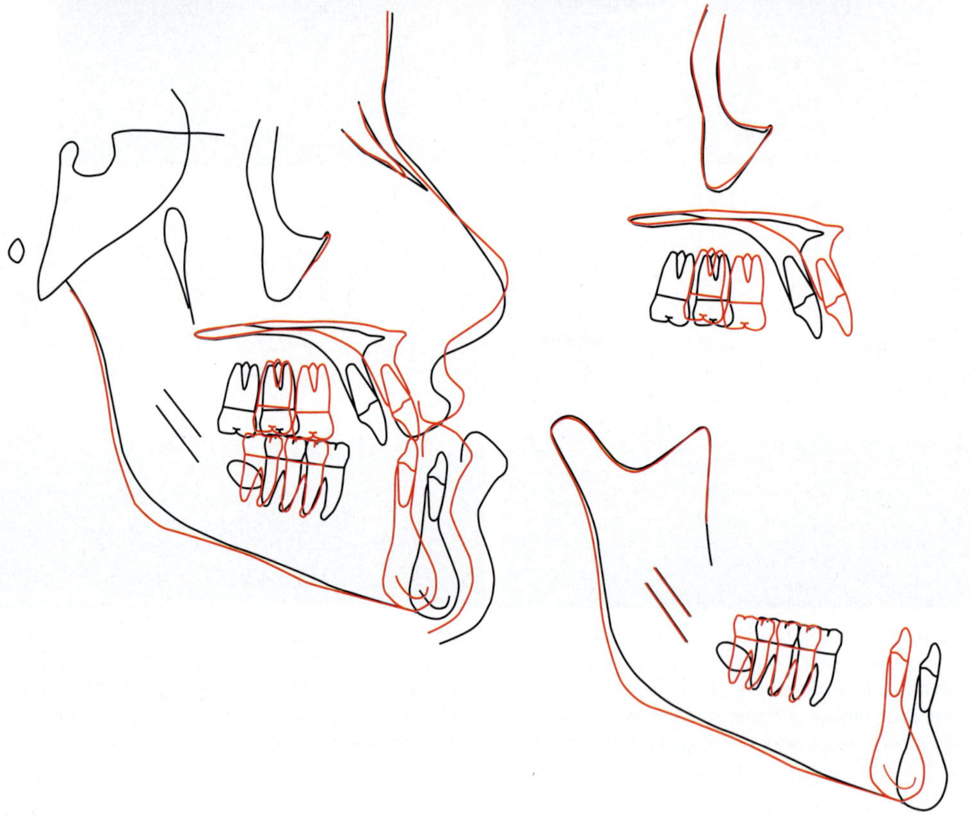

• **Fig. 22.1, cont'd** (J–L) Frontal and oblique smiles and resting profile views at the completion of treatment. (M) Superimposition of pretreatment and posttreatment tracings shows the hard tissue and soft tissue profile changes during treatment. Note in the superimposition tracing and the posttreatment facial views that the nose was tipped forward but the rhinoplasty prevented further upward tipping of the nasal tip and improved tip projection.

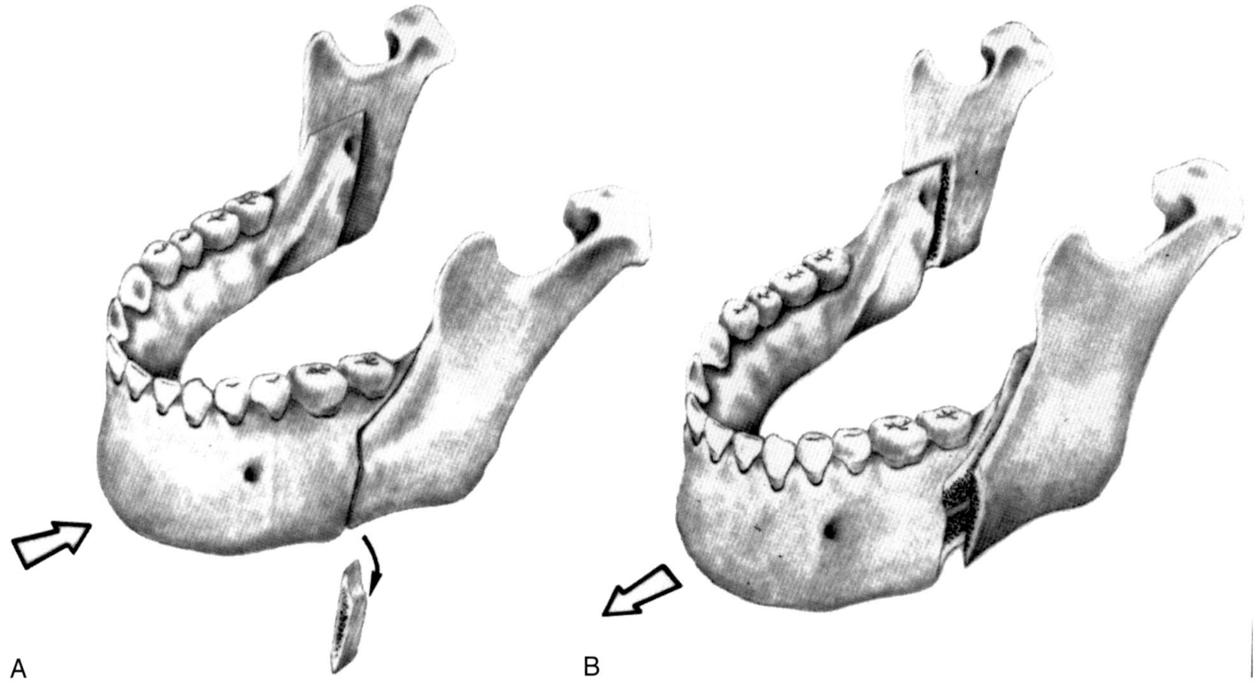

• **Fig. 22.2** The sagittal split osteotomy procedure can be used to set back or advance the mandible, as shown in (A) and (B), respectively.

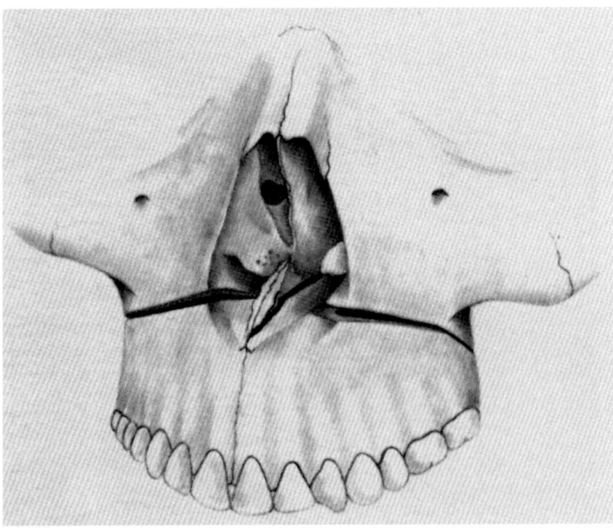

• **Fig. 22.3** The location of the osteotomy cuts for the Le Fort I downfracture technique, which allows the maxilla to be moved up and forward readily. Moving it down is feasible but requires careful retention during healing. Moving it back is very difficult because of the structures behind the maxilla, but moving protruding incisors back can be accomplished easily with a segmental osteotomy to move the canine-to-canine segment back into a premolar extraction space.

Combined surgical and orthodontic treatment can now be carried out successfully for patients with a severe dentofacial problem of any type. This has been made more predictable and accurate with the use of new digital technologies and cone beam imaging for simulations of skeletal and dental changes (Fig. 22.4) and some soft tissue approximated changes (Figs. 22.5). Bone thickness and nerves anatomy can also be illustrated (Fig. 22.6). Digitally printed skeletal structures and teeth (acrylic models) for planning can be produced (Fig. 22.7) as can printed surgical guides (Fig. 22.8A), fixation appliances (see Fig. 22.8B) and intraoral occlusal surgical splints (see Fig. 22.8C). Similar techniques are applied for patient treatment planning later in this chapter. This chapter provides an overview of current orthognathic surgery, which is covered in detail in two well-illustrated texts.[4,5]

The Borderline Patient: Camouflage Versus Surgery

Malocclusion Severity as an Indication for Surgery

One indication for surgery obviously is a malocclusion too severe for orthodontics alone. It is possible now to be at least semiquantitative about the limits of orthodontic treatment in the context of producing normal occlusion. As the diagrams of the "envelope of discrepancy" (Fig. 22.9) indicate, the limits vary according to the tooth movement that would be needed. As the figure shows, teeth can be moved farther in some directions than others at any age (the limits for tooth movement change little if any with age), but growth modification is possible only while active growth is occurring. Because growth modification in children enables greater changes than are possible by tooth movement alone in adults, some conditions that could have been treated with orthodontics alone in children (e.g., a centimeter of overjet) become surgical problems in adults. On the other hand, some conditions that might initially look less severe (e.g., 5 mm of reverse overjet) can be seen even at an early age to require surgery if they are ever to be corrected.

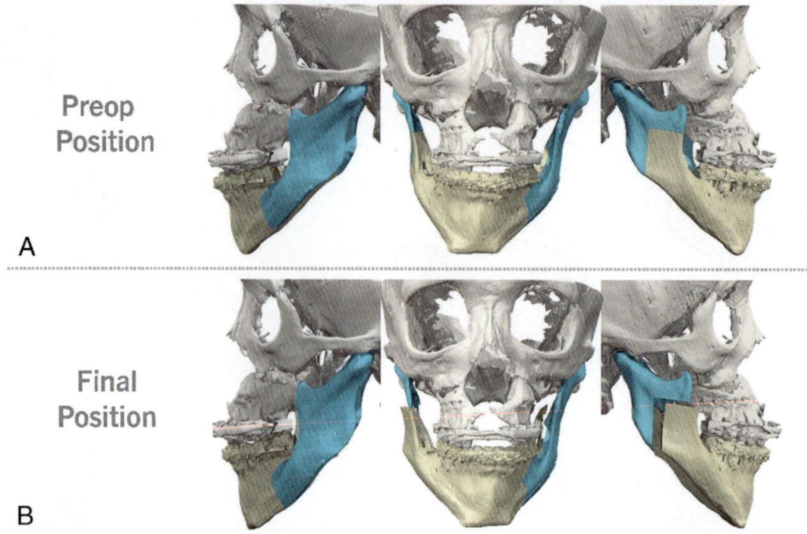

• **Fig. 22.4** (A) These cone beam computed tomography images show the preoperative skeletal and dental relationships of a 39-year-old female with a complete cleft palate, who is post maxillary distraction osteogenesis and has negative overjet and marked mandibular asymmetry. (B) These are the projected postoperative images. Note the ramus osteotomy on the right and the sagittal split osteotomy on the left used to reduce the mandibular asymmetry. (Courtesy Dr. H. Emam.)

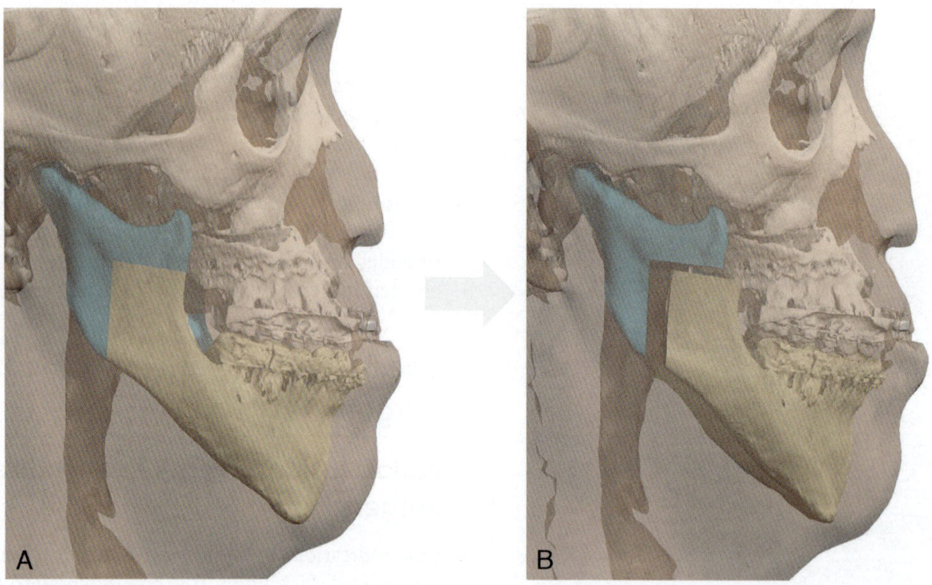

• **Fig. 22.5** (A) Preoperative cone beam computed tomography image with selected soft tissue. (B) Postoperative soft tissue approximation for selected areas. (Courtesy Dr. H. Emam.)

Keep in mind that the envelope of discrepancy outlines the estimated limits of hard tissue change toward ideal occlusion, *if* other limits due to the major goals of treatment do not apply. In fact, soft tissue limitations both physically and esthetically not reflected in the envelope of discrepancy often are a major factor in the decision for orthodontic or surgical-orthodontic treatment. Measuring millimeter distances to the ideal condylar position for normal function and measuring distances to define ideal esthetics are problematic. The diagnostic and treatment planning approach discussed in Chapters 6 and 7 reflects the heavy emphasis on soft tissue considerations in modern treatment and is essential when camouflage versus surgery is considered.

Extraction of Teeth and the Camouflage Versus Surgery Decision

The decision for camouflage or surgery must be made before treatment begins because the orthodontic treatment to prepare for surgery often is just the opposite of orthodontic treatment

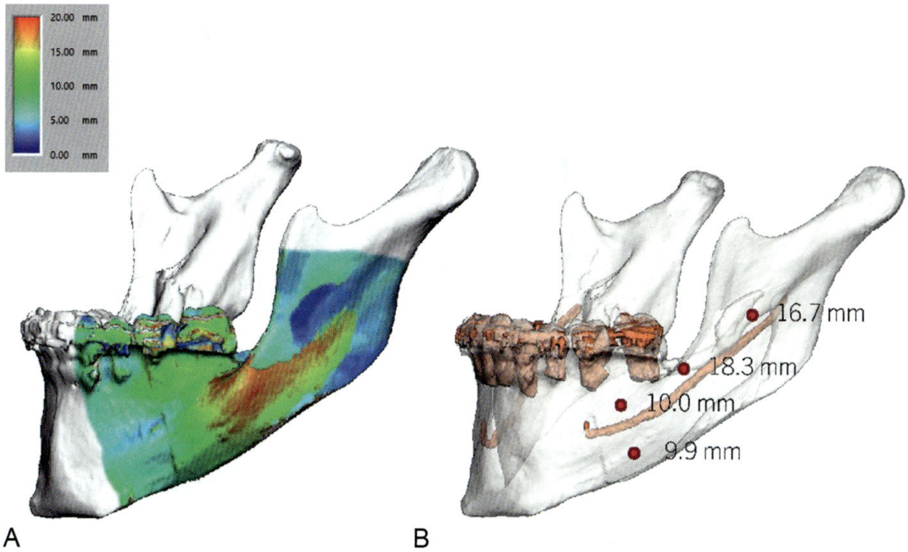

• **Fig. 22.6** Cone beam computed tomography generated (A) bone thickness color map with key and (B) inferior alveolar nerve map with potential bone screw fixation locations and bone thickness. (Courtesy Dr. H. Emam.)

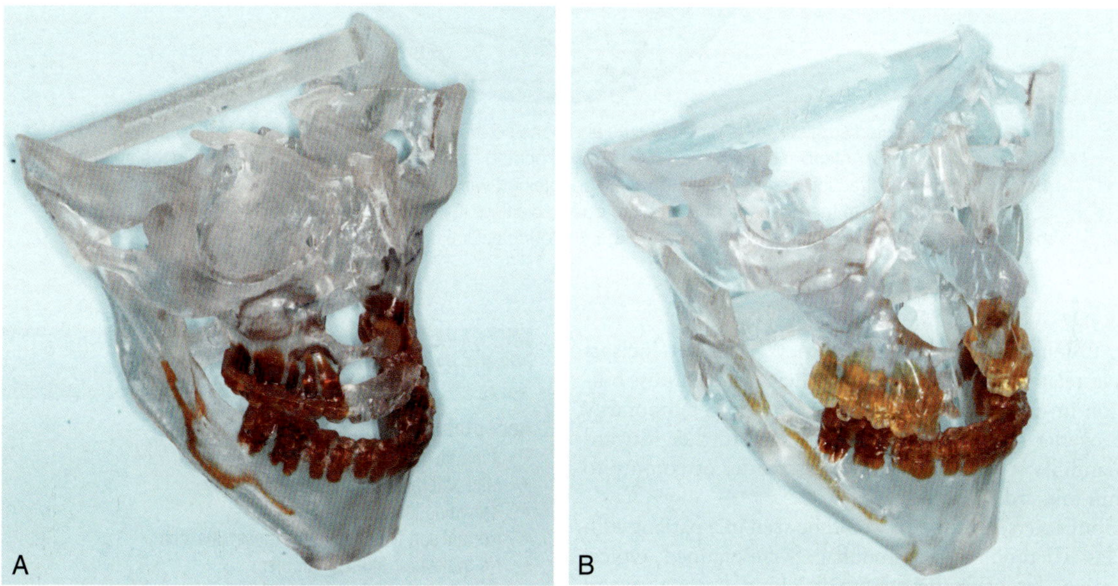

• **Fig. 22.7** (A) Printed preoperative acrylic model printed from the cone beam computed tomography showing the skeletal and dental features for study and treatment planning. (B) Projected postoperative printed model. (Courtesy Dr. H. Emam.)

for camouflage. It is a serious error to attempt camouflage on the theory that if it fails, the patient can then be referred for surgical correction. At that point, another phase of "reverse orthodontics" to eliminate the effects of the original treatment will be required before surgery can provide both normal jaw relationships and normal occlusion (Fig. 22.10).

The critical importance of deciding on camouflage or surgery at the beginning of treatment is illustrated by the difference in extractions needed with the two approaches. In camouflage, extraction spaces are used to produce dental compensations for the jaw discrepancy, and the extractions are planned accordingly. For example, with orthodontic treatment alone, a patient with mandibular deficiency and a Class II malocclusion might have upper first premolars removed to allow the retraction of the protrusive maxillary anterior teeth. Extraction in the lower arch would be avoided, and the lower incisors probably would be tipped facially to help reduce the overjet (see Fig. 16.22).

The extraction pattern for a patient with a similar malocclusion but a more severe mandibular deficiency would be quite different if mandibular advancement were planned (see Fig. 22.11). Instead of creating dental compensation for the jaw deformity, orthodontic treatment now would be planned to remove it. In the upper arch, the position of the incisors relative to the maxilla often is normal or retrusive; if so, upper premolar extraction would be

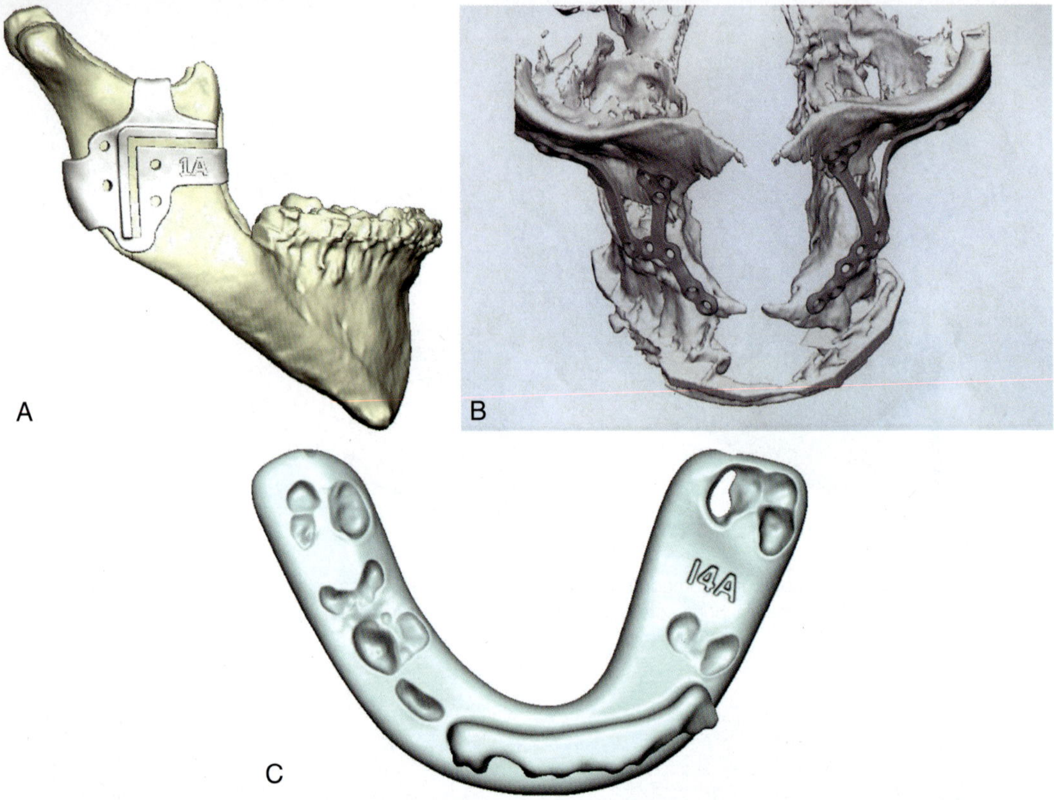

• **Fig. 22.8** (A) Printed surgical guide for bony cuts and bone screws, in this case for the right side to support the ramus osteotomy. (B) Anterior-superior image of the metal printed maxillary fixation appliance to retain the anterior movement of the distraction osteogenesis. This will be retained with bone screws in the zygoma and maxilla on both right and left. Note the absence of the palate due to clefting. (C) Printed splint to help register and stabilize the maxilla and mandible during and following surgery. (Courtesy Dr. H. Emam.)

undesirable. Often in mandibular deficiency the lower incisors are protrusive relative to the chin. Then there are two possibilities: extraction in the lower arch to retract them and temporarily increase the overjet so the chin will be brought further forward when the mandible is advanced, or a lower border osteotomy to move the chin forward.

A similar but reversed situation would be seen in a patient with a skeletal Class III problem. If camouflage were planned, typical extractions might be lower first premolars alone, lower first and upper second premolars, or one lower incisor. Surgical preparation of a patient with a Class III problem often requires moving the lower incisors forward and retracting the upper incisors (which may require extraction of upper first premolars) to correct their axial inclinations and increase the reverse overjet (see Fig. 22.10). As a general rule, Class III problems are less amenable to camouflage than Class II issues because retracting the lower incisors may make the chin appear even more prominent—just the opposite of effective camouflage. If space were needed in the lower arch, second rather than first premolar extraction would be a logical choice so that the lower incisors were not retracted.

It obviously is important for the patient who could be treated with either orthodontics or surgery to understand all these considerations in deciding which to choose. Although the patient can and must make the decision, it remains true that some conditions can be treated better with orthodontics alone than others, simply because the impact on facial esthetics is likely to be better. Some characteristics that can make the difference between satisfactory camouflage treatment and camouflage failure are summarized in Box 22.1.

• BOX 22.1 Orthodontic Camouflage of Skeletal Malocclusion

Acceptable Results Likely

- Average or short facial pattern
- Mild anteroposterior jaw discrepancy
- Crowding less than 4–6 mm
- Normal soft tissue features (nose, lips, chin)
- No transverse skeletal problem

Poor Results Likely

- Long vertical facial pattern
- Moderate or severe anteroposterior jaw discrepancy
- Crowding greater than 4–6 mm
- Exaggerated features
- Transverse skeletal component of problem

Orthognathic Surgery Versus Temporary Skeletal Anchorage

The advent of temporary skeletal anchorage in the form of miniplates or bone screws has led many orthodontists to wonder if this

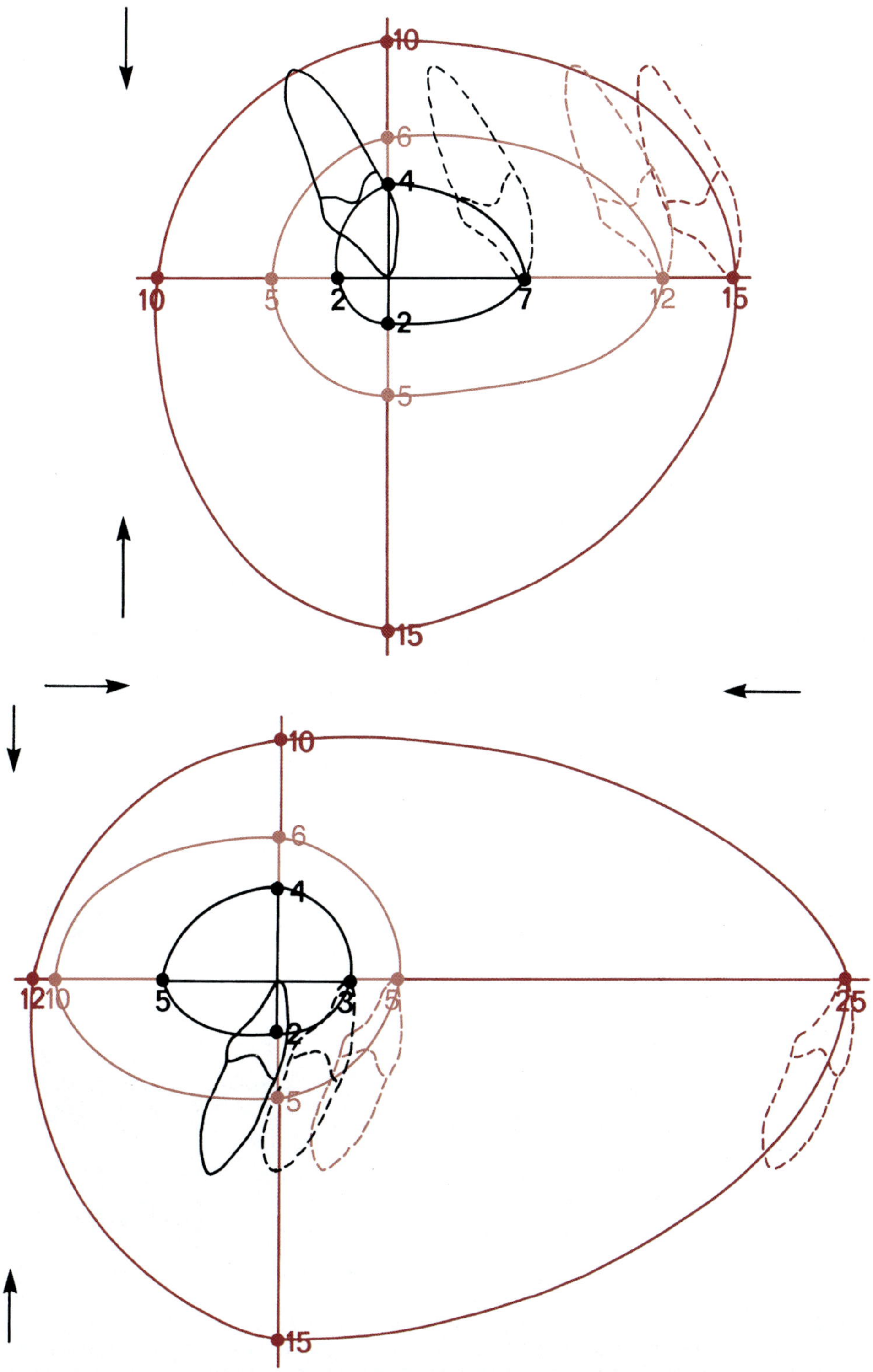

• **Fig. 22.9** With the ideal position of the upper and lower incisors shown by the origin of the x- and y-axes, the envelope of discrepancy shows the amount of change that could be produced by orthodontic tooth movement alone (the inner envelope of each diagram without skeletal anchorage); orthodontic tooth movement combined with growth modification (the middle envelope); and orthognathic surgery (the outer envelope). Note that the possibilities for each direction of movement (noted by the arrows to achieve a normal incisor position) are not symmetric. There is more potential to move teeth forward than back in the mandible and more potential for extrusion than intrusion in the maxilla. Because growth of the maxilla cannot be modified independently of the mandible, the growth modification envelope for the two jaws is the same. Surgery to move the lower jaw back has more potential than surgery to advance it.

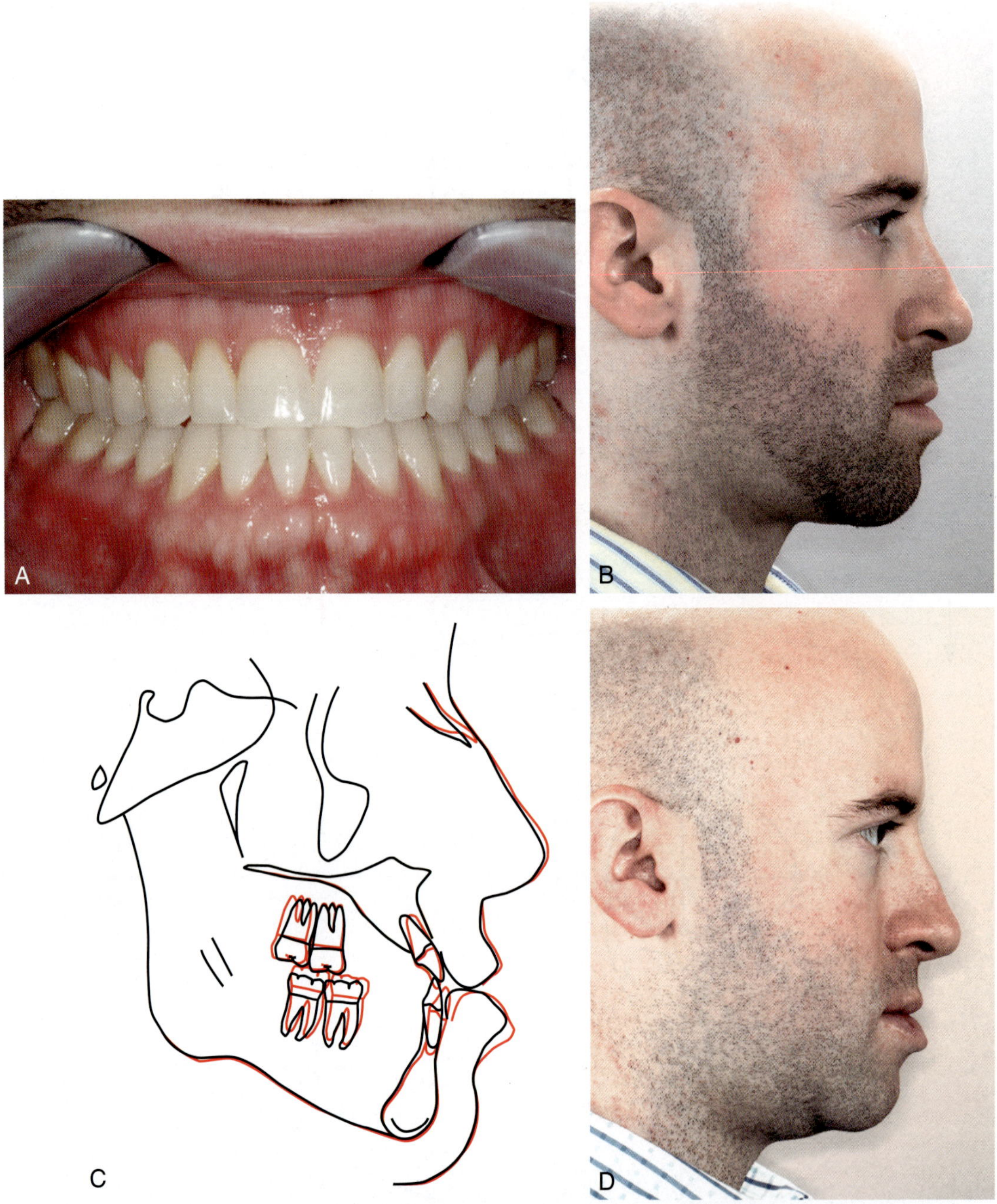

• **Fig. 22.10** (A) This male, who had undergone previous orthodontic treatment to correct his Class III malocclusion, now has minimal reverse overjet but (B) an obvious maxillary deficiency and prominent chin on profile view. This is a Class III camouflage failure as determined by the patient himself, who sought further treatment to improve his facial appearance. The treatment plan was presurgical orthodontics to remove the dental compensation created in the previous treatment, retracting the maxillary incisors and proclining the lower incisors to create reverse overjet similar to what he had before the original orthodontic treatment. (C) The superimposition tracing shows the presurgical changes. (D) The facial appearance before the operation. The "reverse orthodontics" has temporarily made his appearance worse.

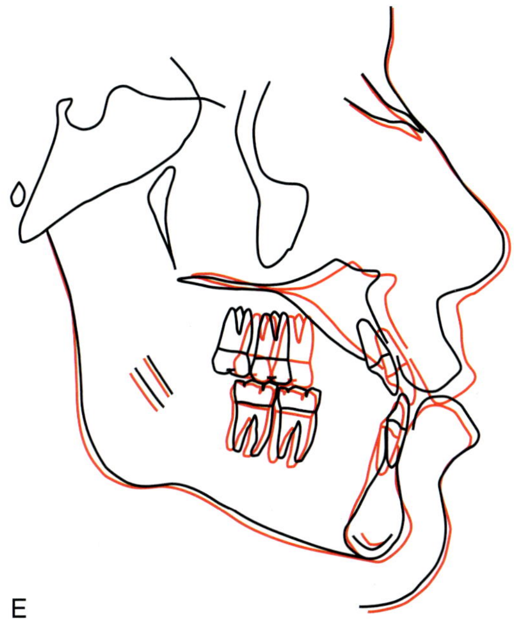

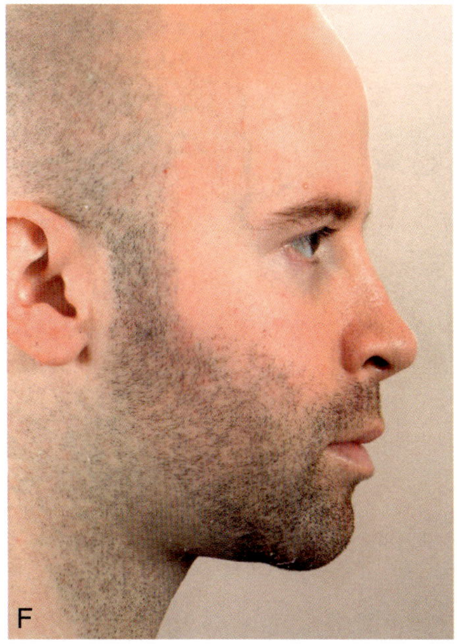

• **Fig. 22.10, cont'd** (E) Cephalometric superimposition showing the changes created by maxillary advancement surgery. (F) The profile at the end of treatment, with the jaw relationship now corrected.

could decrease the number of patients who would need surgery. Applications of skeletal anchorage in treatment of adults have been discussed in detail in Chapter 13 for posterior crossbites after adolescence and in Chapter 20 for anchorage to position individual teeth, retract incisors, distal movement of teeth and intrusion of posterior teeth. Tooth movement for patients with a jaw discrepancy, of course, is camouflage—successful only if the jaw discrepancy is no longer apparent enough to be a problem. It is true that protruding maxillary incisors in a patient with mandibular deficiency can be retracted further with skeletal anchorage. In some cases, this may be a reasonable alternative, but this is as likely to produce a camouflage failure as it is to correct the problem. The limits of orthodontic treatment are much more a matter of facial appearance than anchorage.

There are two circumstances, however, in which skeletal anchorage may be an alternative to orthognathic surgery. Moving the maxilla up with a Le Fort I osteotomy is highly stable and predictable. This has made it possible to correct anterior open bite/long-face problems that previously could not be corrected. Maxillary posterior teeth can be intruded with miniplates at the base of the zygomatic arch, long bone screws reaching into the same area, or palatal anchorage (see Chapter 20). It is clear now that 3 to 4 mm of intrusion can be achieved, with an expected short-term relapse of about 1 mm, and that for the average patient, 2 mm of closure of the open bite occurs for every 1 mm of posterior intrusion. This means that closure of a 6-mm anterior open bite is about the limit unless lower as well as upper molars are intruded, and that a surgical procedure still will be required unless the mandible rotates to the correct position as face height decreases. For example, it can rotate into an anterior crossbite that cannot be managed with either mandibular dental retraction or maxillary proclination.

The other interesting possibility for skeletal anchorage is protraction of the maxilla in preadolescent children (see Chapter 13). It is apparent now that Class III elastics to skeletal anchors in the posterior maxilla and anterior mandible are much more effective than reverse-pull headgear to the teeth in moving the maxilla forward. As with facemask treatment, however, the moment of truth comes during adolescence, when mandibular growth can lead to a return of the Class III problem. Can the maxilla be moved far enough forward at ages 10 to 12 to prevent the need for later surgical advancement? That depends on the severity of the maxillary and midface deficiency, on the amount of dental compensation, and even more on the pattern of adolescent growth.

At present, both intrusion of posterior teeth and maxillary protraction during adolescence are appropriate treatment for the less severe skeletal open bite and maxillary deficiency patients—as long as the patient and parents understand that surgical treatment may still be needed because of posttreatment growth.

Usually, the line between skeletal anchorage and orthognathic surgery is delineated by the amount of change needed and the number of planes of space that involve problems. The bigger the problem and the more problems identified, the more likely orthognathic surgery is the solution.

Esthetic and Psychosocial Considerations

The negative effect on psychic and social well-being from dentofacial disfigurement is well documented[6] and is why most patients seek orthodontic treatment. Those who look different are treated differently, and this becomes a social handicap. This motivation, not surprisingly, is even stronger in patients with the more severe deviations from the norm that might require orthognathic surgery. If an improvement in appearance is a major goal of treatment, it makes sense that in addition to changes in the jaws and teeth, changes in the nose and perhaps other changes in facial soft tissue contours that could be produced by facial plastic surgery should also be considered in the treatment planning. The integration of orthognathic and facial plastic surgery is a current and entirely rational trend.[7]

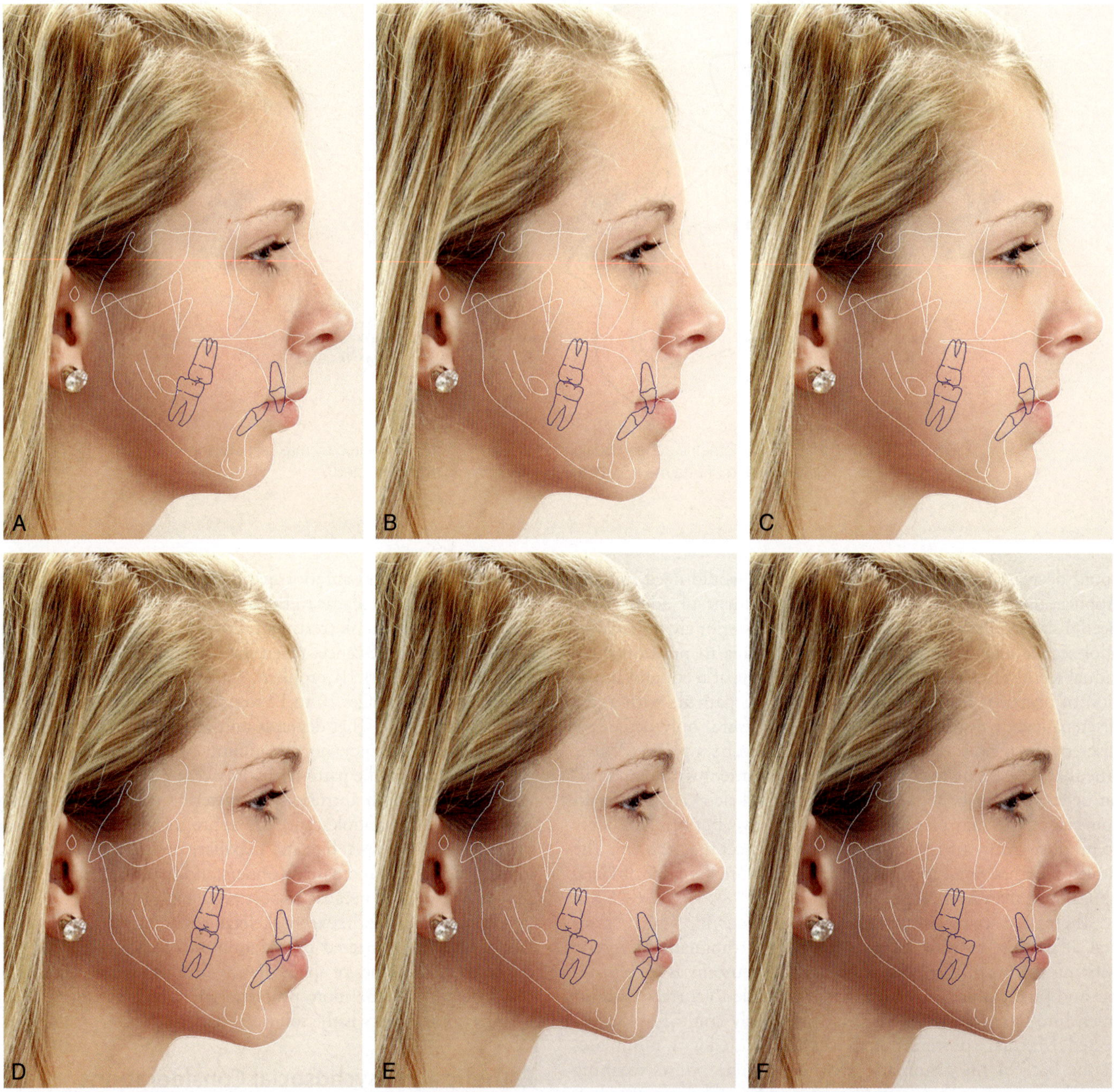

• **Fig. 22.11** Surgical predictions for a patient with mild maxillary retrusion, severe mandibular deficiency, and inadequate projection of the chin. (A) The initial tracing linked to the profile photograph. (B) Simulation of 5 mm of mandibular advancement, an amount of advancement corresponding to the initial overjet. (C) Five millimeters of mandibular advancement plus genioplasty to improve chin projection relative to the lower incisor. (D) 6 mm of maxillary advancement, 11 mm of mandibular advancement, and rhinoplasty. The maxilla was advanced to increase support of the upper lip and allow for greater mandibular advancement. (E) Preoperative retraction of the lower incisors after lower premolar extraction, creating more overjet and allowing a 9 mm mandibular advancement. (F) Retraction of lower incisors, 9 mm of advancement, and rhinoplasty. The rhinoplasty changes were subtle, and rhinoplasty was not recommended. After the patient and her parents viewed the simulations and discussed them with the orthodontist, (E) was selected as the plan.

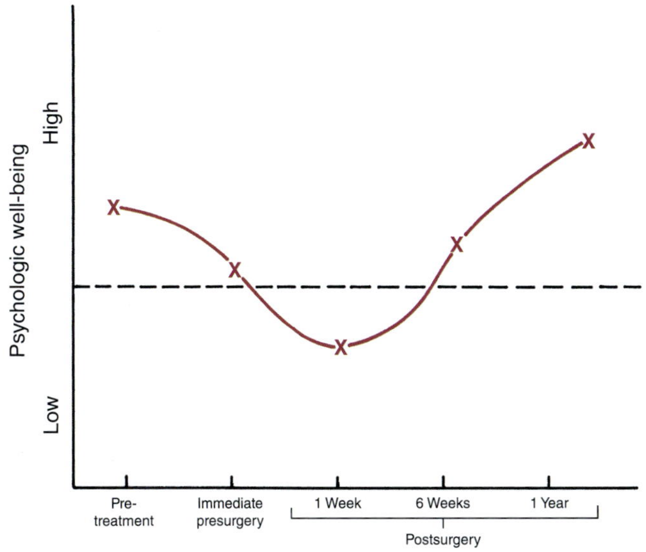

• **Fig. 22.12** A generalized representation of the typical psychologic response to orthognathic surgery, based on the work of Kiyak et al.[20] Before treatment, patients who seek orthognathic surgery tend to have scores above the mean for most psychosocial parameters. Immediately before the operation, patients are not quite so positive, as anxiety and other concerns increase. In the days immediately after the operation, a period of negativism typically occurs (e.g., depression, dissatisfaction). This is related in part to steroid use at the operation and withdrawal afterward but is not totally explained by this. By 6 weeks after the operation the patients usually are on the positive side of normal again, and at 1 year typically rate quite high for satisfaction with treatment and general well-being.

The great majority of patients who undergo orthognathic procedures report long-term satisfaction with the outcome (80%–90%, depending on the type of surgical procedure). A similar number say that, knowing the outcome and what the experience was like, they would recommend such treatment to others and would undergo it again.[8] On long-term recall, patients often comment that the changes produced by their surgical treatment gave them the confidence they needed to succeed in their business or profession.

This does not mean, of course, that there are no negative psychological effects from surgical treatment. First, a few patients or spouses or partners have great difficulty in adapting to significant changes in their facial appearance. This is more likely to be a problem in older individuals. If you are 19, your facial appearance has been changing steadily for all your life, and another change is not a great surprise. If you are 49 and now suddenly see a different face in the mirror, the effect may be unsettling. Psychologic support and counseling therefore are particularly important for older patients, and major esthetic changes in older adults may not be desirable. As we have discussed in Chapter 20, adults seeking treatment fall into two groups: a younger group who seek to improve their lot in life, and an older group whose goal is primarily to maintain what they have. The older group may need orthognathic surgery to achieve their goal, but for them, treatment should often be planned to limit facial change, not maximize it.

Second, whatever the age of the patient, a period of psychologic adjustment following a facial surgical procedure must be expected (Fig. 22.12). In part, this is related to the use of steroids at the operation to minimize postoperative swelling and edema. Steroid withdrawal, even after short-term use, causes mood swings and a drop in most indicators of psychological well-being. The adjustment period lasts longer than can be explained by the steroid effects, however. The surgeon learns to tolerate complaining patients for the first week or two after surgery. By the time orthodontic treatment resumes at 3 to 6 weeks after the operation, the patients are usually—but not always—on the positive side of the psychological scales. Sometimes the orthodontist also has to wait for a patient to make peace with his or her surgical experience.

In the short term, an important influence on the patient's reaction to surgical treatment is how well the actual experience matched what they were expecting. Interestingly, orthognathic surgery does not rate high on discomfort and morbidity scales. Operations involving the mandibular ramus require about the same amount of pain medication as extraction of impacted wisdom teeth; maxillary procedures are tolerated better than that. From a psychological perspective, it is not so much the amount of pain or discomfort you experienced that determines your reaction; it is how this compares with what you thought would happen. This highlights the importance of carefully preparing patients for their surgical experience.

Treatment Planning With Simulation of Alternative Treatment Outcomes

Not only is simulation important in planning treatment, but it has always been a moral and ethical imperative to allow the patient to make important decisions about what treatment he or she will accept, and now it is a legal obligation as well. Involving the patient as decisions about the choice of alternative treatments are made is an essential element of informed consent (see Chapter 7).

Image predictions are particularly valuable in helping patients decide between camouflage and surgery and in planning surgical treatment from the sagittal (profile) perspective. The patient can view the impact on the soft tissue profile of orthodontic camouflage versus surgery when these are realistic treatment alternatives They also can view the effect of varying amounts of surgical change, not just the change in jaw position—more or less mandibular advancement, for example—but also the effect of genioplasty or rhinoplasty in addition to change in jaw position. It is one thing to describe in words what the different outcomes of camouflage and surgery would be and something else to help the patient visualize them by seeing image predictions.

At one point, there was great concern that showing predictions to patients might lead to unrealistic expectations and disappointment with the actual result, but patient responses show that this risk is minimal or nonexistent. In a randomized trial, those who saw the prediction images before the operation were more, not less, likely to be satisfied with their result.[9] Only the patient can decide whether the difference between surgical correction of jaw relationships and orthodontic camouflage would be worth the additional risk and cost of surgery. Computer simulations help them do that.

Early planning and implementation of combined orthodontic and orthognathic surgical cases was conducted using cephalometric head films and acetate tracings to simulate the movements that were anticipated to correct the presenting malocclusion[10] (Fig. 22.13).

While there were quantitative algorithms derived from research available to help predict the resulting soft tissue outcome, they were almost never used. Placement of the dentition was accomplished by hand articulating models, transferring them to an articulator, and handmaking an acrylic splint in the laboratory to guide the

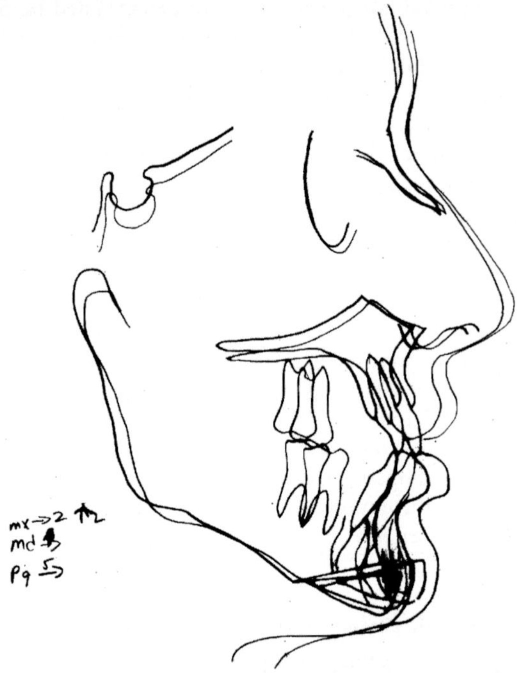

• **Fig. 22.13** Treatment planning was traditionally conducted using acetate tracings of the cephalometric head film, and the movements were planned primarily by correction of the malocclusion. Forecasting the esthetic outcome was limited to the two-dimensional profile view.

surgeon in positioning the jaws and teeth. Anticipation of esthetic outcomes was dependent on the creative eye of the surgeon and/or the orthodontist and was limited to the profile. Naturally, as technology progressed, the use of digital planning of orthognathic cases was developed,[11] evaluated for reliability,[12] accuracy, [13] and validity,[14] by type of surgery[15] and different systems compared.[16]

Algorithms derived from previous cephalometric research were integrated into computerized imaging programs to predict the profile responses more accurately from planned hard tissue movements.[17] However, anticipation of the esthetic outcome was still limited to the profile (Fig. 22.11), while the clinical examination documenting the resting and dynamic hard and soft tissue relationships (primarily such important esthetic items such as incisor size or display at rest, incisor display on smile, smile arc, and buccal corridors), which are a primary determinant in the contemporary approach to planning treatment were largely ignored[18]

Therefore, treatment planning begins with vertical and horizontal placement of the maxillary incisors, and other skeletal movements are driven by that first step in treatment planning. As technology has progressed, three-dimensional (3D) radiography (most frequently cone beam computed tomography [CBCT]) has been incorporated into planning and guiding the osseous surgical movements. The advantage of 3D surgical planning is its accuracy in three dimensions and the manufacturing of positioning splits to guide the surgeon in accurately positioning of the jaws. Currently, the commercially available 3D skeletal placement systems do not incorporate soft tissue responses to hard tissue movements into their programs. This means that what the patient is often most interested in, the esthetic outcome, is only being explored and not commonly used in 3D treatment planning technology. This is primarily due to a lack of research which yields algorithms measuring soft tissue response to hard tissue movements which would provide reliable prediction of facial outcomes in 3-dimensions. This next step is important in the progression of this technology because of the importance that patients place on the facial results of orthodontic/orthognathic surgical treatment. We are confident that with time the appropriate algorithms for soft tissue response to 3D movements will be generated and put to use.

In the meantime, as an interim solution a method utilizing both the profile prediction methods and the 3D skeletal method in a hybrid fashion serves well as this type of technology progresses. The following case provides a good example of the fusion of the two methodologies in planning and executing jaw surgery.

This 15-year-old girl (Fig. 22.14A and B) was previously treated for her Class II malocclusion. The first phase of treatment was discontinued because of lack of progress due to an unfavorable growth in treatment response. The patient was placed into retainers and followed periodically to monitor growth cessation. Only then could a definitive surgical/orthodontic treatment plan be performed.

As a result of that first phase of treatment, her teeth were compensated for the skeletal malocclusion through the use of elastics in an effort to achieve a better occlusal relationship.

Note that her profile (see Fig. 22.14C) reflects marked convexity due to her lack of mandibular growth. However, she had achieved nice dental alignment in her first phase of treatment (see Fig. 22.14D–F) resulting in mild dental compensation and a bilateral Class II malocclusion.

Because of her young age, surgical treatment was not recommended until she reached the point of physical maturity and felt that the surgical approach to her malocclusion was appropriate for her. At age 20, records were updated, and the chief complaint revisited, and both the problems and the positive features were formulated which led to the treatment plan.

Chief complaint: "I have an overbite."

Prioritized Problems:

- Class II malocclusion
- Convex profile
- Deficient chin
- Prominent lower lip with deep labiomental sulcus
- Short lower facial height
- Obtuse nasolabial angle with excessive nasal projection

Positive Features:

- Excellent vertical positioning of the maxillary incisors

Goals:

- Correct the Class II malocclusion
- Idealize anteroposterior maxillary incisor position
- Improve mandibular projection
- Improve upper lip support
- Improve chin projection and labiomental sulcus
- Improve excessive nasal projection, if desired

Tx Plan:

- Attain arch coordination and correction of any alignment issues. Because her previous orthodontic treatment had resulted in good dental alignment and transverse relationships, the initial phase of treatment was begun with clear aligners to correct any rotations and malpositions which may have occurred over the time period since removal of her fixed appliances.

  In the surgical phase of treatment proceed to:
- Le Fort I maxillary advancement (both for esthetics and improvement of potential airway considerations) (discussed in this chapter).

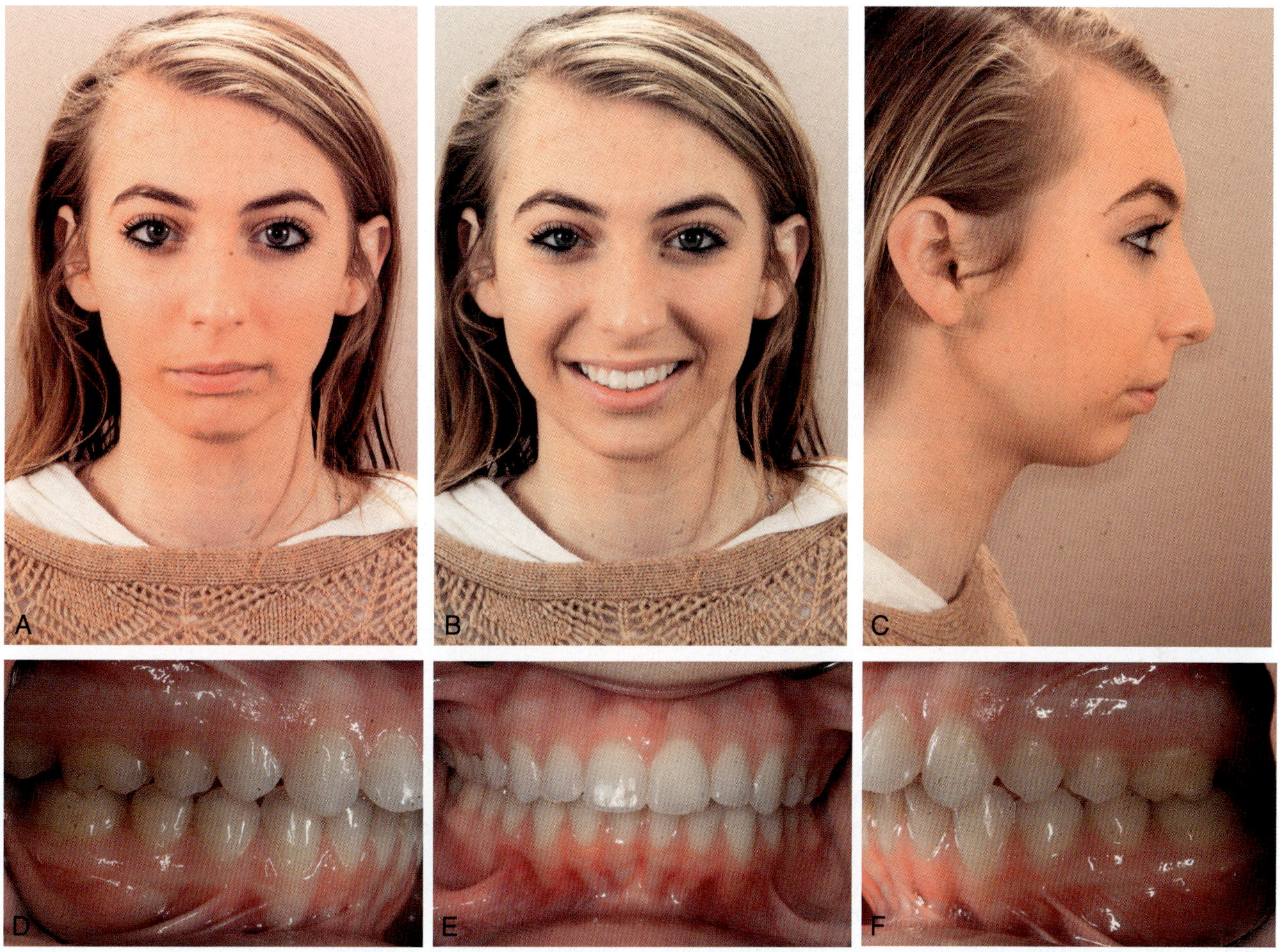

• **Fig. 22.14** (A and B) This 15-year-old girl was referred for surgical consultation after having undergone orthodontic treatment as an adolescent for correction of her class II mandibular deficiency. (B) Her frontal smiling view demonstrates her short lower facial height, the deep labiomental sulcus, and her short lip-chin length with an ideal smile with excellent incisor display and smile arc. (C) Her profile reflected her mandibular deficiency associated with her class II malocclusion. (D–F) Her previous phase of orthodontic treatment resulted in good dental alignment of her teeth, but she had a bilateral Class II malocclusion.

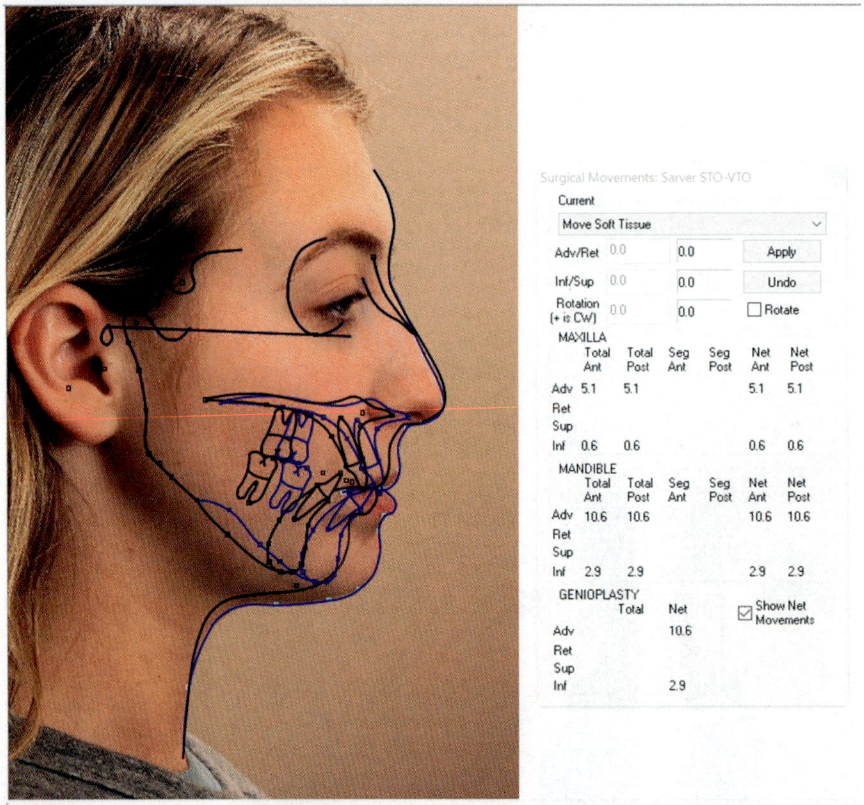

• **Fig. 22.15** In the mid-1990s, sophisticated 2D software for surgical outcome prediction was developed utilizing hard-to-soft-tissue predictive algorithms generated from data gathered from many published studies. This case represents the first phase of a hybrid approach of treatment planning and this image demonstrates the projection of bimaxillary advancement, chin advancement via inferior border osteotomy, and simultaneous rhinoplasty. The quantitative table, reflecting the movements, gives the clinician the desired outcome much as an architect's plan serves as a guide to a builder.

- Simultaneous rhinoplasty.
- Mandibular advancement.
- Inferior border osteotomy to advance the chin.
- Mild downgraft of the chin to increase the lower facial height and provide more pleasing labiomental sulcus.
- Finish dental articulation.

A computer digital approach was used to aid in the planning of her orthognathic surgery combining the use of both 2D (Fig. 22.15) and 3D software (Fig. 22.16). The first step in this computerized planning step was to place her maxillary incisor in ideal vertical and antero- posterior position, resulting in maxillomandibular advancement with a 5 millimeter chin advancement to balance the profile and a 3 mm downward movement of the chin to idealize lower facial height (see Fig. 22.15). The predicted skeletal changes were reflected in the quantitative chart on the right side of the figure. Algorithms derived from previous studies, which were part of the 2D program rendered a forecast of what was expected as the profile changed.

A 3D CBCT was obtained and forwarded for "virtual surgical planning" shown in Fig. 22.16A, and the quantitative numbers generated by the 2D plan were entered into the virtual 3D planner. First, the maxilla was virtually placed in the prescribed 3D position, which was termed the "intermediate position" (Fig. 22.16B). A guiding occlusal wafer (see Fig. 22.16B), termed an "intermediate splint," was then printed to guide the surgeon precisely to the desired position of the maxilla, Therefore, the maxillary osteotomy was performed first and stabilized with plates, using the intermediate wafer matched to the lower arch and guiding the maxillary arch to its precise position using the intermediate splint. The mandibular osteotomy was performed next with a "final splint" (not shown) serving as the guide (see Fig. 22.16C) for its placement based on the stable, plated maxilla. In this case, advancement of the chin with a lower border osteotomy was performed with the inferior border osteotomy guided to its final position with what is termed a "positioning guide."

After 5 months of postoperative orthodontic finishing treatment, her improved facial and smile outcomes are evident (Fig. 22.17A–C). Fig. 22.17B demonstrates her smile improvement with complete incisor display and an ideal smile arc. Her profile (Fig. 22.17C) presented greatly improved alignment with desirable lip balance and nasal esthetics. Her final occlusal relationships were quite good (see Fig. 22.17D–F). Her pretreatment and postoperative cephalograms are shown in Fig. 22.18A and B.

Contemporary Surgical Techniques

The possible jaw movements with orthognathic surgery are shown diagrammatically in Figs. 22.19 and 22.20. As the figures illustrate, both jaws can be repositioned three-dimensionally, but not all directions of movement are feasible. The mandible can be moved forward or backward, rotated, and moved down anteriorly

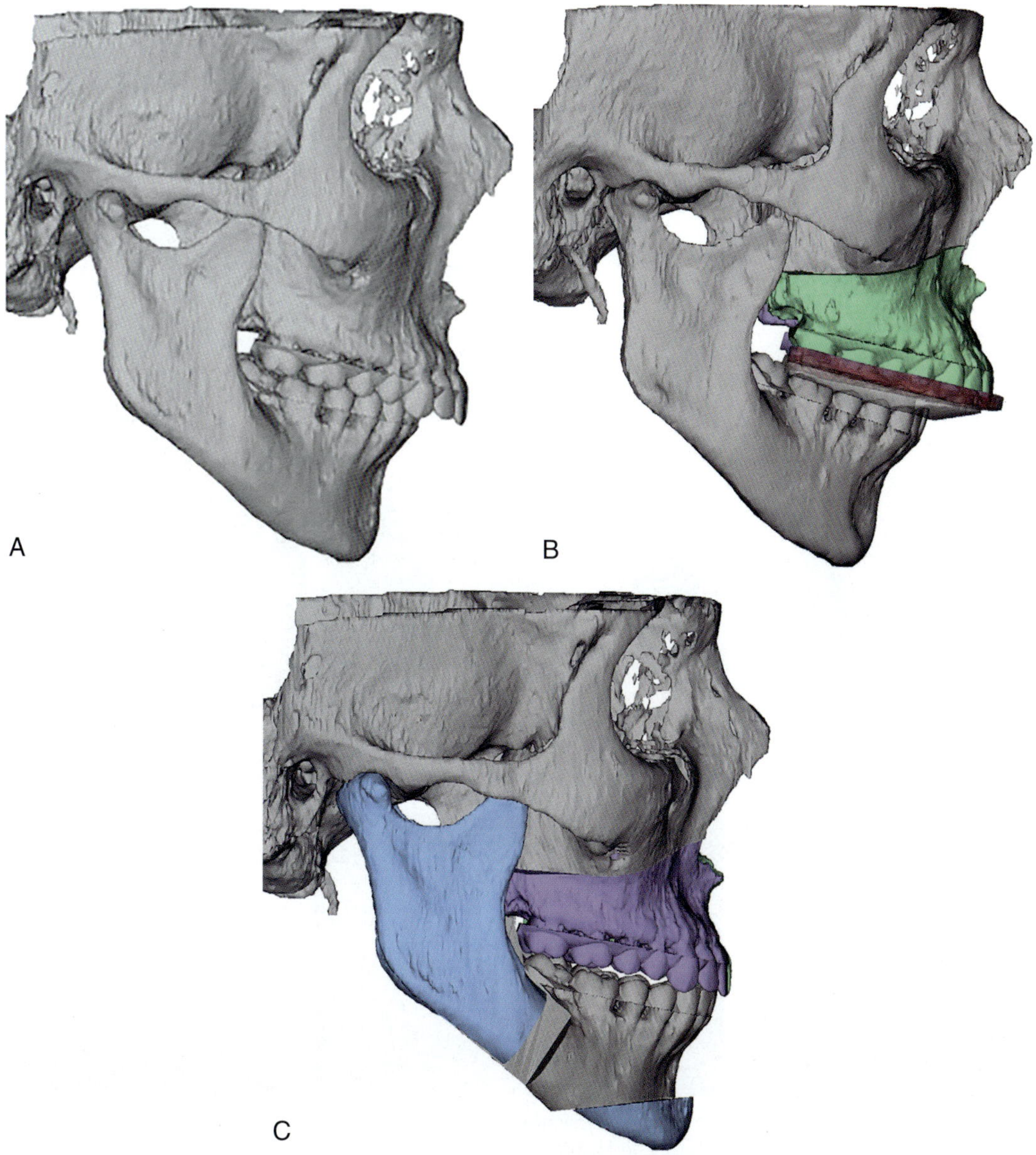

• **Fig. 22.16** (A) From the initial cone beam CT, the surgical planning service rendered an accurate 3D image from the digital data to be used in planning the desired osseous movements. (B) As part of our treatment planning protocols, initial surgical treatment planning starts with virtual positioning both the vertical and horizontal positioning of the maxillary incisors based on the clinical evaluation. In this case, a "maxilla first" approach was planned, so an occlusal wafer was created to guide the surgeon in aiding the precise positioning the maxilla, relative to the mandible, after completion of a Le Fort I osteotomy. (C) This image demonstrates the final surgical plan with the inclusion of bilateral sagittal split osteotomies for advancement of the mandible and an inferior border osteotomy for chin augmentation. With a slight downgraft of the chin, length was added to her chin height to improve the proportion of her lower face. From this final plan an interocclusal splint was printed to guide the surgeon to the desired final occlusal relationships. An additional guide was printed for the chin osteotomy and positioning of the chin segment.

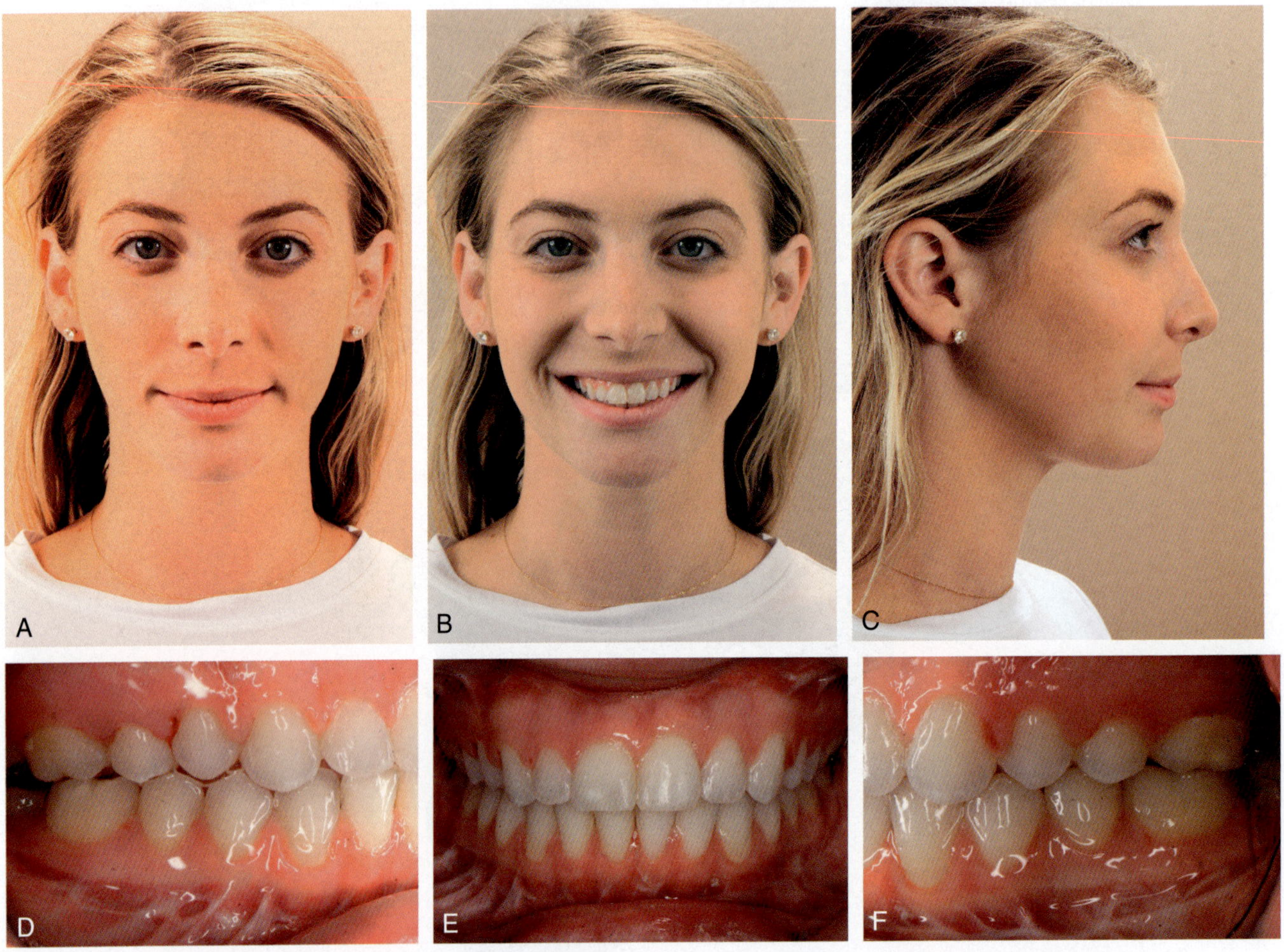

• **Fig. 22.17** (A) After completion of her postoperative surgical and orthodontic treatment, her frontal image reflected the improved lower facial height and improved nasal contour. (B) Her smile outcome was excellent with improvement in her smile projection. Figure (C) Ideal lower facial projection was achieved, and the rhinoplasty helped reduce the nasal projection and idealized her nasal dorsum and tip. (D–F) Ideal overbite and overjet was achieved with Class I occlusion.

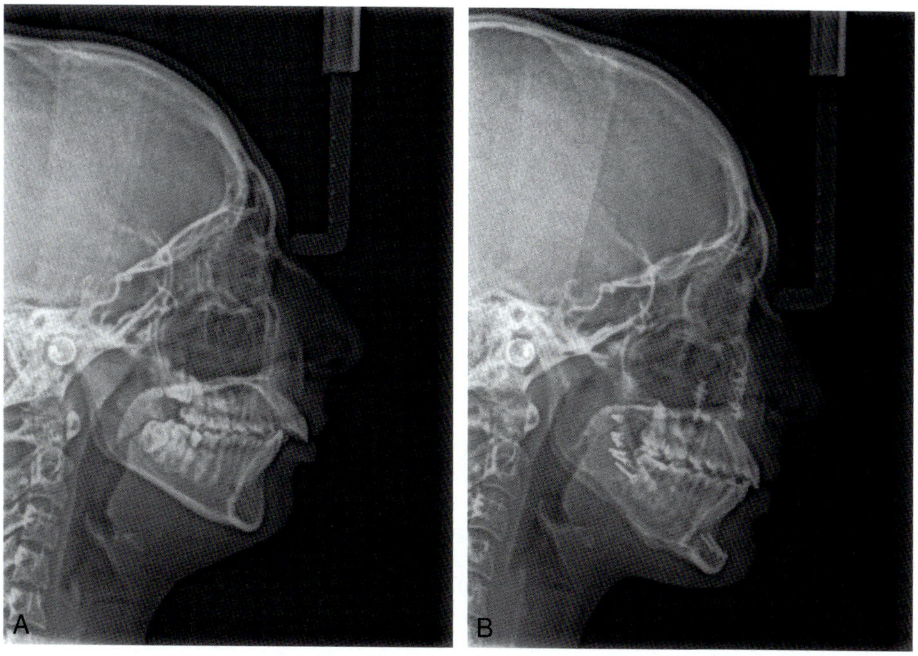

• **Fig. 22.18** (A) The patient's initial cephalometric radiograph from initiation of her surgical/orthodontic phase of treatment reflecting the severe overjet and lower facial retrusion. (B) The final posttreatment cephalogram.

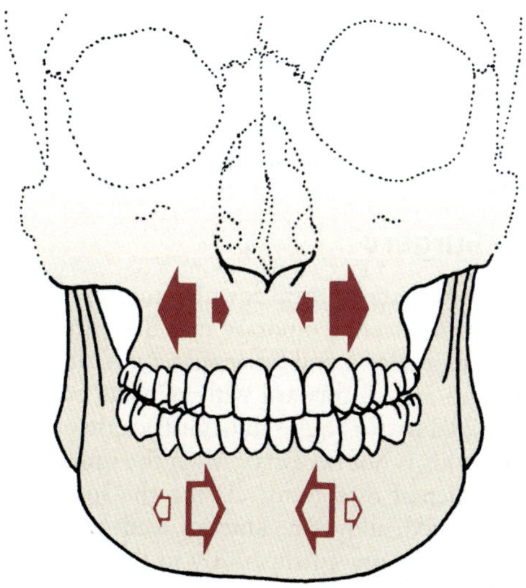

• **Fig. 22.19** The surgical movements that are possible in the transverse dimension are shown on this illustration of the lower face skeleton. The solid arrows indicate that the maxilla can be expanded laterally or constricted with reasonable stability. The smaller size of the arrows pointing to the midline represents the fact that the amount of constriction that is possible is less than the possible amount of expansion. The only transverse movement easily achieved in the mandible is constriction, although limited expansion is now possible with distraction osteogenesis.

to increase the mandibular plane and anterior face height—but rotating it up in a counterclockwise manner with a ramus osteotomy to decrease the mandibular plane angle and decrease anterior face height will create instability unless the maxilla is moved up posteriorly at the same time so that this rotation does not lengthen the ramus and stretch the elevator muscles. The mandible can be narrowed anteriorly but widened only with distraction osteogenesis (discussed later).

The maxilla can be moved up and forward with excellent stability, moved down with difficulty because of instability, and moved back only with great difficulty because of all the structures behind it that are in the way. Fortunately, protruding anterior teeth can be moved back via orthodontics or segmental osteotomy, so there is no reason to move the posterior maxilla back. Segmental osteotomy also allows the maxilla to be widened or narrowed, but widening it tends to be unstable because of the pull of stretched palatal tissues.

Mandibular Surgery

The sagittal split osteotomy (see Fig. 22.2) is now used for almost all mandibular surgery because of several advantages over alternative techniques for ramus surgery:

- The mandible can be moved forward or back as desired, and the tooth-bearing segment can be rotated down anteriorly (increasing the mandibular plane angle) when additional anterior face height is desired.
- This procedure is quite compatible with the use of rigid intraoral fixation (RIF), so immobilization of the jaws during healing is not required.
- Excellent bone-to-bone contact after the osteotomy means that problems with healing are minimized, and postsurgical stability is good.

In contemporary treatment, a lower border osteotomy of the mandible to reposition the chin relative to the mandibular body (Fig. 22.21) is a major adjunct to ramus procedures, especially when the mandible is advanced. It is used in about 30% of the patients who receive a ramus osteotomy and in about the same number of patients with maxillary surgery. The lower border procedure allows the chin to be moved transversely, forward or back, and up or down.

Other mandibular procedures are used primarily for major advancements or surgery involving the condyles. An extraoral approach is often required, and a bone graft is likely to be needed.

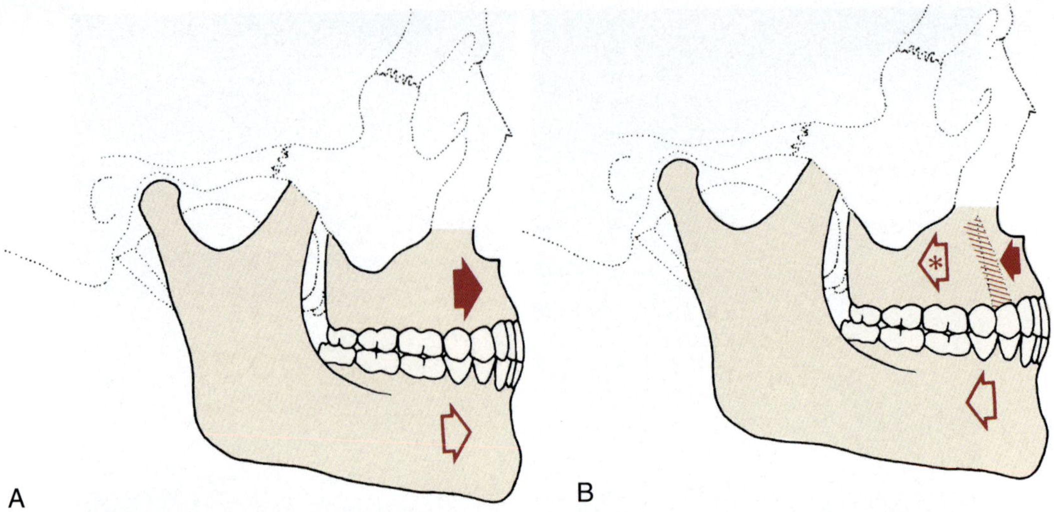

• **Fig. 22.20** The maxilla and mandible can be moved anteriorly and posteriorly as indicated by the red arrows in these line drawings. (A) Anterior movements of the mandible greater than approximately 10 mm create considerable tension in the investing soft tissues and tend to result in increasing instability with greater advancement. Anterior movement of the maxilla is similarly limited to 6–8 mm in most circumstances; the possibility of relapse or speech alteration from nasopharyngeal incompetence increases with larger movements. (B) Posterior movement of the entire maxilla, although possible, is difficult and usually unnecessary. Instead, posterior movement of protruding incisors up to the width of a premolar is accomplished by removal of a premolar tooth on each side, followed by segmentation of the maxilla. The major limitation of posterior movement of the mandible is its effect on the appearance of the throat. When the mandible is moved back, the tongue moves down as the airway is maintained, and a "turkey gobbler" prominence appears below the chin.

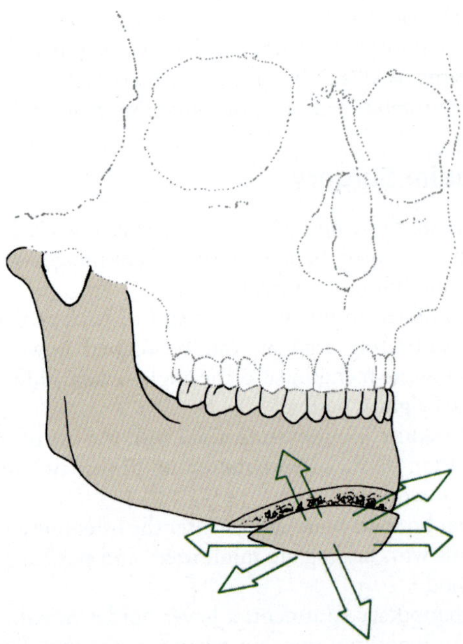

• **Fig. 22.21** The chin can be sectioned anterior to the mental foramen and repositioned in all three planes of space. The lingual surface remains attached to muscles in the floor of the mouth, which provide the blood supply. Moving the chin anteriorly, upward, or laterally usually produces highly favorable esthetic results. Moving it back or down may produce a "boxy" appearance.

Rarely, a midline osteotomy of the mandible with removal of an incisor is used to narrow it anteriorly.[19]

Maxillary Surgery

The Le Fort I osteotomy with downfracture of the maxilla (see Fig. 22.3) dominates contemporary maxillary surgery just as the sagittal split dominates mandibular surgery. It allows the maxilla to be moved up and/or forward with excellent stability. Moving the entire maxilla back is quite difficult because of the structures behind it, but this is not necessary when the upper teeth are protrusive. A segmental osteotomy, closing the space where a premolar was extracted, allows the anterior teeth to be retracted and posterior teeth to be moved superiorly so that anterior open bite is closed as the mandible rotates upward and forward (Fig. 22.22). Segmental osteotomies also allow the posterior maxilla to be widened or (less frequently) narrowed.

Expansion is done with parasagittal osteotomies in the lateral floor of the nose or medial floor of the sinus that are connected by a transverse cut anteriorly. In a two-piece osteotomy, a midline extension runs forward between the roots of the central incisors; this may or may not be included in a three-piece osteotomy (Fig. 22.23). If constriction is desired, bone is removed at the parasagittal osteotomy sites. In expansion, either bone harvested in the downfracture or bank bone is used to fill the void created by lateral movement of the posterior segments.

Skeletal palatal expansion of the type used in adolescents was not feasible in adults because of the increasing resistance from interdigitated midpalatal and lateral maxillary sutures. Recent studies have shown that modest increases in maxillary width can still be achieved when palatal anchorage is used (see Chapter 13). Surgically assisted rapid palatal expansion (SARPE), using bone

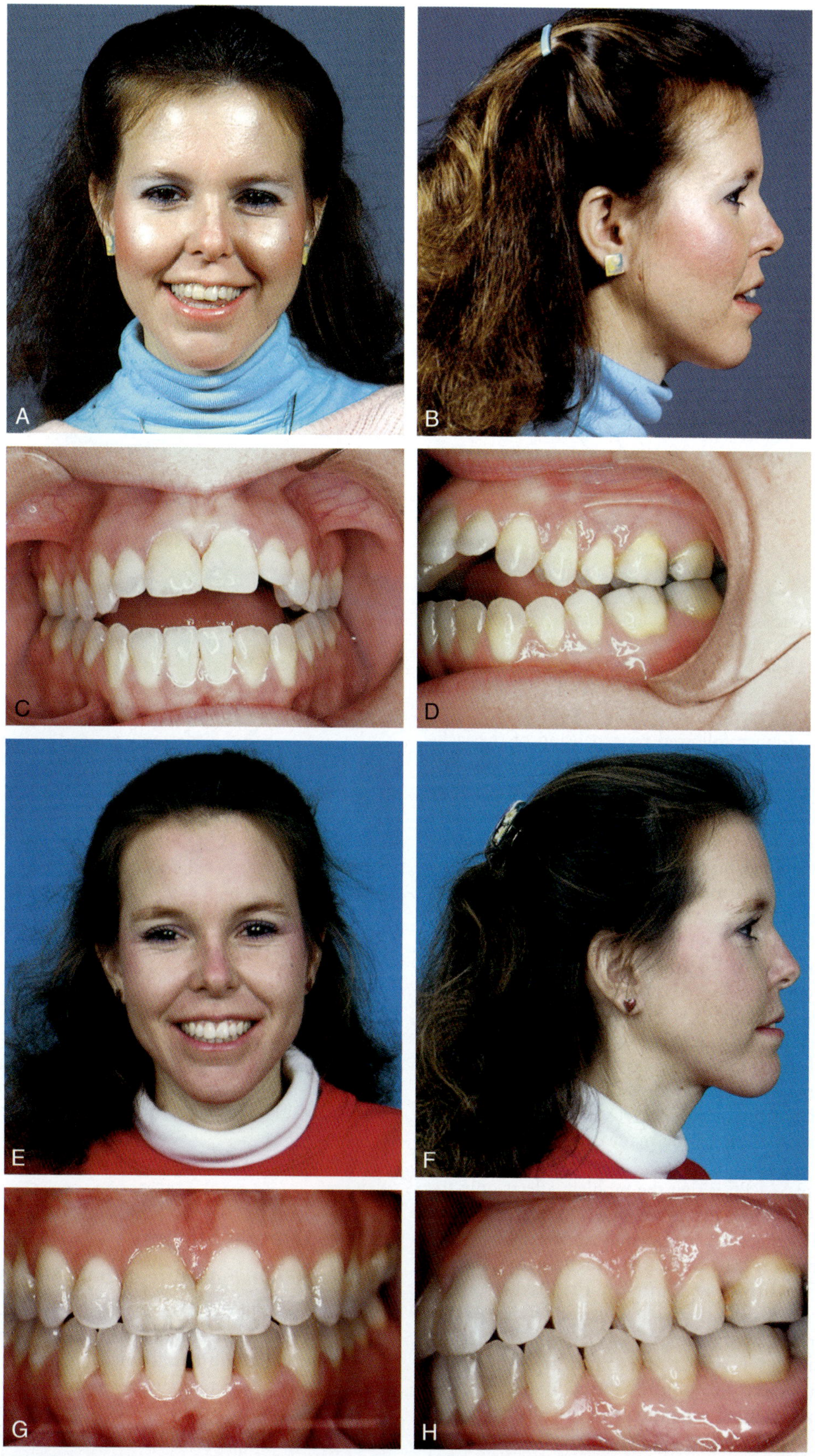

• **Fig. 22.22** Superior repositioning of the maxilla is indicated to correct severe anterior open bite if the lower facial third is long, as in this patient. (A and B) Facial proportions and (C and D) occlusal relationships before treatment. (E and F) Facial proportions and (G and H) occlusal relationships after segmental Le Fort I osteotomy to move the maxillary posterior segments up and the anterior segment down, steepening the occlusal plane. This allowed the mandible to rotate up and forward to close the open bite while providing better incisor display.

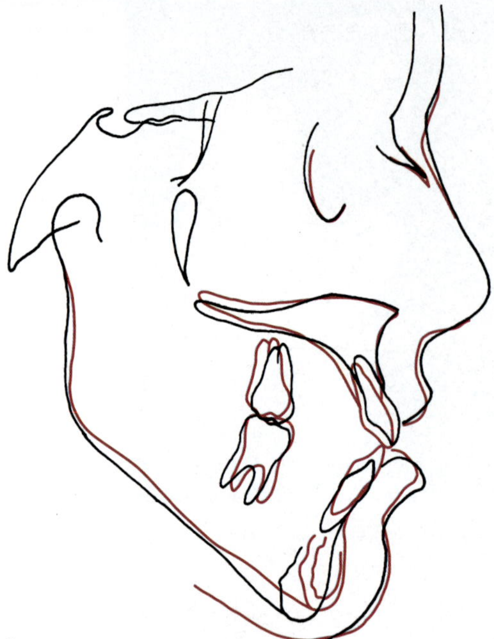

I

• **Fig. 22.22, cont'd** (I) Cephalometric superimposition showing the repositioning of the maxillary segments and the decrease in anterior face height. When the posterior maxilla is repositioned vertically, both the postural (rest) and occlusal positions of the mandible change.

cuts to reduce the resistance followed by expansion of the jackscrew to separate the halves of the maxilla, is another possible treatment approach for adult patients with a narrow maxilla (Fig. 22.24). The original idea of surgically assisted expansion was that cuts in the lateral buttress of the maxilla would decrease resistance to the point that the midpalatal suture could be forced open (i.e., microfractured) in older patients. Although this usually works in patients in their late teens or early 20s, the chance of inadvertent fractures in other areas is a concern, especially for patients in their 30s or older. For SARPE now, surgeons usually make all the cuts needed for a Le Fort I osteotomy, omitting only the final step of downfracture.[20] This allows widening of the maxilla against only soft tissue resistance, manipulating the osteotomy sites with what amounts to distraction osteogenesis. If only expansion is desired, this provides a somewhat less invasive approach than segmental osteotomy. Unfortunately, however, there is no guarantee of symmetric expansion—one of the main disadvantages of this procedure.

The implication of SARPE is that the problem affects only the transverse plane of space, and this is when it is most useful. One of its purported advantages over segmental osteotomy was better stability, and some surgeons advocated a preliminary phase of SARPE before Le Fort I osteotomy to move the maxilla anteroposteriorly or vertically. Current data, however, show that relapse of the dental expansion accompanies SARPE (Fig. 22.25) and that its long-term stability is similar to that with segmental osteotomy.[21] It is difficult, therefore, to justify the additional cost and morbidity of surgically assisted expansion as a first stage of surgical treatment in a patient who would require another operation later to reposition the maxilla in the anteroposterior or vertical planes of space. The primary indication for preliminary SARPE is such severe maxillary constriction that segmental expansion of the maxilla in the Le Fort I procedure might compromise the blood supply to the segments.

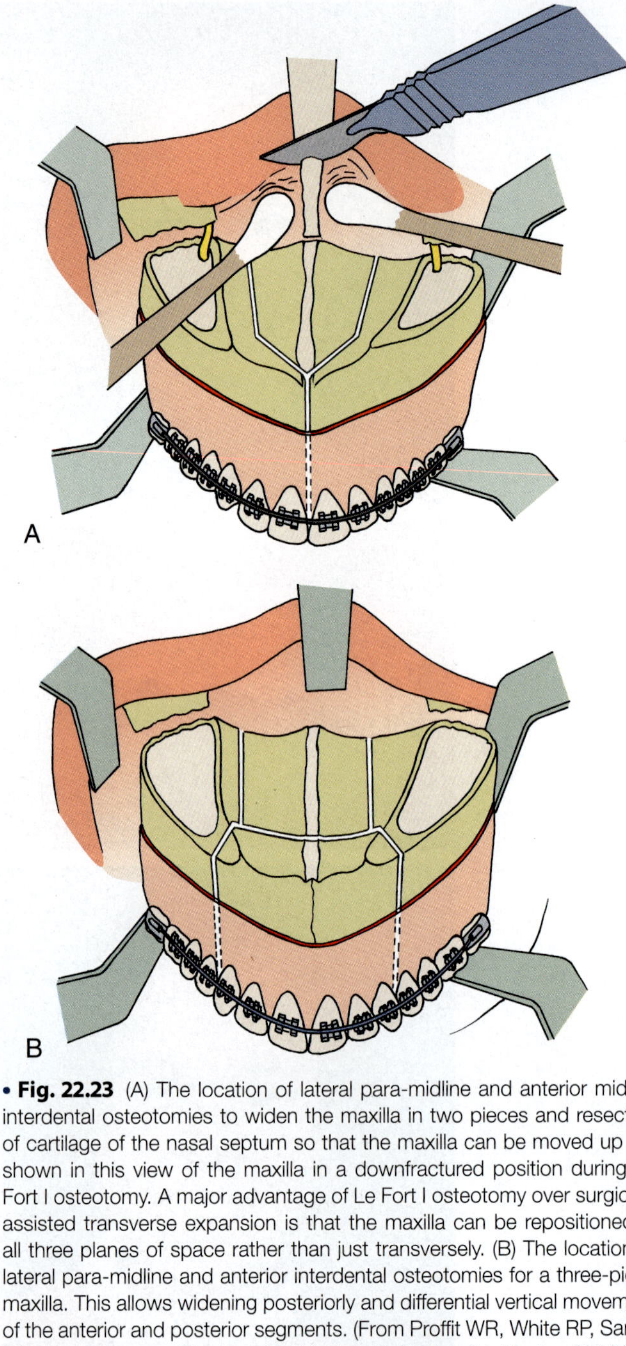

• **Fig. 22.23** (A) The location of lateral para-midline and anterior midline interdental osteotomies to widen the maxilla in two pieces and resection of cartilage of the nasal septum so that the maxilla can be moved up are shown in this view of the maxilla in a downfractured position during Le Fort I osteotomy. A major advantage of Le Fort I osteotomy over surgically assisted transverse expansion is that the maxilla can be repositioned in all three planes of space rather than just transversely. (B) The location of lateral para-midline and anterior interdental osteotomies for a three-piece maxilla. This allows widening posteriorly and differential vertical movement of the anterior and posterior segments. (From Proffit WR, White RP, Sarver DM. *Contemporary Treatment of Dentofacial Deformity*. Mosby; 2003.)

Dentoalveolar Surgery

Recovery From Inadvertent Tooth Movement

Although it is not orthognathic surgery, it is part of orthodontic management of patients to include coordinated periodontal surgery to help with correction of malposed tooth roots, which can happen when teeth undergo unplanned tooth movement after archwires, or fixed retainers break or are distorted (see Fig. 19.16). Induction of new bone formation is now possible with local bone-stimulating hormone therapy and bone grafts so that when displaced roots are repositioned into the alveolar process with torque force, root fenestration can be corrected as well (Fig. 22.26). This requires close coordination between the periodontist and orthodontist.

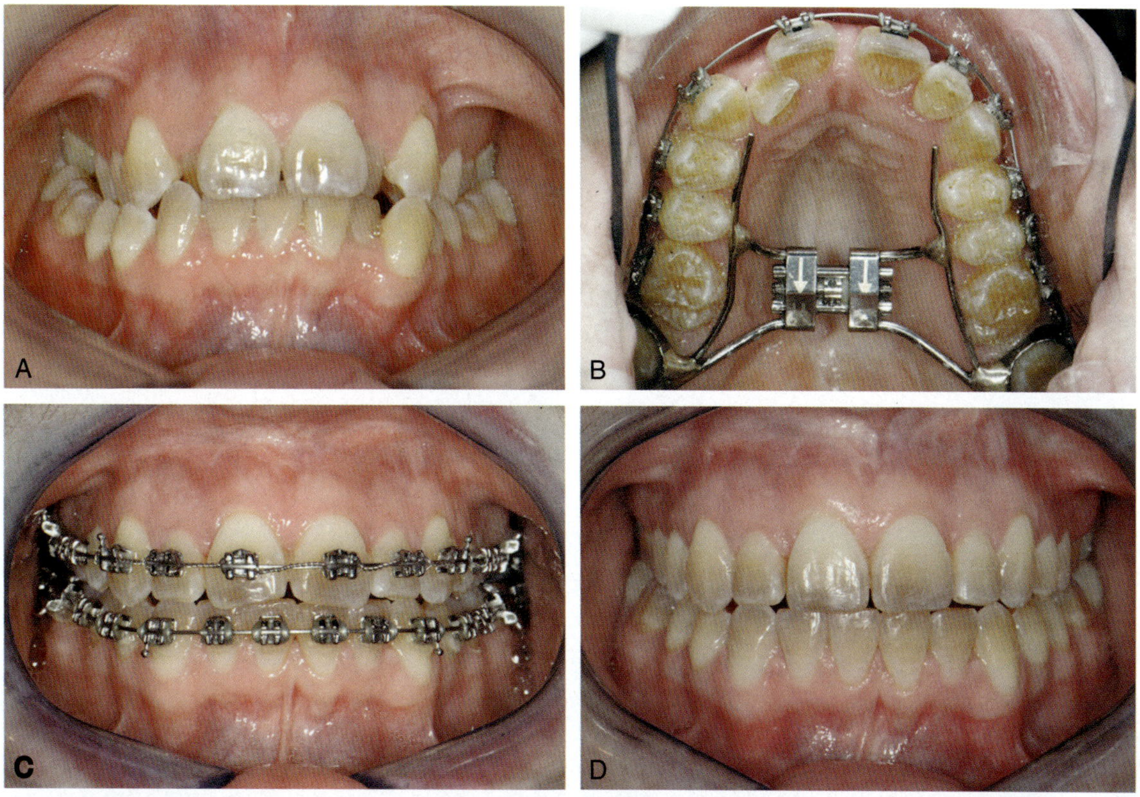

• **Fig. 22.24** In this adult patient with maxillary posterior crossbite and severe crowding, surgically assisted rapid palatal expansion (SARPE) was used to allow transverse expansion. The modern surgical technique includes all the bone cuts for a Le Fort I osteotomy except the downfracture. (A) Narrow maxillary arch, posterior crossbite, and maxillary incisor crowding before treatment. (B) Expansion appliance in place after the operation and activation of the screw over a period of 4 days after a brief latency period, showing the amount of expansion that was obtained. (C) Fixed appliance for completion of alignment. A compressed coil spring that was used to open space for the maxillary left lateral incisor after the palatal expander was removed 3 months after the operation. (D) Widening the maxilla corrected the posterior crossbite and provided space to align the incisors, which made it possible to plan later cosmetic restoration of these stained teeth.

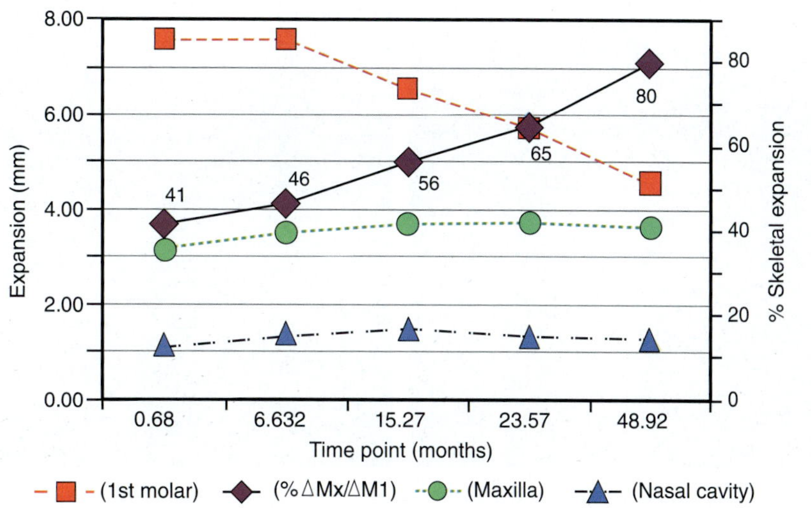

• **Fig. 22.25** Changes in the dental and skeletal dimensions over time after surgically assisted rapid palatal expansion (SARPE) and in the percentages of skeletal versus dental expansion. Squares indicate expansion at the first molar, diamonds indicate percentages of skeletal expansion at each time point, circles indicate maxillary skeletal expansion, and triangles indicate expansion across the nasal cavity. Note that almost all relapse was dental rather than skeletal; the change in the percentage of skeletal change is shown on the right vertical axis. Repeated-measures analysis of variance confirmed a significant relationship between the amount of dental relapse and the time after the operation, whereas skeletal changes were stable and unaffected by time after the operation. (Redrawn from Chamberland S, et al. Short- and long-term stability of SARPE revisited. *Am J Orthod Dentofac Orthop*. 2011;139:815–822.)

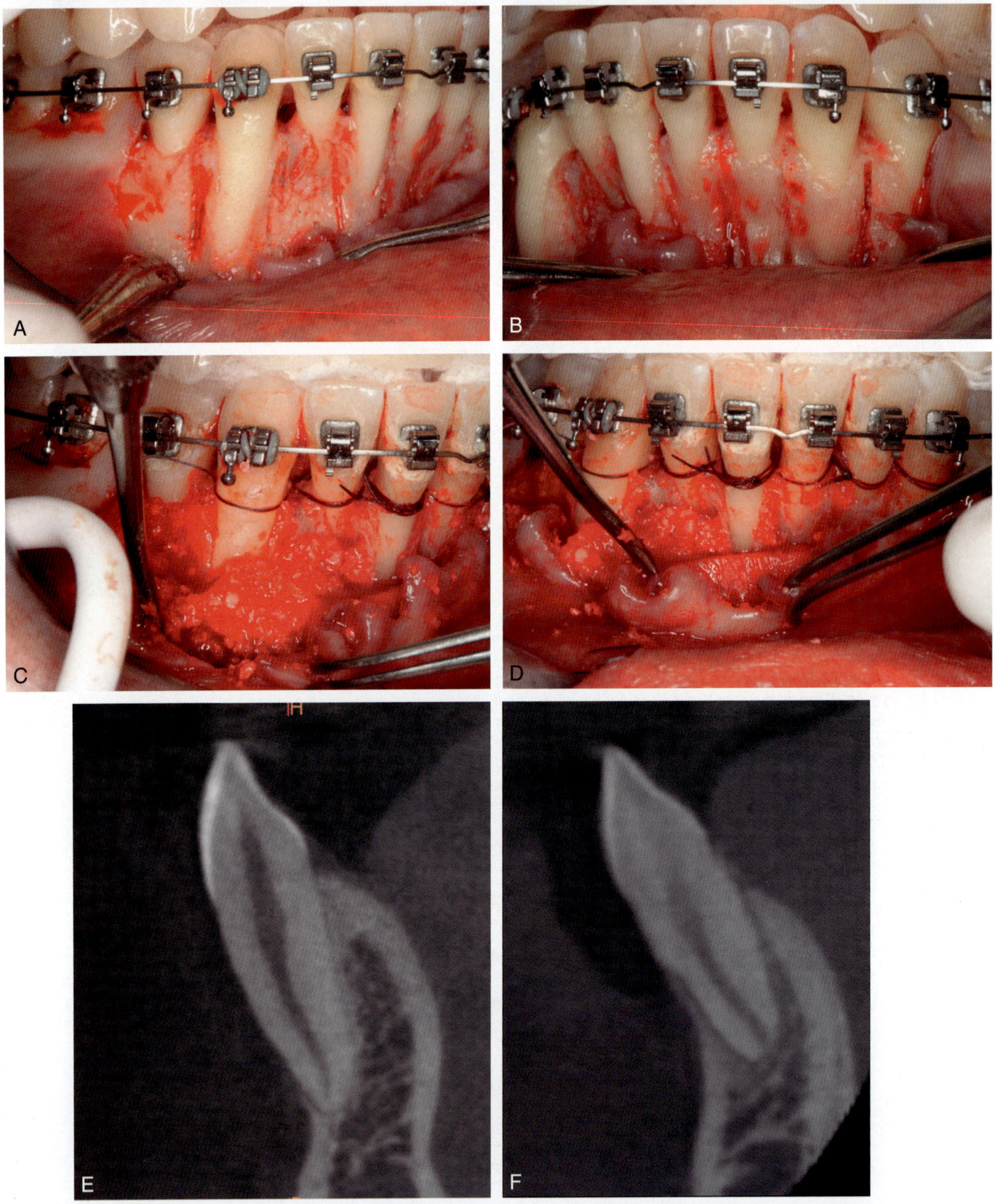

• **Fig. 22.26** (A) Severe root torque and bone fenestration after inadvertent tooth movement from a distorted bonded lingual retainer. (B) Periodontal treatment involved a gingival flap to expose the fenestrated roots and corticotomy cuts to accelerate bone remodeling, then (C) a bone graft slurry to cover the roots and (D) covering of the area as the gingiva was sutured into position. (E) A small-field-of-view three-dimensional image showing the original position of the right canine outside the bone of the root (shown also in A). (F) Active root torque with orthodontic treatment that started immediately after the periodontal surgical procedure succeeded in getting the root back into the alveolar process, and the image shows bone over the lower half of the facial surface of the tooth. (Courtesy Dr. T. Shaughnessy.)

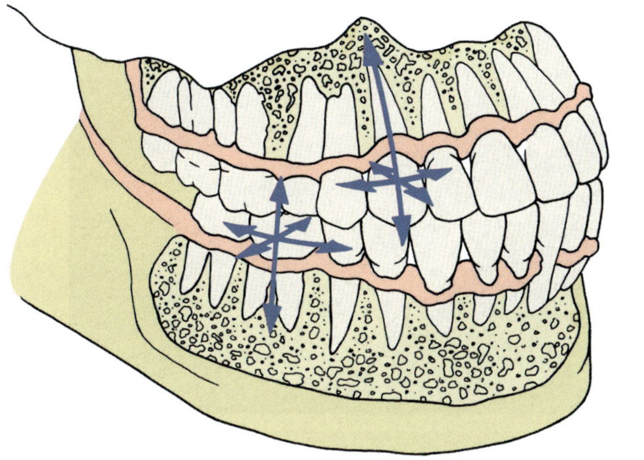

• **Fig. 22.27** The key to surgery to reposition dentoalveolar segments is maintaining an adequate blood supply to the bone and teeth through intact labial or lingual mucosa. In the mandibular posterior area, temporarily lifting the inferior alveolar neurovascular bundle out into the cheek allows cuts to be made safely beneath the teeth. Although the nerve supply to the teeth is interrupted, sensation usually returns and endodontic treatment almost never is required. (From Proffit WR, White RP, Sarver DM. *Contemporary Treatment of Dentofacial Deformity*. Mosby; 2003.)

Repositioning Alveolar Segments

Segments of the dentoalveolar process can be repositioned surgically in all three planes of space (Fig. 22.27), but there are important limitations with this procedure. The principal one is the distance of movement that is possible: in most instances, only a few millimeters. A significant but less important limitation is the size of the segment: a three-tooth or larger segment is preferred, a two-tooth segment is acceptable but less predictable, and a one-tooth segment is a problem waiting to occur.

The reason for both limitations is the same. After an osteotomy beneath the bone segment and teeth, the blood supply is surprisingly good through collateral circulation via the facial and lingual mucosa. This must be preserved to maintain the vitality of the teeth and the integrity of the bone. The further a segment is moved and the smaller it is, the greater the chance of interrupting not only the usual blood supply but also the collateral supply.

An osteotomy below the root apices cuts the nerves to the pulp of the teeth in that segment, and of course there is no collateral innervation. The short-term result is something that dentists rarely observe: a vital but denervated pulp that does not respond to electrical stimulation. At that point, pulp vitality can be demonstrated by the maintenance of either normal pulp temperature (temperature probe) or blood flow (Doppler flow meter), and re-innervation of the pulp often occurs after a few months. Even though the major vessels to the tooth pulp are cut, less than 2% of the involved teeth require endodontic treatment. Even if the apex of a tooth is inadvertently cut off, pulp vitality is likely to be maintained by blood flow through auxiliary foramina.

Distraction Osteogenesis

Distraction osteogenesis is based on manipulation of a healing bone, stretching an osteotomized area before calcification has occurred to generate the formation of additional bone and investing soft tissue (see Chapter 13). For correction of facial deformities, this has two significant advantages and one equally significant disadvantage.

The advantages of distraction are that (1) larger distances of movement are possible than with conventional orthognathic surgery and (2) deficient jaws can be increased in size at an earlier age. The great disadvantage is that precise movements are not possible. With distraction, the mandible or maxilla can be moved forward, but there is no way to position the jaw or teeth in exactly a preplanned place, as can be done routinely with orthognathic procedures. This means that patients with craniofacial syndromes are the prime candidates for distraction of the jaws. They are likely to need intervention at early ages and large distances of movement, and precision in establishing the posttreatment jaw relationship is not so critical for them.

Moderately severe hemifacial microsomia, in which a rudimentary ramus is present on the affected side, is a major indication for distraction because it is the only way to generate new bone to replace the missing part (Fig. 22.28). Distraction is not needed in the milder forms of this syndrome in which mandibular asymmetry exists, but the mandible is reasonably complete (for these patients, growth modification is possible), and it cannot be used as the initial stage of treatment in patients so severely affected that the entire distal portion of the mandible is absent. For them, a bone graft is necessary, and distraction later can be one way to lengthen the graft.

The timing of treatment for patients with moderately severe hemifacial problems remains controversial, but social acceptability becomes a factor in the decision. To improve the child's facial appearance, intervention to advance the mandible on the affected side is often considered at ages 6 to 8, and at that time both of its advantages make distraction a frequent choice. Early distraction, however, is unlikely to be followed by normal growth of the distracted area, and later orthognathic surgery or a second round of distraction will probably be required.

Patients with facial syndromes that include severe maxillary deficiency (e.g., Crouzon, Apert; see Fig. 5.11) are also candidates for early distraction. In these patients, appropriate bone cuts in the posterior and superior areas of the maxilla can allow advancement of the entire midface, similarly to what can be achieved with Le Fort III surgery but without the need for extensive bone grafts. For patients with problems of this type, the precision with which the teeth can be placed in proper occlusion simply becomes a secondary consideration. The fact that later orthodontic and surgical treatment will be required reinforces this attitude toward the initial treatment.

For less severe maxillary or mandibular deficiency, however, distraction offers no advantage over a sagittal split or Le Fort I osteotomy, and after a period of initial enthusiasm about treatment of these patients, it is almost never used now. The orthognathic procedures allow the teeth and jaws to be precisely positioned, and an excellent clinical result can be anticipated. For these patients, distraction is a more difficult way to accomplish a surgical result that requires more extensive postsurgical orthodontics.

One of the things that cannot be done with orthognathic surgery is widening the mandibular symphysis, because there is not enough soft tissue to cover a bone graft in that area. Distraction makes this possible (Fig. 22.29) and provides additional space in the incisor area. Does that make it an acceptable method for nonextraction treatment of lower incisor crowding? Usually, no. When crowded incisors are aligned with orthodontic expansion, this is accomplished at the expense of incisor protrusion and doubtful stability, especially if mandibular canines are expanded

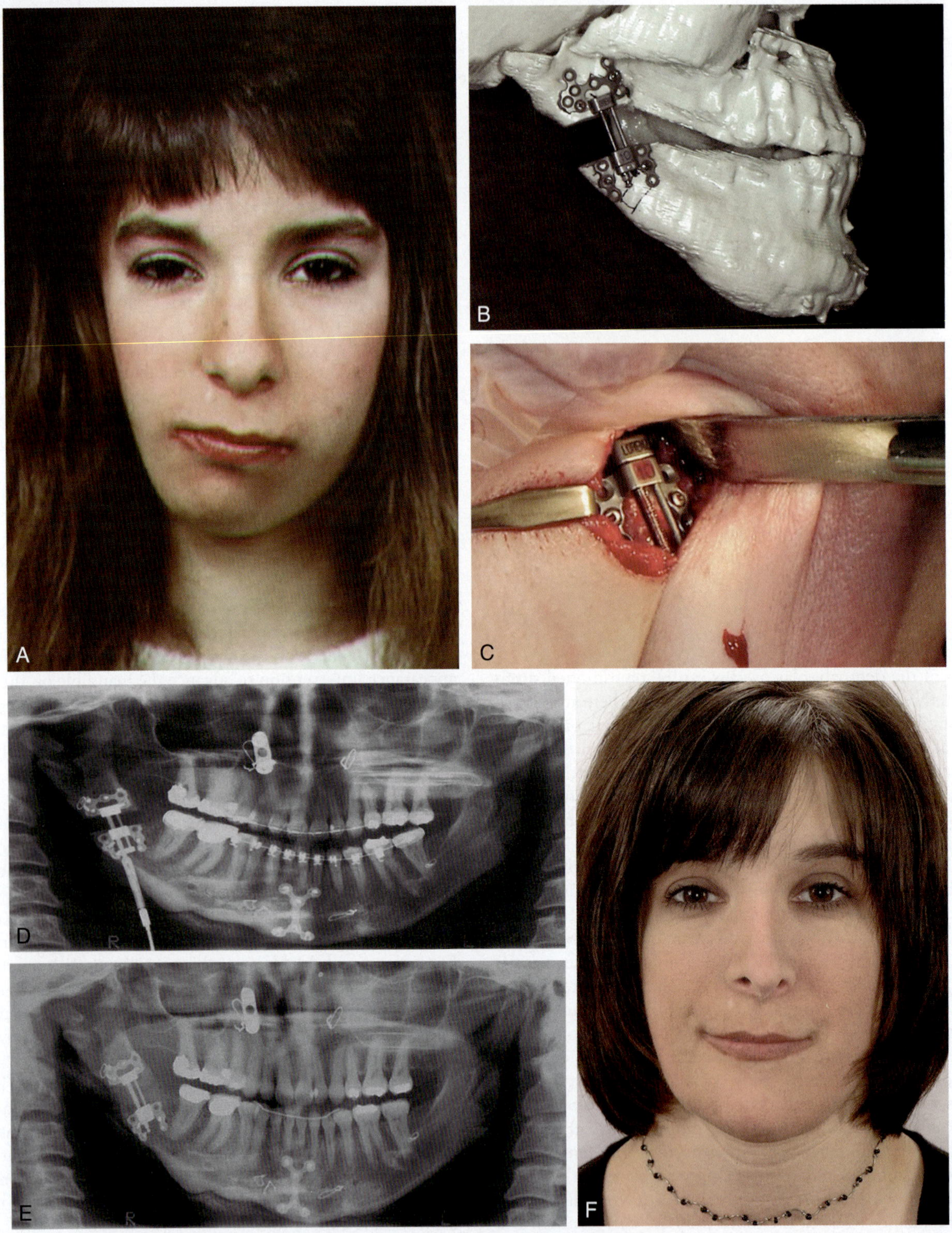

• **Fig. 22.28** Distraction osteogenesis to lengthen the deficient mandibular ramus in a girl with hemifacial microsomia. (A) Facial appearance before treatment. (B) Distractor fitted on stereolithographic models made from a computed tomography scan. (C) Distractor placed at the operation. After the device is in place, cuts are made through the cortical bone of the mandible, and activation of the distractor begins after a latency period to allow initial healing. (D) Panoramic view during distraction showing the opening created by stretching of the healing bone callus. (E) Panoramic view 3 months later, at the end of the postdistraction stabilization period during which the newly formed bone is remodeled and becomes normally calcified. (F) Facial appearance at the completion of treatment. Creating new mandibular bone with distraction, as a general rule, is more effective than placing bone grafts, but distraction cannot be used to replace grafts in all circumstances. (Courtesy Dr. C. Crago.)

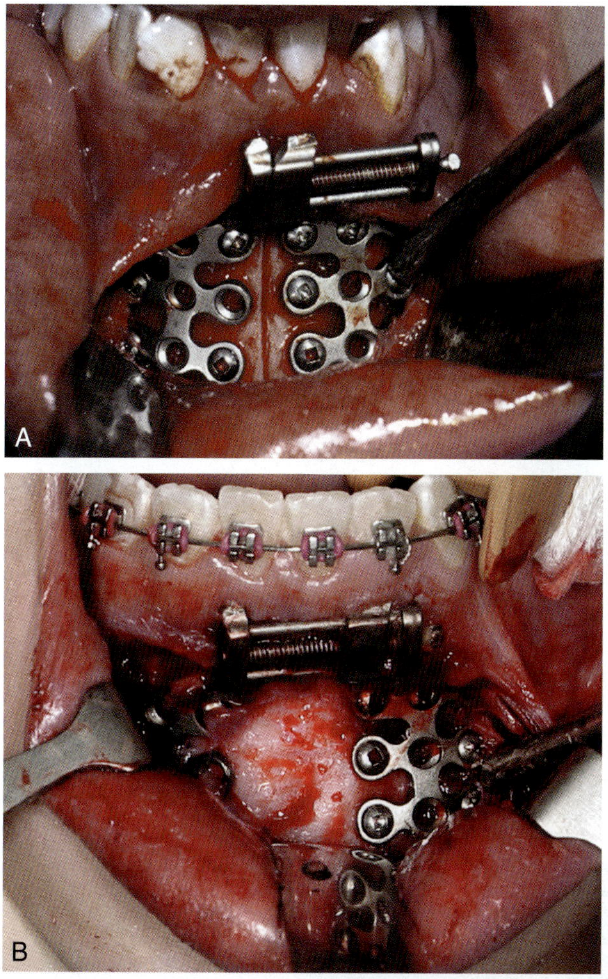

• **Fig. 22.29** Mandibular symphysis distraction to provide greater width to the anterior mandible. (A) Placement of the distraction device. After the device has been contoured to fit and screwed in place, cuts are made through the facial and lingual cortical plates of the mandible, usually extending all the way through the symphysis. Distraction begins after a 5- to 7-day latency period, with the screw activated 2 turns (0.5 mm) twice a day. (B) Intraoperative view when the distractor was removed 16 weeks after the initial surgical procedure. Note the normal appearance of the regenerate bone across the distraction site. (Courtesy Dr. C. Crago.)

without retracting them. The important clinical questions therefore are whether symphysis distraction provides a more stable and less protrusive result than nonextraction orthodontics, and whether either approach to expanding the mandibular dental arch gives a better result than premolar extraction to provide space for alignment.

With distraction at the symphysis, not only osteogenesis (formation of new bone) but also histogenesis (formation of new soft tissue) occurs. The formation of new periosteum over the distracted area is what makes widening of the symphysis possible. To relieve lip and cheek pressure against expanded mandibular canines, however, soft tissue changes would have to extend to the muscles of facial expression at the corners of the mouth. To date, there is no evidence that expansion with distraction is more stable than conventional expansion and given the distance from the osteotomy site to the soft tissues at the corner of the mouth, it seems unlikely that this would be the case. As with distraction for mandibular advancement, symphysis distraction has been abandoned except for patients with what amounts to a midline cleft, with both missing incisors and the bone to support them (see Fig. 13.16).

Adjunctive Facial Procedures

A variety of facial procedures can be used as adjuncts to orthognathic surgery to improve the soft tissue contours beyond what is available from repositioning the jaws.[22] Conceptually, this can be viewed as a form of camouflage, done surgically rather than orthodontically. These procedures can be put into five groups: chin augmentation or reduction, rhinoplasty, facial soft tissue contouring with implants, lip procedures, and submental procedures. We will consider them briefly, in turn.

Chin Augmentation or Reduction

There are two approaches to repositioning the chin relative to the rest of the mandible: a lower border osteotomy to slide it to its new location or (augmentation only) placement of an alloplastic implant.

The lower border osteotomy to advance the chin has the advantages of well-documented predictability and stability, and (because it advances the genial tubercles) it tightens the suprahyoid musculature and produces desirable changes in chin-neck contour. It is particularly advantageous in patients with a combination of vertical excess and anteroposterior deficiency, which results in strain to bring the lips together. Sliding the chin upward and forward in patients with this facial pattern is a "functional genioplasty," in that it allows normal lip function as well as correction of the facial disproportion (Fig. 22.30).[23] Bone modeling thickens the alveolar process below the teeth, and the notch above the repositioned chin fills in with new bone that extends up to the alveolar crest, creating new bone in an area where it is needed for future gingival stability (Fig. 22.31). In later periodontal therapy to control gingival stripping, that area often is bone grafted.

Functional genioplasty, and augmentation with sliding of the chin forward more generally, are more successful when done before age 15 (Fig. 22.32), so this is just the opposite of an orthognathic procedure that should wait until growth is essentially completed. The more the lower incisors erupt after the genioplasty, the better the formation of new bone above the displaced chin. How early can it be done? The practical limit is eruption of the mandibular canines, which would be in the way of the osteotomy until they have moved into the oral cavity. Bone remodeling occurs above and behind the repositioned chin, but the bony chin does not remodel and is remarkably stable over time. Augmentation genioplasty with alloplastic materials is favored by plastic surgeons, who prefer to avoid osteotomy and are often working with late adolescents or adults—although lower border osteotomy still remodels well in older patients. With greater chin advancement in older patients, prominence of the lateral border of the chin that creates a notch along the lower border can become a problem. To compensate for this, there are two possibilities: either splitting the chin so the posterior margins can be moved medially to eliminate the notch, or bone grafts or alloplastic augmentation materials over the lower border to fill in the posterior notch.

A chin implant has two advantages: the possibility of removal if the patient is unhappy with the result, and less risk of decreased sensation in the lower lip (from trauma to the nerve that emerges from the mental foramen to innervate the lip, which must be avoided in any genioplasty). It also has a major disadvantage, particularly with silicone implants: erosion of the implant into the

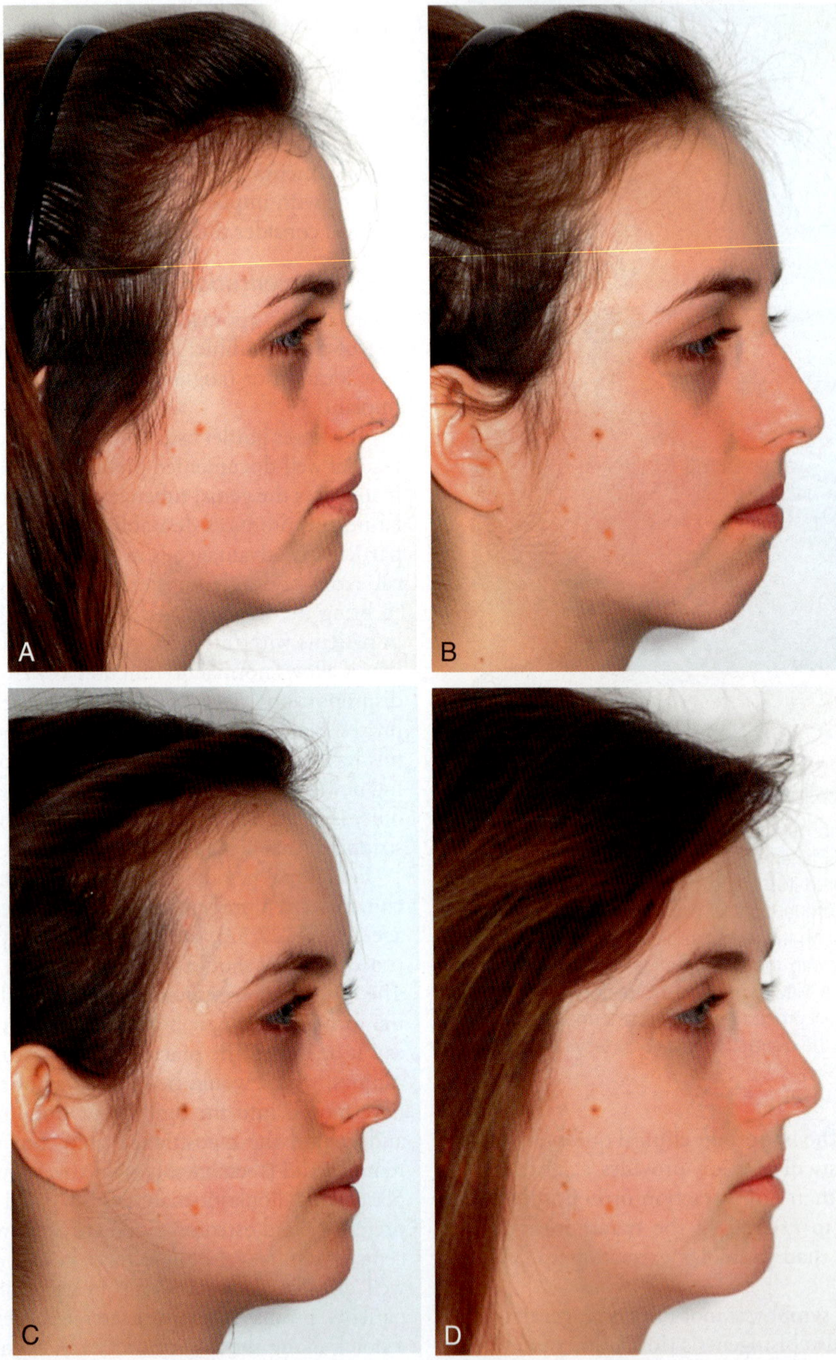

• **Fig. 22.30** (A–D) Profile and (E–H) cephalometric images of a patient who benefited from functional genioplasty after orthodontic treatment to correct her Class II malocclusion. (A) Pretreatment; (B) post orthodontic treatment, (C) post genioplasty and (D) post genioplasty recall. This provides not only improved facial proportions but also normalization of lip function, decreasing lip separation at rest and allowing the lips to be brought into contact without muscle strain. (Courtesy Dr. S. Chamberland.)

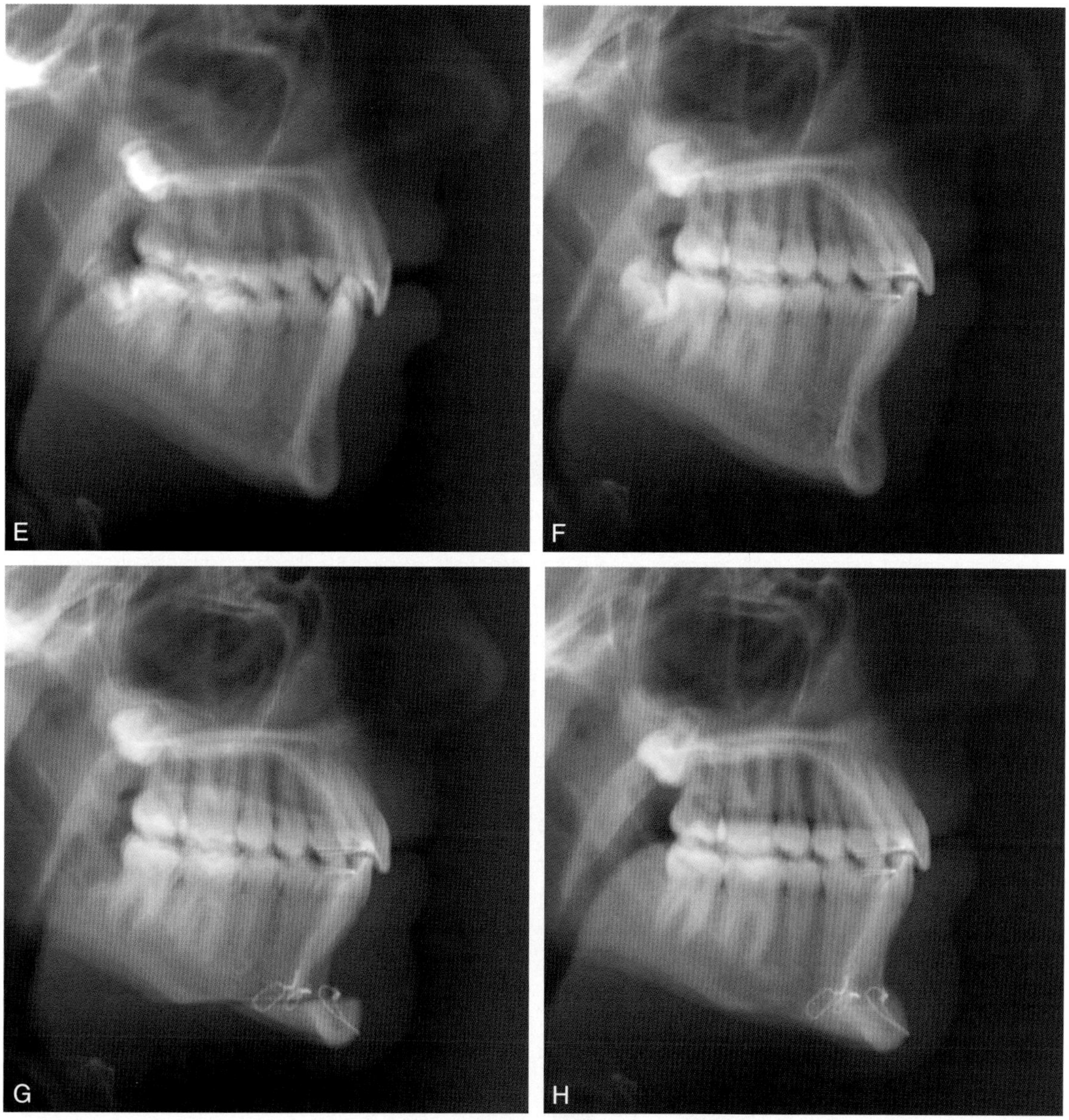

• **Fig. 22.30, cont'd**

surface of the bone or migration into the neck. Newer implant materials placed into a soft tissue pocket rather than directly against the bone provide much better stability and have almost totally replaced silicone. Removal of one of these implants, however, is difficult, and undesirable soft tissue changes may result if this is necessary.[23]

There are two aspects of deformity of the chin in patients with excessive mandibular growth: prominence of the chin relative to the dentition, and excessive height of the chin. In patients with a prominent chin, if a lower border osteotomy is used to simply slide the bony chin backward, and especially if the chin surface is cut away, the soft tissue chin tends to look like an underinflated ball because of the loss of skeletal volume. In patients with excess chin height, however, vertical reduction of the chin by removing a wedge of bone above the chin prominence and then repositioning the chin upward (and often slightly forward) can greatly improve the facial appearance and result in a measurable improvement in the patients' quality of life.[24]

Rhinoplasty

The smile is framed by the chin below and the nose above. It may be necessary to change both to achieve optimal changes in facial appearance. Mandibular surgery repositions the chin relative to the rest of the face, and as we have seen, repositioning the chin relative to the jaw also may be needed. Maxillary surgery via Le Fort I osteotomy rarely has a positive effect on the appearance of the nose and may compromise it. Moving the maxilla up and/or forward can have two major deleterious effects on the nose: rotation of the nasal tip upward, resulting in deepening of the supratip depression, and widening of the alar base. Rhinoplasty, simultaneous with orthognathic surgery or staged to follow it (see Figs. 22.11 and 22.17), can prevent these problems, so it is indicated

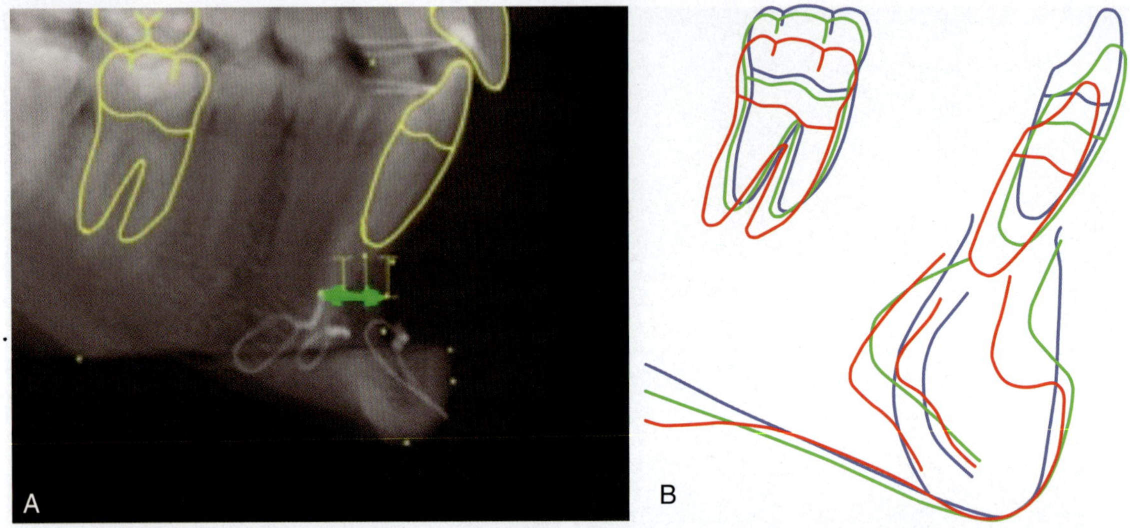

• **Fig. 22.31** When a lower border osteotomy is used to move the chin forward, remodeling along the lower border smooths the bony contour there. New bone formation above the prominence of the chin fills in the notch that is present immediately after the operation, and this extends all the way to the alveolar crest in patients who are still growing vertically. (A) The result is a clinically significant thickening of the symphysis. (B) Cephalometric superimposition tracing shows the change from before *(green)* to after *(red)* and 2 years after *(blue)* the surgical procedure. Note the amount of new bone in the symphysis area and its upward extension toward the alveolar crest accompanying eruption of the incisors in this young patient.

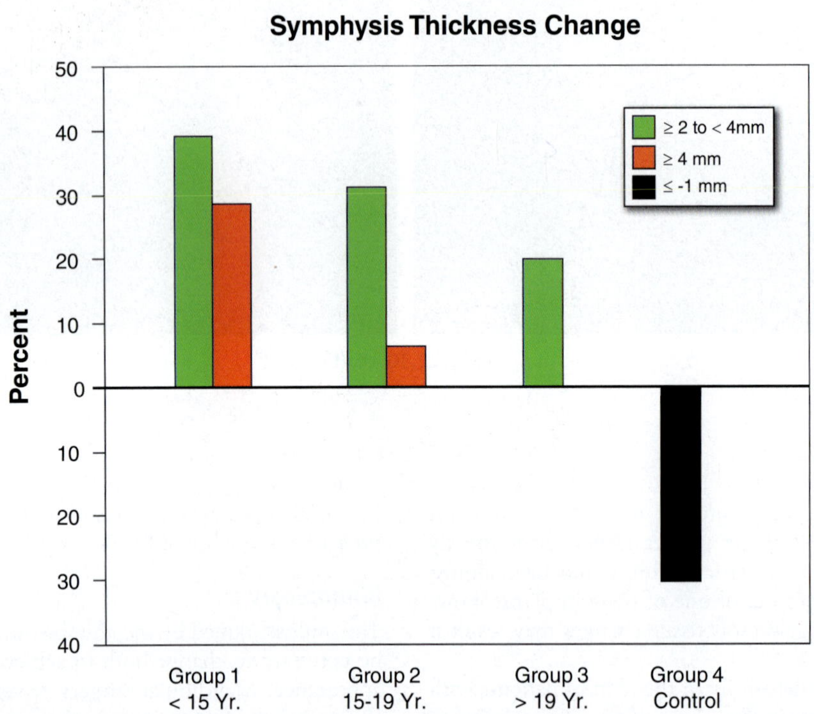

• **Fig. 22.32** This surgical procedure is more effective if it is done before age 15, although it still is applicable to late adolescents and adults. Vertical growth and eruption of the lower incisors increase the amount of new bone formation at the symphysis. A lower border osteotomy should not be done until eruption of mandibular canines has cleared the way for the osteotomy. As in the patient seen in Fig. 22.31, genioplasty at the end of active orthodontics often is the optimum time. (Redrawn from Chamberland et al. Genioplasty in growing patients. *Angle Orthod*. 2015;85:360–373.)

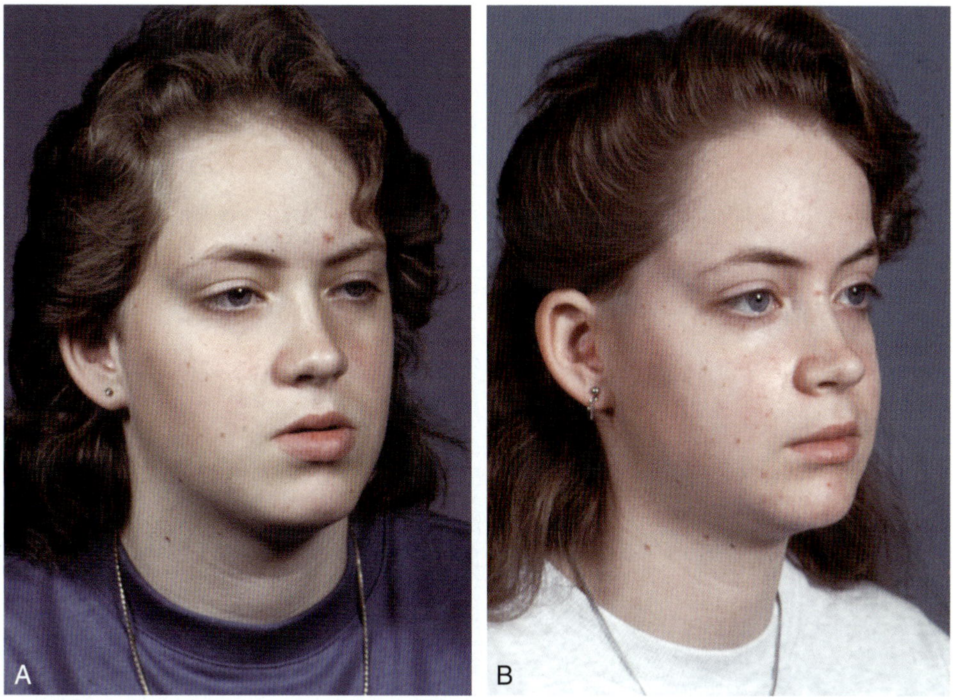

• **Fig. 22.33** In patients with maxillary deficiency who will have the maxilla advanced, surface grafts to augment the paranasal area often are needed, as in this girl. (A) Before the operation. (B) After maxillary advancement and paranasal grafts. Note the increased fullness alongside the nose, which would not have been created just by moving the maxilla.

for this purpose as well as for correction of a preexisting nasal deformity. Although Le Fort II and III procedures do move the nose along with the upper parts of the maxilla, these more extensive and riskier operations are indicated only in the most severe deformities.

Rhinoplasty usually is focused on the contour of the nasal dorsum, the shape of the nasal tip, and the width of the alar base. All these aspects can be significantly improved with modern surgical techniques. Because the soft tissue contours around the nose will be affected by repositioning of the jaws, rhinoplasty follows the orthognathic procedure. It can be done immediately afterward, as part of the same surgical experience, with a switch from nasal to oral intubation after the jaw operation is completed. This is technically more difficult and requires excellent interaction between the orthognathic and rhinoplasty surgeons but greatly increases the chance that the rhinoplasty actually will be accomplished.[25]

Facial Soft Tissue Contouring With Implants

Implants on the surface of the face can greatly improve soft tissue contours and are particularly advantageous for correction of two problems: the paranasal deficiency that often accompanies maxillary deficiency (Fig. 22.33), and the soft tissue deficiencies that accompany facial syndromes such as hemifacial microsomia. Onlay grafts in the paranasal area can be done successfully with use of the patient's own bone, freeze-dried cadaver bone, or alloplastic materials. The more extensive implants needed in patients with congenital anomalies usually are made from alloplastic materials that can be shaped in advance.

Lip Procedures

Instead of changing soft tissue contours indirectly with skeletal surgery, lip procedures directly augment or reduce the lips. Lip augmentation rarely accompanies orthognathic procedures; this is usually done to counteract the loss of lip fullness that accompanies aging. Although injections of collagen or other materials into the lips can be successful, the results tend to be temporary. A more permanent increase in lip projection can be obtained with AlloDerm (human dermis in sheet form), a synthetic material such as Gore-Tex, or the patient's own soft tissue harvested during a simultaneous face lift procedure. These are placed by creating a tunnel beneath the mucosa and threading the material into this space. This approach is preferred when lip augmentation is needed for orthognathic patients.

Lip reduction is rarely performed now but can greatly improve outcomes for the rare patients with extremely thick and prominent lips. It is accomplished via intraoral incisions parallel to the vermilion border and excision of soft tissue, avoiding the removal of muscle but including submucosal glands.

Submental Procedures

Correction of an unesthetic throat form often is needed as an adjunct to orthognathic procedures in older patients. Advancing the mandible improves throat form, and a lower border osteotomy to advance the chin tightens sagging throat tissues even more, but the orthognathic procedures alone are not sufficient to correct a "double chin" or "turkey gobbler" deformity. This often requires a combination of removal of excessive submental fat and tightening of the platysma muscle sling (Fig. 22.34). Both can be done readily at the time of orthognathic surgery. Localized fat deposits superficial to the platysma can be removed with liposuction. Fat below the platysma requires an approach through the muscle that allows direct removal of the fat, then closure of the platysma muscle layer. Loose musculature in the area can be tightened as this is done.

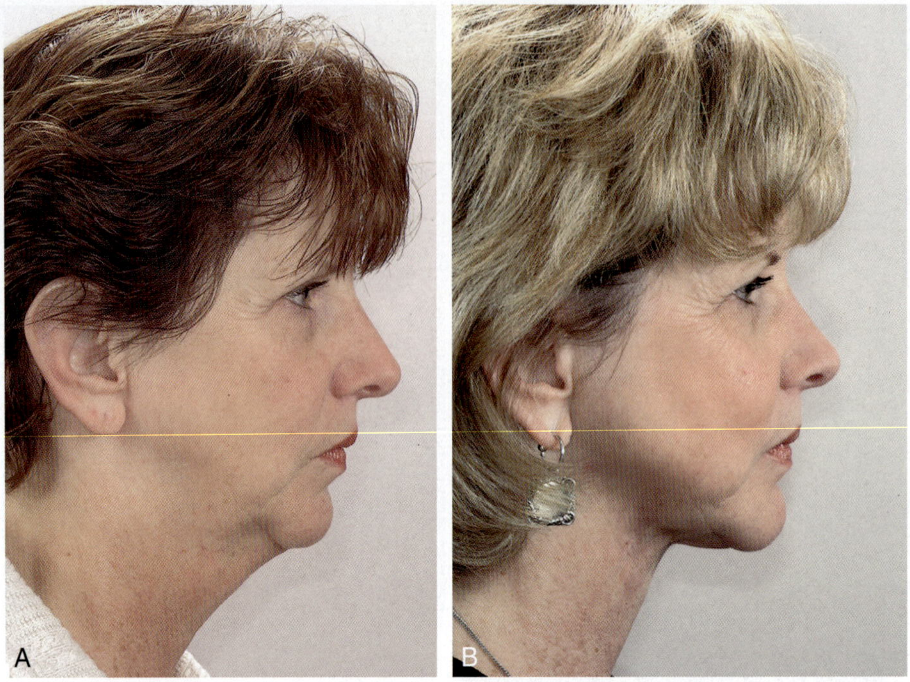

• **Fig. 22.34** (A) This female in her 50s sought treatment because of concern about her protruding maxillary incisors. This issue was due to the mandibular deficiency that is obvious on profile examination. Surgery to advance her mandible was recommended and accepted. At the time of that operation, she also had a submental lipectomy and platysma lift to improve her throat form. (B) Appearance 18 months later, after treatment. Note the contribution of better throat form to the improvement in facial appearance.

Surgical Procedures Related to OSA

Maxillomandibular Surgery

Orthognathic surgery normally has been used to treat significant skeletal discrepancies to improve facial esthetics and dental occlusion. It has also been employed specifically to increase the dimensions of the upper airway as a treatment for obstructive sleep apnea. The goal is to maximize the lumen and minimize the collapsibility of the upper airway, irrespective of the presence of any underlying malocclusion.

Maxillomandibular advancement surgery (MMA) involves the advancement of both upper and lower jaws (usually upwards of 10 mm), depending on the initial occlusion (Fig. 22.35). In the absence of an underlying deformity, esthetics can be compromised and in at least one study 31% of patients self-reported a negative esthetic outcome following MMA.[26] However alternative surgical techniques, which employ a counterclockwise rotation of the occlusal plane with the advancement have improved facial (Fig. 22.36) and dental esthetic and occlusal outcomes (Fig. 22.37), especially in patients with convex pretreatment profiles due to bimaxillary protrusion and weaker chins.[27]

In a systematic review that included data from 518 adult patients who underwent MMA, 85% of patients experienced a more than 50% reduction of their AHI, however a complete resolution or OSA cure occurred less than 40% of the time.[28] Highlighting the significant non-anatomical etiologies to the disease, it should be noted that 73% of the patients in this systematic review also had some form of upper airway soft tissue surgery, which was deemed unsuccessful in treating their OSA, prior to undergoing the MMA procedure. Meaning for some patients, despite multiple and relatively large changes to airway morphology, the disease persists. MMA for OSA is most effective for patients with severe levels (AHI >60) of the disease, ideally with an underlying skeletal discrepancy. In this way, as complete resolution of symptoms is not certain, they will at a minimum appreciate significant improvements to their occlusion and facial profile.

In recognition of the effects of orthognathic surgery on the upper airway, isolated mandibular setback for management of prognathism and a Class III malocclusion have been reconsidered. Is there a greater risk of developing OSA from such procedures? A prospective study of 50 skeletal Class III patients undergoing mandibular set back surgery with or without Le Fort 1 osteotomy had full sleep studies (PSG) performed at baseline and 3 months postoperatively.[29] Roughly half of the sample had mandibular setbacks greater than 10 mm, including some patients with 15 mm or more, which resulted in significant reductions in oropharyngeal, hypopharyngeal, and total airway volumes measured from CBCT imaging. However, despite the substantial magnitude of movement, on average no changes were observed in subjective symptoms of sleep quality, and no significant changes in AHI were reported from the postsurgical sleep studies. It should be noted that three patients were found to have considerable increases in their AHI of greater than 10 events per hour following surgery, and so the potential for deterioration of sleep quality should be discussed with patients planned for such procedures, especially with setbacks greater than 10 mm.

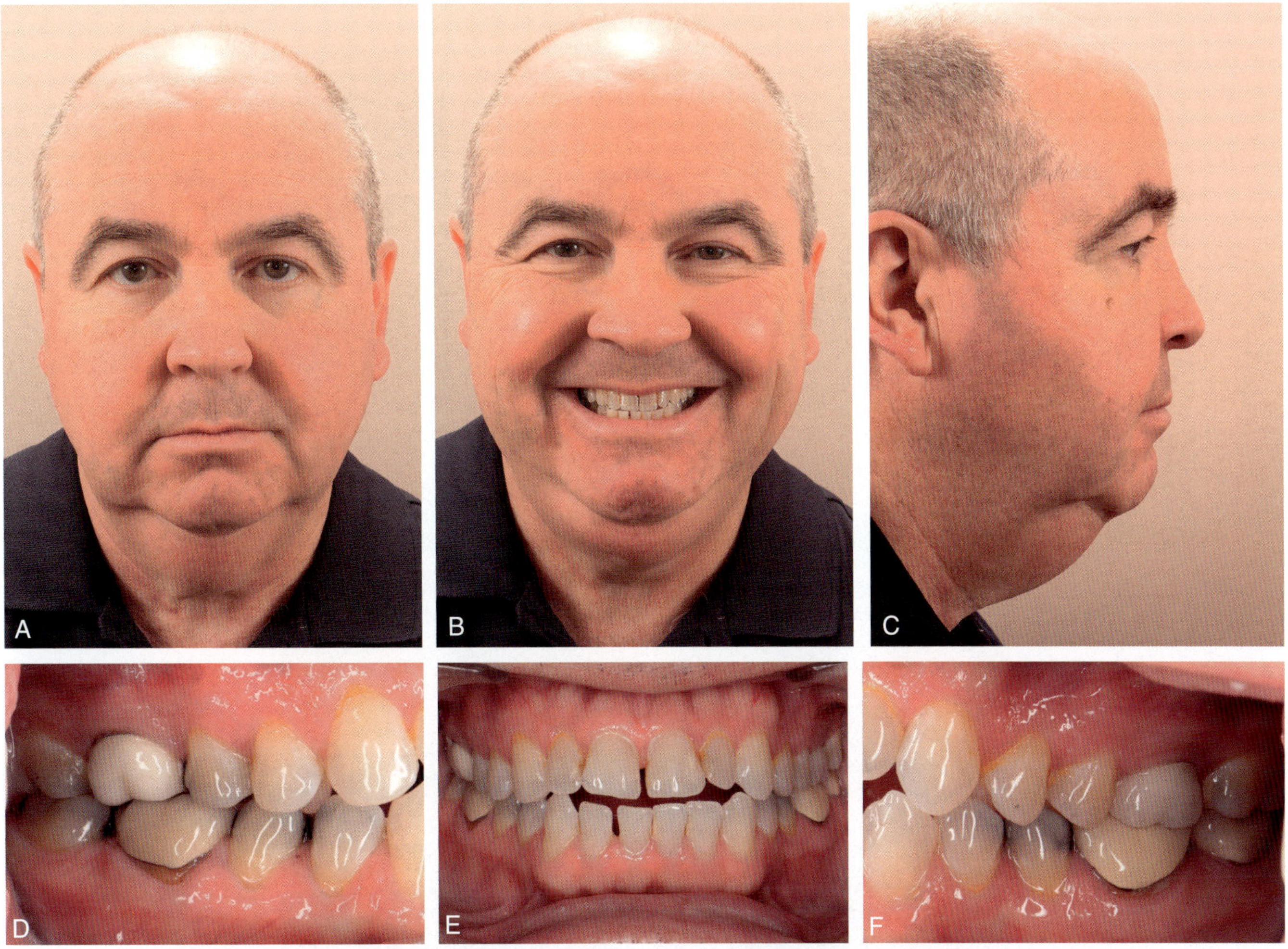

• **Fig. 22.35** Maxillomandibular advancement surgery (MMA) can not only positively alter airway dynamic and sleep apnea, but when planned carefully enhance facial and dental esthetics and occlusion. (A) This 56-year-old male had a history of snoring and poor sleep resulting in fatigue, high blood pressure, and cardiac issues. (B) His facial smile image showed incomplete incisor display and the clinical examination showed only 5 mm of incisor display. (C) The profile image reflected protrusion of both jaws, and an unfavorable chin-neck contour. (D–F) The intraoral images displayed a good posterior occlusion, and an anterior open bite with incisor proclination and spacing.

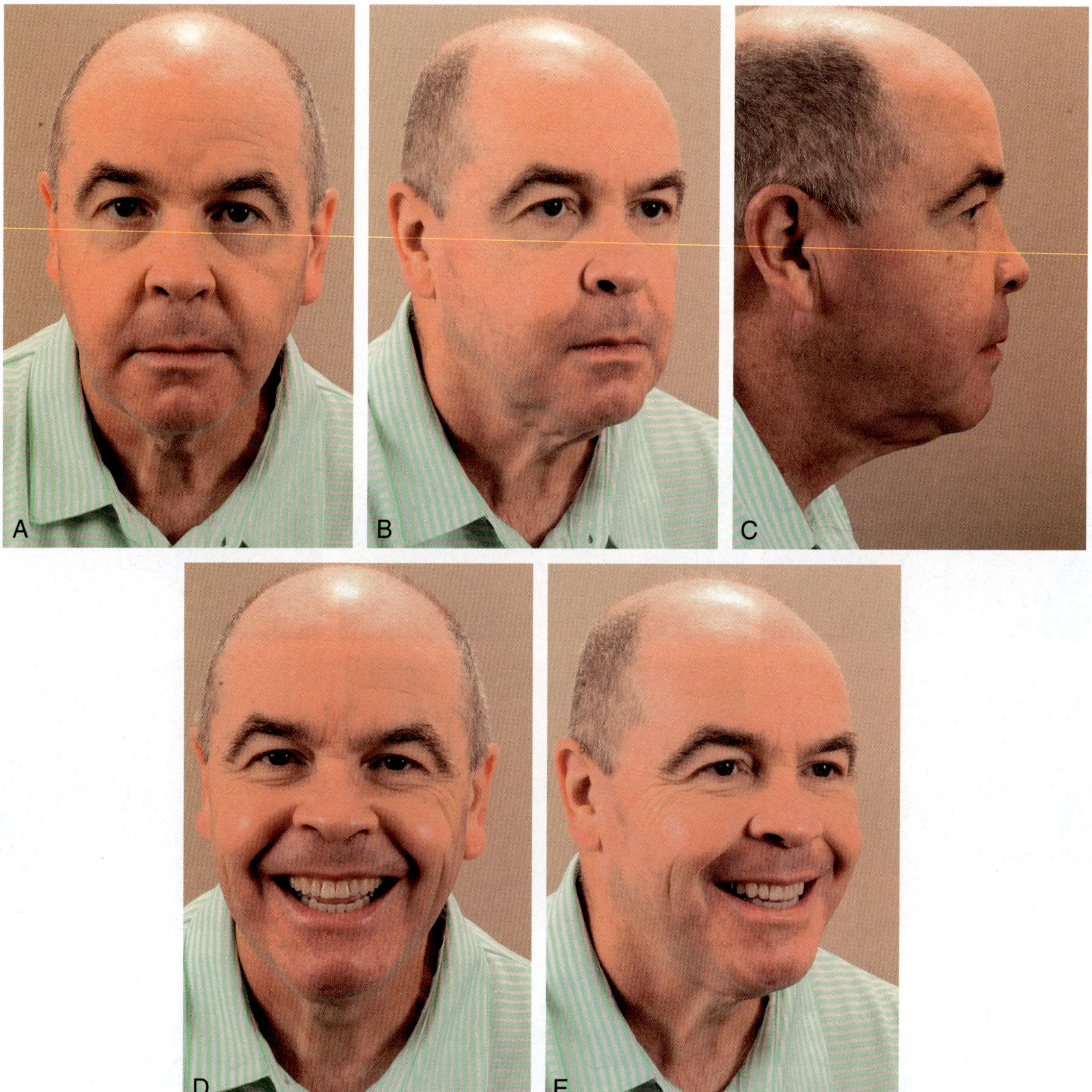

• **Fig. 22.36** (A–C) His final facial images demonstrated a positive esthetic change as a result of the advancements of both jaws and chin, the platysmaplasty, and significant weight loss secondary to his increased exercise regimen. (D–E) As a result of the downgraft of the anterior maxilla, there was a significant improvement in his smile with the increased incisor display.

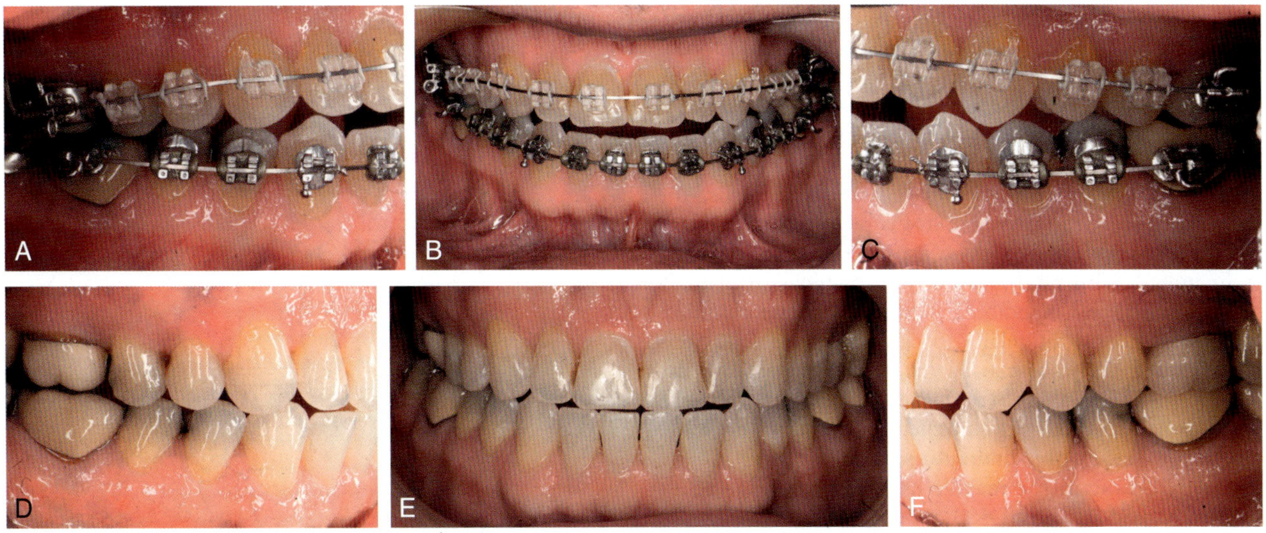

• **Fig. 22.37** For patient in Fig 22.36, (A–C) Presurgical orthodontics resulted in closure of the spacing, uprighting of the maxillary incisors, and had progressed to a full-dimension surgical archwire. (D–F) Once postsurgical orthodontics was complete—the open bite had been corrected with good posterior dental occlusion.

Soft Tissue Surgery

Any anatomical variation of the upper airway from the nasal valves to the larynx may impede normal function of respiration during sleep, and as such several soft tissue surgeries have been employed as treatments for OSA. Among these, nasal turbinate reduction and soft palate procedures such as uvulopalatopharyngoplasty (UPPP) are most common. In isolation these procedures have had variable success rates, and case selection is important to maximize surgical outcomes. A recent RCT investigating the effects of combined UPPP and tongue volume reduction surgery in 102 adults with moderate to severe sleep apnea, reported that on average patients experienced a significant reduction in daytime sleepiness and their apnea-hypopnea index when compared to the control group.[30] Though it is important to note that despite the invasiveness and significant alteration to upper airway anatomy, most patients did not see a complete resolution to their OSA symptoms, with the treatment group still experiencing moderate levels of OSA (AHI >15) at the end of the trial.

Hypoglossal Nerve Stimulation

A relatively new treatment for OSA is the electrical stimulation of the tongue causing it to contract and protrude during inspiration, thereby enlarging the airway. The surgery involves dissecting the specific efferent of the hypoglossal nerve that leads to the genioglossus muscle causing protrusion, to which a small electrode is attached. This is connected to a pacemaker-like device that is implanted subcutaneously on the chest which senses inspiration and matches the timing of tongue protrusion to inhalation. Prior to sleeping the patient activates the device via remote control on a timed delay, allowing it to activate after they have fallen asleep.

Case selection is critical to the success of this technique, which often involves nasendoscopy during drug-induced sleep (DISE) to visualize the pattern of collapse of the upper airway during sleep. Hypoglossal nerve stimulation is contraindicated in patients who experience concentric collapse of the palatal tissues, and who are severely obese (BMI > 35).[31] Though not recommended as a first-line option of treatment due to invasiveness and cost of the procedure, patients fitting these specific criteria can be expected, on average, to see significant reduction in daytime sleepiness and improvements in AHI and other respiration parameters during sleep.[32]

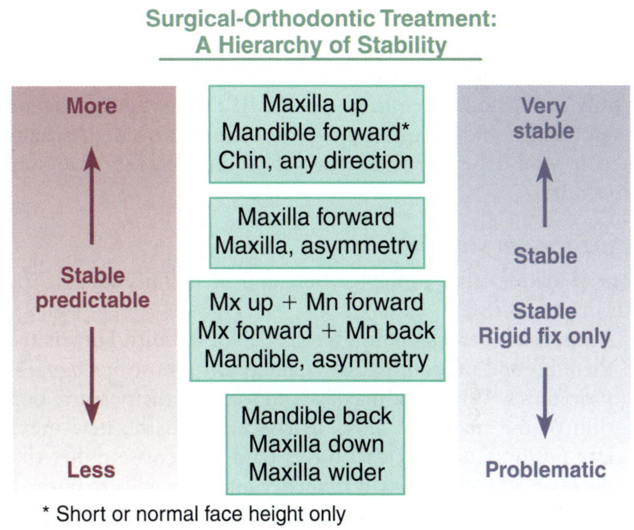

• **Fig. 22.38** The hierarchy of stability during the first postsurgical year, based on data from the University of North Carolina (UNC) Dentofacial Clinic. In this context, "very stable" means a 90% chance of no significant postsurgical change; "stable" means a greater than 80% chance of no change and almost no chance of more than 2 mm of relapse; "problematic" means some degree of relapse is likely and major relapse is possible. It is interesting to note that the key procedures in surgical treatment of Class II problems (superior repositioning of the maxilla, mandibular advancement, and their combination) are quite stable. In Class III treatment, maxillary advancement is the most stable procedure, whereas downward movement of the maxilla and mandibular setback remain problematic.

Postsurgical Stability and Clinical Success

The Hierarchy of Stability and Predictability

Stability after surgical repositioning of the jaws depends on the direction of movement, the type of fixation, and the surgical technique, largely in that order of importance. Enough data exist now to rank different jaw movements in order of stability and predictability (Fig. 22.38).

The most stable orthognathic procedure is superior repositioning of the maxilla, closely followed by mandibular advancement in patients whose anterior facial height is maintained or increased. These procedures, the key ones in correcting severe Class II problems, can be considered to produce a highly stable result even without rigid fixation, and this remains true when they are combined in the treatment of patients with mandibular deficiency and a long face—but only if rigid fixation is used.

In the treatment of patients with Class III problems, the maxilla remains forward just where it was put in about 80% of the patients, and there is almost no tendency for major relapse (4 mm or more). With rigid fixation, the combination of maxillary advancement and mandibular setback is acceptably stable. In contrast, isolated mandibular setback often is unstable. So is downward movement of the maxilla that creates downward-backward rotation of the mandible. For this reason, almost all Class III patients now have maxillary advancement, either alone or (more frequently) combined with mandibular setback.

Surgical widening of the maxilla has the least stable result among the orthognathic surgical procedures. Widening the maxilla stretches the palatal mucosa, and its elastic rebound is the major cause of the relapse tendency. Strategies to control relapse include overcorrection initially and careful retention afterward, with either a heavy orthodontic archwire or a palatal bar during the completion of orthodontic treatment, and then a palate-covering retainer for at least the first postsurgical year. SARPE is preferred over a three-segment maxillary osteotomy if only expansion is required, but SARPE is not advantageous when vertical and/or anteroposterior change is needed, because then it would be the first stage of an unnecessary two-stage procedure.

Influences on Stability

Four principles that influence postsurgical stability help to put this in perspective:

- Neuromuscular adaptation is essential for stability. Fortunately, there is good neuromuscular adaptation to most orthognathic procedures. When the maxilla is moved up, the postural position of the mandible alters in concert with the new maxillary position, and occlusal forces tend to increase rather than decrease. This controls any tendency for the maxilla to immediately relapse downward and contributes to the excellent stability of this surgical movement. Repositioning of the tongue to maintain airway dimensions (i.e., a change in tongue posture) occurs as an adaptation to changes produced by mandibular osteotomy, so surgical reduction of the tongue is not needed when the mandible is set back (Fig. 22.39). When the mandible is moved forward, a similar adaptation in tongue posture can be advantageous in patients with sleep-disordered breathing, and a lower border osteotomy to bring the chin forward also produces forward movement of the tongue because the tongue is attached to the genial tubercles (Fig. 22.40).
- In contrast, neuromuscular adaptation does not occur when the pterygomandibular sling is stretched during mandibular osteotomy, as when the mandible is rotated to close an open bite as it is advanced or set back, so movement of the mandible that stretches the elevator muscles should be avoided.
- Stability is greatest when soft tissues are relaxed during the surgical procedure and least when they are stretched. Moving the maxilla up relaxes tissues. Moving the mandible forward stretches tissues but rotating it up at the gonial angle and down at the chin decreases the amount of stretch. It is not surprising that the most stable mandibular advancements rotate the mandible in this way, whereas the least stable advancements are those that rotate it in the opposite direction, lengthening the ramus and rotating the chin up. The least stable orthognathic surgical procedure, widening the maxilla, stretches the heavy, relatively inelastic palatal mucosa.
- Neuromuscular adaptation affects the length of the masticatory muscles but not their orientation, and adaptation to a new orientation cannot be expected. This concept is best illustrated by the effect of changing the inclination of the mandibular ramus when the mandible is set back or advanced. Successful mandibular advancement requires keeping the ramus in an upright position rather than letting it incline forward as the mandibular body is brought forward. The same is true, in reverse, when the mandible is set back: a major cause of instability appears to be the tendency at the operation to push the ramus posteriorly when the chin is moved back, thus changing its orientation. The orientation is restored when jaw function resumes after the operation, and that moves the jaw forward again. The stability of two-jaw Class III correction is better than mandibular setback alone, apparently because it is easier to avoid pushing the mandible back when a two-jaw operation is done (see Fig. 22.1M).[33]

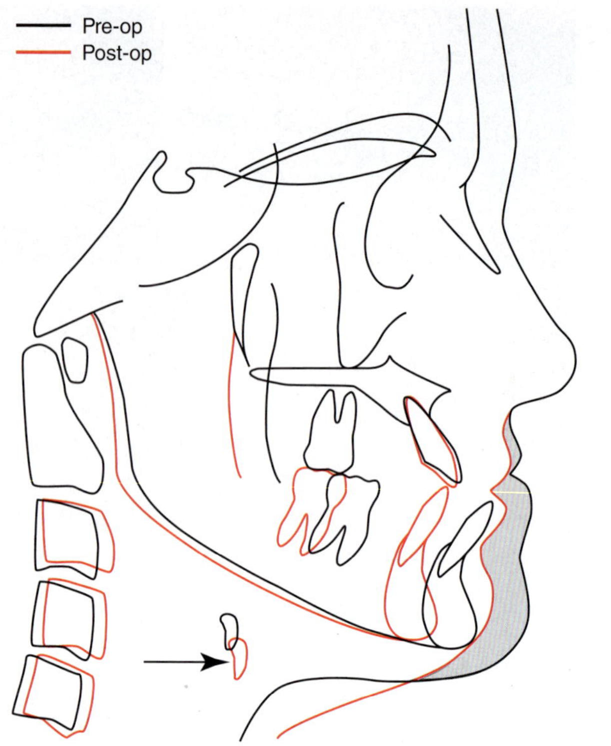

• Fig. 22.39 This cephalometric superimposition shows how the airway is maintained when the mandible is set back in many cases. Although the dentition was moved posteriorly with a ramus osteotomy, the tongue moved down and a little forward rather than back, so the airway was maintained; note the change in position of the hyoid bone, which indicates the position of the base of the tongue. At one time it was routine to remove part of the tongue when the mandible was set back, but this is not necessary because of the physiologic adaptation. The adaptation shows, however, in the form of soft tissue prominence beneath the mandible, the proverbial "double chin."

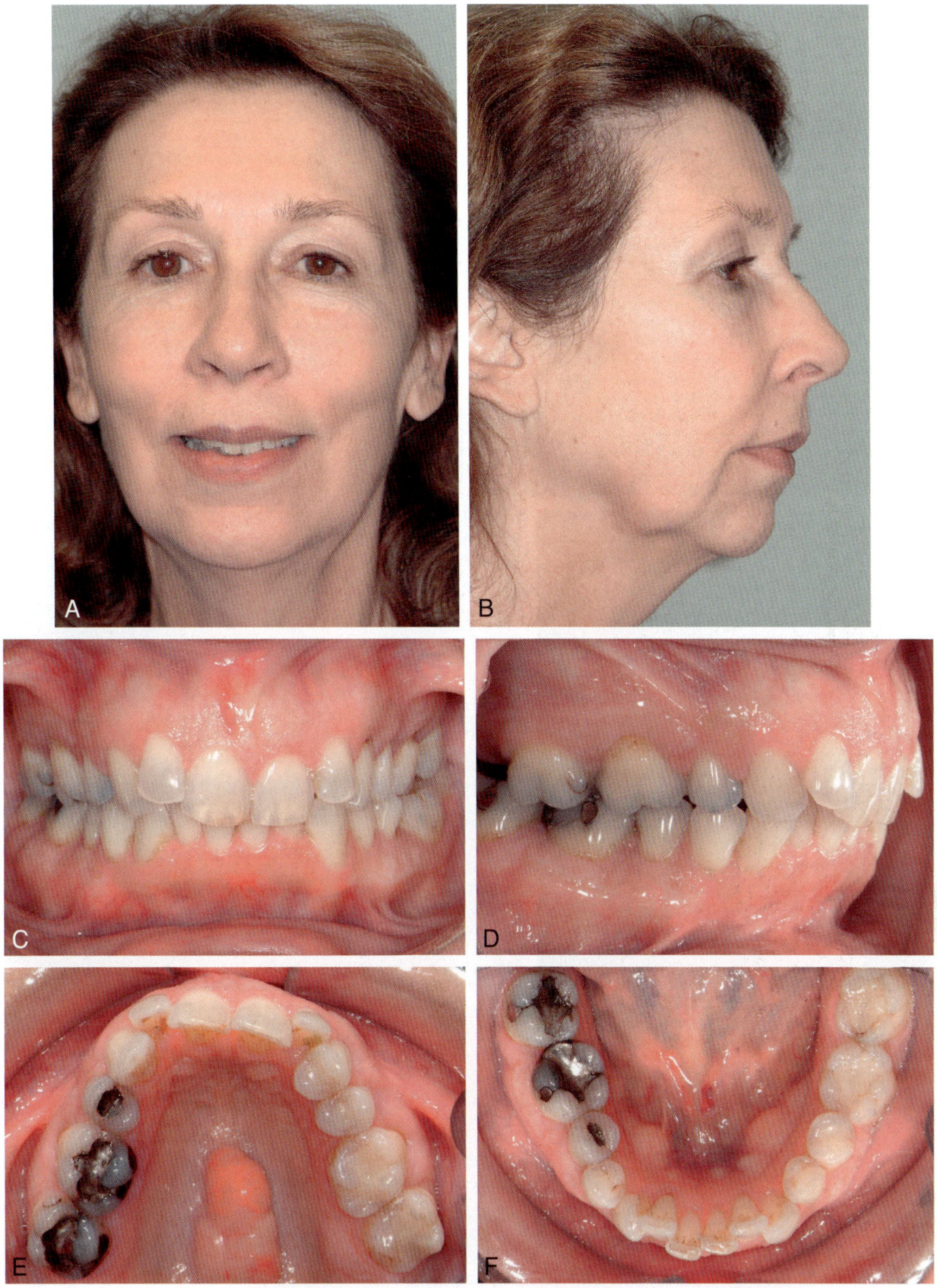

• **Fig. 22.40** This female in her late 50s sought orthodontic consultation about her "crooked teeth" and their effect on her smile. As an adolescent she had undergone extraction of her maxillary right first premolar and left canine and orthodontic treatment to align the teeth; the alignment was lost in the long term without permanent retention. When she was told that her Class II occlusion reflected her jaw relationship, she said she was well aware of her mandibular deficiency and had never liked it. She was referred to an oral and maxillofacial surgeon to discuss the possibility of mandibular advancement, and when he learned that she snored loudly and was chronically tired, he suggested that improving sleep-disordered breathing might be another reason to choose surgery. No sleep study was done, but she agreed that she wanted the esthetic benefit of surgery and the possible airway improvement. (A and B) Frontal smile and lips-together profile; (C–F) intraoral views. Her treatment plan was extraction of the mandibular right first premolar and left second premolar, with an approximately 7 mm mandibular advancement and 6 mm advancement genioplasty.

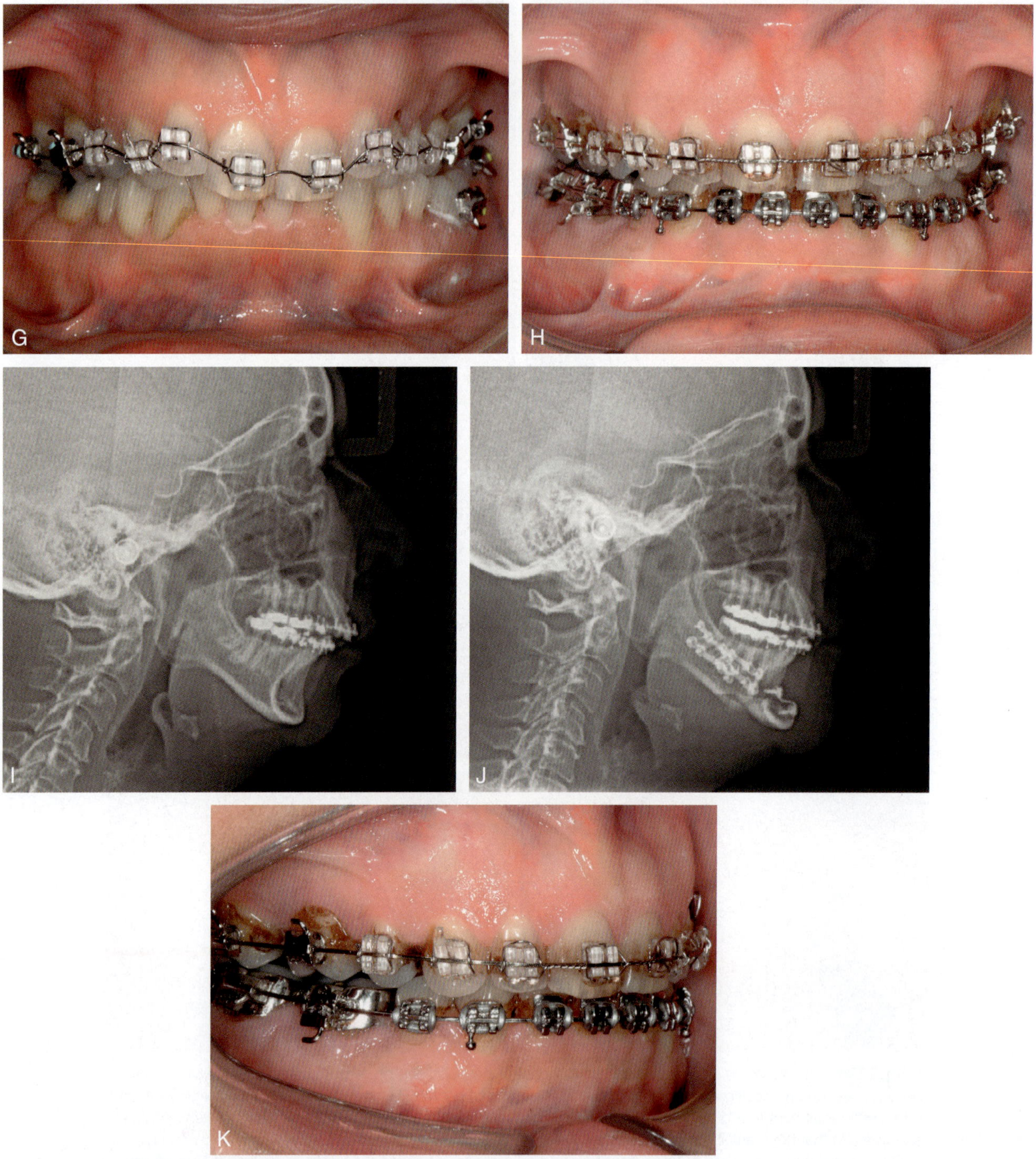

• **Fig. 22.40, cont'd** (G) Initial alignment of the maxillary arch; (H) the mandibular extractions and presurgical preparation of the lower arch followed. (I and J) Cephalometric radiographs before and after the operation. (K) Intraoral views near the end of treatment.

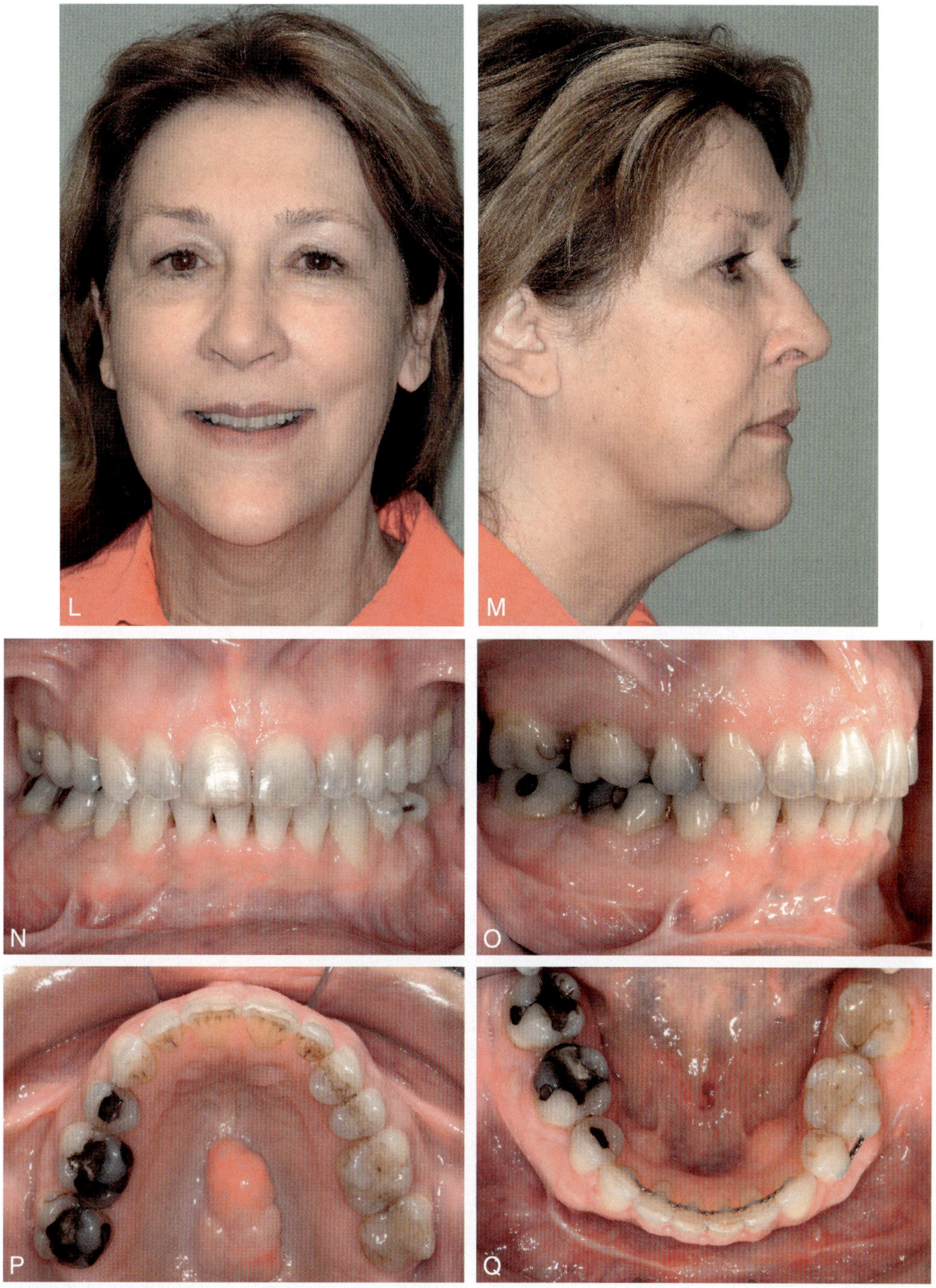

• **Fig. 22.40, cont'd** (L and M) Post surgical facial appearance and (N–Q) intraoral views at debanding. Note the use of a facial bonded retainer wire to keep the second premolar extraction space closed; extending a bonded lingual retainer to the premolar is not recommended.

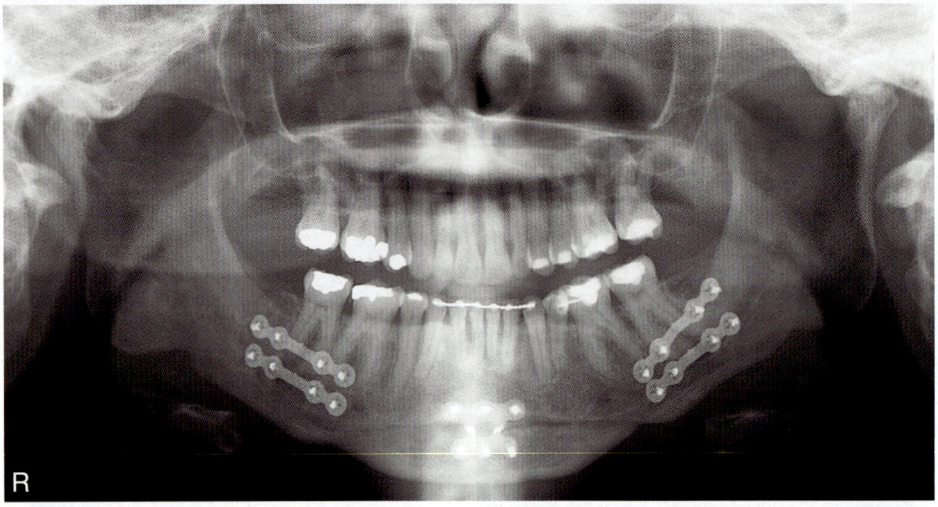

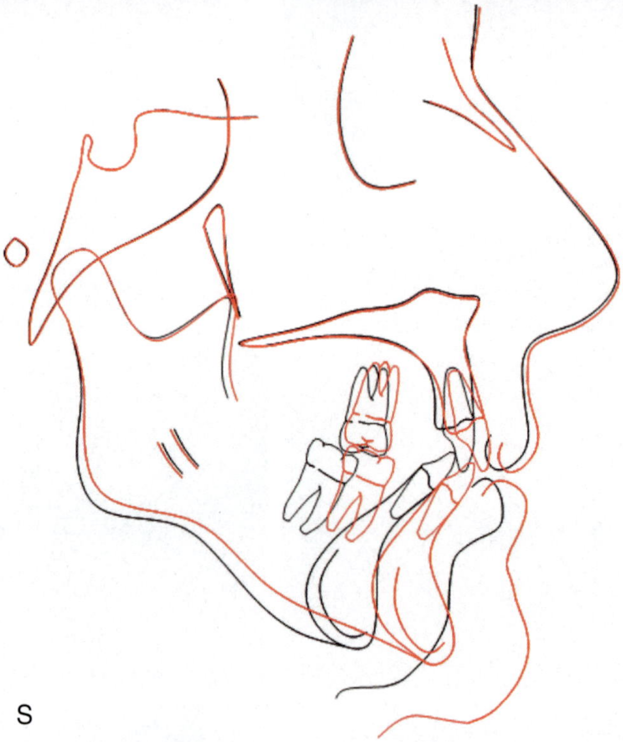

• **Fig. 22.40, cont'd** (R) Panoramic radiograph after placement of bonded mandibular retainers; a removable maxillary retainer was to be worn full-time except for eating. She was quite pleased and reported that she no longer snores and feels that she has more energy, so perhaps there was an airway benefit. (S) Cephalometric superimposition pretreatment to posttreatment. The amount of face height increase was controlled by vertical positioning of the lower incisors. (Courtesy Dr. T. Shaughnessy.)

Special Considerations in Planning Surgical Treatment

Timing of Surgery

Progressive Deformity

In the discussion of growth modification in Chapters 13 and 14, the focus was on what is seen in almost all orthodontic patients with excessive or deficient growth of the jaws: a relatively stable jaw relationship over time, that is, a problem that persists but doesn't rapidly get worse. If growth modification is done early, the problem tends to recur because of later growth in the same pattern, so the usual guidance is to wait until the adolescent growth spurt to start treatment. But rarely, that is not the situation. Instead, the patient has a progressive deformity, one that does get worse over time. Almost always, the problem is asymmetric growth of the mandible, and that is an indication for early surgery. In contrast to orthognathic surgery more generally, the goal of the surgical procedure is not to correct the deformity, but to create an environment in which normal growth is possible.

Asymmetric mandibular deficiency has two major causes: (1) a congenital anomaly, most likely a form of hemifacial macrosomia (see Fig. 22.28), or (2) an old condylar fracture with a limitation on growth from scar tissue that limits translation of the condyle (see Figs. 14.43 and 14.44). Correction of this problem may or may not require surgery, depending on the severity of the limitation. For the more severe forms of hemifacial macrosomia and for failure of translation of the condyles, surgical intervention is indicated when the problem is recognized. Cases of this type are best managed through problem-oriented clinics at a university medical center.

Asymmetric mandibular excess is described by its more scientific name, *hemimandibular hyperplasia*, but the cause is unknown. Important characteristics of this problem include:

- The excessive growth is not a tumor; the histologic diagnosis is normal hard and soft tissue, just too much growth. That means it has the potential to stop growing on its own, which will not correct the asymmetry but would stop it from getting worse.
- Most of the patients are female, about 85% of the total.
- In many adolescent girls, a mild asymmetry develops as one side stops growing and the other continues for a while but then also stops growing. A mild asymmetry created by this last phase of growth is not a problem—but of course if the asymmetric growth continues, there will be problems of both function and facial disproportion.
- The excessive growth occurs in two patterns at the condyles—enlargement of the condyle or lengthening of the condylar neck (Fig. 22.41)—and two patterns in terms of lengthening of the ramus versus the body of the mandible. The more the body of the mandible lengthens, the greater the lateral displacement of the center of the chin; the more the ramus lengthens, the greater the vertical asymmetry, which often includes a lower position of one side of the chin in addition to an asymmetry at the gonial angles. The vertically asymmetric mandibular growth induces a cant in the occlusal plane, and surgical correction is likely to require two-jaw surgery plus genioplasty (Fig. 22.42).
- The clinical impression is that patients whose excessive growth is a lengthening of the condylar process appear to be more likely to stop growing than those who have an enlargement of the condyle, but this has not been documented in a large study.
- Removing the condyle on the affected side stops the excessive growth, even though the deviant growth pattern affects the rest of the mandible, not just the condyle. If the condyle is distorted to the point that it no longer fits into the condylar fossa, condylectomy is indicated. If the excessive growth is an elongation of the condylar neck, a "condylar shave" that removes the superior surface where cellular proliferation occurs can be successful.

For younger patients with either asymmetric deficiency or asymmetric excessive growth, hybrid functional appliances can aid in managing asymmetry before or after orthognathic surgery. These appliances are discussed in Chapter 14.

Symmetric Excess Growth

With the exception of condylectomy in patients with hemimandibular hypertrophy, early jaw surgery has little inhibitory effect on further growth. For this reason, orthognathic surgery should be delayed until growth is essentially completed in patients who have symmetric excessive growth, especially mandibular prognathism. For patients with growth deficiencies, earlier surgery can be considered, but rarely before the adolescent growth spurt.

Actively growing patients with mandibular prognathism can be expected to outgrow early orthodontic or surgical correction and require retreatment (see Fig. 19.2), so the timing of this operation often is a critical consideration. Indirect methods of assessing growth status, such as hand-wrist radiographs or vertebral stages to determine bone age, are not accurate enough for planning the time of the operation. The best method is serial cephalometric radiographs, with the surgical procedure delayed until good superimposition documents that the adult deceleration of growth has occurred. Often the correction of excessive mandibular growth must be delayed until the late teens, unless a second, later surgical correction can be justified because of psychosocial considerations.

The situation is not so clear-cut for patients with the long-face (skeletal open bite) pattern that can be characterized as vertical maxillary excess. There appears to be a reasonable chance for stable surgical correction of this problem before growth is totally completed, but the difference in clinical stability between treatment at, for example, ages 14 and 18 remains incompletely understood. Should patients with a long face have early surgical treatment? Probably not, unless they are willing to have a second later operation if additional growth occurs. Precision planning for cases of this type can produce almost exactly the desired outcome—in the absence of growth. That means delaying the surgical procedure until growth has essentially stopped makes the treatment outcome predictable in a way it cannot be if done early.

Growth Deficiency

Surgery in infancy and early childhood is required for some congenital problems that involve deficient growth. Craniosynostosis and severe hemifacial microsomia are two examples. The major indication for orthognathic surgery before puberty, however, is a progressive deformity caused by restriction of growth. A common cause is ankylosis of the mandible (unilaterally or occasionally bilaterally) after a condylar injury or severe infection (see Chapter 5). An operation to release the ankylosis, followed by functional appliance therapy to guide subsequent growth, is needed in these unusual problems.

A child with a severe and progressive deficiency should be distinguished from one with a severe but stable deficiency, such as a child with a small mandible whose facial proportions are not changing appreciably with growth. A progressive deficiency is an indication for early surgery, whereas a severe but stable deficiency usually is not. The principal exception is an extremely severe problem in which preliminary orthodontic or surgical treatment would improve the patient's quality of life even though an operation would be needed later to deal with the jaw deformity. In keeping with the general principle that orthognathic surgery has surprisingly little impact on growth, early surgery does not improve the growth prognosis unless it relieves a specific restriction on growth, nor does it produce a subsequently normal growth pattern.

Early Mandibular Advancement

In the 1980s, some surgeons advocated early mandibular advancement, assuming that normal growth would occur thereafter, and the problem would not recur. As with early setback and with early distraction osteogenesis for advancement, that is an unwarranted assumption. Many younger patients have further mandibular growth after surgical advancement. Most of this growth is expressed vertically, however, and results in minimal forward movement at the pogonion.[34] To say it differently, the mandible grows no further forward after early advancement, although there is likely to be enough vertical growth to prevent downward and backward rotation. In our view, mandibular advancement before the adolescent growth spurt, with surgery or distraction, is not

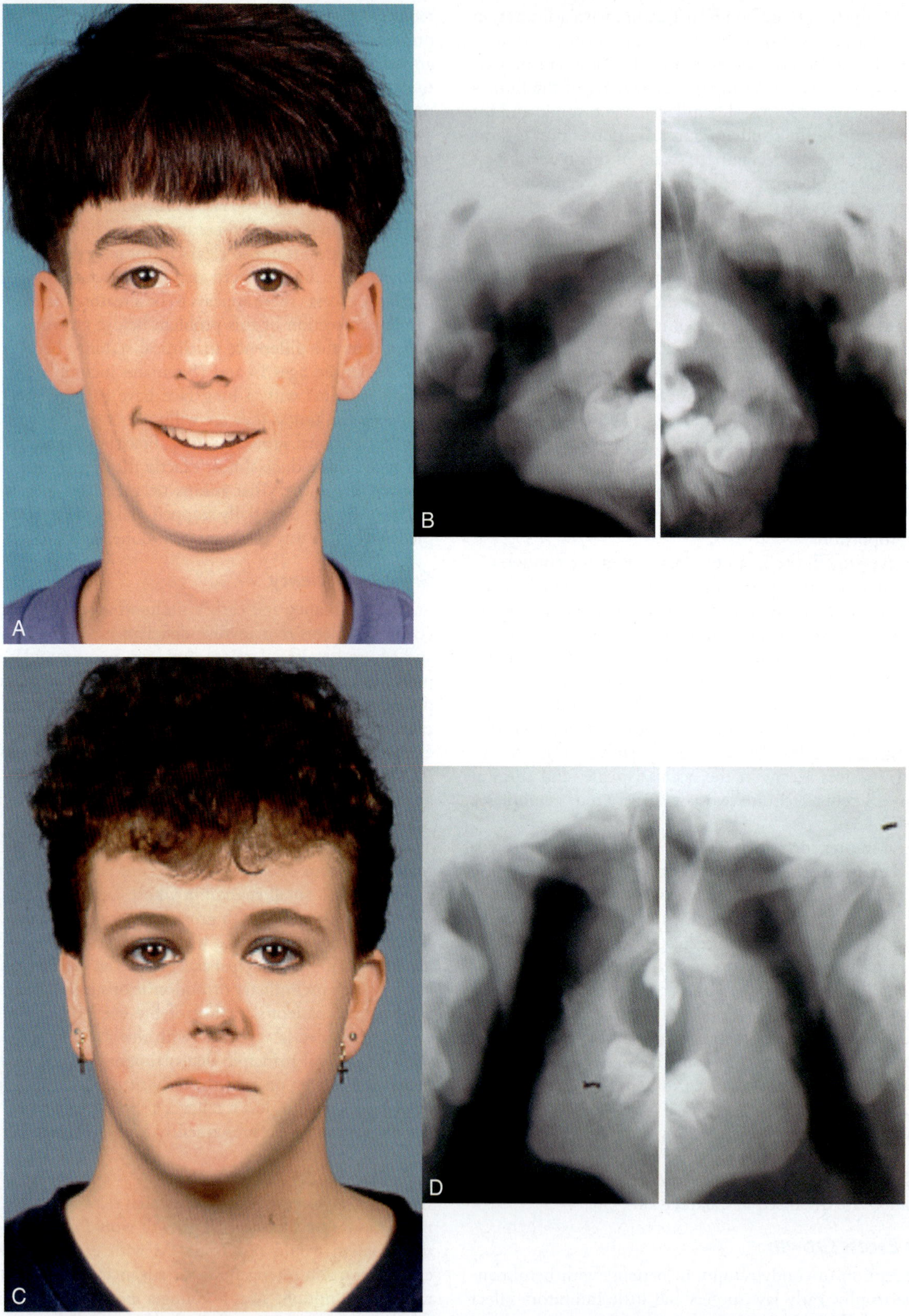

• **Fig. 22.41** Two patterns of growth are seen at the mandibular condyles in patients with hemimandibular hyperplasia: (A) excessive growth on the patient's left side and (B) enlargement of the left condyle. (C) Excessive growth on the patient's left side and (D) lengthening of the left condylar neck but no increase in the size of the condyle. A clinical impression is that patients with elongation of the condylar neck are more likely to stop growing spontaneously than those with enlargement of the condyle, but there are no good data to document this.

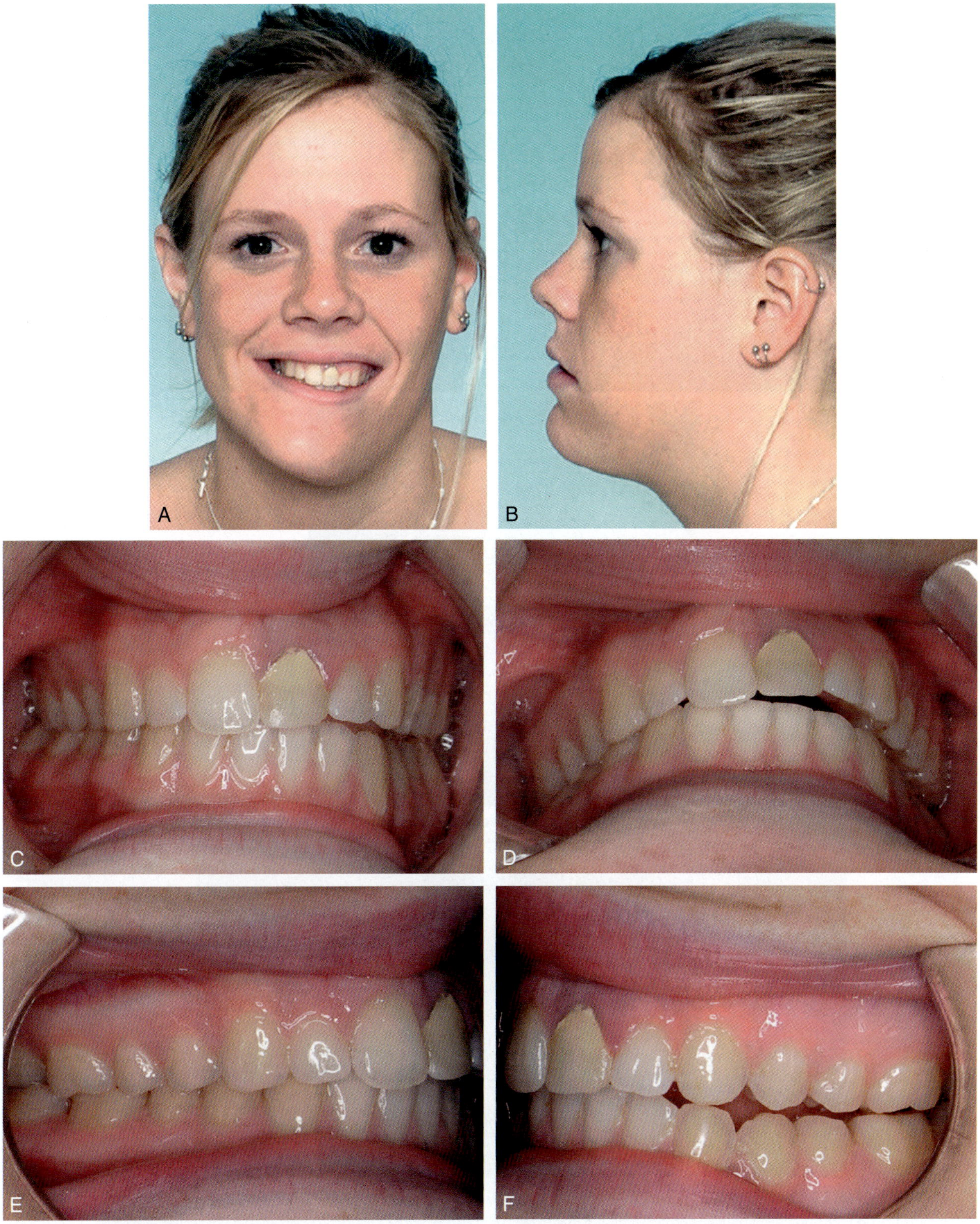

• **Fig. 22.42** Untreated hemimandibular hyperplasia can slowly lead to a major facial asymmetry, as in this 18-year-old college freshman. Her jaw asymmetry was noted at age 11 when she had orthodontic treatment to align crowded teeth. The decision was to wait to see what happened with further growth before any surgical intervention, and the asymmetric growth continued. (A) Frontal and (B) Patient's left profile (C–F) Intraoral views of the teeth. The maxillary left central incisor had been fractured in an accident, but the teeth were still well aligned after the previous orthodontic treatment. Note the normal molar relationship on the right and the half-cusp Class II relationship on the left.

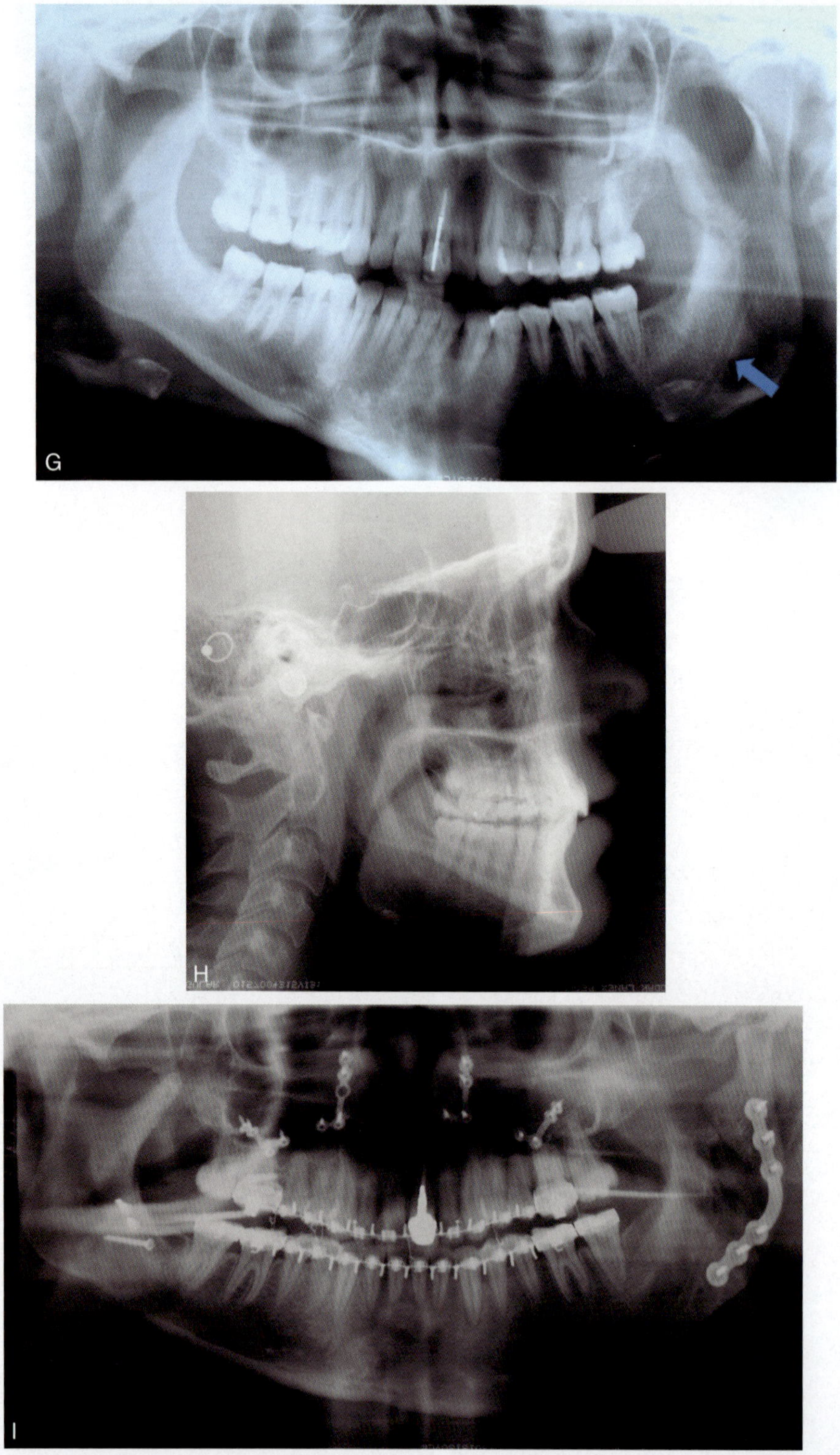

• **Fig. 22.42, cont'd** (G) The panoramic radiograph shows the tremendous enlargement of the left condyle, which can no longer fit into the condylar fossa, the downward path of the mandibular neurovascular bundle on the affected side *(arrow)*, and the excessive bone formation below the mandibular teeth on the left side. Note that this goes all the way to the midline. (H) The cephalometric radiograph shows the vertical lengthening of the ramus on the left. The almost purely vertical excess growth for this patient is unusual; these patients show all possible combinations of excessive vertical versus horizontal growth. At this stage surgical treatment consisted of condylectomy on the right side plus bilateral sagittal split osteotomy (BSSO) on the left side (necessary for correct positioning of that condyle), Le Fort I osteotomy to level the maxillary cant, and lower border osteotomy to remove as much of the excess bone as possible below the teeth on the left side. (I) Panoramic radiograph immediately after the operation. At the operation, first the maxilla was rotated up on the left side to level the occlusal plane to achieve optimum display of the maxillary teeth; then the left condyle was removed, and a cut across the ramus below the condylar stump created a condylar segment that was moved up into the condylar fossa. It is not necessary to bone graft an area the size of the defect seen here on the left side; bone fills in defects of this magnitude during healing.

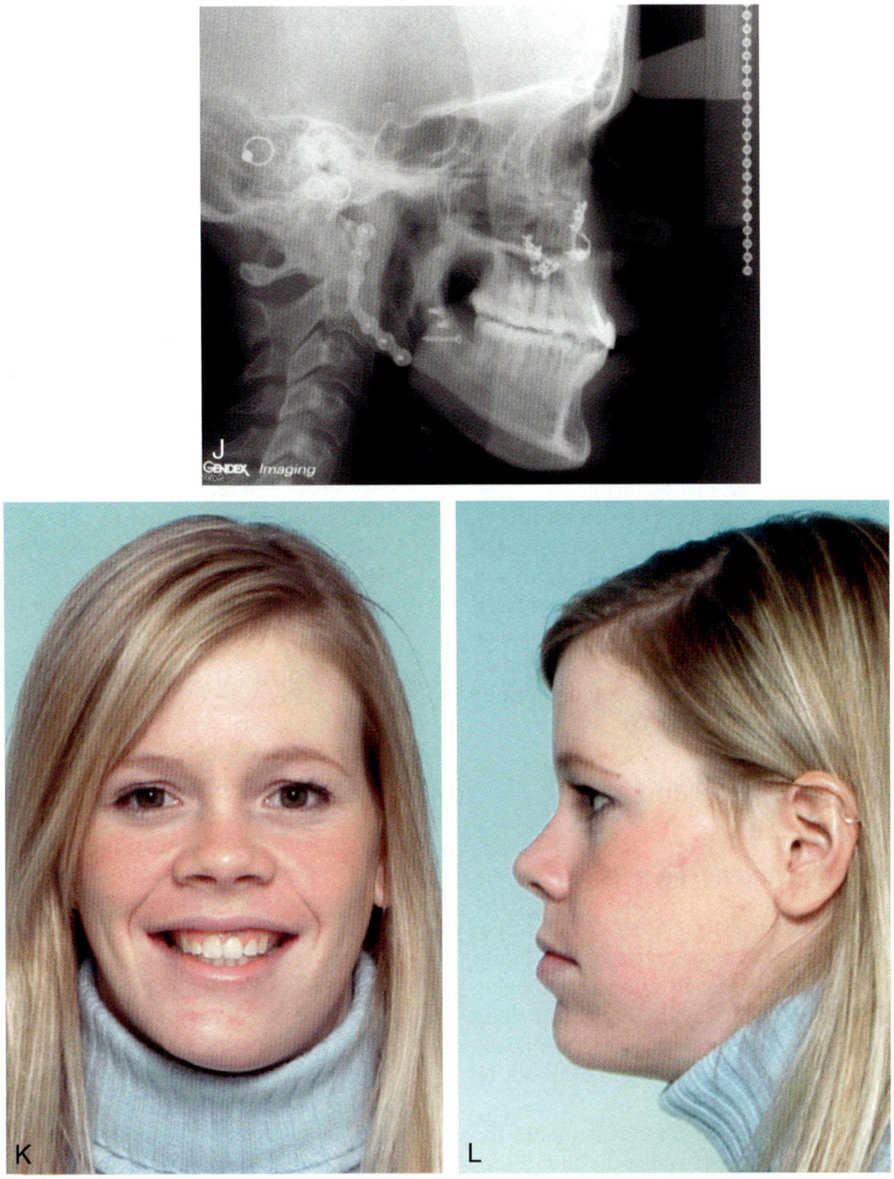

• **Fig. 22.42, cont'd** (J) The cephalometric radiograph at the end of orthodontic treatment, which took only 8 months because minimal use of presurgical and postsurgical orthodontics was needed, shows the leveling of the maxilla and removal of bone along the left lower border up to the level of the neurovascular bundle. (K and L) Frontal and lateral photographs at the end of treatment. The mildly excessive lower border of the mandible on the left side is hardly detectable and would not be noticed unless you were really looking for it.

indicated for patients who do not have a progressive deformity or psychosocial problems severe enough to warrant a second operation later.

On the other hand, if facial growth declines to adult levels at the end of the adolescent growth spurt, there would seem to be no reason to delay mandibular advancement. Minimal facial growth can be expected in patients with severe deficiency during late adolescence, and relapse from that cause is unlikely. However, recent research has shown two interesting findings for patients who underwent mandibular advancement before age 18 compared with those who underwent the surgical procedure at a later age:

1. Some of the adolescent patients had downward and backward rotation of the mandible, which led to a decrease in chin prominence, and a few had shortening of mandibular length that had the same effect. It appears that delaying advancement probably does increase the chance of long-term stability.
2. Both the younger and older patients had high satisfaction levels at 5 years after surgery, but those who had early surgery were even more satisfied with their treatment than those who had surgical treatment at an older age. This was true even though they often recognized that their chin was no longer as prominent as it was shortly after surgery.[35]

How does that translate to informed consent? The data indicate that if a patient really is anxious to have early surgical correction despite knowing that the risk of mild recurrence exists, he or she probably should have it because of the psychosocial benefit. And those who understand the risk and decide they can wait should do so.

Early Maxillary Advancement

Early (adolescent) advancement of a sagittally deficient maxilla or midface remains relatively stable if there is careful attention to detail and grafts are used to combat relapse, but further forward growth of the maxilla is quite unlikely. Subsequent growth of the mandible is likely to result in re-establishment of Class III malocclusion and a concave profile. The patient and parents should be cautioned about the possible need for a second stage of surgical treatment later. In general, maxillary advancement should be delayed until after the adolescent growth spurt unless earlier treatment is needed for psychosocial reasons.

Although surgery to reposition the entire maxilla may affect future growth, this is not necessarily the case for the surgical procedures used to correct cleft lip and palate. In patients with cleft lip and palate, bone grafts to alveolar clefts before eruption of the permanent canines can eliminate the bony defect, which greatly improves the long-term prognosis for the dentition. A review of patients with cleft palate treated with the Oslo protocol (i.e., closure of the lip and hard palate at 3 months, posterior palatal closure at 18 months, and cancellous alveolar bone grafting at 8–11 years) showed no interference with the total amount of facial growth.[36] As surgical methods for initial closure of a cleft palate continue to improve, the number of cleft patients who need maxillary advancement as a final stage of treatment should continue to decrease.

Correction of Combined Vertical and Anteroposterior Problems

Short-Face Class II: Increasing Anterior Face Height

Both mandibular and maxillary deficiencies often are accompanied by short anterior face height, and a goal of treatment should be to increase it. It is important to keep in mind that moving the mandible forward allows a stable increase in face height along with the anteroposterior movement, whereas moving the maxilla down and forcing the mandible to rotate down and back can be problematic.

The most stable type of mandibular advancement rotates the mandibular body segment as it is advanced, so that the chin comes forward and downward and the mandibular plane angle increases. Excellent bony contact after a sagittal split osteotomy easily allows the rotation. The effect is to shorten the mandibular ramus. Although the soft tissues of the anterior lower face are stretched as the chin is advanced and moved down, this is mitigated by relaxation of the posterior soft tissues (which include the mandibular elevator muscles), and the result is little soft tissue pressure in a relapse direction.

In contrast, moving the maxilla down stretches both the anterior and posterior facial soft tissues. Although muscle adaptation appears to occur, there is a strong tendency for the maxilla to relapse upward. Therefore, mandibular ramus surgery is preferred to increase face height, and downward movement of the posterior maxilla, so that the mandible is forced to rotate down and back, is avoided if possible.

Long-Face Class II or Class III Patients: Decreasing Face Height

Moving the maxilla up so that the mandible can rotate up and forward is the most stable orthognathic procedure (see discussion of stability earlier). A Le Fort I osteotomy therefore is the preferred procedure for a patient with an anterior open bite and/or a Class II malocclusion due to downward-backward rotation of the mandible (see Fig. 22.22).

In contrast, although a mandibular ramus osteotomy can be used to decrease anterior face height and decrease the mandibular plane angle, the result is highly unstable because the mandibular elevator muscles are stretched and do not adapt. Moving the maxilla up produces a change in the postural position of the mandible. A ramus osteotomy does not produce the same neuromuscular adaptation, which is why it is unstable. Therefore a Le Fort I osteotomy to elevate the posterior maxilla is preferred to reduce face height. If the mandible is still deficient after it rotates up and forward, a mandibular advancement in combination with the maxillary procedure does not stretch the muscles and is acceptably stable.

For patients with Class III problems, the same guidelines for vertical change are applicable. The recommendations:

- To increase face height, use a mandibular ramus osteotomy in combination with a maxillary osteotomy if downward movement of the maxilla is desired.
- To decrease face height, use a maxillary osteotomy in combination with a mandibular ramus osteotomy if further mandibular advancement or mandibular setback is required.

Special Points in Planning Orthognathic Surgery

Four further special points should be considered when orthognathic surgery is involved:

1. Incision lines contract somewhat as they heal, and when incisions are placed in the vestibule, this can stress the gingival attachment, leading to stripping or recession of the gingiva. This is most likely to be a problem with the lower incisors after the incision for a genioplasty. If the attached gingiva is inadequate, gingival grafting (see Fig. 20.34) should be completed before genioplasty.
2. Many young adults being prepared for orthognathic surgery have unerupted or impacted third molars. If rigid fixation (bone screws) with mandibular ramus surgery is planned, it is desirable to remove the lower third molars at least 6 months before the orthognathic procedure. This allows good bone healing in the area where the screws will be placed.
3. If the patient's primary motivation for treatment is temporomandibular dysfunction (TMD), the unpredictable impact of orthognathic surgery on TMD must be carefully discussed. TMD symptoms usually improve during presurgical orthodontic treatment, just as with any other active orthodontics, and it is important for the patient to understand that this improvement may be transient. If TM joint surgery along with maxillary and/or mandibular surgery will be required, usually it is better to defer this until after the orthognathic surgery because the outcome of joint surgery is more predictable after the new joint positions and occlusal relationships have been established.

   As with all adult orthodontic patients, whether orthognathic or TM joint surgery is or is not involved, definitive restorative and prosthetic treatment is the last step in the treatment sequence. Initial restorative treatment should stabilize or temporize the existing dentition with restorations that will be serviceable and provide patient comfort during the orthodontic and surgical phases. When the final skeletal and dental relationships have been achieved, it is possible to obtain accurate articulator mountings and complete the final occlusal rehabilitation.
4. Speech distortion related to craniofacial problems and their correction.

Patients with Class II, III, and anterior open bite present with qualitative and quantitative speech distortions of various magnitudes. [37–39] These patients have, on average, greater speech distortions than Class I, nonopenbite patients and the greater the anteroposterior problems, the greater the speech distortions. But Cl II patients seem to have smaller distortions.

Although a recent meta-analysis found no consistent improvements in speech distortions for vowels between pre and postoperative orthognathic surgery patients, the most common distortions among these patients are fricatives. The study acknowledged potential confounding variables.[40] New studies found significant changes toward those with Class I malocclusion for selected speech distortion measures following orthognathic surgery.[41] More data should clarify this issue related to orthognathic surgery.

Putting Surgical and Orthodontic Treatment Together: Who Does What and When?

Orthodontic Appliance Considerations

In contemporary surgical-orthodontic treatment, a fixed orthodontic appliance has three uses: to (1) accomplish the tooth movement needed in preparation for surgery; (2) stabilize the teeth and basal bone at the time of the operation and during healing (which is less important now when rigid internal fixation is used almost routinely) and provide attachments for intermaxillary fixation; and (3) produce the necessary postsurgical tooth movement while retaining the surgical change. A fixed appliance should permit the use of full-dimension rectangular archwires for strength and stability during the stabilization phase of treatment.

Any of the variations of the edgewise appliance (including self-ligating brackets), with either 18 or 22 slots, are acceptable for stabilization, but the self-ligating bracket should allow a full-dimension steel wire to be ligated in place for the surgical stabilization. Integral hooks on brackets, however, are not recommended for intermaxillary fixation because tying directly to a bracket increases the chance of dislodging it at a particularly awkward time.

For surgical-orthodontic treatment, ceramic brackets pose a dilemma. Their appearance makes them appealing to esthetically conscious adults who choose surgery, but the brittleness of the ceramic material makes them susceptible to fracture, especially when the jaws are being tied together in the operating room so rigid fixation can be placed. Patients who are told that ceramic brackets might compromise their surgical result usually accept metal brackets instead. If ceramic brackets are used, they should be restricted to the maxillary anterior teeth. The surgeon must treat them gently and be prepared to deal with problems in the operating room.

A modern lingual appliance can be used in surgery patients, as can clear aligners, but with both some attachments on the facial surface of the teeth must be placed for temporary intermaxillary fixation, and patients using Invisalign routinely would have bonded attachments on many teeth for better control. For clear aligner surgical cases, there is a premium on precise internal fixation and accurate construction of splints, especially when segmental osteotomies will be used, because the aligner provides no support at the time of the operation—but excellent results can be obtained with three-dimensional (3D) imaging as the basis for detailed planning of the surgical procedure and splint fabrication (Fig. 22.43).

Presurgical Orthodontics

Goals of Presurgical Treatment

The objective of presurgical treatment is to prepare the patient for the surgical procedure, placing the teeth relative to their own supporting bone without concern for the dental occlusion at that stage. Because some postsurgical orthodontics will be required in any case, it is inefficient to do tooth movement before the operation that could be accomplished more easily and quickly during or after the operation. For example, when a maxillary osteotomy is needed for correction of a vertical or anteroposterior problem, there is no reason to expand the arch transversely during the presurgical orthodontics—this can be done as part of the same maxillary procedure. Most patients with deep overbite before treatment need leveling of the lower arch by extrusion of posterior teeth, and this can be done more quickly and easily during the postsurgical orthodontic treatment (see later).

This means that the amount of presurgical orthodontics can be quite variable, ranging from only appliance placement in a few patients to 12 months or so of treatment in others with severe crowding or protrusion. The presurgical phase should almost never require more than a year, unless it is delayed by waiting for growth to be completed.

The length of the postsurgical phase of treatment depends on the amount of detailing needed. However, when postsurgical treatment extends beyond about 6 months postsurgically, patients tend to become discouraged and satisfaction with treatment decreases.[42] Another way to express the goal of presurgical orthodontics is that it should prepare the patient so that postsurgical treatment can be completed within 6 months.

Steps in Orthodontic Preparation for Surgery

The essential steps in presurgical orthodontics are to arrange the teeth so they will not interfere with placing the jaws in the desired position. This requires aligning the arches or arch segments to make them compatible and establishing the anteroposterior and vertical position of the incisors. Planning exactly how the dental arches will be leveled is particularly important. The guideline is that extrusion generally is done more easily postsurgically, whereas intrusion must be accomplished presurgically or handled surgically. Two common problems require special consideration: how to level an accentuated curve of Spee in the lower arch of a patient with deep overbite and how to level the upper arch in a patient with open bite who has a large vertical discrepancy between anterior and posterior teeth.

Leveling the Mandibular Arch

When an accentuated curve of Spee is present in the lower arch, the decision to level by intrusion of incisors or extrusion of premolars must be based on the desired final face height. In short-face, deep bite patients who need additional face height, ir is almost always advantageous to level the lower arch after surgery. Before surgery, the teeth are aligned and the anteroposterior and vertical position of the incisors is established, but the lower arch is not leveled beyond that point, and steps are needed in all rectangular archwires, including the surgical stabilizing wire. This means the surgical splint will be thicker in the premolar region than anteriorly or posteriorly. At the operation, normal overjet and overbite are created, and the space between the premolar teeth is corrected postoperatively by extruding these teeth with working archwires with a reverse curve of Spee. The leveling occurs rapidly, typically within the first 8 weeks after orthodontic treatment resumes,

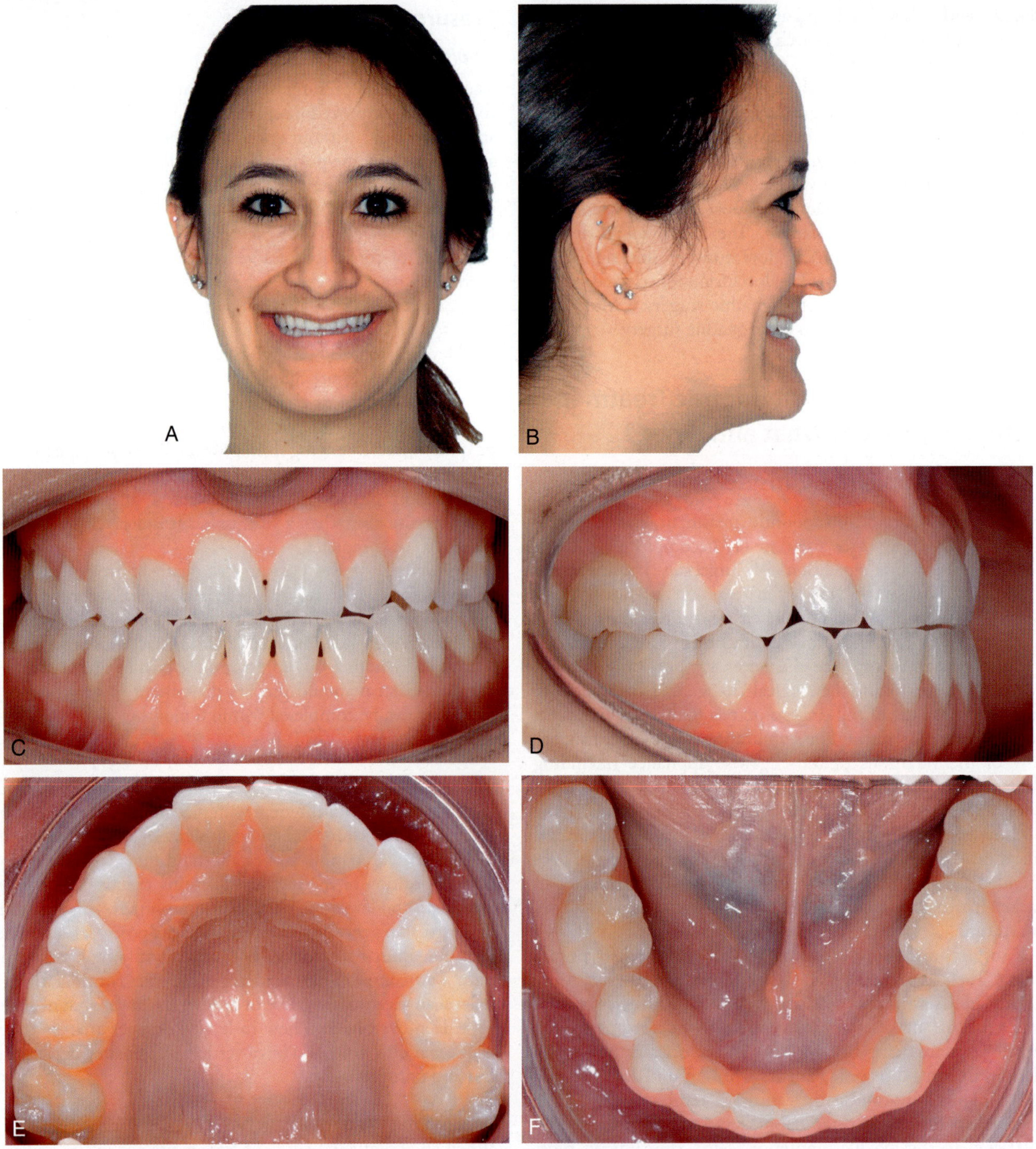

• **Fig. 22.43** Orthognathic surgery cases now can be managed with clear trays rather than a fixed appliance, but temporary attachments for intermaxillary fixation while rigid internal fixation is placed are necessary. A set of aligners for presurgical tooth movement and a second set for postsurgical orthodontics are required. (A and B) This female sought treatment because she was worried about the way her upper teeth were behind her lower teeth, the presence of intermittent temporomandibular (TM) joint pain, and the concave appearance of her mid-face. She had inadequate display of her maxillary incisors on smile. (C–F) Intraoral views before treatment. Note that both maxillary lateral incisors are in a crossbite relationship whereas the other anterior teeth are end-to-end with the lower arch.

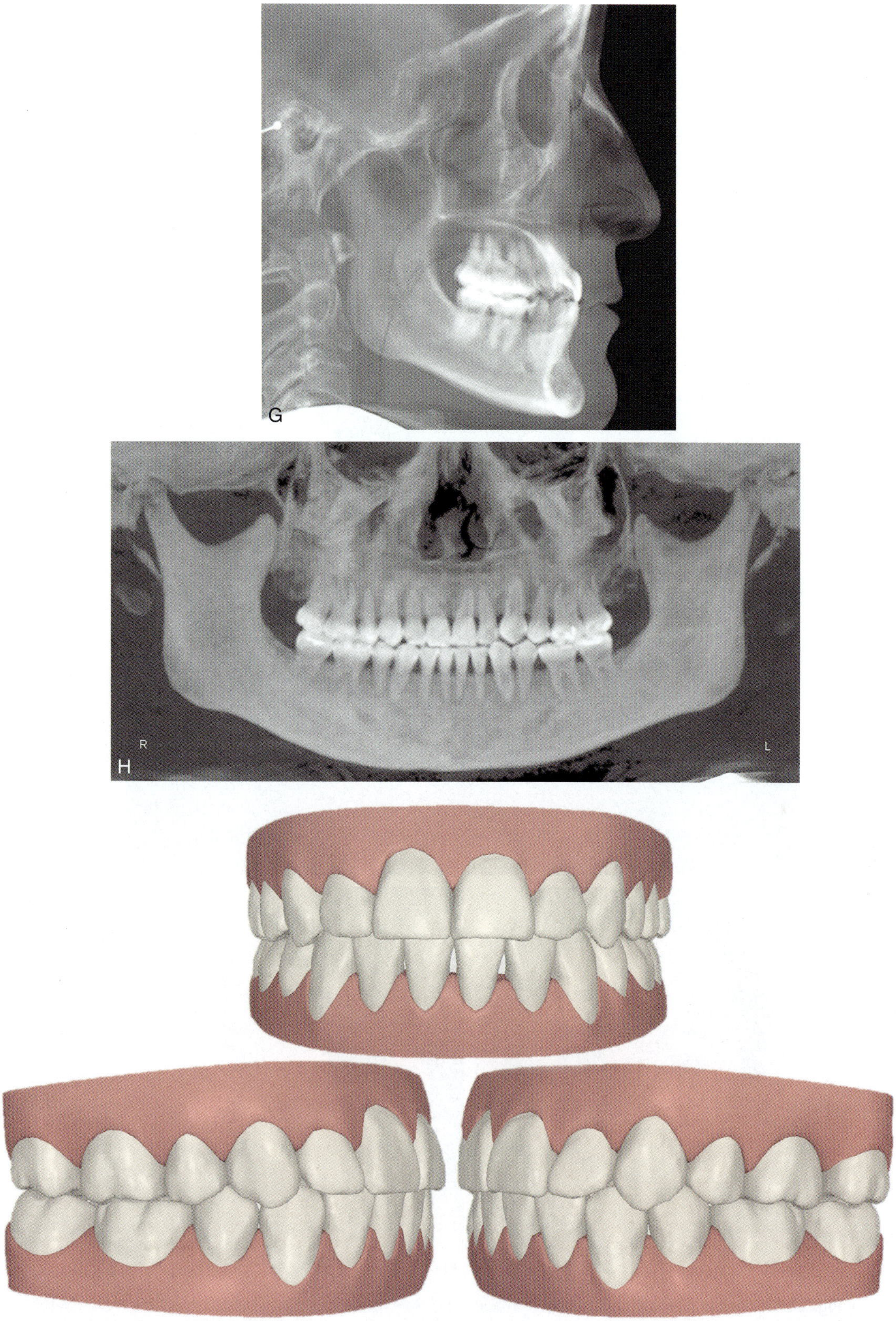

I

• **Fig. 22.43, cont'd** (G) In her diagnostic workup, a large-field-of-view cone beam computed tomography (CBCT) scan was done, and the pretreatment "synthetic ceph" constructed from the 3D data shows the severe maxillary deficiency and protrusion of the maxillary anterior teeth, with the mandibular anterior teeth relatively retruded to the mandible. There was no evidence of TM joint pathology. (H) A "synthetic pan" revealed that all her teeth had short and conical roots, so they were at high risk of root resorption during orthodontics unless force levels could be kept low. Clear tray treatment was offered because it would be quite compatible with work that put her on public display frequently. (I) The first of three plans for her treatment, showing the alignment possible with forward movement of the maxilla and uprighting of the maxillary and mandibular teeth.

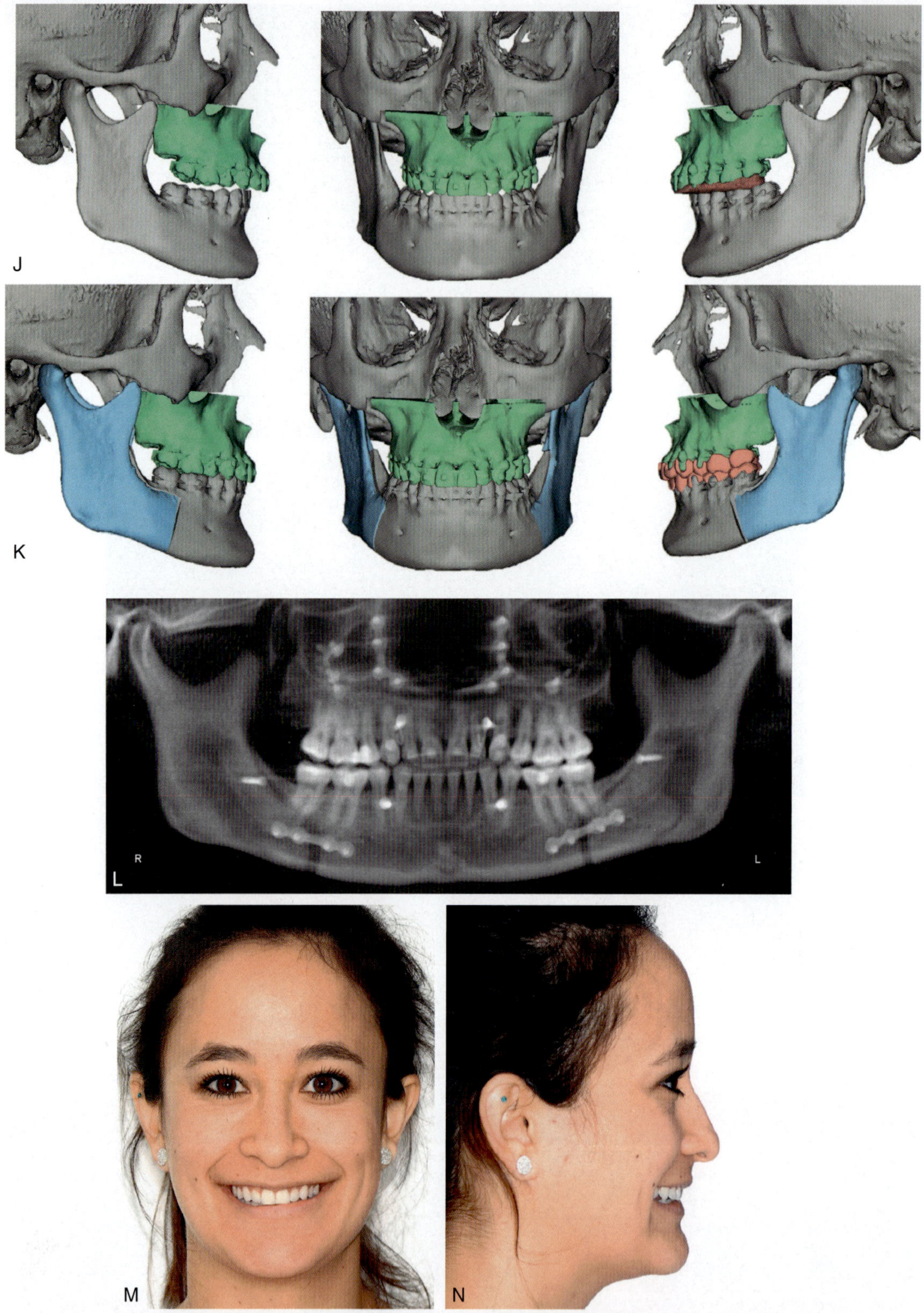

• **Fig. 22.43, cont'd** (J) Based on the CBCT images, the plan included Le Fort I osteotomy of the maxilla with 6 mm of maxillary advancement and rotation of the maxilla to move the anterior teeth down and the posterior teeth up. (K) A mandibular bilateral sagittal split osteotomy (BSSO) would then be used to slightly advance the mandible and fit it with the repositioned maxilla. To do this, an intermediate University of Southern California full-coverage splint with partial coverage of the teeth for better positional control of the bony segments was used to relate the repositioned maxilla to the intact mandible. Then a second final splint was used to relate the mandible to the maxilla after maxillary fixation was completed. Temporary labial attachments shaped to retain wires and/or elastics were placed before the operation for fixation to allow placement of the bone plates for stabilization; these were removed when the postsurgical aligner therapy began. (L) A synthetic panoramic radiograph after the operation shows the maxillary and mandibular bone plates. (M and N) Facial appearance after treatment. The greater prominence of the maxilla and increased display of the maxillary teeth with the teeth at correct inclinations and a compatible smile arc were a major part of the esthetic improvement. (Courtesy Drs. D. Grauer and R. Relle.)

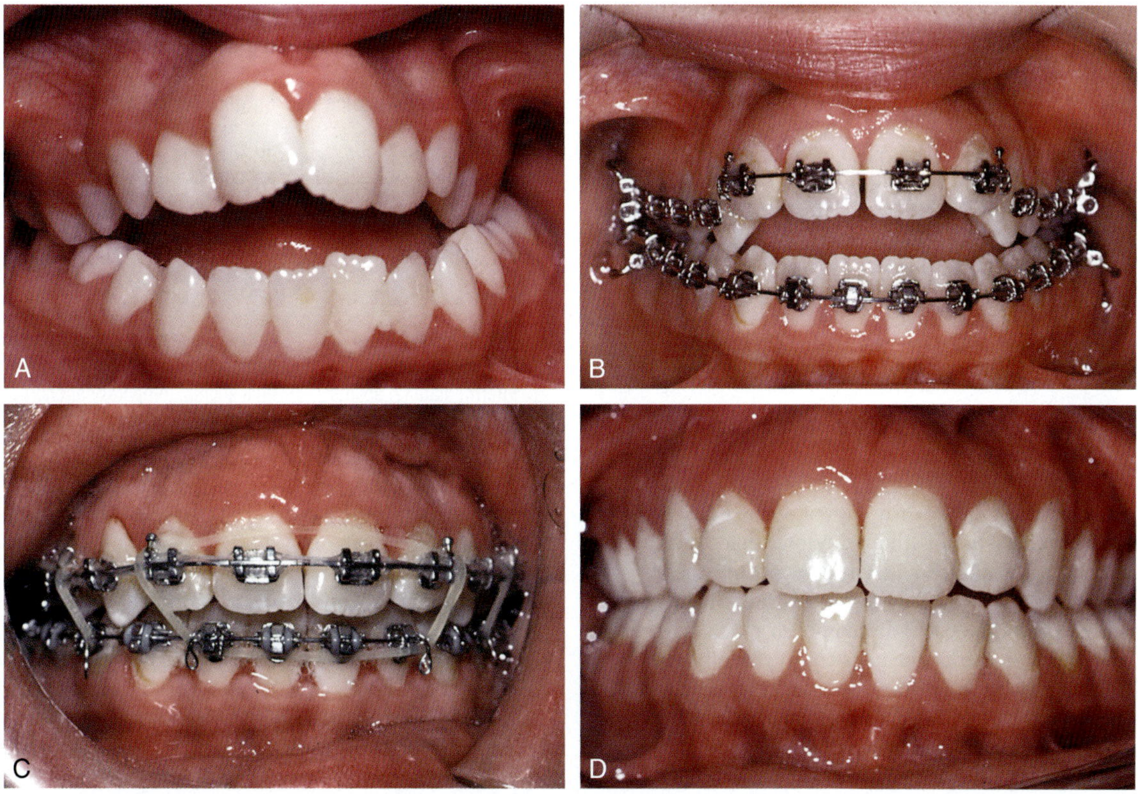

• **Fig. 22.44** In preparation for maxillary segmental surgery, often it is better for the orthodontist to level and align the teeth only within the planned segments, leaving complete leveling of the arch to the surgeon. (A) Pretreatment occlusal relationships in a patient with anterior open bite, a narrow maxilla, and posterior crossbites, in whom treatment with superior repositioning of the maxilla in three segments was planned. (B) Leveling and alignment have been accomplished within the planned anterior and posterior maxillary segments, with archwire segments rather than a continuous archwire. Note that for this patient, the canines are in the posterior segments. (C) Occlusal relationships during postsurgical orthodontic treatment, with light vertical elastics to maintain the vertical position of the teeth. (D) Completion of treatment with reduction in open bite, posterior crossbite, and overjet.

because there are no occlusal contacts to oppose the tooth movement. Some clinicians attribute this to a regional acceleration of bone remodeling due to the ramus osteotomy. That seems unlikely because of the distance from the surgical site. Regional acceleration of tooth movement occurs quite locally, not at distance beyond a few millimeters.

If intrusion is required to keep from increasing face height too much, a segmented arch approach (see Chapter 9) is indicated in the presurgical orthodontics. For the lower arch, surgical leveling rarely is indicated, although a subapical osteotomy to depress the incisor segment is possible.

Leveling the Maxillary Arch

In a patient with open bite who will have vertical repositioning of the maxilla, severe vertical discrepancies within the maxillary arch are an indication for multiple segment surgery. When this is planned, the upper arch should *not* be leveled conventionally. Presurgical leveling should be done only within each segment (Fig. 22.44), and then the segments are leveled at the operation. Extrusion of anterior teeth before surgery must be avoided because even mild orthodontic relapse could cause a problem with postsurgical bite opening.

Establishment of Incisor Position and Space Closure

The anteroposterior position of the incisors determines where the mandible will be placed relative to the maxilla at the operation and therefore is a critical element in planning treatment. This is often the major consideration in planning the closure of extraction sites.

In mandibular advancement, before rigid internal fixation was available, slight overretraction of protruding lower incisors before surgery was the usual plan. This was done because, while the jaws were wired together as initial healing took place, the incisors would be displaced forward relative to the jaw by the pull of stretched soft tissues. In this situation, the occlusal relationship would be maintained, but orthodontic tooth movement would allow the mandible to slip backward. With rigid fixation of the mandibular segments, the jaws are immobilized for only a day or two postsurgically if at all, there is little or no pressure against the teeth, and overcorrection of the incisor positions is unnecessary.

When several surgical segments are planned for the maxilla, a different consideration arises: the axial inclination of the upper incisors and canines should be established presurgically so that major rotation of the anterior segment at the operation can be avoided (Fig. 22.45). Otherwise, establishing correct torque of the incisors surgically will elevate the canines above the occlusal plane, and proper postoperative repositioning of the canines becomes difficult if not impossible. An extraction site that will be the location of an osteotomy cut should not be completely closed before surgery to leave room for the interdental cuts, but most of the extraction space can be closed without creating difficulty for the surgeon.

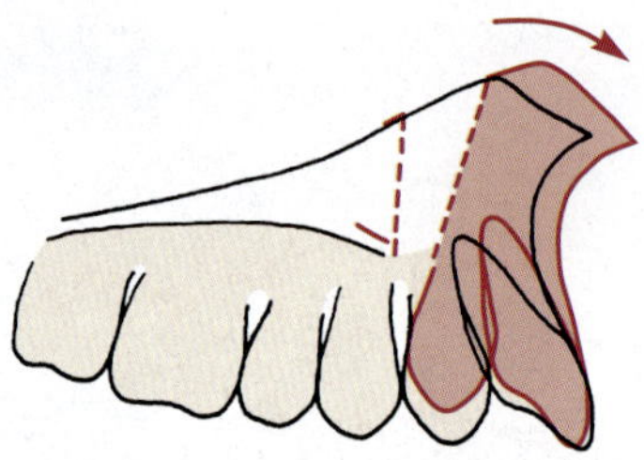

• **Fig. 22.45** In segmental maxillary surgery, it is important to establish the correct inclination of the incisors preoperatively. Otherwise, it will be necessary to rotate the anterior segment at the operation in order to maintain the vertical position of the maxillary incisor while its inclination is changed. This tends to elevate the canine off the occlusal plane and diverge the roots at the osteotomy site.

TABLE 22.1 Sequence of Surgical-Orthodontic Treatment

Consensus Sequence	Surgery First
Orthodontic plan, preliminary surgical plan	3D imaging (?), surgical plan, postsurgical orthodontic plan, splints
Presurgical orthodontics	Orthodontic appliance only, no surgical stabilizing archwire
Final surgical plan	
Orthodontic surgical procedure with final, intermediate (?) splints	Orthognathic surgery, dentoalveolar surgery, corticotomy (?), intermediate and final splints, temporary anchorage devices (TADs) for postsurgical orthodontics
Minimal postsurgical orthodontics, 3–6 months	Extensive (bone screws or miniplates) for postsurgical orthodontics

Recently, an old idea from the early days of orthognathic surgery was reintroduced: surgery first, without any presurgical orthodontics. This method was evaluated and discarded in the 1970s. The presumed advantages now would be faster treatment because segmental osteotomies could be used to accomplish much of the presurgical tooth movement, teeth close to osteotomy sites might move more rapidly, and patients would be more satisfied because their major problem would be addressed first and total treatment time would be shorter.[43] Not surprisingly, both the surgical procedure (with multiple segments and often corticotomy cuts to accelerate healing) and the postsurgical orthodontics would be more difficult. There would be some limitations in anteroposterior changes because of the lack of presurgical decompensation of incisor positions that often requires TAD-supported postsurgical decompensation. In addition, as we have noted, a longer duration of postsurgical orthodontics (9–12 months in most surgery-first patients) has been shown to decrease patient satisfaction with surgical treatment.[42] The treatment sequence with the consensus approach described earlier and surgery first is summarized in Table 22.1.

As of late 2017, most of the limited use of surgery first has been in Asia and Europe, and there still are no good data to document the claimed advantages, but it is generally acknowledged now that patients with severely crowded teeth and deep bites are not good candidates for surgery first.[44] A survey showing that surgery first was less successful in reducing treatment time than many case reports had claimed, and the suggestion that limited presurgical orthodontics would facilitate early surgery, has brought this thinking back closer to the consensus method described earlier.[45]

Stabilizing Archwires

As the patient is approaching the end of orthodontic preparation for surgery, it is helpful to take impressions and examine the hand-articulated models for occlusal compatibility. Minor interferences that can be corrected easily with adjustment of flexible archwires can significantly limit surgical movement.

When final orthodontic adjustments have been made, stabilizing archwires should be placed at least 4 weeks before the operation so that they are passive when the impressions are taken for the surgical splint (usually 1–2 weeks before the operation). This ensures that there will be no tooth movement that would result in a poorly fitting splint and potential compromise of the surgical result.

The stabilizing wires are full-dimension edgewise wires (i.e., 17 × 25 steel in the 18-slot appliance, 21 × 25 TMA or steel in the 22-slot appliance). Hooks as attachments to the archwires are needed to tie the jaws together while rigid fixation is placed. These can be added at the time of the splint impressions. They can be brass wires soldered to a steel stabilizing wire or prefabricated ball-hooks that are soldered or mechanically locked in place on the archwire. Sliding the ball-hooks over the wire without securing them is undesirable because they can slip or rotate when they are used to tie the jaws together during the operation. For patient comfort, tucking the hooks in toward the gingiva is essential and can be accomplished with an optical plier. Tight intermaxillary fixation is necessary at least long enough to place rigid fixation.

With surgery first, often there are no archwires at the operation, but an orthodontic appliance has been placed so that archwires or archwire segments can be placed at the operation or soon afterward. Typically, active orthodontic treatment begins during the first postsurgical week, which is not a happy time for patients undergoing steroid withdrawal.

Patient Management at the Operation

Final Surgical Planning

When the orthodontist considers surgical preparation completed, presurgical records should be obtained. If jaw asymmetry is to be corrected or use of computer-formed archwires is planned, CBCT is indicated. Otherwise, the presurgical records consist of panoramic and lateral cephalometric radiographs, periapical radiographs of interdental osteotomy sites, dental casts, and photographs. Casts should be mounted on a semi-adjustable articulator (or detailed scans oriented to its virtual equivalent) if maxillary surgery is planned. To avoid distortion, it is better to take the impressions with the stabilizing archwires removed. The archwires should be passive by the time these final presurgical impressions for model surgery and splints are taken.

The final planning requires a repetition of the predictions that were done initially. The difference is that the actual rather than predicted orthodontic movements are now available. It frequently is observed that teeth have not been fully decompensated, and this must be considered in the final plan. A current cephalometric radiograph (or the CBCT) is used to simulate surgical movements and evaluate the resulting soft tissue profile. When satisfactory functional and esthetic balance has been achieved, the surgical movements are duplicated in the virtual or actual model surgery, and the surgical splint is fabricated according to the dental relationships it established (Fig. 22.46).

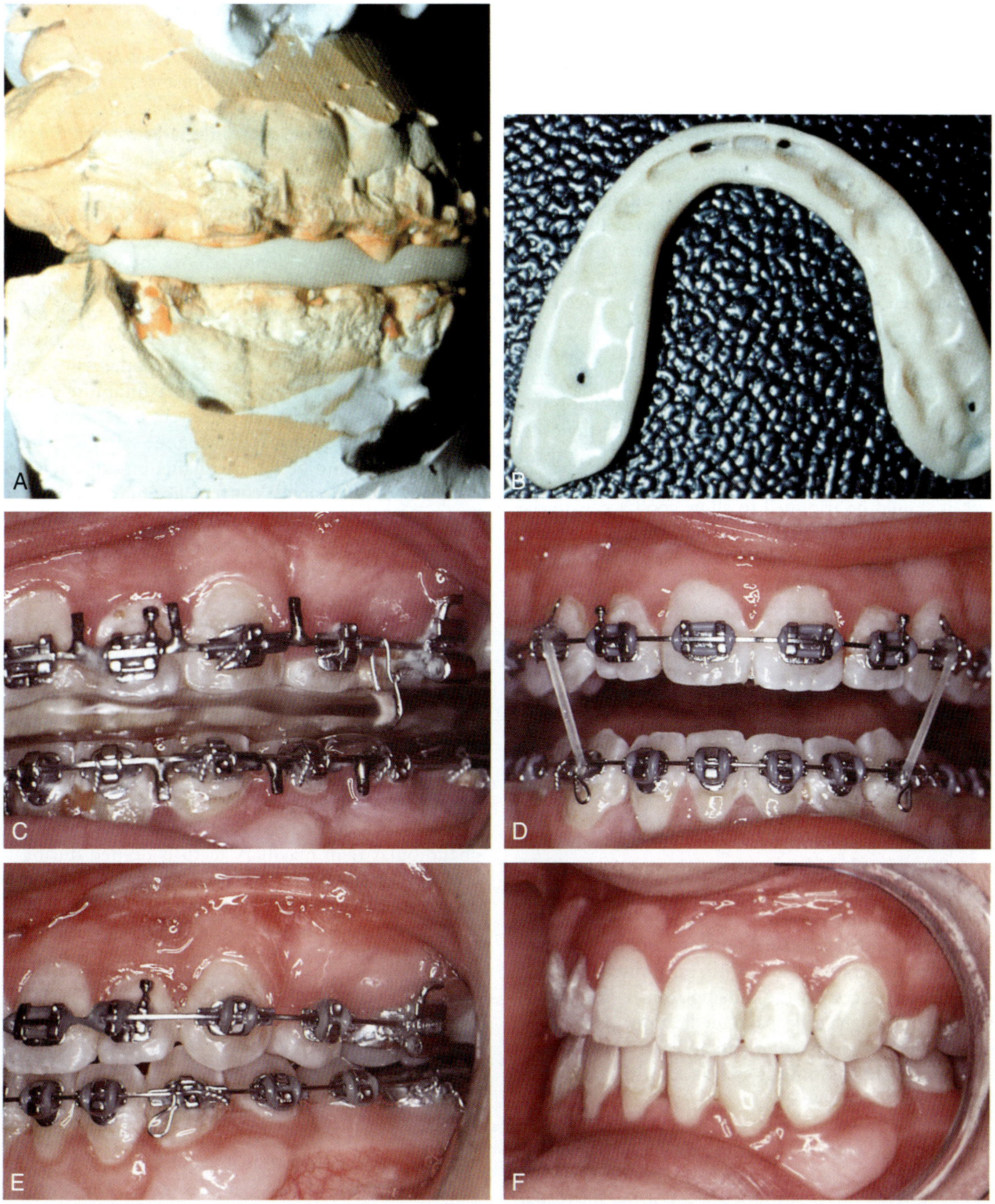

• **Fig. 22.46** Surgical splints play an important role in obtaining the planned surgical outcome. (A) For this patient with mandibular deficiency and a deep bite anteriorly, the plan was to level the mandibular arch after mandibular advancement surgery. An interocclusal splint was fabricated using the model surgery casts, articulated as they would be after the operation. (B) For a patient such as this one, the splint can be quite thin in the anterior and molar areas (note that two incisors and a molar on each side teeth touch through the splint) and thicker in the canine and premolar areas. (C) After the operation the patient functions into the splint, which is tied to either the maxillary (as here) or mandibular archwire, until the surgeon is satisfied with initial healing. (D) At that point the interocclusal splint and the stabilizing archwires are removed (the splint should *not* be removed until the stabilizing archwires also are replaced), and light working archwires are placed. For this patient, the maxillary archwire was 17 × 25 beta-titanium (beta-Ti) and the mandibular archwire was 16-mil steel. Light posterior box elastics are worn full-time, including when eating, for the first month. During the second month, the elastics can be removed during eating, but otherwise are worn full-time. (E) After 2 months, the teeth usually have settled into occlusion, and the vertical elastics can be reduced to night only. (F) Braces removed, 4 months after postsurgical orthodontics began. Note the gingival graft that was placed presurgically to prevent stripping of tissue facial to the mandibular left canine.

Splints and Stabilization

We recommend the routine use of an interocclusal wafer splint made from the casts as repositioned by the virtual or actual model surgery. Because this splint will define the postsurgical result, the orthodontist and surgeon should review the model surgery together. In patients requiring prosthodontic rehabilitation, the dentist responsible for this phase of treatment should be consulted about the acceptability of abutment and ridge relationships. The final planning for the surgical cuts and movements at the operation can be done interactively with Medical Modeling (Denver, CO) or a similar service, and both intermediate and final splints can be fabricated there or printed with other software (see Figs. 22.46 and 22.47).

The splint should be as thin as is consistent with adequate strength. This means that it almost never should be more than 2 mm thick at the thinnest point where teeth are separated minimally. When the lower arch has not been leveled presurgically, some teeth can contact through the splint (see Fig. 22.46B). Because the splint stays in place during initial healing (typically 2 weeks now), it should be trimmed to allow good access to the teeth for hygiene and permit lateral movements during jaw function. It is a mistake to remove the splint immediately after its use in the operating room. It should remain in place until the stabilizing wires also are replaced with lighter and more flexible archwires.

Postoperative Care

With the current emphasis on controlling health care costs, hospital stays for modern orthognathic surgery have been reduced considerably. Sagittal split osteotomies of the mandibular ramus often are performed now at outpatient surgery centers without overnight hospitalization, and lower border osteotomy of the mandible almost never requires an overnight stay. Maxillary osteotomies also can be managed now at outpatient surgery facilities; two-jaw surgery still usually requires an overnight stay, although that can be at a separate surgical center rather than a general hospital. A well-qualified and experienced nursing team is important in providing the postoperative care. With early discharge after jaw surgery, telephone access to the nursing team is important. Patients require surprisingly little pain medication, particularly after maxillary surgery. Rigid fixation and an early return to jaw movements eliminate the discomfort associated with having the jaws wired together for several weeks.

Patients are advised to maintain a soft diet (e.g., milkshakes, potatoes, scrambled eggs, yogurt) for the first week after the operation. Over the next 2 weeks they can progress to foods that require some chewing (soft pasta, meat cut into pieces), using the degree of discomfort as a guide to their rate of progression. By 6 to 8 weeks after the operation, they should be back on a normal diet. Note that this coincides with the time when the orthodontist can allow the patient to eat without the use of elastics (see later).

This progression can be assisted considerably by physical therapy beginning as soon as the postoperative intracapsular joint edema is resolved—typically about 1 week after the operation. For the first week, patients are advised to open and close the jaw gently within comfortable limits. Over the next 2 weeks, three 10- to 15-minute sessions of opening and closing exercises as well as lateral movements are indicated, with the patient closing into the splint. From the third to the eighth weeks, the range of motion is increased. The goal is to achieve optimum function by 8 weeks.

Postsurgical Orthodontics

Some teams prefer an orthodontic visit at 2–3 weeks as a check on occlusion, any broken appliances and satisfactory elastic strength and direction. Once a satisfactory range of motion has been achieved and the surgeon is satisfied with the initial healing, the finishing stage of orthodontics can be started. It is critically important that when the splint is removed, the stabilizing archwires are also removed and replaced by working wires to bring the teeth to their final position. This means that usually the orthodontist, not the surgeon, should remove the splint.

Light vertical elastics are needed initially with these working archwires (see Fig. 22.47P and Q), not so much for tooth movement—the archwires should do that—but to override proprioceptive impulses from the teeth that otherwise would cause the patient to seek a new position of maximum intercuspation. Until the stabilizing archwires are removed, the teeth are held tightly in the presurgical position. Removing the splint without allowing the teeth to settle into better interdigitation can result in the patient adopting an undesirable convenience bite, which in turn complicates orthodontic finishing and could stress recent surgical sites.

The choice of archwires during postsurgical orthodontic treatment is determined by the type and amount of movement needed. The typical settling of teeth into full occlusion can be achieved rapidly with light round wires (typically 16-mil steel) and posterior box elastics with an anterior vector that supports the sagittal correction. A flexible rectangular wire is used in the upper arch to maintain torque control of the maxillary incisors. In 18-slot brackets, this would be 17 × 25 beta-titanium (beta-Ti [TMA]). In 22-slot brackets, 21 × 25 martensitic nickel–titanium (M-NiTi [Nitinol or equivalent]) often is a good choice. A round wire (or a braided rectangular) in the lower arch typically is used because for most patients, more movement of mandibular than maxillary teeth is desired during this settling into occlusion. If that were not the case, it would be better to use a flexible rectangular wire in the lower arch and perhaps a round wire in the upper arch.

Elastics should not be discontinued until a solid occlusion has been established. Typically, patients wear the light elastics full-time, including while they are eating, for the first 4 weeks; full-time except for eating for another 4 weeks; then just at night for a third 4-week period. Elastics can be discontinued during any further detailing of the occlusion. As we have noted, patients are increasingly intolerant of continued treatment after about 6 months, so it is important to finish the postsurgical orthodontic treatment within that time if possible.

Management of two complex cases, one with a customized orthodontic appliance and virtual surgical planning (see Fig. 22.47) and the other with a segmental maxillary osteotomy and adjunctive rhinoplasty and genioplasty (Fig. 22.48), illustrate the application of the principles in surgical-orthodontic treatment that we have emphasized. Details in both cases are provided in the figure captions.

Finally, retention after surgical-orthodontic treatment is no different than for other adult patients (see Chapter 19), with one important exception: if the maxilla was expanded transversely, it is critically important not only to maintain the expansion during the finishing orthodontics, but also to have full-time retainer wear in the maxilla for at least 6 months. If a transpalatal lingual arch was placed after surgery, it should not be removed during the first postsurgical year.

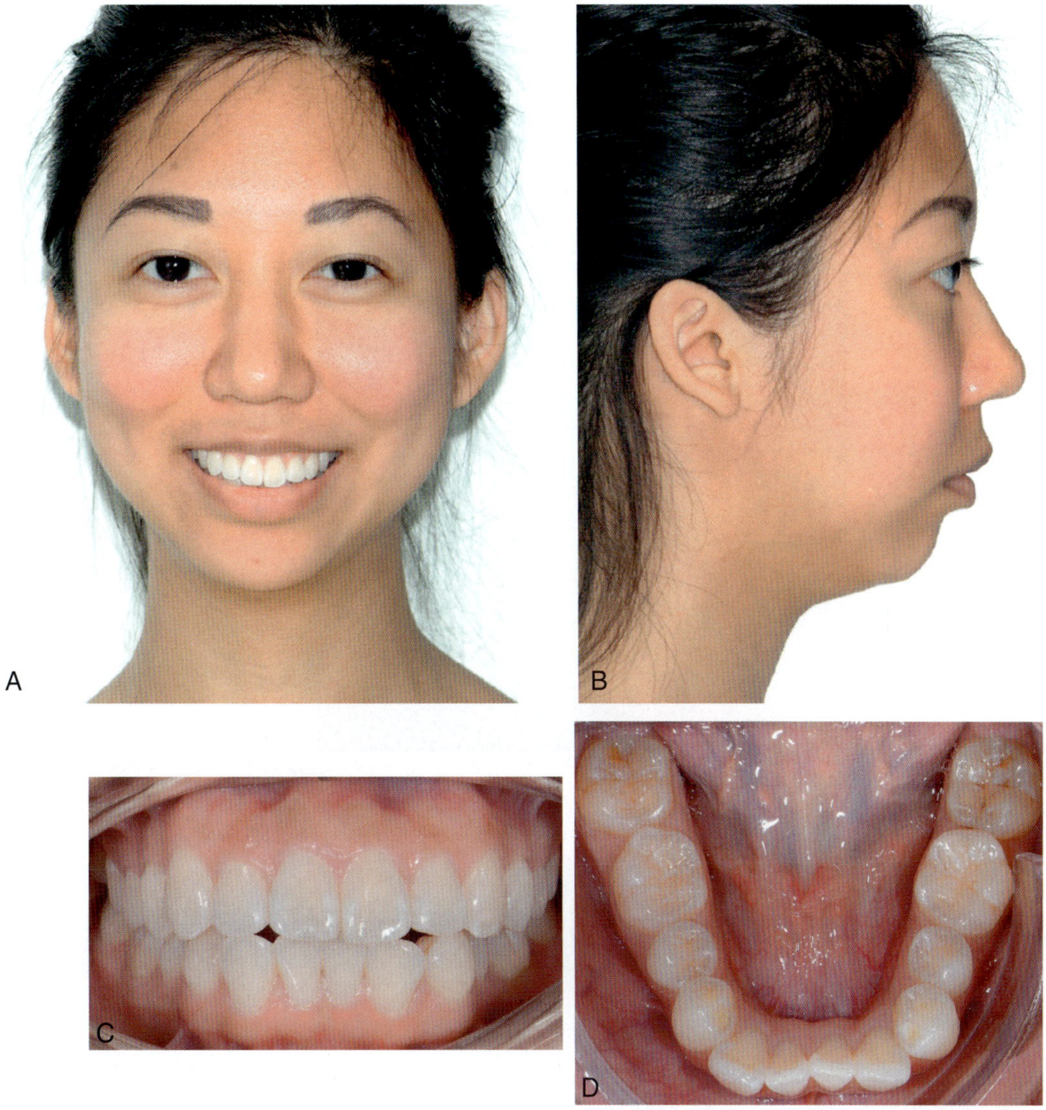

• **Fig. 22.47** Customized orthodontic appliances combined with virtual surgical planning and splints now make it possible now to deliver exceptionally precise treatment outcomes. (A and B) Facial views before treatment for a patient who was concerned about her chin deficiency and its effect on her appearance, the gingival display during smile, and the lack of contact between her anterior teeth. (C and D) Frontal view of occlusion and lower occlusal view. The maxillary incisors were well aligned after previous orthodontic treatment; the lower anterior teeth were protrusive and slightly crowded even though she had congenitally missing lower canines.

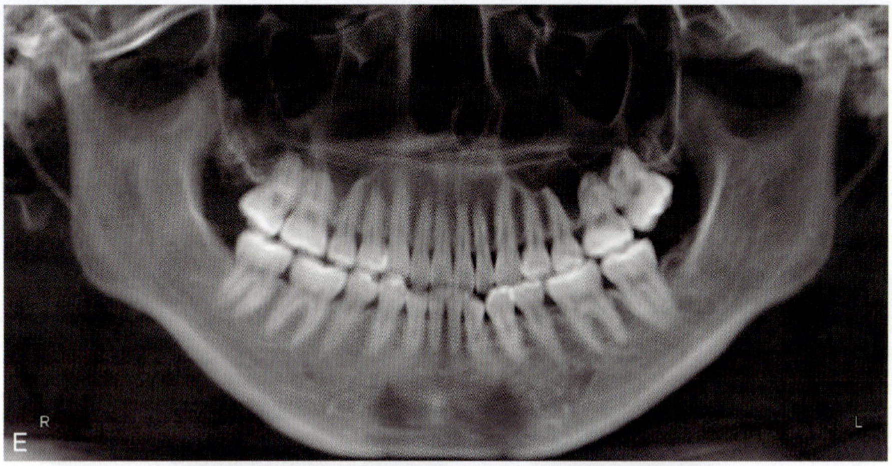

E

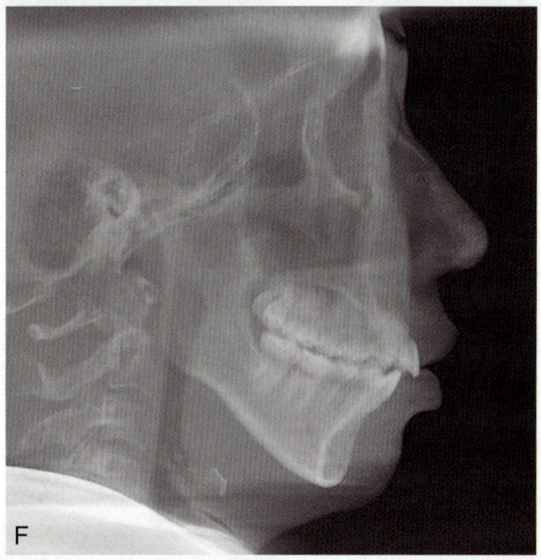

F

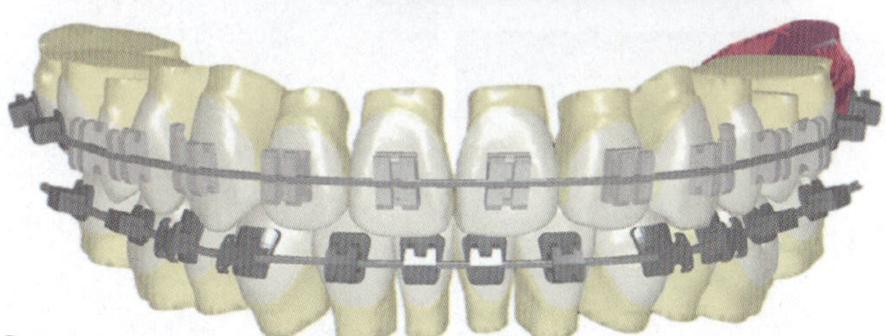

G

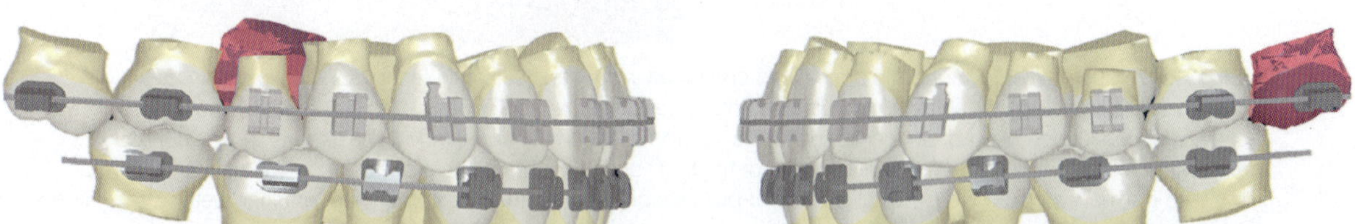

• **Fig. 22.47, cont'd** (E and F) Pretreatment panoramic and cephalometric views reconstructed from the cone beam computed tomography scan. Note the extreme protrusion of the lower anterior teeth relative to the chin but the reasonably normal inclination of maxillary incisors, which was the result of extensive Class II elastic wear during previous treatment but good torque control of the maxillary teeth. This probably also contributed to the mild anterior open bite. The result now would be correctly labeled as an orthodontic camouflage failure. (G) Computer-guided braces are fabricated on a virtual set-up. This allows for assessment of the compatibility of the dental arches, the intra-arch alignment, and the occlusion planned after surgical treatment. The virtual set-up is a diagnostic, treatment planning, treatment delivery, and communication tool. The red second molar in this image was not present in the digital scan and was mirrored from the contralateral one to fabricate its tube.

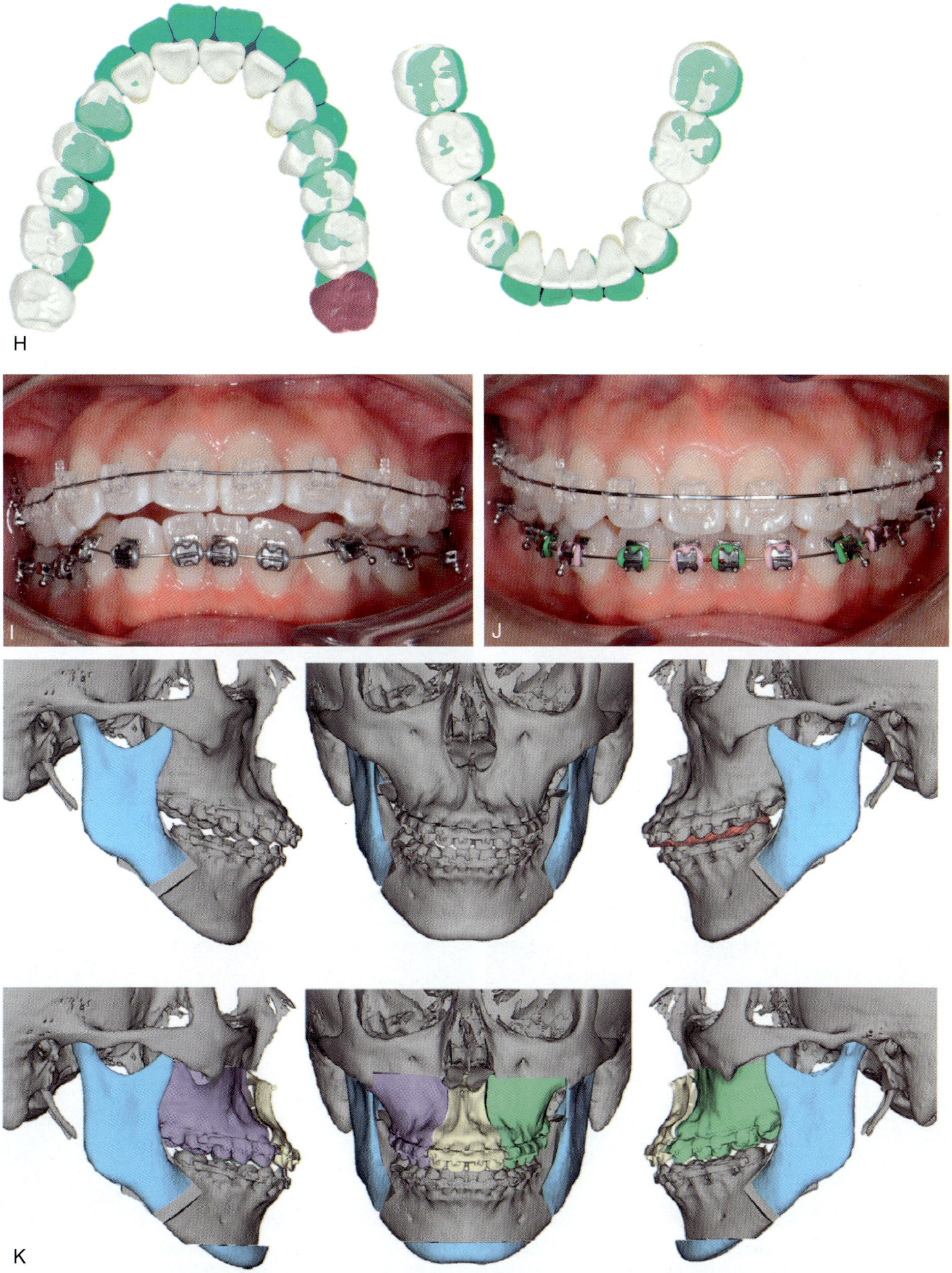

• **Fig. 22.47, cont'd** (H) This image (*green*, final position; *white*, original position) shows a comparison between the initial malocclusion and virtual goals. For the mandible it shows the change in tooth position that will be achieved with the customized fixed appliance. For the maxilla it depicts the tooth movement change and the change in occlusion that will occur at the operation. The patient's treatment plan was (I and J) alignment of the teeth in both arches with preservation of the maxillary incisor vertical position, then (K) an operation to advance the mandible, slightly advance and rotate the maxilla to correct the open bite, and reduce the vertical height of the chin and advance it. These images were produced as part of the virtual planning of the surgical procedure that allowed precise positioning of the jaws and fabrication of intermediate and final splints for use at operation.

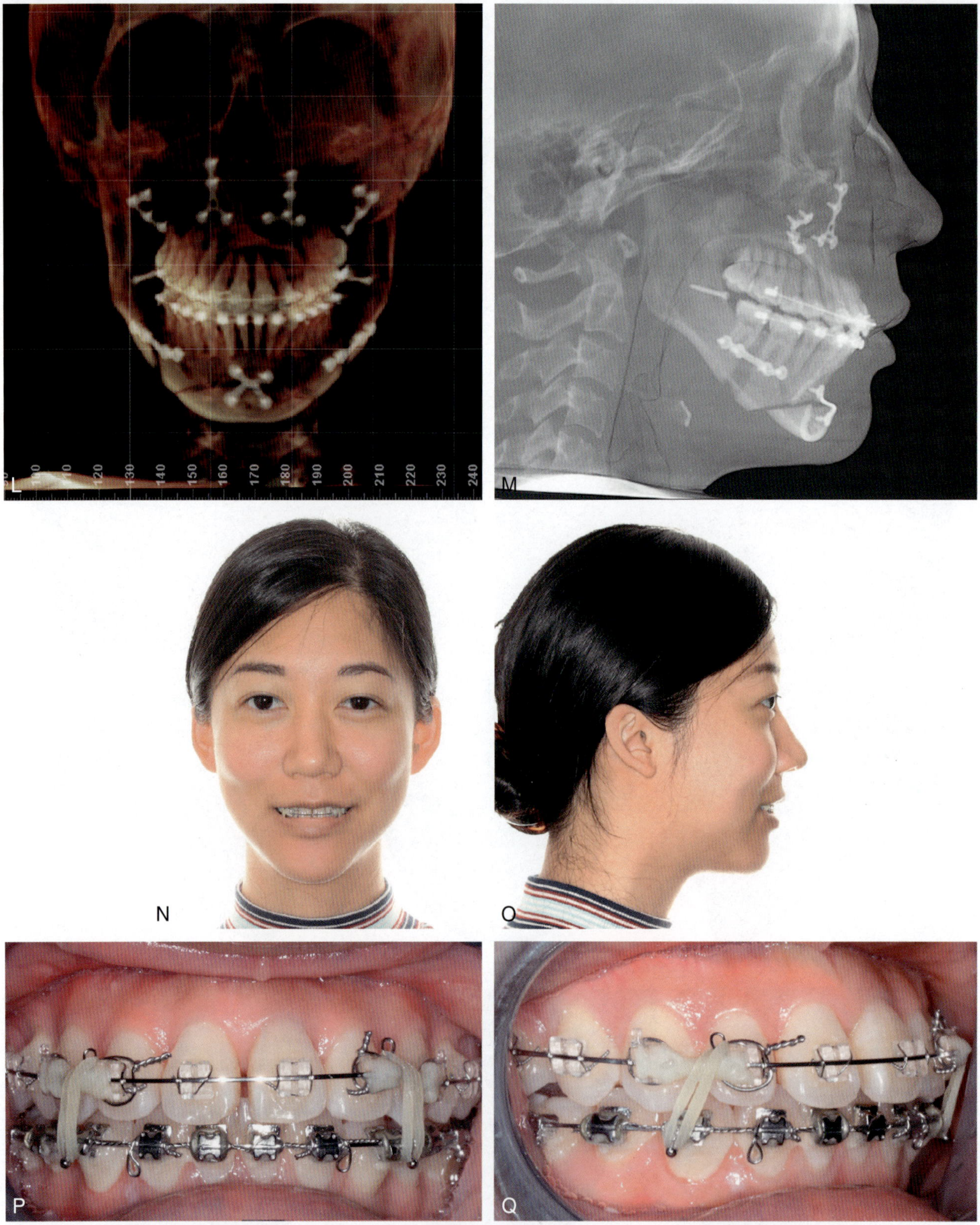

• **Fig. 22.47, cont'd** (L) 3D rendering of the surgical result from cone beam computed tomography images. (M) The postoperative cephalometric image shows the rigid fixation that will remain in place indefinitely. The intermediate and final splints allowed precise placement of the jaws as planned, and the chin also was repositioned as planned. The chin osteotomy angle was established with use of the 3D plan so that the advancement also produced vertical shortening. (N and O) Facial views at 6 weeks after operation, showing the improved facial balance despite some swelling at that point. (P and Q) Vertical elastics were used to stabilize the patient's occlusion in the target position. The final surgical splint was used during the operation to ensure that the position of the jaws matched the 3D virtual plan, then was removed and the patient's occlusion performed the function of a final splint—which is possible only if the occlusion is almost ideal at that point.

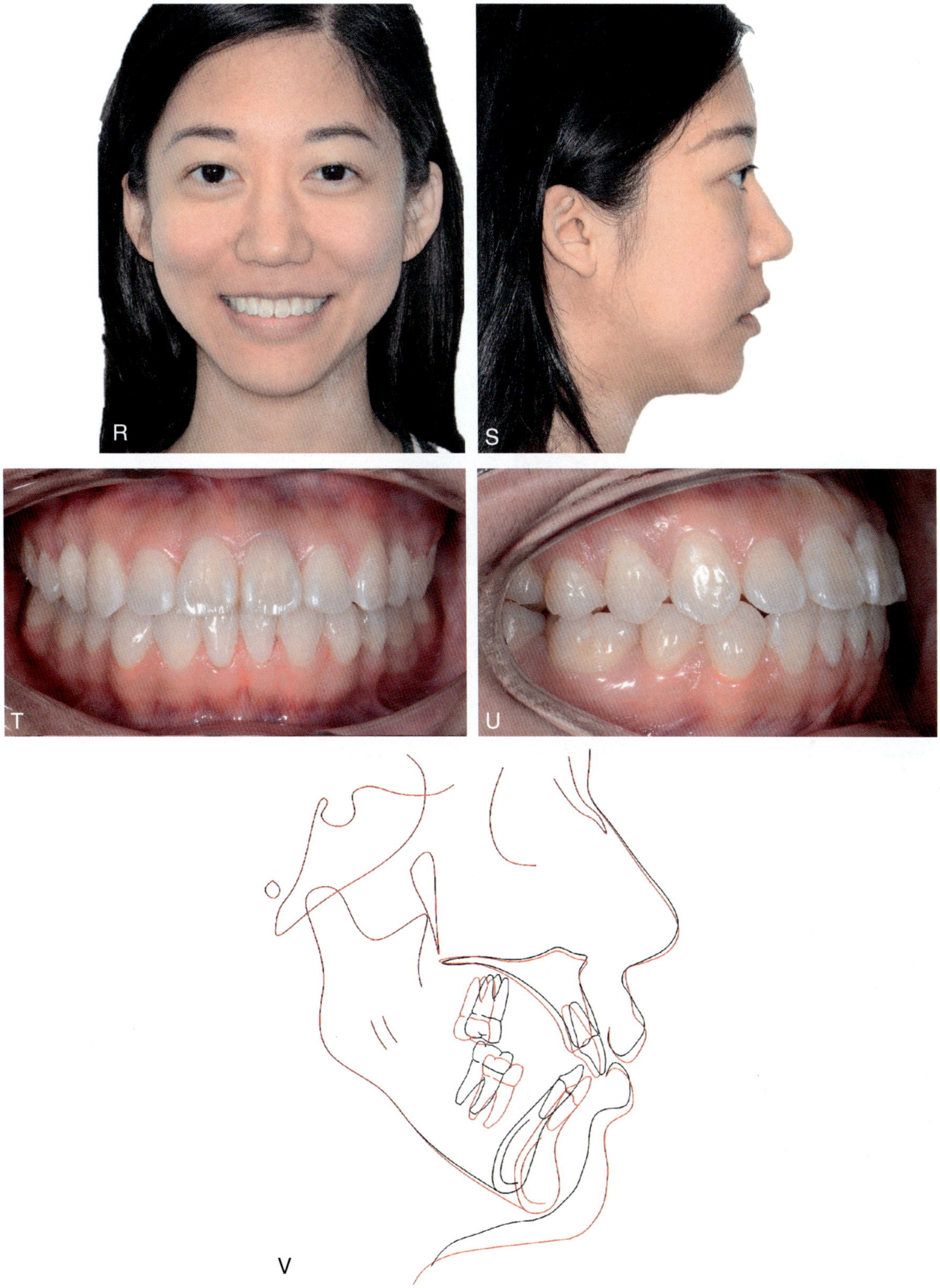

• **Fig. 22.47, cont'd** (R and S) Posttreatment facial images, frontal smile, and profile, with lips at rest. Intraoral views at finish. (T and U) The Class III molar relationship is because of the congenitally missing lower canines but allows perfectly normal function. (V) Superimposition tracing of virtual cephalometric images showing the changes from before to after treatment.

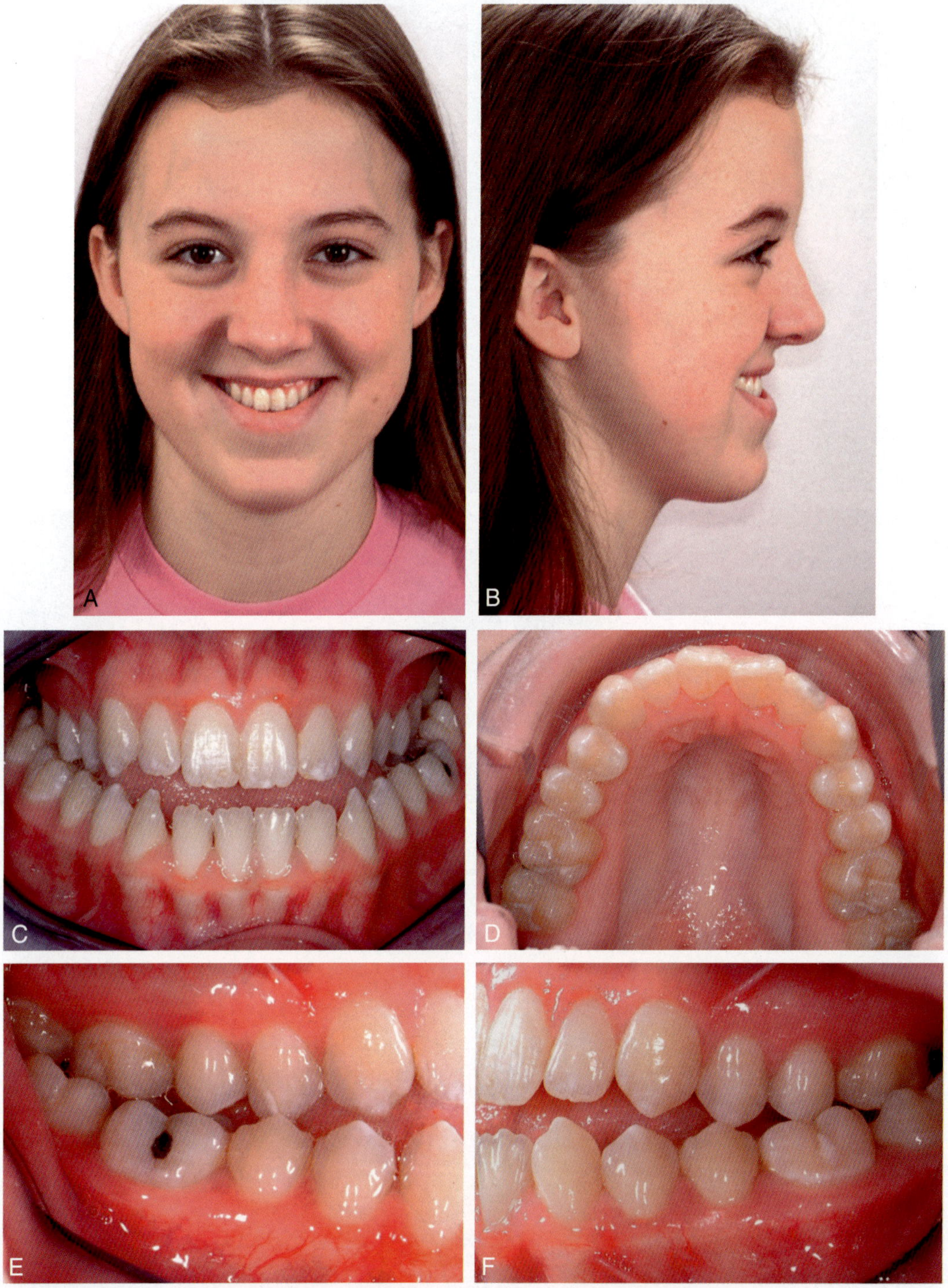

• **Fig. 22.48** For a patient who will need significant maxillary advancement, simultaneous rhinoplasty as well as genioplasty should be considered because advancing the maxilla tends to tip the nasal tip up and widen the nostrils. (A and B) Facial appearance at age 15, for a girl who was followed for several years while waiting for cessation of growth before correction, after it was determined that her problems could not be managed with protraction of the maxilla alone, waiting for cessation of growth before correction. Serial cephalometric radiographs are the best way to do this because other indicators of maturation correlate poorly with the end of growth. (C–F) Pretreatment intraoral views showing a full-cusp molar Class III relationship, anterior and posterior crossbites, anterior open bite, and dental midline discrepancy. If you look carefully at the frontal smile (A), you can see that the maxillary midline is slightly to the left of the midface, and the chin is slightly further left.

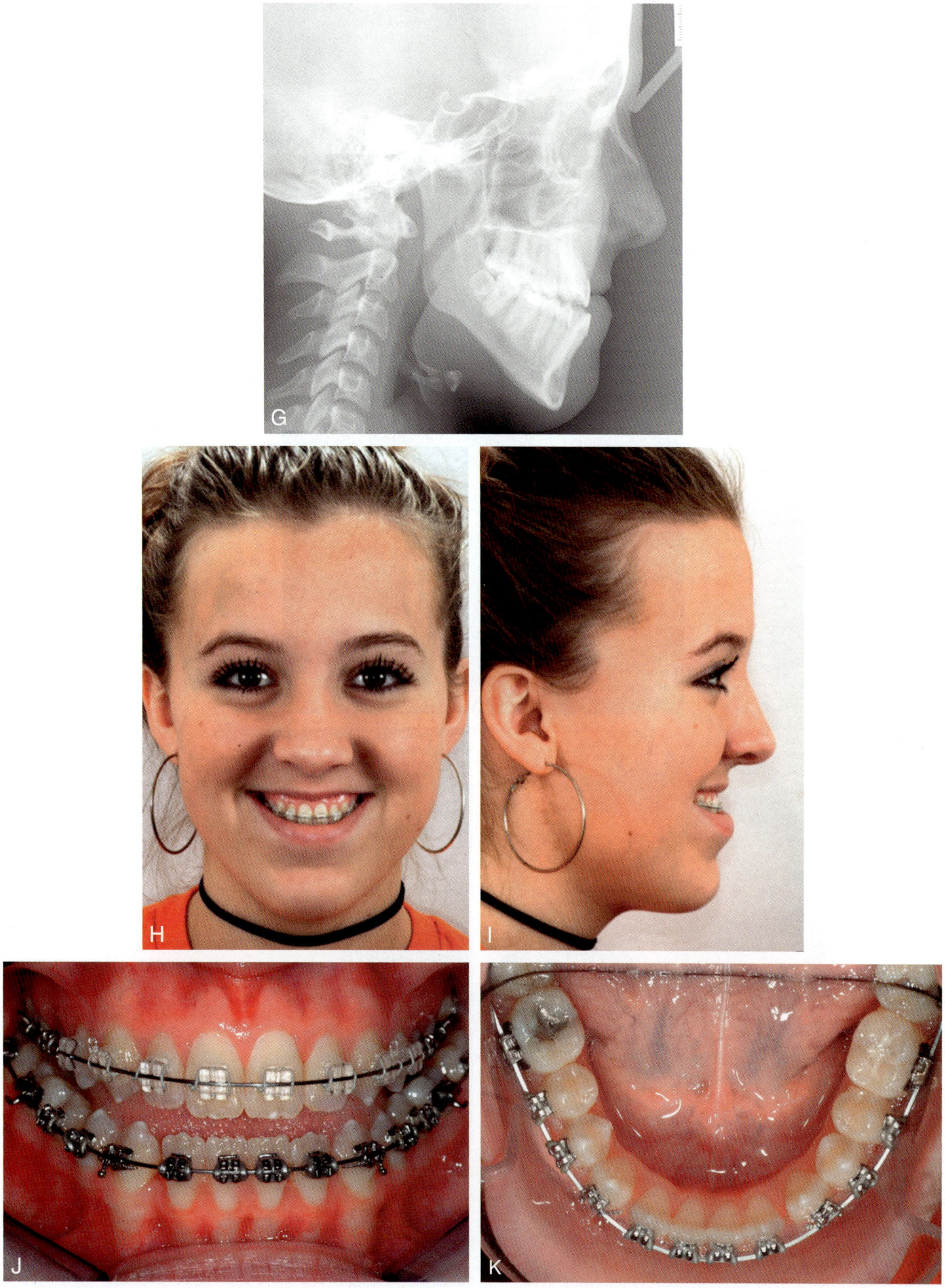

• **Fig. 22.48, cont'd** (G) The cephalometric radiograph shows the skeletal maxillary deficiency, the excess height of the chin (excessive distance from the lower incisors to the bottom of the chin), and the forward position of the lower incisors to the chin. In development of the treatment plan, it was obvious that the maxilla would need to be advanced. The only way to know whether forward movement of the maxilla would also correct the posterior crossbites was to hand-articulate the dental casts. This showed that the posterior expansion would be necessary, so a three-piece maxillary osteotomy was planned along with a lower border osteotomy to remove a wedge of bone above the chin and allow the chin to be moved both up and forward. Because the maxillary advancement would result in some widening of the nasal base, a simultaneous rhinoplasty to maintain nasal width and reposition the nasal tip for optimal esthetics was suggested, and the suggestion was accepted. (H and I) Facial appearance and (J and K) intraoral views.

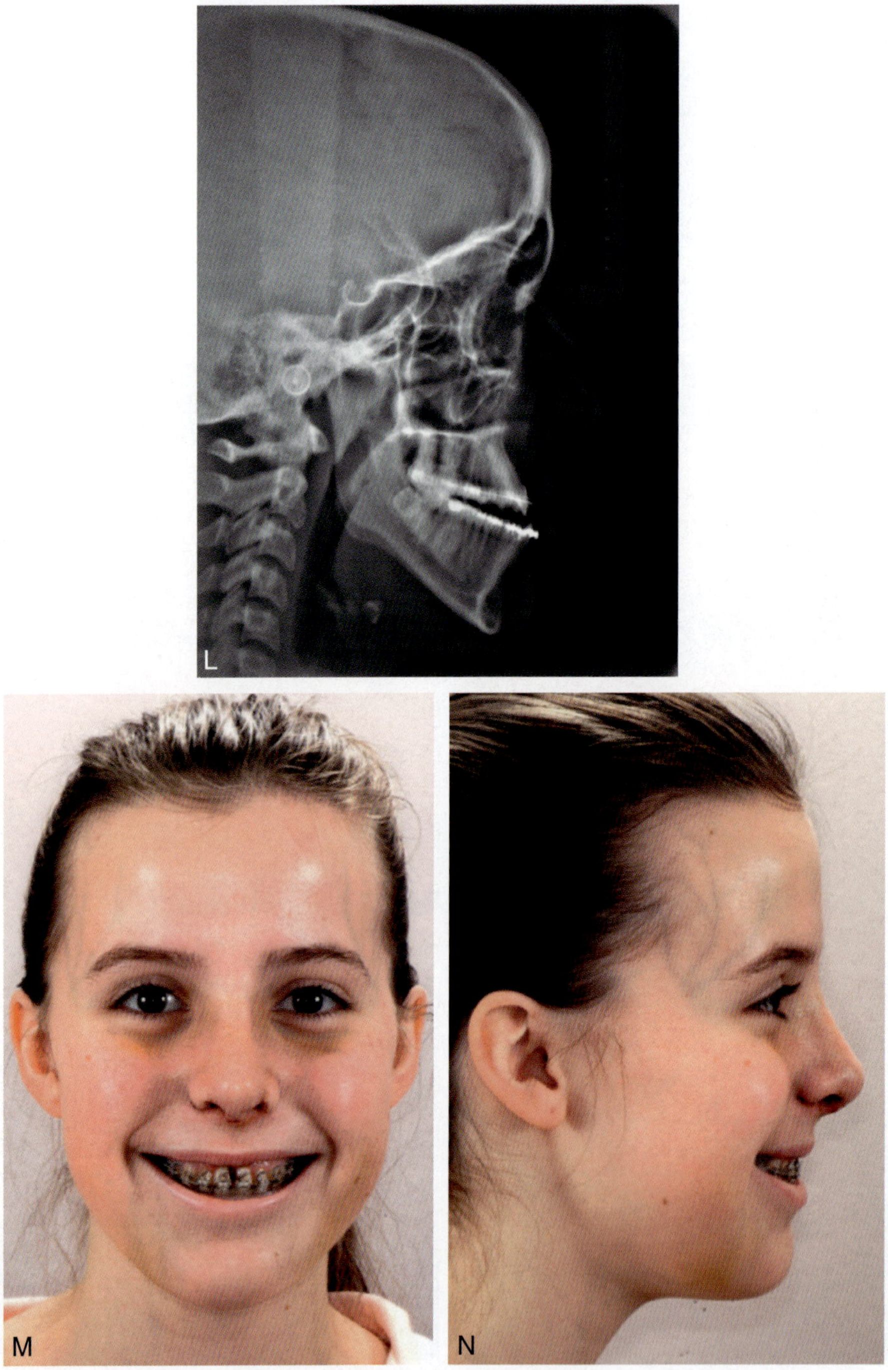

• **Fig. 22.48, cont'd** (L) Cephalometric radiograph just before operation. (M and N) Facial appearance at resumption of orthodontics 3 weeks after operation. The incisions at the base of the nose to control widening and between the nostrils to improve the nasal tip position and contour also can be seen.

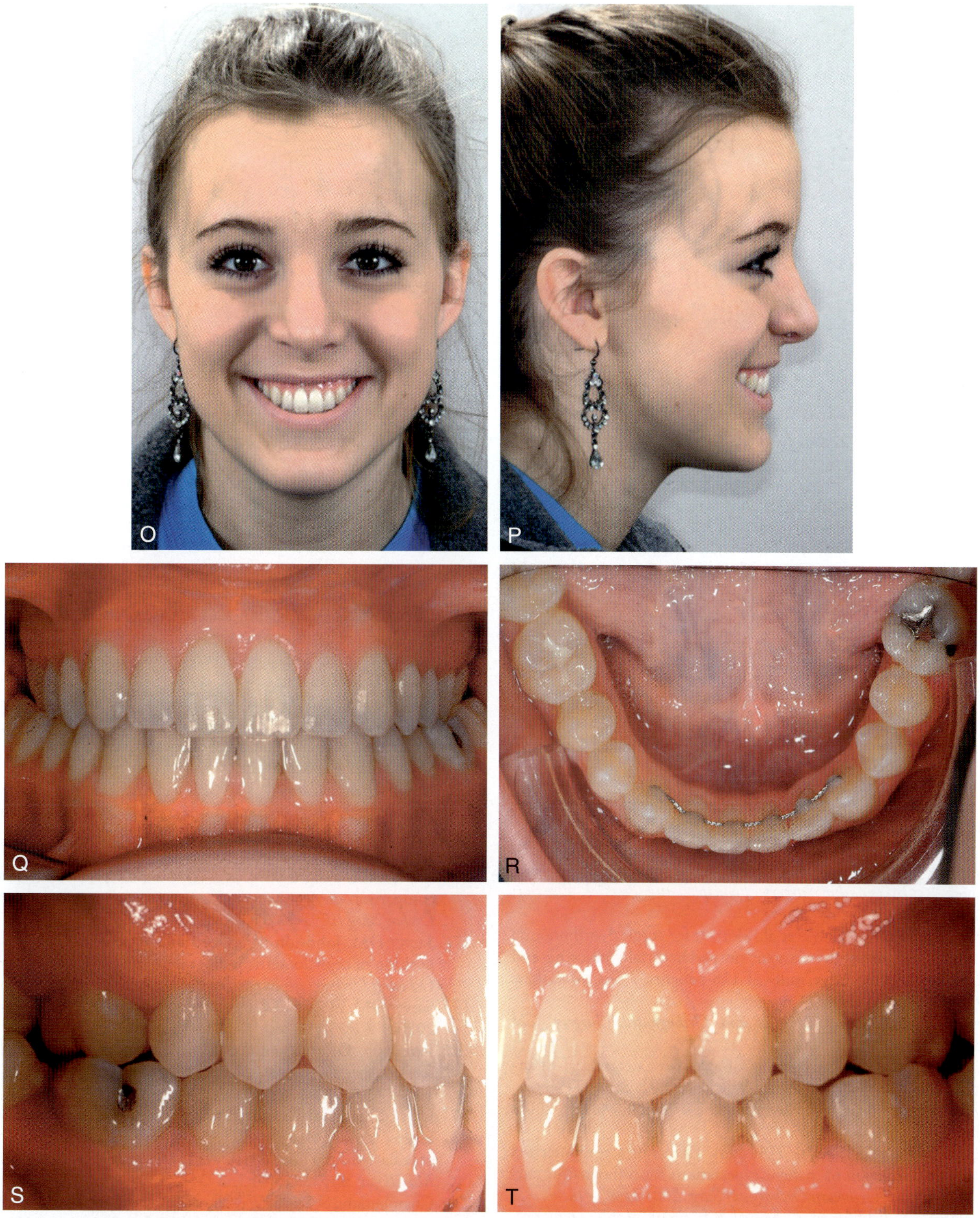

• **Fig. 22.48, cont'd** (O and P) Facial appearance and (Q–T) intraoral views at end of treatment at age 17. Note the correction of the Class III malocclusion and midlines, and the one-half-cusp crossbite for the molars. This was accepted because the lower arch was so wide posteriorly that expanding the posterior maxilla that much would have compromised future dental health.

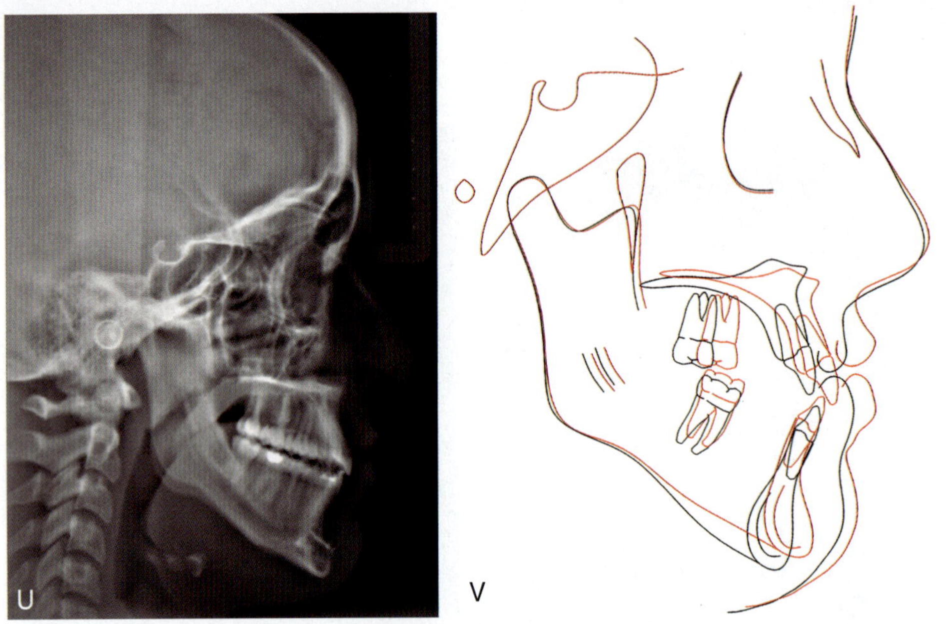

• **Fig. 22.48, cont'd** (U) Posttreatment cephalometric image showing the contribution to the upward-forward movement of the chin to the overall facial balance, and (V) cephalometric superimposition showing the changes from pretreatment to posttreatment. The reduction of face height and anterior positioning of the chin with the genioplasty, and control of nasal tip position and contour with the rhinoplasty, were important components of the treatment outcome.

References

1. Trauner R, Obwegeser H. The surgical correction of mandibular prognathism and retrognathia with consideration of genioplasty. *Oral Surg Oral Med Oral Pathol.* 1957;10:671–692.
2. Bell WH. Le Fort I osteotomy for correction of maxillary deformities. *J Oral Surg.* 1975;33:412–426.
3. Epker BN, Wolford LM. Middle third facial osteotomies: their use in the correction of acquired and developmental dentofacial and craniofacial deformities. *J Oral Surg.* 1975;33:491–514.
4. Proffit WR, White Jr. RP. *Contemporary Treatment of Dentofacial Deformity.* St. Louis: Mosby; 2003.
5. Posnick J. *Orthognathic Surgery: Principles and Practice.* Elsevier; 2013.
6. Oland J, Jensen J, Elklit A, et al. Motives for surgical–orthodontic treatment and effect of treatment on psychosocial well-being and satisfaction: a prospective study of 118 patients. *J Oral Maxillofac Surg.* 2011;69:104–113.
7. Sarver D. *Esthetic Orthodontics and Orthognathic Surgery.* CV Mosby; 1997.
8. Phillips C, Proffit WR. Psychosocial aspects of dentofacial deformity and its treatment. In: Proffit WR, White RP, Sarver DM, eds. *Contemporary Treatment of Dentofacial Deformity.* Mosby; 2003. [Chapter 3].
9. Phillips C, Bailey LJ, Kiyak HA, et al. Effects of a computerized treatment simulation on patient expectations for orthognathic surgery. *Int J Adult Orthodon Orthognath Surg.* 2001;16:87–98.
10. Kolokitha O. Validity of a manual soft tissue profile prediction method following mandibular setback osteotomy. *Eur J Dent.* 2007 Oct;1(4):202–211.
11. Sarver DM, Johnston MW, Matukas VJ. Video imaging in orthognathic surgery. *J Oral Maxillofac Surg.* 1988;46:939–945.
12. Lew KK. The reliability of computerized cephalometric soft tissue prediction following bimaxillary anterior subapical osteotomy. *Int J Adult Orthod Orthog Surg.* 1992;7:97–101.
13. Eales EA, Newton C, Jones ML, Sugar A. The accuracy of computerized prediction of the soft tissue profile: a study of 25 patients treated by means of the Le Fort I osteotomy. *Int J Adult Orthod Orthog Surg.* 1994;9:141–152.
14. Konstiantos KA, O'Reilly MT, Close J. The validity of the prediction of soft tissue profile changes after LeFort I osteotomy using the dentofacial planner (computer software). *Am J Orthod Dentofacial Orthop.* 1994;105:241–249.
15. Upton PM, Sadowsky PL, Sarver DM, Heaven TJ. Evaluation of video imaging prediction in combined maxillary and mandibular orthognathic surgery. *Am J Orthod Dentofacial Orthop.* 1997;112:656–665.
16. Aharon PA, Eisig S, Cisneros GJ. Surgical prediction reliability: a comparison of two computer software systems. *Int J Adult Orthod Orthog Surg.* 1997;12:65–78.
17. Sarver DM, Johnston MJ. Video imaging: techniques for superimposition of cephalometric radiography and profile images. *Int Adult Othodon Orthognath Surg.* 1990;VOL, 5(NO. 4).
18. Sarver DM. *Dentofacial Esthetics: From Macro to Micro. Quintessence*; 2020.
19. Joondeph DR, Bloomquist D. Mandibular midline osteotomy for constriction. *Am J Orthod Dentofacial Orthop.* 2004;126: 268–270.
20. Hamedi Sangsari A, Sadr-Eshkevari P, Al-Dam A, et al. Surgically assisted rapid palatomaxillary expansion with or without pterygomaxillary disjunction: a systematic review and meta-analysis. *J Oral Maxillofac Surg.* 2016;74:338–348.
21. Chamberland S, Proffit WR. Short- and long-term stability of SARPE revisited. *Am J Orthod Dentofacial Orthop.* 2011;139:815–822.
22. Sarver DM, Rousso DR. Plastic surgery combined with orthodontic and orthognathic procedures. *Am J Orthod Dentofacial Orthop.* 2004;126:305–307.
23. Chamberland S, Proffit WR, Chamberland P-E. Genioplasty in growing patients. *Angle Orthod.* 2015;85:360–373.
24. Rustemeyer J, Lehman A. Reduction genioplasty enhances quality of life in female patients with prognathism and maxillary hypoplasia

undergoing bimaxillary osteotomy. *Int J Oral Maxillofac Surg.* 2013;42:1083–1092.
25. Waite PM, Matukas VJ, Sarver DM. Simultaneous rhinoplasty and orthognathic surgery. *Int J Oral Maxillofac Surg.* 1997;17:298–302.
26. Islam S, Aleem F, Ormiston IW. Subjective assessment of facial aesthetics after maxillofacial orthognathic surgery for obstructive sleep apnoea. *British Journal of Oral and Maxillofacial Surgery.* 2015;53:235–238. https://doi.org/10.1016/j.bjoms.2015.11.018.
27. Wei S, Zhang Y, Guo X, et al. Counterclockwise maxillomandibular advancement: a choice for Chinese patients with severe obstructive sleep apnea. *Sleep & Breathing.* 2017;21:853–860. https://doi.org/10.1007/s11325-017-1484-7.
28. Zaghi S, Holty J-EC, Certal V, et al. Maxillomandibular advancement for treatment of obstructive sleep apnea a meta-analysis. *JAMA Otolaryngology - Head and Neck Surgery.* 2016;142:58–66. https://doi.org/10.1001/jamaoto.2015.2678.
29. On SW, Kim HJ, Cho DH, et al. Silent changes in sleep quality following mandibular setback surgery in patients with skeletal class III malocclusion: a prospective study. *Nature Publishing Group.* 2019;9:9737. https://doi.org/10.1038/s41598-019-46166-z.
30. MacKay S, Carney AS, Catcheside PG, et al. Effect of multilevel upper airway surgery vs medical management on the apnea-hypopnea index and patient-reported daytime sleepiness among patients with moderate or severe obstructive sleep apnea: the SAMS randomized clinical trial. *J Am Med Assoc.* 2020;324:1168–1179. https://doi.org/10.1001/jama.2020.14265.
31. Olson MD, Junna MR. Hypoglossal nerve stimulation therapy for the treatment of obstructive sleep apnea. *Neurotherapeutics.* 2021;18:91–99. https://doi.org/10.1007/s13311-021-01012-x. Epub 2021 Feb 8. PMID: 33559036; PMCID: PMC8116425.
32. Costantino A, Rinaldi V, Moffa A, et al. Hypoglossal nerve stimulation long-term clinical outcomes: a systematic review and meta-analysis. *Sleep Breath.* 2020;24:399–411. https://doi.org/10.1007/s11325-019-01923-2.
33. Proffit WR, Phillips C, Turvey TA. Stability after mandibular setback: mandible-only versus 2-jaw surgery. *J Oral Maxillofac Surg.* 2012;70:e408–e414.
34. Snow MD, Turvey TA, Walker D, et al. Surgical mandibular advancement in adolescents: postsurgical growth related to stability. *Int J Adult Orthodon Orthognath Surg.* 1991;6:143–151.
35. Proffit WR, Phillips C, Turvey TA. Long-term stability of adolescent versus adult surgery for treatment of mandibular deficiency. *Int J Oral Maxillofac Surg.* 2010;39:327–332.
36. Roberts HG, Semb G, Hathorn I, et al. Facial growth in patients with unilateral clefts of the lip and palate: a two-center study. *Cleft Palate Craniofac J.* 1996;31:372–375.
37. Oliver S, Keyser MMB, Jhingree S, et al. Impacts of anterior-posterior jaw disproportions on speech of dentofacial disharmony patients. *Eur J Orthod.* 2023 Feb 10;45(1):1–10. https://doi.org/10.1093/ejo/cjac057. PMID: 36308520; PMCID: PMC9912703.
38. Keyser MMB, Lathrop H, Samantha Jhingree S, et al. Impacts of skeletal anterior open bite malocclusion on speech. *FACE.* 2022;3(2):339–349. https://doi.org/10.1177/27325016221082229.
39. Lathrop-Marshall H, Keyser MMB, Jhingree S, et al. Orthognathic speech pathology: impacts of Class III malocclusion on speech. *European Journal of Orthodontics.* 2022;44:340–351. https://doi.org/10.1093/ejo/cjab067.
40. Vilanova ID, Almeida SB, de Araújo VS, et al. Impact of orthognathic surgery on voice and speech: a systematic review and meta-analysis. *Eur J Orthod.* 2023;45:747–763. https://doi.org/10.1093/ejo/cjad025.
41. Jacox LA, Turvey TA, Mielke J, et al. Impacts of jaw disproportions on speech of dentofacial disharmony patients. *J Oral Maxillo Surg.* 2022;80:S26. https://doi.org/10.1016/joms.2022.07.039.
42. Kiyak HA, West RA, Hohl T, et al. The psychological impact of orthognathic surgery: a 9-month follow-up. *Am J Orthod.* 1982;81:404–412.
43. Nagasaka H, Sugawara J, Kawamura H, Nanda R. Surgery first skeletal Class III correction using the skeletal anchorage system. *J Clin Orthod.* 2009;43:97–105.
44. Hernandez-Alfaro F, Guijarro-Martinez R, Piero-Guijarro MA. Surgery first in orthognathic surgery: what have we learned? A comprehensive workflow based on 45 consecutive cases. *J Oral Maxillofac Surg.* 2014;72:376–390.
45. Jeong WS, Choi JW, Kim DY, et al. Can a surgery-first orthognathic approach reduce the total treatment time? *Int J Oral Maxillofac Surg.* 2017;46:473–482.

Index

Page numbers followed by *f* indicate figures; *t*, tables; *b*, boxes.

Q

R

T